Opportunistic Infections

Infectious Disease

SERIES EDITOR: *Vassil St. Georgiev*
National Institute of Allergy and Infectious Diseases,
National Institutes of Health

Opportunistic Infections: *Treatment and Prophylaxis,* **Vassil St. Georgiev,** PhD, 2003

Aging, Immunity, and Infection, edited by ***Joseph F. Albright,*** PhD ***and Julia W. Albright,*** PhD, 2003

Cytokines and Chemokines in Infectious Diseases Handbook, edited by ***Malak Kotb,*** PhD, ***and Thierry Calandra,*** MD, PhD, 2003

Innate Immunity, edited by ***R. Alan B. Ezekowitz,*** MBChB ***and Jules A. Hoffman,*** PhD, 2003

Pathogen Genomics: *Impact on Human Health,* edited by ***Karen Joy Shaw,*** PhD, 2002

Immunotherapy for Infectious Diseases, edited by ***Jeffrey M. Jacobson,*** MD, 2002

Retroviral Immunology: *Immune Response and Restoration,* edited by ***Giuseppe Pantaleo,*** MD and ***Bruce D. Walker,*** MD, 2001

Antimalarial Chemotherapy: *Mechanisms of Action, Resistance, and New Directions in Drug Discovery,* edited by ***Philip J. Rosenthal,*** MD, 2001

Drug Interactions in Infectious Diseases, edited by ***Stephen C. Piscitelli,*** PharmD and ***Keith A. Rodvold,*** PharmD, 2001

Management of Antimicrobials in Infectious Diseases: *Impact of Antibiotic Resistance,* edited by ***Arch G. Mainous III,*** PhD and ***Claire Pomeroy,*** MD, 2001

Infectious Disease in the Aging: *A Clinical Handbook,* edited by ***Thomas T. Yoshikawa,*** MD and ***Dean C. Norman,*** MD, 2001

Infectious Causes of Cancer: *Targets for Intervention,* edited by ***James J. Goedert,*** MD, 2000

Infectious Disease

Opportunistic Infections

Treatment and Prophylaxis

By

Vassil St. Georgiev

*National Institute of Allergy and Infectious Diseases,
National Institutes of Health, Bethesda, MD*

Humana Press Totowa, New Jersey

© 2003 Humana Press Inc.
999 Riverview Drive, Suite 208
Totowa, New Jersey 07512
All rights reserved.

www.humanapress.com

No part of this book may be reproduced, stored in a retrieval system, or transmitted in any form or by any means, electronic, mechanical, photocopying, microfilming, recording, or otherwise without written permission from the Publisher.

Due diligence has been taken by the publishers, editors, and authors of this book to assure the accuracy of the information published and to describe generally accepted practices. The contributors herein have carefully checked to ensure that the drug selections and dosages set forth in this text are accurate and in accord with the standards accepted at the time of publication. Notwithstanding, as new research, changes in government regulations, and knowledge from clinical experience relating to drug therapy and drug reactions constantly occurs, the reader is advised to check the product information provided by the manufacturer of each drug for any change in dosages or for additional warnings and contraindications. This is of utmost importance when the recommended drug herein is a new or infrequently used drug. It is the responsibility of the treating physician to determine dosages and treatment strategies for individual patients. Further it is the responsibility of the health care provider to ascertain the Food and Drug Administration status of each drug or device used in their clinical practice. The publisher, editors, and authors are not responsible for errors or omissions or for any consequences from the application of the information presented in this book and make no warranty, express or implied, with respect to the contents in this publication.

This publication is printed on acid-free paper. ∞
ANSI Z39.48-1984 (American Standards Institute) Permanence of Paper for Printed Library Materials.

Production Editor: Kim Hoather-Potter.

Cover design by Patricia F. Cleary.

For additional copies, pricing for bulk purchases, and/or information about other Humana titles, contact Humana at the above address or at any of the following numbers: Tel: 973-256-1699; Fax: 973-256-8341; E-mail: humana@humanapr.com, or visit our Website: http://humanapress.com

Photocopy Authorization Policy:
Authorization to photocopy items for internal or personal use, or the internal or personal use of specific clients, is granted by Humana Press Inc., provided that the base fee of US $20.00 per copy is paid directly to the Copyright Clearance Center at 222 Rosewood Drive, Danvers, MA 01923. For those organizations that have been granted a photocopy license from the CCC, a separate system of payment has been arranged and is acceptable to Humana Press Inc. The fee code for users of the Transactional Reporting Service is: [1-58829-009-3/03 $20.00].

Printed in the United States of America. 10 9 8 7 6 5 4 3 2 1

Library of Congress Cataloging in Publication Data

Opportunistic infections: treatment and prophylaxis/by Vassil St. Georgiev.
     p. cm. --(Infectious disease)
  Includes bibliographical references and index.
  ISBN 1-58829-009-3 (alk. paper); E-ISBN 1-59259-296-1
    1. Opportunistic infections. I. Georgiev, Vassil St. II. Infectious disease (Totowa, N.J.)

RC112.O676 2003
616.9'0479--dc21

2002027646

Dedication

To my beloved Ellie,
with all my heart.

Preface

The major goal of *Opportunistic Infections: Treatment and Prophylaxis* is to guide clinicians who provide care for patients suffering from an underlying immunodeficiency that may significantly weaken their immune defenses and will complicate the effective treatment of opportunistic infections. In spite of a wealth of isolated data, no single text exists in which all the essential information about various infectious opportunistic infections. Although I make no claim to completeness, it is my hope that the present book will fulfill that need. To achieve this goal, I have endeavored to integrate both results from large-scale clinical trials and trials involving small numbers of patients, as well as reports of single cases—mindful that such an approach has its limitations.

Opportunistic Infections: Treatment and Prophylaxis is organized into four major parts: bacterial, viral, parasitic, and fungal diseases affecting the immunocompromised population. Each part surveys individual infections caused not only by well-known etiologic agents, but also by new and emerging species often taxonomically closely related to a major disease-producing microorganism and until recently not considered to be human pathogens (*Candida* spp. and nontuberculous mycobacteria, for example). For the sake of uniformity, within each part, the species have been arranged according to their taxonomic characteristics.

As the title of the book suggests, the array of diseases included has been broadened to encompass not only opportunistic infections exclusively associated with immunocompromised patients, but also infections commonly benign and self-resolving while affecting immunocompetent hosts, but becoming fulminant or disseminated, and very often life-threatening, in immunosuppressed individuals.

In contrast to normal hosts, where many infectious diseases are usually self-limited, in immunocompromised patients, such infections have the potential of becoming serious illnesses characterized by high morbidity and mortality rates. There are also the opportunistic infections that occur almost exclusively in immunocompromised hosts. Usually widely distributed in the environment, opportunistic pathogens rarely cause serious illness in normal hosts. In this context, it is important to note that prompt and correct diagnosis of a disseminated infection may become crucial as a result of overt differences in the susceptibility to anti-infectious drugs of sometimes closely related opportunistic pathogens. For example, while both *Pseudallescheria boydii* and *Scedosporium prolificans* have been recognized as causes of opportunistic hyalohyphomycoses in immunocompromised patients, diagnosis of disseminated disease caused by *S. prolificans* has been difficult to attain, since its spectrum and symptoms strongly resemble those of pseudallescheriasis and pulmonary aspergillosis. However, early positive identification of *S. prolificans* may prove to be essential because of its extreme drug tolerance and the related poor prognosis of disseminated disease caused by this fungal pathogen.

The information contained in *Opportunistic Infections: Treatment and Prophylaxis* includes—in addition to well-planned, large-scale clinical trials—reports of individual cases or treatment of small numbers of patients. When comparing large-scale clinical trials with therapies of individual cases, a multicenter clinical therapy involving large patient cohorts is unquestionably by far the better means of evaluating the therapeutic efficacy of a drug. A large-scale clinical trial provides the necessary information, clinical experience, as well as the perspective and direction needed for future research. On the other hand, clinical data involving limited numbers of patients or individuals, when well documented, may become useful in evaluating the therapeutic efficacy of a drug that might otherwise go unnoticed by those involved in drug research and development or in clinical practice. However, even with its benefits, such information, because of its limited scope, should be viewed with caution when evaluating the therapeutic efficacy and/or adverse toxicity of a therapeutic modality. Inevitably, in such cases, individual authors will differ and will include their specific (sometimes divergent or controversial) interpretations. It should also be emphasized that in some cases of rare or emerging infections, just the small number of patients and/or their distant geographic distribution would preclude any large-scale clinical trials, thereby leaving reports on treatment of individual cases as the only available data. In addition, there are also those unique cases of immunocompromised patients where an underlying condition may profoundly influence and/or even predicate the treatment of infection.

We trust that in its entirety, the information contained in *Opportunistic Infections: Treatment and Prophylaxis* represents a balanced and accurate account of the current status of opportunistic infections, and will serve as a useful resource for both clinicians and established investigators, as well as for new researchers in the field of drug development and treatment. It will also be especially helpful to those health care practitioners who do not have easy access to medical libraries and journals. We hope, too, that this book will facilitate further understanding of those areas of drug development and treatment that are still not well understood. Our aim is to encourage both scientists and clinicians to explore new avenues in their search for novel, safer, and more effective therapeutic modalities against infectious diseases in immunocompromised patients.

Vassil St. Georgiev, PhD

Contents

Dedication v
Preface vii

PART I. VIRAL INFECTIONS

CHAPTER 1
CYTOMEGALOVIRUS

1. Introduction 3
2. HCMV Infection in Immunocompromised Hosts 4
3. Studies on Therapeutics 5
    3.1. Ganciclovir 5
        3.1.1. Toxicity of Ganciclovir 5
    3.2. Foscarnet 6
        3.2.1. Toxicity of Foscarnet 6
    3.3. Cidofovir 7
    3.4. Fomivirsen 7
    3.5. Valaciclovir 8
4. Treatment of HCMV Infections 8
    4.1. Management of HCMV Disease in AIDS Patients 8
    4.2. Management of HCMV Disease in Solid Organ
           and Bone-Marrow Transplant Recipients 10
5. Prophylaxis and Maintenance Therapy of HCMV Disease 11
6. Ganciclovir Versus Foscarnet in the Treatment of HCMV Infection 13
7. Effects of HAART on HCMV Disease 13
8. Application of Immunotherapy for HCMV Infections 14

CHAPTER 2
VARICELLA-ZOSTER VIRUS (HERPES ZOSTER) INFECTIONS

1. Introduction 23
2. Studies on Therapeutics 24
    2.1. Acyclovir 24
    2.2. Famciclovir 24
    2.3. Sorivudine 25
3. Treatment of Varicella-Zoster Infections 25
    3.1. Herpes Zoster in Organ-Transplant Recipients 26
    3.2. Herpes Zoster in HIV-Infected Patients 27
    3.3. Management of Drug-Resistant Varicella-Zoster Virus Infections 27

3.4. Varicella-Zoster Virus Pneumonitis 27
3.5. Herpes-Zoster Ophthalmicus 27

CHAPTER 3
HERPES SIMPLEX VIRUS
1. Introduction 33
2. Treatment of Herpes Simplex Virus Infections 34
   2.1. Vidarabine 35
   2.2. Acyclovir (Aciclovir) 36
   2.3. Valaciclovir 37
   2.4. Famciclovir/Penciclovir 38
   2.5. Foscarnet 39
   2.6. Cidofovir 40
   2.7. Brivudine (Bromovinyldeoxyuridine, BVDU) 41
   2.8. Drug-Resistant Herpes Simplex Virus
        and Evolving Therapeutic Strategies 41
3. Prophylaxis of Herpesvirus Infections 43

PART II. BACTERIAL INFECTIONS

CHAPTER 4
NOCARDIA SPP.
1. Introduction 55
2. Nocardiosis in Immunocompromised Hosts 55
   2.1. Nocardiosis in HIV-Positive Patients 56
   2.2. Co-Infections With Other Pathogens 57
3. Treatment of Nocardiosis 57
   3.1. Sulfonamides 58
   3.2. Sulfonamide-Trimethoprim Combinations 58
   3.3. Antibiotics 59
   3.4. Acquired Drug Resistance of *Nocardia* spp. 60

CHAPTER 5
OERSKOVIA SSP.
1. Introduction 71
2. Treatment of *Oerskovia* Infections 71

CHAPTER 6
RHODOCOCCUS EQUI
1. Introduction 73
2. Treatment of *Rhodococcus equi* Infection 74

CHAPTER 7
TSUKAMURELLA SSP.
1. Introduction 79
2. Treatment of *Tsukamurella* Infections 79

Contents

CHAPTER 8
MYCOBACTERIUM TUBERCULOSIS
1. Introduction 81
2. *Mycobacterium tuberculosis* Infections
    in AIDS Patients 81
3. Evolution of Therapies and Treatment of *Mycobacterium
    tuberculosis* Infections 82
    3.1. Drug Interactions in HIV-Infected Patients 83
    3.2. Drug Resistance in Tuberculosis 83
    3.3. Highly Active Antiretroviral Therapy (HAART)
        and Mycobacterial Infections in HIV-Infected Patients 84
    3.4. Prophylaxis of Tuberculosis in HIV-Infected Patients 85
    3.5. Adjunctive Immunotherapy of Tuberculosis 85
    3.6. Vaccine Development Against Tuberculosis 85

CHAPTER 9
MYCOBACTERIUM BOVIS
1. Introduction 91
2. Treatment of *Mycobacterium bovis* Infections 92
3. BCG Vector-Based Vaccines in Immunotherapy Against
    HIV Infection 92

CHAPTER 10
NONTUBERCULOUS MYCOBACTERIAL INFECTIONS
1. Introduction 95
2. Nontuberculous Mycobacterial Infections and AIDS 96
3. *Mycobacterium avium* Complex (MAC) 96
    3.1. Introduction 96
    3.2. Treatment of *Mycobacterium avium-intracellulare* Complex
        (MAC) Infections 97
        3.2.1. Immunotherapy of MAC Infections 103
        3.2.2. Prophylaxis of *Mycobacterium avium-intracellulare*
            Infections in AIDS Patients 103
        3.2.3. MAC Infections and Highly Active Antiretroviral
            Therapy (HAART) 107
4. *Mycobacterium kansasii* 107
    4.1. Introduction 107
    4.2. Treatment of *M. kansasii* Infections 108
5. *Mycobacterium xenopi* 110
    5.1. Introduction 110
    5.2. Treatment of *M. xenopi* Infections 111
6. *Mycobacterium haemophilum* 112
    6.1. Treatment of *M. haemophilum* Infections 112
7. *Mycobacterium genavense* 114

CHAPTER 11
LISTERIA MONOCYTOGENES
1. Introduction 129
2. Listeriosis in AIDS Patients 130
3. Treatment of Listeriosis 131

CHAPTER 12
GASTROINTESTINAL INFECTIONS IN THE IMMUNOCOMPROMISED HOST
1. Introduction 135
2. Therapeutic Strategies for Enteric Infections 136
   2.1. Prevention of Enteric Infections 137

PART III. PARASITIC INFECTIONS

CHAPTER 13
CRYPTOSPORIDIUM SPP.
1. Introduction 143
2. Treatment of Cryptosporidiosis 144
   2.1. Macrolide Antibiotics 144
   2.2. Paromomycin 145
   2.3. Rifaximin 146
   2.4. Nitazoxanide (NTZ, Cryptaz) 146
   2.5. Somatostatin and Analogues 147
   2.6. Immunotherapy of Cryptosporidiosis 148
   2.7. Antiretroviral Therapies and Cryptosporidiosis 150
   2.8. Alternative Therapies for Cryptosporidiosis 150

CHAPTER 14
ISOSPORA SPP.
1. Introduction 159
2. Treatment of Isosporiasis 160

CHAPTER 15
TOXOPLASMA GONDII
1. Introduction 163
2. Treatment of Toxoplasmosis 164
   2.1. Pyrimethamine-Sulfonamide Combinations 165
      2.1.1. Acute Renal Failure to Sulfadiazine Therapy
             in AIDS Patients 167
      2.1.2. Adverse Cutaneous Reactions to Pyrimethamine
             Combinations in AIDS Patients 167
   2.2. Trimethoprim-Sulfonamide Combinations 168
   2.3. Antibiotic Therapy of Toxoplasmosis 168
      2.3.1. Spiramycin 168
      2.3.2. Clindamycin and Clindamycin-Pyrimethamine
             Combinations 169
      2.3.3. Clarithromycin 170

         2.3.4. Azithromycin 171
         2.3.5. Doxycycline 171
    2.4. Atovaquone 171
    2.5. Trimetrexate 172
    2.6. Management of Ocular Toxoplasmosis 172
3. Prophylaxis of Cerebral Toxoplasmosis 173
4. Prophylaxis Against Toxoplasmosis and HAART
    in HIV-Infected Patients 175
5. Immunotherapy of Toxoplasmosis 175

CHAPTER 16
MICROSPORIDIA
1. Introduction 183
2. *Enterocytozoon bieneusi* 184
3. *Encephalitozoon* spp. 185
4. *Pleistophora* spp. 185
5. *Trachipleistophora hominis* 185
6. *Nosema* spp. 185
7. *Brachiola vesicularum* 186
8. Treatment of Microsporidiosis 186

CHAPTER 17
STRONGYLOIDES STERCORALIS
1. Introduction 195
2. Strongyloidiasis as Opportunistic Infection
    in Immunocompromised Hosts 195
3. Corticosteroid Therapy as a Predisposing Factor for Strongyloidiasis 197
4. Treatment of Strongyloidiasis 197
    4.1. Comparative Studies 198

CHAPTER 18
CYCLOSPORA SPP.
1. Introduction 205
2. Treatment of Cyclosporiasis 206

PART IV. FUNGAL INFECTIONS

CHAPTER 19
CRYPTOCOCCUS NEOFORMANS
1. Introduction 213
2. Treatment of Cryptococcosis 214
    2.1. Amphotericin B 216
         2.1.1. Toxicity of Amphotericin B 218
    2.2. Combinations of Amphotericin B with 5-Fluorocytosine
         and Other Drugs 218
         2.2.1. Toxicity of Amphotericin B-5-Fluorocytosine
             Combinations 220

  2.3. 5-Fluorocytosine (5-FC) 221
  2.4. Azole Derivatives 221
    2.4.1. Miconazole 221
    2.4.2. Ketoconazole 222
    2.4.3. Fluconazole 222
    2.4.4. Itraconazole 225
3. Prophylaxis and Maintenance Therapy of Cryptococcosis......................226
4. *Cryptococcus neoformans* var. *gattii* 226
5. *Cryptococcus albidus* 227
6. *Cryptococcus laurentii* 227

CHAPTER 20
CANDIDA ALBICANS

1. Introduction 239
2. Human Candidiasis 239
  2.1. Candidal Infections in HIV-Infected Patients 240
3. Treatment of Candidiasis 241
  3.1. Cutaneous Candidiasis 241
  3.2. Chronic Mucocutaneous Candidiasis 242
  3.3. Candidal Onychomycosis 242
  3.4. Oropharyngeal and Esophageal Candidiasis..................................242
  3.5. Systemic Candidiasis 245
    3.5.1. Endogenous (Hematogenous) Candidal
       Endophthalmitis (HCE) 248
    3.5.2. Candidal Meningitis 249
    3.5.3. Candidal Endocarditis 249
    3.5.4. Vulvovaginal Candidiasis 250
    3.5.5. Urinary and Peritoneal Candidiasis 251
    3.5.6. Candidal Arthritis and Osteomyelitis..................................253
    3.5.7. Neonatal Candidiasis 253
4. Azole Drug Resistance and Refractory Candidiasis 255
5. HAART Therapy and Candidiasis..256
6. Drug Activities and *Candida* Virulence 256
7. Prophylaxis of *Candida* Infections 257

CHAPTER 21
EMERGING CANDIDA SPP. INFECTIONS

1. Introduction 269
2. *Candida glabrata* 269
  2.1. Treatment of *C. glabrata* Infections 270
    2.1.1. Fluconazole in the Treatment of *C. glabrata* Infections 271
    2.1.2. *C. glabrata*-Induced Vulvovaginal Candidiasis 271
  2.2. *Candida glabrata* Prophylaxis 272
3. *Candida krusei* 273
  3.1. Prophylaxis Against *C. krusei* Infections
    and Azole Resistance 273

- 4. *Candida lusitaniae* 274
- 5. *Candida dubliniensis* 275
    - 5.1. Molecular and Phenotypic Characterization
      of *C. dubliniensis* 276
    - 5.2. Treatment of *C. dubliniensis* Candidiasis 276
        - 5.2.1. *C. dubliniensis* Resistance to Fluconazole 277
- 6. *Candida rugosa* 277
- 7. *Candida zeylanoides* 278
- 8. *Candida famata* 278
- 9. *Candida guilliermondii* 279
- 10. *Candida norvegensis* 279
- 11. *Candida lipolytica* 280
- 12.. *Candida viswanathii* 280
- 13. *Candida haemulonii* 280
- 14. *Pichia jadinii (Candida utilis)* 281
- 15. *Candida ciferrii* 281

CHAPTER 22
TRICHOSPORON BEIGELII
1. Introduction 291
2. Treatment of Trichosporonosis 292
3. *Blastoschizomyces capitatus* 293
    - 3.1 Treatment of *B. capitatus* Infections 294

CHAPTER 23
RHODOTORULA SPP.
1. Introduction 299
2. Treatment of *Rhodotorula* Infections 299

CHAPTER 24
HANSENULA (PICHIA) SPP.
1. Introduction 303
2. Treatment of *Hansenula* spp. Infections 303

CHAPTER 25
DEMATIACEOUS FUNGAL INFECTIONS: PHAEOHYPHOMYCOSIS
AND CHROMOBLASTOMYCOSIS
1. Introduction 307
2. Phaeohyphomycosis 308
    - 2.1. Treatment of Phaeohyphomycosis 309
        - 2.1.1. *Bipolaris* spp. and *Exserohilum* spp.
          Phaeohyphomycosis 309
        - 2.1.2. *Exophiala (Wangiella) dermatitidis* and *Exophiala* spp.
          Phaeohyphomycosis 311
        - 2.1.3. *Alternaria* spp. Phaeohyphomycosis 313
            - 2.1.3.1. THERAPY OF ALTERNARIOSIS 314
        - 2.1.4. *Phaeosclera dematioides* Phaeohyphomycosis 316

      2.1.5. *Curvularia* spp. Phaeohyphomycosis 316
      2.1.6. *Ochroconis gallopava* Phaeohyphomycosis 318
      2.1.7. *Phialophora* spp. Phaeohyphomycosis 319
      2.1.8. *Phaeoacremonium* spp. Phaeohyphomycosis 320
      2.1.9. *Hormonema dermatioides* Phaeohyphomycosis 320
      2.1.10. *Aureobasidium* spp. Phaeohyphomycosis 320
      2.1.11. *Colletotrichum* spp. Phaeohyphomycosis 321
      2.1.12. *Mycoleptodiscus indicus* Phaeohyphomycosis 321
      2.1.13. *Phoma* spp. Phaeohyphomycosis 321
      2.1.14. *Pleurophomopsis* spp. Phaeohyphomycosis 322
      2.1.15. *Pyrenochaeta* spp. Phaeohyphomycosis 322
      2.1.16. *Geniculosporium* spp. Phaeohyphomycosis 322
      2.1.17. *Veronaea bothryosa* Phaeohyphomycosis 322
  2.2. Cerebral Phaeohyphomycosis 322
      2.2.1. *Nodulisporium* spp. Phaeohyphomycosis 323
      2.2.2. *Scopulariopsis* spp. Phaeohyphomycosis 323
      2.2.3. *Ramichloridium* spp. Phaeohyphomycosis 323
      2.2.4. *Cladophialophora* spp. Phaeohyphomycosis 323
          2.2.4.1. CLADOPHIALOPHORA BANTIANA (XYLOHYPHA BANTIANA,
          CLADOSPORIUM BANTIANUM) 324
  2.3. Fungal Peritonitis in Continuing Ambulatory Peritoneal
      Dialysis (CAPD) 325
3. Chromoblastomycosis 326

CHAPTER 26
HYALOHYPHOMYCOSIS
1. Introduction 343
2. *Pseudallescheria boydii* Infections 343
3. *Scedosporium* spp. Infections 347
  3.1. *Scedosporium apiospermum* 347
  3.2. *Scedosporium prolificans (S. inflatum)* 348
4. *Fusarium* spp. Infections 349
  4.1. Treatment of Fusariosis 350
  4.2. *Fusarium napiforme* 353
5. *Phialemonium* spp. Infections 354
6. *Acremonium* spp. Infections 354
7. *Scopulariopsis* spp. Infections 355
  7.1. *Scopulariopsis brevicaulis* 355
  7.2. *Scopulariopsis acremonium* 357
8. *Microascus* spp. Infections 357
  8.1. *Microascus cinereus* 357
  8.2. *Microascus cirrosis* 357
9. *Paecilomyces* spp. Infections 357
  9.1. Treatment of *Paecilomyces* Infections 359
      9.1.1. *Paecilomyces lilacinus* 359

Contents

   9.1.2. *Paecilomyces variotii* 360
   9.1.3. Post-Transplantation Therapy
      of *Paecilomyces* Infections 360
 10. *Acrophialophora fusispora* Infections 360
 11. *Engyodontium album* Infections 361
 12. *Beauveria bassiana* Infections 361
 13. Non-*Candida* Mycoses After Solid Organ and Bone-Marrow
   Transplantations 362
 14. Pharmacokinetic Interactions of Cyclosporin A with Azole
   Antimycotics 364

CHAPTER 27
HISTOPLASMA SPP.

1. Introduction 383
2. Evolution of Therapies and Treatment of Histoplasmosis 383
  2.1. Prophylaxis in Histoplasmosis 386
  2.2. Histoplasmosis in AIDS Patients 386
  2.3. Histoplasmosis in Transplant Recipients 389
  2.4. Skin Manifestations of Histoplasmosis 389
  2.5. Gastrointestinal Histoplasmosis 390
  2.6. Orofacial Manifestations of Histoplasmosis 390
  2.7. Ocular Histoplasmosis 391
  2.8. Rheumatic Manifestations of Histoplasmosis 391
  2.9. Mediastinal Histoplasmosis 392
  2.10. Pulmonary Histoplasmosis and Pleural Effusions 393
  2.11. Histoplasmosis of the Central Nervous System 393
  2.12. Adrenal Histoplasmosis 394
  2.13. Musculoskeletal Histoplasmosis 394
  2.14. Histoplasmosis of the Thyroid 394
  2.15 Genitourinary Histoplasmosis 394
    2.15.1. Prostatic Histoplasmosis 395
  2.16. Childhood Histoplasmosis 395
3. Host Immune Defense Against Histoplasmosis 396

CHAPTER 28
AFRICAN HISTOPLASMOSIS

1. Introduction 409
2. Management of African Histoplasmosis and Evolution
  of Therapies 409

CHAPTER 29
BLASTOMYCES DERMATITIDIS

1. Introduction 413
2. African Blastomycosis 414
3. Role of Host Immune Response Against *Blastomyces dermatitidis* ... 415
4. Evolution of Therapies and Treatment of Blastomycosis 415

    4.1. Amphotericin B 415
    4.2. Azole Derivatives 418
        4.2.1. Ketoconazole 418
        4.2.2. Itraconazole 419
        4.2.3. Fluconazole 420
        4.2.4. Miconazole 420
    4.3. Treatment of Adult Respiratory Distress Syndrome
        (ARDS) Secondary to Blastomycosis 420

CHAPTER 30
ASPERGILLUS SPP.

1. Introduction 429
    1.1. *Aspergillus*-Related Spondylodiscitis 431
2. Host Immune Response to Aspergillosis 431
3. Therapies and Treatment of Aspergillosis 432
    3.1. Amphotericin B 432
        3.1.1. Liposome-Encapsulated and Lipid-Based Formulations
             of Amphotericin B 434
        3.1.2. Routes of Administration 436
        3.1.3. Combinations of Amphotericin B With Other Drugs 437
    3.2. Azole Derivatives 439
        3.2.1. Clotrimazole 439
        3.2.2. Miconazole 439
        3.2.3. Ketoconazole 441
        3.2.4. Fluconazole 441
        3.2.5. Itraconazole 441
    3.3. Terbinafine 444
    3.4. Caspofungin 444
    3.5. Sodium (Potassium) Iodide Therapy of Aspergilloma 445
    3.6. Therapy of Allergic Bronchopulmonary Aspergillosis (ABPA) 445
    3.7. Therapy of *Aspergillus*-Induced Otomycosis 446
    3.8. Therapy of *Aspergillus*-Induced Onychomycosis 447
4. Prophylaxis Against Aspergillosis 447
5. *Aspergillus chevalieri* 448

CHAPTER 31
COCCIDIOIDES IMMITIS

1. Introduction 461
2. Immune Responses to Human Coccidioidomycosis 462
3. Evolution of Therapies and Treatment of Coccidioidomycosis 462
    3.1. Coccidioidomycosis in Immunocompromised Hosts
        and AIDS Patients 464
    3.2. Cutaneous Manifestations 466
    3.3. Coccidioidomycosis in Pregnancy and Early Infancy 466
    3.4. Coccidioidomycosis in Transplant Recipients 467

   3.4.1. Cardiac Transplant Recipients 467
   3.4.2. Renal Transplant Recipients 468
   3.4.3. Liver Transplant Recipients 468
   3.4.4. Bone-Marrow Transplant Recipients 468
  3.5. Ocular Coccidioidomycosis 469
  3.6. Acute Respiratory Failure 469
  3.7. Coccidioidal Peritonitis and Gastrointestinal Dissemination 469
  3.8. Coccidioidal Infections of Bones and Joints 470
  3.9. Genitourinary Coccidioidomycosis 471
   3.9.1. Coccidioidomycosis of the Prostate 471
   3.9.2. Infection of Intrascrotal Contents With
      or Without Prostatic Involvement 471
   3.9.3. Bladder Involvement 471
   3.9.4. Other Coccidioidal Genitourinary Involvement 471
  3.10. Coccidioidal Infection of Arterial Prosthesis 471
  3.11. Coccidioidal Infections of CNS 471
4. Prophylaxis of Coccidioidomycosis 472
5. Vaccine Studies in Humans 472

CHAPTER 32
PARACOCCIDIOIDES BRASILIENSIS
1. Introduction 483
2. Host Immune Response to Paracoccidioidomycosis 484
3. Paracoccidioidomycosis in the Immunocompromised Host 485
4. Treatment of Paracoccidioidomycosis 486
  4.1. Sulfonamides 486
  4.2. Amphotericin B 486
  4.3. Azole Derivatives 487
   4.3.1. Adrenocortical Dysfunction in Paracoccidioidomycosis
      and Azole Therapy 488
  4.4. Immunostimulants in the Treatment
    of Paracoccidioidomycosis 489

CHAPTER 33
PENICILLIUM MARNEFFEI
1. Introduction 495
2. Treatment of *Penicillium marneffei* Infections 496
3. Prophylaxis and Maintenance Therapy
  Against *Penicillium marneffei* 497

CHAPTER 34
ZYGOMYCOSIS (MUCORMYCOSIS, PHYCOMYCOSIS)
1. Introduction 501
2. Treatment of Zygomycosis 502
  2.1. Amphotericin B Therapy 502

Chapter 35
Pneumocystis carinii

1. Introduction 507
2. Genetic Diversity of *P. carinii* and Clinical Outcome 508
3. Subclinical *P. carinii* Infection 508
4. Atypical *P. carinii* Pulmonary Disease 508
5. Extrapulmonary *P. carinii* Infection 508
6. *P. carinii* Pneumonia Secondary to Methotrexate-Treated
   Rheumatoid Arthritis 509
7. Evolution of Therapies and Treatment of *P. carinii* Pneumonia 510
    7.1. Adjunctive Corticosteroid Therapy for *P. carinii* Pneumonia 514
    7.2. Toxicity of Sulfonamides 515
    7.3. Toxicity of Pentamidine 516
    7.4. Toxicity of Dapsone 516
    7.5. Synergistic Anti-*P. carinii* Activity 517
8. Prophylaxis Against *P. carinii* Pneumonia 517

Index 535

Part I
Viral Infections

1
Cytomegalovirus

1. INTRODUCTION

The cytomegaloviruses are ubiquitous pathogens that commonly infect animals and humans *(1–3)*. Their classification is based on the biological properties of host specificity, length of replication cycle, and the cytopathic effects *(4)*. The genera *Cytomegalovirus* (human cytomegalovirus; HCMV) together with the genera *Muromegalovirus* (murine cytomegalovirus) belong to the subfamily Betaherpesvirinae of the family Herpesviridae. A nonexclusive characteristic of the subfamily Betaherpesvirinae is a restricted host range. Their reproductive cycle is prolonged, with the infection progressing slowly in culture *(4)*.

Also known as betaherpesviruses, the human cytomegaloviruses (CMVs) are highly species-specific both for replication and pathogenesis. Whereas some host cells are more susceptible to infection, others do not succumb to the virus but may play an important role in harboring the pathogen. The latter may persist for longer periods of time, after which it may establish latency. It is likely that the thousands of genetically different strains of HCMV currently in existence, circulate in the general population throughout the world *(5)*. Humans are believed to be the only reservoir for HCMV. Cytomegalovirus infection is acquired throughout life with over 50% of adult population being infected by 50 years of age. Although neonatal HCMV infections can be severe, in healthy populations the disease is usually asymptomatic. Transmission is carried out by direct or indirect person-to-person contact *(2,6)*. Among the various sources of infection, oropharyngeal secretions, cervical and vaginal excretions, spermatic fluids, urine, feces, breast milk, tears, and blood are predominant *(7–9)*. Oral and respiratory spread appear to be the primary routes of transmission during childhood and possibly adulthood. Multiple or large quantities of blood transfusion also convey a greater risk of both primary and recurrent HCMV infections *(2)*.

Infection with HCMV may be acquired throughout the year and does not appear to be seasonal or dependent on climate *(10)*.

HCMV infection in immunocompetent hosts *(11,12)* usually is benign and asymptomatic, although occasionally it may be associated with a heterophile-negative mononucleosis syndrome. In both cases there may be shedding of virus in urine and oral secretions for several months to several years after the primary infection *(13)*.

After primary infection, HCMV remains latent in the cells. However, similarly to other herpesviruses, HCMV can reactivate in immunosuppressed hosts. The primary HCMV infection is frequently followed by persistent and/or recurrent infections. Although most often recurrent infections result from latent viral reactivation, reinfection may also occur possibly because of the antigenic diversity of the cytomegaloviruses *(2,14)*.

From: Opportunistic Infections: Treatment and Prophylaxis
By: Vassil St. Georgiev © Humana Press Inc., Totowa, NJ

In severe disseminated disease, evidence of HCMV presence can be seen in virtually all organs, *(2,15–18),* but ductal epithelial cells are the major site of involvement. In infants and young children, salivary glands are most frequently affected *(16,18).* Viruria resulting from renal infection is consistently observed in all age groups. The lungs are another organ affected by HCMV, especially in immunosuppressed older patients and bone marrow and lung transplant recipients *(19).*

Other organs, although less frequently involved in HCMV infection, include the adrenals, ovaries, bones, pancreas, and the skin *(2,15).* Gisserot et al. *(20)* have described HCMV infection of the submandibular gland in an HIV-infected patient. A case was also presented of an immunocompromised patient with a locally advanced hypopharyngeal carcinoma who developed a severe cytomegalovirus colitis after his first chemotherapy course with 5-fluorouracil (5-FC), decetaxel, and cisplatin *(21).*

It is noteworthy to mention that the term "recurrent infection" is generally used to refer to intermittent excretion of virus from single or multiple sites over a prolonged period of time, and should be differentiated from "chronic" or "prolonged excretion" of virus that characterizes certain forms of HCMV infection *(2).*

The most common clinical manifestations of HCMV infection in immunocompromised hosts include chorioretinitis, gastrointestinal disorders (esophagitis, colitis, cholangitis), Central Nervous Systems (CNS) infection, pneumonitis, and adrenal gland disease. Addison's disease as an unusual manifestation of HCMV-end organ disease in pediatric AIDS has also been reported *(22).*

2. HCMV INFECTION IN IMMUNOCOMPROMISED HOSTS

HCMV has long been considered to be an immunosuppressive agent capable of inhibiting the host immune response and contributing to the persistence of infection *(23).* In a symptomatic primary HCMV infection, the cell-mediated immunity is depressed with T-cell abnormalities most readily defined *(24).* Consequently, the likelihood of CMV infections is markedly increased in the immunocompromised host *(25–30).* By some accounts *(27)* between 46 and 80% of the immunocompromised population may be infected. In renal allograft recipients *(31–39)* the primary infections varies from 22%–100% (average 53%) and recurrent infections from 46%–100% (average 85%). Similar rates of infections have been seen among cardiac and bone marrow transplant recipients *(2,40–43).* HCMV is the most commonly isolated opportunistic pathogen associated with hepatitis following orthotopic liver transplantation *(44–50).* HCMV infection is also a major cause of morbidity following lung transplantation *(51).*

Although HCMV infection is frequently observed in allograft recipients, not all infected individuals will develop disease. In solid organ-transplant recipients, HCMV infection develops largely when a seropositive organ containing the virus is transplanted into a recipient *(44,45).* If the recipient has a pre-existing immunity against HCMV, this can partially ameliorate the disease *(35,52).* However, in bone marrow allograft recipients, HCMV infection usually ensues from reactivation of latent infection in the recipient *(53).*

The fact that after renal transplantation, most patients become productively infected indicates frequent reactivation of latent HCMV *(24,54).* Reactivation occurs despite of the serologic status of donors.

Owing to the high rate of seropositivity (90–100%) among AIDS patients, HCMV was originally thought by some to be the etiologic agent of AIDS *(25,26).* Approximately 40% of patients with AIDS present with HCMV visceral involvement at the advanced stage of the disease *(55,56).* The most common localizations are retinitis and gastrointestinal infection *(57)* and to a lesser extent CNS disorders. When compared to HCMV infection in non- human immunodeficiency virus (HIV) immunosuppressed patients, retinitis in HIV-positive individuals is much more prevalent than pneumonitis. To this end, despite the presence of HCMV in the lungs, Millar et al. *(58)* found no evidence of HCMV-induced pneumonitis in AIDS patients, presumably owing to the inability of the lungs to mount the T-cell response necessary for immunopathology; results from mouse and human studies have lent credence to the hypothesis that the pathogenesis of HCMV pneumonitis is immunopathologically mediated *(59)*.

Because in AIDS patients the coexistence of multiple pathogens is frequent, the diagnosis of HCMV infection may be complicated.

The profound and progressive immune suppression caused by HIV creates optimal conditions for reactivation of a latent intracellular HCMV infection, which becomes chronic with a high frequency of relapses owing to the progression of HIV infection over time. Also, because multiple strains of HCMV have been identified in populations at risk *(14)*, reinfection remains a distinct possibility.

By all accounts, HCMV has become a major opportunistic infection in AIDS patients, with autopsy studies indicating that as high as 90% of patients had active dissiminated infection *(55,60)*.

3. STUDIES ON THERAPEUTICS

3.1. Ganciclovir

Ganciclovir (DHPG, cytovene) is an acyclic analog of 2'-deoxyguanosine that needs to be phosphorylated in order to inhibit the viral synthesis. Its mechanism of action involves suppression of viral DNA synthesis by competitive inhibition of viral DNA polymerases and direct incorporation into viral DNA, resulting in termination of DNA elongation.

Using simple mathematical models, Emery and Griffiths *(61)* showed that the efficacy of ganciclovir against wild-type strains was 91.5% when given intravenously (at 5 mg/kg, b.i.d.), but only 46.5% when given orally (1.0 g, t.i.d.); the corresponding values for a typical ganciclovir-resistant virus were 62 and 35%, respectively. During prolonged periods of ganciclovir therapy, the apparent sudden appearance of ganciclovir resistance has explained by the combination of two exponentially increasing populations (wild-type and mutant) at ganciclovir doses that did not completely inhibit HCMV replication. The modeled and experimental data exhibited excellent agreement over extended period of time (up to 270 d of therapy) and may provide a framework to predict the virulogic course in patients at therapeutic initiation *(61)*.

Although orally given ganciclovir has clear practical advantages over its intravenous administration, the relatively low bioavailability of the drug may be problematic in at-risk patients with malabsorption. Snell et al. *(62)* conducted a pharmacokinetic assessment of oral ganciclovir in lung- transplant recipients with cystic fibrosis (CF) because the bioavailability, and therefore, the therapeutic potential of oral ganciclovir in CF patients post-transplant might be expected to be inadequate given the high incidence of malabsorption in these patients. However, after 3 d of oral ganciclovir and despite a background of general malabsorption, the results demonstrated therapeutically useful plasma drug levels in this population; the mean peak (C_{max}), mean minimum (C_{min}) concentrations, and the mean area under the curve (AUC) were highly correlated, allowing the possibility of steady-state drug monitoring to confirm that the recommended dosing algorithm produced appropriate plasma levels.

3.1.1. Toxicity of Ganciclovir

The major toxic side effect of ganciclovir is its hematoxicity, including neutropenia (40% of the cases), thrombocytopenia, or anemia (20%) *(63)*. In order to reduce the neutropenia, Hardy et al. *(64,65)* recommended the use recombinant human granulocyte-macrophage colony-stimulating factor (GM-CSF) or human granulocyte colony-stimulating factor (G-CSF). Although oral ganciclovir was tolerated at doses of up to 6.0 g daily, at that dose the rate of neutropenia was higher *(66)*.

Another drawback of ganciclovir has been the bone-marrow suppression it has induced when given concomitantly with zidovudine *(67)*. Other side effects included confusion, fever, gastrointestinal disorders (nausea), abnormal liver function, anemia, and cutaneous rash *(55,68–72)*.

Scholz et al. *(73)* provided evidence for an immunosuppressive activity of ganciclovir.

Drugs that inhibit renal tubular secretion or absorption, such as probenicid, may reduce the renal clearance of ganciclovir and exacerbate its toxicity. Similarly, bone marrow-suppressing agents (pentamidine isethionate, trimethoprim-sulfonamide, and amphotericin B) may inhibit bone marrow activity and spermatogenesis and further contribute to genciclovir toxicity.

Generalized seizures have been reported in patients receiving concomitantly ganciclovir and imipenem-cilastin sodium (74). Seizures associated with ganciclovir therapy alone were reported in a patient with AIDS and disseminated CMV disease; despite the administration of phenytoin, the seizure-like activity subsided only after discontinuing of ganciclovir (75).

3.2. Foscarnet

Foscarnet (PFA, foscavir, trisodium phosphonoformate) is a pyrophosphate analog active against wide variety of human herpesviruses including ganciclovir-resistant HCMV strains, by inhibiting viral DNA polymerases (76,77). In addition, foscarnet has been shown to inhibit HIV reverse transcriptase (78).

Contrary to ganciclovir and other nucleosides, foscarnet and other pyrophosphate analogs (phosphonoacetate; PAA) do not require prior phosphorylation in order to inhibit the viral DNA polymerase. These compounds inhibit pyrophosphorolysis competitively with pyrophosphate, but are noncompetitive with dNTPs and uncompetitive with DNA (77).

After a single dose of 90 mg/kg of foscarnet in patients with AIDS, its levels in plasma ranged from 297–1,775 µg/mL (990-5,920 µmol/L), with a mean value of 766 µg/mL (79). The corresponding levels in CSF were 57–225 µg/mL (190–750 µmol/L), with a mean value of 131 µg/mL; the penetration coefficient was 0.05–0.72. At steady-state, the mean foscarnet levels in plasma were 464 µg/mL (1,553 µmol/L), whereas the mean levels in cerebrospinal fluid (CSF) were 308 µg/mL (1,023 µmol/mL); the penetration coefficient was 0.66. Although the penetration coefficients were highly variable after a single administration and at steady-state, the concentrations of foscarnet in the CSF were sufficient for complete inhibition of HCMV replication in vitro (79). The plasma concentrations of foscarnet after twice-daily infusion of 90 mg/kg for 2 wk showed no significant difference between day 1, d 7, and d 14; mean peak and trough concentrations on d 14 were 605 and 52 µM, respectively (80). In all patients, the peak levels of the drug were well above those necessary to inhibit CMV. The property of foscarnet to penetrate well the blood-brain barrier (BBB) would strongly bolster its use in the treatment of HCMV encephalitis.

One unique property of foscarnet has been its ability to inhibit both HIV and HCMV (81–83). In vitro, the combination of foscarnet and zidovudine AZT) produced a moderate synergistic inhibitory effect against HIV-1 at concentrations easily achieved in humans. By using partially purified HIV reverse transcriptase and human CMV DNA polymerase, Eriksson and Schinazi (82) demonstrated significant additive interactions of various combinations of AZT-5'-triphosphate and foscarnet. The synergistic interactions in infected cells and the additive effects seen at the reverese transcriptase level have indicated that mechanisms other than the reverse transcriptase may play a role in the inhibition of HIV replication by these two compounds (81). These in vitro findings suggested that concomitant administration of foscarnet to AIDS patients receiving zidovudine may be appropriate not only to treat CMV disease, but also to control the HIV infection itself.

3.2.1. Toxicity of Foscarnet

The most important side effect of foscarnet is its nephrotoxicity. It may affect as high as 50–60% of patients receiving continuous i.v. administration (84). Intermittent administration (85) and concomitant saline isotonic hydration have decreased foscarnet nephrotoxicity to 15% of cases (86,87).

Electrolyte disorders induced by foscarnet have also been frequently observed. One common side effect is acute ionized hypocalcemia and hypomagnesemia following i.v. administration of the drug (88). Foscarnet-associated hypocalcemia is thought to be responsible for parasthesia, seizure, and nausea. It is caused by the rapid decrease of ionized calcium because of its chelation by foscarnet

(78). Hypophosphatemia and hypomagnesemia, which usually remain asymptomatic, have also been associated with foscarnet *(84,89)*. Foscarnet-induced ionized hypomagnesemia might also contribute to ionized hypocalcemia by impairing excretion of preformed parathyroid hormone or by producing target-organ resistance (88). To this end, concomitant administration of foscarnet with antianxiety medications that may mask the symptoms of electrolyte disorders should bèhundertaken with caution and carefully monitored.

Genital ulcers, owing to high foscarnet concentrations in the urine, have also been reported *(90,91)*. Uvula and esophageal ulcerations caused by foscarnet have been discussed by Saint-Marc et al. *(92)*.

Fan-Harvard et al. *(93)* reported on a possible adverse interaction between foscarnet and ciprofloxacin in patients with AIDS, HCMV retinitis, and *Mycobacterium avium* complex (MAC) infection. The incidence of seizures with foscarnet infusion has been high (13–15%), and is facilitated by predisposing factors, such as renal impairment, electrolyte and metabolic abnormalities, and underlying neurologic disorders. The concurrent administration of ciprofloxacin, a known epileptogenic agent, and foscarnet may predispose patients to the development of seizures and should be applied with caution.

3.3. Cidofovir

Cidofovir [(S)-1-(3-hydroxy-2-[phosphonylmethoxy]propyl)cytosine; HPMPC], an acyclic nucleoside phosphonate analog, was identified as one of the most potent and selective inhibitors of human and murine CMV *(94–99)*. Cidofovir, which was tested in a new assay based on the enhanced esterase activity in CMV-infected cells, specifically inhibited the viral DNA synthesis, with a very long-lasting effect. When compared to genciclovir in a model of murine CMV (MCMV), HPMPC was far superior in preventing MCMV-induced mortality.

Cidofovir has been indicated for i.v. treatment of HCMV retinitis with AIDS *(100,101)*. Its dose regimen, determined in three comparative trials, includes one infusion of 5.0 mg/kg once weekly for 15 d, then once every 15 d. Cidofovir treatment, which has been recommended for patients with relatively low risk of visual deterioration, showed slowing the progression of retinitis on fundoscopy but no effect on visual acuity *(102)*. The most frequent adverse side effects of cidofovir include nephrotoxicity and eye damage.

The most serious ophthalmologic complications of i.v. and intravitreous cidofovir therapy include intraocular inflammation and ocular hypotony *(100,103)*. Anterior uveitis *(100,103–105)* and iritis *(101)* appears to be a frequent side effects during i.v. cidofovir therapy for HCMV retinitis.

3.4. Fomivirsen

Fomivirsen (vitravene, ISIS 2922), an antisense drug, has recently been approved by the U.S. Food and Drug Administration (FDA) for the treatment of HCMV retinitis. The drug, which is injected directly into the eye once or twice monthly, showed efficacy in impending HCMV from replicating locally in the eye without causing any systemic effects *(106)*. The drug is acting by interrupting the viral replication by binding to the virus' genetic material. Fomivirsen cannot suppress HCMV infections elsewhere in the body.

In a 2:1 randomized scheme, fomivirsen was evaluated in 18 AIDS patients with previously untreated unilateral HCMV retinitis in zones 2 and 3 (less than 25% retinal involvement) *(107)*. The drug (150 µg) was administered by intravitreal injection for 3 weekly doses followed by bimonthly maintenance doses; 10 patients were assigned as a deferred treatment group, and were followed to progression before crossover to receive fomivirsen. Intent to treat analysis revealed a median time to observed progression of 71 d for those in the immediate treatment group vs 14 d for those assigned to deferred treatment ($p = 0.0056$).

Retinal toxic side effects associated with intravitreal fomivirsen include the potential for widespread retinal pigment epithelial change *(108)* as well as increased pressure in the eye after injection, a decrease in bone marrow, and inflammation *(109)*.

Table 1
Treatment of HCMV Retinitis

Drug	Regimen
Ganciclovir	5.0 mg/kg, b.i.d., for 2–3 wk[a]
Foscarnet	60 mg/kg, t.i.d. for 2 wk,[b] or 90–100 mg/kg, b.i.d. for 2 wk[b]
Cidofovir	5.0 mg/kg once weekly for 2 wk, then 5.0 mg/kg every 2 wk[c]
Fomivirsen	330 µg (0.5 mL), intravitreal injection on d 1 and d 15, then once a month

[a]The drug is applied in 30-min i.v. infusions; maintenance therapy consists of once daily dose of 5.0 mg/kg.

[b]Foscarnet is applied in 90-min i.v. infusions with 500–1,000 mL isotonic saline; maintenance therapy consists of once daily applications of 90–200 mg/kg of the drug in 90-min infusions *(129)*.

[c]The drug is discontinued if serum creatinine level increases and/or persistent proteinuria appears *(100)*.

3.5. Valaciclovir

Valaciclovir, an acyclovir prodrug, is used to treat infection caused by herpes simplex virus and varicella zoster virus, as well as for prophylaxis against CMV infections *(110)*. Valaciclovir provides significantly better oral bioavailability than acyclovir, thereby contributing to the need for less frequent administration.

The relationship between HCMV viral load, antiviral chemotherapy, and disease progression in 310 HIV-positive patients was investigated as part of the ACTG 204 in a randomized, controlled trial comparing the clinical benefits of valaciclovir with acyclovir *(111)*. In time-updated analyses, the presence of HCMV DNA and elevated viral load throughout the study period in both blood and urine were significantly associated with increased progression to HCMV disease. In contrast, the effect of valaciclovir became of borderline significance. The results demonstrated that high HCMV load in HIV-infected patients increases the risk of disease and adversely impacts on survival, and that the clinical benefit of receiving valaciclovir was directly related to the inhibition of HCMV replication *(111)*.

4. TREATMENT OF HCMV INFECTIONS

4.1. Management of HCMV Disease in AIDS Patients

HCMV infection is common in both homosexual and heterosexual HIV-infected patients, especially in AIDS patients with low CD4$^+$ cell counts *(112)*.

Ganciclovir *(113–117)* and foscarnet *(118–122)* are currently the drugs of choice to treat HCMV retinitis *(123–128)*. Their efficacy is similar, resulting in 90–95% response rate among patients treated for a first episode of HCMV retinitis during induction therapy (Table 1) *(55,74)*.

A number of clinical studies have documented the efficacy of ganciclovir in the treatment of HCMV retinitis *(69–71,113,126,130–138)*. In spite of it, however, retinitis recurred in nearly all cases after cessation of therapy to indicate a virostatic activity for ganciclovir *(130,135–137,139,140)*. Ganciclovir is usually administered intravenously in a 1-hour period infusion with 5.0 mg/kg daily during induction therapy (Table 1) *(55,74)*. Because of its renal excretion, the dosage of ganciclovir should be adjusted to compensate for renal insufficiency. The mean intravitreal concentration of ganciclovir after intravenous administration to AIDS patients with retinal detachments was 0.93 µg/mL

(3.6 µM). This value, which was significantly lower than the concentration of ganciclovir required to achieve 50% of viral plaque formation for many human CMV strains, suggested that the i.v. administration of ganciclovir results in near-steady-state subtherapeutic intravitreal concentrations for many HCMV isolates *(141)*. This may explain the difficulty of long-term complete suppression of HCMV retinitis.

The use of intravenous or intravitreous ganciclovir for treatment of HCMV retinitis has also been associated with the development of antiviral resistant HCMV that is conferred by mutations in the viral UL97 and polymerase genes *(142)*.

Muccioli and Belfort *(143)* reported that a intraocular sustained-release ganciclovir implant proved to be a safe new procedure for the treatment of HCMV retinitis by avoiding the systemic side effects caused by the i.v. medications and improving quality of life of the patients. The intraocular implant was effective in controlling the progression of retinitis for up to 8 mo, even in patients for whom systemic therapy with either ganciclovir or foscarnet or both had failed. However, Williamson et al. *(144)* described a patient who developed oxacillin-resistant *Staphylococcus aureus* endophthalmitis after insertion of a ganciclovir intraocular implant making the case of bacterial endophthalmitis an infrequent but serious complication of ganciclovir intraocular implants.

Patients with AIDS who develop clinically resistant HCMV retinitis may show progression of retinitis despite extended i.v. induction single-drug therapy or alternating therapy with induction doses of ganciclovir or foscarnet. In several clinical experiments *(145–147)*, such patients were treated with a combination of ganciclovir and foscarnet. The recommended dosing regimen for induction combination therapy was ganciclovir (5.0 mg/kg every 12 h) and foscarnet (60 mg/kg, t.i.d.). Maintenance combination therapy was ganciclovir (5.0 mg/kg every 12–24 h) and foscarnet (90–120 mg/kg once daily). All patients exhibited a favorable response to the combination therapy, with complete healing of retinitis in 12 of 14 eyes and partial healing of retinitis with decreased border activity and a cessation of border advancement in 2 of 14 eyes. The combined drug regimen was generally well-tolerated, with no significant toxic effects to require cessation of therapy *(145)*.

An open-pilot, noncomparative, multicenter study was designed to evaluate the efficacy and safety of the foscarnet-ganciclovir combination in induction therapy and maintenance therapy of HCMV-induced central neurological disorders in 31 HIV-infected patients with acute HCMV encephalitis ($n=17$) or myelitis ($n=14$); none of the patients had received HAART *(148)*. All patients received intravenous induction therapy consisting of foscarnet (90 mg/kg) and ganciclovir (5.0 mg/kg) twice daily, followed by maintenance therapy. Clinical efficacy was assessed at the end of the induction phase. Overall, the foscarnet-ganciclovir combination as induction therapy resulted in a 74% clinical improvement or stabilization.

Concurrent therapy of ganciclovir and zidovudine has been shown to significantly enhance the risk of granulocytopenia, and in most cases should be avoided *(67,149,150)*. Results from several vitro studies have also demonstrated the presence of synergistic toxicity between ganciclovir and zidovudine *(151–153)*. The data by Freitas et al. *(154)*, which suggested that zidovudine potentiated the antiviral activity of ganciclovir against a clinical isolate of human CMV and interacted in an additive manner with a laboratory strain, have been questioned by Prichard and Shipman *(155)*.

However, a treatment protocol developed by Causey *(156)* did allow for the co-administration of zidovudine and ganciclovir under certain controlled conditions. Thus, zidovudine may be given concomitantly with ganciclovir if the absolute granulocyte counts are over 750 cells/µL. When the absolute granulocyte counts are initially below 750 cells/iL or fall bellow 750 cells/ µL, zidovudine should be discontinued, while ganciclovir is administered. The Causey's protocol was designed to minimize potential toxicity by avoiding concurrent dosing with zidovudine and ganciclovir when hematologic cytotoxicity becomes evident *(156)*. In patients who were unable to tolerate both drugs, dideoxyinosine (ddI, didanosine) should be used in place of zidovudine; *(157)* alternatively, foscarnet may be used in place of ganciclovir. Carter and Shuster *(158)* reported that combined treatment with oral acyclovir and zidovudine cleared all clinical evidence of active HCMV retinitis.

The tolerance of neutropenia caused by ganciclovir has been increased by adjunctive therapy with (GM-CSF) *(159)*. Hardy et al. *(65)* evaluated in AIDS patients the efficacy and safety of a combination of ganciclovir and GM-CSF.

In a report by Papastamopoulos et al. *(160)*, an AIDS patient with HCMV retinitis was treated with cidofovir for 17 consecutive months without any adverse effects. Initially, the drug was administered at 5.0 mg/kg for 2 wk and maintenance therapy thereafter. In addition, probenicid, hydration, and monitoring for proteinuria were also used to prevent nephrotoxicity. The maintenance therapy was discontinued after the permanent rise of the $CD4^+$ cells over 100 cells/mm^3.

Monkemuller and Wilcox *(161)* reported a case of an HIV-positive patient with HCMV-induced esophageal ulcer and receiving combination antiretroviral therapy. The esophageal symptoms were resolved within 4 d of endoscopy without specific therapy for HCMV.

In a randomized, open-label, Phase II trial involving 42 HIV-infected patients with less than 100 $CD4^+$ cells/mm^3 and persistent asymptomatic HCMV viremia, Salmon-Ceron et al. *(162)* compared the virological and clinical effects on HCMV infection of a 14-day course of intravenous foscarnet (100 mg/kg every 12 h) or no treatment. All HCMV markers (blood culture, pp65 antigenemia, plasma, and leukocyte DNA) either became negative or markedly decreased at d 14 in the foscarnet group. However, after the end of treatment, all markers reappeared or the virus load rapidly increased with a probability of HCMV disease at 6 mo being 43% in both groups. The results of the study suggested that sequential courses of intravenous foscarnet may not constitute a good strategy for preemptive therapy in this population, and that in patients with a positive blood marker, treatment able to induce and maintain negative HCMV blood cultures could be a more effective treatment *(162)*.

4.2. Management of HCMV Disease in Solid Organ and Bone-Marrow Transplant Recipients

Acyclovir, which has displayed poor in vitro efficacy against HCMV in vitro, was found to be beneficial against HCMV infections *(163)* in renal *(31,32)*, liver *(45,164)*, and bone marrow *(165,166)* transplant recipients when given at high doses either parenterally or orally.

Paya et al. *(45)* analyzed the incidence and clinical characteristics of HCMV infection in liver-transplant recipients and conducted a randomized trial to evaluate the efficacy of acyclovir and ganciclovir in the prophylaxis of HCMV infection following orthotopic liver transplantation. Symptomatic HCMV-induced hepatitis, which developed in 25% of patients, was also a major cause of death (21% of all deaths). As prophylaxis therapy, patients received either combination of ganciclovir and acyclovir (group A), or acyclovir alone (group B). Group A patients had a decreased incidence of HCMV infection, mainly owing to decrease in asymptomatic infection. The incidence of symptomatic infection was similar in both groups as well as when compared to control liver-transplant recipients. Overall, the use of acyclovir alone did not appear to have a significant impact in reducing the incidence and severity of HCMV infection *(45)*.

In another study, Martin et al. *(167)* conducted a prospective randomized trial comparing sequential ganciclovir-high dose acyclovir to high-dose acyclovir for prevention of HCMV disease in adult liver-transplant recipients. The patients were randomized to receive either high-dose oral acyclovir (800 mg q.d.i.) alone for 3 mo after transplantation (group A), or intravenous ganciclovir (5.0 mg/kg b.i.d.) for 2 wk followed by high-dose oral acyclovir to complete a 3-mo regimen (group B). Sixty-one percent of the patients from group A developed HCMV infection, as compared to only 24% from group B. Of those randomized, HCMV disease was observed in 28% of group A, but only in 9% of group B. The median time to onset for both HCMV infection and HCMV disease were longer for the ganciclovir-acyclovir group (group B) compared to the acyclovir group (group A) (78 d vs 45 d, and 78 d vs 40 d, respectively). With regard to primary HCMV infection, there was no difference in the rates between the two groups, but tissue-invasive disease and recurrent HCMV disease were less frequent in the ganciclovir-acyclovir group. The overall results of this trial strongly indicated that for prevention of HCMV infection and HCMV disease after liver transplantation, a 2-wk course of ganciclovir immediately after transplantation followed by high-dose of oral acyclovir for 10 wk was superior to a 12-wk course of high-dose oral acyclovir alone.

Based on their results from a randomized trial with liver-transplant recipients, Singh et al. *(168)* concluded that high-dose oral acyclovir (800 mg q.i.d.) is ineffective prophylaxis against HCMV disease. Instead, a preemptive, short-course therapy of intravenous ganciclovir (5.0 mg/kg, b.i.d.) for 7 d in patients with HCMV shedding was well-tolerated and provided effective prophylaxis against subsequent HCMV disease while minimizing toxicity and cost of treatment.

Dunn et al. *(169)* conducted a prospective randomized trial to appraise the efficacy of acyclovir vs ganciclovir plus human immune globulin prophylaxis of HCMV infection after solid organ transplantation. Patients were stratified according to allograft type, age, and presence or absence or diabetes mellitus, and were then randomized to receive either long-duration acyclovir prophylaxis (800 mg orally or 400 mg, q.i.d., i.v. for 12 wk after transplantation or 6 wk after any antirejection therapy), or short-duration ganciclovir (5.0 mg/kg, b.i.d., i.v. for 7 d after transplant or after any antirejection therapy) plus human immune globulin (100 mg, intravenous administration on days 1, 4, and 7 after transplant or after any antirejection therapy. No differences in actuarial patient or allograft survival were observed between the two treatment protocols. Overall, acyclovir prophylaxis appeared to be more effective in reducing the incidence of post-transplant HCMV disease, although this effect was somewhat diminished in high-risk patients. Long-term therapy seemed to better prevent HCMV transmission or reactivation *(169)*.

Results from several studies suggested that combination treatment of ganciclovir and immune globulin *(170)* can increase the number of survivors among bone-marrow transplant recipients *(171–173)*. In a randomized controlled trial, Snydman et al. *(37)* showed that passive immunization with HCMV immune globulin (HCMV-IG) reduced the incidence of HCMV-associated disease by 65% in seronegative recipients of kidney from seropositive donors. The recommended protocol, which was chosen as a result of a pilot study *(174)* consisted of randomly assigned patients receiving intravenously 150 mg/kg HCMV-IG within 72 h of transplantation, then 100 mg/kg at wk 2 and 4 after transplantation, followed by 50 mg/kg at wk 6, 8, 12, and 16 after transplantation. The HCMV-IG was administered initially at a rate of 15 mg/kg/p h; if there were no untoward side effects, the rate was increased to a maximum of 60 mg/kg per hour *(37)*. Overall, the prophylaxis with HCMV-IG was most beneficial to renal transplant recipients at high-risk of HCMV-associated disease *(175)* and was well tolerated by patients in both this and another study involving bone marrow-transplant recipients *(176)*.

The prophylactic (10 mg/kg daily during the 3rd and 4th wk after surgery) vs therapeutic (10 mg/kg daily only after clinical HCMV disease was diagnosed) use of ganciclovir after liver transplantation in adult patients was evaluated by Cohen et al. *(177)* in a prospective, controlled trial of 33 patients. While prophylactic ganciclovir was associated with a lower incidence of serologically diagnosed secondary infection, the development of IgM anti-HCMV antibody, and the absence of leukopenia, the frequency of clinical infections was similar in the two groups *(177)*.

5. PROPHYLAXIS AND MAINTENANCE THERAPY OF HCMV DISEASE

Lifelong maintenance therapy with ganciclovir *(71,133,135)* or foscarnet *(178–183)* can slow the progression of retinitis and minimize vision loss. As an alternative to intravenous infusion, a capsule form of ganciclovir for oral administration has been studied *(184)*. The absolute bioavailability of oral ganciclovir given at a dosage of 1,000 mg t.i.d. with food, averaged 9% *(185)*. Daily doses of 3,000 mg or more yielded average serum ganciclovir concentrations exceeding 0.5 µg/mL *(66)*, a concentration sufficient to inhibit most clinical isolates of HCMV *(186)*.

In an open-label, randomized trial of AIDS patients, Drew et al. *(184)* compared as a maintenance therapy for HCMV retinitis oral (3.0 g daily) versus intravenous (5.0 mg/kg daily) ganciclovir. The results showed a mean time to the progression of retinitis of 62 and 57 d for intravenous and oral ganciclovir, respectively. Overall, oral ganciclovir was safe and effective alternative to intravenous

8. APPLICATION OF IMMUNOTHERAPY FOR HCMV INFECTIONS

Acute and persistent viral diseases such as the HCMV and HIV infections may be limited by the development and maintenance of efficient host T-cell responses to the viral antigens. Recent studies *(229,230)* have provided insights into the nature of the protective T-cell responses and advances in T-cell culture technology have made it possible to evaluate the adoptive transfer of T-cell clones of defined antigen specificity and function to restore deficient responses in the immunocompromised hosts.

In a Phase II, randomized, double-masked, placebo-controlled trial (ACTG 266), Borucki et al. *(231)* compared the effects of standard therapy with standard therapy combined with human monoclonal anti-HCMV antibody (MSL-109) in the treatment of AIDS patients with newly diagnosed HCMV retinitis. MSL-109 was administered intravenously at 15 or 60 mg every 2 weeks. The antibody, which is directed against HCMV gH, was well-tolerated and there was an unexplained survival advantage in the higher-dose recipients.

REFERENCES

1. Weller, T. H. The cytomegaloviruses: ubiquitous agents with protean clinical manifestations. *N. Engl. J. Med.* 285, 203, 1971.
2. Alford, C. A. and Britt, W. J. Cytomegalovirus, in *Fields Virology*, 2nd ed., Fields, B. N., Knipe, D. M., Chanock, R. M., Hirsch, M. S., Melnick, J. L., Monath, T. P., and Roizman, B., Eds. Raven Press, New York, 1981, 1990.
3. Stinski, M. F. Cytomegalovirus and its replication, in *Fields Virology*, 2nd ed., Fields, B. N., Knipe, D. M., Chanock, R. M., Hirsch, M. S., Melnick, J. L., Monath, T. P., and Roizman, B., Eds. Raven Press, New York, 1059, 1990.
4. Roizman, B. Herpesviridae: a brief introduction, in *Fields Virology*, 2nd ed., Fields, B. N., Knipe, D. M., Chanock, R. M., Hirsch, M. S., Melnick, J. L., Monath, T. P., and Roizman, B., Eds. Raven Press, New York, 1787, 1990.
5. Alford, C. A., Stagno, S., Pass, R. F., and Huang, E.-S. Epidemiology of cytomegalovirus, in *The Human Herpesviruses: an Interdisciplinary Perspective*, Nahmias, A., Dowdle, W., and Schinazi, R., Eds. Elsevier, New York, 159, 1981.
6. Lang, D. J. The epidemiology of cytomegalovirus infections: interpretations of recent observations, in *Infections of the Fetus and the Newborn Infant*, vol. 3, Krugman, S. and Gershon, A. A., Eds. Alan R. Liss, New York, 35, 1975.
7. Lang, D. J. and Krammer, J. F. Cytomegalovirus in the semen: observations in selected populations. *J. Infect. Dis.*, 132, 472, 1975.
8. Reynolds, D. W., Stagno, S., Hosty, T. S., Tiller, M., and Alford, C. A. Jr. Maternal cytomegalovirus excretion and perinatal infection. *N. Engl. J. Med.* 289, 1, 1981.
9. Stagno, S., Reynolds, D. W., Pass, R. F., and Alford, C. A. Breast milk and the risk of cytomegalovirus infection. *N. Engl. J. Med.* 302, 1073, 1980.
10. Gold, E. and Nankervis, G. A. Cytomegalovirus, in *Viral Infections of Humans: Epidemiology and Control*, 2nd ed., Evans, A. S., Ed. Plenum Press, New York, 167, 1982.
11. Manian, F. A. and Smith, T. Ganciclovir for the treatment of cytomegalovirus pneumonia in an immunocompetent host. *Clin. Infect. Dis.* 17, 137, 1993.
12. Blair, S. D., Forbes, A., and Parkins, R. A. CMV colitis in an immunocompetent adult. *J. R. Soc. Med.* 85, 238, 1992.
13. Drew, W. L. Diagnosis of cytomegalovirus infection. *Rev. Infect. Dis.*, 10(Suppl. 3), 468, 1988.
14. Drew, W. L., Sweet, E. S., Miner, R. C., and Mocarski, E. S. Multiple infections by cytomegalovirus in patients with acquired immunodeficiency syndrome: documentation by Southern blot hybridization. *J. Infect. Dis.*, 150, 952, 1984.
15. Ho, M. Pathology of cytomegalovirus infection, in *Cytomegalovirus, Biology and Infection: Current Topics in Infectious Disease*, Greenough, W. B. III and Merigan, T. C., Eds. Plenum Press, New York, 119, 1982.
16. Becroft, D. M. O. Prenatal cytomegalovirus infection: epidemiology, pathology and pathogenesis, in *Perspectives in Pediatric Pathology*, Rosenergg, H. S. and Bernstein, J., Eds. Mason Press, New York, 203, 1981.
17. Weiss, D. J., Greenfield, J. W. Jr., O'Rourke, K. S., and McCune, W. J. Systemic cytomegalovirus infection mimicking an exacerbation of Wegener's granulomatosis. *J. Rheumatol.*, 20, 155, 1993.
18. Stagno, S., Pass, R. F., Dworsky, M. E., and Alford, C. A. Congenital and perinatal cytomegalovirus infections. *Semin. Perinatol.*, 7, 31, 1983.
19. Salomon, N. and Perlman, D. C., Cytomegalovirus pneumonia. *Semin. Respir. Infect.*, 14, 353–358, 1999.
20. Gisserot, O., de Jaureguiberry, J. P., Carloz, E., Marlier, S., and Jaubert, D. Soux-maxillite a cytomegalovirus chez un patient infecte par le VIH. *Rev. Med. Interne*, 21, 200–201, 2000.
21. Van den Brande, J., Schrijvers, D., Colpaert, C., and Vermorken, J. B. Cytomegalovirus colitis after administration of docetaxel-5-fluorouracil-cisplatin chemotherapy for locally advanced hypopharyngeal cancer. *Ann. Oncol.* 10, 1369–1372, 1999.

22. Seel, K., Guschmann, M., van Landeghem, F., and Grosch-Worner, I. Addison-disease: an unusual clinical manifestation of CMV-end organ disease in pediatric AIDS. *Eur. J. Med. Res.*, 5, 247–250, 2000.
23. Griffiths, P. D. and Grundy, J. E. Molecular biology and immunology of cytomegalovirus. *Biochem. J.*, 241, 313, 1987.
24. Rinaldo, C. R. Jr., Black, P. H., and Hirsch, M. S. Virus-leukocyte interactions in cytomegalovirus mononucleosis. *J. Infect. Dis.*, 136, 667, 1977.
25. Jacobson, M. A. and Mills, J. Serious cytomegalovirus disease in acquired immune deficiency syndrome (AIDS): clinical findings, diagnosis and treatment. *Ann. Intern. Med.*, 108, 585, 1988.
26. Drew, W. L. and Mintz, L. Cytomegalovirus infection in healthy and immune-deficient homosexual men, in *The Acquired Immune Deficiency Syndrome and Infections of Homosexual Men*, Ma, P. and Armstrong, D., Eds., Yorke Medical Books, New York, 117, 1984.
27. Ho, M. Cytomegalovirus infections in immunosuppressed patients, in *Cytomegalovirus, Biology and Infection: Current Topics in Infectious Disease*, Greenough, W. B. III and Merigan, T. C., Eds., Plenum Press, New York, 171, 1982.
28. Stratta, R. J. Clinical patterns and treatment of cytomegalovirus infection after solid-organ transplantation. *Transplant. Res.* 25(5 suppl. 4), 15, 1993.
29. Pollard, R. B. Cytomegalovirus infections in renal, heart, heart-lung and liver transplantations. *Pediatr. Infect. Dis. J.*, 7, 97, 1988.
30. Holbrook, J. T., Davis, M. D., Hubbard, L. D., et al. Risk factors for advancement of cytomegalovirus retinitis in patients with acquired immunodeficiency syndrome. Studies of Ocular Complications of AIDS Research Group. *Arch. Ophthalmol.* 118, 1196–1204, 2000.
31. Balfour, H. H., Chace, B. A., Stapleton, J. T., Simmons, R. L., and Fryd, D. S. A randomized placebo-controlled trial of oral acyclovir for the prevention of cytomegalovirus disease in recipients of renal allograft. *N. Engl. J. Med.*, 320, 1381, 1989.
32. Legendre, C., Ducloux, D., Ferroni, A., et al. Acyclovir in preventing cytomegalovirus infection in kidney transplant recipients: a case- controlled study. *J. Med. Virol. Suppl.*, 1, 118, 1993.
33. Rubin, R. H., Tolkoff-Rubin, N. E., Oliver, D., et al. Multicenter seroepidemiologic study of the impact of cytomegalovirus infection on renal transplantation. *Transplantation*, 40, 243, 1985.
34. Peterson, P. K., Balfour, H. H., Marker, S. C., Fryd, D. S., Howard, R. J., and Simmons, R.L. Cytomegalovirus disease in renal allograft recipients: a prospective study of the clinical features, risk factors and impact on renal transplantation. *Medicine (Baltimore)*, 59, 283, 1980.
35. Rocha, E., Campos, H. H., Rouzioux, C., et al. Cytomegalovirus infections after kidney transplantation: identical risk whether donor or recipient is the virus carrier. *Transplant. Proc.*, 23, 2638, 1991.
36. Rubin, R. H., Cosimi, A. B., Tolkoff-Rubin, N. E., Russell, P. S., and Hirsch, M. S. Infectious disease syndromes attributable to cytomegalovurus and their significance among renal transplant recipients. *Transplantation*, 24, 458, 1977.
37. Snydman, D. R., Wemer, B. G., Heinze-Lacey, B., et al. Use of cytomegalovirus immune globulin to prevent cytomegalovirus disease in renal-transplant recipients. *N. Engl. J. Med.*, 317, 1049, 1987.
38. Burd, R. S., Gillingham, K. J., Farber, M. S., et al. Diagnosis and treatment of cytomegalovirus disease in pediatric renal transplant recipients. *J. Pediatr. Surg.*, 29, 1049, 1994.
39. Saatci, U., Ozen, S., Ceyhan, M., and Secmeer, G. Cytomegalovirus disease in a renal transplant recipient manifesting with pericarditis. *Int. Urol. Nephrol.*, 25, 617, 1993.
40. Devine, S. M. and Wingard, J. R. Viral infections in severely immunocompromised cancer patients. *Support Care Cancer*, 2, 355, 1994.
41. Goodrich, J. M., Boeckh, M., and Bowden, R. Strategies for the prevention of cytomegalovirus disease after marrow transplantation. *Clin. Infect. Dis.*, 19, 287, 1994.
42. Kirklin, J. K., Naftel, D. C., Levine, T. B., et al. Cytomegalovirus after heart transplantation. Risk factors for infection and death: a multiinstutional study. The Cardiac Transplant Research Database Group. *J. Heart Lung Transplant.*, 13, 394, 1994.
43. Arabia, F. A., Rosado, L. J., Huston, C. L., Sethi, G. K., and Copeland, J. G. III. Incidence and recurrence of gastrointestinal cytomegalovirus infection in heart transplantation. *Ann. Thorac. Surg.*, 55, 8, 1993.
44. Singh, N., Dummer, J. S., Kusne, S., et al. Infections with cytomegalovirus and other herpes viruses in 121 liver transplant recipients: transmission by donated organ and the effect of OKT3 antibodies. *J. Infect. Dis.*, 158, 124, 1988.
45. Paya, C. V., Marin, E., Keating, M., Dickson, R., Porayko, M., and Wiesner, R. Solid organ transplantation: result and implications of acyclovir use in liver transplants. *J. Med. Virol. Suppl.*, 1,123, 1993.
46. Paya, C. V., Hermans, P. E., Wiesner, R. H., et al. Cytomegalovirus hepatitis in liver transplantation: prospective analysis of 93 consecutive orthotopic liver transplantations. *J. Infect. Dis.*, 160, 752, 1989.
47. Paya, C. V., Hermans, P. E., Washington, J. A., et al. Incidence, distribution, and outcome of episodes of infection in 100 orthotopic liver transplantations. *Mayo Clinic Proc.*, 64, 555, 1989.
48. Kusne, S., Dummer, J. S., Singh, N., et al. Infections after liver transplantation: an analysis of 101 consecutive cases. *Medicine (Baltimore)*, 67, 132, 1988.
49. Sano, K., Tanaka, K., Uemoto, S., et al. Cytomegalovirus infection in living related liver transplantation: rapid diagnosis by human monoclonal antibody staining of blood leukocytes. *Transplant. Sci.*, 4, 105, 1994.

50. Wiens, M., Schmidt, C. A., Lohmann, R., Oettle, H., Blumhardt, G., and Neuhaus, P. Cytomegalovirus disease after liver transplantation: diagnostics and therapy. *Transplant. Res.*, 25, 2673, 1993.
51. Mistone, A. P., Brumble, L. M., Loyd, J. E., et al. Active CMV infection before lung transplantation: risk factors and clinical implications. *J. Heart Lung Transplant.*, 19, 744–750, 2000.
52. Griffiths, P. D. Current management of cytomegalovirus disease. *J. Med. Virol. Suppl.*, 1, 106, 1993.
53. Winston, D. J., Huang, E.-S., Miller, M. J., et al. Molecular epidemiology of cytomegalovirus infection associated with bone marrow transplantation. *Ann. Intern. Med.*, 102, 16, 1985.
54. Betts, R. F. The relationship of epidemiology and treatment factors to infection and allograft survival in renal transplantation, in *CMV: Pathogenesis and Prevention of Human Infection*, Plotkin, S. A., Michelson, S., Pagano, J. S., and Rapp, F., Eds. Alan R. Riss, New York, 87, 1984.
55. Katlama, C. Cytomegalovirus infection in acquired immune-deficiency syndrome. *J. Med. Virol. Suppl.* 1, 128, 1993.
56. Salmon, D., Lacassin, F., Harzic, M., et al. Predictive value of cytomegalovirus viremia for the occurence of CMV organ involvement in AIDS. *J. Med. Virol.*, 32, 160, 1990.
57. Haas, C., Marteau, P., Roudiere, L., Gisselbrecht, M., Lowenstein, W., and Durand, H. Severe cytomegalovirus enteritis in AIDS. Favorable outcome of medical treatment. *Presse Med.* 29, 596–597, 2000.
58. Millar, A. B., Patou, G., Miller, R. F., et al. Cytomegalovirus in the lungs of patients with AIDS: respiratory pathogen or passenger? *Am. Rev. Respir. Dis.*, 141, 1474, 1990.
59. Grundy, J. E., Shanley, J. D., and Griffiths, P. D. Is cytomegalovirus interstitial pneumonitis in transplant recipients an immunopathological condition? *Lancet*, 2, 996, 1987.
60. Gallant, J. E., Moore, R. D., Richman, D. D., Keruly, J., and Chaisson, R. E. Incidence and natural history of cytomegalovirus disease in patients with advanced human immunodeficiency virus disease treated with zidovudine: the Zidovudine Epidemiology Group. *J. Infect. Dis.*, 166, 1223, 1992.
61. Emery, V. C. and Griffiths, P. D. Prediction of cytomegalovirus load and resistance patterns after antiviral chemotherapy. *Proc. Natl. Acad. Sci. USA*, 97, 8039–8044, 2000.
62. Snell, G. I., Kotsimbos, T. C., Levvey, B. J., et al. Pharmacokinetic assessment of oral ganciclovir in lung transplant recipients with cystic fibrosis. *J. Antimicrob. Chemother.*, 45, 511–516, 2000.
63. Laskin, O. L., Cederberg, D. M., Mills, J., Eron, L. J., Mildvan, D., and Spector, S. A. Ganciclovir for the treatment and suppression of serious infections caused by cytomegalovirus. *Am. J. Med.*, 83, 201, 1987.
64. Hardy, D. W. Combined ganciclovir and recombinant human granulocyte-macrophage colony-stimulating factor in the treatment of cytomegalovirus retinitis in AIDS patients. *J. Acquir. Immune Defic. Syndr.*, 4(Suppl. 1), S22, 1991.
65. Hardy, D., Spector, S., Polsky, B., et al. Combination of ganciclovir and granulocyte-macrophage colony-stimulating factor in the treatment of cytomegalovirus retinitis in AIDS patients. *Eur. J. Clin. Microbiol. Infect. Dis.*, 13(Suppl. 2), S34, 1994.
66. Spector, S. A., Busch, D. F., Follansbee, S., et al. Pharmacokinetic, safety and antiviral profiles of oral ganciclovir in persons infected with human immunodeficiency virus: a phase I/II study. *J. Infect. Dis.*, 171, 1431, 1995.
67. Hochster, H., Dieterich, D., Bozzette, S., et al. Toxicity of combined ganciclovir and zidovudine for cytomegalovirus disease associated with AIDS. *Ann. Intern. Med.*, 113, 111, 1990.
68. Freeman, W. R., Henderly, D. E., Wan, W. L., et al. Prevalence, pathophysiology, and treatment of rhegmatogenous retinal detachment in treated cytomegalovirus retinitis. *Am. J. Ophthalmol.*, 103, 627, 1987.
69. Collaborative DHPG Treatment Study Group. Treatment of serious cytomegalovirus infections with 9-(1,3-dihydroxy-2-propoxymethyl) guanine in patients with AIDS and other immunodeficiencies. *N. Engl. J. Med.*, 314, 801, 1986.
70. Hooymans, J. M. M., Sprenger, H. G., and Weits, J. Treatment of cytomegalovirus retinitis with DHPG in a patient with AIDS. *Doc. Ophthalmol.*, 67, 5, 1987.
71. Orellana, J., Teich, S. A., Friedman, A. H., Lerebours, F., Winterkorn, J., and Mildvan, D. Combined short- and long-term therapy for the treatment of cytomegalovirus retinitis using ganciclovir (BW B759U). *Ophthalmology*, 94, 831, 1987.
72. Figge, H. L., Bailie, G. R., Briceland, L. L., and Kowalsky, S. F. Possible ganciclovir- induced hepatotoxicity in patients with AIDS. *Clin. Pharm.*, 11, 432, 1992.
73. Scholz, D., Arndt, R., and Meyer, T. Evidence for an immunosuppressive activity of ganciclovir. *Transplant. Proc.*, 26, 3253, 1994.
74. Yoser, S. L., Forster, D. J., and Rao, N. A. Systemic viral infections and their retinal and choroidal manifestations. *Surv. Ophthalmol.*, 37, 313, 1993.
75. Barton, T. L., Roush, M. K., and Dever, L. L. Seizures associated with ganciclovir therapy. *Pharmacotherapy*, 12, 413, 1992.
76. Drew, W. L., Miner, R. C., Busch, D. F., et al. Prevalence of resistance in patients receiving ganciclovir for serious cytomegalovirus infection. *J. Infect. Dis.*, 163, 716, 1991.
77. Öberg, B. Antiviral effects of phosphonoformate (PFA, foscarnet sodium). *Pharmacol. Ther.*, 19, 387, 1983.
78. Sandström, E. G., Kaplan, J. C., Byington, R. E., and Hirsch, M. S. Inhibition of human T cell lymphtropic virus type III by phosphonoformate. *Lancet*, 1, 1480, 1985.
79. Hengge, U. R., Brockmeyer, N. H., Malessa, R., Ravens, U., and Goos, M. Foscarnet penetrates the blood-brain barrier: rational for therapy of cytomegalovirus encephalitis. *Antimicrob. Agents Chemother.*, 37, 1010, 1993.
80. Taburet, A. M., Katlama, C., Blanshard, C., et al. Pharmacokinetics of foscarnet after twice-daily administration for treatment of cytomegalovirus disease in AIDS patients. *Antimicrob. Agents Chemother.*, 36, 1821, 1992.
81. Schinazi, R. F. Combined chemotherapeutic modalities for viral infections: rationale and clinical potential, in *Synergism and Antagonism in Chemotherapy*, Chou, T.-C., and Rideout, D. C., Eds., Academic Press, San Diego, 109, 1991.

82. Eriksson, B. F. H. and Schinazi, R. F. Combinations of 3'-azido-3'-deoxythimidine (zidovudine) and phosphonoformate (foscarnet) against human immunodeficiency virus type 1 and cytomegalovirus in vitro. *Antimicrob. Agents Chemother.*, 33, 663, 1989.
83. Reddy, M. M., Grieco, M. H., McKinley, G. F., et al. Effect of foscarnet therapy on human immunodeficiency virus p24 antigen levels in AIDS patients with cytomegalovirus retinitis. *J. Infect. Dis.*, 166, 607, 1992.
84. Chrisp, P. and Crissold, S. P. Foscarnet: a review of its antiviral activity, pharmacokinetic properties and therapeutic use in immunocompromised retinitis patients with cytomegalovirus retinitis. *Drugs*, 41, 104, 1991.
85. Aweeka, F., Gambertoglio, J., Mills, J., and Jacobson, M. A. Pharmacokinetics of intermittently administered intravenous foscarnet in the treatment of acquired immunodeficiency syndrome patients with serious cytomegalovirus retinitis. *Antimicrob. Agents Chemother.*, 33, 742, 1989.
86. Deray, G., Katlama, C., and Dohin, E. Prevention of foscarnet nephrotoxicity. *Ann. Intern. Med.*, 113, 332, 1990.
87. Deray, G., Martinez, F., Katlama, C., et al. Foscarnet nephrotoxicity: mechanism incidence and prevention. *Am. J. Nephrol.*, 9, 316–321, 1989.
88. Huycke, M. M., Naguib, M. T., Stroemmel, M. M., et al. A double-blind placebo-controlled crossover trial of intravenous magnesium sulfate for foscarnet-induced ionized hypocalcemia and hypomagnesemia in patient with AIDS and cytomegalovirus infection. *Antimicrob. Agents Chemother.*, 44, 2143–2148, 2000.
89. Geahart, M. O. and Sorg, T. B. Foscarnet-induced severe hypomagnesemia and other electrolyte disorders. *Clin. Pharmacother.* 27, 285, 1993.
90. Katlama, C., Dohin, E., Caumes, E., et al. Foscarnet induction therapy for cytomegalovirus retinitis in AIDS: comparison of twice-daily and three times daily regimens. *J. Acquir. Immune Defic. Syndr.*, 5(Suppl. 1), S18, 1992.
91. Evans, L. M. and Grossman, M. E. Foscarnet-induced penile ulcer. *J. Am. Acad. Dermatol.*, 27, 124, 1992.
92. Saint-Marc, T., Fournier, F., Touraine, J. L., and Marneff, E. Uvula and oesophageal ulcerations with foscarnet. *Lancet*, 340, 970, 1992.
93. Fan-Harvard, P., Sanchorawala, V., Oh, J., Moser, E. M., and Smith, S. P. Concurrent use of foscarnet and ciprofloxacin may increase the propensity of seizures. *Ann. Pharmacother.*, 28, 869, 1994.
94. Neyts, J. and De Clercq, E. New inhibitors of cytomegalovirus replication: in vitro evaluation, mechanism of action, and in vivo activity. *Verh. K. Acad. Geneeskd. Belg.*, 56, 561, 1994.
95. Neyts, J., Sobis, H., Snoeck, R., Vandeputte, M., and De Clercq, E. Efficacy of (S)-1-(3- hydroxy-2-phosphonylmethoxypropyl)cytosine and 9-(1,3-dihydroxy-2- propoxymethyl)guanine in the treatment of intracerebral murine cytomegalovirus infections in immunocompetent and immunodeficient mice. *Eur. J. Clin. Microbiol. Infect. Dis.*, 12, 269, 1993.
96. Stals, F. S., Zeytinoglu, A., Havenith, M., De Clercq, E., and Bruggeman, C. A. Rat cytomegalovirus-induced pneumonitis after allogeneic bone marrow transplantation: effective treatment with (S)-1-(3-hydroxy-2-phosphonylmethoxypropyl)cytosine. *Antimicrob. Agents Chemother.* 37, 218, 1993.
97. Stals, F. S., Zeytinoglu, A., Havennith, M., De Clercq, E., and Bruggeman, C. A. Comparative effect of (S)-1-(3-hydroxy-2-phosphonylmethoxypropyl)cytosine and 9-(1,3- dihydroxy-2-propoxymethyl)guanine treatment on cytomegalovirus-induced interstitial pneumonitis in allogeneic bone marrow transplant recipient rats. *Transplant. Proc.* 25(1 Part 2), 1248.
98. Smee, D. F., Morris, J. L., Leonhardt, J. A., Mead, J. R., Holy, A., and Sidwell, R. W. Treatment of murine cytomegalovirus infections in severe combined immunodeficient mice with ganciclovir, (S)-1-[3-hydroxy-2-(phosphonylmethoxy)propyl]cytosine, interferon, and bropirimine. *Antimicrob. Agents Chemother.*, 36, 1837, 1992.
99. Neyts, J., Balzarini, J., Naesens, L., and De Clercq, E. Efficacy of (S)-1-(3-hydroxy-2- phosphonylmethoxypropyl)cytosine and 9-(1,3-dihydroxy-2-propoxymethyl)guanine for the treatment of murine cytomegalovirus infection in severe combined immunodeficiency mice. *J. Med. Virol.*, 37, 67, 1992.
100. Neau, D., Renaud-Rougier, M. B., Villard, J. F., et al. *38th Intersci. Conf. Antimicrob. Agents Chemother.* American Society of Microbiology, Washington DC, 38, 347, abstract H-112, 1998.
101. Berenguer, J. and Mallolas, J. Intravenous cidofovir for compassionate use in AIDS patients with cytomegalovirus retinitis, Spanish Cidofovir Study Group. *Clin. Infect. Dis.*, 30, 182–184, 2000.
102. Anonymous. Cidofovir: new preparation. Of help in CMV retinitis. *Prescrire Int.*, 7, 135–137, 1998.
103. Bainbridge, J. W., Raina, J., Shah, S. M., Ainsworth, J., and Pinching, A. J. Ocular complications of intravenous cidofovir for cytomegalovirus retinitis in patients with AIDS. *Eye*, 13(Part 3a), 353–356, 1999.
104. Cochereau, I., Doan, S., Diraison, M. C., et al. Uveitis in patients treated with intravenous cidofovir. *Ocul. Immunol. Inflamm.*, 7, 223–229, 1999.
105. Ambati, J., Wynne, K. B., Angerame, M. C., and Robinson, M. R. Anterior uveitis associated with intravenous cidofovir use in patients with cytomegalovirus retinitis. *Br. J. Ophthalmol.*, 83, 1153–1158, 1999.
106. Anonymous. Advances in CMV management: fomivirsen (Vitravene) approved. *PI Prospect.*, (No. 28), 7, 1998.
107. Muccioli, C., Goldstein, D. A., Johnson, D. W., et al. (1998) Fomivirsen safety and efficacy in the treatment of CMV retinitis: a phase 3 controlled, multicenter study comparing immediate versus delayed treatment. *5th Conf. Retroviruses Opportunistic Infect.*, Feb.1–5, 224, abstract LB6, 1998.
108. Amin, H. I., Ai, E., McDonald, H. R., and Johnson, R. N. Retinal toxic effects associated with intravitreal fomivirsen. *Arch. Ophthalmol.*, 118, 426–427, 2000.
109. Roehr, B. Fomivirsen approved for CMV retinitis. *J. Int. Assoc. Physicians AIDS Care*, 4, 14–16, 1998.
110. Ormrod, D., Scott, L. J., and Perry, C. M. Valaciclovir: a review of its long term utility in the management of genital herpes simplex virus and cytomegalovirus infections. *Drugs*, 59, 839–863, 2000.

111. Emery, V., Sabin, C., Feinberg, J., Grywacz, M., Knight, S., and Griffiths, P. Quantitative effects of valaciclovir on the replication of cytomegalovirus in patients with advanced HIV disease. *6th Conf. Retroviruses Opportunistic Infect., Jan. 31–Feb. 4*, 153, abstract 459, 1999.
112. Jacobson, M. A. Current management of cytomegalovirus disease in patients with AIDS. *Acquir. Immune Defic. Syndr. Human Retrovir.*, 10, 917, 1994.
113. Markham, A. and Faulds, D. Ganciclovir: an update of its therapeutic use in cytomegalovirus infection. *Drugs*, 48, 455, 1994.
114. Stevens, C. and Roberts, W. B. Jr. Ganciclovir: treatment of cytomegalovirus in immunocompromised individuals. *ANNA J.*, 21, 204, 209, 1994.
115. Bachman, D. M. Treatment of CMV retinitis. *N. Engl. J. Med.* 326, 1702, 1992.
116. Deray, G., Katlama, C., and Jacobs, C. Treatment of CMV retinitis. *N. Engl. J. Med.*, 326, 1702, 1992.
117. Skolnik, P. R. Treatment of CMV retinitis. *N. Engl. J. Med.*, 326, 1701, 1992.
118. Wagstaff, A. J. and Bryson, H. M. Foscarnet: a reapprisal of its antiviral activity, pharmacokinetic properties and therapeutic use in immunocompromised patients with viral infections. *Drugs*, 48, 199, 1994.
119. Greening, J. G. Intravenous foscarnet administration for treatment of cytomegalovirus retinitis. *J. Intraven. Nurs.*, 17, 74, 1994.
120. Wagstaff, A. J., Faulds, D., and Goa, K. L. Aciclovir: a reappraisal of its antiviral activity, pharmacokinetic properties and therapeutic efficacy. *Drugs*, 47, 153, 1994.
121. Polis, M. A., de Smet, M. D., Baird, B. F., et al. Increased survival of a cohort of patients with acquired immunodeficiency syndrome and cytomegalovirus retinitis who received sodium phosphonoformate (foscarnet). *Am. J. Med.*, 94, 175, 1993.
122. Smith, D. G. Jr. and Handy, C. M. A protocol for foscarnet administration. *J. Intraven. Nurs.*, 15, 274, 1992.
123. Moyle, G. and Gazzard, B. G. Foscarnet or ganciclovir for treatment of AIDS and CMV retinitis. *Am. J. Med.* 98, 319, 1995.
124. Colucciello, M. Phosphonoformate for CMV retinitis in AIDS. *Am. J. Med.*, 98, 317, 1995.
125. Balfour, H. H. Jr. Cytomegalovirus retinitis in persons with AIDS: selecting therapy for a sight-threatening disease. *Postgrad. Med. J.*, 97, 109, 1995.
126. Spector, S. A., Weingeist, T., Pollard, R. B., et al. A randomized, controlled study of intravenous ganciclovir therapy for cytomegalovirus peripheral retinits in patients with AIDS. *J. Infect. Dis.*, 168, 557, 1993.
127. AIDS Clinical Trials Group (ACTG). Studies of ocular complications of AIDS foscarnet- ganciclovir cytomegalovirus retinitis trial: 1. Rationale, design, and methods. *Control. Clin. Trials* 13, 22, 1992.
128. Geier, S. A., Klauss, V., Matuschke, A., Kronawitter, U., and Goebel, F. D. 2.5 years survival with sequential ganciclovir/foscarnet treatment in a patient with acquired immune deficiency syndrome and cytomegalovirus retinitis. *Ger. J. Ophthalmol.*, 1, 110, 1992.
129. Jacobson, M. A. Maintenance therapy for cytomegalovirus retinitis in patients with acquired immunodeficiency syndrome: foscarnet. *Am. J. Med.*, 92(Suppl. 2A), 26S, 1992.
130. Henderly, D. E., Freeman, W. R., Causey, D. M., and Rao, N. A. Cytomegalovirus retinitis and response to therapy with ganciclovir. *Ophthalmology*, 94, 425, 1987.
131. Cantrill, H. L., Henry, K., Melroe, N. H., et al. Treatment of cytomegalovirus retinitis with intravitreal ganciclovir: long-term results. *Ophthalmology*, 96, 367, 1989.
132. Felsenstein, D., d'Amico, D. J., Hirsch, M. S., et al. Treatment of cytomegalovirus retinitis with 9-[2-hydroxy- 1-(hydroxymethyl)ethoxymethyl]guanine. *Ann. Intern. Med.*, 103, 377, 1983.
133. Holland, G. N., Sidikaro, Y., Kreiger, A. E., et al. Treatment of cytomegalovirus retinopathy with ganciclovir. *Ophthalmology*, 94, 815, 1987.
134. Jabs, D. A., Enger, C., and Bartlett, J. G. Cytomegalovirus retinitis and acquired immunodeficiency syndrome. *Arch. Ophthalmol.*, 107, 75, 1989.
135. Jabs, D. A., Newman, C., de Bustros, S., and Polk, B. F. Treatment of cytomegalovirus retinitis with ganciclovir. *Ophthalmology*, 94, 824, 1987.
136. Palestine, A. G., Stevens, G. Jr., Lane, H. C., et al. Treatment of cytomegalovirus retinitis with dihydroxy propoxymethyl guanine. *Am. J. Ophthalmol.*, 101, 95, 1986.
137. Rosecan, L. R., Stahl-Bayliss, C. M., Kalman, C. M., and Laskin, O. L. Antiviral therapy for cytomegalovirus retinitis in AIDS with dihydroxy propoxymethyl guanine. *Am. J. Ophthalmol.*, 101, 405, 1986.
138. Holland, G. N. and Shuler, J. D. Progression rates of cytomegalovirus retinopathy in ganciclovir-treated and untreated patients. *Arch. Ophthalmol.*, 110, 1435, 1992.
139. Neuwirth, J., Gutman, I., Hofeldt, A. J., et al. Cytomegalovirus retinitis in a young homosexual male with acquired immunodeficiency. *Ophthalmology*, 89, 805, 1982.
140. Mar, E. C., Cheng, Y. C., and Huang, E.-S. Effect of 9-(1,3-dihydroxy-2-propoxymethyl) guanine on human cytomegalovirus replication in vitro. *Antimicrob. Agents Chemother.*, 24, 518, 1983.
141. Kuppermann, B. D., Quiceno, J. I., Flores-Aguilar, M., et al. Intravitreal ganciclovir concentration after intravenous administration in AIDS patients with cytomegalovirus retinitis: application for therapy. *J. Infect. Dis.*, 168, 1506, 1993.
142. Smith, I. L., Hong, C., Pilcher, M. L., Shapiro, A. M., Jiles, R. E., and Spector, S. A. Development of resistant cytomegalovirus genotypes during oral ganciclovir prophylaxis/preemptive therapy. *38th Intersci. Conf. Antimicrob. Agents Chemother.*, American Society of Microbiology, Washington DC, 38, 349, abstract H-120, 1998.

143. Muccioli, C. and Belfort, R. Jr. Treatment of cytomegalovirus retinitis with an intraocular sustained-release ganciclovir implant. *Braz. J. Med. Biol. Res.*, 33, 779–789, 2000.
144. Williamson, J. C., Virata, S. R., Raasch, R. H., and Kylstra, J. A. Oxacillin-resistant *Staphylococcus aureus* endophthalmitis after ganciclovir intraocular implant. *Am. J. Ophthalmol.*, 129, 554–555, 2000.
145. Kupperman, B. D., Flores-Aguilar, M., Quiceno, J. I., Rickman, L. S., and Freeman, W. R. Combination ganciclovir and foscarnet in the treatment of clinically resistant cytomegalovirus retinitis in patients with acquired immunodeficiency syndrome. *Arch. Ophthalmol.*, 111, 1359, 1993.
146. Flores-Aguilar, M., Kuppermann, B. D., Quiceno, J. I., et al. Pathophysiology and treatment of clinically resistant cytomegalovirus retinitis. *Ophthalmology*, 100, 1022, 1993.
147. Dieterich, D. T., Poles, M. A., Lew, E. A., et al. Concurrent use of ganciclovir and foscarnet to treat cytomegalovirus infection in AIDS patients. *J. Infect. Dis.*, 167, 1184, 1993.
148. Anduze-Faris, B. M., Fillet, A. M., Gozlan, J., et al. Induction and maintenance therapy of cytomegalovirus central nervous system infection in HIV-infected patients. *AIDS*, 14, 517–524, 2000.
149. Jacobson, M. A., de Miranda, P., Gordon, S. M., Blum, M. R., Volberding, P., and Mills, J. Prolonged pancytopenia due to combined ganciclovir and zidovudine therapy. *J. Infect. Dis.*, 158, 489, 1988.
150. Millar, A. B., Miller, R. F., Patou, G., Mindel, A., Marsh, R., and Semple, S. J. G. Treatment of cytomegalovirus retinitis with zidovudine and ganciclovir in patients with AIDS: outcome and toxicity. *Genitourin. Med.*, 66, 156, 1990.
151. Prichard, M. N., Prichard, L. E., Baguley, W. A., Nassiri, M. R., and Shipman, C. Jr. Three-dimensional analysis of the synergistic cytotoxicity between ganciclovir and zidovudine. *Antimicrob. Agents Chemother.*, 35, 1060, 1991.
152. Tian, P. Y., Croutch, J. Y., and Hsiung, G. D. Combined antiviral effect and cytotoxicity of ganciclovir and azidothymidine against cytomegalovirus infection in cultured cells. *Antiviral Res.*, Suppl. 1(April, 1991), 115, abstract 134.
153. Medina, D. J., Hsiung, G. D., and Mellors, J. W. Ganciclovir the anti-human immunodeficiency virus type 1 activity of zidovudine and didanosine in vitro. *Antimicrob. Agents Chemother.*, 36, 1127, 1992.
154. Freitas, V. R., Fraser-Smith, E. B., Chiu, S., Michelson, S., and Schatzman, R. C. Efficacy of ganciclovir in combination with zidovudine against cytomegalovirus in vitro and in vivo. *Antiviral Res.*, 21, 301, 1993.
155. Prichard, M. N. and Shipman, C. Jr. Efficacy of ganciclovir in combination with zidovudine against cytomegalovirus in vitro and in vivo. *Antiviral Res.*, 24, 357, 1994.
156. Causey, D. Concomitant ganciclovir and zidovudine treatment for cytomegalovirus retinitis in patients with HIV infection: an approach to treatment. *J. Acquir. Immune Defic. Syndr.*, 4, 516, 1991.
157. Jacobson, M. A., Owen, W., Campbell, J., Brosgart, C., and Abrams, D. I. Tolerability of combined ganciclovir and didanosine for the treatment of cytomegalovirus disease associated with AIDS. *Clin. Infect. Dis.* 16(Suppl. 1), S69, 1993.
158. Carter, J. E. and Shuster, A. R. Zidovudine and cytomegalovirus retinitis. *Ann. Ophthalmol.*, 24, 186, 1992.
159. Patel, H. D., Anderson, J. R., Duncombe, A. S., Carrington, D., and Murday, A. Granulocyte colony-stimulating factor: a new application for cytomegalovirus-induced neutropenia in cardiac allograft recipients. *Transplantation*, 58, 863, 1994.
160. Papastamopoulos, V., Botsis, C., Paparizos, V. A., Kyriakis, K. P., Zagoraios, Y., and Stavrianeas, N. G. Lack of reactivation of cytomegalovirus retinitis in an AIDS patient, during and after stoping long-term cidofovir treatment: case report. *J. Chemother.*, 12, 258–260, 2000.
161. Monkemuller, K. E. and Wilcox, C. M. Esophageal ulcer caused by cytomegalovirus: resolution during combination antiretroviral therapy for acquired immunodeficiency syndrome. *South. Med. J.*, 93, 818–820, 2000.
162. Salmon-Ceron, D., Fillet, A. M., Aboulker, J. P., et al. Effects of a 14-day course of foscarnet on cytomegalovirus (CMV) blood markers in a randomized study of human immunodeficiency virus-infected patients with persistent CMV viremia. Agence National de Recherche du SIDA 023 Study Group. *Clin. Infect. Dis.*, 28, 901–905, 1999.
163. O'Brien, J. J. and Campoli-Richards, D. M. Acyclovir: an update review of its antiviral activity, pharmacokinetics properties and therapeutic efficacy. *Drugs*, 37, 233, 1989.
164. Mollison, L. C., Richards, M. J., Johnson, P. D., et al. High-dose oral acyclovir reduces the incidence of cytomegalovirus infection in liver transplant recipients. *J. Infect. Dis.*, 168, 721, 1993.
165. Meyers, J. D., Reed, E. C., and Shepp, D. H. Acyclovir for prevention of cytomegalovirus infection and disease after allogeneic marrow transplantation. *N. Engl. J. Med.*, 318, 70, 1988.
166. Ljungman, P., De Bock, R., Cordonnier, C., et al. Practices for cytomegalovirus diagnosis, prophylaxis and treatment in allogeneic bone marrow transplant recipients: a report from the Working Party for Infectious Diseases of the EBMT. *Bone Marrow Transplant.*, 12, 399, 1993.
167. Martin, M., Manez, R., Linden, P., et al. A prospective randomized trial comparing sequential ganciclovir-high dose acyclovir to high dose acyclovir for prevention of cytomegalovirus disease in adult liver transplantation. *Transplantation*, 58, 779, 1994.
168. Singh, N., Yu, V. L., Mieles, L., Wagener, M. M., Miner, R. C., and Gaywski, T. High-dose acyclovir compared with short-course preemptive ganciclovir therapy to prevent cytomegalovirus disease in liver transplant recipients: a randomized trial. *Ann. Intern. Med.*, 120, 375, 1994.
169. Dunn, D. L., Gillingham, K. J., Kramer, M. A., et al. A prospective randomized study of acyclovir versus ganciclovir plus human immune globulin prophylaxis of cytomegalovirus infection after solid organ transplantation. *Transplantation*, 57, 876, 1994.
170. ASHP therapeutic guidelines for intravenous immune globulin. ASHP Commission on Therapeutics. *Clin. Pharm.*, 11, 117, 1992.

171. Reed, E. C., Bowden, R. A., Dandliker, P. S., Lilleby, K. E., and Meyer, J. D. Treatment of cytomegalovirus pneumonia with ganciclovir and intravenous cytomegalovirus immunoglobulin in patients with bone marrow transplants. *Ann. Intern. Med.*, 109, 783, 1988.
172. Emanuel, D., Cunningham, I., Jules-Elysee, K., et al. Cytomegalovirus pneumonia after bone marrow transplantation successfully treated with the combination of ganciclovir and high dose intravenous immune globulin. *Ann. Intern. Med.*, 109, 777, 1988.
173. Dentamaro, T., Volpi, A., Cudillo, L., et al. Effective pre-emptive therapy with ganciclovir and specific immunoglobulins for CMV infection in a bone marrow transplanted patient,. *Haematologica*, 77, 284, 1992.
174. Snydman, D. R., McIver, J., Leszczynski, J., et al. A pilot trial of a novel cytomegalovirus immune globulin in renal transplant recipients. *Transplantation*, 38, 553, 1984.
175. Tsevat, J., Snydman, D. R., Pauker, S. G., Durand-Zaleski, I., Werner, B. G., and Levey, A. S. Which renal transplant patients should receive cytomegalovirus immune globulin? *Transplantation*, 52, 259, 1991.
176. Bowden, R. A., Sayers, M., Flornoy, N., et al. Cytomegalovirus immune globulin and seronegative blood products to prevent primary cytomegalovirus infection after marrow transplantation. *N. Engl. J. Med.*, 314, 1006, 1986.
177. Cohen, A. T., O'Grady, J. G., Sutherland, S., Sallie, R., Tan, K. C., and Williams, R. Controlled trial of prophylactic versus therapeutic use of ganciclovir after liver transplantation in adults. *J. Med. Virol.*, 40, 5, 1993.
178. Walmsley, S. L., Chew, E., Read, S. E., et al. Treatment of cytomegalovirus retinitis with trisodium phosphonoformate (foscarnet). *J. Infect. Dis.*, 157, 569, 1988.
179. Jacobson, M. A., O'Donnell, J. J., Brodie, H. R., Wofsy, C., and Mills, J. Randomized prospective trial of ganciclovir maintenance therapy for cytomegalovirus retinitis. *J. Med. Virol.*, 25, 339, 1988.
180. Jacobson, M. A., Causey, D., Polsky, B., et al. A dose-response study of daily maintenance intravenous foscarnet therapy for cytomegalovirus retinitis in AIDS. *J. Infect. Dis.*, 168, 444, 1993.
181. Jacobson, M. A., O'Donnell, J. J., and Mills, J. Foscarnet treatment of cytomegalovirus retinitis in patients with acquired immunodeficiency syndrome. *Antimicrob. Agents Chemother.*, 33, 736, 1989.
182. Le Hoang, P., Girard, B., Robinet, M., et al. Foscarnet in the treatment of cytomegalovirus retinitis in acquired immune deficiency syndrome. *Ophthalmology*, 96, 865, 1989.
183. Jacobson, M. A. Maintenance therapy for cytomegalovirus retinitis in patients with acquired immunodeficiency syndrome: foscarnet. *Am. J. Med.*, 92(Suppl. 2A), 26S, 1992.
184. Drew, W. L., Ives, D., Lalezari, J. P., et al. Oral ganciclovir as maintenance treatment for cytomegalovirus retinitis in patients with AIDS. Syntex Cooperative Oral Ganciclovir Study Group. *N. Engl. J. Med.*, 223, 615, 1995.
185. Anderson, R. D., Griffy, K. G., Jung, D., Dorr, A., Hulse, J. D., and Smith, R. B. Ganciclovir absolute bioavailability and steady-state pharmacokinetics after oral administration of two 3000-mg/d dosing regimens in human immunodeficiency virus- and cytomegalovirus-seropositive patients. *Clin. Ther.*, 17, 425, 1995.
186. Plotkin, S. A., Drew, W. L., Felsenstein, D., and Hirsch, M. S. Sensitivity of clinical isolates of human cytomegalovirus to 9-(1,3-dihydroxy-2-propoxymethyl)guanine. *J. Infect. Dis.*, 152, 833, 1985.
187. The Oral Ganciclovir European and Australian Cooperative Study Group. Intravenous versus oral ganciclovir: European/Australian cooperative study of efficacy and safety in the prevention of cytomegalovirus retinitis recurrence in patients with AIDS. *AIDS*, 9, 471, 1995.
188. Cochereau, I., Diraison, M. C., Mousalatti, H., et al. Ganciclovir intravitreen a fortes doses pour le traitement de la retinite a CMV. *J. Fr. Ophtalmol.*, 23, 123–126, 2000.
189. Mastroianni, C. M., Ciardi, M., Folgori, F., et al. Cytomegalovirus encephalitis in two patients with AIDS receiving ganciclovir for cytomegalovirus retinitis. *J. Infect.*, 29, 331, 1994.
190. Jacobson, M. A., Kramer, F., Bassiakos, Y., et al. Randomized phase I trial of two different combination foscarnet and ganciclovir chronic maintenance therapy regimens for AIDS patients with cytomegalovirus retinitis: AIDS clinical trials group protocol 151. *J.Infect. Dis.*, 170, 189, 1994.
191. Peters, M., Schürmann, D., Bergmann, F., et al. Safety of alternating ganciclovir and foscarnet maintenance therapy in human immunodeficiency virus (HIV)-related cytomegalovirus infections: an open-labeled pilot study. *Scand. J. Infect. Dis.*, 26, 49, 1994.
192. Balfour, H. H. Jr., Drew, W. L., Hardy, W. D., Heinemann, M. H., and Polsky, B. Therapeutic algorithm for treatment of cytomegalovirus retinitis in persons with AIDS: a roundtable summary. *J. Acquir. Immune Defic. Syndr.*, 5(Suppl. 1), S37, 1992.
193. Polis, M. A. Foscarnet and ganciclovir in the treatment of cytomegalovirus retinitis. *J. Acquir. Immune Defic. Syndr.*, 5(Suppl. 1), S3, 1992.
194. Palestine, A. G., Polis, M. A., De Smet, M., et al. A randomized controlled trial of foscarnet in treatment of cytomegalovirus retinitis in patients with AIDS. *Ann. Intern. Med.*, 115, 665, 1991.
195. Roberts, W. D., Weinberg, K. I., Kohn, D. B., Sender, L., Parkman, R., and Lenarsky, C. Granulocyte recovery in pediatric marrow transplant recipients treated with ganciclovir for cytomegalovirus infection. *Am. J. Pediatr. Hematol. Oncol.*, 15, 320, 1993.
196. Worrell, S., Deayton, J., Hayes, P., Garson, J., Gazzard, B., and Larsson-Sciard, E. Antiretroviral therapy in late stage HIV disease: evidence for immune reconstitution. *6th Conf. Retroviruses Opportunistic Infect., Jan. 31–Feb. 4*, 115, abstract 251, 1999.
197. Mitchell, S. M., Membrey, W. L., Youle, M. S., Obi, A., Worrell, S., and Gazzard, B. G. Cytomegalovirus retinitis after the initiation of highly active antiretroviral therapy: a 2 year prospective study. *Br. J. Ophthalmol.*, 83, 652–655, 1999.
198. Boivin, G. and LeBlanc, R. P. Clearance of cytomegalovirus viremia after initiation of highly active antiretroviral

therapy. *J. Infect. Dis.* 181, 1216–1218, 2000 (see also: *J. Infect. Dis.* 177, 1182–1187, 1998, and *J. Infect. Dis.* 180, 847–849, 1999).
199. Casado, J. L., Arrizabalaga, J., Gutierrez, C. Risk of Cytomegalovirus viremia and disease in HIV-infected patients with protease inhibitor treatment failure. *6th Conf. Retroviruses Opportunistic Infect., Jan. 31–Feb. 4* 153, abstract 458, 1999.
200. Arrizabalaga, J., Casado, J. L., Tural, C., et al. Incidence and risk factors for developing CMV retinitis in HIV- infected patients receiving protease inhibitor therapy. *6th Conf. Retroviruses Opportunistic Infect., Jan. 31–Feb. 4*, 115 abstract 251, 1999.
201. Deayton, J., Mocroft, A., Wilson, P., Emery, V. C., Johnson, M. A., and Griffiths, P. D. Highly active antiretroviral therapy (HAART) including pretease inhibitors can completely suppress asymptomatic CMV viremia in the absence of specific anti-CMV therapy. *38th Intersci. Conf. Antimicrob. Agents Chemother.*, American Society of Microbiology, Washington DC, 38, 448, abstract I-268, 1998.
202. Verbraak, F. D., Boom, R., Wertheim-van Dillen, P. M., van den Horn, G. J., Kijlstra, A., and de Smet, M. D. Influence of highly active antiretroviral therapy on the development of CMV disease in HIV positive patients at high risk for CMV disease. *Br. J. Ophthalmol.* 83, 1186–1189, 1999.
203. Dunn, J. P. Discontinuation of maintenance CMV therapy in HAART responders. *Hopkins HIV Rep.*, 11, 5, 1999.
204. Soriano, V., Dona, C., Rodriguez-Rosado, R., Barreiro, P., and Gonzalez-Lahoz, J. Discontinuation of secondary prophylaxis for opportunistic infections in HIV-infected patients receiving highly active antiretroviral therapy. *AIDS,* 14, 383–386, 2000.
205. MacDonald, J. C., Karavellas, M. P., Torriani, F. J., et al. Highly active antiretroviral therapy-related immune recovery in AIDS patients with cytomegalovirus retinitis. *Ophthalmology*, 107, 877–881, 881–882, 2000.
206. Margolis, T. P. Discontinuation of anticytomegalovirus therapy in patients with HIV infection and cytomegalovirus. *Surv. Ophthalmol.*, 44, 455, 2000.
207. Labetoulle, M., Goujard, C., Frau, E., et al. Cytomegalovirus retinits in advanced HIV- infected patients treated with protease inhibitors: incidence and outcome over 2 years. *J. Acquir. Immune Defic. Syndr.*, 22, 228–234, 1999.
208. Jouan, M., Saves, M., Tubiana, R., et al. Restimop (ANRS 078): a prospective multicentre study to evaluate the discontinuation of maintenance therapy for CMV retinitis in HIV patients receiving HAART. *6th Conf. Retroviruses Opportunistic Infect., Jan. 31–Feb. 4* 153, abstract 456, 1999.
209. Chiller, T., Park, A., Chiller, K., Skiest, D., and Keiser, P. HIV protease inhibitor therapy is associated with increased time to relapse and death in AIDS patients with cytomegalovirus retinitis. *38th Intersci. Conf. Antimicrob. Agents Chemother.*, American Society of Microbiology, Washington DC, 38, 448, abstract I-267, 1998.
210. Whitcup, S. M. Cytomegalovirus retinitis in the era of highly active antiretroviral therapy [clinical conference]. *J. Am. Med. Assoc.*, 283, 653–657, 2000.
211. Maschke, M., Kastrup, O., Esser, S., Ross, B., Hengge, U., and Hufnagel, A. Incidence and prevalence of neurological disorders associated with HIV since the introduction of highly active antiretroviral therapy (HAART). *J. Neurol. Neurosurg. Psychiatry*, 69, 376–380, 2000.
212. Jubault, V., Pacanowski, J., Rabian, C., and Viard, J. P. Interruption of prophylaxis for major opportunistic infections in HIV-infected patients receiving triple combination antiretroviral therapy. *Ann. Med. Interne (Paris)*, 151, 163–168, 2000.
213. Jones, J., Hanson, D., Dworkin, M., and Kaplan, J. Which opportunistic illness occur in the era of HAART and at what CD4 cell counts? *6th Conf. Retroviruses Opportunisctic Infect., Jan. 31–Feb. 4*, 198, abstract 690, 1999.
214. Di Perri, G., Vento, S., Mazzi, R., et al. Recovery of long-term natural protection against reactivation of CMV retinitis in AIDS patients responding to highly active antiretroviral therapy. *J. Infect.*, 39, 193–197, 1999.
215. Postelmans, L., Gerard, M., Sommereijns, B., and Caspers-Velu, L. Discontinuation of maintenance therapy for CMV retinitis in AIDS patients on highly active antiretroviral therapy. *Ocul. Immunol. Inflamm.*, 7, 199–203, 1999.
216. Torriani, F. J., Freeman, W. R., Karavellas, M., et al. Lymphoproliferative responses to CMV predict CMV retinitis reactivation in patients who discontinued CMV maintenance therapy. *6th Conf. Retroviruses Opportunistic Infect., Jan. 31–Feb. 4*, 115, abstract 250, 1999.
217. Torriani, F. J., Freeman, W. R., MacDonald, J. C., et al. CMV retinitis recurs after stopping treatment in virological and immunological failures of potent antiretroviral therapy. *AIDS*, 14, 173–180, 2000.
218. Anonymous. Stopping CMV prophylaxis with HAART. *Treat. Update*, 10, 4–6, 1998.
219. Karavellas, M. P., Lowder, C. Y., MacDonald, C., et al. Immune recovery vitritis associated with inactive cytomegalovirus retinitis: a new syndrome. *Arch. Ophthalmol.*, 116, 169–175, 1998.
220. Silverstein, B. E., Smith, J. H., Sykes, S. O., et al. Cystoid macular edema associated with cytomegalovirus retinitis in patients with the acquired immunodeficiency syndrome. *Am. J. Ophthalmol.*, 125, 411–415, 1998.
221. Zegans, M. E., Walton, R. C., Holland, G. N., et al. Transient vitreous inflammatory reactions associated with combination antiretroviral therapy in patients with AIDS and cytomegalovirus retinitis. *Am. J. Ophthalmol.*, 125, 292–300, 1998.
222. Zafirakis, P., Markomichelakis, N. N., Voudouri, A., Theodossiasis, G. P., and Theodossiasis, P. G. Cystoid macular edema in a patient with acquired immunodeficiency syndrome and past ocular history of cytomegalovirus retinitis after initiation of protease inhibitors. *Doc. Ophthalmol.*, 97, 311-315, 1999.
223. Nguyen, Q. D., Kempen, J. H., Bolton, S. G., Dunn, J. P., and Jabs, D. A. Immune recovery uveitis in patients with AIDS and cytomegalovirus retinitis after highly active antiretroviral therapy. *Am. J. Ophthalmol.*, 129, 634–639, 2000.
224. Postelmans, L., Payen, M. C., De Wit, S., and Caspers-Velu, L. Neovascularization of the optic disc after highly active antiretroviral therapy in an AIDS patient with cytomegalovirus retinitis - A new immune recovery-related ocular disorder? *Ocul. Immunol. Inflamm.*, 7, 237–240, 1999.

225. Badelon, I., Gohier, P., and Chaine, G. Oedeme maculaire cystoide et retinate a cytomegalovirus chez des patients HIV traits par tritherapie antiretrovirale. *J. Fr. Ophtalmol.*, 22, 1034–1041, 1999.
226. Autran, B., Carcelain, G., Li, T. S., et al. Positive effects of combined antiretroviral therapy on CD4$^+$ T cell homeostasis and function in advanced HIV disease. *Science*, 277, 112–116, 1997.
227. Jackson, T. L., Meacock, W., Youle, M., and Graham, E. M. Severe intraocular inflammation after a change of HAART. *Br. J. Ophthalmol.*, 84, 933–934, 2000.
228. Song, M. K., Karavellas, M. P., McDonald, J. C., Plummer, D. J., and Freeman, W. R. Characterization of reactivation of cytomegalovirus retinitis in patients healed after treatment with highly active antiretroviral therapy. *Retina*, 20, 151–155, 2000.
229. Riddell, S. R. and Greenberg, P. D. T-cell therapy of cytomegalovirus and human immunodeficiency virus infection. *J. Antimicrob. Chemother.*, 45(Suppl. T3), 35–43, 2000.
230. Riddell, S. R., Warren, E. H., Lewinsohn, D., et al. Application of T cell immunotherapy for human viral and malignant diseases. *Ernst Schering Res. Found. Workshop*, 30, 53–73, 2000.
231. Borucki, M., Spritzler, J., Gnann, J., et al. A phase II double masked, placebo-controlled evaluation of standard therapy vs. standard therapy combined with human monoclonal anti-cytomegalovirus antibody (MSL-109) in the therapy of AIDS patients with newly diagnosed cytomegalovirus (CMV) retinitis in ACTG 266. *6th Conf. Retroviruses Opportunistic Infect., Jan. 31–Feb. 4,* 154, abstract 460, 1999.

2
Varicella-Zoster Virus (Herpes Zoster) Infections

1. INTRODUCTION

Varicella-zoster virus is one of six herpesviruses isolated from humans. The core of a typical herpesvirus contains a linear, double-stranded DNA, whereas the viral capsid is icosadeltahedral and contains 162 capsomeres with a hole running down the long axis *(1)*.

The varicella-zoster virus (VZV) is associated with two distinct clinical syndromes: varicella (chickenpox) and herpes zoster (shingles). Whereas varicella is a ubiquitous and highly contagious primary infection affecting the general population (especially in childhood), herpes zoster is less common endemic clinical condition that usually occurs in older and/or immunocompromised individuals.

AIDS patients with CD4$^+$ counts of 500 cells/mm^3 or less, or organ-transplant recipients (especially bone-marrow allograft recipients) are at significant risk of VZV infections. Furthermore, patients who have received prior repeated acyclovir treatment have the highest risk of harboring acyclovir-resistant strains *(2,3)*.

Herpes zoster usually is manifested with a painful vesicular eruption customary limited to a single dermatome, although cases of generalized eruptions have also been observed. It does not associate to exogenous exposure but appears to be secondary to reactivation of VZV that remained latent after an earlier attack of varicella *(4)*.

In general, the pathogenesis and mechanism of reactivation of herpes zoster are not well-understood. Predisposing factors associated with the appearance of herpes zoster are generally linked to compromised immune defenses *(5)* and include Hodgkin's disease and other lymphomas, immunosuppressive therapy, trauma to the spinal cord and adjacent structures, and heavy-metal poisoning *(5–8)*. In some instances, the host immune response is still viable enough to halt cutaneous lesions, but not the necrosis and inflammatory response in the ganglion. Such cases, known as zoster sine herpete, are characterized with radicular pain without associated skin lesions *(7,9,10)*.

The disease tends to be more severe in patients with malignancies, those with immune deficiencies, or receiving immunosuppressive therapy. Cutaneous dissemination, which occurs in up to 50% of immunocompromised patients, usually does not affect the morbidity and mortality in this population. However, patients with visceral disease (particularly pneumonitis) have increased mortality rate *(4)*.

The most common complication of herpes zoster is the postherpetic neuralgia that occurs in nearly 50% of patients 60 yr and older; it has been rarely observed in patients under 40 yr. Other complications, especially in immunocompromised hosts include chronic zoster *(11)*, and persistent CNS infection *(12,13)*.

De La Blanchardiere et al. *(14)* conducted a multicenter retrospective study to evaluate the clinical features and prognostic significance of VZV-associated neurological complications. Results of the study showed that encephalitis, myelitis, radiculitis, and meningitis were the most predominant neurological manifestations.

From: Opportunistic Infections: Treatment and Prophylaxis
By: Vassil St. Georgiev © Humana Press Inc., Totowa, NJ

Dolin et al. *(15)* found linkage between increased severity of herpes zoster and compromised status of the cell-mediated response. The presence of VZV-induced lymphocyte blastogenesis and interferon production correlated well with the ability to contain VZV reactivation.

In immunosuppressed patients, varicella infections are common with 50% of patients developing infection after bone-marrow transplantation *(16)*, over 20% following cardiac transplantation *(17)*, and up to 25% of patients receiving chemotherapy for Hodgkin's disease *(18)*. In fact, patients with Hodgkin's disease have been reported to have an increased risk for disseminated herpes zoster virus infection *(19–21)*. Chemotherapeutic regimens consisting of chlorambucil, vinblastin, procarbazine, and prednisone have been associated with increased incidence of herpes zoster infections in patients treated for Hodgkin's disease *(22)*; procarbazine has been suspected to be the cause behind it *(23)*. On several occasions in cancer patients, disseminated herpes zoster infections had been diagnosed concomitant with bacterial and/or fungal infections *(24)*. Varicella infections have also been reported in AIDS-related syndromes *(25)*, especially in Africa *(26)*, but it appears to be less common in patients with established AIDS in spite of their severely immunocompromised state *(27)*.

2. STUDIES ON THERAPEUTICS

2.1. Acyclovir

Acyclovir, a cyclic analog of 2-deoxyguanosine, was introduced into clinic as antiviral drug in 1977 *(28)*. It has highly selective mode of action against both VZV and herpes simplex *(29–32)* resulting in the inhibition of herpesvirus replication at concentrations 300- to 3,000-fold lower than those needed to inhibit mammalian cell functions *(33)*.

A note of caution should be applied when acyclovir is administered orally or even intravenously at lower dosages, because acyclovir-resistant mutant strains of VZV can be readily selected in the presence of the drug *(34)*.

In general, acyclovir is well tolerated in a wide variety of disease states, population types, and age groups *(29)*. However, there have been several reports of acyclovir-associated neurotoxicity *(35)* (confusion, hallucinations, seizures, and coma) in bone-marrow transplant recipients *(36)* and patients with chronic renal failure *(59)*. In the latter case, however, when the dosage regimens of acyclovir had been reduced according to the degree of renal failure, the neurotoxicity was reversed *(38–40)*.

Acute neurotoxicity in patients receiving intravenous acyclovir, although infrequently, has been well-documented *(35)*, especially in patients with renal failure *(37)*. Acute nephrotoxicity has also been observed in patients given oral acyclovir therapy *(41,42,64)*. Davenport et al. *(43)* and Beales et al. *(44)* treated oral acyclovir-induced neurotoxicity in patients with herpes zoster and end-stage renal failure (undergoing continuous ambulatory peritoneal dialysis) with hemodialysis, which by removing the drug *(45)*, effectively reduced the plasma concentrations of acyclovir. It would also seem advisable to recommend dose modification in those patients with end-stage renal failure, by either reducing the dose, increasing the dose intervals, or both *(44)*. A modified acyclovir regimen for intravenous route of admnistration has also been described *(46)*.

However, based on their clinical experience with patients undergoing dialysis, MacDiarmaid-Gordon et al. *(47)* reported that acyclovir-induced neurotoxicity can occur in spite of dose reduction and within the time-course of a standard course of treatment.

Since there is a wide overlap of serum concentrations in patients with and without neurologic side effects, the relation between CNS effects and acyclovir serum concentrations remains unclear *(35,39,48–52)*. Symptoms of neurotoxicity usually appear 24–72 h after acyclovir peak concentrations. Therefore, single drug level measurements may be of little diagnostic value *(52)*.

2.2. Famciclovir

A similar to valaciclovir approach has been taken in the development of famciclovir (famvir), the diacetyl ester of 6-deoxypenciclovir and a prodrug of penciclovir *(53)*. Famciclovir is absorbed in the upper intestine and rapidly metabolized in the intestinal wall and liver to penciclovir by deacetylation and oxidation *(54)*; the bioavailability of penciclovir is about 77% *(55)*. Similar to valaciclovir, famciclovir also reduced the duration of postherpetic neuralgia *(56)*. The primary elimination pathway appeared to be renal excretion of unchanged penciclovir.

In a multicenter, double-blind, controlled trial, 1-wk treatment with oral famciclovir (either 500 mg or 750 mg, t.i.d.) was compared to placebo *(57,58)*. The time to full crusting of zoster lesions was 5 d with the drug and 7 d with placebo. Furthermore, the duration of postherpetic neuralgia was 61 d in patients receiving 750 mg of famciclovir, 63 d in those taking 500 mg, and 119 d in the placebo-receiving group. In another controlled trial, oral famciclovir (administred at doses of either 250, 500, or 750 mg, t.i.d.) was compared to acyclovir (800 mg, 5 times daily) in 545 patients with herpes zoster; the time of crusting, loss of acute pain, and duration of postherpetic neuralgia were similar in all groups. Although there were no significant differences among the three famciclovir dosing regimens, the primary advantage of famciclovir over acyclovir appeared to be its more convenient dosing schedule *(57,59)*.

The recommended dosage of famciclovir for treatment of acute herpes zoster is 500 mg, 3 times daily (every 8 h) for 1 wk. Famciclovir therapy should be initiated within 72 h after the onset of rash *(57)*.

Side effects with famciclovir (given at doses ranging from 125 mg to 2.25 g) during clinical trials occured no more frequently than with the placebo and include headache (9.3% of treated patients), nausea (4.5%), diarrhea (2.4%), and to a lesser extent fatigue, dizziness, abdominal pain, and dyspepsia. When studied for toxicity on testicular functions in male patients with recurrent genital herpes, famciclovir has shown no adverse side effects *(57,60)*. The safety of famciclovir therapy during pregnancy or breast feeding has not yet been established *(57)*.

Aside from fewer doses of medication per day than acyclovir, there appears to be little clinical advantage of famciclovir over acyclovir.

2.3. Sorivudine

The efficacy of sorivudine (BV-araU), a nucleoside antiviral drug has been compared with acyclovir in a double-blind/double-dummy study for the treatment of dermatormal herpes zoster in 170 HIV-infected patients *(61)*. Forty mg of sorivudine were given orally once daily for 10 d, whereas oral acyclovir was administered at 800 mg, 5 times daily for 10 d. Although both drugs were well-tolerated, sorivudine was deemed superior to acyclovir in accelerating the cutaneous healing with the added advantage of once-daily dosing.

3. TREATMENT OF VARICELLA-ZOSTER INFECTIONS

Acyclovir has been the standard therapy for VZV infections for more than a decade. However, it has a relatively short half-life and poor bioavailability necessitating the administration of high doses five times daily in order to maintain adequate plasma concentrations above the IC_{50} for VZV. Nevertheless, its systemic administration has been effective in reducing the severity of acute attack of herpes zoster *(62,63)*. In immunocompromised hosts, infections owing to acyclovir-resistant VZV strains have attained some urgency creating the need for alternative antiviral therapies *(64,65)*. In general, antiviral medications have been most effective when started within 72 h after the onset of rash. The addition of an orally administerd corticosteroid can provide modest benefits in reducing the pain of herpes zoster and the incidence of postherpetic neuralgia. Also, tricyclic antidepressants or anticonvulsants, often administered in low dosages may help in controlling neuropathic pain *(66)*.

In addition to acyclovir, famciclovir and valaciclovir have been used in treating VZV infections *(66)*. Foscarnet has been recommended for treatment of varicella zoster infections in severely immunocompromised patients (such as those with AIDS or bone-marrow transplant recipients) when acyclovir-resistant VZV strains were present *(2,67,68)*. The low incidence of myelosuppression associated with foscarnet allows for the drug to be used in combination with bone marrow-toxic

Table 1
Antiviral Therapy for Varicella-Zoster Infections

Infection	Drug/route of administration	Dose	VZV Duration
Immunocompromised patients	Acyclovir/i.v. divided every 8 h (1500 mg/m² daily divided every 8 h for children <12 yr old)	30 mg/kg daily	5–7 d
	Vidarabine/i.v. infused over 12 h	10 mg/kg daily	5–7 d
	Foscarnet/i.v. divided every 8 h	40 mg/kg daily	5–7 d
Immunocompetent patients	Acyclovir/p.o. q.i.d. for children; 800 mg per dose, q.i.d. for adolescents; 800 mg per dose, 5 times daily for adults	20 mg/kg per dose	5 d

antiretroviral therapies, such as zidovudine. To minimize adverse effects, patients should receive adequate hydration prior to and during foscarnet therapy (69). Nevertheless, patients should be monitored frequently for renal toxicity, electrolyte abnormalities, and alterations in the calcium/phosphorus metabolism during therapy. Chronic maintenance therapy has not been recommended in this situation (2).

In retrospect, the currently available clinical data have established that both acyclovir and vidarabine favorably alter the clinical course of herpes zoster in immunocompromised patients. However, the fact that it is perhaps less toxic and easier to administer have made intravenous acyclovir the drug of choice for treatment of herpes zoster in immunocompromised patients (64) (Table 1).

Studies by Sempere et al. (70) showned that long-term acyclovir prophylaxis delayed but did not prevent VZV infections after autologous blood stem-cell transplantation in patients with acute leukemia.

3.1. Herpes Zoster in Organ-Transplant Recipients

Varicella zoster infections in immunocompromised patients, such as bone-marrow transplant (BMT) recipients can be severe and frequently associated with widespread dissemination reaching mortality rate as high as 50% (71–73).

Reactivation of VZV infections, which has been documented after allogeneic BMT in 30–40% of patients (74), most commonly presents as zoster. Therefore, the prophylactic use of acyclovir in this population has been recommended (75,76).

When compared to vidarabine, acyclovir proved superior in the treatment of BMT recipients (71,77,78).

It has been postulated that when used in organ transplant recipients receiving immunosuppressive cyclosporine A therapy, acyclovir may adversely interact with cyclosporin A by increasing its nephrotoxicity (71,79–82). However, based on several cases of renal-transplant recipients with herpes zoster, Hayes et al. (83) found that acyclovir therapy did not interefere with the concomitant cyclosporin A medication. These results seem to contradict two earlier reports, one by Johnson et al. (84), who suggested a slight improvement in renal functions of renal-allograft recipients while being treated with cyclosporin A and intravenous acyclovir, and by Shepp et al. (71) who observed a deterioration in the renal functions of BMT patients on cyclosporin A therapy following treatment with intravenous acyclovir.

3.2. Herpes Zoster in HIV-Infected Patients

VZV infections are among the most frequent viral opportunistic infections in HIV-infected patients *(85)*. The incidence of herpes zoster among HIV-infected patients is nearly seven times higher as compared to the general population *(86)*.

Snoeck et al. *(87)* described a case of an AIDS patients who developed meningoradiculoneuritis while receiving prophylactically oral acyclovir (400 mg, b.i.d.) for 8 mo following recurrent multidermatomal zoster. A thymidine kinase (TK)-deficient, acyclovir-resistant VZV strain has been isolated from the cerebrospinal fluid (CSF). Upon initiation of foscarnet therapy, the virus became undetectable and the CSF was cleared from mononuclear cells (pleiocytosis) and protein overload (proteinorachia).

3.3. Management of Drug-Resistant Varicella-Zoster Virus Infections

Acyclovir, which is inactive as nucleoside, exerts its antiviral activity after phosphorylation to the nucleotide acyclovir triphosphate *(88)*. The monophosphorylation of the drug is carried out by a virally encoded enzyme, the TK. Viral TK is induced in cells infected with VZV. The acyclovir monophosphate is further phosphorylated to its triphosphate nucleotide form by host-cell enzymes. Decreased or absent induction of virus-encoded TK is one mechanism by which VZV become resistant to acyclovir *(3,89)*. One other potential mode to acquire resistance is alterations in substrate specificity of either viral TK or viral DNA polymerase *(2)*. Acyclovir-resistant VZV infection have been reported exclusively in HIV-seropositive patients, usually in the setting of advanced immunosuppression and previous exposure to acyclovir *(3,90–93)*. One acyclovir-resistant isolate was obtained from a bone marrow transplant recipient who had received the drug intravenously *(89)*.

Intravenous foscarnet has been evaluated as an alternative therapy for acyclovir-resistant VZV at dosage regimens of 60 mg/kg twice-daily or 40 mg/kg (t.i.d.) for 10 d or until the lesion is completely healed *(2)*. At daily doses of 120 mg/kg, i.v. for 10 d, foscarnet produced complete healing in 4 of 5 AIDS patients with TK-deficient VZV strains; the remaining patient developed resistance to foscarnet *(67)*. Smith et al. *(68)* described a patient with chronic hyperkeratoic VZV lesions and acyclovir resistance who responded well to a 3-wk course of foscarnet (120 mg/kg). Adverse effects included nausea, vomiting, bloating, as well as hypokalemia and hyperphosphatemia.

3.4. Varicella-Zoster Virus Pneumonitis

It was not until 1942 that VZV-associated pneumonitis was recognized as a separate clinical entity with potentially lethal outcome in even otherwise healthy adults *(94)*. Currently, VZV-induced pneumonitis is considered to be one of the most serious complications of disseminated VZV infection, especially in immunocompromised individuals *(95)*. Bone-marrow transplant *(73,96,97)*, renal *(98,99)* and liver *(100)* transplant recipients, children with cancer *(101–103)*, and HIV-positive patients *(104)* are at the highest risk of developing VZV pneumonitis.

Corticosteroid therapy administered to patients with underlying disease, such as renal or collagen-vascular disorders, has also been associated with an increased risk of VZV pneumonitis *(95)*. In addition, several reports have indicated that conventional "low-dose" corticosteroid therapy (<2.0 mg/kg daily, or 5.0–20 mg daily) *(105)*, topical nasal corticosteroids for chronic sinusitis *(106)*, and short-course corticosteroid therapy for acute asthma attack when administered during the incubation period of varicella *(107)* may predispose to disseminated varicella infections.

3.5. Herpes-Zoster Ophthalmicus

Herpes-zoster ophthalmicus (HZO) affects the first division of the trigeminal nerve and is associated with a high rate of ocular involvement often leading to serious morbidity *(108–113)*. In the majority of HZO cases, the eye complications appear shortly after the rash and are assumed to be the result by the presence of replicating VZV *(110,114–117)*. The nature of HZO complications are inflammatory and include conjunctivitis, episcleritis, keratitis, and anterior uveitis. Whereas conjunctivitis and episcleritis tend to be transient and self-limiting, the other inflammatory lesions can become chronic or recurrent *(109)*.

Intravenous acyclovir and vidarabine are the mainstay of therapy in patients with VZV retinitis *(118)*. The recommended dose of acyclovir is 1.5 g/m^2 every 8 h for 7 d; intravenous courses of acyclovir are frequently followed by 1–2-wk courses of oral acyclovir as the retinitis regresses. The recommended dose for vidarabine is 10 mg/kg daily in a 12-h infusion for 5 d, both in normal and immunocompromised patients *(118)*.

Recent attention has been centered on the use of acyclovir as both in prophylaxis and disease management *(108,109)*. Current evidence favors the use of topical acyclovir alone in the treatment of established ocular complications *(119)*. There have also been recommendations for topical use of steroids but the precise relationship between antiviral therapy and steroids is still unclear *(120,121)*, and the use of topical steroids should be considered only for most severe cases *(119)*.

When administered orally, acyclovir (800 mg 5 times daily) has only limited therapeutic benefits because it is only partially absorbed, and its plasma levels remaining virtually unchanged at doses over 800 mg *(120)*. In addition, these plasma levels have been only slightly higher than the mean effective dose (ED_{50}) for most strains of VZV *(123,124)*. However, the aqueous humoral levels have been significantly higher if acyclovir had been administered topically to the eye *(108,125)*.

In two studies on the prophylactic use of acyclovir, the beneficial effects have been observed only when the treatment was initiated within 72 h of the onset of rash *(126,127)*. However, the results were conflicting, because in one study the effect was noticed early *(126)*, whereas in the other it occured late *(127)*. To study the possibility of whether ocular treatment with acyclovir provides better efficacy than oral administration, Neoh et al. *(108)* used a multicenter, open, randomized trial to compare the ocular prophylactic effects of topical and oral acyclovir. The patients received prophylactic treatment within 72 h of the onset of rash consisting of either topical acyclovir ointment or 800 mg of oral acyclovir, both 5 times daily for 1 wk; a follow-up examination was carried out 12 mo after completion of treatment. The results have shown that in spite of its better penetration, topical acyclovir apparently did not offer prophylactic value in the management of early HZO *(108)*.

REFERENCES

1. Roizman, B. Herpesviridae: a brief introduction, in *Fields Virology*, 2nd ed., Fields, B. N., Knipe, D. M., Chanock, R. M., et al. Eds., Raven Press, New York, 1787, 1990.
2. Balfour, H. H., Benson, C., Braun, J., et al. Management of acyclovir-resistant herpes simplex and varicella- zoster virus infection. *J. Acquir. Immune Defic. Syndr.*, 7, 254, 1994.
3. Jacobson, M. A., Berger, T. G., Fikrig, S., et al. Acyclovir-resistant varicella-zoster virus infection after chronic oral acyclovir therapy in patients with the acquired immunodeficiency syndrome (AIDS). *Ann. Intern. Med.*, 112, 187, 1990.
4. Gelb, L. D., Varicella-zoster virus, *in Fields Virology*, 2nd ed., Fields, B. N., Knipe, D. M., Chanock, R. M., et al. Eds. Raven Press, New York, 2011, 1990.
5. Hope-Simpson, R. E. Infectiousness of communicable diseases in the household (measles, chickenpox, and mumps). *Lancet*, 2, 549, 1952.
6. Head, H. and Campbell, A. W. The pathology of herpes zoster and its bearing on sensory localization. *Brain*, 23, 353, 1900.
7. Juel-Jensen, B. W. and MacCallum, F. O. *Herpes simplex, Varicella and Zoster*. J. B. Lippincott, Philadelphia, 1972.
8. Schimpff, S., Serpick, A., Stoler, B., et al. Varicella-zoster infection in patients with cancer. *Ann. Intern. Med.*, 76, 241, 1972.
9. Easton, H. G. Zoster sine herpete causing trigeminal neuralgia. *Lancet*, 2, 1065, 1970.
10. Luby, J. P., Ramirez-Ronda, C., Rinner, S., Hull, A., and Vergne-Marini, P. A longitudinal study of varicella zoster infections in renal transplant recipients. *J. Infect. Dis.*, 135, 659, 1977.
11. Gallagher, J. G. and Merigan, T. C. Prolonged herpes-zoster infection associated with immunosuppressive therapy. *Ann. Intern. Med.*, 91, 842, 1977.
12. Horten, B., Price, R. W., and Jimenez, D. Multifocal varicella-zoster virus leukoencephalitis temporarily remote from herpes zoster. *Ann. Neurol.*, 9, 251.
13. Ryder, J. W., Croen, K., Kleinschmidt-DeMasters, B. K., Ostrove, J. M., Straus, S. E., and Cohn, D. L. Progressive encephalitis three months after resolution of cutaneous zoster in a patient with AIDS. *Ann. Neurol.*, 19, 182, 1986.
14. De La Blanchardiere, A., Rozenberg, F., Caumes, E., et al. Neurological complications of varicella-zoster infection in adults with human immunodeficiency virus infection. *Scand. J. Infect. Dis.*, 32, 263–269, 2000.

15. Dolin, R., Reichman, R. C., Masur, M. H., and Whitley, R. J. Herpes zoster-varicella infection in immunocompromised patients. *Ann. Intern. Med.*, 89, 375, 1978.
16. Atkinson, K., Meyers, J. D., Storb, R., Prentice, R. L., and Thomas, E. D. Varicella-zoster virus after marrow transplantation for applastic anaemia or leukaemia. *Transplantation*, 29, 47, 1980.
17. Rand, K. H., Rasmussen, L. E., Pollard, R. B., Arvin, A., and Merigan, T. C. Cellular immunity and herpes virus infections in cardiac-transplant patient. *N. Engl. J. Med.*, 296, 1372, 1976.
18. Guinee, V. F., Guido, J. J., Pfalzgraf, K. A., et al. The incidence of herpes zoster in patients with Hodgkin's disease: an analysis of prognostic factors. *Cancer*, 56, 642, 1985.
19. Correale, J., Monteverde, D. A., Bueri, J. A., and Reich, E. G. Peripheral nervous system and spinal cord involvement in lymphoma. *Acta Neurol. Scand.*, 83, 45, 1991.
20. Rusthoven, J. J., Ahlgren, P., Elhakim, T., et al. Varicella zoster infection in adult cancer patients: a population study. *Arch. Intern. Med.*, 148, 1561, 1988.
21. Sokal, J. E. and Firat, D. Varicella-zoster infection in Hodgkin's disease. *Am. J. Med.* 39, 452, 1965.
22. Norum, J., Bremnes, R. M., and Wist, E. The ChlVPP regimen, a risk factor for herpes zoster virus infection in patients treated for Hodgkin's disease. *Eur. J. Haematol.*, 53, 51, 1994.
23. Feld, R., Evans, W. K., and DeBoer, G. Herpes zoster in patients with carcinoma of the lung. *Am. J. Med.*, 73, 795, 1982.
24. Maiche, A. G., Kajanti, M. J., and Pirhönen, S. Simultaneous disseminated herpes zoster and bacterial infection in cancer patients. *Acta Oncol.*, 31, 681, 1992.
25. Gottlieb, M. S., Wolfe, P. R., Fahey, J. L., et al. The syndrome of persistent generalized lymphadenopathy: experience with 101 patients, in *AIDS-Associated Syndromes*, Gupta, S., Ed. Plenum Press, New York, 85, 1984.
26. Colebunders, R., Francis, H., Izaley, L., et al. Evaluation of a clinical case-definition of acquired immunodeficiency syndrome in Africa. *Lancet*, 1, 492, 1987.
27. Mandal, B. K. Herpes zoster and the immunocompromised. *J. Infect.*, 14, 1, 1987.
28. King, D. H. History, pharmacokinetics, and pharmacology of acyclovir. *J. Am. Acad. Dermatol.*, 18, 176, 1988.
29. Hopefl, A. W. The clinical use of intravenous acyclovir. *Drug Intell. Clin. Pharmacy*, 17, 623, 1983.
30. Whitley, R. J. and Gnann, J. W. Acyclovir: a decade later. *N. Engl. J. Med.*, 327, 782, 1992.
31. Elion, G. B., Furman, P. A., Fyfe, J. A., de Miranda. P., Beauchamp. L., and Schaeffer, H. J. Selectivity of action of an antiherpetic agent, 9-(2-hydroxyethoxymethyl)guanine. *Proc. Natl. Acad. Sci. USA*, 74, 5716, 1977.
32. Schaeffer, H. J., Beauchamp, L., de Miranda, P., Elion, G. B., Bauer, D. J., and Collins, P. 9-(2-Hydroxyethoxymethyl)guanine activity against viruses of the herpes group. *Nature*, 272, 583–585, 1978.
33. Bridgen, D. and Whiteman, P. The mechanism of action, pharmacokinetics and toxicity of acyclovir - a review. *J. Infect. Dis.*, 6(Suppl.1), 3, 1983.
34. Biron, K. K., Fyfe, J. A., Noblin, J. E., and Elion, G. B. Selection and preliminary characterization of acyclovir-resistant mutants of varicella-zoster virus. *Am. J. Med.*, 73(Suppl. A), 383–386, 1982.
35. Wade, J. C. and Meyers, J. D. Neurologic symptoms associated with parenteral acyclovir treatment after marrow transplantation. *Ann. Intern. Med.*, 98, 921, 1983.
36. Keeney, R. E., Kirk, M. S., and Bridgen, D. Acyclovir tolerance in humans. *Am. J. Med.*, 73(Suppl.), 176, 1982.
37. Tomson, C. R. V., Goodship, T. H. J., and Rodger, R. S. C. Psychiatric side-effects of acyclovir in patients with chronic renal failure. *Lancet*, 2, 385, 1985.
38. Wellcome Medical Division. Zovirax in ABPI Data sheet compendium 1991–1992, Datafarm Publishers, London, 1748, 1991.
39. Bataille, P., Devos, P., Noel, J. L., Dautrevaux, C., and Lokiec, F. Psychiatric side-effects with acyclovir. *Lancet*, 2, 724, 1985.
40. Rubin, R. Overdose with acyclovir in a CAPD patient. *Perit. Dial Bull.*, 7, 42, 1987.
41. Swan, S. K. and Bennett, W. M. Oral acyclovir and neurotoxicity. *Ann. Intern. Med.*, 111, 188, 1989.
42. Krigel, R. L. Reversible neurotoxicity due to acyclovir in a patient with chronic lymphatic leukaemia. *J. Infect. Dis.*, 154, 189.
43. Davenport, A., Goel, S., and Mackenzie, J. C. Neurotoxicity of acyclovir in patients with end-stage renal failure treated with continuous ambulatory peritoneal dialysis. *Am. J. Kidney Dis.*, 20, 647, 1992.
44. Beales, P., Almond, M. K., and Kwan, J. T. C. Acyclovir neurotoxicity following oral therapy: prevention and treatment in patients on haemodyalisis. *Nephron*, 66, 362, 1994.
45. Blum, M. R., Liao, S. H. T., and de Miranda, P. Overview of acyclovir pharmacokinetic desposition in adults and children. *Am. J. Med.*, 73(Suppl. 1A), 186, 1982.
46. Laskin, O. L., Longstreth, J. A., Whelton, A., et al. Effect of renal failure on the pharmacokinetics of acyclovir. *Am. J. Med.* 73(Suppl. 1A), 197, 1982.
47. MacDiarmaid-Gordon, A. R., O'Connor, M., Beaman, M., and Ackrill, P. Neurotoxicity associated with oral acyclovir in patients undergoing dialysis. *Nephron*, 62, 280, 1992.
48. Spiegal, D. M. and Lau, K. Acute renal failure and coma secondary to acyclovir therapy,. *J. Am. Med. Assoc.*, 255, 1882, 1986.
49. Johnson, R., Douglas, J., Corey, L., and Krasney, H. Adverse effects with acyclovir and meperidine. *Ann. Intern. Med.*, 103, 962, 1985.
50. Gill, M. J. and Burgess, E. Neurotoxicity of acyclovir in end stage disease. *J. Antimicrob. Chemother.*, 25, 300, 1990.

51. Feldman, S., Rodman, J., and Gregory, B. Excessive serum concentrations of acyclovir and neurotoxicity. *J. Infect. Dis.* 157, 385, 1988.
52. Haefeli, W. E., Schoenenberger, R. A. Z., Weiss, P., and Ritz, R. F. Acyclovir-induced neurotoxicity: concentration-side effect relationship in acyclovir overdose. *Am. J. Med.*, 94, 212, 1993.
53. Gnann, J. W. New antivirals with activity against varicella-zoster virus. *Ann. Neurol.*, 34, S69, 1994.
54. Vere Hodge, R. A. Famciclovir and penciclovir: the mode of action of famciclovir including its conversion to penciclovir. *Antiviral Chem. Chemother.*, 42, 67, 1993.
55. Pue, M. A. and Benet, L. Z. Pharmacokinetics of famciclovir in man. *Antiviral Chem. Chemother.*, 4(Suppl. 1), 47, 1993.
56. Abramowitz, M. Famciclovir for herpes zoster. *Med. Lett. Drugs Ther.*, 36, 97, 1994.
57. Saltzman, R., Jurewicz, R., and Boon, R. Safety of famciclovir in patients with herpes zoster and genital herpes. *Antimicrob. Agents Chemother.*, 38, 2454, 1994.
58. Tyring, S., Nahlik, J., Cunningham, A., and the Collaborative Famciclovir Herpes Zoster Clinical Study Group. Efficacy and safety of famciclovir in the treatment of patients with herpes zoster. *Proc. 33rd Intersci. Conf. Antimicrob. Agents Chemother.*, American Society for Microbiology, Washington, DC, abstract 1540, 1993.
59. Gheeraert, P., and the Famciclovir Herpes Zoster Virus Clinical Study Group. Efficacy and safety of famciclovir in the treatment of uncomplicated herpes zoster,. *Proc. 32nd Intersci. Conf. Antimicrob. Agents Chemother.*, American Society for Microbiology, Washington, DC, abstract 1108, 1992.
60. Sacks, S. L., Bishop, A. M., Fox, R., and Lee, G. C. Y. A double-blind, placebo-controlled trial of the effect of chronically administered oral famciclovir on sperm production in men with recurrent genital herpes infection. *Antiviral Res.*, 23(Suppl. 1), 72, 1994.
61. Gnann, J., Crumpacker, C., Lalezari, J., et al. Sorivudine versus acyclovir for treatment of dermatomal herpes zoster in human immunodeficiency virus-infected patients: results from a randomized, controlled clinical trial. *Antimicrob. Agents Chemother.*, 42, 1139–1145, 1998.
62. Huff, J. C., Bean, B., Balfour, H. H. Jr., et al. Therapy of herpes zoster with oral acyclovir. *Am. J. Med.*, 85(Suppl. 2A), 84, 1988.
63. Wood, M. J., Ogan, P. H., McKendrick, M. W., Care, C. D., McGill, J. I., and Webb, E. M. Efficacy of oral acyclovir treatment of acute herpes zoster. *Am. J. Med.*, 85(Suppl. 2A), 79, 1988.
64. Gnann, J. W. and Whitley, R. J. Natural history and treatment of varicella-zoster in high-risk populations. *J. Hosp. Infect.*, 18(Suppl.), 317, 1991.
65. Balfour, H. H. Jr. Current management of varicella zoster virus infections. *J. Med. Virol.*, Suppl. 1, 74, 1993.
66. Stankus, S. J., Dlugopolski, M., and Packer, D. Management of herpes zoster (shingles) and postherpetic neuralgia. *Am. Fam. Physician*, 61, 2437–2444, 2447–2448, 2000.
67. Safrin, S., Berger, T. G., Gilson, I., et al. Foscarnet therapy in five patients with AIDS and acyclovir-resistant varicella-zoster virus infection. *Ann. Intern. Med.*, 115, 19, 1991.
68. Smith, K. J., Kahlter, D. C., Davis, C., James, W. D., Skelton, H. G., and Angritt, P. Acyclovir-resistant varicella zoster responsive to foscarnet. *Arch. Dermatol.*, 127, 1069, 1991.
69. Deray, G., Martinez, F., Katlama, C., et al. Foscarnet nephrotoxicity: mechanism, incidence and prevention. *Am. J. Nephrol.*, 9, 316, 1989.
70. Sempere, A., Sanz, G. F., Senent, L., et al. Long-term acyclovir prophylaxis for prevention of varicella zoster virus infection after autologous blood stem cell transplantation in patients with acute leukemia,. *Bone Marrow Transplant.*, 10, 495, 1992.
71. Shepp, D. H., Dandliker, P. S., and Meyers, J. D. Treatment of varicella-zoster virus infection in severely immunocompromised patients: a randomized comparison of acyclovir and vidarabine. *N. Engl. J. Med.*, 314, 208, 1986.
72. Paryani, S. G. and Azuin, A. M. Intrauterine infection with varicella-zoster virus after maternal varicella. *N. Engl. J. Med.*, 314, 1542, 1986.
73. Locksley, R. M., Flournoy, N., Sullivan, K. M., and Mayers, J. D. Infection with varicella-zoster virus after marrow transplantation. *J. Infect. Dis.*, 152, 1172, 1985.
74. Bustamantem, C. I. and Wade, J. C. Herpes zoster virus infection in the immunocompromised cancer patient. *J. Clin. Oncol.*, 9, 1903, 1991.
75. Selby, P. J., Jameson, B., and Watson, J. G. Parenteral acyclovir: therapy for herpes virus infection in man. *Lancet*, 2, 1267, 1979.
76. Gluckman, E., Devergie, A., and Melo, R. Prophylaxis of herpes infections after bone marrow transplantation by oral acyclovir. *Lancet*, 2, 706, 1983.
77. Wingard, J. R. Viral infections in leukemia and bone marrow transplant patients. *Leuk. Lymphoma*, 11(Suppl. 2), 115, 1993.
78. Feldman, S. Varicella zoster infections in bone marrow transplants. *Recent Results Cancer Res.*, 132, 177, 1993.
79. Ben, B., Buren, C. T., and Balfour, H. H. Jr. Acyclovir therapy for acute herpes zoster. *Lancet*, 2, 118, 1982.
80. Bridgen, D., Rosling, A. E., and Woods, N. C. Renal function after acyclovir intravenous injection. *Am. J. Med.*, 73(Suppl. 1A), 182, 1982.
81. Stoffel, M., Squifflet, J. P., Pirson, Y., Lamy, M., and Alexandre, G. P. J. Effectiveness of oral acyclovir prophylaxis in renal transplant recipients. *Transplant. Proc.*, 19, 2190, 1987.
82. Meyers, J. D., Wade, J. C., Shepp, D. H., and Newton, B. Acyclovir treatment of varicella-zoster virus infection in the

compromised host. *Transplantation*, 37, 571, 1984.
83. Hayes, K., Shakuntala, V., Pingle, A., Dhawan, I. K., and Masri, M. A. Safe use of acyclovir (zovirax) in renal transplant patients on cyclosporine A therapy: case reports. *Transplant. Proc.*, 24, 1926, 1992.
84. Johnson, P. C., Kumor, K., Welsh, M. S., Woo, J., and Kahan, B. D. Effects of coadministration of cyclosporine and acyclovir on renal function of renal allograft recipients. *Transplantation*, 44, 329, 1987.
85. Glesby, M. J., Moore, R. D., Chaisson, R. E., and the Zidovudine Epidemiology Study Group. Herpes zoster in patients with advanced human immunodeficiency virus infection treated with zidovudine. *J. Infect. Dis.*, 168, 1264, 1993.
86. Friedman-Kien, A. E., Lafleur, F. L., Gendler, E., et al. Herpes zoster: a possible early sign for development of acquired immunodeficiency syndrome in high-risk individuals. *J. Am. Acad. Dermatol.*, 14, 1023, 1986.
87. Snoeck, R., Gérard, M., Sadzot-Delvaux, C., et al. Meningoradiculoneuritis due to acyclovir-resistant varicella zoster in an acquired immune deficiency syndrome patient. *J. Med. Virol.*, 42, 338, 1994.
88. Balfour, H. H. Jr. Acyclovir, in *The Antimicrobial Agents Annual/3*, Peterson, P. K. and Verhoef, J., Eds., Elsevier Science, New York, 345, 1988.
89. Collins, P. Viral sensitivity following the introduction of acyclovir. *Am. J. Med.*, 85, 129, 1988.
90. Janier, M., Hillion, M., Baccard, M., et al. Chronic varicella zoster infection in acquired immunodeficiency syndrome. *J. Am. Acad. Dermatol.*, 18, 584, 1988.
91. Pahwa, S., Biron, K., Lim, W., et al. Continuous varicella-zoster infection associated with acyclovir resistance in a child with AIDS. *J. Am. Med. Assoc.*, 260, 2879, 1988.
92. Linneman, C. C., Biron, K. K., Hoppenjans, W. G., and Solinger, A. M. Emergence of acyclovir-resistant varicella zoster virus in an AIDS patient on prolonged acyclovir therapy. *AIDS*, 4, 577, 1990.
93. Hoppenjans, W. B., Bibler, M. R., Ormer, R. L., and Solinger, A. M. Prolonged cutaneous herpes zoster in acquired immunodeficiency syndrome. *Arch. Intern. Med.*, 126, 1048, 1990.
94. Waring, J. J., Neuburger, K., and Geever, E. F. Severe forms of chickenpox in adults. *Arch. Intern. Med.*, 69, 384, 1942.
95. Feldman, S., Varicella-zoster virus pneumonitis. *Chest*, 106(Suppl.), 22S, 1994.
96. Schuchter, L. M., Wingard, J. R., Piantadosi, S., et al. Herpes zoster infection after autologous bone marrow transplantation. *Blood*, 74, 1424, 1989.
97. Wacker, P., Hartmann, O., Benhamou, E., Salloum, E., and Lemerle, J. Varicella-zoster virus infections after autologous bone marrow transplantation in children. *Bone Marrow Transplant.*, 4, 191, 1989.
98. Feldhoff, C. M., Balfour, H. H. Jr., Simmons, R. L., Najarian, J. S., and Mauer, S. M. Varicella in children with renal transplants. *J. Pediatr.*, 98, 25, 1981.
99. Lynfield, R., Herrin, J. T., and Rubin, R. H. Varicella in pediatric renal transplant recipients. *Pediatrics*, 90, 216, 1992.
100. McGregor, R. S., Zitelli, B. J., Urbach, A. H., Malatack, J. J., and Gartner, J. C. Jr. Varicella in pediatric orthotopic liver transplant recipients. *Pediatrics*, 83, 256, 1989.
101. Feldman, S., Hughes, W. T., and Daniel, C. B. Varicella in children with cancer: 77 cases. *Pediatrics*, 56, 388, 1975.
102. Feldman, S. and Lott, L. Varicella in children with cancer: impact of antiviral therapy and prophylaxis. *Pediatrics*, 80, 465, 1987.
103. Feldman, S., Hughes, W. T., and Kim, H. Y. Herpes zoster in children with cancer. *Am. J. Dis. Child.*, 126, 178, 1973.
104. Jura, E., Chadwick, E. G., Josephs, S. H., et al. Varicella-zoster virus infections in children infected with human immunodeficiency virus. *Pediatr. Infect. Dis. J.*, 8, 586, 1989.
105. Dowell, S. F. and Bresee, J. S. Severe varicella associated with steroid use. *Pediatrics*, 92, 223, 1993.
106. Abzug, M. J. and Cotton, M. F. Severe chickenpox after intranasal use of corticosteroids. *J. Pediatr.*, 123, 577, 1993.
107. Kasper, W. J. and Howe, P. M. Fatal varicella after a single course of corticosteroids. *Pediatr. Infect. Dis. J.*, 9, 729, 1990.
108. Neoh, C., Harding, S. P., Saunders, D., et al. Comparison of topical and oral acyclovir in early herpes zoster ophthalmicus. *Eye*, 8, 688, 1994.
109. Aylward, G. W., Claoué, C. M. P., Marsh, R. J., and Yasseem, N. Influence of oral acyclovir on ocular complications of herpes zoster ophthalmicus. *Eye*, 8, 70, 1994.
110. Womack, L. W. and Leisegang, T. J. Complications of herpes zoster ophthalmicus. *Arch. Ophthalmol.*, 101, 42, 1983.
111. Karbassi, M., Raizman, M. B., and Schuman, J. S. Herpes zoster ophthalmicus. *Surv. Ophthalmol.*, 36, 395, 1992.
112. Harding, S. P., Lipton, J. R., and Wells, J. C. D. Natural history of herpes zoster ophthalmicus: predictors of postherpetic neuralgia and ocular involvement. *Br. J. Ophthalmol.*, 71, 353, 1987.
113. Mader, T. H. and Stulting, R. D. Viral keratitis. *Incet. Dis. Clin. North Am.*, 6, 831, 1992.
114. Harding, S. P., Lipton, J. R., and Wells, J. C. D. Natural history of herpes zoster ophthalmicus, predictors of postherpetic neuralgia and ocular involvement. *Br. J. Ophthalmol.*, 71, 353, 1986.
115. Scheie, H. G. Herpes zoster ophthalmicus. *Trans. Ophthalmol. Soc. U.K.*, 90, 899, 1970.
116. Leisegang, T. J. Corneal complications from herpes zoster ophthalmicus. *Ophthalmology*, 92, 316, 1985.
117. Marsh, R. J. and Cooper, M. Ophthalmic herpes zoster. *Eye*, 7, 350, 1993.
118. Yoser, S. L., Forster, D. J., and Rao, N. A. Systemic viral infections and their retinal and choroidal manifestations. *Surv. Ophthalmol.*, 37, 313, 1993.
119. Harding, S. P. Management of ophthalmic zoster. *J. Med. Virol. Suppl.*, 1, 97, 1993.
120. McGill, J. and Chapman, C. A. A compasrison of topical acyclovir with steroids in the treatment of herpes zoster keratouveitis. *Br. J. Ophthalmol.*, 67, 746, 1983.

121. Marsh, R. J. and Cooper, M. Double-masked trial of topical acyclovir and steroids in the treatment of herpes zoster ocular inflammations. *Br. J. Ophthalmol.*, 75, 542, 1991.
122. Bridgen, D., Foule, A., and Rosling, A. Acyclovir, a new antiherpetic drug: early experience in man with systemically administered drug, in *Developments in Antiviral Therapy*, Collier, L. H. and Oxford, J., Eds. Academic Press, London, 53, 1980.
123. Biron, K. K. and Elion, G. B. In vitro susceptibility of varicella zoster virus to acyclovir. *Antimicrob. Agents Chemother.*, 18, 443, 1980.
124. Crumpacker, C. S., Schnipper, L. E., Zaia, J. A., and Levin, H. J. Growth inhibition by acycloguanosine of herpesvirus isolated from human infections. *Antimicrob. Agents Chemother.*, 15, 642, 1979.
125. Poirier, R. H., Kingham, J. D., de Miranda, P., and Annel, M. Intraocular antiviral penetration. *Arch. Ophthalmol.*, 100, 1964, 1982.
126. Cobo, L. M., Foulks, G. N., Leisegang, T., et al. Oral acyclovir in the treatment of acute herpes zoster ophthalmicus. *Ophthalmology*, 93, 763, 1986.
127. Harding, S. P. and Porter, S. M. Oral acyclovir in herpes zoster ophthalmicus. *Curr. Eye Res.*, 10, 177, 1991.

3
Herpes Simplex Virus

1. INTRODUCTION

The herpesviruses (family Herpesviridae) are highly disseminated in nature. One of these ubiquitous pathogens, herpesvirus hominis, is the etiologic agent of herpes simplex in humans. Forty years after the isolation of the herpes simplex viruses (HSV), Schneweiss *(1)* established the existence of two serotypes, HSV-1 and HSV-2, currently designated under The International Committee on Taxonomy of Viruses (ICTV) rules as human herpes viruses 1 and 2 *(2)*. Type 1 infections are primarily nongenital (e.g., herpes labialis and ocular herpes), whereas type 2 infections are primarily genital (herpes genitales).

Since their discovery, nearly 100 herpesviruses have been, at least partially characterized, and six of them have been isolated from humans: HSV-1 *(3–8)*, HSV-2 *(3–10)*, human cytomegalovirus (HCMV) *(11)*, varicella-zoster virus (VZV) *(12–14)*, Epstein-Barr virus (EBV) *(15,16)*, and human herpesvirus 6 (HHV6) *(17,18)*. Diagnosis of HSV infections may be difficult because of the ability of these viruses to establish latency and often to shed intermittently in the absence of invasive disease *(19)*.

Compared to immunocompetent patients, HSV infections in immunocompromised hosts caused a more severe and invasive illness characterized by prolonged viral shedding and a tendency to heal more slowly. This, coupled with the emergence of resistant strains (isolated exclusively from immunocompromised patients) and frequent reactivation *(20)* requires a more aggressive and targeted antiviral therapy *(21)*.

Prior to the emergence of the AIDS pandemic, chronic mucocutaneous HSV infections have been primarily seen in patients with congenital cellular immune deficiencies, or acquired immune defects associated most often with lymphoproliferative malignancies *(22–24)* and organ transplantations *(22,24–29)*. Thus, 80% of marrow transplant recipients with antibody to HSV before transplantation have reactivated virus after the transplantation *(27,30,31)*. The absence of specific cellular immune response to HSV during the first month after the transplant significantly contributes to the severe, prolonged, and debilitating course of HSV disease *(30)*. Frequent reactivation has been also reported in renal-transplant recipients *(32,33)* and in patients receiving leukemic induction therapy *(34)*.

Currently, HIV-infected patients represent the major population affected by persistent active HSV infections *(35)*. The significant association of HSV-induced genital ulceration and transmission of HIV has been shown in many studies *(36)*. Furthermore, because asymptomatic shedding of HSV can continue despite clinically effective suppression with antiviral chemotherapy, the possibility of person-to-person transmission persists *(37)*.

Mucocutaneous HSV infections in immunocompromised patients may be much more severe than in normal subjects. The lesions tend to be more invasive, slower to heal, and associated with prolonged viral shedding *(38)*.

From: Opportunistic Infections: Treatment and Prophylaxis
By: Vassil St. Georgiev © Humana Press Inc., Totowa, NJ

Because seropositivity for HSV is high in HIV-positive patients, it is very likely that clinical HSV disease is associated with reactivation of latent virus *(39)*. The most common clinical manifestations, usually identified with a high morbidity and mortality rate include orolabial, genital, and anorectal mucocutaneous lesions; esophagitis *(40)*; and less often encephalitis. According to the Centers for Disease Control (CDC) definition *(41)*, ulcerative HSV lesions that have been present for more than 1 mo in an HIV-positive individual, or in persons with no other apparent cause of immunodeficiency, are considered an AIDS-defining condition. However, herpetic esophagitis, although frequent infection in immunocompromised patients, has also been diagnosed in immunocompetent hosts *(42)*.

Chronic perianal HSV lesions causing severe morbidity (pain, itching, and painful defecation), have been considered among the first opportunistic infections associated with AIDS in homosexual men *(43)*. Although HSV perianal infections are common in immunocompromised patients, the cutaneous presentation in these patients may be often atypical (large, chronic, hyperkeratotic ulcers *[44]*) and overlapping with the clinical features of other diseases, thereby posing difficulty in diagnosis *(45)*. The clinical manifestations of orolabial and genital HSV disease in HIV-infected patients (mild to severe tissue-distructive lesions) are usually similar to that observed in other immunosuppressed individuals *(39)*.

HSV-induced encephalitis *(46,47)* (a focal or global inflammation of the brain caused by invasion of the brain parenchyma by viruses, bacteria, parasites, or fungi) is a life-threatening condition with substantial morbidity and mortality despite the use of antiviral therapy *(48,49)*. Cases of HSV encephalitis in AIDS patients usually occur as complications of orolabilal HSV infection. Another orolabial HSV-induced complication is a reported case of inferior alveolar nerve infection *(50)*.

Herpetic geometric glossitis, a recently described form of lingual HSV-1 infection, has been reported in several HIV-positive patients, as well as one cardiac and one pediatric patient with acute myelogenous leukemia (AML) *(31,51)*. Results from a report by Woo and Lee *(52)* demonstrated that oral recrudescent HSV infections may involve any intraoral site in immunocompromised patients with nonkeratinized sites representing nearly half of all cases. Hence, it is advisable that all oral ulcers in immunocompromised patients should be cultured for HSV regardless of their location.

Although HSV disease affects primarily the upper respiratory tract *(53,54)*, lower respiratory tract infections have also been reported *(55)*. In a study by Ramsey et al. *(56)*, mucocutaneous lesions antedated the pneumonia in 17 of 21 patients with HSV pneumonitis. HSV-associated pneumonitis has been diagnosed in immunocompromised patients *(57–60)*, alcoholic hepatitis *(61)*, burn victims *(62,63)*, trauma patients *(64)*, and as a consequence of disseminated HSV infection in neonates *(65,66)*. Although the majority of cases affected adults, HSV pneumonitis has also been described in children *(55–58,62,63,67–69)*. A rare case of disseminated neonatal HSV infection has been reported *(70)*.

Hepatitis is a unusual and often fatal manifestation of HSV infection *(71,72)*. Impaired immunity resulting from pregnancy, malignancy, immunosuppression, or inhalational anesthetics may be predisposing factors. Another unusual site involved is colonic HSV disease *(73)*.

An interesting case of latanoprost-associated recurrent HSV keratitis was reported by Dios Castro and Maquet Dusart *(74)*. The patient (with a past episode of herpetic keratitis 21 yr previously), developed the HSV infection after starting treatment with latanoprost.

2. TREATMENT OF HERPES SIMPLEX VIRUS INFECTIONS

In both immunocompromised and immunocompetent patients, acyclovir demonstrated a high degree of clinical efficacy and no statistically significant differences between acyclovir and placebo for mild or major adverse effects. The availability of acyclovir as a generic preparation will further improve the benefit-to-cost ratio. However, the emergence of HSV resistance to antiviral drugs is of concern, and establishing alternative treatments is very important. Newer drugs (valaciclovir, famciclovir, penciclovir) with high oral bioavailability have the added benefit of less frequent administration and avoidance of intravenous therapy in many cases *(75–78)*.

Table 1
Treatment Regimens for HSV Genital Infections

Drug	Manifestations	Dose/duration	Route of administration
Acyclovir	First-episode genital herpes[a]	200 mg, 5 times daily for 10 (U.S.) or 5 (Europe) d	Oral
	Recurrent genital herpes (episodic treatment)[b]	200 mg, 5 times daily, 5 d	Oral
	Chronic suppression of recurrent genital herpes	400 mg, b.i.d.	
Famciclovir	First-episode genital herpes	250 mg, t.i.d., 5–10 d	Oral
	Recurrent genital herpes, (episodic treatment)	125 mg, b.i.d., 5 d	Oral
	Chronic suppression of recurrent genital herpes	250 mg, b.i.d.	Oral
Penciclovir	Recurrent genital herpes (episodic treatment)	5 mg/kg, t.i.d., 5 d, or 5 mg/kg, b.i.d.[c]	i.v.
Valaciclovir	First-episode genital herpes[d]	1,000 mg, b.i.d., 10 d	Oral
	Recurrent genital herpes (episodic treatment)	500 or 1,000 mg, b.i.d., 5 d	Oral
Foscarnet		40–60 mg, every 8 or 12 h	i.v.

[a]In severe cases with neurologic complications (aseptic meningitis, urinary retention), intravenous acyclovir administered 3 times daily should be considered (108,168,169).

[b]The 1998 Genital Herpes Management Guidelines of the Centers for Disease Control (170) provides several treatment for acyclovir including 200 or 400 mg (3 times daily), or 800 mg (twice daily) for 5 d. Neither of these recommended dose regimens have been properly studied in clinical trials.

[c]In immunocompromised hosts, the 5 mg/kg dose given every 12 h was equally effective to that given every 8 h thereby offering a significant dosing reduction in hospital setting (171).

[d]Based on the pharmacokinetic properties of valaciclovir, several countries have chosen to approve a first-episode treatment consisting of 500 mg given twice daily.

During the past decade, oral administration of antiviral agents such as acyclovir (200 mg, 5 times daily), valaciclovir (1,000 mg b.i.d.), and famciclovir (250 mg, b.i.d.) for 5-10 days has been widely used in treating HSV genital infections in immunocompetent patients (79,80).

Currently accepted treatment regimens for genital herpes are given in Table 1 (40,76,79,80).

2.1. Vidarabine

Vidarabine was the first antiviral agent to be used in the treatment of mucocutaneous HSV infections in the immunocompromised hosts (27,81). However, it proved to be a relatively weak and was quickly displaced by acyclovir.

When applied intravenously (usually in large amounts of liquids), vidarabine has been shown to affect favorably the course of both HSV encephalitis (82) and neonatal HSV infection (83). However, against HSV infection in immunocompromised patients, vidarabine was distinctly inferior to acyclovir (84). One explanation for the observed lack of potency is the need of a modicum of host immune response for efficacy (85), thereby rendering the drug largely ineffective in severely immunocompromised patients. In addition, because of its low solubility, vidarabine has required administration in large fluid volumes over 12–24-h periods, although this should be improved by using the more soluble monophosphate derivative. In several studies vidarabine was found to cause significant central nervous system (CNS) toxicity in some patients (86–89).

2.2. Acyclovir (Aciclovir)

For many years acyclovir remains the drug of choice for the prophylaxis and treatment of HSV infections. After its uptake by virus-infected cells, acyclovir is monophosphorylated initially by HSV-encoded thymidine kinase (TK) followed by the formation of its triphosphate catalyzed by host-cell enzymes. By preferentially inhibiting the viral DNA polymerase over cellular DNA polymerase, acyclovir triphosphate exerts low host-cell toxicity.

The great majority of acyclovir-resistant HSV mutants contain mutations within the TK gene, causing significant decrease in viral TK activity in the HSV-infected host cells.

At present, acyclovir is the most commonly prescribed medication for HSV infections *(90–94)*. Leflore et al. *(95)* did a risk-benefit evaluation of acyclovir for the treatment and prophylaxis of HSV infections summarizing data from 30 randomized, double-blind, placebo-controlled clinical trials involving 3364 patients with genital, oral, and mucocutaneous HSV infections.

Immunocompromised patients receiving acyclovir showed shorter duration of viral shedding and more rapid healing of lesions than patients given placebo *(93,96,97)*. The recommended oral dose for mild to moderate mucocutaneous disease is 200 mg, 5 times daily for 7 d. Higher-dose regimens (400–800 mg, 3–5 times daily over a 10-d period) have also proven beneficial in more severe conditions (marrow-transplant recipients) *(38,91)*, and in patients having frequent recurrences that require continuous suppressive therapy *(98–100)*. In the latter cases, daily administration reduced the frequency of recurrences by up to 80%, with 25–30% of the patients having no further recurrences while taking acyclovir *(101,102)*. The therapy should be initiated within 48 h of onset of rash.

Tod et al. *(103)* studied the pharmacokinetics of acyclovir (given as an oral suspension) and a population analysis in neonates and infants (less than 2 yr of age) with the goal of establishing the most appropriate dosing regimens for treating HSV infections; for neonates (less than 1 mo old) the recommended dose was 24 mg/kg, t.i.d., or four times daily otherwise.

In more serious settings (bone-marrow transplantation, HSV encephalitis, and viscerally disseminated HSV disease in immunocompromised patients) *(104)* or when absorption of oral drug is doubtful, intravenous acyclovir (5.0–10 mg/kg, every 8 h) for 7–10 d may be used in patients without renal insufficiency *(38,92)*. For treatment of first-episode genital herpes, however, a high dose of oral acyclovir (4,000 mg daily) did not prove to be more beneficial than the standard dose of 1,000 mg daily *(105)*.

Intravenous acyclovir (5% solution) is the most effective treatment for a first episode of genital herpes and results in a significant reduction of median duration of viral shedding, pain, and length of time to complete healing *(92,106,107)*. Treatment of mucocutaneous lesions should be continued until they have all crusted *(38)*. In a multicenter, randomized, double-blind, placebo-controlled trial of 97 immunocompromised patients with mucocutaneous HSV infection conducted by Meyers et al. *(93)*, intravenous acyclovir significantly shortened the periods of virus shedding ($p < 0.0002$), lesion pain ($p < 0.01$), lesion scabbing ($p < 0.004$), and lesion healing ($p < 0.04$).

Oral acyclovir (200 mg, 5 times daily) is nearly as effective as intravenous infusions for initial episodes of genital herpes infections *(108,109)* and has become the standard treatment *(38,110)*. The use of oral acyclovir has not been associated with any hepatic, renal, or neurologic toxicity *(111)*.

On average, intravenous or oral acyclovir reduced the incidence of symptomatic HSV infections from about 70% to 5–20% *(99,111–113)*. As demonstrated by Shepp et al. *(114)* in chronically immunocompromised bone-marrow transplant recipients, a sequential regimen of intravenous followed by oral acyclovir for 3–6 mo can virtually eliminate sympromatic HSV disease. The two-part regimen included intravenous infusions of acyclovir (250 mg/m^2, b.i.d.) from 5 d before until 30 d after transplantation; on d 31, in a random and double-blind approach, patients were assigned to receive either oral acyclovir (800 mg, b.i.d.) or an identical placebo until d 75 after transplantation. The results demonstrated that the two-part sequential regimen was effective and convenient for extended prophylaxis of HSV infection following marrow transplantation and should be effective in other chronically immunosuppressed patients as well *(114)*.

Topically applied acyclovir (5% ointment), while reducing the duration of viral shedding and the length of time for lesions to crust, is less effective for genital HSV infections than the orally or intravenously administered drug *(115,116)*. Topical treatment of mucocutaneous HSV infections in normal subjects with vidarabine or other antiviral agents has been largely disappointing *(117–120)*. Topical acyclovir has been neither approved nor recommended for the treatment of recurrent genital herpes in the immunocompetent host *(121)*.

In cases of orolabial herpes, despite promising results in early trials with 5% topical acyclovir *(122)*, subsequent studies showed no clinical benefit *(123,124)* because of the poor drug penetration to the site of viral replication. Current data do not support the use of topical acyclovir for orolabial herpes *(38)*. The recommended treatment is oral acyclovir at 200 mg, 5 times daily for 5 d. While this regimen did not diminish the pain and the time for complete healing, it still reduced the length of time to the loss of crusts by approx 1 d (7 vs 8 d) *(125)*. In another trial, Spruance et al. *(126)* used increased dosing (400 mg, 5 times daily for 5 d) and initiated treatment during the prodromal or erythematous stages of infection; the duration of pain was reduced by 36% and the length of time to the loss of crust by 27%. Although, if started early after recurrence, oral acyclovir may be useful, it still cannot be recommended as a routine therapy for treating orolabial herpes *(38)*.

HIV-positive patients that have developed HSV-1-associated herpetic geometric glossitis responded to 1,000 mg (divided into 5 doses) of acyclovir with complete resolution of tongue fissures *(51)*. However, a pediatric patient with acute myelogenous leukemia and herpetic geometric glossitis needed higher doses of oral acyclovir therapy (3,000 mg daily divided in 5 doses) to treat his HSV-1 lingual infection *(51)*.

For HSV-associated encephalitis, administration of acyclovir at doses of 10 mg/kg, t.i.d, for 10–14 d reduced mortality at 3 mo to 19%, as compared to nearly 50% in patients treated with vidarabine *(48)*. Moreover, 38% treated with acyclovir regained normal function. The therapy was most beneficial when initiated before the development of coma or semicoma *(38)*.

The efficacy of acyclovir treatment (topical and oral) in the treatment of herpetic keratitis has also been studied *(127–129)*. In a randomized, double-blind, clinical trial involving 703 immunocompetent patients (with prior HSV eye disease within the preceding year) receiving 800 mg daily of oral acyclovir, the cumulative probability of a recurrence of any type of ocular HSV infection during the 1-yr treatment period was 19% in the acyclovir group compared to 32% in the placebo group *(129)*.

2.3. Valaciclovir

Valaciclovir is the *L*-valyl ester of acyclovir, and as orally active prodrug it is rapidly and extensively metabolized into acyclovir and *L*-valine. Having its antiviral spectrum and potency similar to that of acyclovir, valaciclovir was developed to overcome the poor bioavailability of acyclovir (54% vs 15–130%). After absorption through the gut wall, valaciclovir is rapidly metabolized after first-pass intestinal and/or hepatic hydrolysis *(130)*.

Valaciclovir has been recommended for the treatment of first-episode genital herpes at 1,000 mg daily dose given for 10 d. Thus, in an international multicenter comparative study involving 643 otherwise healthy adults, valaciclovir (1,000 mg given twice daily) compared favorably against acyclovir (200 mg, 5 times daily): both drugs were equally effective and well-tolerated in accelerating the resolution of the episode *(79)*.

Oral valaciclovir has also been approved and recommended by the Centers for Disease Control (CDC) for the episodic treatment of recurrent genital herpes at 500 mg, b.i.d. for 5 d *(131)*. Thus, when administered at 500 or 1,000 mg b.i.d. for 5 d with 24 h of onset of symptoms, valaciclovir accelerated time-to-episode resolution and lesion healing and time-to-cessation of viral shedding. In a large-scale study of 1,200 immunocompetent patients, 1,000-mg dose of oral valaciclovir given b.i.d., proved equally effective to a standard 200-mg dose of acyclovir (5 times daily) for the treatment of recurrent genital herpes *(132)*.

Rivaud et al. *(133)* reported the development of thrombotic thrombocytopenic purpura in an HIV-infected patient receiving lower-dose valaciclovir (500 mg, b.i.d.) for recurrent ocular HSV infection.

2.4. Famciclovir/Penciclovir

Penciclovir, a novel acyclic nucleoside analog was shown to be effective against HSV infections. The intracellular triphosphate of penciclovir is considerably more stable than the acyclovir triphosphate (in vitro half-life of 10–20 h for penciclovir in HSV-infected cells compared to 0.7–1 h for acyclovir) *(134)*.

Famciclovir is the diacetyl ester of 6-deoxypenciclovir. A nucleoside analog structurally close to acyclovir, famciclovir also shows a similar antiviral spectrum. It has an increased oral bioavailability and is rapidly and extensively absorbed in the upper intestines. After undergoing substantial first-pass metabolism in the intestinal wall and liver (deacetylation and oxidation) degradation, famciclovir is converted into panciclovir *(134,135)*.

In a double-blind, placebo-controlled study, Schacker et al. *(136)* investigated the effects of famciclovir on the suppression of symptomatic and asymptomatic HSV reactivation in HIV-infected patients. Active famciclovir therapy (500 mg, b.i.d. for 8 wk, followed by a washout 1-wk period, and placebo, b.i.d. for 8 wk) reduced the total HSV type 2 shedding from 9.7% of d to 1.3% of d.

In the treatment of first-episode genital herpes, oral famciclovir at 250 mg or 750 mg administered 3 times daily for 5–10 d was equipotent to oral acyclovir given at the standard 200-mg dose (5 times daily for 5 d). Furthermore, in two comparative trials, the effects of oral famciclovir administered at either 125, 250, or 500 mg 3 times daily for 10 d were not significantly different from oral acyclovir (200 mg, 5 times daily for 5 d) *(137)*. Similarly, oral famciclovir at 250, 500, and 750 mg, all three dosages given 3 times daily for 5 d in the treatment of first-episode genital herpes, was found to be equipotent to a standard dose (200 mg, 5 times daily for 5 d) of oral acyclovir *(137)*. Oral famciclovir at doses of 125, 250, or 500 mg, given twice daily and initiated within 6 h of the onset of symptoms, markedly reduced the time-to-healing, time-to-cessation of viral shedding, and the duration of lesion edema in both patient- *(138)* and clinic-initiated *(139)*, placebo-controlled trials.

Romanowski et al. *(140)* conducted a randomized, double-blind, parallel-group study in 293 HIV-positive patients to compare the efficacy and safety of famciclovir (500 mg, b.i.d.) and acyclovir (400 mg, five times daily) in a 7-d treatment of recurrent HSV orolabial or genital infections. Both drugs were equipotent in preventing new lesion formation, time-to-complete healing, cessation of viral shedding, and loss of lesion-associated symptoms, with the added benefit of less frequent dosing with famciclovir.

The efficacy and safety of penciclovir for the treatment of HSV mucocutaneous infections in 342 immunocompromised patients were evaluated in a double-blind, acyclovir-controlled, multicenter study *(78)*. Two drug regimens were applied: 5 mg/kg penciclovir every 12 or 8 h, or 5 mg/kg of acyclovir given every 8 h, both regimens beginning within 72 h of lesion onset and continuing for up to 7 d. Although nearly 20% of patients in each treatment group developed new lesions during therapy, there were no statistically significant differences in the rates of complete healing or the cessation of viral shedding, as well as the resolution of pain. In addition, both drugs were tolerated well. The 12-h administration of penciclovir had the added advantage of reduced frequency of dosing compared to the 8-h acyclovir *(78)*.

In a randomized, double-blind, multicenter, controlled trial, Diaz-Mitoma et al. *(80)* studied acute intravenous therapy of HSV infections with penciclovir in immunocompromised populations, mainly post-transplantation patients and patients with hematologic malignancies (leukemia, lymphoma, multiple myeloma, myelodysplastic syndrome, aplastic anemia, and bone marrow). Penciclovir (5 mg/kg) was compared with intravenous acyclovir (5 mg/kg), with both drugs given over a 7-d period. Penciclovir was infused both at 12-h and 8-h intervals, whereas acyclovir was applied every 8 h. Using the prevention of new lesion formation, time to healing, time to loss of viral shedding, and loss of pain/symptoms as the efficacy parameters, both drugs proved equipotent, including the every 12-h vs every

8-h infusion of penciclovir. The prolonged intracellular half-life of penciclovir could be useful in reducing the frequency of intravenous dosing *(80)*.

Currently, a topical formulation of penciclovir has been in use for the treatment of herpes simplex labialis *(141,142)*. Chen et al. *(36)* described results from a randomized, double-blind, multicenter, Phase II, clinical trial comparing 1% penciclovir cream (5 times daily, up to 7 d) with 3% acyclovir cream against genital herpes in 205 Chinese patients. Although there were significant differences in the clinical efficacy (in terms of clinical cure rate, times to healing, resolution of all symptoms, absence of blisters, cessesation of new blisters, crusting, and loss of crust) between the penciclovir and acyclovir groups, a significantly shorter time to crusting was found in the penciclovir group.

2.5. Foscarnet

Foscarnet (trisodium phosphonoformate) is a pyrophosphate analog with in vitro activity against all human herpesviruses, as well as HIV *(143,144)*. Foscarnet is probably the most effective antiviral agent for treatment of acyclovir-resistant HSV infections *(145,146)*. Because HSV drug resistance is a fast-emerging problem in immunocompromised patients, foscarnet is considered extremely useful in these indications. In several clinical studies of AIDS patients with HSV infections that were refractory to acyclovir therapy, foscarnet proved to be efficacious and well-tolerated *(147–156)*. The antiviral activity of foscarnet is not dependent on its conversion into monophosphate by the viral thymidine kinase or any other viral or cellular enzyme. Foscarnet interferes with the elongation of the viral DNA chain by inhibiting the cleavage of pyrophosphate groups from the deoxynucleoside triphosphates, a crucial step in the DNA chain elongation. However, it should be noted that resistance to foscarnet may also develop owing to viral DNA polymerase mutants that permit viral replication despite the presence of the drug *(157,158)*.

Because it is poorly absorbed orally, the intravenous infusion of foscarnet is the preferred route of administration in order to achieve adequate serum levels *(124,159)*. Intermittent administration of 60 mg/kg every 8 h (infused over 2-h period) produced peak and through serum concentrations of 530 μM and 100 μM, respectively *(160)*. Foscarnet is excreted exclusively through the kidney with a serum half-life between 0.7 and 4.8 h *(160,161)*.

The major side effect of foscarnet is its renal toxicity, causing the formation of tubular interstitial lesions. Even though its renal toxicity is reversible, prolonged treatment with foscarnet may cause progressive impairment of renal functions; dosage adjustments would be necessary in patients with renal dysfunction *(159,161)*. Hydration before and during each infusion reduces the severity of renal dysfunction in most patients *(162)*.

In a controlled, randomized, dose-comparative trial in AIDS patients with acyclovir-resistant HSV infections, two regimens of foscarnet (40 mg/kg each, administered every 8 or 12 h, respectively) have provided evidence supporting its safety and therapeutic efficacy, as well as its usefulness in maintenance therapy to delay recurrence of HSV lesions *(163)*. The analysis of data from this trial, however, was complicated by the extensive variability in the lesion size at initiation of therapy, making any statistically valid comparison of treatment regimens nearly impossible.

Safrin et al. *(147)* conducted a study of 26 consecutive AIDS patients treated with foscarnet for mucocutaneous acyclovir-resistant HSV infections. The drug was administered parenterally over 1–2 h through either a peripheral or a central venous catheter. The initial dosage in patients who had normal creatinine clearance ranged from 40–60 mg/kg every 8 h and was serially adjusted according to calculate creatinine clearance as described previously *(164)*. Clinical response was noted in 81% of patients, with complete re-epithelialization of HSV lesions in 73%. Cessation of viral shedding was documented in all of the 11 patients who were recultured. Even though there were frequent adverse reactions to foscarnet (rise in serum creatinine levels to ≥3.0 mg/dL, decrease in the absolute number of polymorphonuclear leukocytes to ≤750 cells/mm^3, abnormal serum calcium and phosphorous levels), in only 3 patients (12%) did the observed toxicities necessitate discontinuation of therapy. Before the initiation of the foscarnet therapy, 14 of the patients who did receive vidarabine (10–20 mg/kg daily, for 4–21 d) failed to respond and therapy was ceased in 4 patients (29%) owing to unwarranted toxicity *(147)*.

Chatis et al. *(148)* described the use of foscarnet in a patient with AIDS and a severe HSV-2 mucocutaneous infection who did not respond to therapy with acyclovir, but healed completely after a 16-d course of intravenous foscarnet medication (50 mg/kg, t.i.d.). Again, the major side effect was the rise of the serum creatinine from 70–105 $\mu M/L$ on d 15 of therapy, making it necessary to lower the foscarnet dosage to 40 mg/kg, t.i.d. In addition, during the 16-d course of treatment, the serum phosphate level rose gradually from 1.13–1.7 mmol/L—this condition was treated with basic aluminum carbonate gel (Basaljel^R). Although the calcium concentration rose from 2.0–2.6 mmol/L, no specific treatment was given for this effect *(148)*.

In an open-label trial, four AIDS patients with severe progressive, ulcerative mucocutaneous lesions of the genitals, perineum, perianal region, or finger owing to acyclovir-resistant HSV-2 were successfully treated with intravenous foscarnet at 60 mg/kg, t.i.d, for 12–50 d (each infusion was given over 2 h) *(150)*. Clinical findings revealed a significant clearing of mucocutaneous lesions and eradication of HSV from the mucosal surface. Two of the patients also received maintenance foscarnet therapy at 42–60 mg/kg daily, given for 5–7 d weekly.

An allogeneic bone-marrow transplant recipient who acquired severe mucocutaneous HSV-1 infection during acyclovir prophylaxis, and subsequently failed to respond to high-dose acyclovir was completely cured after a 16-d course of intravenous foscarnet at 40 mg/kg, t.i.d *(165)*.

The therapeutic efficacies of foscarnet and vidarabine have been compared in a randomized trial of 14 patients with AIDS and mucocutaneous HSV lesions that had been unresponsive to intravenous acyclovir therapy for a minimum of 10 d *(156)*. The patients were randomly assigned to receive intravenously either foscarnet (40 mg/kg, every 8 h) or vidarabine (15 mg/kg daily) for 10–42 d. The results have shown foscarnet to have superior efficacy and less frequent toxicity. Once the treatment was stopped, however, there were numerous cases of relapse.

Sall et al. *(154)* described the successful treatment of progressive acyclovir-resistant orofacial HSV infection in an AIDS patient using intravenous foscarnet at 40 mg/kg 3 times daily; improvement was noted within 4 d. The patient completed 3 wk of therapy with no clinical complications or abnormal laboratory values, and with complete re-epithelialization except for a residual peripheral crust.

The intermittent administration of foscarnet (every 8 h) usually produces peak and trough serum drug concentrations of 530 and 100 μM, respectively *(166)*. Excretion of the drug occurs solely by renal mechanisms, and with a serum half-life ranging between 0.7 and 4.8 h *(166,167)*. However, progressive impairment of renal functions can take place after its prolonged use, thereby making dosage adjustments essential in patients with renal dysfunction *(163,167)*.

2.6. Cidofovir

Cidofovir (HPMPC) is an acyclic nucleoside phosphonate derivative that is a potent and selective HSV inhibitor as a result of its interaction with the viral DNA polymerase. The diphosphonate metabolite of cidofovir acts during the DNA polymerase reaction either as a competitive inhibitor to terminate the DNA chain elongation, or as an alternative substrate to allow chain growth *(172)*. The intracellular half-life of cidofovir is very long—24 and 65 h, respectively—after its monophosphate and diphosphonate had been removed from the cell culture *(173)*.

The antiviral activity of cidofovir encompases a broad range of DNA viruses, including herpesviruses deficient for viral TK as well as herpesviruses with DNA polymerase mutations emerging under foscarnet pressure. In addition, acyclovir-resistant HSV strains with TK-deficient or TK-altered phenotypes were more susceptible to inhibition by cidofovir than were wild-type viruses *(174–176)*.

There have been recent studies using cidovofir gel formulation for topical treatment of genital herpes *(177,178)*. In one such study conducted in 30 AIDS patients with acyclovir-unresponsive HSV infection, the gel (0.3% and 1%), which was compared to placebo, was applied once daily for 5 d. The results have shown significant antiviral and clinical efficacy with median decrease of lesion areas by 58% for those treated with cidofovir vs 0% for placebo-treated patients *(177)*. However, because the study was not large enough to provide statistical significance this particular treatment was not approved by the U.S. Food and Drug Administration (FDA). To this end, although the efficacy of cidofovir in the treatment of genital herpes has been demonstrated, the maximum strength that can be tolerated must be determined by further studies *(121)*.

2.7. Brivudine (Bromovinyldeoxyuridine, BVDU)

Tricot et al. *(179)* have used brivudine, a highly potent and selective anti-herpes agent, to treat an intercurrent mucocutaneous HSV infection in 14 severely immunosuppressed patients. The drug was administered orally at daily doses of 7.5 mg/kg (divided over 4-4 doses/d) for 5 d. In all but two patients, BVDU arrested progression of the HSV disease within 1–2 d after the start of treatment. The results of this uncontrolled trial indicated that BVDU may be safe and effective for oral treatment of HSV type 1 infections *(179)*. The mechanism of action of BVDU to a great extent is similar to that of acyclovir. Initially, it is specifically phosphorylated by the virus-encoded TK, which limits its further action to the virus-infected cell. In its 5'-triphosphate form, BVDU interacted with the DNA polymerase as either an inhibitor to shut off the DNA synthesis, or as a substrate that is incorporated selectively into the DNA of virus-infected cells *(180)*.

In another report *(181)*, brivudin led to a rapid regression of HSV-2 infection in a HIV-positive immunosuppressed patient presenting with an unusual exophytic tumor on the lateral part of the tongue and persistent facial herpes infection.

2.8. Drug-Resistant Herpes Simplex Virus and Evolving Therapeutic Strategies

First reported in 1982, acyclovir-resistant strains of HSV have been found primarily in immunocompromised patients *(121,157,182,183)*.

Results from phenotypic and genotypic analyses on acyclovir-resistant HSV isolates have shown that although viral acyclovir resistance can be developed by multiple means, in about half of the cases, frameshift mutations in the homopolymer nucleotide stretches of the TK gene did take place *(184)*.

The primary mechanism of acyclovir resistance has been the induction of viral mutants defective or deficient of TK, the viral-encoded enzyme, which catalyzes the rate-limiting step of triphosphorylation of acyclovir to its active form, acyclovir triphosphate. Foscarnet, a potent inhibitor of HSV DNA polymerases, does not require phosphorylation for its antiviral activity, making it a potentially useful therapeutic agent against acyclovir-resistant HSV infections, especially when used at an earlier stage in the management of such infections *(185)*.

The incidence of acyclovir-resistant HSV in immunocompromised patients, although still relatively low, appears to be on the rise *(92,186–196)*; by one estimate, incidence occurs in only 4.7% of patients (7 of 148 immunocompromised patients but none in 59 immunocompetent patients) *(197)*. In another study, Nugier et al. *(198)* detected resistance in 2.5% of HSV strains from more than 800 strains tested.

Acyclovir-resistant mucocutaneous HSV infections have been recognized with increasing frequency in AIDS patients. However, alternative therapies in this setting have not been widely studied with the exception of foscarnet *(147–152)*. A survey of the extent of acyclovir refractory HSV infection in HIV patients in the United Kingdom *(185)* showed that 70% of patients did not respond to acyclovir therapy; however, no respondents reported any evidence of transmission of acyclovir-resistant strains.

Although most acyclovir resistance has been reported among AIDS patients, some cases of lethal disseminated visceral HSV infections caused by acyclovir-resistant mutants have been described in bone-marrow transplant recipients *(199)* and in one case of meningoencephalitis in an AIDS patient *(200)*. In bone-marrow transplant recipients, acyclovir-resistant HSV isolates have been identified more frequently after therapeutic acyclovir administration than during prophylaxis *(187)*.

Acyclovir resistance is even less frequent in immunocompetent patients *(201–204)*. Erlich et al. *(186)* have reported the presence of acyclovir-resistant HSV in patients with AIDS. The major mechanism of resistance appeared to be a deficiency of viral TK *(205–207)*. Contrary to early reports for reduced virulence *(208,209)* TK-deficient HSV not only maintains its virulence undiminished, but has also been shown to be capable of establishing latent infections *(186)*. Acyclovir-resistant isolates with mutation in the DNA polymerase also have been found in a severely immunocompromised patient *(205,206,210,211)*.

Treatment of severe, acyclovir-resistant HSV infections include continuous therapy with intravenous acyclovir, vidarabine, and foscarnet *(186,212–214)*. Foscarnet (trisodium phosphonoformate) is probably the most effective antiviral agent for treatment of acyclovir-resistant HSV infections *(145,146)*. Both vidarabine and foscarnet did not require activation of its active moiety by viral TK *(215)*. Vidarabine (adenine arabinoside), a nucleoside analog, is phosphorylated by host-cell enzymes, whereas foscarnet is an active inhibitor of HSV DNA polymerase in its native form and does not require phosphorylation for antiviral activity *(215,216)*.

Because the oral absorption of foscarnet is poor, its intravenous infusion is the preferred route of administration in order to achieve adequate serum levels *(159)*. Intermittent administration of 60 mg/kg every 8 h (infused over 2-h period) produced peak and through serum concentrations of 530 μM and 100 μM, respectively *(160)*. Foscarnet is excreted exclusively through the kidney with a serum half-life between 0.7 and 4.8 h *(160,161)*. Because a prolonged treatment with foscarnet may cause progressive impairment of renal functions, dosage adjustments would be necessary in patients with renal dysfunction *(159,161)*.

In an uncontrolled trial of AIDS patients with severe acyclovir-resistant HSV type 2 infection, Erlich et al. *(213)* administered foscarnet intravenously at 60 mg/kg every 8 h (with reduced dosage for renal impairment) for 12–50 d. All patients showed dramatic improvement in their clinical condition with a marked clearing of mucocutaneous lesions and eradication of HSV from mucosal surfaces. Chatis et al. *(217)* also observed complete healing of mucocutaneous lesions in an AIDS patient with severe HSV type 2 infection, following a 16-d course with intravenous foscarnet (50 mg/kg, t.i.d.). In another uncontrolled trial *(145)*, 21 of 26 AIDS patients (81%) with acyclovir-resistant HSV infection showed clinical response to foscarnet, with complete re-epithelialization of lesions occurring in 19 of those patients (73%). In the same study, the outcome of vidarabine therapy was also investigated. Even though HSV was found to be susceptible to vidarabine in vitro, clinical benefit was observed in only 2 of 14 patients who received vidarabine, and toxicity required discontinuation of the drug in 4 patients. Safrin et al. *(146)* have compared foscarnet (40 mg/kg every 8 h) with vidarabine (15 mg/kg once daily) in 14 randomly selected AIDS patients with acyclovir-resistant HSV infections. Foscarnet was found to be more effective and less toxic; lesions healed in all eight patients receiving foscarnet compared with none of the six patients who received vidarabine. In addition, three of the patients given vidarabine showed neurologic abnormalities. However, HSV disease recurred in all patients following discontinuation of therapy *(146)*. Vinckier et al. *(196)* also reported a beneficial clinical response to intravenous foscarnet in an immunocompromised patient with severe HSV infection.

HSV strains resistance to acyclovir by virtue of alteration in the substrate specificity of the TK or the viral DNA polymerase, however, may develop concurrent resistance to either foscarnet or vidarabine *(213,215)*. Thus, in two studies by Birch et al. *(218,219)*, HSV strains resistant to both acyclovir and foscarnet, have been described.

For therapy of resistant mucocutaneous HSV infections, topical trifluorothymidine, and topical or intravenous cidofovir have yielded encouraging results *(157)*. Cidofovir was used by Blot et al. *(220)* in a pediatric bone-marrow transplant recipient to overcome the emergence of HSV resistant to both acyclovir and foscarnet.

In recent years, interferon-α (IFN-α) has been proposed as a possible adjunct treatment in cases of refractory HSV infections in immunocompromised patients receiving chronic acyclovir *(221–223)*. In

Herpes Simplex Virus

one such example, interferon-α-2a (IFN-α2a) was added to topical acyclovir therapy for HSV keratitis in patients with cell-mediated immune dysfunction and subsequent lack of endogenous IFN (221).

3. PROPHYLAXIS OF HERPESVIRUS INFECTIONS

For patients with frequent recurrences of genital HSV infections, prophylaxis is the management of choice (224).

Results from several double-blind, placebo-controlled trials have demonstrated that oral acyclovir at 600–1000 mg daily for 3–6 mo suppressed the rate of recurrence of genital herpes (79,80,141,142) as well as reduced the risk of transmission to sexual partners (171).

Management of recurrent HSV disease may also be carried out with a low-dose suppressive therapy with oral acyclovir (111,225). Doses of 200 mg, q.i.d., or 400 mg, b.i.d., appeared to be equally effective; in some patients, however, doses of 400 mg., q.i.d. (or 800 mg, b.i.d.) may be clinically necessary to control HSV recurrences (104). Long-term oral administration of acyclovir effectively suppressed the recurrence of genital HSV infections (98–100).

Acyclovir prophylaxis of HSV infections should be of clinical benefit in severely immunocompromised patients, especially those undergoing induction chemotherapy or organ transplantation. Computer modeling has been used to test different dose schedules in order to determine the optimal total intravenous daily dose of acyclovir; dose regimens of 125 mg/m^2 every 6 h, and 62.5 mg/m^2 every 4 h were found to be highly effective as prophylactic therapy (24). In a randomized, double-blind, controlled trial conducted in bone-marrow transplant recipients, acyclovir prophylaxis (250 mg/m^2, i.v., every 8 h) was carried out for 18 d starting 3 d before transplantation; no patient given acyclovir developed HSV infection. By comparison, 7 of 10 patients receiving placebo developed HSV disease (112). The recommended oral prophylaxis doses of acyclovir have been 400 mg every 4–8 h (111).

Neither intravenous nor oral antiviral therapy of acute HSV infections reduced the frequency of recurrence (92,107,109). It has been suggested that virus reactivation and antigen exposure is necessary to restore the specific immune response to HSV after organ transplantation (30,32). To this end, acyclovir treatment may delay immune reconstitution by limiting the period of antigen esposure. In addition, acyclovir may also be directly immunosuppressive, as found by Levin et al. (143) for lymphocyte transformation responses in vitro; however, similar suppression was not found by Steele et al. (144) using higher concentration of acyclovir.

Continuous suppressive therapy with acyclovir for patients with recurrent genital herpes can be maintained indefinitely with no evidence of marked adverse effect (113). It has been suggested in the past that acyclovir treatment should be interrupted every 12 mo to reassess the need for continued suppression (226). Currently, however, there is disagreement about whether or not such therapy should be interrupted. It is reasoned that continuation of suppressive therapy should depend on and be tailored to the lifestyle and long-term physical and psychosocial needs for suppression. Moreover, a reduction of the psychological morbidity of patients should be considered an important benefit of such suppressive therapy (121).

Continuous suppressive therapy with oral valaciclovir is also recommended in cases of frequent recurrences of genital herpes with doses of 500 mg (once daily, for patients having 10 or fewer recurrences per year), and 1000 mg (once daily, for patients with 10 or more annual recurrences).

Oral famciclovir has also been demonstrated to be effective in the suppression of genital herpes recurrences at a dose of 250 mg, b.i.d. (121).

Results of two randomized, double-blind, placebo-controlled multicenter trials of a recombinant subunit vaccine have been recently reported (9). The vaccine, which contained 30 µg each of two major HSV-2 surface glycoproteins (gB2 and gD2) against which neutralizing antibodies are directed, were administered at mo 0, 1, and 6, with participants were being followed up for 1 yr after the third administration. The time-to-event curves indicated a 50% lower acquisition rate among vaccine vs placebo recipients during the initial 5 mo of the trial with an overall vaccine efficacy of 9%. The disappointing results from the trials indicated that for efficient and sustained protection from sexual acquisition of HSV-2 infection, an effective vaccine should require more than just high titers of specific neutralizing antibodies.

REFERENCES

1. Schneweiss, K. E. Serologische untersuchungen zur typendifferenzierung des herpesvirus hominis. *Z. Immuno-Forsch.*, 124, 24, 1962.
2. Roizman, B., Carmichael, L. E., Deinhardt, F., et al. Herpesviridae: definition, provisional nomenclature and taxonomy. *Intervirology*, 16, 201, 1981.
3. Roizman, B. Herpesviridae: a brief introduction, in *Fields Virology*, 2nd ed., Fields, B. N., Knipe, D. M., Chanock, R. M., et al. Eds. Raven Press, New York, 1787, 1990.
4. Roizman, B. and Sears, A. E. Herpes simplex viruses and their replication, in *Fields Virology*, 2nd ed., Fields, B. N., Knipe, D. M., Chanock, R. M., et al. Eds. Raven Press, New York, 1795, 1990.
5. Whitley, R. Herpes simplex viruses, in *Fields Virology*, 2nd ed., Fields, B. N., Knipe, D. M., Chanock, R. M., et al. Eds., vol. 2. Raven Press, New York, 1843, 1990.
6. Gruter, W. Das herpesvirus, seine aetiologische und klinische bedeutung. *Munch. Med. Wochenschr.*, 71, 1058, 1924.
7. McGeoch, D. J., Dalrymple, M. A., Davison, A. J., et al. The complete DNA sequence of the long unique region of the genome of herpes simplex virus type 1. *J. Gen. Virol.*, 69, 1531, 1988.
8. Roizman, B. The structure and isomerization of herpes simplex virus genomes. *Cell*, 16, 481, 1979.
9. Corey, L., Langenberg, A. G., Ashley, R., et al. Recombinant glycoprotein vaccine for the prevention of genital HSV-2 infection: two randomized controlled trials. Chiron HSV Vaccine Study Group. *J. Am. Med. Assoc.* 282, 331–340, 1999 (see also: *J. Am. Med. Assoc.* 282, 379–380, 1999, and *J. Am. Med. Assoc.* 283, 746–747, 2000).
10. Marques, A. R. and Strauss, S. E. Herpes simplex type 2 infections: an update. *Dis. Mon.*, 46, 325–359, 2000.
11. Smith, M. G. Propagation in tissue cultures of a cytopathogenic virus from human salivary gland virus (SGV) disease. *Proc. Soc. Exp. Biol. Med.*, 92, 424, 1956.
12. Davison, A. J. and Scott, J. E. The complete DNA sequence of varicella-zoster virus. *J. Gen. Virol.*, 67, 1759, 1986.
13. Dumas, A. M., Geelen, J. L. M. C., Maris, W., and Van der Noordas, J. Infectivity and molecular weight of varicella-zoster virus DNA. *J. Gen. Virol.*, 47, 233, 1980.
14. Ludwig, H. O., Biswal, N., and Benyesh-Melnick, M. Studies on the relatedness of herpesviruses through DNA-DNA hybridization. *Virology*, 49, 95, 1972.
15. Baer, R., Bankier, A. T., Biggin, M. D., et al. DNA sequence and expression of the B95-8 Epstein-Barr virus genome. *Nature*, 310, 207, 1984.
16. Epstein, M. A., Henle, W., Achong, B. G., and Barr, Y. M. Morphological and biological studies on a virus in cultured lymphoblasts from Burkitt's lymphoma. *J. Exp. Med.*, 121, 761, 1965.
17. Lopez, C., Pellett, P., Stewart, J., et al. Characteristics of human herpesvirus-6. *J. Infect. Dis.* 157, 1271, 1988.
18. Salahuddin, S. Z., Ablashi, D. V., Markham, P. D., et al. Isolation of a new virus, HBLV, in patients with lymphoproliferative disorder. *Science*, 234, 596, 1986.
19. Chien, J. W. and Johnson, J. L. Viral pneumonias. Infection in the immunocompromised host. *Postgrad. Med.*, 107, 67–70, 73–74, 77–80, 2000.
20. Oakley, C., Epstein, J. B., and Sherlock, C. H. Reactivation of oral herpes simplex virus: implications for clinical management of herpes simplex virus recurrence during radiotherapy. *Oral Surg. Oral Med. Oral Pathol. Oral Radiol. Endod.*, 84, 272–278, 1997.
21. Snoeck, R. Antiviral therapy of herpes simplex. *Int. J. Antimicrob. Agents*, 16, 157–159, 2000.
22. Muller, S. A., Herrmann, E. C. Jr., and Winkelmann, R. K. Herpes simplex infections in hematologic malignancies. *Am. J. Med.*, 52, 102, 1972.
23. Dreizen, S., McCredie, K. B., Bodey, G. P., and Keating, M. J. Mucocutaneous herpetic infections during cancer chemotherapy,. *Postgrad. Med. J.*, 84, 181, 1988.
24. Wingard, J. R. Viral infections in leukemia and bone marrow transplant patients. *Leuk. Lymphoma*, 11(Suppl. 2), 115, 1993.
25. Stone, W. J., Scowden, E. B., Spannuth, C. L., Lowry, S. P., and Alford, R. H. Atypical simplex virus hominis type 2 infection in uremic patients receiving immunosuppressive therapy. *Am. J. Med.*, 63, 511, 1977.
26. Schneidman, D. W., Barr, R. J., and Graham, J. H. Chronic cutaneous herpes simplex. *J. Am. Med. Assoc.*, 241, 542, 1979.
27. Straus, S. E., Smith, H. A., Brickmann, C., de Miranda, P., McLaren, C., and Keeney, R. E. Acyclovir for chronic mucocutaneous herpes simplex virus infections in immunosuppressed patients. *Ann. Intern. Med.*, 96, 270, 1982.
28. Armstrong, D. Opportunistic infections in the acquired immune deficiency syndrome. *Semin. Oncol.*, 14(Suppl. 3), 40, 1987.
29. Levin, M. J. Impact of herpesvirus infections in the future. *J. Med. Virol. Suppl.*, 1, 158, 1993.
30. Meyers, J. D., Flornoy, N., and Thomas, E. D. Infection with herpes simplex virus and cell- mediated immunity after marrow transplant. *J. Infect. Dis.*, 142, 338, 1980.
31. Cohen, P. R., Kazi, S., and Grossman, M. E. Herpetic geometric glossitis: a distinctive pattern of lingual herpes simplex virus infection. *South. Med. J.*, 88, 1231–1235, 1995.

32. Rand, K. H., Rasmussen, L. E., Pollard, R. B., Arvin, A., and Merigan, T. C. Cellular immunity and herpesvirus infections in cardiac transplant patients. *N. Engl. J. Med.*, 296, 1372, 1977.
33. Pass, R. F., Whitley, R. J., Whelchel, J. D., Diethelm, A. G., Reynolds, D. W., and Alford, C. A. Identification of patients with increased risk of infection with herpes simplex virus after renal transplantation. *J. Infect. Dis.*, 140, 487, 1979.
34. Lam, M. T., Pazin, G. J., Armstrong, J. A., and Ho, M. Herpes simplex infection in acute myelogenous leukemia and other hematologic malignancies: a prospective study. *Cancer*, 48, 2168, 1981.
35. Straus, S. E. Treatment of persistent active herpesvirus infections. *J. Virol. Meth.*, 21, 305, 1988.
36. Chen, X.S., Han, G. Z., Guo, Z. P., Lu, N. Z., Chen, J., and Wang, J. B. A comparison of topical application of penciclovir 1% cream with acyclovir 3% cream for treatment of genital herpes: a randomized, double-blind, multicenter trial. Penciclovir Multicenter Genital Herpes Clinical Study Group. *Int. J. STD AIDS*, 11, 568–573, 2000.
37. Straus, S. E., Seidlin, M., Takiff, H. E., et al. Effect of oral acyclovir treatment on symptomatic and asymptomatic virus shedding in recurrent genital herpes. *Sex. Transm. Dis.*, 16, 107, 1989.
38. Whitley, R. J. and Gnann, J. W. Jr. Acyclovir: a decade later. *N. Engl. J. Med.*, 327, 782, 1992.
39. Fletcher, C. V. Treatment of herpesvirus infections in HIV-infected individuals. *Ann. Pharmacother.*, 26, 955, 1992.
40. Ramanathan, J., Rammouni, M., Baran, J. Jr., and Khatib, R. Herpes simplex esophagitis in the immunocompetent host: an overview. *Am. J. Gastroenterol.*, 95, 2171–2176, 2000.
41. Centers for Disease Control. Revision of the CDC surveillance case definition for acquired immunodeficiency syndrome. *Morbid. Mortal. Wkly Rep.*, 36(Suppl.), S1, 1987.
42. Rosa, I., Hagege, H., Sommers, C., et al. Oesophagite herpetique chez le sujet non infecte par le virus de l'immunodeficience humaine. *Gastroenterol. Clin. Biol.*, 23, 1392–1396, 1999.
43. Siegel, F. P., Lopez, C., Hammer, B. S., et al. Severe acquired immunodeficiency in male homosexuals, manifested by chronic perianal ulcerative herpes simplex lesions. *N. Engl. J. Med.*, 305, 1439, 1981.
44. Tyring, S. K., Carlton, S. S., and Evans, T. Herpes. Atypical clinical manifestations. *Dermatol. Clin.* 16, 783–788, xiii, 1998.
45. Brown, T. S. and Callen, J. P. Atypical presentation of herpes simplex virus in a patient with chronic lymphocytic leukemia. *Cutis*, 64, 123–125, 1999.
46. Schiff, D. and Rosenblum, M. K. Herpes simplex encephalitis (HSE) and the immunocompromised: a clinical and autopsy study of HSE in the settings of cancer and human deficiency virus-type 1 infection. *Human Pathol.* 29, 215–222, 1998 (see also: *Human Pathol.* 29, 207–210, 1998).
47. Ruef, C. Die Enzephalitis beim Erwachsenen. *Schweiz. Med. Wochenschr.*, 124, 1109–1116, 1994.
48. Whitley, R. J., Alford, C. A., Hirsch, M. S., et al. Vidarabine versus acyclovir therapy in herpes simplex encephalitis. *N. Engl. J. Med.*, 314, 144, 1986.
49. Sköldenberg, B., Forsgren, M., Alestig, K., et al. Acyclovir versus vidarabin in herpes simplex encephalitis: randomized multicentre study in consecutive Swedish patients. *Lancet*, 2, 707, 1984.
50. Yura, Y., Kusaka, J., Yamakawa, R., Bando, T., Yoshida, H., and Sato, M. Mental nerve neuropathy as a result of primary herpes simplex virus infection in the oral cavity. A case report. *Oral Surg. Oral Med. Oral Pathol. Oral Radiol. Endod.*, 90, 306–309, 2000.
51. Theriault, A. and Cohen, P. R. Herpetic geometric glossitis in a pediatric patient with acute myelogenic leukemia. *Am. J. Clin. Oncol.*, 20, 567–568, 1997.
52. Woo, S. B. and Lee, S. F. Oral recrudescent herpes simplex virus infection. *Oral Surg. Oral Med., Oral Pathol. Oral Radiol. Endod.*, 83, 239–243, 1997.
53. Wilcox, C. M. and Karowe, M. W. Esophageal infections: etiology, diagnosis, and management. *Gastroenterology*, 2, 188–206, 1994.
54. Ahn, B. M., Chung, H. U., Kim, S. Y., et al. Acute herpetic esophagitis - a case report. *Korean J. Intern. Med.*, 9, 120–124, 1994.
55. Hull, H. F., Blumhagen, J. D., Benjamin, D., and Corey, L. Herpes simplex virus pneumonitis in childhood. *J. Pediatr.*, 104, 211, 1984.
56. Ramsey, P. G., Fife, K. H., Hackman, R. C., Meyers, J. D., and Corey, L. Herpes simplex pneumonia: clinical, virulogic and pathologic features in 20 patients. *Ann. Intern. Med.* 97, 813, 1982.
57. Herout, V., Vortel, V., and Vondrackova, A. Herpes simplex involvement of the lower respiratory tract. *Am. J. Clin. Pathol.*, 46, 411, 1966.
58. Morgan, H. R. and Finland, J. Isolation of herpesvirus from a case of atypical pneumonia and erythema multiforme exudativum, with studies of four additional cases. *Am. J. Med. Sci.*, 217, 91, 1949.
59. Douglas, R. G. Jr., Anderson, M. S., Weg, J. G., et al. Herpes simplex virus pneumonia: occurrence in an allotransplanted lung. *J. Am. Med. Assoc.*, 210, 902, 1966.
60. Jordan, S. W., McLaren, L. C., and Crosby, J. H. Herpetic tracheobronchitis: cytologic and virologic detection. *Arch. Intern. Med.*, 135, 784, 1975.
61. Caldwell, J. E. and Porter, D. D. Herpetic pneumonia in alcoholic hepatitis. *J. Am. Med. Assoc.*, 217, 1703, 1971.
62. Nash, G. and Foley, F. D. Herpetic infection of the middle and lower respiratory tract. *Am. J. Clin. Pathol.*, 54, 857, 1970.
63. Nash, G. Necrotizing tracheobronchitis and bronchopneumonitis consistent with herpetic infection. *Human Pathol.*, 3, 283, 1972.
64. Cherr, G. S., Meredith, J. W., and Chang, M. Herpes simplex virus pneumonia in trauma patients. *J. Trauma*, 49, 547–549, 2000.

65. Wheeler, C. E. Jr. and Huffines, W. D. Primary disseminated herpes simplex of the newborn. *J. Am. Med. Assoc.*, 191, 455, 1965.
66. Haynes, R. E., Azimi, P. H., and Cramblett, H. G. Fatal herpesvirus hominis (herpes simplex virus) infection in children. *J. Am. Med. Assoc.*, 206, 312, 1968.
67. Bland, J. D. and Lilleyman, J. S. Fatal pneumonia associated with two viruses in a child with lymphoblastic leukemia. *Br. Med. J.*, 284, 82, 1982.
68. Tucker, E. S. and Scofield, G. F. Hepatoadrenal necrosis: fatal systemic herpes simplex infection: review of the literature and report of two cases. *Arch. Pathol.*, 71, 84, 1961.
69. Kipps, A., Becker, W., Wainwright, J., and McKenzie, D. Fatal disseminated primary herpesvirus in children: epidemiology based on 93 non-neonatal cases. *S. Afr. Med. J.*, 41, 647, 1967.
70. Dhar, S. and Dhar, S. Disseminated neonatal herpes simplex: a rare entity. *Pediatr. Dermatol.*, 17, 330–332, 2000.
71. Kaufman, B., Gandhi, S. A., Louie, E., Rizzi, R., and Illei, P. Herpes simplex virus hepatitis: case report and review. *Clin. Infect. Dis.*, 24, 334–338, 1997.
72. Seksik, P., Gozlan, J., Guitton, C., Galula, G., Maury, E., and Offenstadt, G. Fatal herpetic hepatitis in adult following short corticotherapy: a case report. *Intensive Care Med.*, 25, 415–417, 1999.
73. Naik, H. R. and Chandrasekar, P. H. Herpes simplex virus (HSV) colitis in a bone marrow transplant recipient. *Bone Marrow Transplant.*, 17, 285–286, 1996.
74. Dios Castro, E. and Maquet Dusart, J. A. Latanoprost-associated recurrent herpes simplex keratitis. *Arch. Soc. Esp. Oftalmol.*, 75, 775–778, 2000.
75. Reusser, P. Antiviral therapy: current options and challenges. *Schweiz. Med. Wochenschr.*, 130, 101–112, 2000.
76. Sacks, S. L. and Wilson, B. Famciclovir/penciclovir. *Adv. Exp. Med. Biol.*, 458, 135–147, 1999.
77. Ormrod, D., Scott, L. J., and Perry, C. M. Valaciclovir: a review of its long term utility in the management of genital herpes simplex virus and cytomegalovirus infections. *Drugs*, 59, 839–863, 2000.
78. Lazarus, H. M., Belanger, R., Candoni, A., Aoun, M., Jurewicz, R., and Marks, L. Intravenous penciclovir for treatment of herpes simplex infections in immunocompromised patients: results of a multicenter, acyclovir-controlled trial. *Antimicrob. Agents Chemother.*, 43, 1192–1197, 1999.
79. Fife, K. H., Barbarash, R. A., Rudolph, T., et al. Valaciclovir versus acyclovir in the treatment of first-episode genital herpes infection. *Sex. Transm. Dis.*, 24, 481–486, 1997.
80. Diaz Mitoma, F., Sibbals, R. G., Shafran, S. D., et al. Oral famciclovir for the suppression of recurrent genital herpes: a randomized controlled trial. *J. Am. Med. Assoc.*, 280, 887–892, 1998.
81. Whitley, R. J., Spruance, S., Hayden, F. G., et al. Vidarabine therapy for mucocutaneous herpes simplex virus infections in the immunocompromised hosts. *J. Infect. Dis.*, 149, 1, 1984.
82. Whitley, R. J., Soong, S.-J., Dolin, R., et al. Adenine arabinoside therapy of biopsy-proven herpes simplex encephalitis. *N. Engl. J. Med.*, 297, 289, 1977.
83. Whitley, R. J., Nahmias, A. J., Soong, S.-J., Gallasso, G. H., Fleming, C. L., and Alford, C. A. Vidarabine therapy of neonatal herpes simplex virus infection. *Pediatrics*, 66, 495, 1980.
84. Ch'ien, L. T., Cannon, N. J., Charamella, L. J., et al. Effect of adenine arabinoside on severe herpesvirus hominis infections in man. *J. Infect. Dis.*, 128, 658, 1973.
85. Steele, R. W., Keeney, R. E., Brown, J., and Young, E. J. Cellular immune responses to herpesviruses during treatment with adenine arabinoside. *J. Infect. Dis.*, 135, 893, 1977.
86. Lauter, C. B., Bailey, E. J., and Lerner, A. M. Microbiologic assays and neurological toxicity during use of adenine arabinoside in humans. *J. Infect. Dis.*, 134, 75, 1976.
87. Sacks, S. L., Smith, J. L., Pollard, R. B., et al. Toxicity of vidarabine. *J. Am. Med. Assoc.*, 241, 28, 1979.
88. Marker, S. C., Howard, R. J., Groth, K. E., Mastri, A. R., Simmons, R. L., and Balfour, H. H. Jr. A trial of vidarabine for cytomegalovirus infection in renal transplant patients. *Arch. Intern. Med.*, 140, 1441, 1980.
89. Van Etta, L., Brown, J., Mastri, A., and Wilson, T. Fatal vidarabine toxicity in a patient with normal renal function. *J. Am. Med. Assoc.*, 246, 1703, 1981.
90. Whitley, R. J., Alford, C. A., Hirsch, M. S., et al. Vidarabine versus acyclovir therapy in herpes simplex encephalitis. *N. Engl. J. Med.*, 314, 144, 1986.
91. Shepp, D. H., Newton, B. A., Dandliker, P. S., Flournoy, N., and Meyers, J. D. Oral acyclovir therapy for mucocutaneous herpes simplex virus infection in immunocompromised marrow transplant recipients. *Ann. Intern. Med.*, 102, 783, 1985.
92. Wade, J. C., Newton, B., McLaren, C., Flournoy, N., Keeney, R. E., and Meyers, J. D. Intravenous acyclovir to treat mucocutaneous herpes simplex virus infection after marrow transplantation: a double-blind trial. *Ann. Intern. Med.*, 96, 265, 1982.
93. Meyers, J. D., Wade, J. C., Mitchell, C. D., et al. Multicenter collaborative trial of intravenous acyclovir for treatment of mucocutaneous herpes simplex virus infection in the immunocompromised host. *Am. J. Med.*, 73(Suppl. 1A), 229, 1982.
94. Griffiths, P. D. Future management of herpesvirus infections. *J. Med. Virol. Suppl.*, 1, 165, 1993.
95. Leflore, S., Anderson, P. L., and Fletcher, C. V. A risk-benefit evaluation of aciclovir for the treatment and prophylaxis of herpes simplex virus infections. *Drug Saf.*, 23, 131–142, 2000.
96. Mitchell, D., Bean, B., Gentry, S. R., Groth, K. E., Boen, J. R., and Balfour, H. H. Jr. Acyclovir therapy for mucocutaneous herpes simplex virus infections in immune compromised patients. *Lancet*, 1, 1389, 1981.
97. Chou, S., Gallagher, J. G., and Merigan, T. C. Controlled trial of intravenous acyclovir in heart-transplant patients with mucocutaneous herpes simplex infections. *Lancet*, 2, 1392, 1981.
98. Douglas, J. M., Critchlow, C., Benedetti, J., et al. A double-blind study of oral acyclovir for suppression of recurrences of genital herpes simplex virus infection. *N. Engl. J. Med.*, 310, 1551–1556, 1984.

99. Mertz, G. J., Jones, C. C., Mills, J., et al. Long-term acyclovir suppression of frequently recurring genital herpes simplex virus infection: a multicenter double-blind trial. *J. Am. Med. Assoc.*, 260, 201–206, 1988.
100. Straus, S. E., Takiff, H. E., Seidlin, M., et al. Suppression of frequently recurring genital herpes: a placebo-controlled double-blind trial of oral acyclovir. *N. Engl. J. Med.*, 310, 1545–1550, 1984.
101. Goldberg, L. H., Kaufman, R., Kurtz, T. O., et al. Long-term suppression of recurrent genital herpes with acyclovir: a 5-year benchmark. *Arch. Dermatol.*, 129, 582–587, 1993.
102. Perrin, L. and Hirscel, B. Combination therapy in primary HIV infection. *Antiviral Res.*, 29, 87–89, 1996.
103. Tod, M., Lokiec, F., Bidault, R., De Bony, F., Petitjean, O., and Aujard, Y. Pharmacokinetics of oral acyclovir in neonates and in infants: a population analysis. *Antimicrob. Agents Chemother.*, 45, 150–157, 2001.
104. Drew, W. L., Buhles, W., Dworkin, R. J., and Erlich, K. S. Management of herpes virus infections (CMV, HSV, VZV), in *The Management of AIDS*, 2nd ed., Sande, M. A. and Volberding, P. A., Eds. W. B. Saunders, Philadelphia, 316, 1990.
105. Wald, A., Benedetti, J., Davis, G., et al. A randomized, double-blind, comparative trial comparing high- and standard-dose oral acyclovir for first-episode genital herpes infections. *Antimicrob. Agents Chemother.*, 38, 174–176, 1994.
106. Corey, L., Fife, K. H., Benedetti, J. K., et al. Intravenous acyclovir for the treatment of primary genital herpes. *Ann. Intern. Med.*, 98, 914, 1983.
107. Peacock, J. E. Jr., Kaplowitz, L. G., Sparling, P. F., et al. Intravenous acyclovir therapy of first episodes of genital herpes: a multicenter double-blind, placebo-controlled trial. *Am. J. Med.*, 85, 301, 1988.
108. Bryson, Y. J., Dillon, M., Lovett, M., et al. Treatment of first episodes of genital herpes simplex virus infection with oral acyclovir: a randomized double-blind controlled trial in normal subjects. *N. Engl. J. Med.*, 308, 915–921, 1983.
109. Mertz, G. J., Critchlow, C. W., Benedetti, J., et al. Double-blind placebo-controlled trial of oral acyclovir in first-episode genital herpes simplex virus infection. *J. Am. Med. Assoc.*, 252, 1147–1151, 1984.
110. Clinical Effectiveness Group (Association of Genitourinary Medicine and the Medical Society for the Study of Venereal Diseases). National guideline for the management of genital herpes. *Sex. Transm. Infect.*, 75(Suppl. 1), S24–S28, 1999.
111. Wade, J. C., Newton, B., Flournoy, N., and Meyers, J. D. Oral acyclovir for prevention of herpes simplex virus reactivation after marrow transplantation. *Ann. Intern. Med.*, 100, 823, 1984.
112. Saral, R., Burns, W. H., Laskin, O. L., Santos, G. W., and Lietman, P. S. Acyclovir prophylaxis of herpes-simplex-virus infections: a randomized, double-blind, controlled trial in bone-marrow-transplant recipients. *N. Engl. J. Med.*, 305, 63, 1981.
113. Kaplowitz, L. G., Baker, D., Gelb, L., et al. Prolonged continuous acyclovir treatment of normal adults with frequently recurring genital herpes simplex virus infection. *J. Am. Med. Assoc.*, 265, 747–751, 1991.
113. Kaplowitz, L. G., Baker, D., Gelb, L., et al. Prolonged continuous acyclovir treatment of normal adults with frequently recurring genital herpes simplex virus infection. *J. Am. Med. Assoc.*, 265, 747–751, 1991.
114. Shepp, D. H., Dandliker, P. S., Flournoy, N., and Meyers, J. D. Sequential intravenous and twice-daily oral acyclovir for extended prophylaxis of herpes simplex virus infection in marrow transplant patients. *Transplantation*, 43, 654, 1987.
115. Corey, L., Nahmias, A. J., Guinan, M. E., Benedetti, J. K., Critchlow, C. W., and Holmes, K. K. A trial of topical acyclovir in genital herpes simplex infections. *N. Engl. J. Med.*, 306, 1313, 1982.
116. Corey, L., Benedetti, J., Critchlow, C., et al. Treatment of primary first-episode genital herpes simplex virus infections with acyclovir: results of topical, intravenous and oral therapy. *J. Antimicrob. Chemother.*, 12(Suppl. B), 79, 1983.
117. Adams, H. G., Benson, E. A., Alexander, E. R., Vontver, L. A., Remington, M. A., and Holmes, K. A. Genital herpetic infection in men and women: clinical course and effect of topical application of adenine arabinoside. *J. Infect. Dis.*, 133(Suppl. A), 151, 1976.
118. Spruance, S. L., Crumpacker, C. S., Haines, H., et al. Ineffectiveness of topical adenine arabinoside 5'-monophosphate in the treatment of recurrent herpes simplex labialis. *N. Engl. J. Med.*, 300, 1180, 1979.
119. Corey, L., Reeves, W. C., Chiang, W. T., et al. Ineffectiveness of topical ether for the treatment of genital herpes simplex virus infection. *N. Engl. J. Med.*, 299, 237, 1978.
120. Myers, M. G., Oxman, M. N., Clark, J. E., and Arndt, K. A. Failure of neutral-red photodynamic inactivation in recurrent herpes simplex virus infection. *N. Engl. J. Med.*, 293, 945, 1975.
121. Leung, D. T. and Sacks, S. L. Current recommendations for the treatment of genital herpes. *Drugs*, 60, 1329–1352, 2000.
122. Fiddian, A. P., Yeo, J. M., Stubbings, R., and Dean, D. Successful treatment of herpes labialis with topical acyclovir. *Br. Med. J.*, 286, 1699, 1983.
123. Spruance, S. L., Schnipper, L. E., Overall, J. C. Jr., et al. Treatment of herpes simplex labialis with topical acyclovir in polyethylene glycol. *J. Infect. Dis.*, 146, 85, 1982.
124. Shaw, M., King, M., Best, J. M., Banatvala, J. E., Gibson, J. R., and Klaber, M. R. Failure of acyclovir cream in treatment of recurrent herpes labialis. *Br. Med. J.*, 291, 7–9, 1985.
125. Raborn, G. W., McGaw, W. T., Grace, M., Tyrrell, L. D., and Samuels, S. M. Oral acyclovir and herpes labialis: a randomized, double-blind, placebo-controlled study. *J. Am. Dent. Assoc.*, 115, 38–42, 1987.
126. Spruance, S. L., Stewart, J. C. B., Rowe, N. H., McKeough, M. B., Wenerstrom, G., and Freeman, D. J. Treatment of recurrent herpes simplex labialis with oral acyclovir. *J. Infect. Dis.*, 161, 185–190, 1990.
127. Turlea, M., Raica, D., and Haidar, A. The efficacy of acyclovir treatment in the therapy of herpetic keratitis. *Oftalmologia*, 49, 55–58, 1999.
128. Luu, K. K., Scott, I. U., Chaudhry, N. A., Verm, A., and Davis, J. L. Intravitreal antiviral injections as adjunctive therapy in the management of immunocompetent patients with necrotizing herpetic retinopathy. *Am. J. Ophthalmol.*, 129, 811–813, 2000.
129. Herpetic Eye Disease Study Group. Oral acyclovir for herpes simplex virus eye disease: effect on prevention of epithelial keratitis and stromal keratitis. *Arch. Ophthalmol.*, 118, 1030–1036, 2000.

130. Perry, C. M. and Faulds, D. Valaciclovir. A review of its antiviral activity, pharmacokinetic properties and therapeutic efficacy in herpesvirus infections. *Drugs*, 52, 754–772, 1996.
131. Spruance, S. L., Tyring, S. K., Di Gregorio, B., et al. A large-scale, placebo-controlled, dose-ranging trial of peroral valaciclovir for episodic treatment of recurrent herpes genitalis. *Arch. Intern. Med.*, 156, 1729–1735, 1996.
132. Tyring, S. K., Douglas, J. M., Corey, L., et al. A randomized, placebo-controlled comparison of oral valaciclovir and acyclovir in immunocompetent patients with recurrent genital herpes infections. *Arch. Dermatol.*, 134, 185–191, 1998.
133. Rivaud, E., Massiani, M. A., Vincent, F., Azoulay, E., and Coudrec, L. J. Valacyclovir hydrochloride therapy and thrombotic thrombocytopenic purpurain an HIV-infected patient. *Arch. Intern. Med.*, 160, 1705–1706, 2000.
134. Vere Hodge, R. A. Famciclovir and penciclovir. The mode of action of famciclovir including its conversion to penciclovir. *Antiviral Chem. Chemother.*, 4, 67–84, 1993.
135. Perry, C. M. and Wagstaff, A. J. Famciclovir. A review of its pharmacological properties and therapeutic efficacy in herpesvirus infections. *Drugs*, 50, 396–415, 1995.
136. Schacker, T., Hui-lin, H., Koelle, D. M., et al. Famciclovir for the suppression of symptomatic and asymptomatic herpes simplex virus reactivation in HIV-infected persons. *Ann. Intern. Med.*, 128, 21–28, 1998.
137. Loveless, M., Sacks, S. L., and Harris, J. R. W. Famciclovir in the management of first- episode genital herpes. *Infect. Dis. Clin. Prac.*, 6(1 Suppl.), S12–S16, 1997.
138. Sacks, S. L., Aoki, F. Y., Diaz-Mitoma, F., et al. Patient-initiated, twice daily oral famciclovir for early recurrent genital herpes: a randomized, double-blind multicenter trial. *J. Am. Med. Assoc.*, 276, 44–49, 1996.
139. Sacks, S. L., Martel, A., Aoki, F., et al. Early, clinic-initiated treatment of recurrent genital herpes using famciclovir: results of a Canadian multicentre study. *Clin. Res.*, 42, 300A, 1994.
140. Romanowski, B., Aoki, F. Y., Martel, A. Y., Lavender, E. A., Parsons, J. E., and Saltzman, R. L. Efficacy and safety of famciclovir for treating mucocutaneous herpes simplex infections in HIV-infected individuals. Collaborative Famciclovir HIV Study Group. *AIDS*, 14, 1211–1217, 2000.
141. Spruance, S. L., Rea, T. L., Thoming, C., et al. Penciclovir cream for the treatment of herpes simplex labialis: a randomized, multicenter, double-blind, placebo-controlled trial. *J. Am. Med. Assoc.*, 277, 1374–1379, 1997.
142. Anonymous. Topical penciclovir for herpes labialis. *Med. Lett. Drugs Ther.*, 39, 57–58, 1997.
143. Levin, M. J., Leary, P. L., and Arbeit, R. D. Effect of acyclovir on the proliferation of human fibroblasts and peripheral blood mononuclear cells. *Antimicrob. Agents Chemother.*, 17, 947, 1980.
144. Steele, R. W., Marmer, D. J., and Keeney, R. E. Comparative in vitro immunotoxicology of acyclovir and other antiviral agents. *Infect. Immunol.*, 28, 957, 1980.
145. Safrin, S., Assaykeen, T., Follansbee, S., and Mills, J. Foscarnet therapy for acyclovir- resistant mucocutaneous herpes simplex virus infection in 26 AIDS patients: preliminary data. *J. Infect. Dis.*, 161, 1078, 1990.
146. Safrin, S., Crumpacker, C., Chatis, P., et al. A controlled trial comparing foscarnet with vidarabine for acyclovir-resistant mucocutaneous herpes simplex in the acquired immunodeficiency syndrome. *N. Engl. J. Med.*, 325, 551, 1991.
147. Safrin, S., Assaykeen, T., Follansbee, S., and Mills, J. Foscarnet therapy for acyclovir- resistant mucocutaneous herpes simplex virus infection in 26 AIDS patients: preliminary data. *J. Infect. Dis.*, 161, 1078, 1990.
148. Chatis, P. A., Miller, C. H., Schrager, L. E., and Crumpacker, C. S. Successful treatment with foscarnet of an acyclovir-resistant mucocutaneous infection with herpes simplex virus in a patient with the acquired immunodeficiency syndrome. *N. Engl. J. Med.*, 320, 297, 1989.
149. Causey, D. M., Rarick, M. U., and Melancon, H. Foscarnet treatment of acyclovir- resistant herpes simplex proctitis in an AIDS patient. *Proc. IVth Int. Conf. AIDS*, Stockholm, abstract no. 3589, 1988.
150. Erlich, K. S., Jacobson, M. A., Koehler, J. E., et al. Foscarnet therapy of severe acyclovir-resistant herpes simplex virus infections in patients with the acquired immunodeficiency syndrome. *Ann. Intern. Med.* 110, 710, 1989.
151. Youle, M. M., Hawkins, D. A., Collins, P., et al. Acyclovir-resistant herpes in AIDS treated with foscarnet. *Lancet*, 2, 341, 1988.
152. Vinckier, F., Boogaerts, M., De Clerck, D., and de Clercq, E. Chronic herpetic infection in an immunocompromised patient: report of a case. *J. Oral. Maxillofac. Surg.*, 45, 723, 1987.
153. Hardy, W. D. Foscarnet treatment of acyclovir-resistant herpes simplex virus infection in patients with acquired immunodeficiency syndrome: preliminary results of a controlled, randomized, regimen-comparative trial. *Am. J. Med.*, 92(Suppl. 2A), 30S, 1992.
154. Sall, R. K., Kauffmann, C. L., and Levy, C. S. Successful treatment of progressive acyclovir-resistant herpes simplex virus using intravenous foscarnet in a patient with the acquired immunodeficiency syndrome. *Arch. Dermatol.*, 125, 1549, 1989.
155. Balfour, H. H. Jr., Benson, C., Braun, J., et al. Management of acyclovir-resistant herpes simplex and varicella-zoster virus infection. *J. Acquir. Immune Defic. Syndr.*, 7, 254, 1994.
156. Safrin, S., Crumpacker, C., Chatis, P., et al. A controlled trial comparing foscarnet with vidarabin for acyclovir-resistant mucocutaneous herpes simplex in the acquired immunodeficiency syndrome. *N. Engl. J. Med.*, 325, 551, 1991.
157. Reusser, P. Herpesvirus resistance to antiviral drugs: a review of the mechanisms, clinical importance and therapeutic options. *J. Hosp. Infect.*, 33, 235-248, 1996.
158. Chakrabarti, S., Pillay, D., Ratcliffe, D., Cane, P. A., Collingham, K. E., and Milligan, D. W. Resistance to antiviral drugs in herpes simplex virus infections among allogeneic stem cell transplant recipients: risk factors and prognostic significance. *J. Infect. Dis.*, 181, 2055- 2058, 2000.
159. Hardy, W. D., Chafey, S., Tan, C., Bryson, Y., Mroz, J., and Martin-Manley, S. Randomized trial of foscarnet (PFA) induction and maintenance therapy (Rx) for acyclovir- resistant (ACV-R) herpes simplex (HSV) infections in AIDS. *Int. Conf. AIDS*, 1991, June 16–21, 7, 258, (abstract no. W.B.2304).

160. Aweeka, F. T., Omachi, R., Jacobson, M. A., Schonfeld, P., Munley, S. M., and Gambertoglio, J. Pharmacokinetics (PK) of foscarnet in patients (PTS) with varying degree of renal function. *Int. Conf. AIDS*, 1993, June 6–11, 9, 485, (abstract no. PO-B26-2097).
161. Ringdén, O., Lönnqvist, B., Paulin, T., et al. Pharmacokinetics, safety and preliminary clinical experiences using foscarnet in the treatment of cytomegalovirus infections in bone marrow and renal transplant recipients. *J. Antimicrob. Chemother.*, 17, 373, 1986.
162. Wagstaff, A. J. and Bryson, H. M. Foscarnet. A reappraisal of its antiviral activity, pharmacokinetic properties and therapeutic use in immunocompromised patients with renal infections. *Drugs*, 48, 199–226, 1994.
163. Öberg, B. Antiviral effects of phosphonoformate. *Pharmacol. Ther.*, 19, 387, 1983.
164. Jacobson, M. A., O'Donnell, J. J., and Mills, J. Foscarnet treatment of cytomegalovirus retinitis in patients with the acquired immunodeficiency syndrome. *Antimicrob. Agents Chemother.*, 33, 736, 1989.
165. Verdonck, L. F., Cornelissen, J. J., Smit, J., et al. Successful foscarnet therapy for acyclovir-resistant mucocutaneous infection with herpes simplex virus in a recipient of allogeneic BMT. *Bone Marrow Transplant.*, 11, 177, 1993.
166. Aweeka, F., Gambertoglio, J. G., Mills, J., and Jacobson, M. A. Pharmacokinetics of intermittently administered intravenous foscarnet in the treatment of AIDS patients with serious CMV retinitis. *Proc. IVth Int. Conf. AIDS,* Stockholm, 1988, abstract no. 3591.
167. Ringdén, O., Lönnqvist, B., Paulin, T., et al. Pharmacokinetics, safety and preliminary clinical experiences using foscarnet in the treatment of cytomegalovirus infections in bone marrow and renal transplant recipients. *J. Antimicrob. Chemother.*, 17, 373, 1986.
168. Mindel, A., Adler, M. W., Sutherland, S., et al. Intravenous acyclovir for primary genital herpes. *Lancet*, 1, 697–700, 1982.
169. Corey, L., Fife, K., Benedetti, J. K., et al. Intravenous acyclovir for the treatment of primary genital herpes. *Ann. Intern. Med.*, 98, 914–921, 1983.
170. Centers for Disease Control and Prevention. Guidelines for treatment of sexually transmitted diseases. *Morb. Mortal. Wkly Rep.*, 47(RR-1), 1–118, 2000.
171. Lazarus, H., Belanger, R., Candon, A., et al. PCV IC study group. Efficacy and safety of penciclovir (PCV) for the treatment of HSV infections in immunocompromised (IC) patients (abstract H72), *37th ICAAC Meeting, Toronto, Ontario*, p. 226, 1997.
172. Talarico, C., Stanet, S., Lambe, C, et al. Mode of action studies on the anti-cytomegalovirus nucleoside analog [1-(2-hydroxy-1-hydroxymethyl)ethoxymethyl)cytosine]. *Antiviral Res.*, S1: 87 (abstract no. 92), 1990.
173. Palmer, J., Vogt, P. E., and Kern, E. R. Prevention and treatment of experimental genital herpes simplex virus type 2 (HSV-2) infections with topical HPMPC. *Antiviral Res.*, 26:A334 (abstract no. 205), 1995.
174. Hitchcock, M. J. M., Jaffe, H. S., Martin, J. C., and Stagg, R. J. Cidofovir, a new agent with potent anti-herpesvirus activity. *Antiviral Chem. Chemother.*, 7, 115–127, 1996.
175. Naesens, L., Snoeck, R., Andrei, G., Balzarini, J., Neyts, J., and De Clercq, E. HPMPC (cidofovir), PMEA (adefovir) and related acyclic nucleoside phosphonate analogues: a review of their pharmacology and clinical potential in the treatment of viral infections. *Antiviral Chem. Chemother.*, 8, 1–23, 1997.
176. Snoeck, R., Andrei, G., Gerard, M., et al. Successful treatment of progressive mucocutaneous infection due to acyclovir- and foscarnet-resistant herpes simplex virus with (S)-1-(3-hydroxy-2-phosphonylmethoxypropyl)cytosine (HPMPC). *Clin. Infect. Dis.*, 18, 570–578, 1994.
177. Lalczari, J., Schacker, T., Feinberg, J., et al. A randomized, double-blind, placebo- controlled trial of cidofovir gel for the treatment of acyclovir-unresponsive mucocutaneous herpes simplex virus infection in patients with AIDS. *J. Infect. Dis.*, 176, 892–898, 1997.
178. Sacks, S. L., Shafran, S. D., Diaz-Mitoma, F., et al. A multicenter phase I/II dose escalation study of single-dose cidofovir gel for treatment of recurrent genital herpes. *Antimicrob. Agents Chemother.*, 42, 2996–2999, 1998.
179. Tricot, G., De Clercq, E., Boogaerts, M. A., and Verwilghen, R. L. Oral bromovinyldeoxyuridine therapy for herpes simplex and varicella-zoster virus infections in severely immunosuppressed patients: a preliminary clinical trial. *J. Med. Virol.*, 18, 11, 1986.
180. De Clercq, E. Biochemical aspects of the selective antiherpes activity of nucleoside analogues. *Biochem. Pharmacol.*, 33, 2159, 1984.
181. Husak, R., Tebbe, B., Goerdt, S., et al. Pseudotumour of the tongue caused by herpes simplex virus type 2 in an HIV-1 infected immunosuppressed patient. *Br. J. Dermatol.*, 139, 118–121, 1998.
182. Grodesky, M. J. The emergence of acyclovir resistance in mucocutaneous herpes simplex viral infections: implications for clinical practice. *Nurse Pract.*, 22, 155–156, 1997.
183. Pottage, J. C. Jr. and Kessler, H. A. Herpes simplex virus resistance to acyclovir: clinical resistance. *Infect. Agents Dis.*, 4, 115–124, 1995.
184. Gaudreau, A., Hill, E., Balfour, H. H. Jr., Erice, A., and Boivin, G. Phenotypic and genotypic characterization of acyclovir-resistant herpes simplex viruses from immunocompromised patients. *J. Infect. Dis.*, 178, 297–303, 1998.
185. Scoular, A. and Barton, S. Therapy for genital herpes in immunocompromised patients: a national survey. The Herpes Simplex Advisory Panel. *Genitourin. Med.*, 73, 391–393, 1997.
186. Erlich, K. S., Mills, J., Chatis, P., et al. Acyclovir-resistant herpes simplex virus infections in patients with the acquired immunodeficiency syndrome. *N. Engl. J. Med.*, 320, 293, 1989.
187. Wade, J. C., McLaren, C., and Meyers, J. D. Frequency and significance of acyclovir- resistant herpes simplex virus isolated from marrow transplant patients receiving multiple courses of treatment with acyclovir. *J. Infect. Dis.*, 148, 1077, 1983.

188. Crumpacker, C. S., Schnipper, L. E., Marlowe, S. I., Kowalsky, P. N., Hershey, B. J., and Levin, M. J. Resistance to antiviral drugs of herpes simplex virus isolated from a patient treated with acyclovir. *N. Engl. J. Med.*, 306, 343, 1982.
189. Westheim, A. I., Tenser, R. B., and Marks, J. G. Jr. Acyclovir resistance in a patient with chronic mucocutaneous herpes simplex virus infection. *J. Am. Acad. Dermatol.*, 17, 875, 1982.
190. Collins, P. and Darby, G. Laboratory studies of herpes simplex virus strains resistant to acyclovir. *Rev. Med. Virol.*, 1, 19, 1991.
191. Ljungman, P. Herpes virus infections in immunocompromised patients: problems and therapeutic interventions. *Ann. Med.*, 25, 329, 1993.
192. Burns, W. H., Saral, R., Santos, G. W., et al. Isolation and characterization of resistant herpes simplex virus after acyclovir therapy. *Lancet*, 1, 421, 1982.
193. Sibrack, C. D., Gutman, L. T., Wilfert, C. M., et al. Pathogenicity of acyclovir-resistant herpes simplex virus type 1 from an immunodeficient child. *J. Infect. Dis.*, 146, 673, 1982.
194. Schinazi, R. F., del Bene, V., Scott, R. T., and Dudley-Thorpe, J. B. Characterization of acyclovir-resistant and -sensitive herpes simplex viruses isolated from a patient with an acquired immune deficiency. *J. Antimicrob. Chemother.*, 18(Suppl.), 127, 1986.
195. Norris, S. A., Kessler, H. A., and Fife, K. H. Severe, progressive herpetic whitlow caused by an acyclovir-resistant virus in a patient with AIDS. *J. Infect. Dis.*, 157, 209, 1988.
196. Vinckier, F., Boogaerts, M., De Clercq, D., and De Clercq, E. Chronic herpetic infection in an immunocompromised patient: report of a case. *J. Oral Maxillofac. Surg.*, 45, 723, 1987.
197. Englund, J. A., Zimmerman, M. K., Swierkosz, E. M., Goodman, J. L., Scholl, D. R., and Balfour, H. H. Jr. Herpes simplex virus resistant to acyclovir: a study in a tertiary care center. *Ann. Intern. Med.*, 112, 416, 1990.
198. Nugier, F., Colin, J. N., Aymard, M., and Langlois, M. Ocurrence and characterization of acyclovir-resistant herpes simplex virus isolates: report on a two-year sensitivity screening survey. *J. Med. Virol.*, 36, 1, 1992.
199. Ljungman, P., Ellis, M. N., Hackman, R. C., Sheep, D. H., and Meyers, J. D. Acyclovir- resistant herpes simplex virus causing pneumonia after marrow transplantation. *J. Infect. Dis.*, 162, 244, 1990.
200. Gateley, A., Gander, R. M., Johnson, P. C., Kit, S., Otsuka, H., and Kohl, S. Herpes simplex virus type 2 meningoencephalitis resistant to acyclovir in a patient with AIDS. *J. Infect. Dis.*, 161, 711, 1990.
201. Nisinoff Lehrman, S., Douglas, J. M., Corey, L., and Barry, D. W. Recurrent genital herpes and suppressive oral acyclovir therapy: relation between clinical outcome and in-vitro drug sensitivity. *Ann. Intern. Med.*, 134, 786, 1986.
202. Parris, D. S. and Harrington, J. E. Herpes simplex virus variants resistant to high concentrations of acyclovir exist in clinical isolates. *Antimicrob. Agents Chemother.*, 22, 71, 1982.
203. McLaren, C., Corey, L., Dekket, C., and Barry, D. W. In vitro sensitivity to acyclovir in genital herpes simplex virus from acyclovir-treated patients. *J. Infect. Dis.*, 148, 868, 1983.
204. Lehrman, S. N., Douglas, J. M., Corey, L., and Barry, D. W Recurrent genital herpes and suppressive oral acyclovir therapy: relation between clinical outcome and in-vitro sensitivity. *Ann. Intern. Med.*, 104, 786, 1986.
205. Schnipper, L. E. and Crumpacker, C. S. Resistance of herpes simplex virus to acylguanosine: role of viral thymidine kinase and DNA polymerase. *Proc. Natl. Acad. Sci. USA*, 77, 2270, 1980.
206. Coen, D. and Schaffer, P. A. Two distinct loci confer resistance to acylguanosine in herpes simplex virus type 1. *Proc. Natl. Acad. Sci. USA*, 77, 2265, 1980.
207. Darby, G., Field, H. J., and Salisbury, S. A. Altered substrate specificity of herpes simplex virus thymidine kinase confers acyclovir-resistance. *Nature*, 289, 81, 1981.
208. Field, H. J. and Darby, G. Pathogenicity in mice of strains of herpes simplex virus which are resistant to acyclovir in vitro and in vivo. *Antimicrob. Agents Chemother.*, 17, 209, 1980.
209. Sibrack, C. D., McLaren, C., and Barry, D. W. Disease and latency characteristics of clinical herpes simplex virus isolates after acyclovir therapy. *Am. J. Med.*, 73(Suppl.), 372, 1982.
210. Collins, P., Larder, B. A., Oliver, N. M., Kemp, S., Smith, I. W., and Darby, G. Characterization of a DNA polymerase mutant of herpes simplex virus from a severely immunocompromised patient receiving acyclovir. *J. Gen. Virol.*, 70, 375, 1989.
211. Knopf, K. W., Kaufman, E. R., and Crumpacker, C. Physical mapping of drug resistance mutations defines an active center on the herpes simplex virus DNA polymerase enzyme. *J. Virol.*, 39, 746, 1981.
212. Fletcher, C. V., Englund, J. A., Bean, B., Chinnock, B., Brundage, D. M., and Balfour, H. H. Jr. Continuous infusion high-dose acyclovir for serious herpesvirus infections. *Antimicrob. Agents Chemother.*, 33, 1375, 1989.
213. Erlich, K. S., Jacobson, M. A., Koehler, J. E., et al. Foscarnet therapy for severe acyclovir-resistant herpes simplex virus type-2 infections in patients with the acquired immunodeficiency syndrome. *Ann. Intern. Med.*, 110, 710, 1989.
214. Engel, J. P., Englund, J. A., Fletcher, C. V., and Hill, E. L. Treatment of resistant herpes simplex virus with continuous-infusion acyclovir. *J. Am. Med. Assoc.*, 263, 1662, 1990.
215. Crumpacker, C. Resistance of herpes viruses to nucleoside analogues: mechanisms and clinical importance, in *Antiviral Chemotherapy*, Mills, J. and Corey, L., Eds., Elsevier Press, New York, 226, 1986.
216. Dorsky, D. I. and Crumpacker, C. S. Drugs five years later: acyclovir. *Ann. Intern. Med.* 107, 859, 1987.
217. Chatis, P. A., Miller, C. H., Schrager, L. E., and Crumpacker, C. S. Successful treatment with foscarnet of an acyclovir-resistant mucocutaneous infection with herpes simplex virus in a patient with acquired immunodeficiency syndrome. *N. Engl. J. Med.*, 320, 297, 1989.
218. Birch, C., Tyssen, D., Tachedjian, G., et al. Clinical effects and in vitro studies of trifluorothymidine combined with interferon-alfa for treatment of drug-resistant and -sensitive herpes simplex infections. *J. Infect. Dis.*, 166, 108, 1992.

219. Birch, C., Tachedjian, G., Doherty, R., Hayes, K., and Gust, I. Altered sensitivity to antiviral drugs of herpes simplex virus isolates from a patient with the acquired immunodeficiency syndrome. *J. Infect. Dis.*, 162, 731, 1990.
220. Blot, N., Schneider, P., Young, P., et al. Treatment of an acyclovir and foscarnet-resistant herpes simplex virus infection with cidofovir in a child after an unrelated bone marrow transplant. *Bone Marrow Transplant.*, 26, 903–905, 2000.
221. Minkovitz, J. B. and Pepose, J. S. Topical interferon alpha-2a treatment of herpes simplex keratitis resistant to multiple antiviral medications in an immunosuppressed patient. *Cornea*, 14, 326–330, 1995.
222. Pisani, M. and Bozzi, M. Experimental use of natural interferon alpha by peroral administration in patients affected by recidivant herpes simplex. *Clin. Ter.*, 151(Suppl. 1), 19–22, 2000.
223. Scalvenzi, M. and Ceddia, C. Research in simple blind with natural interferon alpha at low dosage on subjects affected by labialis and genitalis herpes simplex. *Clin. Ter.*, 151(Suppl. 1), 13–18, 2000.
224. Wutzler, P. Antiviral therapy of herpes simplex and varicella-zoster virus infections. *Intervirology*, 40, 343–356, 1997.
225. Straus, S. E., Seidlin, M., Takiff, H., Jacobs, D., Bowen, D., and Smith, H. A. Oral acyclovir for suppression of recurrent herpes simplex virus infections in immunodeficient patients. *Ann. Intern. Med.*, 100, 522, 1984.
226. Straus, S. E., Croen, K. D., Sawyer, M. H., et al. Acyclovir suppression of frequently recurring genital herpes: efficacy and diminishing need during successive years of treatment. *J. Am. Med. Assoc.*, 260, 2227, 1988.

Part II
Bacterial Infections

4
Nocardia spp.

1. INTRODUCTION

Several *Nocardia* species have been known to be pathogenic to humans and animals, among them, *N. asteroides*, *N. brasiliensis*, *N. farcinica*, *N. nova* (1), *N. transvalensis* (2–4), and *N. otitidiscaviarum* (formerly known as *N. caviae*) (5–8). Nocardial infection is usually transmitted through inhalation or by traumatic inoculation of the skin (9,10).

In immunocompetent hosts, primary nocardiosis has been associated most frequently with cutaneous and ocular infections (2).

2. NOCARDIOSIS IN IMMUNOCOMPROMISED HOSTS

Even though invasive pulmonary and disseminated nocardiosis can occur in immunocompetent hosts, these two forms have been increasingly recognized as opportunistic infections associated with immunocompromised patients (2,9,11–14).

Inhalation of infectious airborn *Nocardia* spores or mycelia is considered the major route of invasive pulmonary infection. In addition, there has been evidence that the prevalence of respiratory-tract colonization may be much higher in defined populations of severely immunocompromised patients, such as cardiac transplant recipients. According to Simpson et al. (15), 44–51% of them may be colonized with *Nocardia* spp.

N. asteroides, which has been the major cause of primary pulmonary nocardiosis, has been implicated in as many as 80% of all cases (16). However, *N. brasiliensis* (17), *N. otitidiscaviarum* (5), and *N. transvalensis* (3) have also been related to pulmonary disease in both immunocompromised and immunocompetent hosts.

Patients with impaired local pulmonary defenses, such as those with chronic obstructive pulmonary conditions (chronic bronchitis and emphysema), asthma, and bronchiectasis (18–20), have been at higher risk of developing pulmonary nocardiosis. In addition. *Nocardia* spp. was also reported to cause infections in solid organ (renal [21–33], liver [34–38], cardiac [15,39–42], heart-lung [43]) and bone-marrow transplant (44–47) recipients (48). By some estimates, up to 4% of post-transplant infections are caused by *Nocardia* species (30).

Other populations at risk including patients with lymphoma (49–53), malignant neoplasms (16,54) sarcoidosis (55–57), collagen vascular disease (58,59) (e.g., systemic lupus erythemathosus [SLS] [1,60–65]), dysgammaglobulinemia (66), chronic granulomatous disease (67–71), chronic alcoholism (72), diabetes mellitus (18,73), trauma or surgery (66), patients undergoing continuous ambulatory peritoneal analysis (CAPD) (59,74), patients suffering from severe adrenocorticotropic hormone (ACTH)-dependent Cushing's syndrome (75,76), and patients infected with HIV (18,77–90), all have been reported to develop invasive pulmonary nocardiosis. Another group at risk has been intravenous drug abusers, mostly because of bacterial contamination of needles (91–94). Seggev (95) has described a fatal case of overwhelming pulmonary nocardiosis (10 mo after an apparent cure) complicating chronic mucocutaneous candidiasis.

From: Opportunistic Infections: Treatment and Prophylaxis
By: Vassil St. Georgiev © Humana Press Inc., Totowa, NJ

There have been several reports *(66,96–101)* describing a coexistence between pulmonary nocardiosis and alveolar proteinosis. In view of the well-established association between pulmonary alveolar proteinosis and hematologic malignancies, it is still unclear whether the connection between pulmonary nocardiosis and alveolar proteinosis represents a true independent association, or whether it merely reflects the independent correlation of each of these two conditions with an underlying hematologic malignancy *(97)*.

Systemic immunosuppression from prolonged treatment with corticosteroids and/or cytotoxic drugs has been a major predisposing factor for the development of invasive pulmonary nocardiosis *(2,102–106)*.

In immunocompromised patients, one complication related to invasive pulmonary nocardiosis has been the development of suppurative and/or chronic pericarditis *(107–112)*.

Furthermore, in severely immunocompromised patients, invasive pulmonary nocardial infections have the tendency to progress rapidly and disseminate through the bloodstream. However, in some patients it may follow a gradually progressive indolent course very often mimicking pulmonary involvement associated with tuberculosis *(113)*, fungal disease, sarcoidosis, and neoplasia *(2)*.

Disseminated nocardiosis is frequently a late-presenting and potentially life-threatening infection *(114)*, having originated endogenously (i.e., secondary to hematogenous spread from the lungs) *(115,116)*, but occasionally also from a primary nonpulmonary (cutaneous) infection *(17,117)*. Most often, dissemination results in brain and skin lesions, with mortality rates reaching 7–44% *(16,66)* or even higher (85%), as was the case in severely immunocompromised hosts *(118)*. Nocardial metastatic lesions may occur in nearly every part of the body. Although rare, bacteremic nocardiosis is reported to be often fatal *(119)*.

Carriere et al. *(38)* reported an unusual case of nocardial thyroiditis: the immunosupressed patient (a liver-kidney transplant recipient) had a preexisting nodular goiter that probably was a predisposing factor for the thyroid infection.

In addition to the brain, which is the most frequent nonpulmonary site involved in disseminated disease (25–40% of all cases of nocardiosis) *(116,120–126)*, other organs involved include the kidneys *(127,128)*, spleen *(127)*, liver *(127,129)*, and less often bone *(130–138)*, eyes *(139,140)*, skin *(115,141–144)*, and the joints *(115,145–148)*.

In a retrospective analysis by Barnicoat et al. *(149)*, patients with primary cerebral nocardiosis (that is, cerebral abscess without concurrent pulmonary involvement) *(150)* and an underlying immunosuppressive disorder had an increased rate of mortality, reaching as high as 95%.

Even though nocardiosis has been most often a late-presenting, community-acquired infection, nosocomial outbreaks have also been reported *(15,151–155)*.

2.1. Nocardiosis in HIV-Positive Patients

Of all *Nocardia* spp. *N. asteroides* was the most common species involved as the causative agent of opportunistic nocardiosis in AIDS patients *(18,77–90,156–160)*. Reports of infections by other *Nocardia* spp. were rare and included *N. brasiliensis (77,161–163)*, *N. farcinica (164,165)*, and *N. nova (156)*.

Despite the high degree of cellular immunodeficiency characteristic of patients infected with HIV, opportunistic *Nocardia* spp. infections in this particular population have been relatively infrequent *(77,78,81,83,84,88,89,94,156,161,164–170)*. However, in advanced HIV disease (lymphocyte counts below 266 cells/mm^3), nocardiosis can be fatal *(94)*. By one estimate *(169)*, only 0.19–0.3% of AIDS patients reported to the Centers for Disease Control (CDC), had been found to develop nocardiosis-complicating AIDS. However, this assessment may have underestimated the frequency of infection, owing to the fact that AIDS surveillance techniques rarely take into consideration follow-up information on infections that such patients may acquire after the diagnosis of AIDS. Findings from post-mortem case series on AIDS patients seemed to support the apparent low incidence of opportunistic nocardiosis in HIV-infected patients *(171,172)*. In this regard, one factor that may account for the low incidence of nocardiosis in HIV-infected patients is the widespread prophylactic use of trimethoprim-sulfamethoxazole (TMP-SMX) against *Pneumocystis carinii* since it is known that TMP-SMX has also a protective effect against *Nocardia* spp. *(94,169)*. Nevertheless, this has not always been the case; in bone-marrow recipients with graft-vs-host disease, TMP-SMX prophylaxis for *P. carinii* failed to prevent consistently nocardial infection, although it may have prevented or delayed dissemination *(44,45)*.

2.2. Co-Infections With Other Pathogens

Although pulmonary nocardiosis mimics pulmonary tuberculosis in clinical symptoms, being chronic in nature, and radiological characteristics *(113,173)*, there have also been several reports about simultaneous infections of *N. asteroides* with *Mycobacterium tuberculosis (77,167,174–178)* and nontuberculous mycobacteria (as many as 6% of all cases of nocardiosis) *(179)*. To this end, a statistically significant association has been observed between primary pulmonary nocardial disease and the subsequent development of nontuberculous pulmonary mycobacteriosis caused by *Mycobacterium kansasii* and the *Mycobacterium avium-intracellulare-Mycobacterium scrofulaceum* complex in cardiac-transplant recipients *(180)*. Currently, however, there is no clear evidence that such co-infections represent a true association that may indicate some interrelationship between these microbial agents *(2)*.

Concomitant pulmonary infections by *N. asteroides* and *Pneumocystis carinii* have also been described in patients undergoing immunosuppressive therapy for organ transplantations and cancer *(181,182)*, as well as *N. asteroids* and *Cryptococcus neoformans* lung abscess *(183)*, and disseminated infection caused by *C. neoformans* and *N. transvalensis (4)*.

In another example, a lung infection caused by *Aspergillus fumigatus* and *N. asteroides* has developed as complication of glucocorticoid treatment *(105)*. A case of actinomycetoma caused simultaneously by *N. brasiliensis* and *N. asteroids* has also been reported *(184)*.

An unusual co-infection of phaeohyphomycosis (caused by *Exphiala jeanselmei*) and *N. asteroids* in a renal-transplant recipient is important to be emphasized because in the presence of more than one microorganism in an immunocompromised patient, the correct differentiation and identification of the pathogens involved is essential in determining the appropriate therapy *(29)*.

A disseminated *Rhodococcus equi* and *N. farcinica* infection in a patient with sarcoidosis has also been described *(57)*.

3. TREATMENT OF NOCARDIOSIS

The treatment of nocardiosis remains problematic because there had been no large controlled clinical trials, and the available empiric recommendations for specific antimicrobial agents have been based on a limited number of patients *(2,185)*. As with other infections in which cell-mediated immunity plays a large defensive role, nocardiosis in immunocompromised patients can relapse after an apparent cure and occasionally appear remote from the original infection *(186)*.

In some patients, treatment with antimicrobial drugs for primary infection failed, leading to metastatic spread of the disease or late relapse *(187)*. To improve the clinical outcome of nocardiosis, surgical intervention in addition to antimicrobial therapy often has been recommended *(6,77,81,108–110,121,161,188–191)*.

The spectrum of nocardiosis may also be changing from a predominantly *N. asteroides*-induced infections to increasing incidence of illness owing to *N. farcinica (33,40,57,140,164,165,192)*, including a confirmed nosocomial outbreak that documented the source and person-to-person transmission *(155)*. According to published statistics, *N. farcinica* constituted the prevailing pathogenic actinomycete in Germany from 1979–1991 *(193)*, and in France one-quarter of all *Nocardia* isolates were *N. farcinica (194)*. The changing etiologic pattern of nocardiosis may also affect the way initial therapy is administered *(164)*. Though *N. asteroides* remains sensitive to most antimicrobial agents *(27,195,196)*, *N. farcinica*, which is almost indistinguishable from *N. asteroides* by regular laboratory methods, has been resistant to cephalosporins *(195)*. Therefore, because of the rising incidence of *N. farcinica* and its drug resistance, it is important that third-generation cephalosporins not be used in the initial management of *Nocardia* infections *(164)*.

Currently, there is no known therapy of choice against *N. transvalensis*. Furthermore, clinical isolates of this species have demonstrated high degree of drug resistance, and therapy with TMP-SMX has not always been successful *(3)*.

3.1. Sulfonamides

Treatment with sulfonamides (sulfisoxazole *[15,94]*, sulfadiazine *[94,197]*, sulfadimidine *[198]*) alone *(15,66,199)* or in combination with trimethoprim has been the mainstay of antimicrobial therapy for human nocardiosis *(2,35,94,181,189,200–207)*. Single sulfonamide drugs used most frequently in the treatment of nocardiosis include sulfisoxazole (4–8 g daily) and sulfadiazine (4–6 g daily) *(94,208–210)*.

Sulfonamide dose regimens should be adjusted to achieve the recommended blood levels of 100–150 µg/mL approx 2 h after an oral dose. For effective treatment, generally high doses of sulfonamides (3–6 g daily) should be given for extended periods (6–12 mo) *(2,202)*. Although primary cutaneous disease may be cured within 1–3 mo and uncomplicated pulmonary nocardiosis may respond to therapy for 6 mo or less, the therapy in immunocompromised hosts and for disseminated nocardiosis may have to be carried out for prolonged periods of time (12 mo or more) *(185,211)*.

One of the unwarranted side effects of the sulfonamides (e.g., sulfadiazine *[208]*) has been the development of drug-induced lithiasis, owing to their poor solubility in urine *(212)*. The result may be an obstructive uropathy leading to acute renal failure. Rapid improvement can be achieved by drug discontinuation or decrease of dosage, systemic administration of fluid, and urine alkalinization *(85)*.

3.2. Sulfonamide-Trimethoprim Combinations

While the combination of sulfamethoxazole with trimethoprim (co-trimoxazole) is used frequently either orally or intravenously *(116,149,185,213–216)*, its beneficial therapeutic effect may occur less from the synergistic relationship between these two drugs than from an improved penetration into the cerebrospinal fluid (CSF) and generally favorable pharmacokinetics *(217)*.

Some problems posed by sulfonamide-trimethoprim combinations *(218–221)* included patient's intolerance *(222)* (acute pancreatitis *[223,224]*) and drug incompatibility with cyclosporine, which is used as antirejection agent in organ-transplant recipients. The latter may result in reversible cyclosporine-induced nephrotoxicity *(12,225–228)*. Furthermore, in cases when the concentration of the sulfonamide component has been too high relative to that of trimethoprim, in vitro antagonism has been demonstrated *(9,229)*.

It is important to note that 50% of HIV-infected patients would still experience adverse reactions (fever, severe hypersensitivity reactions, and prolonged myelosuppression) owing to TMP-SMX, which could be of sufficient severity to cause discontinuation *(164,230)*.

Miralles *(164)* has described an AIDS patient presenting with disseminated *N. farcinica* infection diagnosed by percutaneous kidney biopsy. Intravenous therapy with TMP-SMX (350 mg/1750 mg) given 4 times daily (at a dose of 5.0 mg/kg TMP) over 4 wk led to significant clinical improvement.

Although rare, testicular nocardiosis in immunocompromised patients has also been diagnosed *(191,231–234)*. The mortality in such cases was high (3 of 5 reported patients, 60%), and the two survivors required long-term sulfonamide treatment combined with orchiectomy *(191,234)*.

Lopez et al. *(191)* reported a case of epididymo-orchitis owing to *N. asteroides* in an immunocompromised liver-transplant recipient receiving immunosuppressive therapy. Treatment with co-trimoxazole (20 mg/kg trimethoprim daily) for 5 mo, followed by orchiectomy and an additional 4 mo of TMP-SMX therapy, led to clinical resolution of nocardiosis *(191)*.

3.3. Antibiotics

Several reports have indicated that when encountered by sulfonamide resistance, treatment with minocycline *(235–237)*, amikacin, or erythromycin in combination with ampicillin was possible *(202,222,238–240)*. In general, the apparent response to nonsulfonamide agents seemed to have supported published data regarding their in vitro efficacy against *Nocardia* spp. *(241–243)*.

Mycolic acid-containing bacteria, such as *Nocardia* and related taxa, are known to inactivate rifampicin in a variety of species-specific ways including glucosylation, ribosylation, phosphorylation, and decolarization. To this end, *Nocardia* modifies rifampicin by glucosylation (23-OH group) and phosphorylation of the of the antibiotic *(279)*.

Stella et al. *(244)* described a complete cure of a systemic infection owing to *N. asteroides* with a 2-mo course of erythromycin (500 mg, q.i.d.) and amoxicillin/clavulanic acid (500 mg/125 mg, once daily), combined with ultrasound-guided transcutaneous aspiration of multiple subcutaneous metastatic abscesses. In another example, a 15-mo course consisting of minocycline (400–600 mg daily), cefotaxime (1.2–3.0 g daily), and probenicide cured *N. asteroides*-induced pneumonia and brain abscess persisting after therapy with sulfonamides, minocycline, and cefotaxime *(245)*.

A 12-wk course of oral clarithromycin (500 mg twice daily) led to complete resolution of primary cutaneous nocardiosis in a steroid-dependent asthmatic patient who failed to respond to an initial treatment of a 6-wk course of oral cephalexin (500 mg 4 times daily) followed by a 2-wk course of minocycline (100 mg twice daily) *(246)*.

Reports of other antibiotics used in the therapy of nocardiosis included cefuroxime (2.25–4.5 g daily), ceftriaxone (2.0 g daily), cefotaxime, amikacin (1.0 g daily), minocycline (200 mg daily), imipenem, and meropenem *(94,209,235,247–249)*. Drug combinations, such as imipenem-amikacin *(1,20)*, ceftriaxone-amikacin, imipenem-rifampicin, imipenem-cilastatin, imipenem-ciprofloxacin, imipenem-erythromycin *(53)*, ciprofloxacin-doxycycline, cefotaxime-amikacin *(250)*, meropenem-cefotaxime-minocycline, and amoxicillin-clavulanic acid-amikacin have shown evidence of synergy in vitro *(251)* as well as in clinical settings *(56,252–259)*. Metronidazole-flucloxacillin, as well as sulfonamide-ampicillin-clavulanic acid *(42)*, have been used successfully in several cases in Europe *(260,261)*.

Intravenous amikacin and imipenem at doses of 250 mg (q.i.d.) and 1.5 g (q.i.d.), respectively, cured endocarditis of a prosthetic aortic valve caused by *N. asteroides (262)*.

After failure to achieve cure with co-trimoxazole, Overkamp et al. *(56)* effectively treated disseminated nocardiosis in an immunosuppressed patient with a combination of oral rifampicin and intravenous imipenem, followed by oral rifampicin and ampicillin-clavulanic acid.

Bauwens et al. *(263)* described two cases of nocardiosis in immunocompromised renal-transplant recipients successfully treated with amoxicillin (500 mg, q.i.d. for 10 d), and TMP-SMX/cefotaxime (for 6 mo, then followed by TMP-SMX alone for 1 yr), respectively. In another report, a renal-transplant recipient with an unusual case of nocardial psoas and perinephric abscess responded to treatment with ciprofloxacin and cefuroxime combined with surgical drainage *(264)*. Gomez et al. *(265)* treated *N. brasiliensis*-induced mycetoma with bone involvement with oral amoxicillin-clavulanic acid (500 mg and 125 mg, respectively, given 3 times daily for 5–6 mo).

Several cases of concomitant pulmonary nocardiosis and aspergillosis in immunocompromised patients have also been described *(40,266,267)*. In one study, one such patient who also had renal vasculitis was treated successfully with combination of imipenem, co-trimoxazole and a prolonged course of itraconazole *(267)*.

A rare case of pleuropulmonary nocardiosis in an immunosuppressed patient with SLE and receiving chronic treatment with corticosteroids and immunosuppressive drugs was treated successfully with intravenous imipenem (500 mg, b.i.d.); following hospital discharge, the patient continued therapy with oral ciprofloxacin at 500 mg daily *(58)*.

Intravenous imipenem (1.0 g, t.i.d.) combined with oral erythromycin (500 mg, q.i.d.) and roxythromycin (300 mg, b.i.d.) successfully resolved a case of sphenoidal sinusitis due to *N. asteroides* *(198)*.

Zimmerman et al. *(268)* described a case of chronic *N. asteroides* endophthalmitis following extracapsular cataract extraction that was treated with a combination of antibiotics, including intravitreal (200 μg, done twice) and intracameral (200 μg, b.i.d. for 4 wk) injections of amikacin sulfate, topical amikacin sulfate (33 g/L, every 4 h); intravenous imipenem (500 mg, t.i.d. for 6 wk) was also administered after the surgery in addition to oral TMP-SMX, minocycline hydrochloride (100 mg, b.i.d.), and 1% prednisolone (q.i.d.). In spite of the therapy, the patient's clinical course continued to deteriorate, leading to enucleation of the globe *(268)*. The use of intravenous imipenem was also considered after a report *(269)* showing that its aqueous humor concentrations were sufficiently high after intravenous administration.

Abdominal actinomycetoma (a chronic disease that affects subcutaneous tissue) caused by *N. brasiliensis* in a patient with phagocyte immunodeficiency was successfully treated by antibiotic combination given in two 23-d cycles. Each cycle comprised of cefotaxime (1.0 g every 8 h) and amikacin (500 mg every 12 h) *(250)*.

Srinivasan and Sundur *(270)* reported eight cases of nocardial endophthalmitis following posterior chamber intraocular lens implantation, which all responded to various topical antibiotic agents (10% ampicillin sodium, 0.2% trimethoprim sulfate, 30% sulfacetamide sodium, 0.3% norfloxacin, and 0.3% ciprofloxacine hydrochloride) administered according to the sensitivity of the isolates.

Treatment of primary cutaneous nocardiosis had included the use of intravenous (TMP: 240 mg/ SMX: 1.2 g, daily) *(271)* or oral (TMP: 480 mg/SMX: 2.4 g, b.i.d.) *(272)* trimethoprim-sulfamethoxazole, and various antibiotic combinations *(273)*, namely: rifampin (600 mg daily)-clofazimine (300 mg daily)-minocycline (1.0 g daily) *(273)*, cefalexine 500 (1.0 g daily)-gentamicin (1.0 g daily for 5 d) *(273)*, and enoxacin (600 mg daily)-minocycline (200 mg daily)-doxycycline (100 mg daily) *(274)*. Rees et al. *(41)* reported the successful treatment of primary cutaneous *N. farcinica* nocardiosis in an immunosuppressed heart-transplant recipient with oral doxycycline (100- mg daily); prior treatment with imipenem (1.0 g daily, i.v.) and amikacin (1.0 g daily, i.v.) had failed to bring clinical improvement.

Kimura et al. *(275)* reported a dramatic resolution of pulmonary nocardiosis to combined sulfamethoxazole-trimethoprim and sparfloxacin treatment in a patient on a long-term oral prednisolone (15 mg daily) therapy for Evans syndrome. A triple combination comprised of TMP/SMX, ceftriaxone, and amikacin was used to treat successfully nocardial brain abscess in a renal-transplant recipient *(31)*.

3.4. Acquired Drug Resistance of Nocardia spp.

Joshi and Hamory *(276)* reported the development of multiple drug-resistant strain of *N. asteroides* in a patient with AIDS and concomitant disseminated histoplasmosis. The pattern of resistance, known as type 5, has been specific for broad-spectrum cephalosporins, ciprofloxacin, and all aminoglycosides (except amikacin). In another case, a patient with *N. asteroides*-associated brain abscess and ventriculitis had developed resistance to sulfonamides but was susceptible to β-lactams *(277)*.

An acquired resistance to clavulanic acid (as part of a combination with amoxicillin) by *N. brasiliensis* has been attributed to mutational change in the inhibitor and active site(s) in the β-lactamase *(278)*.

REFERENCES

1. Arnal, C., Man, H., Delisle, F., M'Bappe, P., and Cocheton, J. J. *Nocardia* infection of a joint prosthesis complicating systemic lupus erythematosus. *Lupus*, 9, 304, 2000.
2. McNeil, M. M. and Brown, J. M., The medically important aerobic Actinomycetes: epidemiology and microbiology. *Clin. Microbiol. Rev.*, 7, 357, 1994.

3. McNeil, M. M., Brown, J. M., Georghiou, P. R., Allworth, A. M., and Blacklock, Z. M. Infections due to *Nocardia transvalensis*: clinical spectrum and antimicrobial therapy. *Clin. Infect. Dis.*, 15, 453, 1992.
4. Dyer, J. R., Ketheesan, N., Norton, R. E., Ashhurst-Smith, C. I., Keary, P., and La Brooy, J. T. Disseminated infection due to *Nocardia transvalensis* coincident with *Cryptococcus neoformans* variety *gattii* meningitis. *Eur. J. Clin. Microbiol. Infect. Dis.*, 18, 587–590, 1999.
5. Causey, W. A. *Nocardia caviae*: a report of 13 new isolations with clinical correlation. *Appl. Environ. Microbiol.*, 28, 193, 1974.
6. Hartmann, A. Halvorsen, C. E., Jenssen, T., et al. Intracerebral abscess caused by *Nocardia otitidiscaviarum* in a renal transplant patient - cured by evacuation plus antibiotic therapy. *Nephron*, 86, 79–83, 2000.
7. Taniguchi, H., Mukae, H., Ashitani, J., et al. Pulmonary *Nocardia otitidiscaviarum* infection in a patient with chronic respiratory infection. *Intern. Med.*, 37, 872–876, 1998.
8. Petersen, D. L., Hudson, L. D., and Sullivan, K. Disseminated *Nocardia caviae* with positive blood cultures. *Arch. Intern. Med.*, 138, 1164, 1978.
9. Curry, W. A. Human nocardiosis: a clinical review with selected case reports. *Arch. Intern. Med.*, 140, 818, 1980.
10. Kahn, F. W., Gornick, C. C., and Tofte, R. W. Primary cutaneous *Nocardia asteroides* infection with dissemination. *Am. J. Med.*, 70, 859, 1981.
11. Beaman, B. L. and Beaman, L. *Nocardia* species: host-parasite relationships. *Clin. Microbiol. Rev.*, 7, 213, 1994.
12. Arduino, R. C., Johnson, P. C., and Miranda, A. G. Nocardiosis in renal transplant recipients undergoing immunosuppression with cyclosporine. *Clin. Infect. Dis.*, 16, 505, 1993.
13. Bani-Sadr, F., Hamidou, M., Raffi, F., Chamoux, C., Caillon, J., and Freland, C. Aspects cliniques et bactériologiques des nocardioses: 9 observations. *Presse Med.*, 24, 1062, 1995.
14. Ledesma Castano, F., Hernandez Hernandez, J. L. Echevarria Viema, S., and Conde Yague, R., Immunosuppression and pulmonary nocardiosis. *Ann. Med. Intl.*, 13, 50, 1996.
15. Simpson, G. L., Stinson, E. B., Egger, M. J., and Remington, J. S. Nocardial infections in the immunocompromised host: a detailed study in a defined population. *Rev. Infect. Dis.*, 3, 492, 1981.
16. Beaman, B. L., Burnside, J., Edwards, B., and Causey, W. Nocardial infections in the United States, 1972–1974. *J. Med. Vet. Dis.*, 134, 286, 1976.
17. Smego, R. A. Jr. and Gallis, H. A. The clinical spectrum of *Nocardia brasiliensis* infection in the United States. *Rev. Infect. Dis.*, 6, 164, 1984.
18. Georghiou, P. R. and Blacklock, Z. M. Infection with *Nocardia* species in Queensland: a review of 102 clinical isolates. *Med. J. Aust.*, 156, 692, 1992.
19. Murray, J. F., Finegold, S. M., Froman, S., and Will, D. W. The changing spectrum of nocardiosis: a review and presentation of nine cases. *Am. Rev. Respir. Dis.*, 83, 315.
20. Cremades, M. J., Menendez, R., Santos, M., and Gobernado, M. Repeated pulmonary infection by *Nocardia asteroids* complex in a patient with bronchiectasis. *Respiration*, 65, 211–213, 1998.
21. Santamaria Saber, L. T., Figueiredo, J. F., Santos, S. B., et al. *Nocardia* infection in renal transplant recipient: diagnostic and therapeutic considerations. *Rev. Inst. Med. Trop. Sao Paolo*, 35, 417, 1993.
22. Kong, N. C., Morad, Z., Suleiman, A. B., Cheong, I. K., and Lajin, I. Spectrum of nocardiosis in renal patients. *Ann. Acad. Med. Singapore*, 19, 375, 1990.
23. Carpintero, Y., Mendaza, P., Portero, F., et al. *Nocardia asteroides* pneumonia in a patient undergoing a kidney transplant. *Enferm. Infecc. Microbiol. Clin.*, 14, 65, 1996.
24. Gutierrez, H., Salgado, O., Garcia, R., Henriquez, C., Herrera, J., and Rodriguez-Iturbe, B. Nocardiosis in renal transplant patients. *Transplant. Proc.*, 26, 341, 1994.
25. Vilaseca Arroyo, Z., Olive, A., Lauzurica Valdemoros, R., and Jimenez Lasanta, J. A. Pyomyositis caused by *Nocardia asteroids* in a patient with kidney transplant. *Med. Clin. (Barc.)*, 114, 558–559, 2000.
26. Wong, K. M., Chak, W. L., Chan, Y. H., et al. Subcutaneous nodules attributed to nocardiosis in a renal transplant recipient on tacrolimus therapy. *Am. J. Nephrol.*, 20, 138–141, 2000.
27. Rinaldi, S., D'Argenio, P., Fiscarelli, E., Farina, C., and Rizzoni, G. Fatal disseminated *Nocardia farsinica* infection in a renal transplant recipient. *Pediatr. Nephrol.*, 14, 111–113, 2000.
28. Sartoris, K. E., Baillie, G. M., Tiernan, R., and Rajagopalan, P. R. Phaeohyphomycosis from *Exphiala jeanselmei* with concomitant *Nocardia asteroids* infection in a renal transplant recipient: case report and review of the literature. *Pharmacotherapy*, 19, 995–1001, 1999.
29. Magee, C. C., Halligan, R. D., Milford, E. L., and Sayegh, M. H. Nocardial infection in a renal transplant recipient on tacrolimus and mycophenolate mofetil. *Clin. Nephrol.*, 52, 44–46, 1999.
30. Hiller, R., Singh, H., and Crone, M. Left leg paralysis in a renal transplant. *Am. J. Kidney Dis.*, 33, E1, 1999.
31. Sabeel, A., Alrabiah, F., Alfurayh, O., and Hassounah, M. Nocardial brain abscess in a renal transplant recipient successfully treated with triple antimicrobials. *Clin. Nephrol.*, 50, 128–130, 1998.
32. Reddy, S. S. and Holley, J. L. Nocardiosis in a recently transplanted renal patient. *Clin. Nephrol.*, 50, 123–127, 1998.
33. Shimizu, T., Furumoto, H., Asagami, C., Kanaya, K., Mikami, Y., and Muto, M. Disseminated subcutaneous *Nocardia farcinica* abscesses in a nephritic syndrome patient. *J. Am. Acad. Dermatol.*, 38(5 Pt.2), 874–876, 1998.
34. Forbes, G. M., Harvey, F. A., Philpott-Howard, J. N., et al. Nocardiosis in liver transplantation: variation in presentation, diagnosis and therapy. *J. Infect.*, 20, 11, 1990.
35. Weinberger, M., Eid, A., Schreiber, L., et al. Disseminated *Nocardia transvalensis* resembling pulmonary infection in a liver transplant patient. *Eur. J. Clin. Microbiol. Infect. Dis.*, 14, 337, 1995.

36. Lumbreras, C., Lizasoian, M., Moreno, E., et al. Major bacterial infections following liver transplantation: a prospective study. *Hepato-Gastroenterology*, 39, 362, 1992.
37. Raby, N., Forbes, G., and Williams, R. *Nocardia* infection in patients with liver transplants or chronic liver disease: radiologic findings. *Radiology*, 174, 713, 1990.
38. Carriere, C., Marchandin, H., Andrieu, J. M., Vandome, A., and Perez, C. *Nocardia* thyroiditis: unusual location of infection. *J. Clin. Microbiol.*, 37, 2323–2325, 1999.
39. Krick, J. A., Stinson, E. B., and Remington, J. S. *Nocardia* infection in heart transplant patients. *Ann. Intern. Med.*, 82, 18, 1975.
40. Monteforte, J. S. and Wood, C. A. Pneumonia caused by *Nocardia nova* and *Aspergillus fumigatus* after cardiac transplantation. *Eur. J. Clin. Microbiol. Infect. Dis.*, 12, 112, 1993.
41. Rees, W., Schuler, S., Hummel, M., and Hetzer, R. Primary cutaneous *Nocardia farcinica* infection following heart transplantation. *Dtsch. Med. Wochenschr.* 119, 1276, 1994; [correction in *Dtsch. Med. Wochenschr.* 119, 1276, 1994].
42. Merigou, D., Beylot-Barry, M., Ly, S., et al. Primary cutaneous *Nocardia asteroids* infection after heart transplantation. *Dermatology*, 196, 246–247, 1998.
43. Roberts, S. A., Franklin, J. C., Mijch, A.,and Spelman, D. *Nocardia* infection in heart-lung transplant recipients at Alfred Hospital, Melbourne, Australia, 1989–1998. *Clin. Infect. Dis.*, 31, 968–972, 2000.
44. Shearer, C. and Chandrasekar, P. H. Pulmonary nocardiosis in a patient with a bone marrow transplant. Bone Marrow Transplantation Group. *Bone Marrow Transplant.*, 15, 479, 1995.
45. Freites, V., Sumoza, A., Bisotti, R., et al. Subcutaneous *Nocardia asteroides* in a bone marrow transplant recipient. *Bone Marrow Transplant.*, 15, 135, 1995.
46. Hodohara, K., Fujiyama, Y., Hiramita, Y., et al. Disseminated subcutaneous *Nocardia asteroides* abscesses in a patient after bone marrow transplantation. *Bone Marrow Transplant.*, 11, 341, 1993.
47. Bhave, A. A., Thirunavukkarasu, K., Gottlieb, D. J., and Bradstock, K. Disseminated nocardiosis in a bone marrow transplant recipient with chronic GVHD. *Bone Marrow Transplant.*, 23, 519–521, 1999.
48. Chapman, S. W. and Wilson, J. P. Nocardiosis in transplant recipients. *Semin. Respir. Infect.*, 5, 74, 1990.
49. Noto, N., Sugaya, N., Wakabayashi, Y., Hirose, S. A case of pulmonary nocardiosis in malignant lymphoma under VEMP therapy. *Rinsho Ketsueki*, 26, 1140, 1985.
50. Pinkhas, J., Oliver, I., de Vries, A., Spitzer, S. A., and Henig, E. Pulmonary nocardiosis complicating malignant lymphoma successfully treated with chemotherapy. *Chest*, 63, 367, 1973.
51. Shelkovitz-Shilo, L., Feinstein, A., Trau, H., Kaplan, B., Sofer, E., and Schewach-Millet, M. Lymphocutaneous nocardiosis due to *Nocardia asteroides* in a patient with intestinal lymphoma. *Int. J. Dermatol.*, 31, 178, 1992.
52. Taylor, G. D. and Turner, A. R. Cutaneous abscess due to *Nocardia* after "alternative" therapy for lymphoma. *Can. Med. Assoc. J.*, 133, 767, 1985.
53. Sakai, C., Takagi, T., and Satoh, Y. *Nocardia asteroides* pneumonia, subcutaneous abscess and meningitis in a patient with advanced malignant lymphoma: successful treatment based on in vitro antimicrobial susceptibility. *Intern. Med.*, 38, 683–686, 1999.
54. Berkey, P. and Bodey, G. P. Nocardial infection in patients with neoplastic disease,. *Rev. Infect. Dis.*, 11, 407, 1989.
55. Ziza, J. M., Mayaud, C., and Carnot, F. Anatomo-clinical conference. Pitie-Salpetriere Hospital: case n. 1-1988. Degradation of the respiratory function in a patient followed for severe sarcoidosis. *Ann. Med. Interne (Paris)*, 139, 41, 1988.
56. Overkamp, D., Waldmann, B., Lins, T., Lingenfelser, T., Petersen, D., and Eggstein, M. Successful treatment of brain abscess caused by *Nocardia* in an immunocompromised patient after failure of co-trimoxazole. *Infection*, 20, 365, 1992.
57. Mohammedi, I., Vedrinne, J. M., Floccard, B., Reverdy, M. E., Duperret, S., and Motin, J. Disseminated *Rhodococcus equi* and *Nocardia farcinica* infection in a patient with sarcoidoses. *J. Infect.*, 36, 134–135, 1998.
58. Nzeusseu Toukap, A., Hainaut, P., Moreau, M., Pieters, T., Noirhomme, P., and Gigi, J. Nocardiosis: a rare cause of pleuropulmonary disease in the immunocompromised host. *Acta Clin. Belg.*, 51, 161, 1996.
59. Lopes, J. O., Alves, S. H., Benevenga, J. P., Salla, A., and Tatsch, I. *Nocardia asteroides* peritonitis during continuous ambulatory peritoneal dialysis. *Rev. Inst. Med. Trop. Sao Paolo* 35, 377, 1993.
60. Garty, B. Z., Stark, H., Yaniv, I., Varsano, I., and Danon, Y. I. Pulmonary nocardiosis in a child with systemic lupus erythematosus. *Pediatr. Infect. Dis. J.*, 4, 66, 1985.
61. Gorevic, P. D., Katler, E. I., and Agus, B. Pulmonary nocardiosis: occurence in men with systemic lupus erythematosus. *Arch. Intern. Med.* 140, 361, 1980.
62. McNab, P., Fuentealba, C., Ballesteros, F., et al. *Nocardia asteroides* infection in a patient with systemic lupus erythematosus. *Rev. Med. Chil.*, 128, 526–528, 2000.
63. Chantarojanasiri, T., Sittirath, A., Preutthipan, A. Tapaneya-Olarn, W., and Suwanjutha, S. Pulmonary involvement in childhood systemic lupus erythematosus. *J. Med. Assoc. Thai.*, 82(Suppl. 1), S144–S148, 1999.
64. Nakajima, A., Taniguchi, A., Tanaka, M., et al. A case of systemic lupus erythematosus complicated by *Nocardia farcinica*. *Kansenshogaku Zasshi*, 73, 477–481, 1999.
65. Balbir-Gurman, A., Schapira, D., and Nahir, A. M. Primary subcutaneous nocardial infection in a SLE patient. *Lupus*, 8, 164–167, 1999.
66. Palmer, D. L., Harvey, R. L., and Wheeler, J. K. Diagnostic and therapeutic considerations in *Nocardia asteroides* infection. *Medicine (Baltimore)*, 53, 391, 1974.
67. Tirapu, J. M., Alvarez, M., Crespo, J. A., et al. Chronic granulomatous 992)disease and pulmonary nocardiosis. *Med. Clin. (Barcelona)*, 99, 27, 1992.

68. Casale, T. B., Macher, A. M., and Fauci, A. S. Concomitant pulmonary aspergillosis and nocardiosis in a patient with chronic granulomatous disease of childhood. *South. Med. J.*, 77, 274, 1984.
69. Fernandez-Funez, V. A., Solera, J., Castro, C., Beato, J. L., Medrano, F., and Camino, E. Chronic granulomatous disease and infection by *Nocardia*. *Enferm. Infecc. Microbiol. Clin.*, 7, 564, 1989.
70. Johnston, H. C., Shigeoka, A. O., Hurley, D. C., and Pysher, T. J. *Nocardia* pneumonia in a neonate with chronic granulomatous disease. *Pediatr. Infect. Dis. J.*, 8, 526, 1989.
71. Jonsson, S., Wallace, R. J. Jr., Hull, S. I., and Musher, D. M. Reccurent *Nocardia* pneumonia in an adult with chronic granulomatous disease. *Am. Rev. Respir. Dis.*, 133, 932, 1986.
72. Valencia, M. E., Lavilla, P., Lopez Dupla, J. M., and Gil Aguado, A. Disseminated nocardiosis in a patient with chronic alcoholism. *Rev. Clin. Esp.*, 186, 146, 1990.
73. Sahl, B., Fegan, C., Hussain, A., Jaulim, A., Whale, K., and Webb, A. Pulmonary infection with *Nocardia caviae* in a patient with diabetes mellitus and liver cirrhosis. *Thorax,*, 43, 933, 1988.
74. Liassine, N. and Rahal, K. Peritonitis caused by *Nocardia farcinica* in a patient undergoing continuous ambulatory peritoneal analysis. *Arch. Inst. Pasteur Alger.*, 58, 95, 1992.
75. Bakker, R. C., Gallas, P. R., Romijn, J. A., and Wiersinga, W. M. Cushing's syndrome complicated by multiple opportunistic infections. *J. Endocrinol. Invest.*, 21, 329–333, 1998.
76. Dohchin, A., Sato, M., Yamanaka, H. Pulmonary nocardiosis associated with Cushing's syndrome. *Nihon Kokyuki Gakkai Zasshi*, 37, 125–129, 1999.
77. Kim, J., Minamoto, G. Y., and Grieco, M. H. Nocardial infection as a complication of AIDS: report of six cases and a review. *Rev. Infect. Dis.*, 13, 624, 1991.
78. Kramer, M. R. and Uttamchandani, R. B. The radiographic appearance of pulmonary nocardiosis associated with AIDS. *Chest*, 98, 382, 1990.
79. Marin Casanova, P., Garcia-Martos, P., Fernandez Gutierez del Alamo, C., Garcia Herruzo, J., Escribano Moriana, J. C., and Aznar Martin, A. Nocardiosis in a patient with AIDS. *Rev. Clin. Esp.*, 188, 83, 1991.
80. Perez Perez, M., Garcia-Martos, P., Escribano Moriana, J. C., and Marin Casanova, P. *Nocardia caviae* meningitis in a patient with HIV infection. *Rev. Clin. Esp.*, 187, 374, 1990.
81. Rodriguez, J. L., Barrio, J. L., and Pitchenik, A. E. Pulmonary nocardiosis in the acquired immunodeficiency syndrome: diagnosis with bronchoalveolar lavage and treatment with non- sulphur containing drugs. *Chest*, 90, 912, 1986.
82. Allworth, A. M. and Bowden, F. J. Managing HIV. Part 5: treating secondary outcomes. HIV and bacterial infections. *Med. J. Aust.*, 164, 546, 1996.
83. Sanchez Munoz-Torrero, J. F., Yniguez, T. R., Garcia-Onieva, E., et al. Nocardiosis in patients with human immunodeficiency virus infection in Spain. *Rev. Clin. Esp.*, 195, 468, 1995.
84. Meyer, C. N. Nocardiosis in HIV patients. *Ugeskr. Laeger*, 157, 4358, 1995.
85. Farina, L. A., Palou Redorta, J., and Chechile Toniolo, G. Reversible acute renal failure due to sulfonamide-induced lithiasis in an AIDS patient. *Arch. Esp. Urol.*, 48, 418, 1995.
86. Khorrami, P. and Heffeman, E. J. Pneumonia and meningitis due to *Nocardia asteroides* in a patient with AIDS. *Clin. Infect. Dis.*, 17, 1084, 1993.
87. Weiss, D., Bodmer, T., Mathieu, R., and Malinverni, R. Systemic *Nocardia* infection in an AIDS patient. *Schweiz. Med. Wochenschr.*, 122, 1057, 1992.
88. Javaly, K., Horowitz, H. W., and Wormser, G. P. Nocardiosis in patients with human immunodeficiency virus infection: report of 2 cases and review of the literature. *Medicine (Baltimore)*, 71, 128, 1992.
89. Aguilar, P. H., Pahl, F. H., Uip, D. E., et al. Cerebellar abscess by *Nocardia*: a case report. *Arq. Neurosiquiatr.*, 53, 307, 1995.
90. Desfemmes, T., Cadranel, J., Delisle, F., Akoun, G., and Mayaud, C. Pulmonary and cerebral nocardiosis in a patient infected with HIV. *Rev. Mal. Respir.*, 10, 262, 1993.
91. Garcia-Martos, P., Diaz, J., Perez, M., Alvarez, M. M., and Rubin, J. Meningeal syndrome in a patient addicted to parenteral drugs. *Enferm. Infecc. Microbiol. Clin.*, 8, 313, 1990.
92. Hershewe, G. L., Davis, L. E., and Bicknell, J. M. Primary cerebellar brain abscess from nocardiosis in a heroin addict. *Neurology*, 38, 1655, 1988.
93. Vanderstigel, M., Leclercq, R., Brun-Buisson, C., Schaeffer, A., and Duval, J. Blood-borne pulmonary infection with *Nocardia asteroides* in a heroin addict. *J. Clin. Microbiol.*, 23, 175, 1986.
94. Uttamchandani, R. B., Daikos, G. L., Reyes, R. R., et al. Nocardiosis in 30 patients with advanced human immunodeficiency virus infection: clinical features and outcome. *Clin. Infect. Dis.*, 18, 348, 1994.
95. Seggev, J. S. Fatal pulmonary nocardiosis in a patient with chronic mucocutaneous candidiasis. *J. Allergy Clin. Immunol.*, 94, 259, 1994.
96. Andriole, V. T., Baldas, M., and Wilson, G. L. The association of nocardiosis and pulmonary alveolar proteinosis. *Ann. Intern. Med.*, 60, 266, 1964.
97. Anonymous. Case records of the Massachusetts General Hospital. Weekly clinicopathological exercises: case 18 - 1988. A 30-year-old man with bilateral pulmonary consolidation and cavitation. *N. Engl. J. Med.*, 318, 1186, 1988.
98. Burbank, B., Morrione, T. G., and Cutler, S. S. Pulmonary alveolar proteinosis and nocardiosis. *Am. J. Med.*, 28, 1002, 1960.
99. Teleghani-Far, M., Barber, J. B., Sampson, C., and Marsden, K. A. Cerebral nocardiosis and pulmonary alveolar proteinosis. *Am. Rev. Respir. Dis.*, 89, 561, 1964.

100. Pascual, J., Sureda, A., Gomez Aguinaga, M. A., and Vidal, R. Alveolar proteinosis: a report of a case treated by total bronchopulmonary lavage. *Ann. Med. Intl.*, 7, 276, 1990.
101. Oerlemans, W. G., Jansen, E. N., Prevo, R. L., and Eijsvogel, M. M. Primary cerebellar nocardiosis and alveolar proteinosis. *Acta Neurol. Scand.*, 97, 138–141. 1998.
102. Debieuvre, D., Dalphin, J. C., Jacoulet, P., Breton, J. L., Boiron, P., and Depierre, A. Disseminated infection due to an unusual strain of *Nocardia farcinica. Rev. Mal. Respir.*, 10, 356, 1993.
103. Borges, A. A., Krasnow, S. H., Wadleigh, R. G., and Cohen, M. H. Nocardiosis after corticosteroid therapy for malignant thymoma. *Cancer*, 71, 1746, 1993.
104. Borget, C., Gepner, P., Piette, A. M., and Chapman, A. Primary *Nocardia asteroides* deltoid abscess in treated Horton disease. *Rev. Rhum. Mal. Osteoartic.*, 59, 149, 1992.
105. Fernandez Pelaez, J. M., Sanchez Martin, E. Polo Romero, F. J., and Sez Mendez, L. Lung infection caused by *Aspergillus fumigatus* and *Nocardia asteroides* as complication of glucocorticoid treatment. *Med. Clin. (Barc.)* 114, 358, 2000 (see also: *Med. Clin. (Barc.)* 113, 549–555, 1999).
106. Kukurai, M., Hiraga, T., Yamada, T., Usui, K., Kiyosawa, T., and Nakagawa, H. Subcutaneous nocardial abscesses in a patient with bullous pemphigoid during immunosuppressive therapy: report of a case and review of the literature. *J. Dermatol.*, 26, 829–833, 1999.
107. Anonymous. *Nocardia asteroides* pericarditis. *Mayo Clin. Proc.*, 65, 1276, 1990.
108. Kessler, R., Follis, F., Daube, D., and Wernly, J. Constrictive pericarditis from *Nocardia asteroides* infection. *Ann. Thorac. Surg.*, 52, 861, 1991.
109. Leung, W. H., Wong, K. L., Lau, C. P., and Wong, C. K. Purulent pericarditis and cardiac tamponade caused by *Nocardia asteroides* in mixed connective tissue disease. *J. Rheumatol.*, 17, 1237, 1990.
110. Poland, G. A., Jorgensen, C. R., and Sarosi, G. A. *Nocardia asteroides* pericarditis: report of a case and review of the literature. *Mayo Clin. Proc.*, 65, 819, 1990.
111. Hornick, P., Harris, P., and Smith, P. *Nocardia asteroides* purulent pericarditis. *Eur. J. Cardiothorac. Surg.* 9, 468, 1995.
112. Susens, G. P., Al-Shamma, A., Rowe, J. C., Herbert, C. C., Bassis, M., and Coggs, G. C. Purulent constrictive pericarditis caused by *Nocardia asteroides. Ann. Intern. Med.*, 67, 1021, 1967.
113. Gaude, G. S., Hemashettar, B. M., Bagga, A. S., and Chatterji, R. Clinical profile of pulmonary nocardiosis. *Indian J. Chest Dis. Allied Sci.*, 41, 153–157, 1999.
114. Nenoff, P., Kellermann, S., Borte, G., et al. Pulmonary nocardiosis with cutaneous involvement mimicking a metastasizing lung carcinoma in a patient with chronic myelogenous leukaemia. *Eur. J. Dermatol.*, 10, 47–51, 2000.
115. Boudoulas, O. and Camisa, C. *Nocardia asteroides* infection with dissemination to skin and joints. *Arch. Dermatol.*, 121, 898, 1985.
116. Naguib, M. T. and Fine, D. P. Brain abscess due to *Nocardia brasiliensis* hematogenously spread from a pulmonary infection. *Clin. Infect. Dis.*, 21, 459, 1995.
117. Welsh Lozano, O. and Lopez Lopez, J. R. Mycetomas with pulmonary dissemination. *Med. Cutan. Ibero Lat. Am.*, 13, 517, 1985.
118. Presant, C. A., Wiernik, P. H., and Serpick, A. A. Factors affecting survival in nocardiosis. *Am. Rev. Respir. Dis.*, 108, 1444, 1973.
119. Kontoyiannis, D. P., Ruoff, K., and Hooper, D. C. *Nocardia* bacteremia. Report of 4 cases and review of the literature. *Medicine (Baltimore)*, 77, 255–267, 1998.
120. Findley, J. C., Arafah, B. M., Silverman, P., and Aron, D. C. Cushing's syndrome with cranial and pulmonary lesions: necessity for tissue diagnosis. *South. Med. J.*, 85, 204, 1992.
121. Idemyor, V. and Cherubin, C. E. Pleurocerebral *Nocardia* in a patient with human immunodeficiency virus. *Ann. Pharmacother.*, 26, 188, 1992.
122. Ohguni, S., Yamamoto, D., Furuya, H., et al. A case of adult T-cell leukemia (ATL) complicated with multiple nocardial abscesses. *Kansenshogaku Zasshi*, 65, 1459, 1991.
123. Tanaka, M., Sato, Y., Ito, H., Ichikawa, Y., Oizumi, K., and Shigemori, M. A case of Cushing's syndrome associated with *Nocardia* cerebral abscess. *Kansenshogaku Zasshi*, 65, 243, 1991.
124. Buxton, N. and McIntosh, J. Multiple nocardial brain abscesses: report of two patients. *Br. J. Neurosurg.*, 8, 501, 1994.
125. Coutant-Perronne, V., Lutz, V., Mainardi, J. L., Acar, J. F., Kugelstadt, P., and Goldstein, F. Méningite a *Nocardia* sans abscès cérébral a la scanographie. *Presse Med.*, 24, 1271, 1995.
126. Philit, F., Boibieux, A., Coppere, B., Reverdy, M. E., Peyramond, D., and Bertrand, J. L. *Nocardia asteroides* meningitis without brain abscess in a nonimmunodepressed adult. *Presse Med.*, 23, 346, 1994.
127. Kulkarni, S. A. and Kulkarni, A. G. Disseminated nocardiosis. *J. Assoc. Physicians India*, 39, 779, 1991.
128. Raghavan, R., Date, A., and Bhaktaviziam, A. Fungal and nocardial infections of the kidney. *Histopathology*, 11, 9, 1987.
129. Roman, H. O., Vilar, J. H., Corrales, J. L., and Lanari Zubiaur, F. J. Liver abscess caused by *Nocardia*: report of a case. *Rev. Esp. Enferm. Apar. Dig.*, 80, 282, 1991.
130. Almekinders, L. C. and Lechiewicz, P. F. *Nocardia* osteomyelitis: case report and review of the literature. *Orthopedics*, 12, 1583, 1989.
131. Awad, I., Bay, J. W., and Petersen, J. M. Nocardial osteomyelitis of the spine with epidural spinal cord compression - a case report. *Neurosurgery* 15, 254.
132. De Luca, J., Walsh, B., Robbins, W., and Visconti, E. B. *Nocardia asteroides* osteomyelitis. *Postgrad. Med. J.*, 62, 673, 1986.

133. Guiral, J., Refolio, C., Carrero, P., and Carbajosa, S. Sacral osteomyelitis due to *Nocardia asteroides*: a case report. *Acta Orthop. Scand.*, 62, 389, 1991.
134. Laurin, J. M., Resnik, C. S., Wheeler, D., and Needleman, B. W. Vertebral osteomyelitis caused by *Nocardia asteroides*: report and review of the literature. *J. Rheumatol.*, 18, 455, 1991.
135. Masters, D. L., and Lentino, J. R. Cervical osteomyelitis related to *Nocardia asteroides*. *J. Infect. Dis.*, 149, 824, 1984.
136. Petersen, J. M., Awad, I., Ahmad, M., Bay, J. W., and McHenry, M. C. *Nocardia* osteomyelitis and epidural abscess in the nonimmunocompromised host. *Cleve. Clin. Q.*, 50, 453, 1983.
137. Law, B. J. and Marks, M. I. Pediatric nocardiosis. *Pediatrics*, 70, 560, 1982.
138. Schwartz, J. G. and Tio, F. O. Nocardial osteomyelitis: a case report and review of the literature. *Diagn. Microbiol. Infect. Dis.*, 8, 37, 1987.
139. Price, N. C., Frith, P. A., and Awdry, P. N. Intraocular nocardiosis: a further case and review. *Int. Ophthalmol.*, 13, 177, 1989.
140. Lakosha, H., Pavlin, C. J., and Lipton, J. Subretinal abscess due to *Nocardia farsinica* infection. *Retina*, 20, 269–274, 2000.
141. Curley, R. K., Hayward, T., and Holden, C. A., Cutaneous abscesses due to systemic nocardiosis - a case report. *Clin. Exp. Dermatol.*, 15, 459, 1990.
142. Kalb, R. E., Kaplan, M. H., and Grossman, M. E. Cutaneous nocardiosis: case reports and review. *J. Am. Acad. Dermatol.*, 13, 125, 1985.
143. Nishimoto, K. and Ohno, M. Subcutaneous abscesses caused by *Nocardia brasiliensis* complicated by malignant lymphoma: a survey of cutaneous nocardiosis reported in Japan. *Int. J. Dermatol.*, 24, 437, 1985.
144. Yu, C. T., Tsai, Y. H., Leu, H. S., and Shieh, W. B. Pulmonary nocardiosis with skin and subcutaneous dissemination: an imitator mimicking tuberculosis. *Chang Keng I Hsueh*, 15, 54, 1992.
145. Clague, H. W., Harth, M., Hellyer, D., and Morgan, W. K. Septic arthritis due to *Nocardia asteroides* in association with pulmonary alveolar proteinosis. *J. Rheumatol.*, 9, 469, 1982.
146. Cons, F., Trevino, A., and Lavalle, C. Septic arthritis due to *Nocardia brasiliensis*. *J. Rheumatol.*, 12, 1019, 1985.
147. Di Vittorio, G., Carpenter, J. T. Jr., and Bennett, J. C. Arthritis in systemic nocardiosis. *South. Med. J.*, 75, 507, 1982.
148. Koll, B. S., Brown, A. E., Kiehn, T. E., and Armstrong, D. Disseminated *Nocardia brasiliensis* infection with septic arthritis. *Clin. Infect. Dis.*, 15, 469, 1992.
149. Barnicoat, M. J., Wierzbicki, A. S., and Norman, P. M. Cerebral nocardiosis in immunosuppressed patients: five cases. *Q. J. Med.*, 72, 689, 1989.
150. Palomares, M., Martinez, T., Pastor, J., et al. Cerebral abscess caused by *Nocardia asteroids* in renal transplant recipient. *Nephrol. Dial. Transplant.*, 14, 2950–2952, 1999.
151. Cox, F. and Hughes, W. T. Contagious and other aspects of nocardiosis in the compromised host. *Pediatrics*, 55, 135, 1975.
152. Baddour, L. M., Baselski, V. S., Herr, M. J., Christensen, G. D., and Bisno, A. L. Nocardiosis in recipients of renal transplants: evidence for nosocomial acquisition. *Am. J. Infect. Control*, 14, 214, 1986.
153. Hellyar, A. G. Experience with *Nocardia asteroides* in renal transplant recipients. *J. Hosp. Infect.*, 12, 13, 1988.
154. Houang, E. T., Lovett, I. S., Thompson, F. D., Harrison, A. R., Joekes, A. M., and Goodfellow, M. *Nocardia asteroides* infection: a transmissible disease. *J. Hosp. Infect.*, 1, 31, 1980.
155. Wenger, P. N., Brown, J. M., McNeil, M. M., and Jarvis, W. R. *Nocardia farcinica* sternotomy site infections in patients following open heart surgery. *J. Infect. Dis.*, 178, 1539–1543, 1998.
156. Long, P. F. A retrospective study of *Nocardia* infections associated with the acquired immune deficiency syndrome (AIDS). *Infection*, 22, 362, 1994.
157. Lee, C. C., Loo, L. W., and Lam, M. S. Case reports of nocardiosis in patients with human immunodeficiency virus (HIV) infection. *Ann. Acad. Med. Singapore*, 29, 119–126, 2000.
158. Bava, J., Franchi, M., Bellegarde, E., and Negroni, R. Acid fast filaments in stool samples from an AIDS patient. *Medicina (B. Aires)*, 58, 733–735, 1998.
159. Ogg, G., Lynn, W. A., Peters, M., Curati, W., McLaughlin, J. E., and Shaunak, S. Cerebral nocardia abscesses in a patient with AIDS: correlation of magnetic resonance and white cell scanning images with neuropathological findings. *J. Infect.*, 35, 311–313, 1997.
160. Zwerski, S., Witebsky, F. G., Conville, P. S., Gill, V. J., and Freifeld, A. G. Fatal *Nocardia* pulmonary infection in a child with acquired immunodeficiency syndrome and lymphoid interstitial pneumonitis. *Pediatr. Infect. Dis. J.*, 16, 1088–1089, 1997.
161. Bonacini, M. and Walden, J. M. *Nocardia brasiliensis* peritonitis in a patient with AIDS. *Am. J. Gastroenterol.*, 85, 1432, 1990.
162. Sieratzki, H. J. *Nocardia brasiliensis* infection in patients with AIDS. *Clin. Infect. Dis.*, 14, 977, 1992.
163. Sieratzki, H. J. Nocardiosis in patients with AIDS. *Clin. Infect. Dis.*, 15, 370, 1992.
164. Miralles, G. D. Disseminated *Nocardia farcinica* infection in an AIDS patient. *Eur. J. Clin. Microbiol. Infect. Dis.*, 13, 497, 1994.
165. Parmentier, L., Salmon-Ceron, D., and Boiron, P. Pneumonopathy and kidney abscess due to *Nocardia farcinica* in an HIV-infected patient. *AIDS*, 6, 891, 1992.
166. Struillou, L. and Raffi, F. Cerebro-meningeal infections in patients with human immunodeficiency virus infections. *Rev. Prat.*, 44, 2187, 1994.

167. Lynn, W., Whyte, M., and Weber, J. Nocardia, mycobacteria and AIDS. *AIDS*, 3, 766, 1989.
168. Cherubin, C. E. Nocardiosis in patients with AIDS. *Clin. Infect. Dis.*, 15, 370, 1992.
169. Holtz, H. A., Lavery, D. P., and Kapila, R. *Actinomycetales* infection in the acquired immunodeficiency syndrome. *Ann. Intern. Med.*, 102, 203, 1992.
170. Rivero, A. Esteve, A., Santos, J., and Marquez, M. Cardiac tamponade caused by *Nocardia asteroides* in an HIV-infected patient. *J. Infect.*, 40, 206–207, 2000.
171. Niedt, G. W., and Schinella, R. A. Acquired immunodeficiency syndrome: clinicopathologic study of 56 autopsies. *Arch. Pathol. Lab. Med.*, 109, 727, 1985.
172. Schinella, R., Chaitin, B., and Gross, E. The AIDS autopsy: comparison of intravenous drug abusers with non-intravenous drug abusers, in *Progress in AIDS Pathology*, Rotterdam, H. and Sommers, S. C., Eds. Field and Wood, New York, 219, 1989.
173. Laurent, F., Mick, V., and Boiron, P. *Nocardia* infections: clinical and biological aspects. *Ann. Biol. Clin. (Paris)*, 57, 545–554, 1999.
174. Lerner, P. I. Pneumonia due to *Actinomyces*, *Arachnia*, and *Nocardia*, in *Respiratory Infections: Diagnosis and Management*, Pennington, J. E., Ed. Raven Press, New York, 387, 1983.
175. Weed, L. A., Andersen, H. A., Good, A., and Baggenstoss, A. H. Nocardiosis: clinical, bacteriologic and pathological aspects. *N. Engl. J. Med.*, 253, 1137, 1955.
176. Aisu, T. O., Eriki, P. P., Morrisey, A. B., Ellner, J. J., and Daniel, T. M. Nocardiosis mimicking pulmonary tuberculosis in Ugandan AIDS patients. *Chest*, 100, 888, 1991.
177. Bhagat, K., Ibrahim, H., and Naik, K. Not everything acid-fast is *Mycobacterium tuberculosis* - a case of *Nocardia*. *Cent. Afr. J. Med.*, 45, 217–220, 1999.
178. Mousa, H. A. Tuberculosis of bones and joints: diagnostic approaches. *Int. Orthop.*, 22, 245–246, 1998.
179. Georg, L. K., Ajello, L., McDurmont, C., and Hosty, T. S. The identification of *Nocardia asteroides* and *Nocardia brasiliensis*. *Am. Rev. Respir. Dis.*, 84, 337, 1961.
180. Simpson, G. L., Raffin, T. A., and Remington, J. S. Association of prior nocardiosis and subsequent occurence of nontuberculous mycobacteriosis in a defined, immunosuppressed population. *J. Infect. Dis.*, 146, 211, 1982.
181. Ruiz, L. M., Montejo, M., Benito, J. R., et al. Simultaneous pulmonary infection by *Nocardia asteroides* and *Pneumocystis carinii* in a renal transplant patient. *Nephrol. Dial. Transplant.*, 11, 711, 1996.
182. Perschak, H., Gubler, J., Speich, R., and Russi, E. Pulmonary nocardiosis concurent with *Pneumocystis carinii* pneumonia in two patients undergoing immunosuppressive therapy. *J. Infect.*, 23, 183, 1991.
183. Shafiq, M., Schoch, P. E., Cunha, B. A., and Illescu, M. D. *Nocardia asteroides* and *Cryptococcus neoformans* lung abscess. *Am. J. Med.*, 109, 70–71, 2000.
184. Soto-Mendoza, N. and Bonifaz, A. Head actinomycetoma with a double aetiology caused by *Nocardia brasiliensis* and *N. asteroides*. *Br. J. Dermatol.*, 143, 192–194, 2000.
185. Filice, G. A. and Simpson, G. L. Management of *Nocardia* infections, in *Current Clinical Topics in Infectious Diseases*, vol. 5, Remington, J. S. and Swartz, M. N., Eds. McGraw- Hill Book Co., New York, 49, 1984.
186. King, C. T., Chapman, S. W., and Butkus, D. E. Recurrent nocardiosis in renal transplant recipient. *South. Med. J.*, 86, 225, 1993.
187. Byrne, E., Brophy, B. P., and Perrett, L. V. *Nocardia* cerebral abscess: new concepts in diagnosis, management, and prognosis. *J. Neurol. Neurosurg. Psychiatry*, 42, 1038, 1979.
188. Madiba, T. E., Hoosen, A. A., Madaree, A., and Abdool Carrim, A. T. O. Surgical excision of scalp mycetoma due to *Nocardia*. *Trop. Geogr. Med.*, 46, 185, 1994.
189. Granier, F., Kahla-Clemenceau, N., Richardin, F., et al. *Nocardia farcinica* infection: cutaneous form in an immunodepressed patient. *Presse Med.*, 23, 329, 1994.
190. Adair, J. C., Beck, A. C., Apfelbaum, R. I., and Baringer, J. R. Nocardial cerebral abscess in the acquired immunodeficiency syndrome. *Arch. Neurol.*, 44, 548, 1987.
191. Lopez, E., Ferrero, M., Lumbreras, C., Gimeno, C., Gonzalez-Pinto, I., and Palengue, E. A case of transient nocardiosis and literature review. *Eur. J. Clin. Microbiol. Infect. Dis.*, 13, 310, 1994.
192. Terraza, S., Ramos, C., Revillo, M. J., Gracia, M., Vitoria, I., and Moles, B. Pulmonary infection by *Nocardia farcinica*. *Enferme Infecc. Microbiol. Clin.*, 17, 258–259, 1999.
193. Schaal, K. P. and Lee, H. J. Actinomycetes infections in humans - a review. *Gene*, 115, 201, 1992.
194. Boiron, P., Provost, F., Chevrier, G., and Dupont, B. Review of nocardial infections in France 1987 to 1990. *Eur. J. Clin. Microbiol. Infect. Dis.*, 11, 709, 1992.
195. Wallace, R. J. Jr., Tsukamura, M., Brown, B. A., et al. Cefotaxime-resistant *Nocardia asteroides* strains are isolates of the controversial species *Nocardia farcinica*. *J. Clin. Microbiol.*, 28, 2726, 1990.
196. Yazawa, K., Mikami, Y., and Uno, J. In vitro susceptibility of *Nocardia* spp. to a new fluoroquinolone, tosufloxacin (T-3262). *Antimicrob. Agents Chemother.*, 33, 2140, 1989.
197. Frazier, A. R., Rosenow, E. C. III, and Roberts, G. D. Nocardiosis: a review of 25 cases occuring during 24 months. *Mayo Clin. Proc.*, 50, 657, 1975.
198. Roberts, S. A., Bartley, J., Braatvedt, G., and Ellis-Pegler, R. B. *Nocardia asteroides* as a cause of sphenoidal sinusitis: case report. *Clin. Infect. Dis.*, 21, 1041, 1995.
199. Geisler, P. J. and Andersen, B. R. Results of therapy in systemic nocardiosis. *Am. J. Med. Sci.*, 278, 188, 1979.
200. Chosidow, O., Wolkenstein, P., Bagot, M., et al. *Nocardia asteroides* septicemia in a pemphigus patient: successful treatment with trimethoprim-sulfamethoxazole and amikacin association. *Dermatologica*, 181, 311, 1990.

201. Rice, S. A., Barton, L. L., and Gartner, G. S. Fever and skin lesions in a five-year-old boy. *Pediatr. Infect. Dis. J.*, 12, 887, 1993.
202. Mamelak, A. N., Obana, W. G., Flaherty, J. F., and Rosenblum, M. L. Nocardial brain abscess: treatment strategies and factors influencing outcome. *Neurosurgery*, 35, 622, 1994.
203. Casty, F. E. and Wencel, M. Endobronchial nocardiosis. *Eur. Respir. J.*, 7, 1903, 1994.
204. Adams, H. G., Beeler, B. A., Wann, L. S., Chin, C. K., and Brooks, G. F. Synergistic action of trimethoprim and sulfamethoxazole for *Nocardia asteroides*: efficacious therapy in five patients. *Am. J. Med.*, 287, 8, 1984.
205. Welsh, O., Salinas, M. C., and Rodriguez, M. A. Treatment of eumycetoma and actinomycetoma. *Curr. Top. Med. Mycol.*, 6, 47, 1995.
206. Lyos, A. T., Tuchler, R. E., Malpica, A., and Spira, M. Primary soft-tissue nocardiosis. *Ann. Plast. Surg.*, 34, 212, 1995.
207. Huang, C. C., Lee, C. C., and Chu, N. S. A case of cerebral nocardiosis successfully treated with trimethoprim-sulfamethoxazole. *J. Formos. Med. Assoc.*, 90, 407, 1991.
208. de la Hoz Caballer, B., Fernandez-Rivas, M., Fraj Lazaro, J., et al. Management of sulfadiazine allergy in patients with acquired immunodeficiency syndrome. *J. Allergy Clin. Immunol.*, 88, 137, 1991.
209. Jansen, C., Frenay, H. M., Vandertop, W. P., and Visser, M. R. Intracerebral *Nocardia asteroides* abscess treated by neurosurgical aspiration and combined therapy with sulfadiazine and cefotaxime. *Clin. Neurol. Neurosurg.*, 93, 253, 1991.
210. Fraj Lazaro, J., de la Hoz Caballer, B., Davilla Gonzalez, I., Puyana Ruiz, J., and Alvarez Cuesta, E. Desensitization to sulfadiazine in patients with AIDS and opportunistic infection. *Rev. Clin. Esp.*, 185, 167, 1989.
211. Geiseler, P. J. and Andersen, B. R. Results of therapy in systemic nocardiosis. *Am. J. Med. Sci.*, 278, 188, 1979.
212. Portoles, J., Torralbo, A., Prats, D., Blanco, J., and Barrientos, A. Acute renal failure and sulphadiazine crystalluria in kidney transplant. *Nephrol. Dial. Transplant.*, 9, 180, 1994.
213. Baikie, A. G., Macdonald, C. B., and Mundy, G. R. Systemic nocardiosis treated with trimethoprim and sulfamethoxazole. *Lancet*, 2, 261, 1970.
214. Pourmand, G., Jazaeri, S. A., Mehrsai, A., Kalhori, S., and Afshar, K. Nocardiosis: report of four cases in renal transplant recipients. *Transplant. Proc.*, 27, 2731, 1995.
215. Maderazo, E. G. and Quintiliani, R. Treatment of nocardial infection with trimethoprim and sulfamethoxazole. *Am. J. Med.*, 57, 671, 1974.
216. Wallace, R. J. Jr., Septimus, E. J., Williams, T. W., et al. Use of trimethoprim-sulfamethoxazole for treatment of infections due to nocardia. *Rev. Infect. Dis.*, 4, 315, 1982.
217. Stevens, D. A. Clinical and clinical laboratory aspects of nocardial infection. *J. Hyg.*, 91, 377, 1983.
218. Burman, L. G. Significance of the sulfonamide component for the clinical efficacy of trimethoprim-sulfonamide combinations. *Scand. J. Infect. Dis.*, 18, 89, 1986.
219. Burman, L. G. The antimicrobial activities of trimethoprim and sulfonamides. *Scand. J. Infect. Dis.*, 18, 3, 1986.
220. Cockerill, F. R. III and Edson, R. S. Trimethoprim-sulfamethoxazole. *Mayo Clin. Proc.*, 62, 921, 1987.
221. Spehn, J., Grosser, S., Jessel, A., von Essen, J., and Klose, G. High-dosage cotrimoxazole therapy of disseminated *Nocardia brasiliensis* infection. *Dtsch. Med. Wochenschr.*, 111, 215, 1986.
222. Schiff, T. A., McNeil, M. M., and Brown, J. M. Cutaneous *Nocardia farcinica* infection in a nonimmunocompromised patient: case report and review. *Clin. Infect. Dis.* 16, 756, 1993.
223. Simmons, B. P., Gelfand, M. S., and Roberts, G. D. *Nocardia otitidiscaviarum* (*caviae*) infection in a heart transplant patient presented as having a thigh abscess (Madura thigh). *J. Heart Lung Transplant.*, 11, 824, 1992.
224. Antonow, D. R. Acute pancreatitis associated with trimethoprim-sulfamethoxazole. *Ann. Intern. Med.*, 104, 363, 1986.
225. Nyberg, G., Gabel, H., Althoff, P., Bjork, S., Herlitz, H., and Brynger, H. Adverse effect of trimethoprim on kidney function in renal transplant patients. *Lancet*, 1, 394, 1984.
226. Ringdén, O., Myrenfors, P., Klintmalm, G., Tyden, G., and Ost, L. Nephrotoxicity by cotrimazole and cyclosporine in transplanted patients. *Lancet*, 1, 1016, 1984.
227. Sands, M. and Brown, R. B. Interactions of cyclosporine with antimicrobial agents. *Rev. Infect. Dis.*, 11, 691, 1989.
228. Thompson, J. F., Chalmers, D. H. K., Hunnisett, A. G. W., Wood, R. F. M., and Morris, P. J. Nephrotoxicity of trimethoprim and cotrimoxazole in renal allograft recipients treated with cyclosporine. *Transplantation*, 36, 204, 1983.
229. Bennett, J. E. and Jennings, A. E. Factors influencing susceptibility of *Nocardia* species to trimethoprim-sulfamethoxazole. *Antimicrob. Agents Chemother.*, 13, 624, 1978.
230. Gordin, F. M., Simon, G. L., Wofsy, C. B., and Mills, J. Adverse reactions to trimethoprim- sulfamethoxazole in patients with the acquired immunodeficiency syndrome. *Ann. Intern. Med.*, 100, 495, 1984.
231. Young, L. S., Armstrong, D., Blevins, A., and Lieberman, P. *Nocardia asteroides* infection complicating neoplastic disease. *Am. J. Med.*, 50, 356, 1971.
232. Wheeler, J. S., Culkin, D. J., O'Connell, J., and Winters, G. *Nocardia* epididymo-orchitis in an immunosuppressed patient. *J. Urol.*, 136, 1314, 1986.
233. Geelhoed, G. W. and Myers, G. H., Nocardiosis of the testis. *J. Urol.*, 111, 791, 1974.
234. Strong, D. W. and Hodges, C. V. Disseminated nocardiosis presenting as testicular abscess. *Urology*, 1, 57, 1976.
235. Kim, J., Minamoto, G. Y., Hoy, C. D., and Grieco, M. H. Presumptive cerebral *Nocardia asteroides* infection in AIDS: treatment with ceftriaxone and minocycline. *Am. J. Med.*, 90, 656, 1991.
236. Wren, M. V., Savage, A. M., and Alford, R. H. Apparent cure of intracranial *Nocardia asteroides* infection by minocycline. *Arch. Intern. Med.*, 139, 249, 1979.
237. Paredes, B. E., Hunger, R. E., Braathen, L. R., and Brand, C. U. Cutaneous nocardiosis caused by *Nocardia brasiliensis* after an insect bite. *Dermatology*, 198, 159–161, 1999.
238. Avram, M. M., Ramachandran Nair, S., Lipner, H. I., and Cherubin, C. E. Persistent nocardemia following renal transplantation: association with pulmonary nocardiosis. *J. Am. Med. Assoc.*, 239, 2779, 1978.

239. Bach, M. C., Monaco, A. P., and Finland, M. Pulmonary nocardiosis: therapy with minocycline and with erythromycin plus ampicillin. *J. Am. Med. Assoc.*, 224, 1378, 1973.
240. Yogev, R., Greenslade, T., Firlit, C. F., and Lewy, P. Successful treatment of *Nocardia asteroides* infection with amikacin. *J. Paediatr.*, 96, 771, 1980.
241. Berkey, P., Moore, D., and Rolston, K. In vitro susceptibilities of *Nocardia* species to newer antimicrobial agents. *Antimicrob. Agents Chemother.*, 32, 1078, 1988.
242. Gombert, M. E. Susceptibility of *Nocardia asteroides* to various antibiotics, including newer beta-lactams, trimethoprim-sulfamethoxazole, amikacin, and *N*-formimidoyl theinamycin. *Antimicrob. Agents Chemother.*, 21, 1011, 1982.
243. Wallace, R. J. Jr., Steele, L. C., Sumter, G., and Smith, J. M. Antimicrobial susceptibility patterns of *Nocardia asteroides*. *Antimicrob. Agents Chemother.*, 32, 1776, 1988.
244. Stella, P. R., Vermeulen, E. J., Roggeveen, Ch., Overbosch, E. H., and van Dorp, W. T. Systemic infection with *Nocardia asteroides* cured with amoxicillin/clavulanic acid, erythromycin and ultrasound-guided transcutaneous aspiration. *Neth. J. Med.*, 44, 178, 1994.
245. Fried, J., Hinthorn, D., Ralstin, J., Gerjarusak, P., and Liu, C. Cure of brain abscess caused by *Nocardia asteroides* resistant to multiple antibiotics. *South. Med. J.*, 81, 412, 1988.
246. Lee, M. S. and Sippe, J. R. Primary cutaneous nocardiosis. *Australas. J. Dermatol.*, 40, 103–105, 1999.
247. Velasco, N., Farrington, K., Greenwood, R., and Rahman, A. F. Atypical presentation of systemic nocardiosis and successful treatment with meropenem. *Nephrol. Dial. Transplant.*, 11, 709, 1996.
248. Garcia del Palacio, J. I. and Martin Perez, I. Response of pulmonary nocardiosis to ceftriaxone in a patient with AIDS. *Chest*, 103, 1925, 1993.
249. Lo, W. and Rolston, K. V. Use of imipenem in the treatment of pulmonary nocardiosis. *Chest*, 103, 951, 1993.
250. Mendez-Tovar, L. J., Serrano-Jaen, L., and Almeida-Arvizu, V. M. Combined cefotaxime and amikacin for immunomodulation in the treatment of actinomycetoma resistant to conventional treatment. *Gac. Med. Mex.*, 135, 517–521, 1999.
251. Gombert, M. E. and Aulicino, T. M. Synergism of imipenem and amikacin in combination with other antibiotics against *Nocardia asteroides*. *Antimicrob. Agents Chemother.*, 24, 810, 1983.
252. Gombert, M. E., Aulicino, T. M., duBouchet, L., Silverman, G. E., and Sheinbaum, W. M. Therapy of experimental cerebral nocardiosis with imipenem, amikacin, trimethoprim-sulfamethoxazole, and minocycline. *Antimicrob. Agents Chemother.*, 30, 270, 1986.
253. Garlando, F., Bodmer, T., Lee, C., Zimmerli, W., and Pirovino, M. Successful treatment of disseminated nocardiosis complicated by cerebral abscess with ceftriaxone and amikacin: case report. *Clin. Infect. Dis.*, 15, 1039, 1992.
254. Bartels, R. H., van der Spek, J. A., and Oosten, H. R. Acute pancreatitis due to sulfamethoxazole-trimethoprim. *South. Med. J.*, 85, 1006, 1992.
255. Thaler, F., Gotainer, B., Teodori, G., Dubois, C., and Loirat, P. Mediastinitis due to *Nocardia asteroides* after cardiac transplantation. *Intensive Care Med.*, 18, 127, 1992.
256. Krone, A., Schaal, K. P., Brawanski, A., and Schuknecht, B. Nocardial cerebral abscess cured with imipenem/amikacin and enucleation. *Neurosurg. Rev.*, 12, 333, 1989.
257. Bath, P. M., Pettingale, K. W., and Wade, J. Treatment of multiple subcutaneous *Nocardia asteroides* abscesses with ciprofloxacin and doxycycline. *Postgrad. Med. J.*, 65, 190, 1989.
258. Ruppert, S., Reinold, H. M., Jipp, P., Schroter, G., Egner, E., and Schaal, K. P. Successful antibiotic treatment of a pulmonary infection with *Nocardia asteroides* (biovariety A3). *Dtsch. Med. Wochenschr.*, 113, 1801, 1988.
259. Stasiecki, P., Diehl, V., Vlaho, M., Krueger, G. R., and Schaal, K. P. New effective therapy of systemic infection with *Nocardia asteroides*. *Dtsch. Med. Wochenschr.*, 110, 1733, 1985.
260. King, C. T., Chapman, S. W., and Butkus, D. E. Recurrent nocardiosis in a renal transplant recipient. *South. Med. J.*, 86, 225, 1993.
261. Buggy, B. P. *Nocardia asteroides* meningitis without brain abscess. *Rev. Infect. Dis.*, 9, 228, 1987.
262. Ertl, G., Schaal, K. P., and Kochsiek, K. Nocardial endocarditis of an aortic valve prosthesis. *Br. Heart J.*, 57, 384, 1987.
263. Bauwens, M., Hauet, T., Crevel, J., Goujon, J., Patte, D., and Touchard, G. Nocardiosis in recipients of renal transplants: two case reports. *Transplant. Proc.*, 27, 2430, 1995.
264. Shohaib, S. Nocardial psoas and perinephric abscess in a renal transplant treated by surgery and antibiotics. *Nephrol. Dial. Transplant.*, 9, 1209, 1994.
265. Gomez, A., Saul, A., Bonifaz, A., and Lopez, M. Amocillin and clavulanic acid in the treatment of actinomycetoma. *Int. J. Dermatol.*, 32, 218, 1993.
266. Varma, P. P., Church, S., Gupta, K. L., Sakhuja, V., and Chugh, K. S. Invasive pulmonary aspergillosis and nocardiosis in an immunocompromised host. *J. Assoc. Physicians India*, 41, 237, 1993.
267. Holt, R. I., Kwan, J. T., Sefton, A. M., and Cunningham, J. Successful treatment of concomitant pulmonary nocardiosis and aspergillosis in an immunocompromised renal patient. *Eur. J. Clin. Microbiol. Infect. Dis.*, 12, 110, 1993.
268. Zimmerman, P. L., Mamalis, N., Alder, J. B., Teske, M. P., Tamura, M., and Jones, G. R. Chronic *Nocardia asteroides* endophthalmitis after extracapsular cataract extraction. *Arch. Ophthalmol.*, 111, 837, 1993.
269. Denis, F., Adenis, J. P., and Mounier, M. Intraocular passage of imipenem in man. *Pathol. Biol. (Paris)*, 37, 415, 1989.
270. Srinivasan, M. and Sundar, K. Nocardial endophthalmitis. *Arch. Ophthalmol.*, 112, 871–872, 1994.
271. Marck, Y., Meunier, L., Perez, C., and Meynadier, J. Nocardiose cutanée primitive a *Nocardia asteroides* chez un malade immunodéprimé. *Ann. Dermatol. Venereol.*, 122, 675, 1995.

272. Clark, N. M., Braun, D. K., Pasternak, A., and Chenoweth, C. E. Primary cutaneous *Nocardia otitidiscaviarum* infection: case report and review. *Clin. Infect. Dis.*, 20, 1266, 1995.
273. Freland, C., Fur, J. L., Nemirovsky-Trebucq, B., Lelong, P., and Boiron, P. Primary cutaneous nocardiosis caused by *Nocardia otitidiscaviarum*: two case and a review of the literature. *J. Trop. Med. Hyg.*, 98, 395, 1995.
274. Suzuki, Y., Toyama, K., Utsugi, K., et al. Primary lymphocutaneous nocardiosis due to *Nocardia otitidiscaviarum*: the first case report from Japan. *J. Dermatol.*, 22, 344, 1995.
275. Kimura, K., Hiroi, M., Toyama, K., et al. A case report of pulmonary nocardiosis successfully treated with a combination of sulfamethoxazole-trimethoprim (ST) and sparfloxacin. *Nihon Kokyuki Gakkai Zasshi*, 38, 702–705, 2000.
276. Joshi, N. and Hamory, B. H. Drug-resistant *Nocardia asteroides* infection in a patient with acquired immunodeficiency syndrome. *South. Med. J.*, 84, 1155, 1991.
277. Oda, Y., Kamijyo, Y., and Kang, Y. *Nocardia* brain abscess and ventriculitis - resistance of *Nocardia* to sulfonamides and susceptibilities to beta-lactams. *No Shinkei Geka*, 14(3 Suppl.), 340, 1986.
278. Steingrube, V. A., Wallace, R. J. Jr., Brown, B. A., et al. Acquired resistance of *Nocardia brasiliensis* to clavulanic acid related to change in beta-lactamase following therapy with amoxicillin-clavulanic acid. *Antimicrob. Agents Chemother.*, 35, 524, 1991.
279. Tanaka, Y., Yazawa, K., Dabbs, E. R., et al. Different rifampicin inactivation mechanisms in *Nocardia* and related taxa. *Microbiol. Immunol.*, 40, 1–4, 1996.

5
Oerskovia ssp.

1. INTRODUCTION

Oerskovia species are ubiquitous, non-spore-forming, gram-positive bacteria first described by Orkov in 1938 as motile *Nocardia (1)*; in 1957, Erickson designated the organism as *Nocardia turbata (2)*. In the early 1970s, several other groups also described this *Nocardia*-like *actinomycete (3–5)*. On the basis of its ability to fragment into motile rods, its lack of aerial mycelia, and the presence of large amounts of galactose in the cell wall, in 1970 the organism was distinguished from *N. turbata* as *Orskovia turbata* by Prauser et al. *(6,7)*. A second species, *O. xanthineolytica* was identified by ts ability to degrade xanthine and hypoxanthine *(8)*. So far, only two motile species have been described, *O. turbata* and *O. xanthineolytica*. Other nonmotile *Oerskovia*-like strains have also been identified *(4)*.

Oerskovia species are found in organic material, plants, and brewery sewage. When grown on agar- and broth-based media, *Oerskovia* ssp. develop into yellow pigmented colonies without aerial hyphae, which differentiate them from *Nocardia (5,9)*.

2. TREATMENT OF *OERSKOVIA* INFECTIONS

With the exception of *Corynebacterium diphtheriae*, these species possess a low tendency of pathogenicity in humans. *Oerskovia*-related infections have been described only sporadically mainly in immunocompromised hosts *(2,10–24)* including those with AIDS *(16,23)*. Very often infections have occured in patients with indwelling access devices that allow the organism to bypass nonspecific host defenses *(10–14,25,26)*. In immunocompromised patients even a relatively avirulent bacteria like *Oerskovia* species can cause a severe infection, especially in the presence of a foreign body *(25)*.

Although all patients so far described had survived *Oerskovia* infection, response to antibiotic therapy has been variable. The removal of the access device, if present, was almost always required *(11)*. Vancomycin and trimethoprim-sulfamethoxazole appear to be the only antibiotics to which *Oerskovia* ssp. have been consistently susceptible *(10–14,17,18)* and are, therefore, recommended as the antibiotic treatment of choice *(20,22)*. Vancomycin has been used at 1.0-g dose twice daily for 14 d *(22)*.

Ellerbroek et al. *(25)* described the first *Oerskovia* infection in a bone-marrow transplant recipient with non-Hodgkin lymphoma. The uncertainty of the ensuing antibiotic treatment reflected on the difficulties of treating relapsing bacteremia in the presence of underlying severe immunosuppression with incomplete repopulation after bone-marrow transplant, and the presence of indwelling central venous catheters for prolonged periods of time. The patient responded well after initial treatment with meropenem (2.0 g three times daily); the antibiotic regimen was changed after 3 wk into trimethoprim-sulfamethoxazole (960 mg twice daily) and amoxicillin (6 times, a 2.0-g dose; i.v. then oral). Because of unacceptable side effects, the antibiotic treatment was changed to imipenem-cilastatin (500 mg twice daily) and amikacin (600 mg twice daily; i.v. for 3 wk), followed by clarithromycin and rifampicin orally, and penicillin. The patient died 2 wk later after developing neurological symptoms based on intracerebral relapse of the nonHodgkin's lymphoma.

From: Opportunistic Infections: Treatment and Prophylaxis
By: Vassil St. Georgiev © Humana Press Inc., Totowa, NJ

REFERENCES

1. Orskov, J. Untersuchungen über Strahlenpilze, reingezüchtet aus dänischen Erd-proben. *Zentralbl. Bakteriol. Parasitenkd. Infectionskr. Hyg. Abt.*, 98, 344–357, 1938.
2. Erickson, D. Factors promoting cell division in a soft mycelial type of *Nocardia*: *Nocardia turbata* n. sp. *J. Gen. Microbiol.*, 11, 198–208, 1954.
3. Sottnek, F. O., Brown, J. M., Weaver, R. E., and Caroll, G. F. Recognition of *Oerskovia* species in the clinical laboratory: characterization of 35 isolates. *Int. J. Syst. Bacteriol.* 72, 263–270, 1977.
4. Lechevalier, M. P. Description of a new species, *Orskovia xanthineolytica*, and emendation of *Oerskovia*. *Int. J. Syst. Bacteriol.*, 22, 260–264, 1972.
5. McNeil, M. M. and Brown, J. M. The medically important aerobic actinomycetes: epidemiology and microbiology. *Clin. Microbiol. Rev.*, 7, 357–417, 1994.
6. Prauser, H., Lechevalier, M. P., and Lechevalier, H. Description of *Oerskovia* gen. n. to harbor Orskov's motile *Nocardia*. *Appl. Microbiol.*, 19, 534, 1970.
7. Sukapure, R. S., Lechevalier, M. P., Reber, H., Higgins, M. L., Lechevalier, H. A., and Prauser, H. Motile nocardoid *Actinomycetales*. *Appl. Microbiol.*, 19, 527–533, 1970.
8. Lechevalier, M. P. Description of a new species, *Oerskovia xanthineolytica*, and emendation of *Oerskovia* Prauser et al. *Int. J. Syst. Bacteriol.*, 22, 260–262, 1972.
9. Soto, A., Zapardiel, J., and Soriano, F. Evaluation of API Coryne system identifying coryneform bacteria. *Clin. Pathol.*, 47, 756–759, 1994.
10. Cruickshank, J. G., Gawler, A. H., and Shaldon, *Oerskovia* species: rare opportunistic pathogens. *J. Med. Microbiol.*, 12, 513–515, 1979.
11. Guss, W. J. and Ament, M. E. *Oerskovia* infection caused by contaminated home parenteral nutrition solution. *Arch. Intern. Med.*, 149, 1457–1458, 1989.
12. Hussain, Z., Gonder, J. R., Lannigan, R., and Stoakes, L. Endophthalmitis due to *Oerskovia xanthineolytica*. *Can. J. Ophthalmol.*, 22, 234–236, 1987.
13. Kailath, E. J., Goldstein, E., and Wagner, F. K. Case report: meningitis caused by *Oerskovia xanthineolytica*. *Am. J. Med. Sci.*, 295, 216–217, 1988.
14. Le Prowse, C. R., McNeil, M. M., and McCarty, J. M. Catheter-related bacteremia caused by *Oerskovia turbata*. *J. Clin. Microbiol.*, 27, 571–572, 1989.
15. McDonald, C. L., Chapin-Robertson, K., Dill, S. R., and Martino, R. L. *Oerskovia xanthineolytica* bacteremia in an immunocompromised patient with pneumonia. *Diagn. Microbiol. Infect. Dis.*, 18, 259–261, 1994.
16. Reina, J., Llompart, I., and Altes, J. An auxillary abscess produced by *Oerskovia turbata* in an AIDS patient. *Rev. Clin. Esp.*, 188, 485–486, 1991.
17. Reller, L. B., Maddoux, G. L., Eckman, M. R., and Pappas, G. Bacterial endocarditis caused by *Oerskovia turbata*. *Ann. Intern. Med.*, 83, 664–666, 1975.
18. Rihs, J. D., McNeil, M. M., Brown, J. M., and Yu, V. L. *Oerskovia xanthineolytica* implicated in peritonitis associated with peritoneal dialysis: case report and review of *Oerskovia* infections in humans. *J. Clin. Microbiol.*, 28, 1934–1937, 1990.
19. Truant, A. L., Satishchandran, V., Eisenstaedt, R., Richman, P., and McNeil, M. M. *Oerskovia xanthineolytica* and methiciline resistant *Staphylococcus aureus* in a patient with cirrhosis and variceal hemorrhage. *Eur. J. Clin. Microbiol. Infect. Dis.*, 11, 950–951, 1992.
20. Harrington, R. D., Lewis, C. G., Aslanzadeh, J., Stelmach, P., and Woolfrey, A. E. *Oerskovia xanthineolytica* infection of a prosthetic joint: case report and review. *J. Clin. Microbiol.*, 34, 1821–1824, 1996.
21. Borra, S. and Kleinfeld, M. Peritonitis caused by *Oerskovia xanthineolytica* in a patient on chronic ambulatory dialysis. *Am. J. Kid. Dis.*, 27, 458, 1996.
22. Maguire, J. D., McCarthy, M. C., and Decker, C. F. *Oerskovia xanthineolytica* bacteremia in an immunocompromised host: case report and review. *Clin. Infect. Dis.*, 22, 554–556, 1996.
23. Lair, M. I., Bentolila, S., Grenet, D., et al. *Oerskovia turbata* and *Comamonas acidovorans* in a patient with AIDS. *Eur. J. Clin. Microbiol. Infect. Dis.*, 15, 424–426, 1996.
24. Shah, M., Gentile, R. C., McCormick, S. A., and Rogers, S. H. *Oerskovia xanthineolytica* keratitis. *CLAO*, 22, 96, 1996.
25. Ellerbroek, P., Kuipers, S., Rozenberg-Arska, M., Verdonck, L. F., and Petersen, E. J. *Oerskovia xanthineolytica*: a new pathogen in bone marrow transplantation. *Bone Marrow Transplant.*, 22, 503–505, 1998.
26. Lujan-Zilbermann, J., Jones, D., and De Vincenzo, J. *Oerskovia* xanthineolytica peritonitis: case report and review. *Pediatr. Infect. Dis. J.*, 18, 738–739, 1999.

6
Rhodococcus equi

1. INTRODUCTION

Rhodoccocus equi is a well-recognized bacterial pathogen in veterinary medicine *(1)*. Inhalation or ingestion appears to be the major route of infection in foals, and the primary source of infection is believed to be the soil *(2)*. The taxonomic history of *R. equi* has been rather confusing. Currently, this pathogen is being described *(3)* as either *R. equi* or *Corynebacterium equi*.

In humans, *R. equi* infections are relatively rare, with the first case reported in 1963 *(4)*. Prior to 1983, only 12 cases of human *R. equi* infections were described *(5)*, including cases in immunocompetent patients *(6,7)*. However, with the growing immunocompromised population, *R. equi* has increasingly emerged as an opportunistic pathogen in patients with underlying immunosuppression, and in most cases in people that have a history of contact with farm animals, contaminated soil, and manure *(8)*. The first description of *R. equi* infection in a patient with AIDS was reported in 1986 *(9)*.

In general, impairment of cell-mediated immunity is considered to be the major predisposing factor in humans to *R. equi* infections. In many renal and bone-marrow transplant recipients, and in patients with lymphatic leukemias, treatment with imunosuppressive drugs (cyclosporin A, corticosteroids, antimetabolites) can be inhibitory to mitogen-induced production of interferon-α (IFN-α) by CD4$^+$ lymphocytes *(1)*.

The ability of *R. equi* to remain in and to destroy the macrophages has been the basic feature of its pathogenicity.

Mastroianni et al. *(10)* studied in AIDS patients the antibody response to *R. equi* infection and its correlation with the clinical outcome of the disease. The results indicated that patients who recovered from *R. equi* pneumonia showed a pronounced antibody response to all major bacterial protein antigens; by comaprison, the clinical course was more severe in patients who exhibited a negligible humoral response. The findings of Mastroianni et al. *(10)* may prove to be important because they suggest that a specific antibody production in AIDS patients infected with *R. equi* might be a needed function in the protection against and recovery from *R. equi* pneumonia, possibly by enhancing the uptake and killing the bacteria by alveolar macrophages and neutrophils. In a related study, Catarino-de-Araujo et al. *(11)* searched for an antibody profile of *R. equi* infection in AIDS patients. Because of the diversity of virulence-associated antigens of *R. equi* and host immune dysfunction, these investigators did not detect a characteristic antibody profile among the patients studied, although the presence of specific antibodies in serum samples suggested prognostic value. Positive patient outcome and recovery from pneumonia were correlated with *R. equi* antibody detection, whereas the lack or disappearance of specific antibodies, mainly those to low molecular-weight antigens, was correlated with disease progression and patient death *(11)*.

The increased number of human *R. equi* infections has been associated primarily with underlying immunosuppressive disorders *(4,12–20)*, immunosuppressive chemotherapy (organ-transplant recipients [17,18,22–32], sarcoidosis [33,34]), and with the spread of AIDS *(4,9,11,35–90)*.

From: Opportunistic Infections: Treatment and Prophylaxis
By: Vassil St. Georgiev © Humana Press Inc., Totowa, NJ

The usual manifestations of *R. equi* pneumonia include gradually developing fever (several days to several weeks in duration), malaise, dyspnea, and nonproductive cough; hemoptysis has also been noticed *(1, 91)*. The *R. equi* infection is most often diagnosed as cavitary pneumonia, which is characterized by a high mortality rate despite prolonged antibiotic chemotherapy *(1,10,51,54,65,69,72,92)*. In several reports, *R. equi* infections were associated with penetrating eye injuries *(93,94)*, inflammatory mass in the pelvis *(37)*, bloody diarrhea and cachexia *(39)*, pleural effusion *(95)*, osteomyelitis secondary to a pneumonic episode *(23,29)*, thyroid abscess *(89)*, paraspinal abscess *(17)*, meningitis *(76)*, psoas abscess *(37)*, lung abscess *(12)*, and cervical lymphadenitis *(96)*. Otomastoiditis due to *R. equi* has been rare *(80)*, and disseminated *R. equi* with otomastoiditis has been reported once in an AIDS patient *(79)*.

Cases of pulmonary malacoplakia secondary to *R. equi*-associated pneumonia in AIDS patients have also been described *(52,61,76,81,84,86)*. The occurence of these two conditions was apparently due to a deficiency in cellular immunity and macrophage cellular activity as well as failure of the intracellular bactericidal and phagolysosomal functions *(52)*.

Hamrock et al. *(82)* described disseminated *R. equi* infection in an AIDS patient involving the large intestine; histological examination of colon biopsies showed appearance mimicking Whipple's disease and *Mycobacterium avium-intracellulare* infection.

R. equi infections in children, although rare, have been described, but no pediatric death has thus far been reported *(97)*. Treatment with multiple antibiotics seems to be successful.

2. TREATMENT OF *RHODOCOCCUS EQUI* INFECTION

Treatment of *R. equi* infection in nonHIV-infected patients has comprised either multiple antibiotics alone or a combination of antibiotics and surgery *(43,60,98)*. Relapses have been common, requiring a second course of antibiotics. Dissemination of infection (subcutaneous abscesses *[1,15]*, multiple brain abscesses *[5,72,99]*, lung, kidneys, brain, bloodstream *[70]*, and osteomyelitis *[23]*) following discontinuation of antimicrobial therapy has been reported on several occasions. By one account *(43)*, the overall mortality from *R. equi* infection in nonHIV-infected patients may reach 20%.

Mycolic acid-containing bacteria, such as *Nocardia* and related taxa (*Rhodococcus*), are known to inactivate rifampicin in a variety of species-specific ways including glucosylation, ribosylation, phosphorylation, and decolarization. To this end, *Rhodococcus* modifies rifampicin by phosphorylation of the 21-OH group of the antibiotic *(110)*.

A review of the treatment of *R. equi* disease in HIV-infected patients showed that patients had received multiple antibiotic treatments comprising, on average, 4.1 antibiotics during the course of their illness *(43)*. Relapses were frequent after discontinuation of therapy *(71,100)*. Mortality rates for patients undergoing surgery was 50%, a value similar to the 57% of those receiving antibiotics alone *(43)*.

The selection of lipid-soluble antibiotics capable of intracellular penetration has been considered to be critical for the successful treatment of *R. equi* disease. Antibiotic susceptibilities of 24 *R. equi* isolates tested showed the following values (in %): vancomycin *(100)*, rifampin *(100)*, tobramycin *(100)*, streptomycin *(100)*, erythromycin *(95)*, chloramphenicol *(92)*, gentamicin *(95)*, kanamycin *(86)*, trimethoprim-sulfamethoxazole *(80)*, tetracycline (53), and carbenicillin *(50)*; there was little sensitivity towards ampicillin *(25)*, clindamycin *(22)*, oxacillin *(14)*, cephalothin *(13)*, and penicillin *(9,43)*. In general, there were no differences in the susceptibility patterns between isolates from HIV-infected individuals and those from non-HIV-infected patients. The emergence of multidrug-resistance strains of *R. equi* has been reported *(101)*.

According to Colebunders et al. *(102)*, in three cases of AIDS complicated by *R. equi* infection, despite the fact that the pathogen was susceptible to tetracycline, erythromycin, amikacin, co-trimoxazole, rifampicin, and vancomycin, these antibiotics were not clinically successful. Clinical improvement was noticed only in one patient following teicoplanin and imipenem-cilastatin therapy. Dabbs and Quan *(103)* reported that *R. equi* monooxygenase inactivated rifampicin.

In the experience of Mascellino et al. *(104)*, the combinations of erythromycin-rifampin and imipenem-teicoplanin were the most effective treatments of *R. equi* infections. Resistance to imipenem *(47)*, rifampicin *(66)*, and rifampin-fluoroquinolone *(105)* has been reported.

Combination antibiotic treatments that included clarithromycin *(55)*, imipenem-vancomycin *(56,57)*, imipenem-teicoplanin *(68)*, and erythromycin-rifampin *(98,106,107)*, have also been recommended *(107)*. *R. equi* lung abscess in a patient with Evan's syndrome (autoimmune hemolytic anemia and thrombocytopenia) receiving high-dose corticosteroids, was successfully treated with a combination of clarithromycin, vancomycin, ciprofloxacin and imipenem *(21)*. Frequent relapses (as high as 87.5%) necessitated longer duration of treatment *(107)*.

In addition to using antimicrobial drugs, surgical treatment of human *R. equi* infections included drainage of suppurative lesions and resection of granulomatous tissue. Control of predisposing factors by decreasing the dosage of concurrent immunosuppressive therapy, or controlling underlying malignancies, also have been recommended to prevent *R. equi* infections *(1,43)*.

Scotton et al. *(108)* reported the successful cure of *R. equi*-associated nosocomial meningitis with levofloxacin and shunt removal.

Spark et al. *(109)* have stressed the importance of using biochemical profiles of known non-*equi* strains and ribosomal DNA analysis to identify unequivocally the *Rhodococcus* species.

REFERENCES

1. Prescott, J. F. *Rhodococcus equi*: an animal and human pathogen. *Clin. Microbiol. Rev.*, 4, 20–34, 1991.
2. Barton, M. D. and Hughes, K. L. *Corynebacterium equi*: a review. *Vet. Bull.*, 50, 65, 1980.
3. Skerman, V. D. B., McGowan, V., and Sneath, P. H. A. Approved list of bacterial names. *Int. J. Syst. Bacteriol.*, 30, 225, 1980.
4. Golub, B., Falk, G., and Spink, W. W. Lung abscecess due to *Corynebacterium equi*: report of first human infection. *Ann. Intern. Med.*, 66, 1174, 1967.
5. Van Etta, L. L., Filice, G. A., Ferguson, R. M., and Gerding, D. N. *Corynebacterium equi*: a review of 12 cases of human infection. *Rev. Infect. Dis.*, 5, 1012, 1983.
6. Blanco, J., Yebra, M., Munoz, R., and Burillo. A. Cerebral abscess caused by *Rhodococcus equi* in an immunocompetent patient. *Enfer. Infecc. Microbiol. Clin.*, 16, 294–295, 1998.
7. Sigler, E., Miskin, A., Shtlarid, M., and Berrebi. A. Fever of unknown origin and anemia with *Rhodococcus equi* infection in an immunocompetent patient. *Am. J. Med.*, 104, 510, 1998.
8. Verville, T. D., Huycke, M. M., Greenfield, R. A., Fine, D. P., Kuhls, T. L., and Slater, L. N. *Rhodococcus equi* infections in humans: 12 cases and a review of the literature. *Medicine (Baltimore)*, 73, 119, 1994.
9. Sane, D. C. and Durack, D. T. Infection with *Rhodococcus equi* in AIDS. *N. Engl. J. Med.*, 314, 56, 1986.
10. Mastroianni, C. M., Lichtner, M., Vullo, V., and Delia, S. Humoral immune response to *Rhodococcus equi* in AIDS patients with *R. equi* pneumonia. *J. Infect. Dis.*, 169, 1179, 1994.
11. Caterino-de-Araujo, A., de Los Santos-Fortuna, E., Zandona-Meleiro, M. C., et al. Search for an antibody profile of *Rhodococcus equi* infection in AIDS patients despite the diversity of isolates and patient immune dysfonction. *Microbes. Infect.*, 1, 663–670, 1999.
12. Elissalde, G. S. and Renshaw, H. W. *Corynebacterium equi*: an interhost review with emphasis on the foal. *Comp. Immunol. Microbiol. Infect. Dis.*, 3, 433, 1980.
13. Borleffs, J. C., Petersen, E. J., Kaasjager, K., Teding van Berkhout, F., and Rozenberg-Arska, M. *Rhodococcus equi* pneumonia in patients with immunodeficiency. *Ned. Tijdschr.Geneeskd.*, 138, 2587, 1994.
14. Marsch, J. C. and von Graevenitz, A. Recurrent *Corynebacterium equi* infection with lymphoma. *Cancer*, 32, 147, 1973.
15. Berg, R., Chmel, H., Mayo, J., and Armstrong, D. *Corynebacterium equi* infection complicating neoplastic disease. *Am. J. Clin. Pathol.*, 68, 73, 1977.
16. Gardner, S. E., Pearson, T., and Hughes, W. T. Pneumonitis due to *Corynebacterium equi*. *Chest*, 70, 92, 1976.
17. Jones, M. R., Say, P. J., Neale, T. J., and Horne, J. G. *Rhodococcus equi*: an emerging opportunistic pathogen? *Aust. NZJ. Med.*, 19, 103, 1989.
18. Williams, G. D., Flanigan, W. J., and Campbell, G. S. Surgical management of localized thoracic infections in immunosuppressed patients. *Ann. Thor. Surg.*, 12, 471, 1971.
19. Carpenter, J. L. and Blom, J. *Corynebacterium equi* pneumonia in a patient with Hodgkin's disease. *Am. Rev. Respir. Dis.*, 114, 235, 1987.
20. Akan, H., Akova, M., Ataoglu, H., Aksu, G., Arslan, O., and Koc, H. *Rhodococcus equi* and *Nocardia brasiliensis* infection of the brain, and liver in a patient with acute nonlymphoblastic leukemia. *Eur. J. Clin. Microbiol. Infect. Dis.*, 17, 737–739, 1998.
21. Tsang, K. W., Lam, P. S., Yuen, K. Y., Ooi, C. C., Lam, W., and Ip, M. *Rhodococcus equi* lung abscess complicating Evan's syndrome treated with corticosteroid. *Respiration*, 65, 327–330, 1998.

22. Gainsford, S. A. and Frater, E. Two cases of infection involving *Rhodococcus equi*. *N. Z. J. Med. Lab. Technol.*, 40, 100, 1986.
23. Novak, R. M., Polisky, E. L., Janda, W. M., and Libertin, C. R. Osteomyelitis caused by *Rhodococcus equi* in a renal transplant recipient. *Infection*, 16, 186, 1988.
24. Rubin, R. H. Pneumonia in the compromised host, in *Update: Pulmonary Disease and Disorders*, Fishman, A. P., Ed. McGraw-Hill Book Co., New York, 1, 1982.
25. Savdie, E., Pigott, P., and Jennis, F. Lung abscess due to *Corynebacterium equi* in a renal transplant recipient. *Med. J. Aust.*, 1, 817, 1977.
26. Segovia, J., Pulpón, L. A., Crespo, M. G., et al. *Rhodococcus equi*: first case in a heart transplant recipient. *J. Heart Lung Transplant.*, 13, 332, 1994.
27. Szabo, B., Miszti, C., Majoros, L., Nabradi, Z., and Gomba, S. Isolation of rare opportunistic pathogens in Hungary: case report and short review of the literature. *Acta Microbiol. Immnunol. Hung*, 47, 9–14, 2000.
28. Gallen, F., Kernaonet, E., Foulet, A., Goldstein, A., Lebon, P., and Babinet, F. Pulmonary infection from *Rhodococcus equi* after renal transplantation. Review of the literature. *Nephrologie*, 20, 383–386, 1999.
29. Fischer, L., Sterneck, M., Albrecht, H., Krupski, G., Polywka, S., Rogiers, X., and Broelsch, C. E. Vertebral osteomyelitis due to *Rhodococcus equi* in a liver transplant recipient. *Clin. Infect. Dis.*, 26, 749–752, 1998.
30. Munoz, P., Burillo, A., Palomo, J., Rodriguez-Creixems, M., and Bouza, E. *Rhodococcus equi* infection in transplant recipients: case report and review of the literature. *Transplantation*, 65, 449–453, 1998.
31. La Rocca, E., Gesu, G., Caldara, R., et al. Pulmonary infection caused by *Rhodococcus equi* in a kidney and pancreas transplant recipient: a case report. *Transplantation*, 65, 1524–1525, 1998.
32. Marsh, H. P., Bowler, I. C., and Watson, C. J. Successful treatment of *Rhodococcus equi* pulmonary infection in a renal transplant recipient. *Ann. R. Coll. Surg. Engl.*, 82, 107–108, 2000.
33. Hillerdal, G., Riesenfeldt-örn, I., Pedersen, A., and Ivanicova, E. Infection with *Rhodococcus equi* in a patient with sarcoidosis treated with corticosteroids. *Scand. J. Infect. Dis.*, 20, 673, 1988.
34. Mohammedi, I., Vedrinne, J. M., Floccard, B., Reverdy, M. E., Duperret, S., and Motin, J. Disseminated *Rhodococcus equi* and *Nocardia farcinica* infection in a patient with sarcoidosis. *J. Infect.*, 36, 134–135, 1998.
35. Takai, S., Koike, K., Ohbushi, S., Izumi, C., and Tsubaki, S. Identification of 15- to 17- kilodalton antigens associated with virulent *Rhodococcus equi*. *J. Clin. Microbiol.*, 29, 439, 1991.
36. Bishopric, G. A., d'Agay, M. F., Schlemmer, B., Sarfati, E., and Brocheriou, C. Pulmonary pseudotumour due to *Corynebacterium equi* in a patient with the acquired immunodeficiency syndrome. *Thorax*, 43, 486, 1988.
37. Flerer, J., Wolf, P., Sood, L., Gay, T., Noonan, K., and Haghighi, P. Non-pulmonary *Rhodococcus equi* infections in patients with acquired immune deficiency syndrome (AIDS). *Clin. Pathol.*, 40, 556, 1987.
38. Kunke, P. J. Serious infection in an AIDS patient due to *Rhodococcus equi*. *Clin. Microbiol. Newslett.*, 9, 163, 1987.
39. Samies, J. H., Hathaway, B. N., Echols, R. M., Veazey, J. M. Jr., and Pilon, V. A. Lung abscess due to *Corynebacterium equi*: report of the first case in a patient with acquired immune deficiency syndrome. *Am. J. Med.*, 80, 685, 1986.
40. Sonnet, J., Wauters, G., Zech, F., and Gigi, J. Opportunistic *Rhodococcus equi* infection in an African AIDS case (1976–1981). *Acta Clin. Belg.*, 42, 215, 1987.
41. Wang, H. H., Tollerud, D., Danar, D., Hanff, P., Gottesdiener, K., and Rosen, S. Another Whipple-like disease in AIDS? *N. Engl. J. Med.*, 314, 1577, 1986.
42. Weingarten, J. S., Huang, D. Y., and Jackman, J. D. Jr. *Rhodococcus equi* pneumonia: an unusual early manifestation of the acquired immunodeficiency syndrome (AIDS). *Chest*, 94, 195, 1988.
43. Harvey, R. L. and Sunstrom, J. C. *Rhodococcus equi* infection in patients with and without human immunodeficiency virus infection. *Rev. Infect. Dis.*, 13, 139, 1991.
44. Haglund, L. A., Trotter, J. A., Slater, L. N., Harris, S. L., Rettig, P. J., and Harkess, J. R. Case 9-1989: AIDS and a cavitary pulmonary lesion. *N. Engl. J. Med.*, 321, 395, 1989.
45. MacGregor, J. H., Samuelson, W. M., Sane, D. C., and Godwin, J. D. Opportunistic lung infection caused by *Rhodococcus (Corynebacterium) equi*. *Radiology*, 160, 83, 1986.
46. Marco, M. L., Remacha, A., and Echevarri, B. *Rhodococcus equi* pneumonia in patients with AIDS. *Arch. Bronconeumol.*, 30, 519, 1994.
47. Fernandez, A., Santos, J., Sanchez, M. A., and Alfaro, C. *Rhodococcus equi* pneumonia in a patient with AIDS. *Enferm. Infecc. Microbiol. Clin.* 12, 471, 1994.
48. Legras, A., Lemmens, B., Dequin, P. F., Cattier, B., and Besnier, J. M. Tamponade due to *Rhodococcus equi* in acquired immunodeficiency syndrome. *Chest* 106, 1278, 1994.
49. Figueras Villalba, M. P., Martinez Alvarez, R. M., and Munoz Marco, J. J. Pneumonia by *Rhodococcus equi* in patients with HIV infection. *Ann. Med. Intl.*, 11, 238, 1994.
50. Heudier, P., Taillan, B., Garnier, G., et al. L'infection a *Rhodococcus equi* au cours du sida: un cas avec abcès pulmonaire. Revue de la littérature. *Rev. Med. Interne*, 15, 268, 1994.
51. Nzerue, C. *Rhodococcus equi* infection: a cause of cavitary pulmonary disease in immuno- compromised patients. *Cent. Afr. J. Med.*, 39, 262, 1993.
52. Lemmens, B., Besnier, J. M., Diot, P., et al. Malacoplasie pulmonaire et pneumonie a *Rhodococcus equi* chez un patients infecté par le virus de l'immunodépression humaine: a propos d'un cas avec revue de la littérature. *Rev. Mal. Respir.*, 11, 301, 1994.
53. Fiaccadori, F. Emergent pathologies: *Rhodococcus equi* infection in the acquired immunodeficiency syndrome. *Ann. Ital. Med. Int.*, 9, 10, 1994.

54. Frame, B. C. and Petcus, A. F. *Rhodococcus equi* pneumonia: case report and literature review. *Ann. Pharmacother.*, 27, 1340, 1993.
55. Pialoux, G., Goldstein, F., Dupont, B., Gonzalez Canali, G., and Sansonetti, P. Combination antibiotic treatment with clarithromycin for human immunodeficiency virus-associated *Rhodococcus equi* infection. *Clin. Infect. Dis.*, 17, 513, 1993.
56. Javaloyas, M., Garcia, D., and Ruffi, G. Recurrent abscess of the lung caused by *Rhodococcus equi* in an HIV-positive patient: response to a combination imipenem/vancomycin. *Med. Clin. (Barcelona)*, 100, 759, 1993.
57. Gazquez, I., Garcia Gonzalez, M., Pena, J. M., Rubio, M., and Nogues, A. A pulmonary abscess due to *Rhodococcus equi* in an AIDS patient. *Rev. Clin. Esp.*, 192, 152, 1993.
58. Clotet, B., Sirera, G., and Erice, A. *Rhodococcus equi* infection in HIV-infected patients. *J. Acquir. Immune Defic. Syndr.*, 6, 429, 1993.
59. Piersantelli, N., Casini-Lemmi, M., Cavanna, E., et al. *Rhodococcus equi* infections in AIDS: personal cases. *Pathologica*, 84, 517, 1992.
60. Curry, J. D., Harrington, P. T., and Hosein, I. K. Successful medical therapy of *Rhodococcus equi* pneumonia in a patient with HIV infection. *Chest*, 102, 1619, 1992.
61. Rouveix, E., Dupont, C., Ichai, P., et al. Two particular aspects of *Rhodococcus equi* infection: malacoplakia and acquisition of resistance to antibiotics. *Presse Med.*, 21, 1086, 1992.
62. Pialoux, G. and Dupont, B. Lung abscess caused by *Rhodococcus equi* in HIV infection: two cases. *Presse Med.*, 21, 1086, 1992.
63. Pialoux, G., Fournier, S., Dupont, B., et al. Lung abscess caused by *Rhodococcus (Corynebacterium) equi* in HIV infection: two cases. *Presse Med.*, 21, 417, 1992.
64. Gray, B. M. Case report: *Rhodococcus equi* pneumonia in a patient infected by the human immunodeficiency virus. *Am. J. Med. Sci.*, 303, 180, 1992.
65. Drancourt, M., Bonnet, E., Gallais, H., Peloux, Y., and Raoult, D. *Rhodococcus equi* infection in patients with AIDS. *J. Infect.*, 24, 123, 1992.
66. Nordman, P., Chavanet, P., Caillon, J., Duez, J. M., and Portier, H. Recurrent pneumonia due to rifampicin-resistant *Rhodococcus equi* in a patient infected with HIV. *J. Infect.*, 24, 104, 1992.
67. Rouquet, R. M., Clave, D., Massip, P., Moatti, N., and Leophonte, P. Imipenem/vancomycin for *Rhodococcus equi* pulmonary infection in HIV-positive patient. *Lancet*, 337, 375, 1991.
68. Chavanet, P., Bonnotte, B., Caillot, D., and Portier, H. Imipenem/teicoplanin for *Rhodococcus equi* pulmonary infection in AIDS patient. *Lancet*, 337, 794, 1991.
69. Roca, V., Vinuelas, J., Perez-Cecilia, E., et al. Bacteremic pneumonia caused by *Rhodococcus equi* and HIV infection: report of a new case and review of the literature. *Enferm. Infecc. Microbiol. Clin.*, 9, 627, 1991.
70. Sirera, G., Romeu, J., Clotet, B., et al. Relapsing systemic infection due to *Rhodococcus equi* in a drug abuser seropositive for human immunodeficiency virus. *Rev. Infect. Dis.*, 13, 509, 1991.
71. Flepp, M., Luthy, R., Wust, J., Steinke, W., and Greminger, P. *Rhodococcus equi* infection in HIV disease. *Schweiz. Med. Wochenschr.*, 119, 566, 1989.
72. Daley, C. L. Bacterial pneumonia in HIV-infected patients. *Semin. Respir. Dis.*, 8, 104, 1993.
73. de Los Santos-Fortuna, E., Mastroianni, C. M., Lichtner, M., Mengoni, F., Vullo, V., and Caterino-De-Araujo, A. Search for virulence-associated antigens of *Rhodococcus equi* in strains isolated from patients with acquired immunodeficiency syndrome. *Braz. J. Infect. Dis.*, 3, 184-188, 1999.
74. Hulsewe-Evers, H. P., Jansveld, C. A., Jansz, A. R., Schneider, M. M., and Bravenboer, B. HIV-infected patient with *Rhodococcus equi* pneumonia. *Neth. J. Med.* 57, 25-29, 2000
75. Schneider, M. M. Change in natural history of opportunistic infections in HIV-infected patients. *Neth. J. Med.*, 57, 1-3, 2000.
76. Caterino-de-Araujo, A., de Los Santos-Fortuno, E., Zandona-Meleiro, M. C., Calore, E. E., and Perez Calore, N. M. Detection of the 20-kDa virulence-associated antigen of *Rhodococcus equi* in malakplakia-like lesion in pleural tissue obtained from an AIDS patient. *Pathol. Res. Pract.*, 196, 321–327, 328, 2000.
77. Fang, C. T., Hung, C. C., Chang, S. C., et al. Pulmonary infection in human immunodeficiency virus-infected patients in Taiwan. *J. Formos. Med. Assoc.*, 99, 123–127, 2000.
78. Sanchez, J. F., Ojeda, I., Martin, C., Sanchez, F., and Vinuelas, J. Bacteremic pneumonia due to *Rhodococcus equi* in a patient with human immunodeficiency virus infection and visceral leishmaniasis. *Enfer. Infecc. Microbiol. Clin.*, 17, 532–533, 1999.
79. Kim, S. C., Jorgensen, J., Graybill, J. R., and Smith, J. Otomastoiditis caused by *Rhodococcus equi* in a patient with AIDS. *P. R. Health Sci. J.*, 18, 285-288, 1999.
80. Ibarra, R. and Jinkins, J. R. Severe otitis and mastoiditis due to *Rhodococcus equi* in a patient with AIDS. Case report. *Neuroradiology*, 41, 699-701, 1999.
81. Guerrero, M. F., Ramos, J. M., Renedo, G., Gadea, I., and Alix, A. Pulmonary malacoplakia associated with *Rhodococcus equi* infection in patients with AIDS: case report and review. *Clin. Infect. Dis.*, 28, 1334–1336, 1999.
82. Hamrock, D., Azmi, F. H., O'Donnell, E., Gunning, W. T., Philips, E. R., and Zaher, A.. Infection by *Rhodococcus equi* in a patient with AIDS: histological appearance mimicking Whipple's disease and *Mycobacterium avium-intracellulare* infection. *J. Clin. Pathol.*, 52, 68–71, 1999.
83. Canizares, R., Esparcia, A. M., Roig, P., et al. Cavitated pulmonary lesions in a patient with human immunodeficiency virus infection. *Enferm. Infecc. Microbiol. Clin.*, 17, 141-142, 1999.

84. Shin, M. S., Cooper, J. A., Jr., and Ho, K. J. Pulmonary malacoplakia associated with *Rhodococcus equi* infection in a patient with AIDS. *Chest*, 115, 889–892, 1999.
85. Rodriguez Arrondo, F., von Wichmann, M. A., Arrizabalaga, J., Iribarren, J. A., Garmendia, G., and Idigoras, P. Pulmonary cavitation lesions in patients infected with the human immunodeficiency virus: an analysis of the series of 78 cases. *Med. Clin. (Barc.)*, 111, 725–730, 1998.
86. Alcalde Encinas, M. M., Garcia Garcia, J., Martinez, Madrid, O. J., and Garcia Henarejos, J. A. Bronchial malacoplakia associated with *Rhodococcus equi* pneumonia in a patient with acquired immunodeficiency syndrome. *Rev. Clin. Esp.*, 198, 630–631, 1998.
87. Chiewchanvit, S., Mahanupab, P., Baosoung, V., and Khawan, C. Uncommon manifestations of opportunistic infections in an HIV infected patient. *J. Med. Assoc. Thai.*, 81, 923–926, 1998.
88. Talanin, N. Y., Donabedian, H., Kaw, M., O'Donnell, E. D., and Zaher, A. Colonic polyps and disseminated infection associated with *Rhodococcus equi* in a patient with AIDS. *Clin. Infect. Dis.*, 26, 1241–1242, 1998.
89. Martin-Davila, P., Quereda, C., Rodriguez, H., et al. Thyroid abscess due to *Rhodococcus equi* in a patient infected with the human immunodeficiency virus. *Eur. J. Clin. Microbiol. Infect. Dis.*, 17, 55–57, 1998.
90. Baraia-Etxaburu, J., Malero, P., Unzaga, M. J., et al. Pneumonia caused by *Rhodococcus equi* in a patients with AIDS: difficulty in defining the most appropriate initial treatment. *Enferm. Infecc. Microbiol. Clin.*, 15, 274–275, 1997.
91. Cornish, N. and Washington, J. A. *Rhodococcus equi* infections: clinical features and laboratory diagnosis. *Curr. Clin. Top. Infect. Dis.*, 19, 198–215, 1999.
92. Zink, M. C., Yager, J. A., Prescott, J. F., and Wilkie, B. N. In vitro phagocytosis and killing of *Corynebacterium equi* by alveolar macrophages of foals. *Am. J. Vet. Res.*, 46, 2171, 1985.
93. Ebersole, L. L. and Paturzo, J. L. Endophthalmitis caused by *Rhodococcus equi* Prescott serotype 4. *J. Clin. Microbiol.*, 26, 1221, 1988.
94. Hillman, D., Garretson, B., and Fiscella, R. *Rhodococcus equi* endophthalmitis. *Arch. Ophthalmol.*, 107, 20, 1989.
95. LeBar, W. D. and Pensler, M. I. Pleural effusion due to *Rhodococcus equi*. *J. Infect. Dis.*, 154, 919, 1986.
96. Thomsen, V. F., Henriques, U., and Magnusson, M. *Corynebacterium equi* Magnussson isolated from a tuberculoid lesion in a child with adenitis coli. *Dan. Med. Bull.*, 15, 135, 1968.
97. McGowan, K. L. and Mangano, M. F. Infections with *Rhodococcus equi* in children. *Diagn. Microbiol. Infect. Dis.*, 14, 347, 1991.
98. Sladek, G. G. and Frame, J. N. *Rhodococcus equi* causing bacteremia in an adult with acute leukemia. *South. Med. J.*, 86, 244, 1993.
99. Obana, W. G., Scannell, K. A., Jacobs, R., Greco, C., and Rosenblum, M. L. A case of *Rhodococcus equi* brain abscess. *Surg. Neurol.*, 35, 321, 1991.
100. Jablonowski, H., Armbrecht, C., Mauss, S., et al. *Rhodococcus equi* pneumonia in an HIV-infected patient. *Bildgebung*, 61, 206, 1994.
101. Hsueh, P. R., Hung, C. C., Teng, L. J., et al. Report of invasive *Rhodococcus equi* infections in Taiwan, with an emphasis on the emergence of multidrug-resistant strains. *Clin. Infect. Dis.*, 27, 370-375, 1998
102. Colebunders, R., De Roo, A., Verstraeten, T., et al. *Rhodococcus equi* infection in 3 AIDS patients. *Acta Clin. Belg.*, 51, 101, 1996.
103. Dabbs, E. R. and Quan, S. Light inhibits rifampicin inactivation and reduces rifampicin resistance due to a cloned mycobacterial ADP-ribosylation gene. *FEMS Microbiol. Lett.*, 182, 105–109, 2000.
104. Mascellino, M. T., Iona, E., Ponzo, R., Mastroianni, C. M., and Delia, S. Infections due to *Rhodococcus equi* in three HIV-infected patients: microbiological findings and antibiotic susceptibility. *Int. J. Clin. Pharmacol. Res.*, 14, 157, 1994.
105. Nordman, P., Rouveix, E., Guenounou, M., and Nicolas, M. H. Pulmonary abscess due to a rifampin and fluoroquinolone resistant *Rhodococcus equi* strain in a HIV infected patient. Eur. J. Clin. Microbiol. Infect. Dis., 11, 557, 1992.
106. Hillidge, C. J. Use of erythromycin-rifampin combination in treatment of *Rhodococcus equi* pneumonia. *Vet. Microbiol.*, 14, 337, 1987.
107. Arrizabalaga, J., Hernandez, J., Iribarren, J. A., et al. *Rhodococcus equi* infection in immunocompromised host: 11 cases. *Proc. 36th Intersci. Conf. Antimicrob. Agents Chemother.*, American Society for Microbiology, Washington DC, abstract # I24, 1996.
108. Scotton, P. G., Tonon, E., Giobbia, M., Gallucci, M., Rigoli, R., and Vaglia, A. *Rhodococcus equi* nosocomial meningitis cured by levofloxacin and shunt removal. *Clin. Infect. Dis.*, 30, 223-224, 2000.
109. Spark, R. P., McNeil, M. M., Brown, J. M., Lasker, B. A., Montano, M. A., Garfield, M. D. *Rhodococcus* species fatal infection in an immunocompetent host, *Arch. Pathol. Lab. Med.*, 117, 515, 1993.
110. Tanaka, Y., Yazawa, K., Dabbs, E. R., et al. Different rifampicin inactivation mechanisms in *Nocardia* and related taxa. *Microbiol. Immunol.*, 40, 1-4, 1996.

7
Tsukamurella ssp.

1. INTRODUCTION

Tsukamurella ssp., which belong to the family Nocardiaceae, are Gram-positive, weakly or variably acid-fast, nonmotile, non-sporoforming, rod-shaped, obligate, aerobic actinomycetes. They are environmental saprophytes; soil, sludge, and arthropods are their natural habitats. *Tsukamurella* ssp. pathogenic to humans include *T. paurometabolum (1,2)*, *T. inchonensis (3,4)*, *T. pulmonis (5)*, and *T. tyrosinosolvens (6)*.

Tsukamurella paurometabolum is known albeit rarely, to be an opportunistic pathogen for humans, specifically in patients with predisposing conditions, such as immunosuppression (leukemia, solid tumors, HIV infection), chronic lung pathology (tuberculosis), and foreign bodies (long-term use of indwelling catheters) *(1,7)*. So far, only a few cases of human disease caused by *T. paurometabolum* have been described: pneumonia in a patient with tuberculosis *(8)*, meningitis in a patient with hairy cell leukemia *(9)*, necrotizing fasciitis in a previously healthy patient *(10)*, and peritonitis in a patient undergoing peritoneal dialysis with an indwelling catheter *(11)*. In addition, central venous catheter-related infections owing to *Gordona rubropertincta* and *G. terrae* have also been reported in two immunocompetent patients who had been receiving total perenteral nutrition in their homes *(12)*. Auerbach et al. *(13)* described a hospital outbreak of pseudoinfection with *T. paurometabolum* that was traced to laboratory contamination *(14)*.

Shapiro et al. *(15)* and Lai *(16)* described central venous catheter-related sepsis due to *T. paurometabolum* in immunocompromised cancer patients.

In a recent report, Rey et al. *(7)* reported what appeared to be the first described case of *T. paurometabolum* infection in an HIV-infected individual.

2. TREATMENT OF *TSUKAMURELLA* INFECTIONS

The treatment of choice for *Tsukamurella* infections, in spite of lack of adequate guidelines, is antibiotic therapy combining a β-lactam and an aminoglycoside; catheter removal appears to be essential for cure *(1)*.

Mycolic acid-containing bacteria, such as *Nocardia* and related taxa (*Tsukamurella*), are known to inactivate rifampicin in a variety of species-specific ways including glucosylation, ribosylation, phosphorylation, and decolorization. To this end, *Tsukamurella* modifies rifampicin by ribosylation of the 23-OH group of the antibiotic *(17)*.

Shapiro et al. *(15)* tested in vitro the susceptibilities of an ATCC type strain 25938 of *T. paurometabolum* and three clinical isolates and found them highly susceptible to sulfamethoxazole, imipenem, third-generation of cephalosporins (three of four isolates), amikacin, and ciprofloxacin, but resistant to the penicillins and second-generation of cephalosporins. However, the results of in vitro testing may not always correlate with the outcome in vivo, as evidenced by a case of a patient with subcutaneous abscesses and necrotizing tenosynovitis, who despite amputation and treatment with a four-drug regimen (to which *T. paurometabolum* was susceptible in vitro), did not improve *(10)*.

Lai *(16)* successfully used a combination of erythromycin and gentamicin (i.v. administration for 4 wk) to treat an immunosuppressed cancer patient with central venous catheter-associated sepsis caused by *T. paurometabolum*. In this, as well as other similar cases *(1,15)*, because of prolonged bacteremia, removal of the catheter was essential for cure.

Jones et al. *(18)* treated effectively a patient with persistent *T. paurometabolum* bacteremia with a 6-wk course of vancomycin (1.0 g/wk).

Therapeutic regimens used by Shapiro et al. *(15)*, to treat three cases of *T. paurometabolum* bacteremia included: a 2-wk intravenous therapy with trimethoprim-sulfamethoxazole (TMX-SMZ), followed by 2 wk with oral TMP-SMZ; a 4-wk course of intravenous erythromycin and gentamicin; and intravenous vancomycin and ceftazidime for 4 d, followed by intravenous ceftriaxone for 10 d.

A *Tsukamurella* infection of a knee prosthesis was treated with a course of vancomycin and pipercillin-tazobactam, followed by a course of clarithromycin, ciprofloxacin, and ethambutol *(19)*.

REFERENCES

1. Rey, D., Fraisse, P., Riegel, P., Piemont, Y., and Lang, J. M. *Tsukamurella* infections. Review of the literature apropos of a case. *Pathol. Biol. (Paris)*, 45, 60–65, 1997.
2. Granel, F., Lozniewski, A., Barbaud, A., et al. Cutaneous infection caused by *Tsukamurella paurometabolum*. *Clin. Infect. Dis.*, 23, 839–840, 1996.
3. Yassin, A. F., Rainey, F. A., Burghardt, J., et al. *Tsukamurella* tyrosinosolvens sp. nov. *Int. J. Syst. Bacteriol.* 607–614, 1997.
4. Yassin, A. F., Rainey, F. A., Brzezinka, H., Burghardt, J., Lee, H. J., and Schaal, K. P. *Tsukamurella inchonensis* sp. nov. *Int. J. Syst. Bacteriol.*, 45, 522–527, 1995.
5. Yassin, A. F., Rainey, F. A., Brzezinka, H., et al. *Tsukamurella pulmonis* sp. nov. *Int. J. Syst. Bacteriol.*, 46, 429–436, 1996.
6. Chong, Y., Lee, K., Chon, C. Y., Kim, M. J., Kwon, O. H., and Lee, H. J. *Tsukamurella inchonensis* bacteremia in a patient who ingested hydrochloric acid. *Clin. Infect. Dis.*, 24, 1267–1268, 1997.
7. Rey, D., De Briel, D., Heller, R., et al. *Tsukamurella* and HIV infection. *AIDS*, 9, 1379, 1995.
8. Tsukamura, M. and Kawakami, K. Lung infection caused by *Gordona aurantiaca* (*Rhodococcus auranticus*). *J. Clin. Microbiol.*, 16, 604, 1982.
9. Prinz, G., Ban, E., Fekete, S., and Szabo, Z. Meningitis caused by *Gordona aurantiaca* (*Rhodococcus aurantiacus*). *J. Clin. Microbiol.*, 22, 472, 1985.
10. Tsukamura, M., Hikosaka, K., Nishimura, K., and Hara, S. Severe progressive subcutaneous abscesses and necrotizing tenosynovitis caused by *Rhodococcus aurantiacus*. *J. Clin. Microbiol.*, 26, 201, 1987.
11. Casella, P., Tommasi, A., and Tortorano, A. M. Peritonie da *Gordona aurantiaca* (*Rhodococcus aurantiacus*) in dialisi peritoneale ambulatorie continua. *Microbiologica Medica*, 2, 47, 1987.
12. Buchman, A. L., McNeil, M. M., Brown, J. M., Lasker, B. A., and Ament, M. E. Central venous catheter sepsis caused by unusual *Gordona* (*Rhodococcus*) species: identification with a digoxigenin-labeled rDNA probe. *Clin. Infect. Dis.*, 15, 694, 1992.
13. Auerbach, S. B., McNeil, M. M., Brown, J. M., Lasker, B. A., and Jarvis, W. R. Outbreak of pseudoinfection with *Tsukamurella paurometabolum* traced to laboratory contamination: efficacy of joint epidemiological and laboratory investigation. *Clin. Infect. Dis.*, 14, 1015- 1022, 1992.
14. Haft, R. F., Shapiro, C. L., Gantz, C. L., Christenson, J. C., and Wallace, R. J., Jr. Pseudoinfection due to *Tsukamurella paurometabolum* [comment]. *Clin. Infect. Dis.*, 15, 883, 1992.
15. Shapiro, C. L., Haft, R. F., Gantz, N. M., et al. *Tsukamurella paurometabolum*: a novel pathogen causing catheter-related bacteremia in patients with cancer. *Clin. Infect. Dis.*, 14, 200, 1992.
16. Lai, K. K. A cancer patient with central venous catheter-related sepsis caused by *Tsukamurella paurometabolum* (*Gordona aurantiaca*). *Clin. Infect. Dis.*, 17, 285, 1993.
17. Tanaka, Y., Yazawa, K., Dabbs, E. R., et al. Different rifampicin inactivation mechanisms in *Nocardia* and related taxa. *Microbiol. Immunol.*, 40, 1-4, 1996.
18. Jones, R. S., Fekete, T., Truant, A. L., and Satishchandran, V. Persistent bacteremia due to *Tsukamurella paurometabolum* in a patient undergoing hemodyalisis: case report and review. *Clin. Infect. Dis.*, 18, 830, 1994.
19. Larkin, J. A., Lit, L., Sinnott, J., Wills, T., and Szentivanyi, A. Infection of a knee prosthesis with *Tsukamurella* species. *South. Med. J.*, 92, 831-832, 1999.

8
Mycobacterium tuberculosis

1. INTRODUCTION

Pulmonary tuberculosis (consumption, phthisis) is considered to be one of the most devastating human diseases causing death and prolonged disability among people over many centuries. Following a decline in the prevalence during the latter part of the 20th century, the incidence of tuberculosis has substantially risen in recent years *(1,2)*. Currently, *Mycobacterium tuberculosis* is the greatest single infectious cause of mortality worldwide, causing the death of approximately two million people annually. This, coupled with the AIDS pandemic and the surge in multidrug-resistant clinical isolates of *M. tuberculosis*, have reaffirmed tuberculosis as a primary public health threat.

The pattern of tuberculosis has also changed and in recent years the incidence of extrapulmonary tuberculosis (laryngeal *[3]* and cerebral tuberculosis *[4]*, tuberculous osteomyelitis *[5]*, cervical tuberculous lymphadenitis *[6]*) has become more common *(7)*. Among the various contributing factors responsible for this disturbing trend, special attention has been given to the continuously increasing population of immunocompromised patients, such as organ-transplant recipients *(8–13)*, patients on immunosuppressive therapy *(14)*, patients with idiopathic $CD4^+$-lymphocytopenia *(15)*, severe combined immunodeficiency (SCID) *(16)*, and especially patients who are HIV-positive or already have AIDS *(17–21)*, as well as patients with chronic renal failure undergoing continuous ambulatory peritoneal dialysis *(5)*.

Outbreaks of multiple drug-resistant tuberculosis among HIV-infected and AIDS patients, which have been reported to occur in hospitals and prisons, were characterized by high mortality rates, disease transmission within the institutions, and high transmission rates to health-care workers *(22–25)*. Data reported by Pearson et al. *(26)* also underscored the possibility that nosocomial transmission of multiple drug-resistant tuberculosis may occur both from patient to patient, and from patient to health-care worker.

In the context of HIV infection, tuberculosis has been the only bacterial infection to which HIV-positive subjects are prone that can be readily transmitted to non-HIV-infected individuals. Githui et al. *(27)* examined various aspects associated with HIV-related tuberculosis in a cohort study of HIV-positive and HIV-negative patients from Kenya. Also, the 2-yr incidence of tuberculosis in cohorts of HIV-infected and uninfected urban Rwandan women has shown the rate ratio for development of tuberculosis among HIV-positive patients to be 22% *(28)*.

Small, but a statistically significant increase of tuberculosis in intravenous drug users has also been observed recently.

2. *MYCOBACTERIUM TUBERCULOSIS* INFECTIONS IN AIDS PATIENTS

It has been well-documented that HIV-infected persons are at particular risk of infection with *M. tuberculosis*, and the course of the disease in such patients is accelerated *(29–33)*. It is believed that tuberculosis may be the most common opportunistic infection and the leading cause of death among

From: Opportunistic Infections: Treatment and Prophylaxis
By: Vassil St. Georgiev © Humana Press Inc., Totowa, NJ

patients infected with the HIV worldwide (as high as 30% *[34]*), even though a number of retrospective and prospective studies have shown that the disease may be treatable and often preventable *(35)*. To this end, failure to suspect tuberculosis and to perform appropriate diagnostic tests in HIV-infected persons is the most common reason for diagnostic delays. Furthermore, with advancing HIV infection, the tuberculin skin test reactivity decreases along with reactivity to nonspecific antigens such as mumps, tetanus toxoid, and *Candida (33)*.

Although the disease affects predominantly the alveoli of the lung *(36)*, extrapulmonary involvement is not unusual in HIV-positive patients, especially those with low $CD4^+$ counts, where the extrapulmonary manifestations may occur in as many as half of the cases *(32,37,38)*. In this regard, the lymphatic system has been frequently involved *(39)*. Disseminated cutaneous tuberculosis with concurent pulmonary infection in AIDS patients have been rare and may present as a febrile illness and an abnormal chest radiograph, as well as with the development of widespread cutaneous tuberculous pustules *(40)*.

Berenguer et al. *(41)* found that although the incidence of tuberculous meningitis has been higher among HIV-infected persons, the clinical outcome of the disease has been similar to that in nonHIV-infected patients. Nevertheless, Fortun et al. *(42)* reported a fatal outcome following treatment failure for tuberculous meningitis of two HIV-positive patients.

Although most of the clinical symptoms of tuberculosis (cough, weight loss, fever, night sweats, fatigue) *(43,44)* may be present, they are not always indicative of tuberculosis in patients with AIDS. Calpe et al. *(45)* used routine fibrobronchoscopy to determine the frequency of endobronchial tuberculosis in HIV-positive patients.

Recurrence of HIV-related tuberculosis may be owing to either relapse to the original infection *(46)*, subtherapeutic concentrations of antituberculosis agents, or reinfection with a different strain of *M. tuberculosis (47–49)*.

One serious problem confronting clinicians treating tuberculosis in HIV-infected patients has been the high incidence of multiple drug-resistant strains of *M. tuberculosis* compounding the high mortality rate *(50)*. In addition, such cases usually progress very rapidly. Infection with HIV has emerged as the most important predisposing factor for developing of overt tuberculosis in patients co-infected with *M. tuberculosis (34)*. Furthermore, inadequate treatment has been thought to be one major reason for the development of multidrug-resistant tuberculosis, especially likely to occur when single drugs have been added to a failing regimen *(51)*.

3. EVOLUTION OF THERAPIES AND TREATMENT OF *MYCOBACTERIUM TUBERCULOSIS* INFECTIONS

Specific chemotherapy for tuberculosis was started in the early 1940s. Soon after its discovery as an antituberculosis agent, isoniazid became an essential part of any antimycobacterial therapy. Next, the introduction of rifampicin antibiotics, streptomycin, pyrazinamide, and the fluoroquinolones made it possible that such therapy not only could be relatively short in duration, but also could be given intermittently, thus allowing for closer supervision and monitoring. Izoniazid, rifampin, rifabutine, pyrazinamide, and ethambutol are the major agents currently used to treat tuberculosis *(52)*.

The mechanisms of action of various antimycobacterial drugs are different as are their primary sites of action *(53)*. Thus, isoniazid and rifampin exert bactericidal activity against all populations of mycobacteria. By comparison, streptomycin is most effective against bacilli found in open cavities, whereas the bactericidal activity of pyrazinamide is most pronounced against pathogens within the macrophages.

In therapeutic doses, isoniazid, rifampin, and pyrazinamide usually achieve adequate tissue and body fluid concentrations to kill *M. tuberculosis* in all body sites. Ethambutol, ethionamide, and *p*-aminosalicylic acid (PAS) are all bacteriostatic.

Resistance against drugs is very common in mycobacteria, and the number of drug-resistant mutants is usually proportional to the size of the mycobacterial population. The main rationale for antituberculosis treatment is to give a regimen combining drug(s) with bactericidal activity with bacteriostatic agent(s) that suppress the emergence of drug-resistant mutants. Microbiologic cure usually requires between 18 and 24 mo of therapy. It is generally accepted that using at least two bactericidal drugs against susceptible isolates is likely to provide a cure in 6–9 mo *(54)*.

One of the recommended chemotherapeutic regimens for newly diagnosed patients (both children and adults) involves a 6-mo daily course of isoniazid and rifampicin, supplemented with pyrazinamide for the first 2 mo *(55,56)*. At least nine studies of 6-mo (short-course) antituberculosis chemotherapy have demonstrated promising results in children *(57–65)*. However, variation from a standard 6-mo treatment may become necessary when there has been a high level of initial drug resistance, particularly against isoniazid. After taking into account results from recent clinical trials, recommendations have been made on antituberculosis chemotherapy in infants and children *(54)*.

The optimal treatment of tuberculosis in HIV-positive patients is still being defined because patients' responses to treatment of pulmonary tuberculosis may vary considerably. Although several studies have indicated that adverse outcomes are more likely to occur in patients with delayed sputum sterilization, there is limited methodology to identify such patients prospectively. To this end, Wallis et al. *(66)* developed multivariate models to predict the response to therapy in a prospectively recruited cohort of 42 HIV-negative subjects with drug-sensitive tuberculosis.

Small et al. *(67)* conducted a retrospective study of 132 patients listed in both the AIDS and tuberculosis case registries in San Francisco from 1981–1988. In HIV-infected patients who complied with conventional multidrug therapy, the results indicated a rapid sterilization of sputum, radiographic improvement, and low rates of relapse. In contrast, in patients with advanced HIV infection, the disease caused significantly high mortality. It has been reported that prophylactic medication with isoniazid by far is more beneficial to both HIV-infected, tuberculin-positive patients, and anergic HIV-infected patients, than the risks of potential isoniazid side effects *(68)*.

Since 1986, powerful short-course regimens have also been commonly used *(69)*. One preferred combination has been isoniazid, rifampin, and pyrazinamide administered on a daily basis for 2 mo, followed by isoniazid and rifampin for an additional 4 mo. Also, a 9-mo regimen of isoniazid and rifampin has been found equally effective. However, supplementation (in case of drug resistance) or extension (when immunosuppression has been present) of short-course regimens has been strongly recommended.

3.1. Drug Interactions in HIV-Infected Patients

In cases of rifampin (rifampicin, rifadin, rimactane), although true intolerance to this antibiotic have been rare even among HIV-infected patients, discontinuation owing to thrombocytopenia, creatinine over 2.0 mg/mL, bilirubin over 2.0 mg/mL, or severe reactions (generalized rash, persistent drug fever, or severe interference with methadone metabolism), has been reported *(70)*. In general, rifampin should not be administered with protease inhibitors or non-nucleoside reverse transcriptase inhibitors *(71,72)*. Although rifabutin is an acceptable alternative, certain precautions must be taken into account. In particular, rifabutin should not be used with the hard-gel protease inhibitor saquinavir and the non-nucleoside reverse transcriptase inhibitor delavirdine, and caution applied when co-administered with the soft-gel saquinavir. In addition, rifabutin should be given to HIV-infected persons at one-half the usual daily dose (from 300–150 mg daily) when co-administered with indinavir, nelfinavir, or amprenavir, and at one-fourth the usual daily dose (i.e., 150 mg every other day, or 3 times weekly) with ritonavir. Adding ritonavir facilitated the combined therapy of rifampin and saquinavir *(73)*. Based on pharmacokinetic data, rifabutin may be applied at an increased dose (450 mg daily) when co-administered with efavirenz *(72)*.

3.2. Drug Resistance in Tuberculosis

With the emergence of drug-resistant strains of *M. tuberculosis (74)*, the effective chemotherapy of the disease will require rapid assessment of drug resistance *(75)*. The currently available methodology will not allow determination of drug susceptibility for 2–18 wk because of the 20–24-h doubling time of *M. tuberculosis*. However, some new techniques in development (e.g., firefly luciferase-based assay) may remedy this situation by significantly shortening the ascertainment times. Phenotypic methods to identify drug-resistant *M. tuberculosis* are based on the measurement of the microbial growth on nutritional supplement with antimicrobial agents. However, using this methodology (e.g., the Bactec radiometric method, mycobacterial growth indicator tube, and the method in solid medium) is time-consuming and requires 5–21 d to complete. In contrast, the genotype-based methodology, which uses the knowledge of genes involved in the resistance to identify the different mutations conferring the antimicrobial resistance, reduces the time to detection of resistance from weeks to days *(76)*.

To avoid potential pitfalls when initiating treatment in patients with confirmed multiple drug-resistant tuberculosis, both the treatment history and the in vitro susceptibilities of the patient's tuberculous strains should be thoroughly evaluated. The selected regimen should include between four and seven antimycobacterial agents, including such drugs as pyrazinamide, ethambutol, streptomycin, ofloxacin, ciprofloxacin, ethionamide, cycloserine, capreomycin, and *p*-aminosalicylic acid (PAS) *(77)*. Based on tuberculosis-susceptibility patterns, predictors of multidrug resistance, and implications for initial therapeutic regimens, a theoretically effective antituberculosis regimen was assumed to contain at least two drugs to which an *M. tuberculosis* isolate was susceptible *(78)*.

Historically, the majority of multiple-drug antituberculosis regimens contained isoniazid and rifampin as part of the same regimen *(79)*. As a consequence of this combined therapy, acquired rifampin resistance without preexisting isoniazid resistance *(80)* is highly unusual in patients with tuberculosis *(81)*, and strains resistant only to rifampin rarely have been recovered. However, there has been an increased incidence of HIV-positive patients infected with mono-rifampin-resistant *M. tuberculosis* strains *(82)*. Nolan et al. *(81)* described an unusual pattern of acquired rifampin resistance in three HIV-infected patients who initially had *M. tuberculosis* strains susceptible to both rifampin and isoniazid. During treatment in two patients and after completion of therapy in the remaining one, each patient developed active, rifampin-resistant but isoniazid-susceptible tuberculosis. (One patient subsequently developed isoniazid resistance also.)

Data from studies involving South African gold miners with culture-positive pulmonary tuberculosis (as high as 48.7% also being HIV-positive *[83]*) showed that the primary and acquired drug-resistance rates were stable in this population and not affected by the high prevalence of HIV infection *(83,84)*.

3.3. Highly Active Antiretroviral Therapy (HAART) and Mycobacterial Infections in HIV-Infected Patients

Since its introduction, HAART has reduced significantly the incidence of opportunistic infections in HIV-positive patients in general, and mycobacterial infections in particular *(85)*. This, coupled with continuing prophylaxis against specific opportunistic infections, would definitely increase the survival benefits in this population *(86)*.

Assessment of the incidence of mycobacterial infections among HIV-infected patients following the introduction of HAART has been performed by several groups. In a European report *(87)* using data from an EuroSIDA study (1994–1999) involving a multicenter observational cohort of more than 7000 patients, there has been a marked decrease in the incidence of *M. tuberculosis* infections, and even a larger one for MAC infections. These decreases have been attributed to favorable changes in the CD4$^+$ cell count following the introduction of HAART.

Although the use of HAART exerted a remarkable impact on the course of HIV disease, because of potential drug interactions it also has raised several issues with respect to HIV-related tuberculosis and its treatment. In particular, such drug interactions will necessitate the need of either a nonrifamycin-based regimens or a rifabutin-based regimen in patients receiving HAART and treated for tuberculosis *(33)*.

3.4. Prophylaxis of Tuberculosis in HIV-Infected Patients

In a recent report *(88)*, the Advisory Council for the Elimination of Tuberculosis has recommended a model for tuberculosis control programs to be implemented in the U S, including three priority strategies for prevention and control: 1) identifying and treating persons with active tuberculosis; 2) finding and screening persons who had contact with patients with tuberculosis to determine whether they have been infected with *M. tuberculosis* or have active disease, and providing appropriate treatment if necessary; and 3) screening populations at high risk for tuberculosis and providing therapy to prevent progression of active disease.

Preventive therapy of patients exposed to multiple drug-resistant *M. tuberculosis* has been and is still somewhat controversial and of unknown efficacy *(2)*.

In general, although prophylaxis with isoniazid for 6–12 mo has been very important, it is often a neglected preventive measure for patients latently infected but still without active disease *(69)*. Daily therapy with 300 mg of isoniazid for at least 9 mo has been recommended for patients at high risk for tuberculosis *(89)*.

In a prospective observational cohort study conducted among 2960 community-based injecting drug users (including 942 HIV-seropositive persons) from 1988–1994, Graham et al. *(90)* evaluated the expanded access to isoniazid chemoprophylaxis on the tuberculosis incidence. Directly observed chemoprophylaxis with twice-weekly isoniazid (10–15 mg/kg) was offered to purified protein derivative (PPD) tuberculine-positive individuals, but not to those with cutaneous anergy; disease incidence was monitored by using Poisson regression. Following preventive therapy, there has been a dramatic decrease in incidence from a peak of 6 per 1,000 person-years in 1991 to only one case in 1992 and 0 cases for 24 mo thereafter (mid-1992 to mid-1994), for an overall 83% drop in tuberculosis incidence. The obtained results were consistent with those observed in clinical trials of isoniazid prophylaxis and were obtained without offering chemoprophylaxis to HIV-infected patients with cutaneous anergy.

In HIV-infected pregnant women, when the patients has not been exposed to drug-resistant tuberculosis, daily or twice-weekly prophylaxis with isoniazid is the regimen of choice. However, because of concerns regarding teratogenicity, prophylaxis should be initiated after the first trimester. In addition, to reduce the danger of neurotoxicity, preventive therapy with isoniazid should be accompanied by pyridoxine *(71)*.

3.5. Adjunctive Immunotherapy of Tuberculosis

Modulation of the host response promises to become a powerful tool in treating tuberculosis *(91)*.

In a randomized, placebo-controlled trial, 120 HIV-negative Ugandan patients with newly diagnosed pulmonary tuberculosis were subjected to adjunctive immunotherapy with a heat-killed *M. vaccae*. Patients were randomized to a single dose of *M. vaccae* or placebo 1 wk after beginning of chemotherapy, and were followed up for 1 yr. The results demonstrated an early increase in sputum-culture conversion after 1 mo of chemotherapy and greater radiographic improvement (91 vs 77% for placebo recipients at 6 mo) among patients receiving *M. vaccae*, which was safe and well-tolerated *(92)*.

Adjuvant cytokines such as interlukin (IL)-2, IL-12, interferon-γ (IFN-γ), and granulocyte-macrophase colony-stimulating factor (GM-CSF) may also prove useful in shortening the duration of treatment and overcoming drug resistance *(91)*.

3.6. Vaccine Development Against Tuberculosis

Using microarray DNA-chip technology, Tallat et al. *(93)* initiated a study to determine the best candidate for a therapeutic *M. tuberculosis* vaccine. In another study, the cell-mediated and protective immune responses to DNA vaccines encoding the *M. tuberculosis* proteins ESAT-6, MPT-64, Antigen85A, and KatG administered intranasally or intramuscularly were evaluated *(94)*. At d 28 after a low-dose aerosol challenge with *M. tuberculosis* Erdman, several of the DNA vaccine constructs demonstrated protective immune responses as measured by reducing lung and spleen colony-forming units (CFUs).

Jagannath et al. *(95)* found a mutant of *M. tuberculosis* H37Rv deficient in antigen 85A expression that acted as vaccine against experimental tuberculosis in mice.

A Phase I trial was conducted to assess the safety and immunogenicity of inactivated *M. vaccae* as a candidate vaccine to prevent tuberculosis in AIDS patients *(96,97)*. The trial, which was conducted in Zambia, involved 22 HIV-positive patients with lymphocyte counts at or below 200 cells/mm^3 and 31 healthy subjects (BCG immunized and naive). The patients received either a three-dose (HIV-negative) or a five-dose (HIV-positive) schedule of intradermal *M. vaccae* at 0, 2, 4, 11, and 13 mo. The five-dose series of vaccination was safe and induced lymphocyte proliferation responses to the vaccine antigen *(96)*.

REFERENCES

1. Fry, D. E. The reemergence of mycobacterial infections. *Arch. Surg.*, 131, 14, 1996.
2. Peloquin, C. A. and Berning, S. E. Infection caused by *Mycobacterium tuberculosis*. *Ann. Pharmacother.*, 28, 72, 1994.
3. Yencha, M. W., Linfesty, R., and Blackmon, A. Laryngeal tuberculosis. *Am. J. Otolaryngol.*, 21, 122-126, 2000.
4. Labhard, N., Nicod, L., and Zellweger, J. P. Cerebral tuberculosis in the immunocompetent host: 8 cases observed in Switzerland. *Tuber. Lung Dis.*, 75, 454, 1994.
5. Yalcinkaya, F., Tumer, N., Akar, N., Ekim, M., and Bildirici, Y. Tuberculous osteomyelitis: an unusual case of tuberculous infection in a child undergoing continuous ambulatory peritoneal dialysis. *Pediatr. Nephrol.*, 9, 485, 1995.
6. Weiler, Z., Nelly, P., Baruchin, A. M., and Oren, S. Diagnosis and treatment of cervical tuberculous lymphadenitis. *J. Oral Maxillofac. Surg.*, 58, 477-481, 2000.
7. Huebner, R. E. and Castro, K. G. The changing face of tuberculosis. *Annu. Rev. Med.*, 46, 47, 1995.
8. Park, S. B., Joo, I., Park, Y. I., et al. Clinical manifestations of tuberculosis in renal transplant patients. *Transplant. Proc.*, 28, 1520, 1996.
9. Munoz, P., Palomo, J., Munoz, R., Rodriguez-Creixems, M., Pelaez, T., and Bouza, E. Tuberculosis in heart transplant recipients. *Clin. Infect. Dis.*, 21, 398, 1995.
10. Ahsan, N., Blanchard, R. L., and Mai, M. L. Gastrointestinal tuberculosis in renal transplantation. *Clin. Transplant*, 9, 349, 1995.
11. Miller, R. A., Lanza, L. A., Kline, J. N., and Geist, L. J. *Mycobacterium tuberculosis* in lung transplant recipients. *Am. J. Respir. Crit. Care Med.*, 152, 374, 1995.
12. Tantawichien, T., Suwangool, P., and Suvanapha, R. Tuberculosis in renal transplant recipients. *Transplant. Proc.*, 26, 2187, 1994.
13. Chen, C. H., Hsieh, H., and Lai, M. K. Pulmonary tuberculosis or MOTT infection in kidney transplant recipients. *Transplant. Proc.*, 26, 2136, 1994.
14. Anders, N. and Wollensak, G. Ocular tuberculosis in systemic lupus erythematosus and immunosuppressive therapy. *Klin. Monatsbl. Augenheilkd.*, 207, 368, 1995.
15. Neukirch, B. and Kremer, G. J. Disseminated extrapulmonary tuberculosis in idiopathic CD4-lymphocytopenia. *Dtsch. Med. Wochenschr.*, 120, 23, 1995.
16. Nagasawa, M., Maeda, H., Okawa, H., and Yata, J. Pulmonary miliary tuberculosis and T- cell abnormalities in a severe combined immunodeficient patient reconstituted with haploidentical bone marrow transplantation. *Int. J. Hematol.*, 59, 303, 1994.
17. Phair, J. P., Gross, P. A., Kaplan, J. E., et al. Quality standard for the identification and treatment of persons coinfected with human immunodeficiency virus and *Mycobacterium tuberculosis*. *Clin. Infect. Dis.*, 21(Suppl. 1), S130, 1995.
18. Molina-Gamboa, J. D., Ponce-de-Leon, S., Sifuentes-Osornio, J., Bobadilla del Valle, M., and Ruiz-Palacios, G. M. Mycobacterial infection in Mexican AIDS patients. *J. Acquir. Immune Defic. Syndr. Hum. Retrovirol.*, 11, 53, 1996.
19. Drobniewski, F. A., Pozniak, A. L., and Uttley, A. H. Tuberculosis and AIDS. *J. Med. Microbiol.*, 43, 85, 1995.
20. Kritski, A., Dalcolmo, M., del Bianco, R., et al. Association of tuberculosis and HIV infection in Brasil. *Bol. Oficina Sanit. Panam.*, 118, 542, 1995.
21. Waxman, S., Gang, M., and Goldfrank, L. Tuberculosis in the HIV-infected patient. *Emerg. Med. Clin. North Am.*, 13, 179, 1995.
22. Farley, T. A. AIDS and multidrug-resistant tuberculosis: an epidemic transforms an old disease. *J. La. State Med. Soc.*, 144, 357, 1992.
23. Bagg, J. Tuberculosis: a re-emerging problem for health care workers. *Br. Dent. J.*, 180, 376, 1996.
24. Moroni, M., Gori, A., Rusconi, S., Franzetti, F., and Antinori, S. Mycobacterial infections in AIDS: an overview of epidemiology, clinical manifestations, therapy and prophylaxis. *Monaldi Arch. Chest Dis.*, 49, 432, 1994.
25. Fraser, V. J., Kilo, C. M., Bailey, T. C., Medoff, G., and Dunagan, W. C. Screening of physicians for tuberculosis. *Infect. Control Hosp. Epidemiol.*, 15, 95, 1994.
26. Pearson, M. L., Jereb, J. A., Frieden, T. R., et al. Nosocomial transmission of multidrug-resistant *Mycobacterium tuberculosis*: a risk to patients and health care workers. *Ann. Intern. Med.*, 117, 191, 1992.

27. Githui, W., Nunn, P., Juma, E., et al. Cohort study of HIV-positive and HIV-negative tuberculosis, Nairobi, Kenya: comparison of bacteriological results. *Tuber. Lung Dis.*, 73, 203, 1992.
28. Allen, S., Batungwanayo, J., Kerlikowske, K., et al. Two- year incidence of tuberculosis in cohorts of HIV-infected and uninfected urban Rwandan women. *Am. Rev. Respir. Dis.*, 146, 1439, 1992.
29. Daley, C. L., Small, P. M., Schecter, G. F., et al. An outbreak of tuberculosis with accelerated progression among persons infected with HIV. *N. Engl. J. Med.*, 326, 231, 1992.
30. Churchyard, G. J. and Grant, A. D. HIV infection, tuberculosis and non-tuberculous mycobacteria. *S. Afr. Med. J.*, 90, 472–476, 2000.
31. Subcommittee of the Joint Tuberculosis Committee of the British Thoracic Society. Management of opportunistic mycobacterial infections: Joint Tuberculosis Committee Guidelines 1999. *Thorax*, 55, 210–218, 2000 [see also: *Thorax*, 55, 722, 2000]
32. Chiu, C. P., Wong, W. W., Kuo, B., Tiao, T. M., Fung, C. P., and Liu, C. Y. Clinical analysis of *Mycobacterium tuberculosis* infection in patients with acquired immunodeficiency syndrome. *J. Microbiol. Immunol. Infect.*, 32, 250–256, 1999.
33. Perlman, D. C., El-Helon, P., and Salomon, N. Tuberculosis in patients with human immunodeficiency virus infection. *Semin. Respir. Infect.*, 14, 344–352, 1999.
34. Zumla, A., Malon, P., Henderson, J., and Grange, J. M., Impact of HIV infection on tuberculosis. *Postgrad. Med. J.*, 76, 259–268, 2000.
35. Shafer, R. W. and Edlin, B. R., Tuberculosis in patients infected with human immunodeficiency virus: perspective on the past decade. *Clin. Infect. Dis.*, 22, 683, 1996.
36. Wada, M., Yamamoto, S., Ogata, H., Sugita, N., Kino, T., and Hayashi, A. Two pulmonary tuberculosis cases with HIV infection. *Kekkaku*, 69, 367, 1994.
37. Jones, E., Young, S. M. M., Antoniskis, D., Davidson, P. T., Kramer, F., and Barnes, P. F. Relationship of the manifestations of tuberculosis to CD4 cell counts in patients with human immunodeficiency virus infections. *Am. Rev. Respir. Dis.*, 148, 1292, 1993.
38. Dupon, M., Texier-Maugein, J., Leroy, V., et al. Tuberculosis and HIV infection: a cohort study of incidence and susceptibility to antituberculous drugs, Bordeaux, 1985–1993. *AIDS*, 9, 577, 1995.
39. Greten, T., Hautmann, H., Trauner, A., and Huber, R. M. Esophagomediastinal fistulae as a rare complication of tuberculosis in an HIV-infected patient. *Dtsch. Med. Wochenschr.*, 119, 1613, 1994.
40. Corbett, E. L., Crossley, I., De Cock, K. M., and Miller, R. F. Disseminated cutaneous *Mycobacterium tuberculosis* infection in a patient with AIDS. *Genitourin. Med.*, 71, 308, 1995.
41. Berenguer, J., Moreno, S., Laguna, F., et al. Tuberculous meningitis in patients infected with the human immunodeficiency virus. *N. Engl. J. Med.*, 326, 668, 1992.
42. Fortun, J., Gomez-Mampaso, E., Navas, E., Hermida, C. M., Antela, A., and Guerrero, A. Tuberculous meningitis caused by resistant microorganisms. *Enferm. Infecc. Microbiol. Clin.*, 12, 150, 1994.
43. Moreno, S., Baraia, J., Parras, F., Solera, J., Bernacer, B., Meana, A., and Bouza, E. Fever evolution after treatment in patients with tuberculosis and HIV infection. *Rev. Clin. Esp.*, 195, 150, 1995.
44. Albrecht, H., Stelbrink, H. J., Eggers, C., Rusch-Gerdes, S., and Greten, H. A case of disseminated *Mycobacterium bovis* infection in an AIDS patient. *Eur. J. Clin. Microbiol. Infect. Dis.*, 14, 226, 1995.
45. Calpe, J. L., Chiner, E., and Larramendi, C. H. Endobronchial tuberculosis in HIV-infected patients. *AIDS*, 9, 1159, 1995.
46. Schaaf, H. S., Gie, R. P., van Rie, A., Seifart, H. I., van Helden, P. D., and Cotton, M. F. Second episode of tuberculosis in an HIV-infected child: relapse or reinfection? *J. Infect.*, 41, 100–103, 2000.
47. Dronda, F., Fernandez-Martin, I., Chaves, F., and Gonzalez-Lopez, M. Recurrent *Mycobacterium tuberculosis* bacteremia in AIDS: subtherapeutic concentrations of antitubercular agents? *Med. Clin. (Barcelona)*, 103, 478, 1994.
48. Godfrey-Faussett, P., Githui, W., Batchelor, B., et al. Recurrence of HIV- related tuberculosis in an endemic area may be due to relapse or reinfection. *Tuber. Lung Dis.*, 75, 199, 1994.
49. Small, P. M., Shafer, R. W., Hopewell, P. C., et al. Exogenous reinfection with multidrug-resistant *Mycobacterium tuberculosis* in patients with advanced HIV infection. *N. Engl. J. Med.*, 328, 1137, 1993; [see also comments in *N. Engl. J. Med.*, 329, 811, 812, 1993].
50. Ashley, E. A., Johnson, M. A., and Lipman, M. C. Human immunodeficiency virus and respiratory infection. *Curr. Opin. Pulm. Med.*, 6, 240–245, 2000.
51. Mahmoudi, A. and Iseman, D. Pitfalls in the care of patients with tuberculosis: common errors and their association with the acquisition of drug resistance. *J. Am. Med. Assoc.*, 270, 65, 1993.
52. Van Scoy, R. E. and Wilkowske, C. J. Antimycobacterial therapy. *Mayo Clin. Proc.*, 74, 1038–1048, 1999.
53. Georgiev, V. St. Treatment and developmental therapeutics of *Mycobacterium tuberculosis* infections. *Int. J. Antimicrob. Agents*, 4, 157, 1994.
54. Committee on Infectious Diseases. Chemotherapy for tuberculosis in infants and children. *Pediatrics*, 89, 161, 1992.
55. Blom-Bülow, B. Dosing regimens in the treatment of tuberculosis. *Scand. J. Infect. Dis. Suppl.*, 74, 258, 1990.
56. Doganay, M., Calangu, S., Turgut, H., Bakir, M., and Aygen, B. Treatment of tuberculous meningitis in Turkey. *Scand. J. Infect. Dis.*, 27, 135, 1995.
57. Ibanez, S. and Ross, G. Quimioterapia abreviada de 6 meses en tuberculosis pulmonar infantil. *Rev. Chil. Pediatr.*, 51, 249, 1980.
58. Anane, T., Cernay, J., and Bensenovci, A. Resultats compares des regimens et des regimens long dans la chimiotherapie de la tuberculose de l'enfant en Algerie, *African Regional Meeting of International Union Against Tuberculosis*, Tunis, Tunisia, 1984.

59. Varudkar, B. L. Short-course chemotherapy for tuberculosis in children. *Indian J. Pediatr*, 52, 593, 1985.
60. Pelosi, F., Budani, H., Rubinstein, C., et al. Isoniazid, rifampin and pyrazinamide in the treatment of childhood tuberculosis with duration adjusted to the clinical status. *Am. Rev. Respir. Dis.*, 131(Suppl.), A229, 1985.
61. Starke, J. R. and Taylor-Watts, K. T. Six-month chemotherapy of intrathoracic tuberculosis in children. *Am. Rev. Respir. Dis.*, 139(Suppl.), A314, 1989.
62. Medical Research Council Tuberculosis and Chest Disease Unit. Management and outcome of chemotherapy for childhood tuberculosis. *Arch. Dis. Child.*, 64, 1004, 1989.
63. Biddulph, J. Short-course chemotherapy for childhood tuberculosis. *Pediatr. Infect. Dis. J.*, 9, 794, 1990.
64. Khubchandani, R. P., Kumta, N. B., Bharucha, N. B., and Ramakantan, R. Short-course chemotherapy in childhood pulmonary tuberculosis. *Am. Rev. Resp. Dis.*, 141(Suppl.), A338, 1990.
65. Kumar, L., Dhand, R., Singhi, P. D, Rao, K. L., and Katariya, S. A randomized trial of fully intermittent vs. daily followed by intermittent short-course chemotherapy for childhood tuberculosis. *Pediatr. Infect. Dis. J.*, 9, 802, 1990.
66. Wallis, R. S., Perkins, M. D., Phillips, M., et al. Predicting the outcome of therapy for pulmonary tuberculosis. *Am. J. Respir. Crit. Care Med.*, 161(4 Pt.1), 1076-1080, 2000.
67. Small, P. M., Schecter, G. F., Goodman, P. C., et al. Treatment of tuberculosis in patients with advanced human immunodeficiency virus infection. *N. Engl. J. Med.*, 324, 289, 1991.
68. Rose, D. N., Schechter, C. B., and Sacks, H. S. Preventive medicine for HIV-infected patients: an analysis of isoniazid prophylaxis for tuberculin reactors and for anergic patients. *J. Gen. Intern. Med.*, 7, 589, 1992.
69. Pust, R. E., Tuberculosis in the 1990's: resurgence, regimens, and resources. *South. Med. J.*, 85, 584, 1992.
70. Cook, S. V., Fujiwara, P. I., and Frieden, T. R. Rates and risk factors for discontinuation of rifampicin. *Int. J. Tuberc. Lung Dis.*, 4, 118–122, 2000.
71. U.S. Public Health Service and Infectious Diseases Society of America. 1999 USPHS/IDSA guidelines for the prevention of opportunistic infections in persons infected with human immunodeficiency virus. *Infect. Dis. Obstet. Gynecol.*, 5–74, 2000.
72. Centers for Disease Controls. Prevention and treatment of tuberculosis among patients infected with human immunodeficiency virus: principles of therapy and revised recommendations. *Morb. Mortal. Wkly Rep.*, 47(RR-20), 1998.
73. Veldkamp, A. I., Hoetelmans, R. M., Beijinen, J. H., Mulder, J. W., and Meenhorst, P. L. Ritonavir enables combined therapy with rifampin and saquinavir. *Clin. Infect. Dis.*, 29, 1586, 1999.
74. Riska, P. F., Jacobs, W. R. Jr., and Alland, D. Molecular determinants of drug resistance in tuberculosis. *Int. J. Tuberc. Lung Dis.*, 4(2 Suppl. 1), S4–S10, 2000.
75. Kuaban, C., Bercion, R., Jifon, G., Cunin, P., and Blackett, K. N. Acquired anti-tuberculosis drug resistance in Yaounde, Cameroon, *Int. J. Tuberc. Lung Dis.*, 4, 427–432, 2000.
76. Loiez-Durocher, C., Vachee, A., and Lamaitre, N. Drug resistance in *Mycobacterium tuberculosis*: diagnostic methods *Ann. Biol. Clin. (Paris)*, 58, 291–297, 2000.
77. Iseman, M. D. Treatment of multidrug-resistant tuberculosis. *N. Engl. J. Med.*, 329, 784, 1993.
78. Weltman, A. C. and Rose, D. N. Tuberculosis susceptibility patterns, predictors of multidrug resistance, and implication for initial therapeutic regimens at a New York City hospital. *Arch. Intern. Med.*, 154, 2161, 1994.
79. Ouedraogo, M., Ouedraogo, S. M., Diagbouga, S., et al. Simultaneous resistance to rifampicin and isoniazid in patients with pulmonary tuberculosis. *Rev. Mal. Respir.*, 17, 477-480, 2000.
80. Ausina, V., Riutort, N., Vinado, B., et al. Prospective study of drug-resistant tuberculosis in a Spanish urban population including patients at risk for HIV infection. *Eur. J. Clin. Microbiol. Infect. Dis.*, 14, 105, 1995.
81. Nolan, C. M., Williams, D. L., Cave, M. D., et al. Evolution of rifampin resistance in human immunodeficiency virus-associated tuberculosis. *Am. J. Respir. Crit. Care Med.*, 152, 1067, 1995.
82. Lutfey, M., Della-Latta, P., Kapur, V., et al. Independent origin of mono- rifampin-resistant *Mycobacterium tuberculosis* in patients with AIDS. *Am. J. Respir. Crit. Care Med.*, 153, 837, 1996.
83. Murray, J., Sonnenberg, P., Shearer, S., and Godfrey-Faussett, P. Drug-resistant pulmonary tuberculosis in a cohort of southern African gold miners with a high prevalence of HIV infection. *S. Afr. Med. J.*, 90, 381–386, 2000.
84. Churchyard, G. J., Corbett, E. L., Kleinschmidt, I., Mulder, D., and De Cock, K. M. Drug- resistant tuberculosis in South African gold miners: incidence and associated factors. *Int. J. Tuberc. Lung Dis.*, 4, 433–440, 2000.
85. Centers for Disease Controls. Report of the NIH Panel to define Principles of Therapy of HIV infection and guidelines for use of antiretroviral agents in HIV-infected adults and adolescents. *Morb. Mortal. Wkly Rep.*, 47(No. RR-5), 1998.
86. McNaghten, A. D., Hanson, D. L., Jones, J. L., Dworkin, M. S., Ward, J. W. and the Adult/Adolescent Spectrum of Disease group. Effects of antiretroviral therapy and opportunistic illness primary chemoprophylaxis on survival after AIDS diagnosis. *AIDS*, 13, 1687–1695, 1999.
87. Kirk, O., Gatell, J. M., Mocroft, A., et al. Infections with *Micobacterium tuberculosis* and *Mycobacterium avium* among HIV-infected patients after the introduction of highly active antiretroviral therapy, EuroSIDA Study Group JD. *Am. J. Respir. Crit. Care Med.*, 162(3 pt. 1), 865–872, 2000.
88. Essential components of a tuberculosis prevention and control program. Recommendation of the Advisory Council for the Elimination of Tuberculosis. *Morb. Mortal. Wkly Rep.*, 44(RR- 11), 1, 1995.
89. Stearn, B. F. and Polis, M. A. Prophylaxis of opportunistic infections in persons with HIV infection. *Cleve. Clin. J. Med.*, 61, 187, 1994.
90. Graham, N. M., Galai, N., Nelson, K. E., et al. Effect of isoniazid chemoprophylaxis on HIV-related mycobacterial disease. *Arch. Intern. Dis.*, 156, 889, 1996.
91. Holland, S. M. Cytokine therapy of mycobacterial infections. *Adv. Intern. Med.*, 45, 431–452, 2000.

92. Johnson, J. L., Kamya, R. M., Okwera, A., et al. Randomized controlled trial of *Mycobacterium vaccae* immunotherapy in nonhuman immunodeficiency virus-infected Ugandan adults with newly diagnosed pulmonary tuberculosis. The Ugandan-Case Western Reserve University Research Collaboration. *J. Infect. Dis.*, 181, 1304–1312, 2000.
93. Tallat, A. M., Lyons, R., and Johnston, S. A. Towards therapeutic *Mycobacterium tuberculosis* vaccine using DNA microarray technology. *Abstr. Gen. Meet. Am. Soc. Microbiol.*, May 30–June 3, 1999, 652, abstract U-98.
94. Howard, A., Li, Z., Kelley, C., Collins, F., and Morris, S. Protection and cytokine production associated with DNA vaccines against tuberculosis. *Abstr. Gen. Meet. Am. Soc. Microbiol.*, May 30–June 3, 1999, 651, abstract U-93.
95. Jagannath, C., Copenhanver, R., Armitige, L., et al. A mutant of *Mycobacterium tuberculosis* H37Rv deficient in antigen 85A expression, acts as vaccine against experimental tuberculosis in mice. *Abstr. Gen. Meet. Am. Soc. Microbiol.*, May 30–June 3, 1999, 652, abstract U-96.
96. Waddell, R. D., Chintu, C., Lein, A. D., et al. Safety and immunogenicity of a five-dose series of inactivated *Mycobacterium vaccae* vaccination for the prevention of HIV-associated tuberculosis. *Clin. Infect. Dis.*, 30(Suppl. 3), S309–315, 2000.
97. Lein, A. D., Waddell, R. D., Chintu, C., et al. Phase I trial of *Mycobacterium vaccae* immunization in HIV infected and healthy adults in Lusaka, Zambia. *5th Conf. Retroviruses Opportunistic Infect.*, Feb. 1–5, 1998, 217, abstract 736.

9
Mycobacterium bovis

1. INTRODUCTION

Mycobacterium bovis is a virulent organism that was first isolated from cattle infected with tuberculous tubercles. *M. bovis* was found together with *M. tuberculosis* and *M. africanum* to cause tuberculosis in humans and lower animals. Most of the cases reported in the literature were affected by the Bacille Calmette-Guérin (BCG) strain, a live attenuated strain of *M. bovis* that has been used to prepare the BCG vaccine since 1921. Disseminated BCG infection may also occur in some well-defined immunodeficiencies, such as severe combined immunodeficiency (SCID), chronic granulomatous disease (CGD), and pediatric HIV infection. This severe complication of immunization against tuberculosis has been lethal in the majority of immunized children who had primary immunodeficiency such as hyperimmunoglobulin E syndrome *(1)*.

Because of the possibility of developing progressive disease, the BCG vaccination of asymptomatic HIV-positive patients *(2)* and infants born of HIV-seropositive mothers *(3–5)* is still controvercial *(6–9)* and should be considered with caution *(9–11)*. Cases of immunocompetent and previously healthy children who developed infections owing to *M. bovis*-BCG inoculation have also been reported *(11–14)*. Whereas patients with normal immunity generally recover completely and usually do not require antibiotic therapy, in immunosuppressed patients disseminated BCG infection may not only develop but can also be fatal. Such patients, in addition to treatment of their underlying immunologivc disorder, should receive a full course of antituberculosis chemotherapy *(11)*.

M. bovis often does not produce acute illness, persists in the carrier stage, has multiple non-human reservoirs, and easily crosses species *(15)*.

In recent years, human tuberculosis caused by *M. bovis* has been rare in developed countries *(16)* (0.5% proportion of human tuberculosis by some accounts *[17]*), and when they occurred such infections were most likely the result of either reactivation of a latent infection *(18–21)*, or acquired in developing countries or regions where the pathogen is still endemic *(22–24)*.

Although in humans the disease is usually seen in children *(25,26)* and acquired mainly through infected milk, an increase in the incidence among adult patients has been reported *(25,27)*. Dankner et al. *(28)* have described 73 mostly Hispanic patients with *M. bovis* infection that were identified in the San Diego, California area during a 12-yr period between 1980 and 1991. Of these, 13 were HIV-positive, with one patient having pulmonary disease, four having mesenteric adenitis, and eight having disseminated disease; there were no cases of meningitis. Of the 60 HIV-negative patients, only one presented with disseminated disease, and three of the patients had meningitis, as documented by positive cerebrospinal fluid (CSF) cultures. Glintborg and Wandall *(29)* reported a rare case of a chronic *M. bovis* infection causing lytic bone destruction (osteomyelitis) in the wrist.

With the spread of the AIDS epidemic, *M. bovis*-associated tuberculosis in this population has been steadily growing *(6,22,30–35)*. The majority of reported cases have been on disseminated infections *(3,6,30)*. Although the BCG strain was the commonly isolated *(6,10,30)*, AIDS patients with *M. bovis* infections not caused by the BCG strain have also been reported *(22,31)*. Bouvet et al. *(35)*

From: Opportunistic Infections: Treatment and Prophylaxis
By: Vassil St. Georgiev © Humana Press Inc., Totowa, NJ

described a nosocomial outbreak of multidrug-resistant *M. bovis* tuberculosis among HIV-infected patients in what appeared to be a single-strain source.

2. TREATMENT OF *MYCOBACTERIUM BOVIS* INFECTIONS

An HIV-positive intravenous drug user with a non-BCG *M. bovis* infection was successfully treated with a daily regimen consisting of isoniazid (300 mg) and rifampin (450 mg) given over a 12-wk period *(22)*.

In the first case of disseminated *M. bovis* (non-BCG) infection with meningitis in AIDS, the patient presented with fever, weight loss, inappetence, fatigue, and malaise. A five-drug antituberculosis therapy consisting of isoniazid (300 mg daily), rifampin (600 mg daily), ethambutol (400 mg, t.i.d.), streptomycin (1.0 g daily for a total of 20 g), and pyrazinamide (1.0 g daily) plus prednisone (50 mg daily) resulted in complete recovery *(31)*.

M. bovis sepsis in an HIV-positive infant was treated with intravenous isoniazid (20 mg/kg daily) and rifampin (20 mg/kg daily) *(10)*. After steady clinical improvment from the therapy, which was given for 1 yr, and despite a prophylactic treatment with trimethoprim-sulfamethoxazole (TMP-SMX), the patient's condition worsened dramatically, resulting in death from what was interpreted as a relapse of *Pneumocystis* pneumonia.

Modrego Pardo et al. *(36)* described a case of isoniazid resistance by *M. bovis* leading to meningitis and myelitis. In another report, multidrug-resistant tuberculosis caused by *M. bovis* was diagnosed in an HIV-positive patient *(37)*. Signorini et al. *(38)* described the management of a case of pulmonary and extra-pulmonary tuberculosis caused by an isoniazid/pyrazinamide-resistant strain of *M. bovis* in a pregnant woman. The patient was treated initially with rifampin, isoniazid, and ethambutol; pre-term delivery was induced and streptomycin was added to the regimen. To this end, Mshana et al. *(39)* used 3-(4,5-dimethylthiazol-2-yl)-2,5-diphenyl tetrazolium bromide for rapid detection of rifampin-resistant mycobacteria.

In a randomized, placebo-controlled prospective trial, Noah et al. *(40)* have evaluated the efficacy of oral erythromycin and local isoniazid instillation therapy in infants with BCG lymphadenitis and abscesses. When patients who developed subsequent regional abscesses were excluded, erythromycin caused significantly earlier resolution of lymphadenitis compared with placebo (5.1 mo vs 5.7 mo for placebo; $p < 0.01$). There was no marked difference in the percentage of patients who developed subsequent regional abscesses between the two groups (47% for erythromycin vs 60% for placebo; $p = 0.14$). Local isoniazid instillation caused significantly earlier resolution of abscesses compared with erythromycin therapy (3.9 mo for isoniazid versus 5.2 mo for erythromycin; $p < 0.001$) *(40)*.

The management of a pregnant patient with active multidrug-resistant *M. bovis* tuberculosis was carried out successfully despite concerns over teratogenicity of the second-line antituberculosis medications; the careful timing of treatment initiation resulted in clinical cure for the mother *(41)*.

Lin et al. *(42)* treated an immunodeficient infant with progressive BCG infection with thymostimulin, a specific bovine thymic extract.

A short-course chemotherapy for pulmonary infection owing to *M. bovis* was effective in three alcoholic patients suffering from malnutrition *(20)*.

The therapeutic efficacy of erythromycin in the treatment of BCG infection was examined by Singh *(43)*.

3. BCG VECTOR-BASED VACCINES IN IMMUNOTHERAPY AGAINST HIV INFECTION

A recombinant *M. bovis* bacillus Calmette-Guérin vector-based vaccine capable of secreting the V3 principal neutralizing epitope of human immunodeficiency virus (HIV) was shown to induce immune response to the epitope and prevent HIV infection in guinea pigs *(44)*. Furthermore, immunization of mice with the rBCG resulted in induction of cytotoxic T lymphocytes. Administration of serum IgG from vaccinated guinea pigs was found effective in completely blocking the HIV infection in thymus/liver transplanted severe combined immunodeficiency (SCID)/hu or SCID/PBL mice. In addition, the immune serum IgG was shown to neutralize primary field isolates of HIV that match the neutralizing sequence motif by a peripheral blood mononuclear cell-based virus neutralization assay. The obtained information has supported the concept that the antigen-secreting rBCG system may be used as a tool for the development of HIV vaccines *(44)*.

However, in a study conducted in rhesus monkeys, Yasutomi et al. *(45)* demonstrated that a vaccine-elicited, single viral epitope-specific cytotoxic T-lymphocyte response did not protect against intravenous, cell-free, simian immunodeficiency virus challenge.

REFERENCES

1. Pasic, S., Lilic, D., Pejnovic, N., Vojvodic, D., Simic, R., and Abinun, M. Disseminated Bacillus Calmette-Guerin infection in a girl with hyperimmunoglobulin E syndrome. *Acta Paediatr.,* 87, 702–704, 1998.
2. Lumb, R. and Shaw, D. *Mycobacterium bovis* (BCG) vaccination: progressive disease in a patient asymptomatically infected with the human immunodeficiency virus. *Med. J. Aust.* 156, 286, 1992.
3. Ninane, J., Grymonprez, A., Burtonboy, G., Francois, A., and Cornu, G. Disseminated BCG in HIV infection. *Arch. Dis. Child.* 63, 1268, 1988.
4. Anonymous. BCG vaccination and pediatric HIV infection: Rwanda, 1988–1990. *Morbid. Mortal. Wkly Rep.,* 40, 833, 1991.
5. Sharp, M. J. and Mallon, D. F. Regional bacillus Calmette-Guerin lymphadenitis after initiating antiretroviral therapy in an infant with human immunodeficiency virus type 1 infection. *Pediatr. Infect. Dis. J.,* 17, 660–662, 1998.
6. Boudes, P., Sobel, A., Deforges, L., and Leblic, E. Disseminated *Mycobacterium bovis* infection from BCG vaccination and HIV infection. *J. Am. Med. Assoc.,* 262, 2386, 1989.
7. TenDam, H. G. and Hitze, K. L. Does BCG vaccination protect the newborn and young infants? *Bull. W.H.O.,* 58(part 1), 37, 1980.
8. Reichman, L. B. Why hasn't BCG proved dangerous in HIV-infected patients? *J. Am. Med. Assoc.,* 261, 3246, 1989.
9. Streeton, J. A. *Mycobacterium bovis* (BCG) vaccination. *Med. J. Aust.,* 156, 812, 1992.
10. Houde, C. and Dery, P. *Mycobacterium bovis* species in an infant with human immunodeficiency virus infection. *Pediatr. Infect. Dis. J.,* 7, 810, 1988.
11. al-Bhlal, L. A. Pathologic findings for bacilli Calmette-Guerin infections in immunocompetent and immunocompromised patients. *Am. J. Clin. Pathol.,* 113, 703–708, 2000.
12. Tardieu, M., Truffot-Pernot, C., Carriere, J. P., Dupic, Y., and Landrieu, P. Tuberculous meningitis due to BCG in two previously healthy children. *Lancet,* 1, 440, 1988.
13. Murugasu, B., Quah, T. C., Quak, S. H., Low, P. S., and Wong, H. B. Disseminated BCG infection a case report. *J. Singapore Paediatr. Soc.,* 30, 139, 1988.
14. Marik, I., Kubat, R., Filipsky, J., and Galliova, J. Osteitis caused by BCG vaccination. *J. Pediatr. Orthop.,* 8, 333, 1988.
15. Nelson, A. M. The cost of disease eradication. Smallpox and bovin tuberculosis. *Ann. N. Y.Acad. Sci.,* 894, 83-91, 1999.
16. Long, R., Nobert, E., Chomye, S., et al. Transcontinental spread of multidrug-resistant Mycobacterium bovis. *Am. J. Respir. Crit. Care Med.,* 159, 2014–2017, 1999.
17. Robert, J., Boulahbal, F., Trystram, D., et al. A national survey of human *Mycobacterium bovis* infection in France. Network of Microbiology laboratories in France. *Int. J. Tuberc. Lung Dis.,* 3, 711–714, 1999.
18. Hardie, R. M. and Watson, J. M. *Mycobacterium bovis* in England and Wales: past, present and future. *Epidemiol. Infect.,* 109, 23, 1992.
19. Stoller, J. K. Late recurrence of *Mycobacterium bovis* genitourinary tuberculosis: case report and review of literature. *J. Urol.,* 134, 565, 1985.
20. O'Donohue, W. J. Jr., Bedi, S., Bittner, M. J., and Preheim, L. C. Short-course chemotherapy for pulmonary infection due to Mycobacterium bovis. *Arch. Intern. Med.,* 145, 703, 1985.
21. du Buf-Vereijken, P. W., van der Ven, A. J., Meis, J. F., Lemmens, J. A.,and van der Meer, J. W. Swelling of hand and forearm caused by Mycobacterium bovis. *Neth. J. Med.,* 54, 70–72, 1999.
22. Cornuz, J., Fitting, J. W., Beer, V., and Chave, J. P. *Mycobacterium bovis* and AIDS. *AIDS,* 5, 1038, 1991.
23. Collins, C. H. and Grange, J. M. A review: the bovine tubercle bacillus. *J. Applied Bact.,* 55, 13, 1983.
24. Moda, G., Daborn, C. J., Grange, J. M., and Cosivi, O. The zoonotic importance of Mycobacterium bovis. *Tuber. Lung Dis.,* 77, 103, 1996.
25. Waecker, N. J., Jr., Stefanova, R., Cave, M. D., Davis, C. E., and Dankner, W. M. Nosocomial transmission of *Mycobacterium bovis* bacile Calmette-Guérin to children receiving cancer therapy and to their health care providers. *Clin. Infect. Dis.,* 30, 356–362, 2000.
26. Stone, M. M., Vannier, A. M., Storch, S. K., Peterson, C., Nitta, A, T., and Zhang, Y. Brief report: meningitis due to iatrogenic BCG infection in two immunocompromised children. *N. Engl. J. Med.,* 333, 561–563, 1995.
27. Sauret, J., Jolis, R., Ausina, V., Castro, E., and Cornudella, R. Human tuberculosis due to Mycobacterium bovis: report of 10 cases. Tuber. *Lung Dis.,* 73, 388, 1992.
28. Dankner, W. M., Waecker, N. J., Essey, M. A., Moser, K., Thompson, M., and Davis, C. E. *Mycobacterium bovis*

infections in San Diego: a clinicoepidemiologic study of 73 patients and a historical review of a forgotten pathogen. Medicine (Baltimore), 72, 11, 1993.
29. Glintborg, D. and Wandall, J. H. A rare case of osteomyelitis. A case of *Mycobacterium bovis* in a wrist. *Ugeskr. Laeger,* 162, 1747–1748, 2000.
30. Centers for Disease Control. Disseminated *Mycobacterium bovis* infection from BCG vaccination of a patient with acquired immunodeficiency syndrome. *Morbid. Mortal. Wkly Rep.,* 234, 227, 1985.
31. Albrecht, H., Stellbrink, H. J., Eggers, C., Rusch-Gerdes, S., and Greten, H. A case of disseminated *Mycobacterium bovis* infection in an AIDS patient. *Eur. J. Clin. Microbiol. Infect. Dis.,* 14, 226, 1995.
32. Grange, J. M., Daborn, C., and Cosivi, O. HIV-related tuberculosis due to Mycobacterium bovis. *Eur. Respir. J.,* 7, 1564, 1994.
33. Daborn, C. J. and Grange, J. M. HIV/AIDS and its implications for the control of animal tuberculosis. *Br. Vet. J.,* 149, 405, 1993.
34. Kitching, R. P. Tuberculosis and AIDS: a deadly combination. *Br. Vet. J.,* 149, 405, 1993.
35. Bouvet, E., Casalino, E., Mendoza-Sassi, G., et al. A nosocomial outbreak of multidrug-resistant *Mycobacterium bovis* among HIV-infected patients: a case-control study. *AIDS,* 7, 1453, 1993.
36. Modrego Pardo, P. J., Perez Trullen, J. M., and Pina Latorre, M. A. Meningitis and myelitis by *Mycobacterium bovis* resistant to isoniazid. *Eur. Neurol.,* 40, 113–114, 1998.
37. Hermida Lazcano, I., Lezcano Carrera, M. A., Garcia Diez, F., Ramos Paesa, C., Martin, C., and Aguirre Errasti, J. N. Multidrug-resistant tuberculosis caused by *M. bovis* in a patient with human immunodeficiency virus infection. *Rev. Clin. Esp.,* 198, 261–262, 1998.
38. Signorini, L., Matteelli, A., Bombana, E., et al. Tuberculosis due to drug-resistant *Mycobacterium bovis* in pregnancy. *Int. J. Tuberc. Lung Dis.,* 2, 342–343, 1998.
39. Mshana, R. N., Tadesse, G., Abate, G., and Miorner, H. Use of 3-(4,5-dimethylthiazol-2-yl)- 2,5-diphenyl tetrazolium bromide for rapid detection of rifampin-resistant Mycobacterium tuberculosis. *J. Clin. Microbiol.,* 36, 1214–1219, 1998.
40. Noah, P. K., Pande, D., Johnson, B., and Ashley, D. Evaluation of oral erythromycin and local isoniazid instillation therapy in infants with Bacillus Calmette-Guérin lymphadenitis and abscesses. *Pediatr. Infect. Dis. J.,* 12, 136, 1993.
41. Nitta, A. T. and Milligan, D. Management of four pregnant women with multidrug-resistant tuberculosis. *Clin. Infect. Dis.,* 28, 1298–1304, 1999.
42. Lin, C. Y., Hau, H. C., and Hsieh, H. C. Treatment of progressive Bacillus Calmette-Guérin infection in an immunodeficient infant with a specific bovine thymic extract (thymostimulin). *Pediatr. Infect. Dis. J.,* 4, 402, 1985.
43. Singh, G. Erythromycin for BCG infections. *Clin. Pediatr. (Philadelphia),* 24, 470, 1985.
44. Honda, M., Matsuo, K., Nakasone, T., et al. Protective immune responses induced by secretion of a chimeric soluble protein from a recombinant *Mycobacterium bovis* bacillus Calmette-Guérin vector candidate vaccine for human immunodeficiency virus type 1 in small animals. *Proc. Natl. Acad. Sci. USA,* 92, 10693, 1995.
45. Yasutomi, Y., Koenig, S., Woods, R. M., et al. A vaccine-elicited, single viral epitope-specific cytotoxic T lymphocyte response does not protect against intravenous, cell-free simian immunodeficiency virus challenge. *J. Virol.,* 69, 2279, 1995.

10
Nontuberculous Mycobacterial Infections

1. INTRODUCTION

The incidence of infections caused by mycobacteria other than *Mycobacterium tuberculosis* (MOTT) has increased dramatically over the last decade or so *(1–23)*. In some areas and patient populations, the isolation of nontuberculous (also referred to as "atypical" or "anonymous") *(24–26)* mycobacteria, such as *Mycobacterium avium-intracellulare* complex (MAI) have surpassed even that of of *M. tuberculosis*. In addition to MAI, other nontuberculous mycobacteria (NTM) species that have been implicated in human disease include, among others, *M. haemophilium, M. kansasii, M. fortuitum, M. chelonae, M. bovis, M. malmoense, M. neoaurum, M. gordonae, M. terrae-triviale,* and *M. scrofulaceum*.

Because of antigenic similarities between *M. scrofulaceum* and MAI, occasional isolates identified biochemically as *M. scrofulaceum* have been serotyped as MAI and vice versa. For this reason some investigators have classified MAI and *M. scrofulaceum* together as a new pathogenic entity, the *M. avium-intracellulare scrofulaceum* complex (MAC) *(1,27,28)*.

Infections caused by NTM include chronic pulmonary disease *(29–31)*, lymphadenitis, skin and soft-tissue involvement *(11)*, and are seen in patients on continuous ambulatory peritoneal dialysis (CAPD) *(32)*, and infections of the skeletal system *(33)*. Since the 1980s, disseminated NTM disease has become common, especially in association with opportunistic infections in AIDS patients *(34)*, and also has appeared in an increasingly growing population of immunocompromised patients, such as those with malignancies, organ-transplant recipients, and those receiving immunosuppressive (e.g., corticosteroid *[35]*) therapies *(36)*.

Patients with NTM infections usually have been started on conventional multiple-drug antituberculosis therapy once acid-fast bacilli (AFB) has been detected, and before the exact type of mycobacteria has been identified *(11,37,38)*. In general, combinations containing rifampicin and ethambutol have been effective *(39)*. Dautzenberg et al. *(13)* treated AIDS patients with fever and AFB on microscopic examination of bacteriologic samples or mycobacteria isolated by culture with a daily four-drug combination consisting of rifabutine (7–10 mg/kg), isoniazid (5.0 mg/kg), ethambutol (20 mg/kg), and clofazimine (100 mg).

Based on in vitro susceptibility testing, Tsukamura and Yamori *(40)* recommended the following drug regimens for the treatment of various atypical mycobacteria: rifampicin-enviomycin-ethambutol for *M. avium-intracellulare*, ofloxacin-enviomycin-rifampicin for *M. kansasii*, enviomycin-ethambutol-isoniazid for *M. szulgai*, and ofloxacin for *M. fortuitum*.

However, the therapy of NTM infections may often be difficult in patients with severe underlying conditions and the natural resistance of most of the nontuberculous mycobacteria to currently available antituberculosis drugs. In addition, as opposed to *M. tuberculosis*, the nontuberculous mycobacteria, although sharing generally reduced sensitivity to antimycobacterial agents, may also differ in terms of drug specificity *(41)*.

From: Opportunistic Infections: Treatment and Prophylaxis
By: Vassil St. Georgiev © Humana Press Inc., Totowa, NJ

In general, in order to avoid the development of resistant strains *(42)*, and based on the frequently found synergism in vitro, nearly all NTM infections may have to be treated by combined chemotherapy *(43)*. The latter, coupled with surgical debridement *(44,45)* has been found especially beneficial in the therapy of difficult to treat infections owing to *M. ulcerans*, *M. scrofulaceum*, and *M. fortuitum/chelonae (41)*

2. NONTUBERCULOUS MYCOBACTERIAL INFECTIONS AND AIDS

Although less pathogenic than *M. tuberculosis*, in AIDS patients a number of nontuberculous mycobacteria have caused unexpectedly severe mycobacteriosis similar to that seen previously in cancer patients and transplant recipients. In general, during the time of their illness as many as 50% of AIDS patients may be infected with acid-fast bacilli *(46)*, with an estimated 5% of them developing life-threatening disseminated disease as a result of infection with MAC serovars 4 and 8 *(47)*. The virtual absence in the US AIDS population of some of the other virulent MAC serotypes (types 2, 6, 9, 12, 14, and 16), given their presence in other patients living within the same communities has been surprising *(48–50)*. Furthermore, about 10% of the mycobacterial isolates have been identified as *M. kansasii* (mostly coming from AIDS patients living in the midwest US), with another 6–9% being attributed to *M. chelonae*, *M. scrofulaceum*, *M. gordonae*, and *M. fortuitum (49)*.

In contrast to the United States and Europe, there has not been detailed epidimiological data on nontuberculous mycobacteriosis in African AIDS patients *(51,52)*. Most of the information currently available, which has been accumulated from African AIDS patients treated in Europe *(53)*, showed the preponderance of *M. tuberculosis* in these patients *(54)*. In European AIDS patients, there has been an increasing incidence of MAC serotypes 4 and 8 *(55)*, especially during the development of clinical AIDS *(52)*.

3. *MYCOBACTERIUM AVIUM* COMPLEX (MAC)

3.1. Introduction

M. avium, *M. intracellulare*, and *M. scrofulaceum* are the three major pathogens comprising the *Mycobacterium avium* complex (MAC). *M. avium* and *M. intracellulare* are the most commonly isolated nontuberculous mycobacteria and are often referred to as *M. avium-intracellulare* (MAI).

In 1982, for the first time, disseminated MAC disease was described in AIDS patients *(56,57)*. Presently, the disease, which may start as gastrointestinal infection *(58,59)*, affects approximately one-third of these patients *(60,61)*. In the U.S., *M. avium* is recognized as one of the most common opportunistic infections in HIV-positive patients *(62–65)*. The frequency of disseminated MAC infections in AIDS patients have risen significantly with diagnosis rates ranging from 18–56% *(66)*. Environmental risk factors, such as soil, water, and especially consumption of hard cheese, have been associated with an increased risk of acquisition of disseminated MAC infections in persons with AIDS *(67)*.

Compared to *M. tuberculosis*, infections with MAC tend to occur later in the course of AIDS, when immunosuppression is more advanced *(66)*. Autopsy studies *(68)* have indicated that between 30 and 50% of AIDS patients have evidence of disseminated MAC infection at their death.

One striking feature of *M. avium* infections in AIDS patients is the fact that the majority of isolates belong to serotype 4, and over 95% belong to one of three serotypes (1, 4, and 8) *(69)*. The latter finding suggests not only that serotypes 1, 4, and 8 may have a more virulent nature, but also that in the context of HIV disease, *M. avium* isolates are more virulent than those of *M. intracellulare*. Other unusual features of serotypes 1, 4, and 8 include the observation that most strains are pigmented *(69)*, and that nearly all of them contained one or more small plasmids showing some degree of homology in their DNA content *(70)*.

In a retrospective study conducted in a cohort of 702 HIV-infected patients, Flegg et al. *(71)* analyzed 46 cases of disseminated MAC infection. While concomitant colonization of the respiratory and gastrointestinal tracts was common (61 and 48%, respectively), dissemination was diagnosed antemortem in 18% of AIDS patients, and was the AIDS-defining diagnosis in 6% of all AIDS cases. Even though the overall survival from AIDS was not significantly different between patients who did or did not develop disseminated MAC disease, the latter markedly contributed to AIDS morbidity, and its incidence increased with prolonged AIDS survival *(71)*.

Assessing the relative risks associated with a history of prior opportunistic infections, changes in the CD4$^+$ levels, and baseline prognostic factors, Finkelstein et al. *(72)* found that the occurence of each opportunistic infection increased the risk of subsequent opportunistic infection, even after adjusting for the CD4$^+$ count. Specifically, the occurence of *Pneumocystis carinii* pneumonia significantly increased the risk of MAC and cytomegalovirus (CMV) infections, and to a certain degree the risk of systemic mycoses. Thus, diagnosis of MAC was associated with an increased risk of subsequent cytomegalovirus infection, where the occurence of the latter increased the risk of a MAC infection *(72)*.

Claass et al. *(73)* described a case of opportunistic disseminated MAC disease in a pediatric patient following chemotherapy for acute myeloid leukemia. The patient's cellular immunity was severely immunocompromised, with a marked depression of the CD4$^+$ counts.

In another report, a fatal case of maxillary sinusitis caused by *M. avium-intracellulare* was described in a pediatric patient with AIDS *(74)*.

3.2. Treatment of Mycobacterium avium-intracellulare *Complex (MAC) Infections*

The present questions regarding chemotherapy of MAC infection, especially in immunocompromised patients, is still far from being answered. Although in recent years some progress has been made in treating such infections, there is still no viable drug and/or combinations of drugs effective against them. The chemotherapy of the MAC infection still remains a formidable challenge because of the resistance of MAI isolates to the majority of conventional antimycobacterial agents. Results from controlled clinical trials are scarce, and a significant part of the published reports provide recommendations for therapies that are limited in scope, often anecdotal, and based mainly on empirical data *(75)*.

In general, because of drug resistance, all *M. avium-intracellulare* infections should be treated using combined chemotherapy. The first-line antimycobacterial agents currently in clinical use against *M. tuberculosis* are 10-100 times less active in vitro against MAC isolates. Such a marked decline in therapeutic potency is considered to result from the highly lipophilic nature of the *M. avium* cell wall which would prevent adequate drug penetration *(76)*. Antimycobacterial agents that have a better in vitro activity against MAC isolates (cycloserine, ethionamide) are usually considered second-line chemotherapeutics because of their more pronounced toxicity.

Thoracic infection caused by MAC typically occur in patients with underlying lung disease or immunologic abnormality. However, immunocompetent hosts have also been diagnosed with the disease *(77,78)*.

Current therapies for pulmonary *M. avium-intracellulare* infections include the use of multiple drug combinations *(79–81)*. Such regimens, however, because of their multiple-drug involvement may create a relatively high risk of toxic side effects (e.g., gastrointestinal intolerance) and their early withdrawal. The U.S. Public Health Service has provided some guidelines for treatment of MAC infection in both adults and children. It has been recommended that active disseminated MAC infections be treated with regimens that include at least two drugs, one of which is either clarithromycin or azithromycin; ethambutol may be considered as the second drug. Other potentially useful drugs include clofazimine, rifabutin, rifampin, amikacin, and ciprofloxacin. Although clinical response may be observed within 4–6 wk, sterilization of blood cultures usually takes longer.

The development of two new macrolide antibiotics, clarithromycin and azithromycin, may have signaled the turning point in the treatment of *M. avium* infection *(82–99)*. Currently, clarithromycin and azithromycin represent the cornerstone of disseminated MAC bacteremia therapy in AIDS patients *(100,101)*.

Results from controlled clinical trials have indicated the high efficiency of clarithromycin in both AIDS patients with disseminated disease and non-AIDS patients having localized pulmonary infection *(95,102,103)*. When given alone, or as part of antimycobacterial combinations, clarithromycin at doses of 0.5–2.0 g (usually administered twice daily) was found effective in controlling MAC bacteremia in AIDS patients *(104)*.

In a randomized, double-blind, dose-ranging study *(95)*, 154 AIDS patients with symptomatic MAC disease were treated for 12 wk with clarithromycin at dosages of 500 mg, 1.0 g, or 2.0 g, given twice daily. Clarithromycin decreased the mycobacterial colony-forming units (CFU) counts from 2.7–2.8 $\log_{10}$/mL of blood at baseline to less than 0 $\log_{10}$/mL during the follow-up examination ($p < 0.0001$), and at 6 wk, the median CFU counts per mL of blood was 0 or 1 for all three dose regimens. Although clarithromycin-resistant isolates of MAC developed in 46% of patients at a median of 16 wk, the median survival rate was longer in patients receiving the 500-mg dose (249 d) than in patients given 1.0 g or 2.0 g dosages. Overall, the 500-mg dose of clarithromycin was well-tolerated and associated with better survival *(95)*. To this end, Cohn et al. *(105)* found excess mortality in patients receiving 1.0 g clarithromycin (as part of three-drug combinations for treatment of disseminated MAC infections) compared to the 500-mg, b.i.d. dose.

Even though monotherapy with clarithromycin may result in the elimination of bacteremia in nearly all patients, relapse of disease inevitably will occur in patients who survive long enough to reach this event. In addition, short-term clarithromycin monotherapy may lead to bacterial resistance (within 12–16 wk), underscoring the importance of long-term treatment with a combination of antimycobacterial drugs *(95,97,100,104)*. Comparison of clarithromycin-sensitive and clarithromycin-resistant *M. avium* strains isolated from AIDS patients during therapeutic regimens containing clarithromycin showed that strains isolated during bacteremic relapses were epidemiologically related to the initial strain and did not show changes in the rate of intracellular entry and in terms of tumor necrosis factor-α (TFN-α) induction *(106)*.

Dautzenberg et al. *(107)* studied the therapeutic efficacy of clarithromycin in a randomized, double-blind, placebo-controlled trial involving 15 male AIDS (late-stage) patients with disseminated *M. avium* infection. The patients were divided into two groups. The first one received clarithromycin alone for 6 wk, then placebo plus rifampin, isoniazid, ethambutol, and clofazimine for 6 wk; the second group was treated with placebo alone, then clarithromycin plus the other four drugs. The MIC value of clarithromycin for 90% of the strains isolated from patients at baseline (as measured on 7H11 agar at pH 6.6) was 8.0 µg/mL. Eight eligible patients from the first group with initial positive culture responded with a marked decline in the number of *M. avium* CFU; in six cases, CFUs decreased to zero. When seven of the patients were switched to placebo plus the other four drugs, the CFU counts rose in four patients and remained undetectable in three. The five eligible patients from the second group initially treated with placebo had progressive increase in the CFU counts; when three were switched to clarithromycin plus the other four drugs, their CFU counts declined.

Because MAC is a major cause of chronic lymphadenitis in young children, and because complete surgical excision (which is usually curative) is not always possible, the efficacy of clarithromycin-based combination therapy of MAC lymphadenitis in otherwise healthy children has been studied. Clarithromycin in combination with either ethambutol or rifamycin was found to be effective *(108)*.

The side effects of clarithromycin were generaly mild and included a transient hypoacusis. Elevation of the serum glutamic-pyruvic transaminase and/or alkaline phosphatase levels was observed in two patients, one on clarithromycin medication and the other one receiving placebo *(107)*. Price and Tuazon *(109)* reported the existence of clarithromycin-induced thrombocytopenia. Nightingale et al. *(110)* observed acute psychosis in two AIDS patients with disseminated MAC infection after therapy with clarithromycin. The psychosis resolved when the treatment was discontinued and recurred when it was resumed. Clarithromycin has also been associated with a case of corneal opacity in an AIDS patient *(111)*. A report by Auclair et al. *(112)* indicated the presence of potential interaction between clarithromycin and the antifungal drug itraconazole, presumably through the itraconazole's effects on cytochrome P450 3A4 activity; patients experienced an increase in both the clarithromycin concentration and clarithromycin:14-OH-clarithromycin ratio, but no clinical side effects.

Using combination of clarithromycin and rifabutin for 8 mo, Malessa et al. *(113)* described the the first case of successful treatment of MAC-induced meningoencephalitis in an AIDS patient.

Benson et al. *(114)* conducted an open, prospective, randomized study to compare the efficacy and safety of clarithromycin (500 mg, b.i.d.) and ethambutol (15 mg/kg, daily), or rifabutin (450 mg, daily) (or both) against disseminated MAC infections in AIDS patients. Overall, the triple combination of clarithromycin, ethambutol, and rifabutin was associated with survival and microbiologic efficacy compared with either clarithromycin-ethambutol or clarithromycin-rifabutin. The combination of clarithromycin (1.0 g, daily), rifabutin (300–600 mg), and ethambutol (25 mg/kg) administered three times weekly was also studied in a prospective noncomparative trial in HIV-negative patients with MAC infection *(117)*. When data was compared with results from previous studies involving a regimen of daily clarithromycin and regimens including intermittent (three times weekly) azithromycin with the same companion drugs, no differences in treatment responses were evident *(115)*.

The effect of a combination of clarithromycin, ciprofloxacin, and amikacin was evaluated in 12 AIDS patients with *M. avium-intracellulare* infection *(116)*. Mycobacteremia was cleared and symptoms were resolved in all patients after 2–8 wk of therapy. Although four of the patients died, disseminated *M. avium-intracellulare* disease was not considered the primary cause of death *(116)*. Adding ciprofloxacin to a combination of clarithromycin and ethambutol had improved survival over treatmen with clarithromycin-ethambutol alone *(117)*.

In another combination, rifampicin and ethambutol were used in addition to clarithromycin for more than 12 mo of treatment; streptomycin was part of the combination for the initial 2–3 mo of therapy *(118)*. Although this regimen was found safe and tolerable even in elderly outpatients, it was not as effective against MAC pulmonary disease control compared with results of recent reports from U. S. and Europe: five bacteriologically converted cases did not show radiologic improvement.

Because rifampin and rifabutin have been known to induce the hepatic cytochrome P450 system *(119)*, Wallace et al. *(120)* examined their impact on the metabolism of clarithromycin. The serum levels of clarithromycin and its major major metabolite, 14-hydroxyclarithromycin were measured in the sera of patients receiving 500 mg twice daily before and after the addition of other antimycobacterial drugs, including 600 mg daily of either rifampin or rifabutin. The mean serum levels of clarithromycin when given as a single drug (5.4 ± 2.1 µg/mL) decreased to 0.7 ± 0.6 and 2.0 ± 1.5 µg/mL in patients receiving rifampin and rifabutin, respectively. However, the mean serum levels of 14-hydroxyclarithromycin were not influenced and remained similar in all three groups (1.8–1.9 µg/mL). Overall, rifampin and, to a lesser extent, rifabutin appeared to induce the metabolism of clarithromycin and reduce its serum concentrations when applied as part of the same regimen.

Clinical studies conducted in AIDS patients have shown that azithromycin was active against disseminated MAC infection at daily doses of 600 or 1200 mg for 6 wk *(86,101,121)*. Gastrointestinal side effects (diarrhea, nausea, and abdominal pain) were most common and more frequent in patients receiving 1200 mg of the antibiotic *(101,121)*. Wallace at al. *(122)* reported sensorineural ototoxicity associated with azithromycin during treatment of MAC infection.

An initial therapy of pulmonary MAC diseases, which has been recommended by the American Thoracic Society (ATS) *(58)*, consisted of daily administration of isoniazid (300 mg), rifampin (600 mg), and ethambutol (25 mg/kg for the first 2 mo, then 15 mg/kg), with streptomycin also given during the initial 3–6 mo of therapy *(58,123,124)*. Although the optimal dose or duration of streptomycin medication is still not well defined, daily treatment for 5 d weekly is preferred for patients younger than 70 yr of age and with normal renal function; after 6 mo of treatment, the streptomycin therapy should become intermittent. The length of the ATS-recommended treatment is also not well-defined. It has been suggested *(58)* that patients who failed to convert their sputum cultures after 12 mo of treatment should be reassessed, although earlier changes in the course of therapy may still be necessary. Subsequent therapies of such patients are difficult to manage because of the higher risk of drug toxicity.

With regard to the ATS four-drug regimen, Heifets and Iseman *(125)* objected to the inclusion of isoniazid because of its toxicity and negligible in vitro efficacy against *M. avium-intracellulare*. To this end, Tsukamura *(126)* has studied the bacteriostatic and bactericidal activity of isoniazid against various MAC strains. At concentrations of 0.1–25 µg/mL, the drug was bactericidal for several relatively susceptible strains. Overall, *M. avium* strains were more resistant to isoniazid than *M. intracellulare* strains. Although frequently used in various drug combinations, since isoniazid has been essentially inactive against MAC at achievable serum concentrations, its usefulness in combined treatment of MAC infections has been seriously questioned *(125,127,128)*.

In a Canadian HIV Trial Network Protocol 010 (CTN010), in which two regimens were compared in the treatment of *M. avium* complex bacteremia, 229 AIDS patients were randomly assigned to receive either rifampin (600 mg, daily), ethambutol (approx 15 mg/kg, daily), clofazimine (100 mg, daily), and ciprofloxacin (750 mg, b.i.d.) (regimen A); or rifabutin (600 mg, daily, amended to 300 mg daily in mid-trial), ethambutol (same as above), and clarithromycin (1.0 g, b.i.d.) (regimen B) *(129,130)*. In the regimen B group, the dose of rifabutin was reduced by half after 125 patients were randomized because 24 of 63 patients developed uveitis. Overall, among the 187 evaluable patients, the three-drug regimen B (rifabutin-ethambutol-clarithromycin) was superior than its four-drug counterpart (regimen A) in several evaluation criteria: blood cultures became negative more often in the regimen B group than in the regimen A group (69 and 29%, respectively; $p < 0.001$); in patients treated at least 4 wk, the bacteremia resolved more frequently in the regimen B group (78 vs 40%; $p < 0.001$); in the regimen B group, bacteremia resolved more often with the 600-mg dose of rifabutin than with the 300-mg dose ($p = 0.025$), but the latter regimen was still more effective than regimen A ($p < 0.05$); and the median survival time was 8.6 mo and 5.2 mo for regimens B and A, respectively ($p = 0.001$). The incidence rate of mild uveitis that developed in 3 of 53 patients receiving the 300-mg dose of rifabutin was about one-quarter that observed with the 600-mg dose ($p < 0.001$) *(129)*.

The individual effects of clofazimine, ethambutol, and rifampin on MAC bacteremia in AIDS patients were investigated by Kemper et al. *(131)*. Patients were randomized to receive daily doses of either 200 mg clofazimine, 15 mg/kg ethambutol, or 600 mg rifampin for 4 wk. Only ethambutol resulted in a statistically significant reduction in the level of mycobacteremia: the median range in individual baseline colony counts was $-0.60 \log_{10}$ CFU/mL after 4 wk of treatment ($p = 0.046$). By comparison, the median changes in individual baseline colony counts were $-0.2 \log_{10}$ CFU/mL and $+0.2 \log_{10}$ CFU/mL for clofazimine and rifampin, respectively (both, $p > 0.4$).

Jorup-Ronstrom et al. *(132)* evaluated the clinical efficacy of ethambutol (15 mg/kg), rifabutin (6.0 mg/kg), and amikacin (15 mg/kg, i.v. for 2–4 wk) in 31 HIV-infected patients with severe immunodeficiency and MAC infection. Clinical response was observed in 22 of 31 patients after a median time of 14 d; 5 patients had relapses that were successfully treated with another course of amikacin. Similarly, intravenous administration of amikacin (15 mg/kg), ethambutol (20 mg/kg), and ciprofloxacin (400 mg daily) associated with either clarithromycin or azithromycin provided encouraging results in the treatment of disseminated MAC infections in AIDS patients *(100)*.

Another recommended multiple-drug regimen involved cycloserine (250 mg, b.i.d.), ethionamide (250 mg twice daily, then increased to three times daily if tolerated), and prolonged use of streptomycin (3–5 times weekly) *(58)*. The use of clofazimine and ciprofloxacin has also been reported *(133)*.

Because the disseminated form of *M. avium-intracellulare* disease is more likely to affect immunocompromised patients *(134–136)* the severity of infection usually depends on the degree of immunosuppression, extent of mycobacterial involvement, and the therapeutic regimen. To this end, recurrence is not unusual *(137)*. Whereas in non-AIDS patients the four-drug regimen recommended for pulmonary infections appears to be beneficial *(58)*, in patients with a severely suppressed immune system during the late stages of AIDS, the response and long-term prognosis are generally poor *(62,138)*. In several reports, multiple-drug therapy that included ethambutol, rifampin (or rifabutin), clofazimine, and an injectable aminoglycoside (streptomycin, amikacin) has provided symptomatic and clinical improvement to some *(137,139,140)* but not all *(141)* patients. Thus, using a combination of rifabutin (150 or 300 mg daily) and clofazimine (100 mg daily), Mazur et al. *(141)* described a rather insignificant response to long-term therapy: a sustained clearing of mycobacteremia was observed in only 4 of 13 patents with MAC infection. Similarly, Hawkins et al. *(62)* reported that treatment of mycobacteremia with a three-drug combination of rifabutin/clofazimine/ethionamide or ethambutol was successful in only 2 of 26 patients.

One example of recurring mycobacteremia has been reported in the aftermath of a clinical trial involving 25 HIV-positive patients with MAC infection. A combination of rifabutin (300–600 mg daily), clofazimine (100 mg daily), isoniazid (300 mg daily), and ethambutol (15 mg daily) was administered for 6–74 wk (average of 38 wk) *(142)*. The results have been encouraging: mycobacteremia was cleared in 22 of 25 patients. On the negative side, however, 6 of the 22 patients involved eventually had a recurrence, most often in the group receiving 300 mg daily of rifabutin. Some of the adverse side effects associated with high-dose rifabutin in macrolide-containing regimens for the treatment of *M. avium* complex lung disease have been discussed by Berning and Peloquin *(143)*.

Rifabutin, a macrophage-penetrating lipophilic rifamycin derivative with long half-life, although showing dose-limiting toxic side effects (mainly arthralgia/arthritis and uveitis) *(144–155)*, can reduce the incidence of MAC infection when given either alone or in combination with other drugs *(67)*. Rifabutin-associated uveitis, which is characterized by anterior segment inflammation along with vitreous infiltrate, may resolve by topical steroid therapy *(154)*. Other adverse side effects included gastrointestinal symptoms (nausea, vomiting, or diarrhea) and abnormal liver enzyme levels *(156)*.

Compared to those of its structural analog, rifampicin, the clinical pharmacokinetics of rifabutin showed important differences *(157)*. Thus, rifabutin has relatively low oral bioavailability—about 20% after a single dose administration. Although its elimination half-life is long (45 h), because of the very large volume of distribution (over 9.0 L/kg), the average plasma concentrations remained relatively low after repeated administration of conventional doses *(158)*.

In a prospective study conducted by Sullam et al. *(159)*, rifabutin (600 mg, daily) or placebo were evaluated, each in combination with clofazimine and ethambutol, in AIDS patients with MAC bacteremia. The patients in the rifabutin group had a significantly higher rate of microbiological response, as defined by either sterilization of the blood, or at least a 2-$\log_{10}$ reduction in mycobacterial titers.

Griffith et al. *(156)* conducted a multiple-drug trial that included high-dose rifabutin for the treatment of MAC disease. Twenty-six patients received 600 mg daily of rifabutin in combination with ethambutol, streptomycin, and either clarithromycin (500 mg, b.i.d.; 15 patients) or azithromycin (600 mg, daily; 11 patients). Rifabutin-related adverse side effects occured in 77% of patients, with 58% requiring either dosage adjustment or discontinuation of rifabutin therapy. The most common toxicity was the reduction of the mean total white blood cell count, which decreased from 8600 ± 2800 cells/mm^3 before treatment to 4500 ± 2100 cells/mm^3 during treatment ($p = 0.0001$), followed by diffuse polyarthralgia syndrome, and anterior uveitis.

A recommended dose of 300 mg daily of rifabutin is considered to be safe in multidrug regimens containing a macrolide component for the treatment of MAC lung disease *(156)*. Results from two double-blind, randomized, placebo-controlled trials involving 1,100 patients with AIDS and AIDS-related complex have confirmed the safety and efficacy of rifabutin when given at low doses: the therapy decreased in half the rate of MAC bacteremia and significantly reduced symptoms associated with disseminated MAC disease *(160)*.

The results of several European trials of rifabutin alone or in multiple-drug combinations for treatment of infections owing to *M. avium* complex in patients with AIDS have been discussed by Dautzenberg *(161,162)*. Thus, in a prospective open study in France involving 50 patients, treatment with rifabutin, isoniazid, ethambutol, and clofazimine was well-tolerated, and the rate of conversion of cultures from positive to negative reached 70% at 6 mo. Another randomized, double-blind, placebo-controlled, prospective trial (the NTMT01 trial) has assessed the role of rifabutin in treatment with a combination containing clofazimine, isoniazid, and ethambutol; the culture conversion rate was 74% for the rifabutin group and 53% for the placebo-given patients at the last valid observation for evaluable patients. In the ongoing Curavium study, patients have been receiving clarithromycin in addition to either clofazimine or both rifabutin and ethambutol. Overall results have indicated that the best treatment for MAC infection in AIDS patients will require multiple-drug regimens, and rifabutin can be used as part of such combinations *(162)*.

Microcalorimetric studies of the initial interaction between *M. avium* and ethambutol suggested that the latter may potentiate the effect of other antimycobacterial drugs on MAI by increasing the permeability of the bacterial cell wall *(163)*. For example, in a case report involving a 57-yr-old female patient with recurring tenosynovitis due to MAI infection, treatment with a combination of ethambutol and rifabutin proved successful *(164)*. Hoffner et al. *(165)* found combinations of ethambutol with fluorinated quinolones, such as ciprofloxacin, ofloxacin, and norfloxacin, to be synergistic because of the enhanced penetration of quinolones caused by ethambutol.

The potentiating effect of ethambutol, which is thought to be mediated through a specific ethambutol receptor(s) located in the outer cell envelope of MAC *(165)*, may be the result of interference with the cell wall-permeability barrier of MAC to other drugs *(165,166)*.

Sullam *(144)* has observed a markedly enhanced efficacy of ethambutol-clofazimine combination after rifabutin had been added to the regimen. However, in combination with clarithromycin, rifabutin at daily dosages of 450 mg or more has been associated with a high incidence of uveitis, thus prompting the recommendation that only 300 mg of the drug be given daily with this macrolide.

Another four-drug combination consisting of rifampin (600 mg daily, orally), ethambutol (15 mg/kg, daily), clofazimine (100–200 mg, daily), and ciprofloxacin (750 mg b.i.d., orally) was tried for 12 wk in 31 patients; in addition, 6 of the patients also received amikacin *(167)*. At the end of the treatment period, the majority of patients showed improved clinical signs.

Peloquin *(168)* has found that in some non-AIDS patients infected with MAC, rifampin at 600 mg daily, and ciprofloxacin at 750 mg b.i.d. failed to produce serum drug concentrations (SDCs) that would have exceeded the pathogen's minimum inhibitory concentration (MIC), and therefore, may require doubling of these dosages to attain SDCs similar to those observed in patients without the absorption problem.

Ciprofloxacin-induced acute renal dysfunction has also been observed 8–10 d after commencement of therapy; the patients recovered spontaneously following cessation of therapy for 2–8 wk, and toxicity did not recur when treatment was restarted with regimens that did not contain ciprofloxacin *(169)*. In another study *(170)*, a possible interaction between foscarnet and ciprofloxacin in two patients with AIDS, CMV retinitis, and MAC infection has been examined. The incidence of seizures with foscarnet infusion is high, ranging from 13–15%, and predisposing factors, such as renal impairment, electrolyte and metabolic abnormalities, and underlying neurologic disorders have been associated with seizures during foscarnet therapy. The two patients developed generalized tonic-clonic seizures while receiving both drugs, with neither of them having any of the aforementioned risk factors.

Wormser et al. *(171)* recommended the use of a low-dose dexamethasone (typically 2.0 mg daily) as adjunctive therapy for disseminated MAC infections in AIDS patients. All patients experienced substantial and sustained weight gain (12–50% of pre-steroid treatment weight; $p < 0.03$), reduction of fever, and increased serum albumin; the serum alkaline phosphatase level, however, fell from 368 ± 247 U/L to 128 ± 43.6 U/L ($p < 0.04$).

Osteomyelitis in immunocompetent patients due to dissemination of *M. avium* complex has been reported on several occasions *(65,94,172–174)*. Jones et al. *(172)* described a case of MAC-associated osteomyelitis and septic arthritis in an immunocompetent patient. The infection, which was derived from an injury sustained 13 yr earlier and had spread through the bone, joint, and soft tissue emerging at the medial aspect, was treated successfully with surgical debridement, drainage, arthrodesis, and 18 mo of chemotherapy consisting of clarithromycin, rifampin, ethambutol, and ciprofloxacin, with an initial 2 wk of amikacin. However, in another case of MAI-induced osteomyelitis involving the patella, distal femur, and the proximal tibia, the patient failed to respond to arthroscopic synovectomy and combination therapy. The need for aggressive surgical intervention has been stressed *(94)*. Pirofsky et al. *(102)* described a case of spinal osteomyelitis due to *M. avium-intracellulare* in an immunocompromised elderly patient undergoing corticosteroid therapy.

It is important to note that therapy of HIV-positive patients with zidovudine during treatment of MAC infections may result in bone-marrow depression and high risk of toxicity. Protionamide (also prothionamide), although effective, often caused nausea. A low-maintenance dose of corticosteroids was instituted in order to suppress fever and malaise *(175)*. Table 1 lists toxic side effects caused by drugs currently used to treat MAC infections.

Results from studies of HIV-infected patients with newly diagnosed MAC bacteremia has shown that treatment of MAC infection was associated with decreases in the plasma TNF-α and interleukin (IL)-6 levels *(176,177)*.

3.2.1. Immunotherapy of MAC Infections

Recently, it was shown that human alveolar macrophages can be selectively activated without systemic effect by the use of aerosolized IFN-α, a cytokine capable of enhancing the oxidative and antimicrobial activities of macrophages. In this context, Chatte et al. *(178)* used IFN-α to treat an HIV-negative patient with silicosis and advanced MAI cavitary lung disease with three courses of aerosolized interferon-α (IFN-α) (500 µg 3 d weekly for 5 wk in two courses, and 200 µg 3 d weekly for 5 wk after a short single trial of subcutaneous IFN-α). The numbers of MAI decreased in the sputum during therapy, but cultures remained positive (at the same levels) for the first two treatment periods. However, the patient's sputum became AFB smear negative and the number of colonies decreased significantly after the third course of IFN-α therapy. Cessation of IFN-α treatment led to a rapid increase in the number of MAI in the sputum *(178)*. Previously, Holland et al. *(179)* treated a refractory MAC infection with combination of subcutaneous IFN-α (administered 2–3 times weekly at 25–50 µg/m² of body-surface area) and antimycobacterial medication. All patients showed marked clinical and radiologic improvement, abatement of fever, clearing of lesions, and reduced need for paracentesis *(179)*.

Tsukada et al. *(134)* have reported a case of an opportunistic disseminated MAI infection in an immunosuppressed patient with myelodysplastic syndrome (refractory anemia) on a long-term corticosteroid therapy. Although the patient responded initially to a combination of antimycobacterial drugs and recombinant human GM-CSF, spike fever recurred and the pantocytopenia progressed. Furthermore, the presence of hepatosplenomegaly and marked retroperitoneal lymphadenopathy indicated further dissemination of MAI. Additional treatment with human rGM-CSF and a very low-dose of cytosine arabinoside failed to bring any improvement.

Neutrophils isolated from AIDS patients following a 5-d treatment with G-CSF (but not rifabutin) demonstrated enhanced killing of *M. avium* added ex vivo *(180)*. However, G-CSF did not have significant effect on the HIV viral load.

Studies by Kang et al. *(181)* in mice have shown that fibroblasts secreting IL-12, which stimulates resistance to *M. avium* complex, may serve as a vehicle for paracrine secretion of IL-12 for immunotherapy of MAC infection.

3.2.2. Prophylaxis of Mycobacterium avium-intracellulare Infections in AIDS Patients

Guidelines have been established by the U.S. Public Health Service for the prophylactic treatment of MAC infections in HIV-positive patients (Table 2). It is recommended that AIDS patients with CD4⁺ cell counts below 100 cells/mm³ should receive such therapy. However, medication adherence by patients should be considered essential for the treatment and prophylaxis of MAC infections, especially in HIV-infected patients *(182)*.

A proposed dose regimen of 300 mg daily of rifabutin has been based on results from two clinical trials showing the beneficial effect of prophylactic rifabutin in delaying or preventing MAC bacter-

Table 1
Toxic Side Effects of Drugs Used to Treat MAC Infections

Drug	Toxicities
Isoniazid	Fever, rash, hepatitis, central nervous system (CNS) disorders, peripheral neuropathy
Ethionamide	Gastrointestinal intolerances (vomiting, abdominal pain, nausea), hepatitis, CNS disorders (depression, seizures, hallucinations), peripheral neuritis
Ethambutol	CNS disorders (optic neuritis, peripheral neuritis, dizziness, disorientation, hallucinations)
Clofazimine	Discoloration of tissue and body fluids, gastrointestinal toxicity (abdominal pain, diarrhea, malabsorption)
Cycloserine	Peripheral neuropathy (dizziness, insomnia, nervousness)
Ciprofloxacin	Gastrointesinal disorders (nausea, vomiting, diarrhea), CNS toxicity (headache, insomnia), hypersensitivity (fever, rash), acute renal dysfunction
Tetracyclines (doxycycline, minocycline)	Gastrointestinal toxicity (nausea, vomiting, diarrhea), CNS disorders (minocycline: dizziness, vertigo), hypersensitivity (rash, photosensitivity, hyperpigmentation), hematologic disturbancies (anemia, leukopenia)
Sulfonamides (trimethoprime/ sulfamethoxazole)	Gastrointestinal intolerance (nausea, vomiting, diarrhea), leukopenia, anemia thrombocytopenia, hypersensitivity (rash, fever, Stevens-Johnsone syndrome)
Cefoxitine	Hypersensitivity (fever, rash, eosinophilia), anemia, leukopenia
Rifabutin	Arthralgia, arthritis, uveitis, transient rash, jaundice, pseudojaundice hepatitis, hemolytic anemia, leukopenia, thrombocytopenia
Clarithromycin	Transient hypoacusis, thrombocytopenia, acute psychosis, elevated glutamic- pyruvic transferase and/or alkaline phosphatase levels, corneal opacity
Azithromycin	Sensorineural ototoxicity
Streptomycin, amikacin	Vestibulary/auditory disturbancy (dizziness, vertigo, ataxia, tinnitus, hearing loss), nephrotoxicity (tubular necrosis, nonoliguric azotemia, neuromuscular blockade, hypersensitivity (streptomycin: rash, fever, eosinophilia)
Rifampin	Gastrointestinal intolerance (nausea, vomiting), rash, fever, hepatitis, "flu-like" syndrome, thrombocytopenia, renal failure associated with intermittent therapy, discoloration of secretion and urine, increased hepatic metabolism of drugs administered concomitantly (contraceptives, ketoconazole, oral hypoglycemics, prednisolone, quinidine, warfarine, methadone)

Table 2
Prophylaxis for MAC Infections[a]

Patients	Indication	Prophylactic drug regimens	
		First line	Alternative line
Adults and adolescents	First episode: CD4+ counts of <50 µL	Clarithromycin 500 mg, p.o., b.i.d.; or Azithromycin 1.2. g, p.o., weekly	Rifabutin, 300 mg, p.o., daily; or Azithromycin 1.2. g, p.o., weekly + rifabutin 300 mg, p.o., daily
	Prior disseminated disease	Clarithromycin 500 mg, p.o., b.i.d. + ethambutol 15 mg/kg, p.o., daily (with or without rifabutin) 300 mg p.o., daily	Azithromycin 500 mg, p.o., daily + ethambutol 15 mg/kg (with or without rifabutin) 300 mg, p.o., daily
Infants and children	First episode[b]	Clarithromycin 7.5 mg/kg (max 1.2 g), p.o., b.i.d.; or Azithromicin 20 mg/kg (max 1.2 g), p.o., weekly	Azithromycin 5 mg/kg (max 250 mg), p.o., daily; or Rifabutin 300 mg p.o., daily[c]
	Prior disease	Clarithromycin 7.5. mg/kg (max 500 mg), p.o., b.i.d. + ethambutol 15 mg/kg (max 900 mg), p.o., daily (with or without rifabutin 5 mg/kg [max. 300 mg], p.o., daily	Azithromycin 5 mg/kg (max 250 mg), p.o., daily + ethambutol 15 mg/kg (max 900 mg), p.o., daily (with or without rifabutin 5 p.o., daily

[a]Adapted from the 1999 U.S. Public Health Service and Infectious Diseases Society of America *Guidelines for the Prevention of Opportunistic Infections in HIV-Infected Patients.*
[b]For children aged ≥6 yr, CD4+ count <50/µL; aged 2–6 yr, CD4+ count <75/µL; aged 1–2 yr, CD4+ count <500/µL; aged <1 yr, CD4+ count <750/µL.
[c]For children aged ≥6 yr.

emia in AIDS patients with low CD4+ counts *(160,183–188)*. In both studies, rifabutin was given at 300 mg daily. The first trial involved 590 patients with mean baseline CD4+ cell counts of 65.9 (rifabutin group) and 56.5 (placebo). Only 9% (26 of 292 patients) of the rifabutin recipients developed *M. avium-intracellulare* bacteremia compared to 16% (47 of 298 patients) for the placebo group. In the second trial, which enrolled 556 patients, the mean baseline CD4+ cell counts were 61.8 for rifabutin recepients and 52.8 for the placebo group; 30 of 274 patients (11%) of the rifabutin-treated patients and 53 of 282 (19%) of the placebo-receiving patients developed MAI bacteremia. Adverse side effects (urine discoloration), although similar in both groups, have been more frequent in the rifabutin-treated recipients. There was no difference in the survival rates of the rifabutin and placebo groups, and MAI isolated from breakthrough bacteremia cases was not rifabutin-resistant. Although the overall results of both trials demonstrated that prophylaxis with rifabutin was effective in reducing *M. avium-intracellulare* bacteremia, the probability of AIDS patients (especially those with CD4+ cell counts below 100 cell/mm^3) to develop MAI bacteremia 2 yr thereafter was still greater than 20%. Special concerns about rifabutin prophylaxis include its interactions with metadone, ketoconazole, zidovudine, and hepatically metabolized drugs. Although less potent inducer than rifampin, rifabutin was found to induce hepatic cytochrome P450, which may enhance the clearance of some types of drugs *(189)*. In addition, studies by Pulik et al. *(190)* showed that rifabutin prophylaxis in HIV-infected patients reduced the incidence of campylobacter infections.

The prophylactic efficacies of clarithromycin and azithromycin (alone or in combinations with other drugs) in preventing *M. avium-intracellulare* bacteremia have been the subjects of several reports *(86,191–193)*. In one randomized study, 108 patients received either 500 mg, 1,000 mg, or 2,000 mg of clarithromycin twice daily *(194)*. Interim results for the first 72 patients have shown a 2.6–2.8 log decline in CFUs of MAI in the blood over a 3-mo period. The median sterilization times were 55, 43, and 27 d for 500 mg, 1,000 mg, and 2,000 mg dosage regimens, respectively. However, a substantial drug intolerance was observed in patients receiving 2.0 g of the drug.

Similar to azithromycin, one significant drawback of clarithromycin as a single-drug prophylactic therapy has been the emergence of resistance. Hewitt et al. *(195)* conducted a nonrandomized retrospective chart review of all patients at their center who had $CD4^+$ counts below 200 cells/mm^3. Ninety of 148 patients treated had received for at least 4 wk, clarithromycin (500 mg, daily), rifabutin (300 mg/daily), dapsone (50 mg or 100 mg three times weekly), or clarithromycin and dapsone in combination. Although MAI bacteremia was not evident in 22, 11, and 11 patients receiving clarithromycin, dapsone, and dapsone/clarithromycin combination, respectively, 1 of 18 patients receiving rifabutin, and 14 of 58 patients who did not receive treatment have showed bacteremia *(195)*.

The efficacy and safety of clarithromycin and rifabutin alone and in combination for prevention of MAC disease were compared in a randomized, double-blind, placebo-controlled trial involving 1178 AIDS patients with $CD4^+$ cell counts of 100 cells/μL or less *(191)*. Combination therapy was no more effective than clarithromycin; failures to either combination or clarithromycin alone were associated with MAC strains resistant to clarithromycin. Although both clarithromycin and combination therapy were more effective for prevention of MAC than rifabutin alone, combination therapy was associated with more adverse side effects (31%; $p < .001$) *(191)*.

Abrams et al. *(196)* investigated the efficacy of clofazimine as prophylaxis for disseminated *M. avium-intracellulare* disease. A trial was conducted involving 109 patients randomized to receive either clofazimine at 50 mg daily or no treatment. After a mean follow-up of 299 d, 7 of 53 clofazimine recipients, and 6 of 46 no-treatment patients had developed disseminated MAI infection ($p = 0.76$). The size of the trial was too small to allow for any definitive conclusions about the prophylactic efficacy of clofazimine.

Reconstitution of the immune system after long-term use of antiretroviral therapy such as highly active antiretroviral therapy (HAART) raises the question of whether anti-infectious prophylaxis should be maintained. According to several reports *(197–199)*, prophylaxis agains MAC infections can be safely withdrawn or withheld in HIV-infected adults who experienced immune reconstitution (increases in $CD4^+$ cell counts) while receiving antiretroviral therapy such as 1.2 g of azithromycin once weekly *(197,200)* and protease inhibitor-containing regimens *(201)*. However, it is important to emphasize that possible reactions to earlier pathogens after restoration of specific immunity would warrant *secondary prophylaxis* even in patients responding to powerful HAART regimens *(193,202)*. Consistent with the new U.S. Public Health Service guidelines, azithromycin prophylaxis, started after the $CD4^+$ count has fallen to 50 cells/mm^3, has been the most effective MAC prophylaxis strategy in terms of both survival rate and cost-effectiveness *(203)*.

Scharfstein et al. *(204)* developed a simulation model to project costs, life expectancy, and cost-effectiveness of prophylaxis to prevent MAC in AIDS patients.

Noncompliance with MAC prophylaxis due to use of numerous other medications, drug interactions, and lack of knowledge of the condition by patients is still a problem *(205)*. Data from a crossover study of MAC prophylaxis adherence by McNabb et al. *(206)* comparing azithromycin (2×600 mg tablets, once weekly) with clarithromycin (500 mg, every 12 h) for 2 mo, suggested that the azithromycin administration schedule maximized the benefit of MAC prophylaxis because patients receiving complicated medication have been more willing/able to adhere to once-weekly than twice-daily dosing.

3.2.3. MAC Infections and Highly Active Antiretroviral Therapy (HAART)

The impact of highly active antiretroviral therapy (HAART) among HIV-positive patients in decreasing the incidences of mycobacterial infections by improving the immune function (even in more advance disease) has been the subject of several recent reports *(207–215)*. Usually, the Cox's model is used to calculate the relative hazards of MAC occurrence according to the age and time-dependent variables, such as CD4$^+$ below 50 cells/mm^3, previous occurrence of tuberculosis, CMV infection and other AIDS-defining disease, nature of antiretroviral treatment, and MAC prophylaxis *(208)*. In general, due to increases in the CD4$^+$ cell counts following HAART, there have been significant documented decreases in the incidence of tuberculosis (TB) and to an even larger extent of MAC infections among HIV-positive patients *(207–210)*.

Using data from the EuroSIDA study involving 7000 patients enrolled in an European multicenter observational cohort, the overall incidence of *M. tuberculosis* (TB) and MAC infections were 0.8 and 1.4 cases/100 person-years of follow-up (PYF), decreasing from 1.8 (TB) and 3.5 cases/100 PYF (MAC) before September 1995 to 0.3 and 0.2 cases/100 PYF after March 1997 *(207)*.

One criteria for discontinuing primary prophylaxis in adult HIV-positive patients is increase of the CD4$^+$ count over 100 cells/μL for over 3–6 mo and sustained suppression of HIV plasma RNA. There has been no criteria established for stopping secondary prophylaxis of MAC infection.

However, a HAART-associated improvement of the immune status might convert a clinically silent MAC infection into an active mycobacterial disease *(216)*. Thus, Nalaboff et al. *(217)* and Kaplan *(218)* described an unusual manifestation of infection with MAC ("*M. avium-intracellulare* reversal syndrome") in AIDS patients after the initiation of HAART, which included protease inhibitors and two new nucleoside analogs. Patients experienced a febrile illness and developed mass lesions containing mycobacterial microorganisms in various organ systems (bone, skin, and mesenteric and mediastinal nodes) coinciding with improvement in their immunologic status (decreased viral loads and increased CD4$^+$ cell counts). It has been postulated that the observed complications may represent a response of the recovering immune system to a new or previously subclinical infection with MAC *(217)*.

Furthermore, MAC infection may also recur as a generalized or focal disease in those patients experiencing HAART-associated CD4$^+$ cell recovery, which, although significant, has not been optimal *(219,220)*.

4. MYCOBACTERIUM KANSASII

4.1. Introduction

Buhler and Pollack *(221)* were the first to describe a *M. kansasii* infection in 1953. Initially characterized as the "yellow bacillus," *M. kansasii* is a photochromogenic mycobacterium, with nearly all of its strains being yellow-orange; only occasionally, strains may become nonpigmented or scotochromogenic.

The most common *M. kansasii* infection has been chronic pulmonary disease, which may resemble that caused by MAI (e.g., caseating granulomas *[222]*), except that fewer patients had preexisting lung disease and the response to chemotherapy was stronger *(223–234)*. Chronic pulmonary caused by *M. kansasii* can range from mild, self-limiting disease to severe progressive and sometimes fatal illness with extensive cavitation *(24,235–237)*. Pleural effusions and lymphadenopathy have been rare *(1)*.

Disseminated *M. kansasii* usually involved immunosuppressed patients with impaired cellular immunity *(35,228,238–241)*. Characteristic manifestations, such as fever, constitutional symptoms, pulmonary symptoms, hepatosplenomegaly, and hematologic abnormalities (leukopenia, pancytopenia) have been common. Lymphadenopathy, diffuse bone involvement, skin lesions *(242,243)*, genitourinary involvement *(244,245)*, pericarditis *(246,247)*, myelodysplastic syndrome *(248)*, and gastrointestinal involvement have been observed less frequently *(1)*. Development of cervical lymphadenitis caused by *M. kansasii*, particularly in immunosuppressed children and patients, is growing in importance and should be considered in the differential diagnosis in cervical masses *(507)*.

Clinically similar to that of *M. tuberculosis* meningitis, *M. kansasii*-related meningitis has been rare but with higher mortality rate *(250)*.

The first incidence of *M. kansasii* infection in AIDS patients has been reported by Woods and Washington *(1)*. Later, more cases of both pulmonary and disseminated disease followed to parallel the rise of the AIDS epidemic *(10,251–274)*.

In patients with advanced HIV-related immunosuppression, *M. kansasii* may cause serious and potentially life-threatening pulmonary disease *(261,263,275)*. Boudon et al. *(256)* conducted a retrospective study of 12 HIV-positive patients (10 of them with AIDS) who had developed *M. kansasii* pulmonary infections characterized by nodular, interstitial or diffuse parenchymal infiltrates, and mediastinal and hilar adenopathies, but no cavitary lung disease. Valainis et al. *(264)* also did not observed cavitary formation at the time of initial presentation. In contrast, based on chest radiografts, Levine and Chaisson *(261)* and Bamberger et al. *(257)* reported the presence of pulmonary cavitation in AIDS patients with *M. kansasii* mycobacteriosis. In fact, the latter group has found radiographic evidence of either pulmonary cavitation or predominantly upper-lobe disease in 8 of 22 patients with *M. kansasii* pulmonary disease *(257)*. To explain these discrepancies, it has been suggested that pulmonary cavitations in patients with *M. kansasii* infection may instead be the result of zidovudine medication, which is known to lead to partial reconstitution of the cellular immune responses, thereby increasing the hypersensitivity reaction (e.g., exudative reaction) and resulting in tissue necrosis and cavitation *(262)*. In the experience of Chaisson and Levine *(275)*, however, the higher prevalence of of pulmonary cavities in AIDS patients with *M. kansasii* disease cannot be explained by zidovudine therapy because in their study, only 2 of 8 patients receiving zidovudine at the time of the diagnosis had pulmonary cavitation compared with 5 of 11 patients not receiving zidovudine therapy.

Several reports *(254,276,277)* have presented cases of patients who developed septic arthritis due to *M. kansasii*.

In a retrospective study involving 49 AIDS patients, *M. kansasii* was isolated at a mean CD4$^+$ cell count of 62 cells/mm^3 and at a mean interval of 17 mo after the diagnosis of AIDS; 17 patients had disseminated disease *(274)*. In contrast, Urkijo et al. *(258)* reported that in all but two of 13 AIDS cases, the CD4$^+$ cell counts were lower than 200 cells/mm^3 when *M. kansasii* was diagnosed.

4.2. Treatment of M. kansasii *Infections*

Most strains of *M. kansasii* were found susceptible in vitro to rifampin, cyclosporine, rifabutin, davercin, and ofloxacin, and only slightly resistant to isoniazid, ethambutol, augmentin, and streptomycin *(1,278)*.

In clinical settings, most patients with *M. kansasii* infections (both pulmonary and extrapulmonary) have been responsive to combinations of two or more antimycobacterial drugs, one of which was rifampin *(28,224,227,228,279)*. However, Wallace et al. *(280)* have identified 36 rifampin-resistant *M. kansasii* isolates, with 32% of them recovered from HIV-positive patients. Previously, Dautzenberg et al. *(259)* reported on acquired rifampicin resistance during *M. kansasii* infection in an AIDS patient; the minimal inhibitory concentrations of rifampicin against the *M. kansasii* strain were 0.2 µg/mL at the onset and 128 µg/mL after the treatment, respectively. Meynard et al. *(281)* have described a rifampin-resistant *M. kansasii* infection in an AIDS patient receiving rifabutin.

Antimicrobial combinations containing clarithromycin or azithromycin have been shown to be effective against nontuberculous mycobacterial infections *(282,283)*. However, an AIDS patient with severe *M. kansasii* infection failed to respond to a treatment with clarithromycin and ethambutol; the initial isolate was found to be highly resistant to clarithromycin *(284)*. Nucleotide sequencing of the 23S rRNA gene of this isolate showed a single base mutation at position 2058, the same that was found for clarithromycin-resistant *M. avium*.

Five weeks after treatment consisting of rifampin, isoniazid, and streptomycin, a patient with pulmonary *M. kansasii* infection suddenly developed acute renal failure (rapidly developing glomerulonephritis); after antirifampin antibody was detected, the cessation of rifampin treatment led to rapid spontaneous recovery of the patient's renal function *(285)*.

Although pulmonary infections have responded well to therapy *(3,286,287)*, relapses have occurred *(280,286,288)*, and although rarely, fatal outcomes due to progression of disease have also been reported *(237,257,263)*. Surgical treatment of pulmonary *M. kansasii* infections was reported to be beneficial in certain specific cases, including localized disease with persistent cavitation in which the organism has not been eradicated from sputum after a 6-mo follow-up period, acquired drug resistance resulting from poor compliance, and severe drug intolerance.

With the exception of disseminated disease where despite adequate therapy *(239)*, the outcome may be uncertain (and even fatal *[289]*), the prognosis of extrapulmonary disease when treated appropriately has been generally favorable *(1)*. In this respect, reducing the dose of corticosteroids may be a beneficial adjunct to the therapy *(290)*. Combination of rifampin and ethambutol (but not isoniazid as previously suggested) is recommended *(273)*.

When *M. kansasii* has been confined to the skin *(291)*, the disease was usually indolent *(292)*, and chemotherapy with traditional antituberculosis agents as well as erythromycin, minocycline, and doxycycline has been successful *(290)*. However, Delaporte et al. *(242)* found treatment with minocycline followed by ciprofloxacin to be ineffective in a case of immunocompetent patient with cutaneous infection due to *M. kansasii*. Because erythromycin was well-tolerated and showed adequate tissue penetration with excellent activity against *M. kansasii*, its use in the therapy of cutaneous infections has been recommended *(293)*.

Patel et al. *(7)* have described *M. kansasii* infections in solid transplant recipients presenting as a cutaneous lesion and a pulmonary nodule that responded well to surgery, reduction in doses of immunosuppressive medication, and/or therapy with antimycobacterial drugs.

Treatment with conventional antituberculosis drugs (including isoniazid and pyridoxine at 300 and 150 mg daily, respectively) of *M. kansasii*-induced cavitating pneumonia in a patient with rheumatoid arthritis had to be stopped because of exacerbation of isoniazid-induced peripheral neuropathy; clinical improvement was observed only after both isoniazid and pyridoxine have been withdrawn *(294)*. Trimethoprime-sulfamethoxazole combination does not offer protection against *M. kansasii* infection *(269)*.

A fatal outcome due to *M. kansasii* pneumonia was reported in a case of an HIV-positive patient despite treatment with isoniazid, rifampin, ethambutol, and clofazimine *(263)*.

Sauret et al. *(295)* evaluated the therapeutic response of *M. kansasii* pulmonary disease to 12- and 18-mo course of daily chemotherapy consisting of rifampicin-isoniazid-ethambutol (ethambutol only for the first 6 mo). Because patients from both groups showed essentially the same degree of clinical improvement based on radiographic examination and sputum conversion, the 12-mo course (with ethambutol given only during the first 6 mo of therapy) has been recommended as adequate *(295)*. Campbell *(31)* has disagreed with the role of isoniazid as presented by Sauret et al. *(295)* and concurred with the finding of the prospective study by the British Thoracic Society *(296)* that isoniazid may be of no benefit whatsoever in the treatment of *M. kansasii* pulmonary infection.

In a retrospective multicenter study conducted by the British Thoracic Society the optimal duration of treatment of *M. kansasii* pulmonary infections with rifampicin and ethambutol, and whether isoniazid should also be given, were found to be uncertain *(257)*. The results have shown that although, overall a 9-mo course of treatment with rifampicin and ethambutol appeared to be adequate, patients who contracted *M. kansasii* pulmonary infections nevertheless had a high mortality rate resulting from other causes. In addition, it seemed that isoniazid (which had been recommended at a potentially harmful daily dose of 600 mg *[297]*) did not appear to be necessary as part of a drug regimen for *M. kansasii* infection, especially when most strains have been resistant to isoniazid and pyrazinamide *(24,296)*.

Umeda et al. *(298)* described a case of *M. kansasii* lung infection associated with myelofibrosis that had been refractory to treatment with conventional antituberculosis drugs, and leading to hilar and mediastinal lymph node enlargement and finally their calcification.

Ahn et al. *(299)* tested 14 wild strains and 14 relapse or treatment failure isolates of *M. kansasii*, and found them to be highly susceptible to sulfamethoxazole, with 26 of 28 isolates having MICs of less than or equal to 4.0 µg/mL in a broth microdilution assay. In addition, treatment failure isolates frequently exhibited acquired resistance to rifampin (MIC > 2.0 µg/mL), isoniazid (MIC > 4.0 µg/mL), and ethambutol (MIC > 4.0 µg/mL) not seen among the wild isolates. Eight patients with cavitary disease induced by rifampin-resistant *M. kansasii* were treated successfully with a 4–10-wk course of sulfamethoxazole-containing regimens that also included high-dose isoniazid (900 mg), ethambutol (25 mg/kg), and an aminoglycoside (either streptomycin or amikacin)

In another report *(300)*, a patient with *M. kansasii* pulmonary infection developed severe aplastic anemia (hypoplastic marrow and pancytopenia) after treatment with a conventional regimen of antituberculosis drugs. Changing to ofloxacin, to which the pathogen was sensitive, did not bring any clinical improvement because of complete resistance after several months of treatment. The disease was cured by lobectomy and postoperative administration of sparfloxacin.

Matthiessen et al. *(302)* have cultured *M. kansasii* from the sputum of a patient with the Swyer-James syndrome. The lung infection, which responded well to daily administration of rifampicin (600 mg), ethambutol (1.6 g), and protionamide (0.5 g), recurred after 2 yr. The recurrence again responded well to the same drug regimen with additional sulfamethoxazole (1.6 g). Kramers et al. *(302)* grew *M. kansasii* from blood samples of a patient with Sweet's syndrome and leukopenia related to hairy cell leukemia. The patient recovered after treatment with recombinant IFN-α and tuberculostatic drugs. Remarkably, the skin lesions completely regressed within 1 wk after the start of rIFN-α therapy. Previously, Bennett et al. *(303)* reported the development of disseminated atypical mycobacteriosis (*M. kansasii*, *M. avium-intracellulare*, and *M. chelonae*) in 9 of 186 patients with hairy cell leukemia.

According to Kurasawa et al. *(304)* the use of isoniazid, rifampicin, ethambutol, and/or streptomycin (or kanamycin) was highly effective in the treatment of *M. kansasii* and *M. szulgai* infections. *M. kansasii*-produced β-lactamase can be inhibited by clavulanic acid *(305)*.

5. MYCOBACTERIUM XENOPI

5.1. Introduction

Although it was first isolated in 1957 *(306)*, *M. xenopi* was not recognized as a human pathogen until 1965 *(222)*. It is a scotochromogenic organism producing a yellow pigment that varies in intensity.

Human infections by *M. xenopi* have been associated mainly with pulmonary disease, with adult males being more frequently affected than females *(5,14,307–322)*. Most patients had either preexisting lung disease *(323)* or another predisposing factor, such as immunosuppression due to extrapulmonary malignancies *(324)*, alcoholism *(325)*, diabetes mellitus *(1)*, solid organ *(326,327)* and bone-marrow *(328)* transplatations, or AIDS *(320,329–335)*.

The *M. xenopi* infection may be chronic, subacute, or acute. Clinical symptoms, which for the most part have been nearly indistinguishable from pulmonary tuberculosis *(17,314,318,336)* or illness caused by MAI or *M. kansasii*, included nodular or mass lesions, single or multiple cavities, multifocal nodular densities, apical shadowing, consolidation, and fibrosis *(1)*.

Extrapulmonary infections induced by *M. xenopi* have been rare and involved bone and joints *(312,337–346)* tenosynovitis *(347)*, lymph node, epididymis, a sinus tract, urogenital infection *(348)*, psoas muscles *(349)*, and a prosthetic temporomandibular joint *(222)*.

Disseminated disease has been reported on several occasions *(330,331,350,351)*, including in patients with AIDS *(161,331–333)*, in an immunocompromised patient with myelogenous leukemia and diabetes mellitus *(350)*, and in a patient who was not known to be immunosuppressed *(352)*.

A newly described species of mycobacteria, *M. celatum*, rarely has been diagnosed as the cause of localized and disseminated human disease, and can be mistaken easily for *M. xenopi* when identification is based on biochemical testing alone. Zurawski et al. *(353)* reported two such cases in AIDS patients where pneumonia and bacteremia due to *M. celatum* was diagnosed as *M. xenopi* infection.

5.2. Treatment of M. xenopi Infections

Results from in vitro susceptibility testing and clinical management of *M. xenopi* disease have been inconsistent *(1,6)*. There have been reports in which in vitro sensitivities against antimycobacterial agents such as isoniazid, ethambutol, streptomycin, and rifampin correlated well with their clinical efficacy when applied in combinations (such as rifampin-ethambutol *[336]*) *(39,316)*. However, in other studies *(310)*, although resistance to the aforementioned drugs has been observed, there have been uniform susceptibility to cycloserine and ethionamide. Even so, relapses were not infrequent *(39)*, and response to retreatment was poor *(310)*. Baugnee et al. *(354)* found little evidence of correlation between in vitro sensitivity to antimycobacterial drugs and their therapeutic efficacies.

Because of frequent unreability of antimycobacterial drug therapy against *M. xenopi* infections, complications of treatment, and the risk of recurrence after treatment, in most cases, surgical debridement has been beneficial *(319,355)*. To this end, preliminary results from collapse therapy with plombage for pulmonary disease caused by multidrug-resistant *M. xenopi* was reported *(356)*. Collapse therapy is a conservative alternative therapy in patients with pulmonary disease caused by multidrug-resistant mycobacteria at high risk of treatment failure considered to be unsuitable for pulmonary resection *(356)*.

In a double-blind, randomized, placebo-controlled, 12-wk trial involving AIDS patients with disseminated disease due to either *M. avium* or *M. xenopi*, Dautzenberg et al. *(161)* evaluated the therapeutic efficacy of rifabutin (450 or 600 mg, daily). Companion drugs used in both the infection and placebo arms included ethambutol, clofazimine, and isoniazid. Although no significant difference was observed in clinical improvement, mortality, or toxicity between the two treatment arms, it has been suggested that the addition of rifabutin to a triple-drug combination may contribute to the clearance of disseminated mycobacterial infection in AIDS patients without causing additional toxicity. In a previously conducted French study on mycobacterial infections resistant to rifampin, a treatment protocol for *M. xenopi* infection was proposed *(357)*. The suggested daily regimen consisted of 5.0–7.0 mg/kg rifabutin, 20 mg/kg ethambutol, 3.0–5.0 mg/kg isoniazid, and 400 mg of ofloxacin (or 800 mg of pefloxacin). Seventy-seven percent (10 out of 13) of *M. xenopi* cultures were negative, 3 mo after commencing therapy.

A case of *M. xenopi* pulmonary infection was treated with a combination of isoniazid (400 mg), streptomycin (0.75 g), and rifampicin (450 mg); 2 mo after treatment, transbronchial biopsy specimens showed development of a new lesion, which was subsequently resolved by the same antimycobacterial drugs *(358)*.

Huber et al. *(329)* described a case of an AIDS patient with *M. xenopi* pneumonia who was successfully treated with an antituberculosis drug regimen consisting of daily administration of isoniazid (300 mg), rifampicin (600 mg), streptomycin (900 mg), and pyrizinamide (2.0 g). In another case, pulmonary *M. xenopi* infection in a natural killer (NK) cell-deficient patient was treated successfully with a combination of clarithromycin, rifabutin, and sparfloxacin *(359)*.

Relapsing peritonitis due to *M. xenopi* in a patient undergoing continuous peritoneal dialysis was treated with oral antibiotics in combination with intraperitoneal streptomycin, permitting peritoneal dialysis to be continued with satisfactory clearance and ultrafiltration capacity. The streptomycin pharmacokinetics revealed that 75% of the intraperitoneally administered dose was absorbed from the dialysate *(317).*

Miller et al. *(337)* linked a case of Pott's disease with *M. xenopi* infection. Also known as "tuberculosis of the spine," the Pott's disease (osteitis or carries of the vertebrae) usually occurs as complication of tuberculosis of the lungs *(360).* Previously, two reports by Prosser *(338)* and Rahman et al. *(339)* have described vertebral (lumber spine) infection due to *M. xenopi.*

Kiehl et al. *(361)* have described a rare lupus-vulgaris-like infection caused by *M. xenopi* in an immunocompetent female patient, which responded well to treatment with isoniazid.

A case of fulminant hepatic encephalopathy and renal failure in a patient with *M. xenopi* infection resulted in death despite combination therapy with isoniazid, rifampin, and prothionamide *(362).* This fatal outcome may not be so unusual because there has been a widespread recognition that isoniazid can cause fulminant hepatic failure *(363,364),* as well as previous fatalities from hepatic failure after its administration (bilirubin levels exceeding 340 µmol/L) *(365).*

Consideration should be given to regular clinical monitoring of liver function, especially when patients continue to take isoniazid during the prodromal phase (usually lasting for 1–4 wk and often characterized by vague and nonspecific symptoms) of their illness when the severity of hepatitis correlates with continued drug use during this phase *(366).*

AIDS patients may show significant rise of their mycobacteria-specific lymphoproliferative responses shortly after initiation of HAART treatment; this was temporarily associated with elevations of the CD4$^+$ cell counts and the subsequent resolution of *M. xenopi* infection without antimycobacterial therapy *(367).*

6. MYCOBACTERIUM HAEMOPHILUM

First described in 1978 *(368), Mycobacterium haemophilum* is the etiologic agent of a rare but rapidly emerging infection *(369)* associated mainly with the development of ulcerating cutaneous lesions *(369–387).*

Initially, *M. haemophilum* disease has been observed in patients receiving immunosuppressive therapy *(388),* such as renal-transplant recipients *(370,372,376,386).* However, in the last several years, the infection has been diagnosed with increased frequency in patients with AIDS *(369,371,375,377–379,381,384,389–391).* In addition, *M. haemophilum* has also been identified in immunocompetent children with cervical and perihilar lymphadenitis *(374,383,384,387),* as well as in patients with lymphoma *(368,386,392),* renal, bone marrow and cardiac transplant recipients, rheumatoid arthritis, marrow hypoplasia, and Crohn's disease *(392,393).*

M. haemophilum is known to cause disseminated cutaneous lesions; bacteremia; and disease of the bones, joints, lymphatics, and the lungs. Cutaneous lesions are found most often on the extremities (frequently overlying joints), and less commonly on the trunk and face. Patients with severe immune deficiencies caused by AIDS, immunosuppressive therapy (such as organ-transplant recipients), and lymphoma, in addition to skin lesions, had the pathogen isolated from vitreous fluid, synovial fluid, bronchoalveolar lavage fluid, lung tissue, blood, lymph nodes, wound specimens, bone marrow, and sputum, which suggests hematogenous spread of the organism *(378,379,381,385,394).*

Recently, *M. haemophilum* was also recognized as a newly emerging cause of osteomyelitis in immunocompromised patients; its incidence has increased significantly with the growing AIDS epidemic *(395–400)* and organ transplantations *(398,401,402).*

6.1. Treatment of M. haemophilum Infections

M. haemophilum appears to be an emerging opportunistic pathogen in AIDS patients and should be considered in the differential diagnosis of suspected mycobacterial infections in HIV-positive patients. There have been a number of cases described where the initial response to therapy was favorable, only to be followed by a recurrence of infection *(375).* Complete resolution was only observed when the antimycobacterial therapy was combined with antiretroviral therapy *(389).*

Careful surgical drainage of lesions and antimycobacterial therapy have been used to treat *M. haemophilum* infections *(403)*. Ward et al. *(404)* have reported on the rare but difficult-to-treat nontuberculous mycobacterial infections (*M. haemophilum* and *M. chelonae*) associated with the tunnel of Hickman-Broviac central venous catheter in immunosuppressed patients with hematologic malignancies undergoing high-dose chemotherapy supported by bone-marrow transplantation. In their experience, even early wide surgical excision of the infected tunnel site and prolonged antibiotic therapy considered to be necessary may still result in recurrence.

Most studies have demonstrated in vitro susceptibility of *M. haemophilum* to rifampin and *p*-aminosalicylic acid *(368,372,379,380,382,405)*. When tested for susceptibility, *M. haemophilum* isolates have been found variously susceptible to amikacin, streptomycin, kanamycin, ethionamide, cycloserine, capreomycin, cefotaxin, minocycline, doxycycline, ciprofloxacine, rifabutin, and trimethoprim-sulfamethoxazole *(396,406)*, whereas the majority of isolates were resistant to ethambutol, isoniazid, and pyrazinamide *(368,369,379,380,385,391)*. However, the correlation between data from in vitro susceptibility tests and results from antimycobacterial therapy were not very clear. In one case described by Dever et al. *(375)*, a patient responded dramatically to a regimen of isoniazid, rifampin, ethambutol, and ciprofloxacin. However, the infection still recurred to respond markedly to a subsequent treatment with izoniazid, rifampin, ethambutol, ciprofloxacin, amikacin, and clofazimine. To this end, development of resistance to rifamycins has been demonstrated after patients were treated for several months *(391)*.

Various treatment regimens have been used including combinations of antimycobacterial drugs, such as isoniazid, rifampin *(399)*, and ethambutol *(368,399)*, isoniazid and rifampin *(373)*, trimethoprim-sulfamethoxazole *(380)*, minocycline *(372,376)*, erythromycin *(376,407)*, rifampine and minocycline *(372)*, rifampine and *p*-aminosalicylic acid *(378)*, rifampin and erythromycin *(377)*, as well as doxycycline *(399)*, clarithromycin, ciprofloxacin *(387,399)*, amikacine *(399)*, clofazimine *(399)*, streptomycin, and pyrazinamide*(369)*.

Minocycline administered as either adjunctive therapy with surgery, or combined with rifampin, has produced some response *(372,376)*. Improvement has been observed also by using sulfamethoxazole alone *(380)*. Thus, treatment with sulfamethoxazole at a dose of 1.0 g given twice daily resulted in slow but steady regression of lesions in a patient with *M. haemophilum* infection *(380)*.

McBride et al. *(387)* reported a case of a postoperative (coronary artery bypass surgery) *M. haemophilum* infection in an immunocompetent patient who responded with nearly complete resolution of skin lesions to ciprofloxacin given at 500 mg twice daily, for 5 mo.

Branger et al. *(372)* have reported a case involving a renal-transplant recipient who developed a *M. haemophilum* infection associated with *M. xenopi* infection. Initial therapy with isoniazid and rifampin had no clinical effect. After surgical drainage of the lesion and administration of minocycline, the patient recovered. In another case involving an immunosuppressed renal-transplant recipient *(382)*, treatment with rifampin (450 mg daily), isoniazid (300 mg daily), and ethambutol (400 mg daily), as well as reduction of immunosuppressive prednisolone therapy to a maintenance level (20 mg daily), did not bring any regression of lesions; eventually the lesions began to regress and later resolved fully. A cardiac transplant recipient showed excellent response to a prolonged treatment with clarithromycin and rifampin; it is noteworthy to report the interaction between these two antibiotics and cyclosporine, including the offsetting effects of clarithromycin-rifampin therapy on the blood levels of cyclosporine *(401)*.

An AIDS patient who developed tenosynovitis caused by *M. haemophilum* was the first documented case in AIDS *(379)*. Of the several antimycobacterial drugs tested for susceptibility, only rifampin exhibited significant activity against the isolate of the patient. In another report *(381)*, two AIDS patients failed to respond to any of the applied antimycobacterial therapy (isoniazid, rifampin) against *M. haemophilum* lesions; there was also evidence of hematogenous dissemination of disease (positive blood cultures, and distant sites of involvement). Thibert et al. *(385)* also reported similar hematogenous dissemination in an AIDS patient.

7. MYCOBACTERIUM GENAVENSE

In 1992, Hirschel et al. *(408)* described the first *M. genavense* infection in a severely immunocompromised AIDS patient. The patient, who died from the infection, presented with fever, hepatosplenomegaly, and gastrointestinal symptoms. The pathogen was present in massive quantities in nearly all tissues examined (duodenum, feces, urine, and bone marrow). The infection probably begins in the gastrointestinal tract after oral contamination *(409)*. The pathogenicity of *M. genavense* in AIDS patients was described as similar to that of disseminated infection caused by *M. avium-intracellulare (409–420)*. The use of corticosteroids by these patients possibly favored colonization and dissemination of atypical mycobacteria *(409,414,416,417,421)*. In a study conducted by Pechère et al. *(412)*, the median CD4$^+$ count of infected patients was 0.016×10^9/L (16 cells/mm^3).

In a study of 18 AIDS patients with disseminated *M. genavense* disease, Böttger et al. *(410)* described the main clinical features in the majority of patients as relentless loss of weight, fever, and diarrhea resulting from the massive infection of the intestine and liver as well as lungs, bone marrow, and lymph nodes.

From 1990–1992, 12.8% of disseminated mycobacterial infections in AIDS patients from Switzerland were attributed to *M. genavense (412)*. Because of such high incidence, it has been suggested that this mycobacterial species should be considered seriously in the differential diagnosis of patients with AIDS with CD4$^+$ counts below 100 cells/mm^3, and presenting with diarrhea, weight loss, and fever *(410,412,419,420,422,423)*. In addition, biopsies of liver, duodenum, bone marrow, or lymph nodes should reveal acid-fast rods that cannot be cultured on solid media, although blood cultures in Middlebrook 13A liquid medium may show some growth. In a case report by Albrecht et al. *(424) M. genavense* was identified as the cause of pseudo-Whipple's disease and sclerosing cholangitis.

Berman et al. *(425)* described a rather unusual case of *M. genavense* infection in an AIDS patient who presented with grand mal seizures and a mass brain lesion, with evidence of dissemination.

Krebs et al. *(426)* described the first case of disseminated *M. genavense* infection in an HIV-seronegative patient with lymphocytic anemia, a chronic hematologic disorder. The patient had been receiving chlorambucil (partially in combination with prednisone) for his condition when the infection developed. Treatment with clarithromycin, ethambutol, and rifabutin resulted in improvement in anemia and general health, as well as in regression of lymphadenopathy and splenomegaly. In another case, an HIV-seronegative woman with chronic lymphopenia presented with a localized *M. genavense* soft-tissue infection *(427)*. The lesion resolved after treatment with clarithromycin, ethambutol, and ciprofloxacin. Figueras et al. *(428)* reported hyperpigmentation in an AIDS patient receiving rifabutin for disseminated *M. genavense*.

The optimum treatment of *M. genavense* has yet to be determined, although by analogy with *M. avium-intracellulare* and antibiotic sensitivity tests *(429,430)*, amikacin, clofazimine, ethambutol, rifabutin, clarithromycin, azithromycin, and ciprofloxacin (as well as other fluoroquinolones) may be considered *(410)*. According to Bessesen et al. *(413)*, and Matsiota-Bernard et al. *(431)*, the best clinical response and clearance of bacteremia were associated with clarithromycin therapy. Among patients who had been treated with at least two antimycobacterial drugs for 1 mo or more, the median survival was 263 d (95% confidence interval, 144–382 d), compared with 81 d (95% confidence interval, 73–89 d) for those not treated ($p = 0.0009$) *(412)*.

REFERENCES

1. Woods, G. L. and Washington, J. A. II. (1987) Mycobacteria other than *Mycobacterium tuberculosis*: review of microbiologic and clinical aspects. *Rev. Infect. Dis.*, 9, 275, 1987.
2. Xia, X. X. Clinical analysis of 41 cases of pulmonary atypical mycobacteriosis. *Chung Hua Chieh Ho Ho Hsi Tsa Chih*, 15, 200, 1992.
3. Boggs, D. S. The changing spectrum of pulmonary infections due to nontuberculous mycobacteria. *J. Okla. State Med. Assoc.*, 88, 373, 1995.
4. Choudhri, S., Manfreda, J., Wolfe, J., Parker, S., and Long, R. Clinical significance of nontuberculous mycobacteria isolates in a Canadian tertiary care center. *Clin. Infect. Dis.*, 21, 128, 1995.

5. Hoffner, S. E. Pulmonary infections caused by less frequently encountered slow-growing environmental mycobacteria. *Eur. J. Clin. Microbiol. Infect. Dis.*, 13, 937, 1994.
6. Dautzenberg, B. and Mercat, A. Atypical mycobacterial infections. *Presse Med.*, 23, 1483, 1994.
7. Patel, R., Roberts, G. D., Keating, M. R., and Paya, C. V. Infections due to nontuberculous mycobacteria in kidney, heart, and liver transplant recipients. *Clin. Infect Dis.*, 19, 263, 1994.
8. Kozin, S. H. and Bishop, A. T. Atypical *Mycobacterium* infections of the upper extremity. *J. Hand Surg. [Am]*, 19, 480, 1994.
9. Kennedy, T. P. and Weber, D. J. Nontuberculous mycobacteria: an underappreciated cause of geriatric lung disease. *Am. J. Respir. Dis.*, 149, 1654, 1994.
10. Idigbe, E. O., Nasidi, A., Anyiwo, C. E., et al. Prevalence of human immunodeficiency virus (HIV) antibodies in tuberculosis patients in Lagos, Nigeria. *J. Trop. Med. Hyg.*, 97, 91, 1994.
11. Georgiev, V. St. Treatment and developmental therapeutics of *Mycobacterium avium* complex (MAC) infections. *Int. J. Antimicrob. Agents*, 4, 247, 1994.
12. Bonafe, J. L., Grigorieff-Larrue, N., and Bauriaud, R. Atypical cutaneous mycobacterium diseases: results of a national survey. *Ann. Dermatol. Venereol.*, 119, 463, 1992.
13. Dautzenberg, B., Truffot, C., Mignon, A., et al. Rifabutin in combination with clofazimine, isoniazid and ethambutol in the treatment of AIDS patients with infections due to opportunistic mycobacteria. *Tubercle*, 72, 168, 1991.
14. Clague, H. W., el-Ansary, E. H., Hopkins, C. A., and Roberts, C. Pulmonary infection with opportunist mycobacteria on Merseyside 1974–1983. *Postgrad. Med. J.*, 62, 363, 1986.
15. Griffith, D. E., Girard, W. M., and Wallace, R. J. Jr. Clinical features of pulmonary disease caused by rapidly growing mycobacteria: an analysis of 154 patients. *Am. Rev. Respir. Dis.*, 147, 1271, 1993.
16. Wallace, R. J. Jr. The clinical presentation, diagnosis, and therapy of cutaneous and pulmonary infections due to the rapidly growing mycobacteria, *M. fortuitum* and *M. chelonae*. *Clin. Chest Med.*, 10, 419, 1989.
17. Contreras, M. A., Cheung, O. T., Sanders, D. E., and Goldstein, R. S. Pulmonary infection with nontuberculous mycobacteria. *Am. Rev. Respir. Dis.*, 137, 149, 1988.
18. Martinez Moragon, E., Menendez, R., Santos, M., Lorente, R., and Marco, V. Lung diseases due to opportunistic environmental *Mycobacteria* in patients uninfected with human immunodeficiency virus. *Arch. Bronconeumol.*, 32, 170, 1996.
19. Kurasawa, T., Ikeda, N., Sato, A., et al. A clinical study of non-tuberculous pulmonary mycobacteriosis. *Kekkaku*, 70, 621, 1995.
20. Skogberg, K., Ruutu, P., Tukiainen, P., and Valtonen, V. V. Nontuberculous mycobacterial infection in HIV-negative patients receiving immunosuppressive therapy. *Eur. J. Clin. Microbiol. Infect. Dis.*, 14, 755, 1995.
21. Molina-Gamboa, J. D., Ponce-de-Leon, S., Sifuentes-Osornio, J., Bobadilla del Valle, M., and Ruiz-Palacios, G. M. Mycobacterial infection in Mexican AIDS patients. *J. Acquir. Immune Defic. Syndr. Hum. Retrovirol.*, 11, 53, 1996.
22. Raszka, W. V. Jr., Skillman, L. P., McEvoy, P. L., and Robb, M. L. Isolation of nontuberculous, non-*avium* mycobacteria from patients infected with human immunodeficiency virus. *Clin. Infect. Dis.*, 20, 73, 1995.
23. Furrer, H., Bodmer, T., and von Overbeck, J. Disseminated nontuberculous mycobacterial infections in AIDS patients. *Schweiz. Med. Wochenschr.*, 124, 89, 1994.
24. Davies, P. D. Infection with *Mycobacterium kansasii*. *Thorax*, 49, 435, 1994.
25. Grange, J. M. and Yates, M. D. Infections caused by opportunistic mycobacteria: a review. *J. R. Soc. Med.*, 79, 226, 1986.
26. Runyon, E. H. Anonymous mycobacteria in pulmonary disease. *Med. Clin. North Am.*, 43, 273, 1959.
27. Noel, S. B., Ray, M. C., and Greer, D. L. Cutaneous infection with *Mycobacterium avium- intracellulare scrofulaceum* intermediate: a new pathogenic entity. *J. Am. Acad. Dermatol.*, 19, 492, 1988.
28. Gruft, H., Falkinham, J. O. III, and Parker, B. C. Recent experience in the epidemiology of disease caused by atypical mycobacteria. *Rev. Infect. Dis.*, 3, 990, 1981.
29. Wongwatana, S. and Sriyabhaya, N. Nontuberculous mycobacterial infection of the lung in a chest hospital in Thailand. *J. Med. Assoc. Thai.*, 75, 1, 1992.
30. Zvetina, J. R., Maliwan, N., Frederick, W. E., and Reyes, C. *Mycobacterium kansasii* infection following primary pulmonary malignancy. *Chest*, 102, 1460, 1992.
31. Campbell, I. A. Treatment of pulmonary disease caused by *Mycobacterium kansasii*, results of 18 vs. 12 mo' chemotherapy [comment]. *Tuber. Lung Dis.*, 76, 583, 1995.
32. White, R., Abreo, K., Flanagan, R., et al. Nontuberculous mycobacterial infections in continuous ambulatory peritoneal dialysis patients. *Am. J. Kidney Dis.*, 22, 581, 1993.
33. O'Brien, R. J., Geiter, L. J., and Snider, D. E. Jr. The epidemiology of nontuberculous mycobacterial diseases in the United States: results from a national survey. *Am. Rev. Respir. Dis.*, 135, 1007, 1987.
34. Joint Position Paper of the American Thoracic Society and the Centers for Disease Control. Mycobacteriosis and the acquired immunodeficiency syndrome. *Am. Rev. Respir. Dis.*, 136, 492, 1987.
35. Veale, D., Fishwick, D., White, J. E., Gascoigne, A. D., Gould, K., and Corris, P. A. Culture of *Mycobacterium kansasii* in the blood of an HIV-negative patient. *Thorax*, 48, 672, 1993.
36. Wolinsky, E. Mycobacterial diseases other than tuberculosis. *Clin. Infect. Dis.*, 15, 1, 1992.
37. Heurlin, N. and Petrini, B. Treatment of non-tuberculous mycobacterial infections in patients without AIDS. *Scand. J. Infect. Dis.*, 25, 619, 1993.
38. Hornick, D. B., Dayton, C. S., Bedell, G. N., and Fick, R. B. Jr. Nontuberculous mycobacterial lung disease: substantiation of a less aggressive approach. *Chest*, 93, 550, 1988.
39. Al Jarad, N., Demertzis, P., Jones, D. J., et al. Comparison of characteristics of patients and treatment outcome for pulmonary non-tuberculous mycobacterial infection and pulmonary tuberculosis. *Thorax*, 51, 137, 1996.

40. Tsukamura, M. and Yamori, S., Chemotherapeutic regimens for nontuberculous mycobacterial infection based on invitro susceptibility test results. *Kekkaku*, 65, 349, 1990.
41. Brodt, H. R., Current therapy of atypical mycobacterial infections. *Immun. Infekt.*, 20, 39, 1992.
42. Neubert, R., Resistant behavior of atypical mycobacteria to antibiotics and sulfonamides. *Z. Erkr. Atmungsorgane*, 167, 47, 1986.
43. Vandiviere, H. M., Dillon, M., and Melvin, I. G., Atypical mycobacteria causing pulmonary disease: rapid diagnosis using skin test profiles. *South. Med. J.*, 80, 5, 1987.
44. Inagaki, K., Arai, T., Yano, M., et al. Role of surgical treatment in atypical mycobacteriosis of the lung. *Kekkaku*, 66, 769, 1991.
45. Plaus, W. J. and Hermann, G. The surgical management of superficial infections caused by atypical mycobacteria. *Surgery*, 110, 99, 1991.
46. Collins, F. M., *M. avium*-complex infections and development of the acquired immunodeficiency syndrome: casual opportunist or casual cofactor. *Int. J. Leprosy*, 54, 458, 1986.
47. Horsburgh, C. R. and Selik, R. M. The epidemiology of disseminated tuberculous mycobacterial infection in the acquired immunodeficiency syndrome (AIDS). *Am. Rev. Respir. Dis.*, 139, 4, 1989.
48. Good, R. C. and Snider, D. E. Jr. Isolation of nontuberculous mycobacteria in the United States, 1980. *J. Infect. Dis.*, 146, 829, 19982.
49. Good, R. C. Opportunistic pathogens in the genus *Mycobacterium*. *Annu. Rev. Microbiol.*, 39, 347, 1986.
50. McClatchy, J. K. The seroagglutination test in the study on nontuberculous mycobacteria. *Rev. Infect. Dis.*, 3, 867, 1981.
51. Quinn, T. C., Mann, J. M., Curran, J. W., and Piot, P. AIDS in Africa: an epidimiological paradigm. *Science*, 234, 955, 1986.
52. Lamoureux, G., Davignon, L., Turcotte, R., Leverdier, M., Mankiewicz, E., and Walker, M. C. Is prior mycobacterial infection a common predisposing factor to AIDS in Haitians and Africans? *Ann. Inst. Pasteur*, 138, 521, 1987.
53. Anonymous. Clinical features of AIDS in Europe. *Eur. J. Cancer Clin. Oncol.*, 20, 165, 1984.
54. Pinching, A. J. Acquired immune deficiency syndrome: with special reference to tuberculosis. *Tubercle*, 68, 65, 1987.
55. Goldman, K. P. AIDS and tuberculosis. *Tubercle*, 69, 71, 1988.
56. Macher, A.M., Kovacs, J. A., Gill, V., et al. Bacteremia due to *Mycobacterium avium- intracellulare* in the acquired immunodeficiency syndrome. *Ann. Intern. Med.*, 99, 782, 1983.
57. Greene, J. B., Sidhu, G. S., Lewin, S., et al. *Mycobacterium avium-intracellulare*: a cause of disseminated life-threatening infection in homosexuals and drug abusers. *Ann. Intern. Med.*, 97, 539, 1982.
58. Wallace, R.J. Jr., O'Brien, R., Glassroth, J., Raleigh, J., and Dutt, A. Diagnosis and treatment of disease caused by nontuberculosis mycobacteria. *Am. Rev. Respir. Dis.*, 142, 940, 1990.
59. Damsker, B. and Bottone, E. J. *Mycobacterium avium-Mycobacterium intracellulare* from the intestinal tracts of patients with acquired immunodeficiency syndrome: concepts regarding acquisition and pathogenesis. *J. Infect. Dis.*, 151, 179, 1985.
60. Lerner, C. W. and Tapper, M. L. Opportunistic infection complicating acquired immunodeficiency syndrome. *Medicine (Baltimore)*, 63, 155, 1984.
61. Fauci, A. S., Masur, H., Gelmann, E. P., Markham, P. B., Hahn, B. H., and Lane, H. C. The acquired ammunodeficiency syndrome: an update. *Ann. Intern. Med.*, 102, 800, 1965.
62. Hawkins, C. C., Gold, J. W. M., Whimbey, E., et al. *Mycobacterium avium*-complex infections in patients with acquired immunodeficiency syndrome. *Ann. Intern. Med.*, 105, 184, 1986.
63. Snider, D. E., Hopewell, P. C., Mills, J., and Reichman, L. B. Mycobacteriosis and the acquired immunodeficiency syndrome. *Am. Rev. Respir. Dis.*, 136, 492, 1987.
64. Moroni, M., Gori, A., Rusconi, S., Franzetti, F., and Antinori, S. Mycobacterial infections in AIDS: an overview of epidemiology, clinical manifestations, therapy and prophylaxis. *Monaldi Arch. Chest Dis.*, 49, 432, 1994.
65. Benson, C. Disseminated *Mycobacterium avium* complex disease in patients with AIDS. *AIDS Res. Hum. Retroviruses*, 10, 913, 1994.
66. Mehta, J. B. and Morris, F. Impact of HIV infection on mycobacterial disease. *Am. Fam. Physician*, 45, 2203, 1992.
67. Anwar, D., Sudre, P., and Horsburgh, B. Disseminated *Mycobacterium avium* complex disease (DMAC): environmental risk factors in persons with human immunodeficiency virus infection. *38th Intersci. Conf. Antimicrob. Agents Chemother.*, American Society of Microbiology, Washington DC, 404, abstract I-133, 1998.
68. Wallace, J. M. and Hannah, J. B. *Mycobacterium avium* complex infection in patients with the acquired immunodeficiency syndrome. *Chest*, 93, 926, 1988.
69. Kiehn, T. E., Edwards, F. F., Brannon, P., et al. Infections caused by *Mycobacterium avium* complex in immunocompromised patients: diagnosis by blood culture and fecal examination, antimicrobial susceptibility tests, and morphological and seroagglutination characteristics. *J. Clin. Microbiol.*, 21, 168, 1985.
70. Crawford, J. T. and Bates, J. H. Analysis of plasmids in *Mycobacterium avium-intracellulare* isolates from persons with acquired immunodeficiency syndrome. *Am. Rev. Respir. Dis.*, 134, 659, 1986.
71. Flegg, P. J., Laing, R. B., Lee, C., et al., Disseminated disease due to *Mycobacterium avium* complex in AIDS. *Q. J. Med.*, 88, 617, 1995.
72. Finkelstein, D. M., Williams, P. L., Molenberghs, G., et al. Patterns of opportunistic infections in patients with HIV infection. *J. Acquir. Immune Defic. Syndr. Hum. Retrovirol.*, 12, 38, 1996.
73. Claass, A., Claviez, A., Westphal, E., Rusch-Gerdes, S., and Schneppenheim, R., First case of disseminated *Mycobacterium avium* infection, Infection, 23, 301, 1995.
74. Sussman, S. J. Sinusitis caused by *Mycobacterium avium-intracellulare* in a patient with human immunodeficiency virus. *Pediatr. Infect. Dis. J.*, 14, 726, 1995.

75. Horsburgh, C. R. Jr. Advances in the prevention and treatment of *Mycobacterium avium* disease. *N. Engl. J. Med.*, 335, 428, 1996.
76. Rastogi, N., Frehel, C., Ryter, A., Ohayon, H., Lesourd, M., and David, H.L. Multiple drug resistance in *Mycobacterium avium*: is the wall architecture responsible for the exclusion of antimicrobial agents? *Antimicrob. Agents Chemother.*, 20, 666, 1981.
77. Sanchez Munoz, M. C., Barrio Gomez de Aguero, M. I., Martinez Carrasco, M. C., and Antelo Landeira, M. C. Primary *Mycobacterium avium* respiratory infection in nonimmunocompromised children. *Arch. Bronconeumol.*, 31, 246, 1995.
78. Patz, E. F. Jr., Swensen, S. J., and Erasmus, J. Pulmonary manifestations of nontuberculous *Mycobacterium*. *Radiol. Clin. North Am.*, 33, 719, 1995.
79. Kalayjian, R. C., Toossi, Z., Tomashefski, J. F. Jr., et al. Pulmonary disease due to infection by *Mycobacterium avium* complex in patients with AIDS. *Clin. Infect. Dis.*, 20, 1186, 1995.
80. Kissinger, P., Clark, R., Morse, A., and Brandon, W. Comparison of multiple drug therapy regimens for HIV-related disseminated *Mycobacterium avium* complex disease. *J. Acquir. Immune Defic. Syndr. Hum. Retrovirol.*, 9, 133, 1995.
81. Calzetti, C., Magnani, G., Elia, G., Avanzi, M., Pasetti, G., and Fiaccadori, F. Retrospective study of *Mycobacterium avium* complex infection in the acquired immunodeficiency syndrome. *Ann. Ital. Med. Int.*, 8, 166, 1993.
82. Wallace, R. J. Jr., Brown, B. A., Griffith, D. E., Girard, W. M., and Murphy, D. T., Clarithromycin regimens for pulmonary *Mycobactrium avium* complex: the first 50 patients. *Am. J. Respir. Crit. Care Med.*, 153, 1766, 1996.
83. Frothingham, R. Clarithromycin treatment for *Mycobacterium avium-intracellulare* complex lung disease. *Am. J. Respir. Crit. Care Med.*, 153, 1990, 1996.
84. Bates, J. H. *Mycobacterium avium* disease: progress at last. *Am. J. Respir. Crit. Care Med.*, 153, 1737, 1996.
85. Young, L. S. Treatment and prophylaxis of *Mycobacterium avium* complex. *Int. J. STD AIDS*, 7(Suppl. 1), 23, 1996.
86. Perronne, C. Azithromycin and *Mycobacterium avium* infection. *Pathol. Biol. (Paris)*, 43, 565, 1995.
87. Coulaud, J. P. Azithromycin: new orientation. *Pathol. Biol. (Paris)*, 43, 547, 1995.
88. Singh, N. and Yu, V. L. Clarithromycin therapy for *Mycobacterium avium* complex bacteremia. *Ann. Intern. Med.*, 123, 154, 155, 1995; [see also: *Ann. Intern. Med.*, 121, 905, 1994].
89. van der Meer, J. T. and Danner, S. A. Clarithromycin therapy for *Mycobacterium avium* complex bacteremia. *Ann. Intern. Med.*, 123, 154, 1995.
90. Musher, D. M. Clarithromycin therapy for *Mycobacterium avium* complex bacteremia. *Ann. Intern. Med.*, 123, 154, 1995.
91. Ives, D. V., Davis, R. B., and Currier, J. S. Impact of clarithromycin and azithromycin on patterns of treatment and survival among AIDS patients with disseminated *Mycobacterium avium* complex. *AIDS*, 9, 261, 1995.
92. Dautzenberg, B., Piperno, D., Diot, P., Truffot-Pernot, C., and Chauvin, J. P. Clarithromycin in the treatment of *Mycobacterium avium* lung infections in patients without AIDS. Clarithromycin Study Group of France. *Chest*, 107, 1035, 1995.
93. Havlir, D. V. *Mycobacterium avium* complex: advances in therapy. *Eur. J. Clin. Microbiol. Infect. Dis.*, 13, 915, 1994.
94. Rapp, R. P., McCraney, S. A., Goodman, N. L., and Shaddick, D. J. New macrolide antibiotics: usefulness in infections caused by mycobacteria other than *Mycobacterium tuberculosis*. *Ann. Pharmacother.*, 28, 1255, 1994.
95. Chaisson, R. E., Benson, C. A., Dube, M. P., et al. Clarithromycin therapy for bacteremic *Mycobacterium avium* complex disease: a randomized, double-blind, dose-ranging study in patients with AIDS. *Ann. Intern. Med.*, 121, 905–911, 1994.
96. Dautzenberg, B., Saint-Marc, T., Durant, J., et al. Treatment with clarithromycin of 173 HIV+ patients with disseminated *Mycobacterium avium intracellulare* infection. *Rev. Mal. Respir.*, 11, 271, 1994.
97. Husson, R. N., Ross, L. A., Sandelli, S., et al. Orally administered clarithromycin for the treatment of systemic *Mycobacterium avium* complex infection in children with acquired immunodeficiency syndrome. *J. Pediatr.*, 124, 807, 1994.
98. Wallace, R. J. Jr., Brown, B. A., Griffith, D. E., et al. Initial clarithromycin monotherapy for *Mycobacterium avium-intracellulare* complex lung disease. *Am. J. Respir. Crit. Care Med.*, 149, 1335, 1994.
99. Dautzenberg, B., Saint Marc, T., Meyohas, M. C., et al. Clarithromycin and other antimicrobial agents in the treatment of disseminated *Mycobacterium avium* infections in patients with acquired immunodeficiency syndrome. *Arch. Intern. Med.*, 153, 368, 1993.
100. Roger, P. M., Carles, M., Pandiani, L., Keita-Perse, O., Mondain, V., De Salvador, F., and Dellamonica, P. Efficacy and safety of an intravenous induction therapy for treatment of disseminated *Mycobacterium avium* complex infection in AIDS patients: a pilot study. *38th Intersci. Conf. Antimicrob. Agents Chemother.*, American Society of Microbiology, Washington DC, 402, abstract I-126, 1998.
101. Koletar, S. L., Berry, A. J., Cynamon, M. H., et al. Azithromycin as treatment for disseminated *Mycobacterium avium* complex in AIDS patients. *Antimicrob. Agents Chemother.*, 43, 2869–2872, 1999.
102. Pirofsky, J. G., Huang, C. T., and Waites, K. B. Spinal osteomyelitis due to *Mycobacterium avium-intracellulare* in an elderly man with steroid-induced osteoporosis. *Spine*, 18, 1926, 1993.
103. Goldberger, M. and Masur, H. Clarithromycin therapy for *Mycobacterium avium* complex disease in patients with AIDS: potential and problems. *Ann. Intern. Med.*, 121, 974, 1994.
104. Barradell, L. B., Plosker, G. L., and McTavish, D. Clarithromycin: a review of its pharmacological properties and therapeutic use in *Mycobacterium avium-intracellulare* complex infection in patients with acquired immune deficiency syndrome. *Drugs*, 46, 289, 1993.
105. Cohn, D., Fisher, E., Franchino, B., et al. A prospective, randomized trial of four 3-drug regimens for treatment (Rx) of disseminated MAC disease in AIDS(DM): excess mortality with high-dose clarithromycin. *4th Conf. Retroviruses Opportunistic Infect., Jan. 22–26*, 186, abstract 659, 1997.
106. Matsiota-Bernard, P., Zinzendoerf, N., Onody, C., and Guenounou, M. Comparison of clarithromycin-sensitive and clarithromycin-resistant *Mycobacterium avium* strains isolated from AIDS patients during therapy regimens including clarithromycin. *J. Infect.*, 40, 49–54, 2000.

107. Dautzenberg, B., Truffot, C., Legris, S., et al. Activity of clarithromycin against *Mycobacterium avium* infection in patients with the acquired immune deficiency syndrome: a controlled clinical trial. *Am. Rev. Respir. Dis.*, 144, 564, 1991.
108. Johnson, M., Pavia, A. T., Kendall, M., and Christenson, J., Clarithromycin-based combination therapy for *Mycobacterium avium-intracellulare* complex (MAC) lymphadenitis in children. *38th Intersci. Conf. Antimicrob. Agents Chemother.*, American Society of Microbiology, Washington DC, 552, abstract L-19, 1998.
109. Price, T. A. and Tuazon, C. U. Clarithromycin-induced thrombocytopenia. *Clin. Infect. Dis.*, 15, 563, 1992.
110. Nightingale, S. D., Koster, F. T., Mertz, G. J., and Loss, S. D. Clarithromycin-induced mania in two patients with AIDS. *Clin. Infect. Dis.*, 20, 1563, 1995.
111. Dorrell, L., Ellerton, C., Cottrell, D. G., and Snow, M. H. Toxicity of clarithromycin in the treatment of *Mycobacterium avium* complex infection in a patient with AIDS. *J. Antimicrob. Chemother.*, 34, 605, 1994.
112. Auclair, B., Berning, S. E., Huitt, G. A., and Peloquin, C. A. Potential interaction between itraconazole and clarithromycin. *Pharmacotherapy*, 19, 1439–1444, 1999.
113. Malessa, R., Diener, H. C., Olbricht, T., Bohmer, B., and Brockmeyer, N. H. Successful treatment of meningoencephalitis caused by *Mycobacterium avium* intracellulare in AIDS. *Clin. Investig.*, 72, 850, 1994.
114. Benson, C., Williams, P., Currier, J., et al. ACTG 223: an open, prospective, randomized study comparing efficacy and safety of clarithromycin(c) plus ethambutol (E), rifabutin(r) or both for treatment (Rx) of MAC disease in pts. with AIDS. *6th Conf. Retroviruses Opportunistic Infect., Jan. 31–Feb. 4.*, 114, abstract 249, 1999.
115. Griffith, D. E., Brown, B. A., Cegielski, P., Murphy, D. T., and Wallace, R. J. Jr. Early results (at 6 months) with intermittent clarithromycin-including regimens for lung disease due to *Mycobacterium avium* complex. *Clin. Infect. Dis.*, 30, 288–292, 2000.
116. de Lalla, F., Maserati, R., Scarpellini, P., Marone, P., Nicolin, R., Caccamo, F., and Rigoli, R. Clarithromycin-ciprofloxacin-amikacin for therapy of *Mycobacterium avium- Mycobacterium intracellulare* bacteremia in patients with AIDS. *Antimicrob. Agents Chemother.*, 36, 1567, 1992.
117. Keiser, P., Nassar, N., Skiest, D., Rademacher, S., and Smith, J. W. A retrospective study of the addition of ciprofloxacin to clarithromycin and ethambutol in the treatment of disseminated *Mycobacterium avium* complex infection. *Int. J. STD AIDS*, 10, 791–794, 1999.
118. Sato, K. and Ebe, T. A study on the effect of combined chemotherapy on *Mycobacterium avium* complex pulmonary disease. *Kekkaku*, 75, 471–476, 2000.
119. Grange, J. M., Winstanley, P. A., and Davies, P. D. Clinically significant drug interactions with antituberculosis agents. *Drug Saf.*, 11, 242, 1994.
120. Wallace, R. J. Jr., Brown, B. A., Griffith, D. E., Girard, W., and Tanaka, K. Reduced serum levels of clarithromycin in patients treated with multidrug regimens including rifampin or rifabutin for *Mycobacterium avium-M. intracellulare* infection. *J. Infect. Dis.*, 171, 747, 1995.
121. Anonymous. Azithro once a week for MAC. *Treat. Update*, 10, 3–4, 1998.
122. Wallace, M. R., Miller, L. K., Nguyen, M. T., and Shields, A. R. Ototoxicity with azithromycin. *Lancet*, 343, 241, 1994.
123. Ahn, C. H., Ahn, S. S., Anderson, R.A., Murphy, D.T., and Mammo, A. A four-drug regimen for initial treatment of cavitary disease caused by *M. avium* complex. *Am. Rev. Respir. Dis.*, 134, 438, 1986.
124. Seibert, A.F. and Base, J. B. Four drug therapy of pulmonary disease caused by *Mycobacterium avium* complex. *Am. Rev. Respir. Dis.*, 139, A399, 1989.
125. Heifets, L. B. and Iseman, M. D. Individualized therapy versus standard regimens in the treatment of *Mycobacterium avium* infections. *Am. Rev. Respir. Dis.*, 144, 1, 1991.
126. Tsukamura, M. In-vitro bacteriostatic and bactericidal activity of isoniazid on the *Mycobacterium avium-Mycobacterium intracellulare* complex. *Tubercle*, 71, 199, 1990.
127. Agins, B. D., Berman, D. S., Spicehandler, D., Al-Sadr, W., Simberkoff, M. S., and Rahal, J. J. Effect of combined therapy with ansamycin, clofazimine, ethambutol, and isoniazid for *Mycobacterium avium* infection in patients with AIDS. *J. Infect. Dis.*, 159, 784, 1989.
128. Heifets, L. B. and Iseman, M. D. Choice of antimicrobial agents of *M. avium* disease based on quantitative tests of drug susceptibility. *N. Engl. J. Med.*, 323, 419, 1990.
129. Shafran, S. D., Singer, J., Zarowny, D. B., et al., A comparison of two regimens for the treatment of *Mycobacterium avium* complex bacteremia in AIDS: rifabutin, ethambutol, and clarithromycin versus rifampin, ethambutol, clofazimine, and ciprofloxacin. Canadian HIV Trials Network Protocol 010. *N. Engl. J. Med.*, 335, 377, 1996.
130. Singer, J., Thorne, A., Khorasheh, S., et al. Symptomatic and health status outcomes in the Canadian randomized MAC treatment trial (CTN010). Canadian HIV Trials Network Protocol 010 Study Group. *Int. J. STD AIDS*, 11, 212–213, 2000.
131. Kemper, C. A., Havlir, D., Haghighat, D., et al. The individual microbiologic effect of three antimycobacterial agents, clofazimine, ethambutol, and rifampin, on *Mycobacterium avium* complex bacteremia in patients with AIDS. *J. Infect. Dis.*, 170, 157, 1994.
132. Jorup-Ronstrom, C., Julander, I., and Petrini, B., Efficacy of triple drug regimen of amikacin, ethambutol and rifabutin in AIDS patients with symptomatic *Mycobacterium avium* complex infection. *J. Infect.*, 26, 67, 1993.
133. Davidson, P.T., Khanijo, V., Goble, M., and Moulding, T. S., Treatment of disease due to *Mycobacterium intracellulare*. *Rev. Infect. Dis.*, 3, 1052, 1981.
134. Tsukada, H., Chou, T., Ishizuka, Y., et al. Disseminated *Mycobacterium avium-intracellulare* infection in a patient with myelodysplastic syndrome (refractory anemia). *Am. J. Hematol.*, 45, 325, 1994.
135. Schelonka, R. L., Ascher, D. P., McMahon, D. P., Drehner, D. M., and Kuskie, M. R. Catheter-related sepsis caused by *Mycobacterium avium* complex. *Pediatr. Infect. Dis. J.*, 13, 236, 1994.

136. Clark, D., Lambert, C. M., Palmer, K., Strachan, R., and Nuki, G. Monoarthritis caused by *Mycobacterium avium* complex in a liver transplant recipient. *Br. J. Rheumatol.*, 32, 1099, 1993.
137. Darouiche, R. O., Koff, A., Rosen, T., Darnule, T. V., Lidsky, M. D., and El-Zaatari, A. K. Recurrent disseminated infection with *Mycobacterium avium* complex identified in tissues by molecular analysis. *Clin. Infect. Dis.*, 22, 714, 1996.
138. Rathbun, R. C., Martin, E. S. III, Eaton, V. E., and Matthew, E. B. Current and investigational therapies for AIDS-associated *Mycobacterium avium* complex disease. *Ther. Revs.*, 10, 280, 1991.
139. Baron, E. J. and Young, L. S. Amikacin, ethambutol and rifampin for treatment of disseminated *Mycobacterium avium-intracellulare* infections in patients with acquired immune deficiency syndrome. *Diagn. Microbiol. Infect. Dis.*, 5, 215, 1986.
140. Bach, M.C. Treating disseminated *Mycobacterium avium-intracellulare* infection. *Ann. Intern. Med.*, 110, 169, 1989.
141. Masur, H., Tuazon C., Gill, V., Grimes, G., Baird, B., Fauci, A. S., and Lane, H. C. Effect of combined clofazimine and ansamycin therapy on *Mycobacterium avium-intracellulare* bacteremia in patients with AIDS. *J. Infect. Dis.*, 155, 127, 1987.
142. Hoy, J., Mijch, A., Sandland, M., Grayson, L., Lucas, R., and Dwyer, B. Quadruple-drug therapy for *Mycobacterium avium-intracellulare* bacteremia in AIDS patients. *J. Infect. Dis.*, 161, 801, 1990.
143. Berning, S. E. and Peloquin, C. A. Adverse events associated with high-dose rifabutin in macrolide-containing regimens for the treatment of *Mycobacterium avium* complex lung disease. *Clin. Infect. Dis.*, 22, 885, 1996.
144. Sullam, P. M. Rifabutin therapy for disseminated *Mycobacterium avium* complex infection. *Clin. Infect. Dis.*, 22(Suppl. 1), S37, S41, 1996.
145. Lowe, S. H., Kroon, F. P., Bollemeyer, J. G., Stricker, B. H., and van't Wout, J. W. Uveitis during treatment of disseminated *Mycobacterium avium-intracellulare* complex infection with the combination of rifabutin, clarithromycin and ethambutol. *Neth. J. Med.*, 48, 211, 1996.
146. Tseng, A. L. and Walmsley, S. L. Rifabutin-associated uveitis. *Ann. Pharmacother.*, 29, 1149, 1995.
147. Frau, E., Gregoire-Cassoux, N., Hannouche, D., et al., Uveitis with hypopyon in patients with acquired immunodeficiency syndrome, treated with rifabutin. *J. Fr. Ophthalmol.*, 18, 435, 1995.
148. Chevalley, G. F., Kaiser, L., Bouchenaki, N., Baglivo, E., and Kress, O. Uveitis associated with rifabutin treatment: apropos of 3 patients. *Klin. Monatsbl. Augenheilkd.*, 206, 388, 1995.
149. Rifai, A., Peyman, G. A., Daun, M., and Wafapoor, H. Rifabutin-associated uveitis during prophylaxis for *Mycobacterium avium* complex infection. *Arch. Ophthalmol.*, 113, 707, 1995.
150. Dunn, A. M., Tizer, K., and Cervia, J. S. Rifabutin-associated uveitis in a pediatric patient. *Pediatr. Infect. Dis. J.*, 14, 246, 1995.
151. Jacobs, D. S., Piliero, P. J., Kuperwaser, M. G., et al. Acute uveitis associated with rifabutin use in patients with human immunodeficiency virus infection. *Am. J. Ophthalmol.*, 118, 716, 1994.
152. Saran, B. R., Maguire, A. M., Nichols, C., et al. Hypopyon uveitis in patients with acquired immunodeficiency syndrome treated for systemic *Mycobacterium avium* complex infection with rifabutin. *Arch. Ophthalmol.*, 112, 1159, 1994.
153. Frank, M. O., Graham, M. B., and Wispelway, B. Rifabutin and uveitis. *N. Engl. J. Med.*, 330, 868, 1994.
154. Khan, M. A., Singh, J., and Dhillon, B. Rifabutin-induced uveitis with inflammatory vitreous infiltrate. *Eye*, 14(Part 3a), 344–346, 2000.
155. Arevalo, J. F. and Freeman, W. R. Corneal endothelial deposits in children positive for human immunodeficiency virus receiving rifabutin prophylaxis for *Mycobacterium avium* complex bacteremia. *Am. J. Ophthalmol.*, 129, 410–411, 2000 [see also: *Am. J. Ophthalmol.*, 127, 164–169, 1999].
156. Griffith, D. E., Brown, B. A., Girard, W. M., and Wallace, R. J. Jr. Adverse events associated with high-dose rifabutin in macrolide-containing regimens for the treatment of *Mycobacterium avium* complex lung disease. *Clin. Infect. Dis.*, 21, 594, 1995.
157. Brogden, R. N. and Fitton, A. Rifabutin: a review of its antimicrobial activity, pharmacokinetic properties and therapeutic efficacy. *Drugs*, 47, 983, 1994.
158. Skinner, M. H. and Blaschke, T. F. Clinical pharmacokinetics of rifabutin. *Clin. Pharmacokinet.*, 28, 115, 1995.
159. Sullam, P. M., Gordin, F. M., and Wynne, B. A. Efficacy of rifabutin in the treatment of disseminated infection due to *Mycobacterium avium* complex. The Rifabutin Treatment Group. *Clin. Infect. Dis.*, 19, 84, 1994.
160. Siegal, F. P. Rifabutin prophylaxis for *Mycobacterium avium* complex infection in patient with AIDS. *Clin. Infect. Dis.*, 22(Suppl. 1), S23, S30, 1996.
161. Dautzenberg, B., Olliaro, P., Ruf, B., et al. Rifabutin versus placebo in combination with three drugs in the treatment of nontuberculous mycobacterial infection in patients with AIDS. *Clin. Infect. Dis.*, 22, 705–708, 1996.
162. Dautzenberg, B. Rifabutin in the treatment of *Mycobacterium avium* complex infection: experience in Europe. *Clin. Infect. Dis.*, 22(Suppl.1), S33, 1996.
163. Hoffner, S. E., Svenson, S. B., and Beezer, A. E. Microcalorimetric studies of the initial interaction between antimycobacterial drugs and *Mycobacterium avium*. *J. Antimicrob. Chemother.*, 25, 353, 1990.
164. Eggelmeijer, F., Kroon, F. P., Zeeman, R. J., Dijkmans, B. A., and van't Wout, J. W. Tenosynovitis due to *Mycobacterium avium-intracellulare*: case report and a review of the literature. *Clin. Exp. Rheumatol.*, 10, 169, 1992.
165. Hoffner, S. E., Kratz, M., Olsson-Liljequist, B., Svenson, S. B., and Källenius, G., In vitro synergistic activity between ethambutol and fluorinated quinolones against *Mycobacterium avium* complex. *J. Antimicrob. Chemother.*, 24, 317, 1989.
166. Källenius, G., Svenson, S. B., and Hoffner, S. E., Ethambutol: a key for *Mycobacterium avium* complex chemotherapy? *Am. Rev. Respir. Dis.*, 140, 264, 1989.
167. Kemper, C. A., Chiu, J., Meng, T. C., et al., Microbiologic and clinical response of patients with AIDS and MAC bacteremia to a four oral drug regimen. *30th Intersci. Conf. Antimicrob. Agents Chemother.*, American Society for Microbiology, Washington, DC, abstract 1267, 1990.

168. Peloquin, C. A. Dosage of antimycobacterial agents. *Clin. Pharm.*, 10, 664, 1991.
169. Yew, W. W., Chau, C. H., Wong, P. C., and Choi, H. Y. Ciprofloxacin-induced renal dysfunction in patients with mycobacterial lung infection. *Tuber. Lung. Dis.*, 76, 173, 1995.
170. Fan-Harvard, P., Sanchorawala, V., Oh, J., Moser, E. M., and Smith, S. P. Concurrent use of foscarnet and ciprofloxacin may increase the propensity for seizures. *Ann. Pharmacother.*, 28, 869, 1994.
171. Wormser, G. P., Horowitz, H., and Dworkin, B. Low-dose dexamethasone as adjunctive therapy in AIDS patients. *Antimicrob. Agents Chemother.*, 38, 2215, 1994.
172. Jones, A. R., Bartlett, J., and McCormack, J. G. *Mycobacterium avium* complex (MAC) osteomyelitis and septic arthritis in an immunocompetent host. *J. Infect.*, 30, 59, 1995.
173. King, B. F. Disseminated *Mycobacterium avium* complex in an immunocompetent previously healthy woman. *J. Am. Board Fam. Pract.*, 7, 145, 1994.
174. Jouan, M., Olivier, C., Truffot, C., Fourniols, E., Carcelain, G., Katlama, C., and Bricaire, F. *38th Intersci. Conf. Antimicrob. Agents Chemother.*, American Society of Microbiology, Washington DC, 430, abstract I-205, 1998.
175. Weits, J., Sprenger, H. G., Ilic, P., van Klingeren, B., Elema, J. D., and Steensma, J. T. *Mycobacterium avium* disease in AIDS patients; diagnosis and therapy. *Ned. Tijdschr. Geneeskd.*, 135, 2485, 1991.
176. MacArthur, R. D., Lederman, M. M., Benson, C. A., et al. Effects of *Mycobacterium avium* complex-infection treatment on cytokine expression in human immunedeficiency virus-infected persons: results of AIDS clinical trials group protocol 853. *J. Infect. Dis.*, 181, 1486–1490, 2000.
177. MacArthur, R. D., Lederman, M., Benson, C. A., et al. *38th Intersci. Conf. Antimicrob. Agents Chemother.*, American Society of Microbiology, Washington DC, 403, abstract I-130, 1998.
178. Chatte, G., Panteix, G., Perrin-Fayolle, M., and Pacheco, Y. Aerosolized interferon gamma for *Mycobacterium avium*-complex lung disease. *Am. J. Respir. Crit. Care Med.*, 152, 1094–1096, 1995.
179. Holland, S. M., Eisenstein, E. M., Kuhns, D. B., Turner, M. L., Fleisher, T. A., Strober, W., and Gallin, J. I. Treatment of refractory disseminated nontuberculous mycobacterial infection with interferon gamma: a preliminary report. *N. Engl. J. Med.*, 330, 1348, 1994.
180. George, S., Coffey, M., Cinti, S., et al. Neutrophils from AIDS patients treated with G-CSF demonstrate enhanced killing of *M. avium*. *5th Conf. Retroviruses Opportunistic Infect.*, Feb. 1–5, 214, abstract 724, 1998.
181. Kang, B. Y., Chung, S. W., Lim, Y. S., et al. Interleukin-12-secreting fibroblasts are more efficient than free recombinant interleukin-12 in inducing the persistent reesistance to *Mycobacterium avium* complex infection. *Immunology*, 97, 474–480, 1999.
182. Rimland, D. and St. John, A. Trends in disseminated *Mycobacterium avium* infection (DMAC) in AIDS patients since the availability of primary prophylaxis. *5th Conf. Retroviruses Opportunistic Infect.*, Feb. 1–5, 215, abstract 727, 1998.
183. Nichols, C. W. *Mycobacterium avium* complex infection, rifabutin, and uveitis - is there a connection? *Clin. Infect. Dis.*, 22(Suppl. 1), S43, S47, 1996.
184. American Foundation for AIDS Research. MAC (*Mycobacterium avium* complex). *AIDS/HIV Treatment Directory*, 6(4), 88, 1993.
185. Wynne, B., et al. The development of *Mycobacterium avium* complex (MAC) bacteremia in AIDS patients in the placebo (PLAC)-controlled MAC prophylaxis studies (087023 & 087027). *32nd Intersci. Conf. Antimicrob. Agents Chemother.*, American Society for Microbiology, Washington, DC, abstract 890, 1992.
186. Eccles, E. and Ptak, J. *Mycobacterium avium* complex infection in AIDS: clinical features, treatment, and prevention. *J. Assoc. Nurses AIDS Care*, 6, 37, 1995.
187. Hoy, J. F., Marriott, D., and Gottlieb, T. Managing HIV. Part 5: Treating secondary outcomes. 5. 15 HIV and non-tuberculous mycobacterial infection. *Med. J. Aust.*, 164, 543, 1996.
188. Stearn, B. F. and Polis, M. A. Prophylaxis of opportunistic infections in persons with HIV infection. *Cleve. Clin. J. Med.*, 61, 187, 1994.
189. Chaisson, R. E., McCutchan, J. A., Nightingale, S., and Young, L. S. Managing *Mycobacterium avium* complex infection. *AIDS Clin. Care*, 5, 1, 1993.
190. Pulik, M., Genet, P., Leturdu, F., Lionnet, F., Louvel, D., and Touahri, T. Rifabutin prophylaxis against *Mycobacterium avium* complex infections in HIV-infected patients: impact on the incidence of campylobacteriosis. *AIDS Patient Care STDS*, 13, 467–472, 1999.
191. Benson, C. A., Williams, P. L., Cohn, D. L., et al. Clarithromycin or rifabutin alone or in combination for primary prophylaxis of *Mycobacterium avium* complex disease in patients with AIDS: A randomized, double-blind, placebo-controlled trial. The AIDS Clinical Trials Group 196/Terry Beirn Community Programs for Clinical Research on AIDS 009 Protocol Team. *J. Infect. Dis.*, 181, 1289–1297, 2000.
192. Cohn, S. E., Kammann, E., Williams, P., Chesney, M. A., and Currier, J. Predictors of adherence to azithromycin prophylaxis for prevention of *Mycobacterium avium* complex (MAC) disease. *6th Conf. Retroviruses Opportunistic Infect.*, Jan. 31–Feb. 4., 151, abstract 444, 1999.
193. Moyle, G. J., Gill, J., and Nelson, M. Secondary prophylaxis for mycobacterial infections with once weekly azithromycin. *5th Conf. Retroviruses Opportunistic Infect.*, Feb. 1–5, 215, abstract 728, 1998.
194. Chaisson, R. E., Benson, C. A., Dube, M. P., et al., Clarithromycin therapy for disseminated *Mycobacterium avium* complex (MAC) in AIDS. *32nd Intersci. Conf. Antimicrob. Agents Chemother.*, American Society for Microbiology, Washington, DC, abstract 891, 1992.
195. Hewitt, R. G., Maliszewski, M., Goldberg, M., and Harmon, B. Prevention of *M. avium* complex (MAC) bacteremia in patients with CD4[+] <200 by rifabutin, clarithromycin or dapsone. *Proc. IXth Int. Conf. AIDS*, Berlin, 1993, abstract PO-B07-1184.

196. Abrams, D. I., Mitchell, T. F., Child, C. C., et al. Clofazimine as prophylaxis for disseminated *Mycobacterium avium* complex infecion in AIDS. *J. Infect. Dis.*, 167, 1459, 1993.
197. Currier, J. S., Williams, P. L., Koletar, S. L., et al. Discontinuation of *Mycobacterium avium* complex prophylaxis in patients with antiretroviral therapy-induced increase in CD4$^+$ cell counts. A randomized, double-blind, placebo-controlled trial. AIDS Clinical Trials Group 362 Study Team. *Ann. Intern. Med.*, 133, 493–503, 2000.
198. Dworkin, M. S., Hanson, D. L., Kaplan, J. E., Jones, J. L., and Ward, J. W. Risk for preventable opportunistic infections in persons with AIDS after antiretroviral therapy increases CD4$^+$ T lymphocyte counts above prophylaxis treshholds. *J. Infect. Dis.*, 182, 611–615, 2000.
199. Soriano, V., Dona, C., Rodriguez-Rosado, R., Barreiro, P., and Gonzalez-Lahoz, J. Discontinuation of secondary prophylaxis for opportunistic infections in HIV-infected patients receiving highly active antiretroviral therapy. *AIDS*, 14, 383–386, 2000.
200. El-Sadr, W. M., Burman, W. J., Grant, L. B., et al. Discontinuation of prophylaxis for *Mycobacterium avium* complex disease in HIV-infected patients who have a response to antiretroviral therapy. Terry Bairn Community Programs for Clinical Research on AIDS. *N. Engl. J. Med.*, 342, 105–1092, 2000.
201. Sullivan J. H., Moore, R. D., Keruly, J. C., and Chaisson, R. E. Effect of antiretroviral therapy on the increase of bacterial pneumonia in patients with advanced HIV infection. *Am. J. Respir. Crit. Care Med.*, 162, 64–67, 2000.
202. Fonquernie, L., Meynard, J. L., Kirstetter, M., et al. Granulome abdominal pseudo-tumoral contemporain de la reconstitution immunitaire sous traitmenet anti-retroviral. *Presse Med.*, 29, 186–187, 2000.
203. Sendi, P. P., Craig, B. A., Meier, G., et al. Cost-effectiveness of azithromycin for preventing *Mycobacterium avium* complex infection in HIV-positive patients in the era of highly active antiretroviral therapy. The Swiss HIV Cohort Study. *J. Antimicrob. Chemother.*, 44, 811–817, 1999.
204. Scharfstein, J. A., Paltiel, A. D., Weinstein, M. C., et al. The cost-effectiveness of prophylaxis for *Mycobacterium avium* complex in AIDS. *Int. J. Technol. Asses. Health Care*, 15, 531–547, 1999.
205. Minor, S., Tseng, A., and Salit, I. E. Prophylaxis against *Mycobacterium avium* complex (MAC) in HIV: application of guidelines. *38th Intersci. Conf. Antimicrob. Agents Chemother.*, American Society of Microbiology, Washington DC, 409, abstract I-143h, 1998.
206. McNabb, J. C., Lacy, M. K., Ross, J. W., Rousseau, M., Nightingale, C. H., and Nicolau, D. P. Randomized, cross-over adherence trial of azithromycin and clarithromycin for MAC prophylaxis in AIDS patients. *38th Intersci. Conf. Antimicrob. Agents Chemother.*, American Society of Microbiology, Washington DC, 407, abstract I-142, 1998.
207. Kirk, O., Gatell, J. M., Mocroft, A., et al. Infections with *Mycobacterium tuberculosis* and *Mycobacterium avium* among HIV-infected patients after the introduction of highly active antiretroviral therapy. EuroSIDA Study Group JD. *Am. J. Respir. Crit. Care Med.*, 162(3 Part 1), 865–872, 2000.
208. Mary-Krause, M., Rabaud, C., Jouan, M., Obadia, M., de la Blanchardiere, A., Raffi, F., and May, T. *Mycobacterium avium* complex chez les sujets seropositifs pour le VIH: incidence et facteurs de risqué avant et apres l'introduction des traitements antiretroviraux hautement actifs. Groupe d'epidemiologie clinique des centres d'information et de soins de l'immunodeficience humaine (CISIH). *Pathol. Biol. (Paris)*, 48, 495–504, 2000.
209. Kaplan, J. E., Hanson, D., Dworkin, M. S., et al. Epidemiology of human immunodeficiency virus-associated opportunistic infections in the United States in the era of highly active antiretroviral therapy. *Clin. Infect. Dis.*, 30(Suppl. 1), S5–S14, 2000.
210. Jones, J., Hanson, D., Dworkin, M., and Kaplan, J. Which opportunistic illness occur in the era of HAART and at what CD4 cell counts? *6th Conf. Retroviruses Opportunistic Infect.*, Jan. 31–Feb. 4, 198, abstract 690, 1999.
211. Schrier, R., Torriani, F., Durand, D., Jeffrey, D., Drew, L., and Lalazari, J. Immune reconstitution of advanced HIV patients (following HAART). *6th Conf. Retroviruses Opportunistic Infect.*, Jan. 31–Feb. 4, 129, abstract 325, 1999.
212. Havlir, D. V., Schrier, R., Torriani, F., Chervenak, K., and Boom, H. Reconstitution of *M. avium* complex (MAC) immune responses after highly active antiretroviral therapy (HAART). *6th Conf. Retroviruses Opportunistic Infect.*, Jan. 31–Feb. 4, 114, 248, 1999.
213. Aberg, J. A., Yajko, D. M., and Jacobson, M. A., Eradication of disseminated *Mycobacterium avium* complex (DMAC) in four patients after twelve mo anti-mycobacterial therapy and response to highly active antiretroviral therapy (HAART). *5th Conf. Retroviruses Opportunistic Infect.*, Feb. 1–5, 215, 729, 1998.
214. Cooper, D. A. Immunological effects of antiretroviral therapy. *Antivir. Ther.*, 3(Suppl. 4), 19–23, 1998.
215. Currier, J. S., Williams, P. L., Grimes, J. M., Squires, K. S., Fischl, M. A., and Hammer, S. M., Incidence rates and risk factors for opportunistic infections in a phase III trial comparing Indinavir + ZDV + 3TC to ZDV +3TC. *5th Conf. Retroviruses Opportunistic Infect.*, Feb. 1–5, 127, abstract 257, 1998.
216. Girmenia, C., Martino, P., Mazzucconi, M. G., Bizzoni, L., and Cassone, A. HAART and *Mycobacterium avium* complex in an HIV infected patient with severe factor VII deficiency. *Haemophilia*, 6, 116–117, 2000.
217. Nalaboff, K. M., Rozenshtein, A., and Kaplan, M. H., Imaging of *Mycobacterium avium-intracellulare* infection in AIDS patients on highly active antiretroviral therapy: reversal syndrome. *AJR A. J. Roentgenol.*, 175, 387–390, 2000.
218. Kaplan, M. H. Mycobacteria avium intracellulare (MAIS) reversal syndrome set off by highly active anti retroviral therapy (HAART). Improved immunity is not always good but it is better than no immunity. *5th Conf. Retroviruses Opportunistic Infect.*, Feb. 1–5, 215, abstract 726, 1998.
219. Cinti, S. K., Kaul, D. R., Sax, P. E., Crane, L. R., and Kazanjian, P. H. Recurrence of *Mycobacterium avium* infection in patients receiving highly active antiretroviral therapy and antimycobacterial agents. *Clin. Infect. Dis.*, 30, 511–514, 2000.
220. Pelgrom, J., Bastian, I., Van den Enden, E., Portaels, F., and Colebunders, R. Cutaneous ulcer caused by *Mycobacterium avium* and recurrent genital herpes after highly active antiretroviral therapy. *Arch. Dermatol.*, 136, 129, 2000.
221. Buhler, V. B. and Pollack, A. Human infection with atypical acid-fast organisms. *Am. J. Clin. Pathol.*, 23, 363, 1953.
222. Wolinsky, E. Nontuberculous mycobacteria and associated diseases. *Am. Rev. Respir. Dis.*, 119, 107, 1979.

223. Ahn, C. H., McLarty, J. W., Ahn, S. S., Ahn, S. I., and Hurst, G. A. Diagnostic criteria for pulmonary disease caused by *Mycobacterium kansasii* and *Mycobacterium intracellulare*. *Am. Rev. Respir. Dis.*, 125, 388, 1982.
224. Kin, T. C., Arora, N. S., Aldrich, T. K., and Rochester, D. F. Atypical mycobacterial infections: a clinical study of 92 patients. *South. Med. J.*, 74, 1304, 1981.
225. Christensen, E. E., Dietz, G. W., Ahn, C. H., Chapman, J. S., Murry, R. C., and Hurst, G. A. Radiographic manifestations of pulmonary *Mycobacterium kansasii* infections. *Am. J. Radiol.*, 131, 985, 1978.
226. Banks, J., Hunter, A. M., Campbell, I. A., Jenkins, P. A., and Smith, A. P. Pulmonary infection with *Mycobacterium kansasii* in Wales, 1970–9: review of treatment and response. *Thorax*, 38, 271, 1983.
227. Johanson, W. G. Jr. and Nicholson, D. P. Pulmonary disease due to *Mycobacterium kansasii*: an analysis of some factors affecting prognosis. *Am. Rev. Respir. Dis.*, 99, 73, 1989.
228. Lillo, M., Orengo, S., Cernoch, P., and Harris, R. L., Pulmonary and disseminated infection due to *Mycobacterium kansasii*: a decade of experience. *Rev. Infect. Dis.*, 12, 760, 1990.
229. Zenone, T., Boibieux, A., Tigaud, S., et al. Non-tuberculous mycobacterial tenosynovitis: a review. *Scand. J. Infect. Dis.*, 31, 221–228, 1999.
230. Corbett, E. L., Blumberg, L., Churchyard, G. J., et al. Nontuberculous mycobacteria: defining disease in a prospective cohort of South African miners. *Am. J. Respir. Crit. Care Med.*, 160, 15–21, 1999.
231. Corbett, E. L., Hay, M., Churchyard, G. J., et al. *Mycobacterium kansasii* and *M. scrofulaceum* isolates from HIV-negative South African gold miners: incidence, clinical significance and radiology. *Int. J. Tuberc. Lung Dis.*, 3, 501–507, 1999.
232. Reparaz, J. Disease from *Mycobacterium kansasii*. *Enferm. Infecc. Microbiol. Clin.*, 17, 85–90, 1999.
233. Evans, S. A., Colville, A., Evans, A. J., Crisp, A. J., and Johnston, I. D. Pulmonary *Mycobacterium kansasii* infection: comparison of the clinical features, treatment and outcome with pulmonary tuberculosis. *Thorax*, 51, 1248–1252, 1996.
234. Tietz, A., Tamm, M., and Battegay, M. *Mycobacterium kansasii* abscess of the chest wall after drainage of bacterial empyema. *Eur. J. Clin. Microbiol. Infect. Dis.*, 19, 71–73, 2000.
235. Iwata, H., Kinoshita, M., Sumiya, M., et al. Emergence of erosive polyarthritis coincident with *Mycobacterium kansasii* pulmonary infection in a patient with systemic sclerosis-rheumatoid arthritis overlap syndrome. *Clin. Exp. Rheumatol.*, 17, 757–758, 1999.
236. Carballal Regidor, J. M., Montero Martinez, C., and Verea Hernando, H. *Mycobacterium kansasii* pulmonary infection: atypical presentation. *Arch. Bronconeumol.*, 35, 410–411, 1999.
237. Yamada, H., Kohyama, T., Terashi, K., et al. Fatal pulmonary infection due to multidrug-resistant *Mycobacterium kansasii* which developed in an immunocompetent young man. *Intern. Med.*, 36, 298–300, 1997.
238. Mead, G. M., Dance, D. A. B., and Smith, A. G. Lymphadenopathy complicating hairy cell leukemia: a case of disseminated *Mycobacterium kansasii* infection. *Acta Haematol. (Basel)*, 70, 335, 1983.
239. McGeady, S. J. and Murphey, S. A. Disseminated *Mycobacterium kansasii* infection. *Clin. Immunol. Immunopathol.*, 20, 87, 1981.
240. Oermann, C. M., Starke, J. R., and Seilhemer, D. K. Pulmonary disease caused by *Mycobacterium kansasii* in a patient with cystic fibrosis. *Pediatr. Infect. Dis.*, 16, 257–259, 1997.
241. Anzalone, G., Cei, M., Vizzaccaro, A., and Tramma, B., and Bisetti, A. *M. kansasii* pulmonary disease in idiopathic CD4+ T-lymphocytopenia. *Eur. Respir. J.*, 9, 1754–1756, 1996.
242. Delaporte, E., Savage, C., Alfandari, S., Piette, F., Leclerc, H., and Bergoend, H. *Mycobacterium kansasii* cutaneous infection. *Ann. Dermatol. Venereol.*, 120, 289, 1993.
243. Czelusta, A. and Moore, A. Y. Cutaneous *Mycobacterium kansasii* infection in a patient with systemic lupus erythematosus: case report and review. *J. Am. Acad. Dermatol.*, 40(2 Pt. 2), 359–363, 1999.
244. Stewart, C. and Jackson, L. Spleno-hepatic tuberculosis due to *Mycobacterium kansasii*. *Med. J. Aust.*, 2, 99, 1976.
245. Hepper, N. G. G., Karlson, A. G., Leary, F. J., and Soule, E. H. Genitourinary infection due to *Mycobacterium kansasii*. *Mayo Clin. Proc.*, 46, 387, 1971.
246. Palmer, J. A. and Watanakunakorn, C. *Mycobacterium kansasii* pericarditis. *Thorax*, 39, 876, 1984.
247. Bacon, M. E., Whelan, T. V., Mahoney, M. D., Patel, T. G., and Judson, P. L. Pericarditis due to *Mycobacterium kansasii* in a patient undergoing dialysis for chronic renal failure. *J. Infect. Dis.*, 152, 846, 1985.
248. Komeno, T., Itoh, T., Ohtani, K., et al. Disseminated nontuberculous mycobacteriosis caused by *Mycobacterium kansasii* in a patient with myelodysplastic syndrome. *Intern. Med.*, 35, 323–326, 1996.
249. Garcia, F. J., Atienza, M. P., and Calvo, J. Cervical lymphadenitis caused by non- tuberculous mycobacteria. A case report. *Acta Otorrinolaringol. Esp.*, 48, 595–598, 1997.
250. Flor, A., Capdevila, J. A., Martin, N., Gavalda, J., and Pahissa, A. Nontuberculous mycobacterial meningitis: report of two cases and review. *Clin. Infect. Dis.*, 23, 1266–1273, 1996.
251. Nandwani, R., Shanson, D. C., Fisher, M., Nelson, M. R., and Gazzard, B. G. *Mycobacterium kansasii* scalp abscesses in an AIDS patient. *J. Infect. Dis.*, 31, 79, 1995.
252. Mandal, D., Curless, E., and Ostick, D. G. Pyogenic abscess caused by *Mycobacterium kansasii* in advanced AIDS. *Int. J. STD AIDS*, 3, 362, 1992.
253. Naguib, M. T., Byers, J. M., and Slater, L. N. Paranasal sinus infection due to atypical mycobacteria in two patients with AIDS. *Clin. Infect. Dis.*, 19, 789, 1994.
254. Friedman, A. W. and Ike, R. W. *Mycobacterium kansasii* septic arthritis in a patient with acquired immune deficiency syndrome. *Arthritis Rheum.*, 36, 1631, 1993.
255. Weinroth, S. E., Pincetl, P., and Tuazon, C. U. Disseminated *Mycobacterium kansasii* infection presenting as pneumonia and osteomyelitis of the skull in a patient with AIDS. *Clin. Infect. Dis.*, 18, 261, 1994.

256. Boudon, P., Le Pennec, M. P., Malbec, D., et al., *Mycobacterium kansasii* infection in patients with human immunodeficiency virus infection. *Rev. Med. Interne*, 16, 747, 1995.
257. Bamberger, D. M., Driks, M. R., Gupta, M. R., et al. *Mycobacterium kansasii* among patients infected with human immunodeficiency virus in Kansas City. Kansas City AIDS Research Consortium. *Clin. Infect. Dis.*, 18, 395, 1994.
258. Urkijo, J. C., Montejo, M., Aguirrebengoa, K., Urra, E., and Aguirre, C. Disease caused by *Mycobacterium kansasii* in patients with HIV infection. *Enferm. Infecc. Microbiol. Clin.*, 11, 120, 1993.
259. Dautzenberg, B., Antoun, F., and Truffot, C. Acquired rifampicin resistance during *M. kansasii* infection in a patient with AIDS. *Rev. Mal. Respir.*, 9, 464, 1992.
260. Naher, R. and Peters, B. *Mycobacterium kansasii* seroma of the skin in HIV infection. *Hautarzt*, 43, 361, 1992.
261. Levine, B. and Chaisson, R. E. *Mycobacterium kansasii*: a cause of treatable pulmonary disease associated with advanced human immunodeficiency virus (HIV) infection. *Ann. Intern. Med.*, 114, 861, 1991.
262. Valainis, G. T. *Mycobacterium kansasii* infection. *Ann. Intern. Dis.*, 115, 496, 1991.
263. Jost, P. M. and Hodges, G. R. *Mycobacterium kansasii* infection in a patient with AIDS. *South. Med. J.*, 84, 1501, 1991.
264. Valainis, G. T., Cardona, L. M., and Greer, D. L. The spectrum of *Mycobacterium kansasii* disease associated with HIV-1 infected patients. *J. Acquir. Immune Defic. Syndr.*, 4, 516, 1991.
265. Pintado, V., Gomez-Mampaso, E., Martin-Davila, P., et al. *Mycobacterium kansasii* infection in patients infected with the human immunodeficiency virus. *Eur. J. Clin. Microbiol. Infect. Dis.*, 18, 582–586, 1999.
266. Corbett, E. L., Churchyard, G. J., Hay, M., et al. The impact of HIV infection on *Mycobacterium kansasii* disease in South African gold miners. *Am. J. Respir. Crit. Care Med.*, 160, 1014, 1999.
267. Klein, J. L., Corbett, E. L., Slade, P. M., Miller, R. F., and Coker, R. J. *Mycobacterium kansasii* and human immunodeficiency virus co-infection in London. *J. Infect.* 37, 252-259, 1998.
268. Enani, M. A., Frayha, H. H., and Halim, M. A. An appendiceal abscess due to *Mycobacterium kansasii* in a child with AIDS. *Clin. Infect. Dis.*, 27, 891–892, 1998.
269. van der Meer, J. T., Kerssemakers, S. P., van Steenwijk, R. P., and Kuijper, E. J. Infections with *Mycobacterium kansasii* in the Academic Medical Center in Amsterdam: the changing clinical spectrum since the tart of the HIV epidemic. *Ned. Tijdschr. Geneeskd.*, 142, 965–969, 1998.
270. Sasaki, Y., Yamagushi, F., Suzuki, K., Saitoh, M., and Izumizaki, M. A case of AIDS with disseminated *Mycobacterium kansasii* infection in which *Mycobacterium avium* complex was also detected from his sputum repeatedly. *Kekkaku*, 72, 573–577, 1997.
271. Fishman, J. E., Schwartz, D. S., and Sais, G. J. *Mycobacterium kansasii* pulmonary infection in patients with AIDS: spectrum of chest radiographic findings. *Radiology*, 204, 171–175, 1997.
272. Campo, R. E. and Campo, C. E. *Mycobacterium kansasii* disease in patients infected with human immunodeficiency virus. *Clin. Infect. Dis.*, 24, 1233–1238, 1997.
273. Rooney, G., Nelson, M. R., and Gazzard, B. *Mycobacterium kansasii*: its presentation, treatment and outcome in HIV infected patients. *J. Clin. Pathol.*, 49, 821–823, 1996.
274. Witzig, R. S., Fazal, B. A., Mera, R. M., et al. Clinical manifestations and implications of coinfection with *Mycobacterium kansasii* and human immunodeficiency virus type 1. *Clin. Infect. Dis.*, 21, 77, 1995.
275. Chaisson, R. E. and Levine, B. *Mycobacterium kansasii* infection: a reply. *Ann. Intern. Med.*, 115, 496, 1991.
276. Singh, G. Treatment of septic arthritis due to *Mycobacterium kansasii*. *Br. Med. J. (Clin. Res. Ed.)*, 290, 857, 1985.
277. Bernard, L., Vincent, V., Lortholary, O., et al. *Mycobacterium kansasii* septic arthritis: French retrospective study of 5 years and review. *Clin. Infect. Dis.*, 29, 1455–1460, 1999.
278. Zwolska-Kwiek, Z., Augustynowicz-Kopec, E., and Zalewska-Schontaler, N. Drug sensitivity of bacillus strains *M. avium-intracellulare* (MAIC), *M. kansasii* cultured from patients with mycobacteriosis before treatment. *Pneumonol. Alergol. Pol.*, 61, 248, 1993.
279. Hopewell, P., Cynamon, M., Starke, J., Iseman, M., and O'Brien, R. Evaluation of new anti- infective drugs for the treatment of disease caused by *Mycobacterium kansasii* and other mycobacteria. *Clin. Infect. Dis.*, 15(Suppl. 1), S307, 1992.
280. Wallace, R. J. Jr., Dunbar, D., Brown, B. A., et al. Rifampin-resistant *Mycobacterium kansasii*. *Clin. Infect. Dis.*, 18, 736, 1994.
281. Meynard, J. L., Lalande, V., Meyohas, M. C., Petit, J. C., and Frottier, J. Rifampin-resistant *Mycobacterium kansasii* infection in a patients with AIDS who was receiving rifabutin *Clin. Infect. Dis.*, 24, 1262–1263, 1997.
282. Tartaglione, T. Treatment of nontuberculous mycobacterial infections: role of clarithromycin and azithromycin. *Clin. Ther.*, 19, 726–638, 603, 1997.
283. Mizutani, S. Chemotherapy of pulmonary *Mycobacterium kansasii* infection. *Kekkaku*, 71, 527–531, 1996.
284. Burman, W. J., Stone, B. L., Brown, B. A., Wallace, R. J., Jr., and Bottger, E. C. AIDS- related *Mycobacterium kansasii* infection with initial resistance to clarithromycin. *Diagn. Microbiol. Infect. Dis.*, 31, 369–371, 1998.
285. Ogata, H., Kubo, M., Tamaki, K., Hirakata, H., Okuda, S., and Fujishima, M. Crescentic glomerulonephritis due to rifampin treatment in a patient with pulmonary atypical mycobacteriosis. *Nephron*, 78, 319–322, 1998.
286. Echevarria, M. P., Martin, G., Perez, J., and Urkijo, J. C. Pulmonary infection by *Mycobacterium kansasii*: presentation of 27 cases. *Enferm. Infecc. Microbiol. Clin.*, 12, 280, 1994.
287. Nakazono, T., Sugie, T., Ogata, H., et al. Investigation on the treatment of infection due to *Mycobacterium kansasii*. *Kekkaku*, 69, 587, 1994.
288. Domej, W., Maier, A., Schmidt, F., Dimai, H. P., and Wirnsberger, G. H. Relapse of pulmonary *Mycobacterium kansasii* disease associated with large-cell cancer of the lung: a case report. *Incol. Rep.*, 5, 853–856, 1998.
289. Delclaux, C., Laederich, J., Adotti, F., and Kleinknecht, D. Fatal disseminated *Mycobacterium kansasii* infection in a hemodialysis patient. *Nephron*, 64, 155, 1993.

290. Breathnach, A., Levell, N., Munro, C., Natarajan, S., and Pedler, S. Cutaneous *Mycobacterium kansasii* infection: case report and review. *Clin. Infect. Dis.*, 20, 812, 1995.
291. Bolivar, R., Satterwhite, T. K., and Floyd, M. Cutaneous lesions due to *Mycobacterium kansasii*. *Arch. Dermatol.*, 116, 207, 1980.
292. Curco, N., Pagerols, X., Gomez, L., and Vives, P. *Mycobacterium kansasii* infection limited to the skin in a patient with AIDS. *Br. J. Dermatol.*, 135, 324–326, 1996.
293. Groves, R. W., Newton, J. A., and Hay, R. J. Cutaneous *Mycobacterium kansasii* infection - treatment with erythromycin. *Clin. Exp. Dermatol.*, 16, 300, 1991.
294. Nisar, M., Watkin, S. W., Bucknall, R. C., and Agnew, R. A. Exacerbation of isoniazid induced peripheral neuropathy by pyridoxine. *Thorax*, 45, 419, 1990.
295. Sauret, J., Hernandez-Flix, S., Castro, E., Hernandez, L., Ausina, V., and Coll, P. Treatment of pulmonary disease caused by *Mycobacterium kansasii*: results of 18 vs. 12 months' chemotherapy. *Tuber. Lung Dis.*, 76, 104, 1995.
296. Research Committee, British Thoracic Society. *Mycobacterium kansasii* pulmonary infection: a prospective study of the results of nine mo of treatment with rifampicin and ethambutol. *Thorax*, 49, 442, 1994.
297. Ahn, C. H., Lowell, J. R., Ahn, S. I., and Hurst, G. A. Short-course chemotherapy for pulmonary disease caused by *Mycobacterium kansasii*. *Am. Rev. Respir. Dis.*, 128, 1048, 1983.
298. Umeda, A., Asano, K., Kawai, A., et al. *Mycobacterium kansasii* lung infection associated with myelofibrosis—a case refractory to treatment with antitubercular agents. *Nippon Kyobu Shikkan Gakkai Zasshi*, 32, 1170, 1994.
299. Ahn, C. H., Wallace, R. J. Jr., Steele, L. C., and Murphy, D. T. Sulfonamide-containing regimens for disease caused by rifampin-resistant *Mycobacterium kansasii*. *Am. Rev. Respir. Dis.*, 135, 10, 1987.
300. Yoshimoto, S., Konishi, H., Kawahara, S., et al. A case of pulmonary atypical mycobacteriosis comlicated with aplastic anemia, treated with surgical resection and postoperative sparfloxacin. *Nippon Kyobu Shikkan Gakkai Zasshi*, 30, 1345, 1992.
301. Matthiessen, W., Schonfeld, N., Mauch, H., Wahn, U., and Grassot, A. Nontuberculous mycobacteriosis as a complication of the Swyer-James syndrome, *Dtsch. Med. Wochenschr.*, 118, 139, 1993.
302. Kramers, C., Raemaekers, J. M., van Baar, H. M., de Pauw, B. E., and Horrevorts. A. M. Sweet's syndrome as the presenting symptom of hairy cell leukemia with concomitant infection by *Mycobacterium kansasii*. *Ann. Hematol.*, 65, 55, 1992.
303. Bennett, C., Vardiman, J., and Golomb, H. Disseminated atypical mycobacterial infection in patients with hairy cell leukemia. *Am. J. Med.* , 80, 891, 1986.
304. Kurasawa, T., Ikeda, N., Sato, A., et al., A clinical study of non-tuberculous pulmonary mycobacteriosis. *Kekkaku*, 70, 621, 1995.
305. Segura, C. and Salvado, M. Beta-lactamases of *Mycobacterium tuberculosis* and *Mycobacterium kansasii*. *Microbiologia*, 13, 331–336, 1997.
306. Bullin, C. H., Tanner, E. I., and Collins, C. H. Isolation of *Mycobacterium xenopi* from water taps. *J. Hyg. (Cambridge)*, 68, 97, 1970.
307. Costrini, A. M., Mahler, D. A., Gross, W. M., Hawkins, J. E., Yesner, R., and D'Esopo, N. D. Clinical and roentgenographic features of nosocomial pulmonary disease due to *Mycobacterium xenopi*. *Am. Rev. Respir. Dis.* , 123, 104, 1981.
308. Stewart, C. J., Dixon, J. M. S., and Curtis, B. A. Isolation of mycobacteria from tonsils, naso-pharyngeal secretions and lymph nodes in East Anglia. *Tubercle*, 51, 178, 1970.
309. Engbaek, H. C., Vergmann, B., Baess, I., and Will, D. W. *M. xenopi*: a bacteriological study of *M. xenopi* including case reports of Danish patients. *Acta Pathol. Microbiol. Scand.* , 69, 576, 1967.
310. Banks, J., Hunter, A. M., Campbell, I. A., Jenkins, P. A., and Smith, A. P. Pulmonary infection with *Mycobacterium xenopi*: review of treatment and response. *Thorax*, 39, 376, 1984.
311. Galblum, L. I. and Abraham, A. A. *Mycobacterium xenopi* mycobacteriosis. *South. Med. J.*, 74, 1026, 1981.
312. Simor, A. E., Salit, I. E., and Vellend, H. The role of *Mycobacterium xenopi* in human disease. *Am. Rev. Respir. Dis.* , 129, 435, 1984.
313. Platia, E. V. and Vosti, K. L. *Mycobacteria xenopi* pulmonary disease. *West. J. Med.* , 138, 102, 1983.
314. Smith, M. J. and Citron, K. M. Clinical review of pulmonary disease caused by *Mycobacterium xenopi*. *Thorax*, 38, 373, 1983.
315. Koizumi, J. H. and Sommers, H. M. *Mycobacterium xenopi* and pulmonary disease. *Am. J. Clin. Pathol.* , 73, 826, 1980.
316. Terashima, T., Sakamaki, F., Hasegawa, N., Kanazawa, M., and Kawashiro, T. Pulmonary infection due to *Mycobacterium xenopi*. *Intern. Med.* , 33, 536–539, 1994.
317. Sennesael, J. J., Maes, V. A., Pierard, D., Debeukelaer, S. H., and Verbeelen, D. L. Streptomycin pharmacokinetics in relapsing *Mycobacterium xenopi* peritonitis. *Am. J. Nephrol.* , 10, 422, 1990.
318. Thomas, P., Liu, F., and Weiser, W. Characteristics of *Mycobacterium xenopi* disease. *Bull. Int. Union Tuberc. Lung Dis.* , 63, 12, 1988.
319. Parrot, R. G. and Grosset, J. H. Post-surgical outcome of 57 patients with *Mycobacterium xenopi* pulmonary infection. *Tubercle*, 69, 47, 1988.
320. Froidure, M., Massin, F., Duez, J. M., Baudouin, N., Camus, P., and Jeannin, L. Lung disease due to *Mycobacterium xenopi* excluding AIDS. Apropos of 8 cases. *Rev. Mal. Respir.* , 17, 481–487, 2000.
321. Jiva, T. M., Jacoby, H. M., Weymouth, L. A., Kaminski, D. A., and Portmore, A. C. *Mycobacterium xenopi*: innocent bystander or emerging pathogen? *Clin. Infect. Dis.* , 24, 226–232, 1997 [see also: *Clin. Infect. Dis.* , 24, 233–234, 1997].
322. Hoffner, S. E. Pulmonary infections caused by less frequently encountered slow-growing environmental mycobacteria. *Eur. J. Clin. Microbiol. Infect. Dis.*, 13, 937–941, 1994.

323. Cynamon, M. H. and Klemens, S. P. Activity of azithromycin against *Mycobacterium avium* infection in beige mice. *Antimicrob. Agents Chemother.*, 36, 1611, 1992.
324. Levendoglu-Tugal, O., Munoz, J., Brudnicki, A., Fevzi Ozkaynak, M., Sandoval, C., and Jayabose, S. Infections due to nontuberculous mycobacteria in children with leukemia. *Clin. Infect. Dis.*, 27, 1227–1230, 1998.
325. Kawamura, M., Kusanagi, Y., Satou, Y., Itou, S., Honma, M., and Shimoide, H. A case of pulmonary infection with *Mycobacterium xenopi*. *Nihon Kokyuki Gakkai Zasshi*, 36, 86–89, 1998.
326. Branger, B., Gouby, A., Oulès, R., et al. *Mycobacterium haemophilum* and *Mycobacterium xenopi* associated infection in a renal transplant patient. *Clin. Nephrol.*, 23, 46, 1985.
327. Kesten, S. and Chaparro, C. Mycobacterial infections in lung transplant recipients. *Chest*, 115, 741–745, 1999.
328. Busch, F. W., Bautz, W., Dierkesmann, R., et al. Lung changes caused by *Mycobacterium xenopi* infection in a patient with bone marrow transplantation: problems in differential diagnosis. *Pneumologie*, 45, 340, 1991.
329. Huber, W., Bautz, W., Holzmann, B., Classen, M., and Schepp, W., Pneumonia due to a rare atypical *Mycobacterium* in AIDS, *Dtsch. Med. Wocheschr.*, 118, 1636–1640, 1993.
330. Eng, R. H. K., Forrester, C., Smith, S. M., and Sobel, H. *Mycobacterium xenopi* infection in a patient with acquired immunodeficiency syndrome. *Chest*, 86, 145, 1984.
331. Tecson-Tumang, F. T. and Bright, J. L. *Mycobacterium xenopi*, and the acquired immunodeficiency syndrome. *Ann. Intern. Med.*, 100, 461, 1984.
332. Ausina, V., Barrio, J., Luquin, M., et al. *Mycobacterium xenopi* infections in the acquired immunodeficiency syndrome. *Ann. Intern. Med.*, 109, 927, 1988.
333. Shafer, R. W. and Sierra, M. F. *Mycobacterium xenopi, Mycobacterium fortuitum, Mycobacterium kansasii,* and other nontuberculous mycobacteria in an area of endemicity for AIDS. *Clin. Infect. Dis.*, 15, 161, 1992.
334. Juffermans, N. P., Verbon, A., Danner, S. A., Kuijper, E. J., and Speelman, P. *Mycobacterium xenopi* in HIV-infected patients: an emerging pathogen. *AIDS*, 12, 1661–1666, 1998.
335. El-Solh, A. A., Nopper, J., Abdul-Khoudoud, M. R., Sherif, S. M., Aquilina, A. T., and Grant, B. J. Clinical and radiographic manifestations of uncommon pulmonary nontuberculous mycobacterial disease in AIDS patients. *Chest*, 114, 138–145, 1998.
336. Sniadack, D. H., Ostroff, S. M., Karlix, M. A., et al. A nosocomial pseudo-outbreak of Mycobacterium xenopi due to a contaminated potable water supply: lessons in prevention. *Infect. Control Hosp. Epidemiol.*, 14, 636–641, 1993.
337. Miller, W. C., Perkins, M. D., Richardson, W. J., and Sexton, D. J. Pott's disease case by *Mycobacterium xenopi*: case report and review. *Clin. Infect. Dis.*, 19, 1024–1028, 1994.
338. Prosser, A. J. Spinal infection with *Mycobacterium xenopi*. *Tubercle*, 67, 229, 1986.
339. Rahman, M. A. A., Phongsathorn, V., Hughes, T., and Bielawska, C. Spinal infection by *Mycobacterium xenopi* in a non-immunosuppressed patient. *Tuber. Lung Dis.*, 73, 392, 1992.
340. Feyen, J., Martens, M., and Mulier, J. C. Infection of the knee joint with *Mycobacterium xenopi*. *Clin. Orthop.*, 179, 189, 1983.
341. Marks, J., Cook, J., and Pringle, J. A. S. Bone abscess due to *Mycobacterium xenopi*. *Tubercle*, 56, 157, 1975.
342. Libbrecht, E., Bressieux, J. M., Chelius, P., et al. *Mycobacterium xenopi* osteoarthritis of the ankle in a patient followed for psoriatic rheumatism. *Presse Med.*, 29, 539–540, 2000.
343. Danesh-Clough, T., Theis, J. C., and van der Linden, A. *Mycobacterium xenopi* infection of the spine: a case report and literature review. *Spine*, 25, 626–628, 2000.
344. Kely, M., Thibert, L., and Sinave, C. Septic arthritis in the knee due to *Mycobacterium xenopi* in a patient undergoing hemodialysis. *Clin. Infect. Dis.*, 29, 1342–1343, 1999.
345. Ollagnier, E., Fresard, A., Guglielminotti, C., et al. Osteoarticular *Mycobacterium xenopi* infection. *Presse Med.*, 27, 800–803, 1998.
346. Martinez-Roig, A., Elizari, M. J., Puente, M., Bonet, M., and Brill, W. Osteitis of the calcaneus by *Mycobacterium xenopi*. *Pediatr. Infect. Dis.*, 16, 77-79, 1997 [see also: *Pediatr. Infect. Dis.*, 16, 1011, 1997].
347. Zenone, T., Boibieux, A., Tigaud, S., et al. Non-tuberculous mycobacterial tenosynovitis: a review. *Scand. J. Infect. Dis.*, 31, 221–228, 1999.
348. Lovodic-Sivcev, B. and Vukelic, A. Changes in the kidney in patients with successive findings of *Mycobacterium xenopi* and *Mycobacterium fortuitum* in the urine: report of 16 cases. *Med. Pregl.*, 52, 334–342, 1999.
349. Prigogine, T., Stoffels, G., Fauville-Dufaux, M., Trolin, C., and Raftopoulos, C. Primary psoas muscle abscess due to *Mycobacterium xenopi*. *Clin. Infect. Dis.*, 26, 221–222, 1998.
350. Damsker, B., Bottone, E. J., and Deligdisch, L. *Mycobacterium xenopi*: infection in an immunocompromised host. *Human Pathol.*, 13, 866, 1982.
351. Price, A. B., Owen, R., Sowter, G., Einberg, J., and Smith, H. Disseminated *Mycobacterium xenopi* infection. *Lancet*, 2, 383, 1985.
352. Weinberg, J. R., Dootson, G., Gertner, D., Chambers, S. T., and Smith, H. Disseminated *Mycobacterium xenopi* infection. *Lancet*, 1, 1033, 1985.
353. Zurawski, C. A., Cage, G. D., Rimland, D., and Blumberg, H. M. Pneumonia and bacteremia due to *Mycobacterium celatum* masquerading as *Mycobaterium xenopi* in patients with AIDS: an underdiagnosed problem? *Clin. Infect. Dis.*, 24, 140–143, 1997.
354. Baugnee, P. E., Pouthier, F., and Dalaunois, L. Pulmonary mycobacteriosis due to *Mycobacterium xenopi*: in-vitro sensitivity to classical antitubercular agents and clinical development. *Acta Clin. Belg.*, 51, 19–27, 1996.
355. Bellamy, J., Leroy-Terquem, E., Duhamel, J. P., et al. *Mycobacterium xenopi* infection in emphysematous bulla: appropos of 4 cases operated on. *Rev. Mal. Respir.*, 4, 261, 1987.

356. Jouveshomme, S., Dautzenberg, B., Bakdach, H., and Derenne, J. P. Preliminary results of collapse therapy with plombage for pulmonary disease caused by multidrug-resistant mycobacteria. *Am. J. Respir. Crit. Care Med.*, 157(5 Pt.1), 1609–1615, 1998.
357. Group for the Study and Treatment of Resistant Mycobacterial Infections (GETIM). Rifabutine in the treatment of mycobacterial infections resistant to rifampicin: preliminary results. *Rev. Mal. Respir.*, 6, 335, 1989.
358. Shirayama, R., Hamada, K., Hayashi, H., et al. Atypical mycobacteriosis (*Mycobacterium xenopi*) with "initial aggravation". *Nihon Kyobu Shikkan Gakkai Zasshi*, 34, 1035-1039, 1996.
359. Schmitt, H., Schnitzler, N., Riehl, J., Adam, G., Sieberth, H. G., and Haase, G. Successful treatment of pulmonary *Mycobacterium xenopi* infection in a natural killer cell-deficient patient with clarithromycin, rifabutin, and sparfloxacin. *Clin. Infect. Dis.*, 29, 120–124, 1999.
360. Jones, P. G., Schrager, M. A., and Zabransky, R. J. Pott's disease caused by *Mycobacterium xenopi*. *Clin. Infect. Dis.*, 21, 1352, 1995.
361. Kiehl, P., Eicher, U., and Vakilzaden, F. A lupus-vulgaris-like atypical mycobacteriosis caused by *Mycobacterium xenopi* (*lupus xenopi*). *Hautarzt*, 43, 569–575, 1992.
362. Crantock, L., Crawford, D., and Powell, L. Fulminant hepatic failure complicating the treatment of *Mycobacterium xenopi*. *Med. J. Aust.*, 155, 723, 1991.
363. Thompson, J. E. Fulminant hepatic failure complicating the treatment of *Mycobacterium xenopi*. *Med. J. Aust.*, 156, 811–812, 1992.
364. Garibaldi, R. A., Kaplan, H. S., and Brittingham, T. E. Jaundice and death from isoniazid. *J. Tenn. Med. Assoc.*, 63, 23, 1970.
365. Black, M., Mitchell, J., Zimmermann, H., Ishak, K. G., and Epler, G. R. Isoniazid associated hepatitis in 114 patients. *Gastroenterology*, 69, 289, 1975.
366. Powell, L. W. and Crawford, D. H. G. Fulminant hepatic failure complicating the treatment of *Mycobacterium xenopi*: a reply. *Med. J. Aust.*, 156, 812, 1992.
367. Foudraine, N. A., Hovenkamp, E., Notermans, D. W., et al. Immunopathology as a result of highly active antiretroviral therapy in HIV-1-infected patients. *AIDS*, 13, 177–184, 1999.
368. Sompolinsky, D., Lagziel, A., Naveh, D., and Yankilevitz, T. *Mycobacterium haemophilum* sp. nov., a new pathogen of humans. *Int. J. Syst. Bacteriol.*, 28, 67, 1978.
369. Strauss, W. L., Ostroff, S. M., Jernigan, D. B., et al. Clinical and epidemiologic characteristics of *Mycobacterium haemophilum*, an emerging pathogen in immunocompromised patients. *Ann. Intern. Med.*, 120, 118–125, 1994.
370. Walder, B. K., Jeremy, D., Charlesworth, J. A., MacDonald, G. J., Pussell, B. A., and Robertson, M. R. The skin and immunosuppression. *Australas. J. Dermatol.*, 17, 94, 1976.
371. Becherer, P. and Hopfer, R. L. Infection with *Mycobacterium haemophilum*. *Clin. Infect. Dis.*, 14, 793, 1992.
372. Branger, B., Gouby, A., Oules, R., et al. *Mycobacterium haemophilum* and *Mycobacterium xenopi* associated infection in a renal transplant recipient. *Clin. Nephrol.*, 23, 46–49, 1985.
373. Davis, B. R., Brumbach, J., Sanders, W. J., and Wolinsky, E. Skin lesions caused by *Mycobacterium haemophilum*. *Ann. Intern. Med.*, 97, 723–724, 1982.
374. Dawson, D. J., Blacklock, Z. M., and Kane, D. W. *Mycobacterium haemophilum* causing lymphadenitis in an otherwise healthy child. *Med. J. Aust.*, 2, 289, 1981.
375. Dever, L. L., Martin, J. W., Seaworth, B., and Joegensen, J. H. Varied presentations and responses to treatment of infections caused by *Mycobacterium haemophilum* in patients with AIDS. *Clin. Infect. Dis.*, 14, 1195–1200, 1992.
376. Gouby, A., Branger, B., Oules, R., and Ramuz, M. Two cases of *Mycobacterium haemophilum* infection in a renal-dialysis unit. *J. Med. Microbiol.*, 25, 299–300, 1988.
377. Holton, J., Nye, P., and Miller, R. *Mycobacterium haemophilum* infection in a patient with AIDS. *J. Infect. Dis.*, 23, 303–306, 1991.
378. Kristjansson, M., Bieluch, V. M., and Byeff, P. D. *Mycobacterium haemophilum* infection in immunocompromised patients: case report and review of the literature. *Rev. Infect. Dis.*, 13, 906–910, 1991.
379. Males, B. M., West, T. E., and Bartholomew, W. R. *Mycobacterium haemophilum* infection in a patient with acquired immune deficiency syndrome. *J. Clin. Microbiol.*, 25, 186, 1987.
380. Moulsdale, M. T., Harper, J. M., Thatcher, G. N., and Dunn, B. L. Infection by *Mycobacterium haemophilum*, a metabolically fastidious acid-fast bacillus. *Tubercle*, 64, 29, 1983.
381. Rogers, P. L., Walker, R. E., Lane, H. C., et al. Disseminated *Mycobacterium haemophilum* infection in two patients with the acquired immunodeficiency syndrome. *Am. J. Med.*, 84, 640, 1988.
382. Ryan, C. G. and Dwyer, B. W. New characteristics of *Mycobacterium haemophilum*. *J. Clin. Microbiol.*, 18, 976, 1983.
383. Saubolle, M. A., Rudinsky, M., Merritt, E. S., et al. *Mycobacterium haemophilum* infection in two otherwise normal pediatric patients. *91st Annu. Mtg. Am. Soc. Microbiol.*, American Society for Microbiology, Washington, DC, 391, 1991.
384. Thilbert, L., Lebel, F., Martineau, B., and Chicoine, L. *Mycobacterium haemophilum* in Quebec. *Can. Dis. Wkly Rep.*, 14, 196, 1988.
385. Thibert, L., Lebel, F., and Martineau, B. Two cases of *Mycobacterium haemophilum* infection in Canada. *J. Clin. Microbiol.*, 28, 621, 1990.
386. Mezo, A., Jennis, F., McCarthy, S. W., and Dawson, D. J. Unusual mycobacteria in 5 cases of opportunistic infections. *Pathology*, 11, 377, 1979.
387. McBride, J. A., McBride, M. E., and Wolf, J. E. Jr. Evaluation of commercial blood-containing media for cultivation of *Mycobacterium haemophilum*. *Am. J. Clin. Pathol.*, 98, 282, 1992.

388. Shih, J. Y., Hsueh, P. R., Chang, Y. L., Lin, S. F., Teng, L. J., and Luh, K. T. Pyomyositis due to *Mycobacterium haemophilum* in a patient with polymyositis and long-term steroid use. *Clin. Infect. Dis.*, 26, 505–507, 1998.
389. Friedli, A., Krischer, J., Hirschel, B., Saurat, J. H., and Pechere, M. An annular plaque due to *Mycobacterium haemophilum* infection in a patient with AIDS. *J. Am. Acad. Dermatol.*, 43(5 Pt. 2), 913–915, 2000.
390. Bachmann, S., Schnyder, U., Pfyffer, G. E., Luthy, R., and Weber, R. *Mycobacterium haemophilum* infection in a patient with AIDS. *Dtsch. Med. Wochenschr.*, 121, 1189–1192, 1996.
391. Kiehn, T. E. and White, M. *Mycobacterium haemophilum*: an emerging pathogen. *Eur. J. Clin. Microbiol. Infect. Dis.*, 13, 925–931, 1994.
392. Saubolle, M. A., Kiehn, T. E., White, M. H., Rudinsky, M. F., and Armstrong, D. *Mycobacterium haemophilum*: microbiology and expanding clinical and geographic spectra of disease in humans. *Clin. Microbiol. Rev.*, 9, 435–447, 1996.
393. White, M. H., Papadopoulos, E. B., Small, T. N., Kiehn, T. E., and Armstrong, D. *Mycobacterium haemophilum* infections in bone marroe transplant recipients. *Transplantation*, 60, 957–960, 1995.
394. Armstrong, D., Kiehn, T., Boone, N., et al. *Mycobacterium haemophilum* infections—New York City metropolitan area, 1990–1991. *Morb. Mortal. Wkly Rep.*, 40, 636, 1991.
395. Lefkowitz, R. A. and Singson, R. D. Considering *Mycobacterium haemophilum* in the differential diagnosis for lytic bone lesions in AIDS patients who present with ulcerating skin lesions. *Skeletal Radiol.*, 27, 334–336, 1998.
396. Soubani, A. O., al-Marri, M., and Forlenza, S. Successful treatment of disseminated *Mycobacterium haemophilum* infection in a patient with AIDS. *Clin. Infect. Dis.*, 18, 475–476, 1994.
397. Sowden, D., Kemp, R., and Dawson, D. Osteomyelitis due to *Mycobacterium haemophilum* in a patient with AIDS. *Pathology*, 25, 308–309, 1993.
398. Kiehn, T. E., White, M., Pursell, K. J., et al. A cluster of four cases of *Mycobacterium haemophilum* infection. *Eur. J. Clin. Microbiol. Infect. Dis.*, 12, 114–118, 1993.
399. Yarrish, R. L., Shay, W., LaBombardi, V. J., Meyerson, M., Miller, D. K., and Larone, D. Osteomyelitis caused by *Mycobacterium haemophilum*: successful therapy in two patients with AIDS. *AIDS*, 6, 557–561, 1992.
400. Gupta, I., Kocher, J., Miller, A. J., Weisholtz, S. J., Perz, J., and Scully, M. *Mycobacterium haemophilum* osteomyelitis in an AIDS patient. *N. J. Med.*, 89, 201–202, 1992.
401. Plemmons, R. M., McAllister, C. K., Garces, M. C., and Ward, R. L. Osteomyelitis due to *Mycobaterium haemophilum* in a cardiac transplant patient: case report and analysis of interactions among clarithromycin, rifampin, and cyclosporin. *Clin. Infect. Dis.*, 24, 995–997, 997.
402. Branger, B., Oules, R., Gouby, A., et al. Cutaneous *Mycobacterium haemophilum* mycobacteriosis in a kidney transplant patient. *Presse Med.*, 12, 2699, 1983.
403. McGovern, J., Bix, B. C., and Webster, G. *Mycobacterium haemophilum* skin disease successfully treated with excision. *J. Am. Acad. Dermatol.*, 30(2 Pt. 1), 269–270, 1994.
404. Ward, M. S., Lam, K. V., Cannell, P. K., and Herrmann, R. P. Mycobacterial central venous catheter tunnel infection: a difficult problem. *Bone Marrow Transplant.*, 24, 325–329, 1999.
405. Dawson, D. J. and Jennis, F. Mycobacteria with a growth requirement for ferric ammonium citrate identified as *Mycobacterium haemophilum*. *J. Clin. Microbiol.*, 11, 190, 1980.
406. McBride, M. E., Rudolph, A. H., Tschen, J. A., et al. Diagnostic and therapeutic considerations for cutaneous *Mycobacterium haemophilum* infections. *Arch. Dermatol.*, 127, 276–277, 1991.
407. Armstrong, K. L., James, R. W., Dawson, D. J., Francis, P. W., and Masters, B. *Mycobacterium haemophilum* causing perihilar or cervical lymphadenitis in healthy children. *J. Pediatr.*, 121, 202–205, 1992.
408. Hirschel, B., Chang, H. R., Mach, N., et al. Fatal infection with a novel unidentified mycobacterium in a man with the acquired immunodeficiency syndrome. *N. Engl. J. Med.*, 323, 109, 1990.
409. Kuijper, E. J., de Witte, M., Verhagen, D. W., Kolk, A. H., van der Meer, J. T., and Dankert, J. *Mycobacterium genavense* infection of 2 HIV seropositive patients in Amsterdam. *Ned. Tijdschr. Geneeskd.*, 142, 970–972, 1998.
410. Böttger, E. C., Teske, A., Kirschner, P., et al. Disseminated "*Mycobacterium genavense*" infection in patients with AIDS. *Lancet*, 340, 76, 1992.
411. Pechère, M. and Hirschel, B. Infections a *Mycobacterium genavense* fréquence et présentation clinique. *Presse Med.*, 24, 239, 1995.
412. Pechère, M., Opravil, M., Wald, A., et al. Clinical and epidemiological features of infection with *Mycobacterium genavense*. *Arch. Intern. Med.*, 155, 400, 1995.
413. Bessesen, M. T., Shlay, J., Stone-Venohr, B., Cohn, D. L., and Reves, R. R. Disseminated *Mycobacterium genavense* infection: clinical and microbiological features and response to therapy. *AIDS*, 7, 1357, 1993.
414. Van der Ven, A. J., Jacobs, J. A., and Schrey, G. Infection with *Mycobacterium genavense* in 2 HIV-seropositive patients in Amsterdam. *Ned. Tijdschr. Geneeskd.*, 142, 2537–2538, 1998.
415. Vergnaud, M., Dauga, C., Dompmartin, A., Malbruny, B., Bazin, C., and Grimont, P. A. Genital infection due to *Mycobacterium genavense* in a patient with AIDS. *Clin. Infect. Dis.*, 27, 1531, 1998.
416. Hillebrand-Haverkort, M. E. Infection with *Mycobacterium genavense* in 2 HIV- seropositive patients in Amsterdam. *Ned. Tijdschr. Geneeskd.*, 142, 2165–2166, 1998.
417. van Ginneken, E. E. and Koopmans, P. P. Infection with *Mycobacterium genavense* in 2 HIV-seropositive patients in Amsterdam. *Ned. Tijdschr. Geneeskd.*, 142, 1629, 1998.
418. Fournier, S., Pialoux, G., and Vincent, V. *Mycobacterium genavense* and cutaneous disease in AIDS. *Ann. Intern. Med.*, 128, 409, 1998.
419. Rodriguez, P., March, F., Garrigo, M., Moreno, C., Barrio, J., and Gurgui, M. Disseminated *Mycobacterium genavense*

infection in patients with HIV infection. Description of 5 cases and review of the literature. *Enferm. Infecc. Microbiol. Clin.*, 14, 220–226, 1996.
420. Glesby, M. J. and Hoover, D. R. *Mycobacterium genavense* infection and survival. *Arch. Intern. Med.*, 155, 2128–2129, 1995 [see.also: *Arch. Intern. Med.*, 155, 400–404, 1995].
421. Hillebrand-Haverkort, M. E., Kolk, A. H., Kox, L. F., Ten Velden, J. J., and Ten Veen, J. H. Generalized *Mycobacterium genavense* infection in HIV-infected patients: detection of the *Mycobacterium* in hospital tap water. *Scand. J. Infect. Dis.*, 31, 63–68, 1999.
422. Collins, F. M., Morrison, N. E., and Montalbine, V. Immune response to persistent mycobacterial infection in mice. *Infect. Immun.*, 19, 430, 1978.
423. Heiken, H., Kirschner, P., Stoll, M., Böttger, E. C., and Schmidt, R. E., *Mycobacterium genavense* infection in AIDS. *Dtsch. Med. Wochenschr.*, 118, 296, 1993.
424. Albrecht, H., Rusch-Gerdes, S., Stellbrink, H. J., Greten, H., and Jackle, S., Disseminated *Mycobacterium genavense* infection as a cause of pseudo-Whipple's disease and sclerosing cholangitis. *Clin. Infect. Dis.*, 25, 742-743, 1997.
425. Berman, S. M., Kim, R. C., Haghighat, D., Mulligan, M. E., Fierer, J., and Wyle, F. C. *Mycobacterium genavense* infection presenting as a solitary brain mass in a patient with AIDS: case report and review. *Clin. Infect. Dis.*, 19, 1152, 1994.
426. Krebs, T., Zimmerli, S., Bodmer, T., and Lammle, B., *Mycobacterium genavense* infection in a patient with long-standing chronic lymphocytic leukaemia. *J. Intern. Med.*, 248, 343- 348, 2000.
427. Laeutez, S., Boutoille, D., Bemer-Melchior, P., Ponge, T., and Raffi, F., Localized *Mycobacterium genavense* soft tissue infection in an immunodeficient HIV-negative patient. *Eur. J. Clin. Microbiol. Infect. Dis.*, 19, 51-52, 2000.
428. Figueras, C., Garcia, L., and Bertran, J. M. Hyperpigmentation in a patient with AIDS, receiving rifabutin for disseminated *Mycobacterium genavense* infection. *Eur. J. Pediatr.*, 157, 612, 1998.
429. Dionisio, D., Tortoli, E., Simonetti, M. T., et al. Intestinal mycobacterial infections in AIDS: clinical course and treatment of infections caused by *Mycobacterium avium*, *Mycobacterium kansasii*, *Mycobacterium genavense*. *Recent Prog. Med.*, 85, 526, 1994.
430. Albrecht, H., Rusch-Gerdes, S., Stellbrink, H. J., and Greten, H., Treatment of disseminated *Mycobacterium genavense* infection. *AIDS*, 9, 659–660, 1995.
431. Matsiota-Bernard, P., Thierry, D., De Truchis, P., Saillour, M., and Paraire, F. *Mycobacterium genavense* infection in a patient with AIDS who was successfully treated with clarithromycin. *Clin. Infect. Dis.*, 20, 1565–1566.

11
Listeria monocytogenes

1. INTRODUCTION

Listeria monocytogenes (also referred to as *Corinebacterium infantisepticum* and *Corinebacterium parvulum*) is a motile gram-positive bacillus with pathogenic activity in mammals, birds, and fish. It belongs to the genus *Listeria*, which has uncertain affiliation but closely resembles the organisms of the family Corinebacteriaceae *(1)*.

In humans, the *L. monocytogenes*, a food-borne pathogen *(2–5)*, exhibits marked tropism for the central nervous system (CNS) and the placenta *(6)*. A preceding gastrointestinal infection or disruption causing inflamed bowel mucosa may facilitate blood stream invasion by the pathogen *(7)*. In immunocompromised hosts, listeriosis is a rare but serious infectious disease, which, if not recognized and treated appropriately, may reach a mortality rate of 20–30% *(8–13)*. As many as 5% of the general population harbor *Listeria* in their intestinal tract *(14,15)*.

In cases of central nervous system (CNS) involvement, transcellular penetration (transcytosis) of *L. monocytogenes* across the blood-brain barrier (BBB) has been demonstrated *(16)*. The epithelial cells of the choroid plexus, ependymal cells, macrophages/microglia, and the neurons are the target cells of the pathogen *(17)*. *L. monocytogenes* infection of CNS is often not recognized and treated appropriately in the early stages of the disease, therefore, making early diagnosis and treatment critical for reducing its morbidity and high mortality rate *(18,19)*. In addition to meningitis and meningoencephalitis, cerebritis and abscess *(20)* may also occur, whereas infection of the brainstem (rhomboencephalitis) *(21)* is challenging to recognize, and therefore, initiate appropriate early therapy *(18)*.

Primarily, listeriosis affects individuals with deficient cell-mediated immunity *(7)*, often the very young *(22–24)*; the elderly; patients on immunosuppressive therapy such as transplant recipients *(25–28)*, cancer patients *(13,29–32)* and pregnant women *(33)*. Thus, *L. monocytogenes* has been the most common cause of bacterial meningitis in cancer patients *(29)* such as those with hematologic malignancies (leukemia) where predisposition to infections is compounded by both immunodeficiency related to leukemia itself (humoral and cellular immune dysfunction) and the results of cumulative immunosuppression related to treatment *(30,34)*.

AIDS patients because of their severe immunodeficiency may be higly susceptible to invasive *Listeria* infections *(7,35–41)*, especially those patients with CD4$^+$ cell counts below 50 µL *(42)*. By comparison with the general population, HIV-infected patients are 60 times more likely to acquire listeriosis *(42)*. Because of serious immunodeficiencies, in patients with full-blown AIDS, the risk has been even higher (150–280 times) *(8,14,35)*. Surprisingly though, the overall incidence of listeriosis in HIV-positive patients has been relatively low. The risk in such patients can be best determined from large population-based studies.

Listeriosis during pregnancy is not uncommon and may occur even in the absence of overt immune deficiency *(33)*. During pregnancy, listeriosis can lead to congenital infection, neonatal sepsis and meningitis, or fetal death *(11,43,44)*. However, it is usually mild and rarely fatal unless other risk

From: Opportunistic Infections: Treatment and Prophylaxis
By: Vassil St. Georgiev © Humana Press Inc., Totowa, NJ

factors are present. Reinfection is possible *(45)*. The first maternal death by listerial bacteremia of a pregnant woman with AIDS was reported by Wetli et al. *(46,47)*. In utero infections by *L. monocytogenes* have occurred transplacentally resulting in abortions, stillbirths, or premature births. When acquired during birth, listeriosis can cause cardiorespiratory distress, diarrhea, vomiting, and menengitis.

In adults, *Listeria* infection either as the result of an outbreak or sporadic, has been primarily foodborne *(14,48–51)*. It is typically associated with meningitis, endocarditis *(52)*, and disseminated granulomatous lesions, but also with endogenous endophthalmitis *(53,54)*, peritonitis *(55)*, liver abscess *(56)*, arterial aneurysms *(57)*, and pneumonia *(13)*. In an extremely rare case, Heikinen et al. *(58)* described a case of infrarenal endoluminal bifurcated stent graft infected with *L. monocytogenes*.

Morelli and Wilson *(59)* have discussed the possibility that infliximab (a new monoclonal antibody used to block the activity of tumor necrosis factor [TNF] that is causing increased inflammation and tissue damage in Crohn's disease and rheumatoid arthritis) may increase the susceptibility to listeriosis.

2. LISTERIOSIS IN AIDS PATIENTS

In AIDS patients, *Listeria*-induced infections are seldom diagnosed and most often observed in the late stages of the disease when CD4$^+$ cell counts are usually well below normal *(7,35–37,40,42,60–69)*. In 1984, the first case of *L. monocytogenes* infection in HIV-infected patient was reported by Real et al. *(61)*. At least 16 different serotypes have been isolated from HIV-infected patients with serotypes 1/2a, 1/2b, and 4b being the most prevalent (in over 90% of the population) *(70)*. Listeriosis usually presented as meningitis *(7,37,40,65)*, meningoencephalitis *(7,62)*, primary bacteremia *(7,36,60,61,63,66,67)*, and/or infection of the contents of the pregnant uterus; other manifestations have been rare *(9,35,64,69)*.

In general, the clinical symptoms of listeriosis in HIV-infected patients did not differ significantly from those in other patients, except for the high incidence of brain abscesses and cerebritis seen in renal-transplant recipients *(29,71,72)*. In one report, meningitis accounted for 71% of listerial infections among HIV-positive patients *(14)*.

Several hypothesis have been proposed to explain the rare occurence of listeriosis in AIDS patients. It is possible that multiple courses of prophylactic antibiotic medications taken by AIDS patients to prevent the progression of HIV and prevent other opportunistic infections might alter the gastrointestinal flora and even eradicate the microorganism. Thus, trimethoprim-sulfamethoxazole, commonly given to prevent *Pneumocystis carinii* infections, has also been very effective treatment against *L. monocytogenes (73)*. In another hypothesis, it has been postulated that contrary to predisposed immunocompromised patients who receive corticosteroid therapy that impair random movement, chemotaxis, and bactericidal activity of macrophages and polymorphonuclear cells, in AIDS patients the activity of nonimmune macrophages and granulocytes has been retained relatively intact *(65,74)*. Another factor could be the possibility that a T-cell subset other than CD4$^+$ cells may be responsible for the antilisterial immune response *(74)*.

It was also thought possible that genetic factors may play a role in the human defense against listeriosis *(74)*. Thus, it was postulated that one reason for the inability of AIDS patients to resist opportunistic infections has been their impaired (decreased) expression of class II histocompatibility gene proteins (such as HLA-DR), which are needed for successful antigen presentation and antigen-induced T lymphocyte activation *(75)*. It is relevant to mention that studies in experimental animals have demonstrated that protection against *Listeria* appeared restricted not by class II, but class I antigens *(76)*.

Furthermore, most opportunistic infections in HIV-positive patients are caused by either endogenous reactivation of latent pathogens (*Pneumocystis carinii*, *Toxoplasma gondii*, cytomegalovirus, mycobacteria, and herpes simplex virus), or from the inability of the host immune defenses to resist pathogens to which exposure is common *(35)*. However, *Listeria* is not known to remain latent in

Table 1
Recommended Therapies of Listeriosis

Listeria Infection	Treatment	Refs.
Meningitis	Ampicillin (2.0 g every 4 h, i.v.)	(37)
	Ampicillin (2.0 g every 4 h, i.v.)	(63)
	TMP-SMX (160 mg of TMP) every 6 h	
Meningoencephalitis	Amoxycillin (12 g daily, i.v.;	
	then 6 g daily, i.v.)	(62)
	Ampicillin (15 g daily, i.v.)	(60)
Brain abscess	Penicillin, chloramphenicol	(69)
Bacteremia	Ampicillin (3.0 g every 4 h, i.v.)	(40)
	Gentamicin (80 mg every 8 h, i.v.)	
	Ampicillin (12 g daily, i.v.)	(61)
	Amoxycillin, gentamicin, sulfadiazine, pyrimethamine	(66)
	Penicillin	(61)
	Vancomycin	(68)
Endocarditis	Penicillin, netilmicin	(64)

human macrophages for prolonged periods of time after the initial asymptomatic infection, and widespread exposure to *L. monocytogenes* in nonepidemic situations has been infrequent and of transitory nature *(9)*.

3. TREATMENT OF LISTERIOSIS

Listeriosis usually respond to antimicrobial therapy with no reports of recurrent infection *(1,33,35)*. In general, treatment with antibiotics (penicillin, ampicillin, amoxicillin), alone or in combination with aminoglycoside (gentamicin), is usually recommended (Table 1) *(21,35,45,77)*. Although a variety of antibiotics have shown activity, ampicillin alone or in combination with gentamicin *(78)* remains the treatment of choice as first-line agents against listeriosis *(79)*. Second-line antilisteriosis agents include trimethoprim-sulfamethoxazole, erythromycin, vancomycin, and fluoroquinolones. The cephalosporins are not active against *Listeria (28,79)*.

On several occasions, trimethoprim-sulfamethoxazole (TMP-SMX) was reported to be effective when administered at concentrations attainable in serum and cerebrospinal fluid (CSF) *(80–82)*. Berenguer et al. *(35)* treated successfully an HIV-positive patient with a 21-d course of intravenous trimethoprim-sulfamethoxazole (5.0 mg of TMP/25 mg of SMX, q.i.d.).

Wacker et al. *(31)* have reported a case of a 5-yr-old boy with acute lymphoblastic leukemia (ALL) and intolerance to oral TMP-SMX who had *L. monocytogenes* bacteremia and meningitis developed during maintenance chemotherapy. In spite of a prompt 7-d course of intravenous amoxicillin-gentamicin and microbiologic clearance of the bloodstream, the patient failed to respond to therapy. However, the addition of intravenous TMP-SMX (10 mg/kg daily of TMP) after desensitization led to a rapid resolution of meningitis and fever and ultimate cure of the patient.

One patient with a brain abscess caused by *L. monocytogenes* was treated with penicillin, chloramphenicol, and surgical drainage of the abscess *(69)*. *Listeria*-induced endocarditis responded to penicillin and netilmicin, combined with surgery *(64)*.

Meropenem was used successfully to treat *L. monocytogenes* meningitis in a penicillin-allergic pediatric renal-transplant patient *(28)*.

At high concentrations, the antimicrobial peptide enterocin-35 *(83,84)*, a new class II bacteriocin was found to produce localized holes in the wall and cellular membrane of *L. monocytogenes* resulting in bacterial death *(85)*.

REFERENCES

1. Kales, C. P. and Holzman, R. S. Listeriosis in patients with HIV infection: clinical manifestations and response to therapy. *J. Acquir. Immun.*, 3, 139, 1990.
2. Schlech III, W. F. Foodborne listeriosis. *Clin. Infect. Dis.*, 31, 770–773, 2000.
3. Mandel, Y., Freed, M., Shpilberg, O., and Ashkenazi, I. *Listeria* monocytogenes: the bacterium, mode of transmission and relation to food consumption. *Harefuah*, 136, 713–717, 1999.
4. Inoue, S., Nakama, A., Arai, Y., et al. Prevalence and contamination levels of *Listeria monocytogenes* in retail foods in Japan. *Int. J. Food Microbiol.*, 59, 73–77, 2000.
5. Wong, S., Street, D., Delgado, S. I., and Klontz, K. C. Recalls of foods and cosmetics due to microbial contamination reported to the U.S. Food and Drug Administration. *J. Food Prot.*, 63, 1113–1116, 2000.
6. Rainis, T. and Potasman, I. *Listeria monocytogenes* infections: ten years' experience: *Harefuah*, 137, 436–440, 512.
7. Mascola, L., Lieb, L., Chiu, J., Fannin, S. L., and Linnan, M. J. Listeriosis: an uncommon opportunistic infection in patients with acquired immunodeficiency syndrome: report of five cases and a review of the literature. *Am. J. Med.*, 84, 162, 1988.
8. Angulo, F. J. and Swerdlow, D. L. (1995) Bacterial enteric infections in patients infected with human immunodeficiency virus. *Clin. Infect. Dis.*, 21(Suppl.1), S84.
9. Armstrong, D. Listeria monocytogenes, in *Principles and Practice of Infectious Diseases*, 3rd ed., Mandell, G. L., Douglas, R. G., and Bennett, J.E., Eds. Churchill Livingstone, New York, NY, 1587, 1990.
10. Staundiger, R., Levine, D., Swaminathan, B., and Zagzag, D. Neurolisteriosis presenting as recurrent transient ischemic attacks. *Ann. Neurol.*, 48, 661–665, 2000.
11. de Valk, H., Vaillant, V., and Goulet, V. Epidemiologie des listerioses humaines en France. *Bull. Acad. Natl. Med.*, 184, 267–274, 2000.
12. Tobalina Larrea, I., Lopez Legarra, G., Martinez Odriozola, P., et al. Pleural effusion due to *Listeria monocytogenes*. A case report and review of the literature. *An. Med. Interna*, 16, 463–465, 1999.
13. Ruiz Lopez, F. J., Mendez Martinez, P., Ortiz Romero, M. M., Martinez Garceran, J. J., Bolarin Lopez, J., and Sanchez Gascon, F. *Listeria monocytogenes* pneumonia: a severe complication in a patient with neoplasia. *Ann. Med. Intl*, 16, 420–422, 1999.
14. Schuchat, A., Deaver, K. A., Wenger, J. D., et al. Role of foods in sporadic listeriosis. I. Case-control study of dietary risk factors. *J. Am. Med. Assoc.*, 267, 2041, 1992.
15. Schlech, W. F., III. New perspectives on the gastrointesinal mode of transmission in invasive *Listeria monocytogenes* infection. *Clin. Invest. Med.*, 7, 321, 1984.
16. Huang, S., Stins, M. F., and Kim, K. S. Bacterial penetration across the blood-brain barrier during the development of neonatal meningitis. *Microbes Infect.*, 2, 1237–1244, 2000.
17. Schluter, D., Buck, C., Reiter, S., Meyer, T., Hof, H., and Deckert-Schluter, M. Immune reactions of *Listeria monocytogenes* in the brain. *Immunobiology*, 201, 188–195, 1999.
18. Bartt, R. *Listeria* and atypical presentation of *Listeria* in the central nervous system. *Semin. Neurol.*, 20, 361–373, 2000.
19. Taege, A. J. Listeriosis: recognizing it, treating it, preventing it. *Cleve. Clin. J. Med.*, 66, 375–380, 1999.
20. Erny, O., Rousseaux, M., Pruvo, J. P., Guarouaou, D., and Savage, C. A case of listeriosis revealed by voluminous cerebral abscesses. *Rev. Med. Interne*, 20, 541–542, 1999.
21. Bravo, M., Ferrer, S., and Trujillo, S. *Listeria monocytogenes* rhomboencephalitis. Clinical case. *Rev. Med. Chil.*, 126, 828–832, 1998.
22. McLure, J. M. A 9-month-old boy with fever and lethargy. *Clin. Pediatr. (Phila.)*, 39, 295–296, 296–298.
23. Economou, M., Karyda, S., Kansouzidou, A., and Kavaliotis, J. *Listeria* meningitis in children: report of two cases. *Infection*, 28, 121–123, 2000.
24. Boga, A. S., Montero, R. B., Garcia, F. S., and Valcarcel, G. R. *Listeria monocytogenes* meningitis during the incubation period of hepatitis A disease. *Pediatr. Infect. Dis.*, 19, 265–266, 2000.
25. Girmenia, C., Iori, A. P., Bernasconi, S., et al. Listeriosis in recipients of allogeneic bone marrow transplants from unrelated donors. *Eur. J. Clin. Microbiol. Infect. Dis.*, 19, 711–714, 2000.
26. Jost, L., Jost, L., Nogues, M., Davalos, M., Turin, M., Manes, F., and Leiguarda, R. Neurological complications of renal transplant. *Medicina (B. Aires)*, 60, 161–164, 2000.
27. Reek, C., Tenschert, W., Elsner, H. A., Kaulfers, P. M., and Huland, H. Pulsed-field gel electrophoresis for the analysis of *Listeria monocytogenes* infection clusters after kidney transplantation. *Urol. Res.*, 28, 93–96, 2000.
28. Weston, V. C., Punt, J., Vloebeghs, M., Watson, A. R., and Ispahani, P. *Listeria monocytogenes* meningitis in a penicillin-allergic paediatric renal transplant patient. *J. Infect.*, 37, 77–78, 1998.
29. Niemen, R. E. and Lorber, B., Listeriosis in adults: a changing pattern: report of eight cases and review of the literature 1968-1978. *Rev. Infect. Dis.*, 2, 2–7, 1980.
30. Tsiodras, S., Samonis, G., Keating, M. J., and Kontoyiannis, D. P., Infection and immunity in chronic lymphocytic leukemia. *Mayo Clin. Proc.*, 75, 1039–1054, 2000.
31. Wacker, P., Ozsahin, H., Groll, A. H., Gervaix, A., Reinhard, L., and Humbert, J., Trimethoprim-sulfamethoxazole salvage for refractory listeriosis during maintenance chemotherapy for acute lymphoblastic leukemia. *J. Pediatr. Hematol. Oncol.*, 22, 340–343, 2000.
32. Adeonigbagbe, O., Khademi, A., Karowe, M., Gualtieri, N., and Robilotti, J., *Listeria monocytogenes* peritonitis: an unusual presentation and review of the literature. *J. Clin. Gastroenterol.*, 30, 436–437, 2000.

33. Decker, C. F., Simon, G. L., DiGioia, R. A., and Tuazon, C. U. *Listeria monocytogenes* infections in patients with AIDS: report of five cases and review. *Rev. Infect. Dis.,* 13, 413, 1991.
34. Morra, E., Nosari, A., and Montillo, M. Infectious complications in chronic lymphocytic leukaemia. *Hematol. Cell Ther.,* 41, 145–151, 1999.
35. Berenguer, J., Solera, J., Diaz, M. D., Moreno, S., Lopez-Herce, J. A., and Bouza, E. Listeriosis in patients infected with human immunodeficiency virus. *Rev. Infect. Dis.,* 13, 115, 1991.
36. Read, E. J., Orenstein, J. M., Chorba, T. L., et al. *Listeria monocytogenes* sepsis and small cell carcinoma of the rectum: an unusual presentation of the acquired immunodeficiency syndrome. *Am. J. Clin. Pathol.,* 83, 385, 1985.
37. Gould, I. A., Belok, L. C., and Handwerger, S. *Listeria monocytogenes*: a rare cause of opportunistic infection in the acquired immunodeficiency syndrome (AIDS) and a new cause of meningitis in AIDS: a case report. *AIDS Res.,* 2, 231, 1986.
38. Whimbley, E., Gold, J. W. M, Polsky, B., et al. Bacteremia and fungemia in patients with the acquired immunodeficiency syndrome. *Ann. Intern. Med.,* 104, 511, 1986.
39. Qayyum, Q. J., Scerpella, E. G., Moreno, J. N., and Fischl, M. A. Report of 24 cases of *Listeria monocytogenes* infection at the University of Miami Medical Center. *Rev. Invest. Clin.,* 49, 265–270, 1997.
40. Koziol, K., Rielly, K. S., Bonin, R. A., and Salcedo, J. R. *Listeria monocytogenes* meningitis in AIDS. *Can. Med. Assoc. J.,* 135, 43, 1986.
41. Centers for Disease Control and Prevention. 1993 Revised classification system for HIV infection and expanded surveillance case definition for AIDS among adolescents and adults. *Morb. Mortal. Wkly Rep.,* 41(RR-17), 1, 1992.
42. Jurado, R. L., Farley, M. M., Pereira, E., et al. Increased risk of meningitis and bacteremia due to *Listeria monocytogenes* in patients with human immunodeficiency virus infection. *Clin. Infect. Dis.,* 17, 224–227, 1993.
43. Dawson, K. G., Emerson, J. C., and Burns, J. L. Fifteen years of experience with bacterial meningitis. *Pediatr. Infect. Dis.,* 18, 816–822, 1999.
44. Pong, A. and Bradley, J. S. Bacterial meningitis and the newborn infant. *Infect. Dis. Clin. North Am.,* 13, 711–733, 1999.
45. Lurie, S., Feinstein, M., and Mamet, Y. *Listeria monocytogenes* reinfection in a pregnant woman. *Br. J. Obstet. Gynaecol.,* 106, 509–510, 1999.
46. Wetli, C. V., Roldan, E. O., and Fojaco, R. M. Listeriosis as a cause of maternal death: an obstetric complication of the acquired immunodeficiency syndrome (AIDS). *Am. J. Obstet. Gynecol.,* 147, 7, 1983.
47. Wetli, C. V., Roldan, E. O., and Fojaco, R. M. Listeriosis in AIDS: an unfounded assumption. *Am. J. Obstet. Gynecol.,* 149, 805, 1984.
48. Schlech, W. F., Lavigne, P. M., Bortolussi, R. A., et al. Epidemic listeriosis: evidence for transmission by food. *N. Engl. J. Med.,* 308, 203, 1983.
49. Pinner, R. W., Schuchat, A., Swaminathan, B., et al. Role of foods in sporadic listeriosis. II. Microbiologic and epidemiologic investigation. *J. Am. Med. Assoc.,* 267, 2046, 1992.
50. Farber, J. M., Daley, E. M., MacKie, M. T., and Limerick, B. A small outbreak of listeriosis potentially linked to the consumption of imitation crab meat. *Lett. Appl. Microbiol.,* 31, 100–104, 2000.
51. Centers for Disease Control, Multistate outbreak of listeriosis - United States, 1998. *MMWR Morb. Mortal. Wkly Rep.,* 47, 1085–1086, 1998.
52. Hood, S. and Baxter, R. H. *Listeria* endocarditis causing aortic root abscess and a fistula to the left atrium. *Scott. Med. J.,* 44, 117–118, 1999.
53. Deramo, V. A., Shah, G. K., Garden, M., and Maguire, J. I. Good visual outcome after *Listeria monocytogenes* endogenous endophthalmitis. *Retina,* 19, 566–568, 1999.
54. Lohmann, C. P., Gabel, V.P., Heep, M., Linde, H. J., and Reischl, U. *Listeria monocytogenes*-induced endogenous endophthalmitis in an otherwise healthy individual: rapid PCR-diagnosis as the basis for active treatment. *Eur. J. Ophthalmol.,* 9, 53–57, 1999.
55. Jorquera Plaza, F., Espinel Diez, J., Fernandez Gundin, M. J., et al. Spontaneous bacterial peritonitis caused by *Listeria monocytogenes*. *Gastroenterol. Hepatol.,* 21, 489–491, 1998.
56. Bronnimann, S., Baer, H. U., Malinverni, R., and Buchler, M. W. *Listeria monocytogenes* causing solitary liver abscess. Case report and review of the literature. *Dig. Surg.,* 15, 364–368, 1998.
57. Paccalin, M., Amoura, Z., Brocheriou, I., et al. Infectious aneurysm due to *Listeria monocytogenes*: a new case and review of the literature. *Rev. Med. Interne,* 19, 661–665, 1998.
58. Heikkinen, L., Valtonen, M., Lepentalo, M., Saimanen, E., and Jarvinen, A. Infrarenal endoluminal bifurcated stent graft infected with *Listeria monocytogenes*. *J. Vasc. Surg.,* 29, 554–556, 1999.
59. Morelli, J. and Wilson, F. A. Does administration of infliximab increase the susceptibility to listeriosis? *Am. J. Gastroenterol.,* 95, 841–842, 2000.
60. Thiel, M., Kindt, R., Schmidt, H., Schassan, H., and Horst-Schmidt-Kliniken Potel, J. Listerien sepsis bei AIDS. *Dtsch. Med. Wochenschr.,* 111, 316, 1986.
61. Real, F. X., Gold, J. W. M., Krown, S. E., and Armstrong, D. *Listeria monocytogenes* bacteremia in the acquired immunodeficiency syndrome. *Ann. Intern. Med.,* 101, 883, 1984.
62. Schattenkerk, J. K. M. E., Klöpping, C., Speelman, J. D., Van Ketel, R. J., and Danner, S. A. Complications of the acquired immunodeficiency syndrome. *Ann. Intern. Med.,* 104, 726, 1986.
63. Harvey, R. L. and Chandrasekar, P. H. Chronic meningitis caused by *Listeria* in a patient infected with human immunodeficiency virus. *J. Infect. Dis.,* 157, 1091, 1988.

64. Riancho, J. A., Echevarria, S., Napal, J., Duran, R. M., and Macias, J. G. Endocarditis due to *Listeria monocytogenes* and human immunodeficiency virus infection. *Am. J. Med.*, 85, 737, 1988.
65. Beninger, P. R., Savoia, M. C., and Davis, C. E. *Listeria monocytogenes* meningitis in a patient with AIDS-related complex. *J. Infect. Dis.*, 158, 1396, 1988.
66. Bizet, C., Mechali, D., Rocourt, J., and Fraisse, F. *Listeria monocytogenes* bacteraemia in AIDS. *Lancet*, 1, 501, 1989.
67. Patey, O., Nedelec, C., Emond, J. P., Mayorga, R., N'Go, N., and Lafaix, C. *Listeria* monocytogenes septicemia in an AIDS patient with a brain abscess. *Eur. J. Clin. Microbiol. Infect. Dis.*, 8, 746, 1989.
68. Katner, H. P. and Joiner, T. A. *Listeria monocytogenes* sepsis from an infected indwelling I.V. catheter in a patient with AIDS. *South. Med. J.*, 82, 94, 1989.
69. Harris, J. O., Marquez, J., Swerdlow, M. A., and Magana, I. A. *Listeria* brain abscess in the acquired immunodeficiency syndrome. *Arch. Neurol.*, 46, 250, 1989.
70. Gellin, B. G. and Broome, C. V. Listeriosis. *J. Am. Med. Assoc.*, 261, 1313, 1989.
71. Stamm, A. M., Desmukes, W. E., Simmons, B. P., et al. Listeriosis in renal transplant recipients: report of an outbreak and review of 1-2 cases. *Rev. Infect. Dis.*, 4, 665, 1982.
72. Louria, D. B., Hensle, T., Armstrong, D., et al. Listeriosis complicating malignant disease: a new complication. *Ann. Intern. Med.*, 67, 261, 1967.
73. Spitzer, P. G., Hammer, S. M., and Karchmer, A. W. Treatment of *Listeria monocytogenes* infection with trimethoprim-sulfamethoxazole: case report and review of the literature. *Rev. Infect. Dis.*, 8, 427, 1986.
74. Jacobs, J. L. and Murray, H. W. Why is *Listeria monocytogenes* not a pathogen in the acquired immunodeficiency syndrome? *Arch. Intern. Med.*, 146, 1299, 1986.
75. Fahey, J. L. Immunologic alterations, in Gotlieb, M. S. (moderator), The acquired immunodeficiency syndrome. *Ann. Intern. Med.*, 99, 208, 1983.
76. Jungi, T. W., Gill, T. J., Kunz, H. W., and Jungi, R. Genetic control of cell-mediated immunity in the rat. *J. Immunogenetics*, 9, 445, 1982.
77. Fanos, V. and Dall'Agnola, A. Antibiotics in neonatal infections: a review. *Drugs*, 58, 405–427, 1999.
78. Blanot, S., Boumaila, C., and Berche, P. Intracerebral activity of antibiotics against *Listeria monocytogenes* during experimental rhombencephalitis. *J. Antimicrob. Chemother.*, 44, 565–568, 1999.
79. Temple, M. E. and Nahata, M. C. Treatment of listeriosis. *Ann. Pharmacother.*, 34, 656–661, 2000.
80. Tuazon, C. U., Shamsuddin, D., and Miller, H. Antibiotic susceptibility and synergy of clinical isolates of *Listeria monocytogenes*. *Antimicrob. Agents Chemother.*, 21, 525, 1982.
81. Winslow, D. L. and Pankey, G. A. In vitro activities of trimethoprim and sulfamethoxazole against *Listeria monocytogenes*. *Antimicrob. Agents Chemother.*, 22, 51, 1982.
82. Larsson, S., Walder, M. H., Cronberg, S. N., Forsgren, A. B., and Moestrup, T. Antimicrobial susceptibilities of *Listeria monocytogenes* strains isolated from 1958 to 1982 in Sweden. *Antimicrob. Agents Chemother.*, 28, 12, 1985.
83. Concha, R., Farias, M. E., Kummerlin, R., and Sesma, F. Enterocin-35, a bacteriocin with activity against *Listeria monocytogenes*. Possible use in the food industry. *Rev. Latinoam. Microbiol.*, 41, 133–138, 1999.
84. Ennahar, S., Deschamps, N., and Richard, J. Natural variation in susceptibility of *Listeria* strains to class IIa bacteriocins. *Curr. Microbiol.*, 41, 1–4, 2000.
85. Minahk, C. J., Farias, M. E., Sesma, F., and Morero, R. D. Effect of enterocin CRL35 on *Listeria monocytogenes* cell membrane. *FEMS Microbiol. Lett.*, 192, 79–83, 2000.

12
Gastrointestinal Infections in the Immunocompromised Host

1. INTRODUCTION

The gastrointestinal (GI) tract is the largest lymphoid organ in the human body and, therefore, any defects in the cellular and/or humoral immune responses may be a strong predisposing factor to a multitude of enteric viral, fungal, bacterial, and protozoan pathogens as seen in some of the preceding chapters (1–18).

The identification of enteric pathogens in the GI tract has been especially important in patients with AIDS where the HIV-induced immunodeficiency would greatly facilitate the possibility of opportunistic infections (19–21). For example, gastrointestinal disorders have occurred in 30–50% of North American and European AIDS patients, and in nearly 90% of patients in developing countries. In AIDS patients, the initial symptoms of diarrhea include nausea, anorexia, malaise, and other mononucleosis-like manifestations at the time of seroconversion (22). In full-blown AIDS, depending on the particular pathogen, diarrhea is manifested with large stool volumes, presence of blood, and abdominal pain (23). In cases of chronic diarrhea, often the illness is accompanied by inanition and cachexia. In African patients with AIDS, this condition, referred to as "slim disease," could be superimposed on underlying gastrointestinal infections caused by some tropical pathogens (24).

Several viruses have been identified as enteric pathogens in patients with T-cell deficiencies from causes other than AIDS, such as chemotherapy before bone-marrow transplantation or severe combined immunodeficiency syndrome (SCID) (25–27). Novel viruses such as rotavirus, adenovirus, calicivirus, and astrovirus have been diagnosed in chronic diarrheal disease in children with SCID (28,29) and in bone-marrow transplant recipients. In the latter case, rotaviral and adenoviral infections were associated with markedly increased mortality (30).

In the majority of AIDS patients, the causative agent(s) of GI infections can be identified (Table 1), and appropriate treatment may reduce the severity and frequency of gastrointestinal infections (31,32). Although less often and with minimal inflammation, the human immunodeficiency virus (HIV) itself has also been found to infect mononuclear cells in lamina propria of the intestine in 30–39% of patients (33–35), and in lamina propria of the esophagus in 36% of patients (1). This, coupled with the fact that several studies of AIDS patients with GI manifestations have demonstrated the presence of villous atrophy, crypt hyperplasia, the occurence of lactase deficiency and malabsorption, all in the absence of identifiable pathogens (3,31,34,36–39), has raised the possibility that patients with AIDS may still develop an HIV-associated enteropathy caused by functional changes in the small bowel mucosa (34) as well as malabsorption (3,36,37).

From: Opportunistic Infections: Treatment and Prophylaxis
By: Vassil St. Georgiev © Humana Press Inc., Totowa, NJ

Table 1
Gastrointestinal Pathogens in Immunocompromised Hosts[a]

Pathogen	Clinical site/manifestations
Fungi	
Candida albicans	Esophagus
Histoplasma capsulatum	Colon
Penicilliosis marnefei	Intestines
Viruses	
Cytomegalovirus	Esophagus, stomach, colon, enterocolitis
Herpes simplex virus	Esophagus, rectum
Adenovirus	Colon
Rotavirus	Small intestine
Astravirus	Small intestine
Calicivirus	Small intestine
Bacteria	
Mycobacterium avium-intracellulare (MAC)	Stomach, small intestine, colon
Campylobacter spp.	Diarrhea, possible bacteremia
Salmonella spp.	Diarrhea, septicemia
Shigella spp.	Diarrhea
Clostridium difficile	Colon
Listeria monocytogenes	Meningitis, bacteremia
Vibrio spp. (non-cholerae)	Possible bacteremia
Protozoa	
Cryptosporidium	Diarrhea
Isospora belli	Diarrhea
Microsporidia (Enterocytozoon bieneusi)	Diarrhea
Giardia lamblia	Diarrhea
Entameba histolytica	Diarrhea
Blastocystis	Diarrhea
Balantidium	Diarrhea
Dientamoeba	Diarrhea

[a]Data collected from refs. *(1,6,7,9,13,20,27,40–45)*.

2. THERAPEUTIC STRATEGIES FOR ENTERIC INFECTIONS

The evolution of therapies and current recommendations for treatment of various enteric infections in immunocompromised patients are described in details throughout this treatise in the corresponding chapters discussing individual enteric infections.

It should be strongly emphasized that enteric diseases in severely ill patients, such as those with AIDS, could be caused by a wide array of pathogens, which will make empirical antimicrobial therapy difficult to implement. It is important, therefore, that patients while being evaluated, be given supportive therapy with rehydration, electrolyte supplementation, and drug regimens to inhibit intestinal secretion or motility. Although treatment with anti-motility drugs may be considered controversial for certain bacterial diarrheas (bloody diarrhea, fecal leukocytes, abdominal pain), in the majority of cases, significant symptomatic benefit may result from therapy with loperamide, diphenoxylate, paregoric, or Kaopectate® *(1)*.

In patients with AIDS, major problems that need to be addressed are the recurrence of diarrheal infection after termination of therapy, and the emergence of drug-resistant pathogens (cytomegalovirus [CMV] *[6,9,16,43,44,46]*, herpes simplex virus [HSV] *[47,48]*, *Campylobacter* spp. *[49]*, and *Shigella* spp. *[50]*). Other enteric pathogens, such as *Cryptosporidium*, *Microsporidia*, and to a great extent *Mycobacterium avium-intracellulare* (MAC) cannot be cured with the currently available antimicrobial agents.

Even though in 80–87% of AIDS-associated diarrhea, the causative pathogen(s) of the diarrhea is identified, enteropathies characterized with malabsorption, small-bowel mucosal abnormalities, and no identifiable pathogens have been observed in patients with profuse diarrhea *(34)*. Two drugs, octreotide and 5-acetylsalicylic acid (5-ASA), have been reported to be of some benefit in treating profuse diarrheal disease.

Octreotide, a synthetic cyclic octapeptide congener of somatostatin, was found to be effective in the treatment of patients with severe refractory diarrhea caused by pancreatic cholera (the Vipoma syndrome), carcinoid syndrome, and diabetic diarrhea *(51–53)*, as well as AIDS-associated diarrhea *(54–58)*. In these situations, the drug was reported to decrease the jejunal secretion of water and electrolytes, and to increase the absorption of water and electrolytes by the jejunal mucosa.

In a prospective, multicenter clinical trial, Cello et al. *(59)* studied the efficacy and safety of octreotide in the treatment of 51 AIDS patients with profuse refractory diarrhea (over 500 mL liquid stool daily). The patients received subcutaneously 50 µg of octeotride every 8 h for 48 h; when the stool volume was not reduced to less than 250 mL/daily, the dose was increased stepwise to 100, 250, and 500 µg. The results of this short-term therapy were somewhat disappointing, with a response rate reaching only 41%. However, because 61% of the patients with no identifiable enteric pathogens responded partially or completely to octreotide, the drug may still be of some benefit to such patients.

Tierney et al. *(60)* investigated the efficacy of 5-ASA in the treatment of HIV-associated inflammatory bowel disease (mucosal inflammation) in the absence of identifiable enteric pathogens. The patients received orally 6 g of 5-ASA for 2 mo. Diarrheal symptoms stabilized or improved in 7 of 9 patients, and the mucosal production of p24 antigen decreased significantly over a 2-mo period.

2.1. Prevention of Enteric Infections

In immunocompetent patients, antimicrobial therapy can lengthen the shedding period of *Salmonella* spp. in the stool and, therefore, is not usually recommended *(41)*. There have been no controlled studies on the antimicrobial treatment of HIV-positive patients with *Salmonella* gastroenteritis. However, it has been recommended that HIV-infected patients receive antimicrobial therapy with ciprofloxacin (500–750 mg twice daily) to prevent extraintestinal infection *(41)*. In case of *Campylobacter* infections, again ciprofloxacin (500 mg twice daily) has been recommended instead of erythromycin *(41)*. HIV-infected patients with *Salmonella* septicemia would require long-term therapy with ciprofloxacin (500–750 mg twice daily) to prevent recurrence. Possible preventive therapy in children include trimethoprime-sulfamethoxazole, ampicillin, cefotaxime, ceftriaxone, or chloramphenicol.

The use of ganciclovir and foscarnet in treating and prophylaxis for CMV disease is recommended, although dose-limiting adverse effects and the need for long-term maitenance therapy may hinder their use in many patients *(61)*.

REFERENCES

1. Smith, P. D., Quinn, T. C., Strober, W., Janoff, E. N., and Masur, H. Gastrointestinal infections in AIDS. *Ann. Intern. Med.*, 116, 63, 1992.
2. Malebranche, R., Arnoux, E., Guérin, J. M., et al. Acquired immunodeficiency syndrome with severe gastrointestinal manifestations in Haiti. *Lancet*, 2, 873, 1983.
3. Dworkin, B., Wormser, G. P., Rosenthal, W. S., et al. Gastrointestinal manifestations of the acquired immunodeficiency syndrome: a review of 22 cases. *Am. J. Gastroenterol.*, 80, 774, 1985.
4. Colebunders, R., Francis, H., Mann, J. M., et al. Persistent diarrhea, strongly associated with HIV infection in Kinshasa.

Am. J. Gastroenterol., 82, 859, 1987.
5. Janoff, E. N. and Smith, P. D. Perspectives on gastrointestinal infections in AIDS. *Gastroenterol. Clin. North Am.*, 17, 451, 1988.
6. Zvizdic, S., Beslagic, E., Kapic, E., and Zvizdic-Karahodzic, M. Cytomegalovirus disease in immunocompromised patients. *Med. Arch.*, 54, 9–11, 2000.
7. Weiss, L. M. and Keohane, E. M.The uncommon gastrointestinal Protozoa: Microsporidia, Blastocystis, Isospora, Dientamoeba, and Balantidium. *Curr. Clin. Top. Infect. Dis.*, 17, 147–187, 1997.
8. Scott-Conner, C. E. H., and Fabrega, A. J. Gastrointestinal problems in the immunocompromised host. A review for surgeons. *Surg. Endosc.*, 10, 959–964, 1996.
9. Toogood, G. J., Gillespie, P. H., Gujral, S., et al. Cytomegalovirus infection and colonic perforation in renal transplant patients. *Transpl. Int.*, 9, 248–251, 1996.
10. Rotterdam, H. and Tsang, P. Gastrointestinal disease in the immunocompromised patient. *Hum. Pathol.*, 25, 1123–1140, 1994.
11. Deveikis, A. Gastrointestinal disease in immunocompromised children. *Pediatr. Ann.*, 23, 562–569, 1994.
12. Cornalba, G. P., Dore, R., and Colombo, E. Abdominal manifestations in immunocompromised patients. *Radiol. Med. (Torino)*, 87(5 Suppl. 2), 52–61, 1994.
13. Cheung, A. N. and Ng, I. O. Cytomegalovirus infection of the gastrointestinal tract in non-AIDS patients. *Am. J. Gastrointerol.*, 88, 1882–1886, 1993.
14. Buckner, F. S. and Pomeroy, C. Cytomegalovirus disease of the gastrointestinal tract in patients without AIDS. *Clin. Infect. Dis.*, 17, 644–656, 1993.
15. Wall, S. D. and Jones, B. Gastrointestinal tract in the immunocompromised host: opportunistic infections and other complications. *Radiology*, 185, 327–335, 1992.
16. Lorenzo Patino, M. J., Arnal Monreal, F., Armesto Perez, A., Bello Giz, J. A., and Gomez Balado, M. Gastrointestinal infection caused by cytomegalovirus in immunodepressed patients. *Rev. Esp. Enferm. Dig.*, 82, 109–112, 1992.
17. Arora, A. Gastrointestinal tract infection in immunocompromised hosts. *Trop. Gastroenterol.*, 10, 9–22, 1989.
18. Nylander, W. A., Jr. The acute abdomen in the immunocompromised host. *Surg. Clin. North Am.*, 68, 457–470, 1988.
19. Redvanly, R. D. and Silverstein, J. E. Intra-abdominal manifestations of AIDS. *Radiol. Clin. North Am.*, 35, 1083–1125, 1997.
20. Wilcox, C. M. and Monkmuller, K. E. Review article: the therapy of gastrointestinal infections associated with the acquired immunodeficiency syndrome. *Aliment. Pharmacol. Ther.*, 11, 425–443, 1997.
21. Anthony, S. J. HIV enteropathy: a challenge in diagnosis and management. *J. Natl. Med. Assoc.*, 86, 347–351, 1994.
22. Cooper, A. D., Gold, J., Maclean, P., et al. Acute AIDS retrovirus infection: definition of a clinical illness associated with seroconversion. *Lancet*, 1, 537, 1985.
23. Smith, P. D. and Janoff, E. N. Infectious diarrhea in human immunodeficiency virus infection. *Gastroenterol. Clin. North Am.*, 17, 587, 1988.
24. Serwadda, D., Mugerwa, R. D., Sewankambo, N. K., et al. Slim disease: a new disease in Uganda and its association with HTLV-III infection. *Lancet*, 2, 849, 1985.
25. Saulsbury, F. T., Winkelstein, J. A., and Yolken, R. H. Chronic rotavirus infection in immunodeficiency. *J. Pediatr.*, 97, 61, 1980.
26. Yolken, R. H., Bishop, C. A., Townsend, T. R., et al. Infectious gastroenteritis in bone-marrow-transplant recipients. *N. Engl. J. Med.*, 306, 1010, 1982.
27. LeBaron, C. W., Furutan, N. P., Lew, J. F., et al. Viral agents of gastroenteritis. Public health importance and outbreak management. *Morb. Mortal. Wkly Rep.*, 39(RR-5), 1, 1990.
28. Chrystie, I. L., Booth, I. W., Kidd, A. H., Marxhall, W. C., and Banatvala, J. E., Multiple faecal virus excretion in immunodeficiency. *Lancet*, 1, 282, 1982.
29. Madeley, C. R. Epidemiology of gut viruses, in *Viruses and the Gut*, Farthing, M. J. G., Ed. Smith Kline & French Laboratories, Welwyn Garden City, UK, 5, 1988.
30. Yolken, R. H., Bishop, C. A., Townsend, T. T., et al. Infectious gastroenteritis in bone-marrow-transplant recipients. *N. Engl. J. Med.*, 306, 1010, 1982.
31. Smith, P. D., Lane, H. C., Gill, V. J., Quinnan, G. V., Fauci, A. S., and Masur, H. Intestinal infections in patients with the acquired immunodeficiency syndrome (AIDS): etiology and response to therapy. *Ann. Intern. Med.*, 108, 328, 1988.
32. Laughon, B. E., Druckman, D. A., Vernon, A., et al. Prevalence of enteric pathogens in homosexual men with and without acquired immunodeficiency syndrome. *Gastroenterology*, 94, 984, 1988.
33. Fox, C. H., Kotler, D. P., Tierney, A. R., Wilson, C. S., and Fauci, A. S. Detection of HIV-1 RNA in the lamina propria of patients with AIDS and gastrointestinal disease. *J. Infect. Dis.*, 159, 467, 1989.
34. Ullrich, R., Zeitz, M., Heise, W., L'age, M., Höffken, G., and Riecken, E. O. Small intestinal structure and function in patients infected with human immunodeficiency virus (HIV): evidence for HIV-induced enteropathy. *Ann. Intern. Med.*, 111, 15, 1989.
35. Jarry, A., Cortez, A., Rene, E., Muzeau, F., and Brousse, N. Infected and immune cells in the gastrointestinal tract of AIDS patients: an immunohistochemical study of 127 cases. *Histopathology*, 16, 133, 1990.
36. Gillin, J. S., Shike, M., Alcock, N., et al. Malabsorption and mucosal abnormalities of the small intestine in the acquired immunodeficiency syndrome. *Ann. Intern. Med.*, 102, 619, 1985.
37. Kotler, D. P., Gaetz, H. P., Lange, M., Klein, E. B., and Holt, P. R. Enteropathy associated with the acquired immunodeficiency syndrome. *Ann. Intern. Med.*, 101, 421, 1984.

38. Harriman, G. R., Smith, P. D., Horne, M. K., et al. Vitamin B 12 malabsorption in patients with acquired immunodeficiency syndrome. *Arch. Intern. Med.,* 149, 2039, 1989.
39. Heise, W., Mostertz, P., Arasteh, K., Skörde, J., and L'age, M. Gastrointestinale befunde bei der HIV-infektion. *Deutsch. Med. Wochensshr.,* 113, 1588, 1988.
40. Grohmann, G. S., Glass, R. I., Pereira, H. G., et al. Enteric viruses and diarrhea in HIV-infected patients. *N. Engl. J. Med.,* 329, 14, 1993.
41. Angulo, F. J. and Swerdlow, D. L. Bacterial enteric infections in persons infected with human immunodeficiency virus. *Clin. Infect. Dis.,* 31(Suppl.1), S84, 1995.
42. Ko, C. I., Hung, C. C., Chen, M. Y., Hsueh, P. R., Hsiao, C. H., and Wong, J. M. Endoscopic diagnosis of intestinal penicilliosis marnefei: report of three cases and review of the literature. *Gastrointest. Endosc.,* 50, 111–114, 1999.
43. Kaufman, H. S., Kahn, A. C., Iacobuzio-Donahue, C., Talamini, M. A., Lillemoe, K. D., and Hamilton, S. R. Cytomegalovirus enterocolitis: clinical association and outcome. *Dis. Colon Rectum,* 42, 24–30, 1999.
44. Tarng, Y. W., Shih, D. F., Liu, S. I., Wang, B. W., and Mok, K. T. Cytomegalovirus appendicitis in a patient with acquired immunodeficiency syndrome: a case report. *Chung Hua I Hsieh Tsa Chih (Taipei)*, 60, 48–51, 1997.
45. Flanigan, T. P. Human immunodeficiency virus infection and cryptosporidiosis: protective immune responses. *Am. J. Trop. Med. Hyg.,* 50(5 Suppl.), 29-35, 1994.
46. Erice, A., Chou, S., Biron, K. K., Stanat, S. C., Balfour, H. A. Jr., and Jordan, M. C. Progressive disease due to ganciclovir-resistant cytomegalovirus in immunocompromised patients. *N. Engl. J. Med.,* 320, 289, 1989.
47. Oliver, N. M., Collins, P., Van der Meer, J., and Van't Wout, J. W. Biological and biochemical characterization of clinical isolates of herpes simplex virus type 2 resistant to acyclovir. *Antimicrob. Agents Chemother.,* 33, 635, 1989.
48. Sacks, S. L., Wanklin, R. J., Reece, D. E., Hicks, K. A., Tyler, K. L., and Coen, D. M. Progressive esophagitis from acyclovir-resistant herpes simplex. *Ann. Intern. Med.,* 111, 893, 1989.
49. Dworkin, B., Wormser, G. P., Abdoo, R. A., Cabello, F., Aguero, M. E., and Sivak, S. L. Persistence of multiply antibiotic-resistant *Campylobacter jejuni* in a patient with the acquired immunodeficiency syndrome. *Am. J. Med.,* 80, 965, 1986.
50. Gander, R. M. and LaRocco, M. T. Multiple drug-resistance in *Shigella flexneri* isolated from a patient with human immunodeficiency virus. *Diagn. Microbiol. Infect. Dis.,* 8, 193, 1987.
51. Vinik, A. I., Tsai, S. T., Moattari, A. R., Cheung, P., Ackhauser, F. E., and Cho, K. Somatostatin analogue (SMS 201-995) in the management of gastroenteropancreatic tumors and diarrhea syndromes. *Am. J. Med.,* 81(Suppl. 6B), 23, 1986.
52. Kvols, L. K. Metastatic carcinoid tumors and the carcinoid syndrome: a selective review of chemotherapy and hormonal therapy. *Am. J. Med.,* 81(Suppl. 6B), 49, 1986.
53. Williams, S. T., Woltering, E. A., O'Dorisio, T. M., and Fletcher, W. S. Effect of octeotride acetate on pancreatic exocrine function. *Am. J. Surg.,* 157, 459, 1989.
54. Katz, M. D., Erstad, B. L., and Rose, C. Treatment of severe cryptosporidium-related diarrhea with octeotride in a patient with AIDS. *Drug Intell. Clin. Pharm.,* 22, 134, 1988.
55. Clotet, B., Sirera, G., Cofan, F., Monterola, J. M., Tortosa, F., and Fox, M. Efficacy of the somatostatin analogue (SMS-201-995), sandostatin for cryptosporidial diarrhoea in patients with AIDS. *AIDS,* 3, 857, 1989.
56. Füessl, H. S., Zoller, W. G., Kochen, M. M., et al. Treatment of secretory diarrhea in AIDS with the somatostatin analogue SMS 201-995. *Klin. Wochenschr.,* 67, 452, 1989.
57. Robinson, E. N. Jr. and Fogel, R. SMS 201-995, a somatostatin analogue, and diarrhea in the acquired immunodeficiency syndrome (AIDS). *Ann. Intern. Med.,* 109, 680, 1988.
58. Cook, D. J., Kelton, J. G., Stanisz, A. M., and Collins, S. M. Somatostatin treatment for cryptosporidial diarrhea in a patient with the acquired immunodeficiency syndrome. *Ann. Intern. Med.,* 108, 708, 1988.
59. Cello, J. P., Grendell, J. H., Basuk, P., et al. Effect of octeotride on refractory AIDS-associated diarrhea: a prospective, multicenter clinical trial. *Ann. Intern. Med.,* 115, 705, 1991.
60. Tierney, A. R., Reka, S., Hecker, L., Cohen, S., Clayton, F., and Kotler, D. P. Treatment of HIV-associated inflammatory bowel disease with oral 5-ASA. *Proc. VIIIth Int. Conf. AIDS,* Amsterdam, 1992, abstract no. PoB 3725.
61. Levinson, M. L. and Jacobson, P. A. Treatment and prophylaxis of cytomegalovirus disease. *Pharmacotherapy,* 12, 300–318, 1992 [see also: *Pharmacotherapy,* 13, 167–168, 1993].

PART III
PARASITIC INFECTIONS

13
Cryptosporidium spp.

1. INTRODUCTION

Over the last 10 years or so, the reported incidence of cryptosporidiosis and isosporiasis, two invasive opportunistic/nosocomial infections in man, has risen dramatically. Large populations of immunocompromised patients—as a result of underlying diseases such as hematologic malignancies and acquired immunodeficiency syndrome (AIDS), or patients undergoing cancer chemotherapy or immunosuppressive therapy—are particularly susceptible to the effects of these infections. With the spread of the AIDS epidemic, the subject of actual and potential therapy of cryptosporidiosis became increasingly important and of considerable interest to clinicians. The causative agents of cryptosporidiosis and isosporiasis are two parasites, *Cryptosporidium* spp. and *Isospora belli*, respectively. The pathogens represent two genera of coccidian protozoans classified in the suborder Eimeriina, order Eucoccidiida. Taxonomically both coccidian protozoa are related to *Toxoplasma gondii* and *Plasmodium* spp.

Prior to 1982, cryptosporidiosis was considered to be an infrequent parasitic disease occuring mainly in animals and with only 8 reported cases in humans *(1–5)*. In the last several years, however, because of improved diagnostic techniques and the raising tide of the AIDS epidemic, and immunosuppressed population in general, *Cryptosporidium*-induced infections are considered to be one of the world's most commonly found causes of diarrheal illness in humans, especially infants and children *(6–8)*, the elderly *(9,10)*, and AIDS patients in particular *(11–22)*.

Cryptosporidial infections are not limited to gastrointestinal illness only. Respiratory, conjunctival, gastric and gall blader infections caused by *Cryptosporidium* have also been reported *(23–30)*, whereas Ito and Kawata *(31)* have presented a case of liver cryptosporidiosis. Acute pancreatitis in HIV-infected patients due to *Cryptosporidium* infection has also been described *(32)*.

Rose *(33)* described three outbreaks of waterborne disease attributed to *Cryptosporidium* with two of them linked to drinking water, and the third to surface water. Other investigators *(34–41)* have also reported outbreaks of cryptosporidiosis associated with water. Experiments by Fayer and Nerad *(42)* demonstrated that oocysts of *C. parvum* in water can retain viability and infectivity after freezing and that oocysts may survive longer at freezing temperatures as low as –20°C *(43)*.

Based on environmental occurence, the risk of *Cryptosporidium* transmission by the water route may be equal to, or greater than, that of *Giardia*. Shepherd and Wyn-Jones *(44)* evaluated and optimized methods for the simultaneous detection of *C. parvum* and *Giardia* cysts from water including cartridge or membrane filtrations, and calcium carbonate flocculation. The knowledge of the hydrophobic and cell surface charge properties of *C. parvum* is important for the appropriate choice of various flocculation treatments, membrane filters, and cleaning agents in connection with the oocyst recovery *(45)*. Rochelle et al. *(46)* have developed a rapid procedure for detection of *Cryptosporidium* using in vitro cell culture combined with polymerase chain reaction (PCR).

From: Opportunistic Infections: Treatment and Prophylaxis
By: Vassil St. Georgiev © Humana Press Inc., Totowa, NJ

Because it invades surface epithelial cells that line the intestinal tract, but not the deeper layers of the intestinal mucosa, *C. parvum* can be regarded as a minimally invasive mucosal pathogen in the immunocompetent host. In such patients, cryptosporidial infections result in a self-limited, flu-like gastrointestinal disorder *(47–51)* and mucosal inflammation, which resolves spontaneously in 1–4 wk *(50–53)*. Patients will develop immunity and recover completely from the infection. The highest incidence of cryptosporidiosis has been reported in infant populations of the tropical and subtropical zones during the warmer months of the year *(54,55)*.

In immunocompromised hosts, however, *Cryptosporidium* usually produces a severe and prolonged illness with high morbidity, which in AIDS patients has been clearly associated with the $CD4^+$ counts *(13,56–59)*. The mortality rate of cryptosporidiosis in immunocompromised patients is also high *(60)*: in adults, it is associated mainly with AIDS patients *(1,61,62)* and children having hypogammaglobulinemia *(63,64)*, severe combined immunodeficiency (SCID) *(65,66)*, or patients receiving immunosuppressive therapy for malignancies *(67–70)* or renal-transplant recipients *(71)*.

2. TREATMENT OF CRYPTOSPORIDIOSIS

Currently, there is no clinically effective chemotherapy of cryptosporidial diarrhea in immunocompromised patients *(72–78)*. Moreover, the lack of clinical improvement in such patients following chemotherapy alone may be the result, at least partially, of the presence of multiple concurrent infections and therapies aggravating the already-existing immune deficiencies *(79,80)*. Prophylaxis has been equally ineffective, although in one report *(81)* rifabutin or clarithromycin, when taken for *Mycobacterium avium* complex (MAC) prophylaxis, were associated with a reduced risk for cryptosporidiosis.

There is also no known treatment for pulmonary cryptosporidiosis, a rare complication of intestinal cryptosporidiosis in AIDS patients.

Over the years, a number of therapeuic approaches to cure cryptosporidiosis have been attempted using different agents, including macrolide antibiotics, peptides, and immunotherapy. So far, the results have been rather disappointing.

2.1. Macrolide Antibiotics

Among the macrolide antibiotics most notably, spiramycin has been tested extensively both in vitro and in vivo for its clinical efficacy against cryptosporidiosis *(82)*. In several anecdotal reports *(83–93)*, spiramycin was described as useful against cryptosporidial diarrhea and with relatively low incidence of toxic side effects, most often gastrointestinal irritation and hypersensitivity reaction *(92,94)*. With regard to data reporting anticryptosporidial efficacy of spiramycin *(95–97)*, especially in immunocompromised hosts *(98)*, it is important to emphasize that, so far, all results about its clinical efficacy have originated mainly from uncontrolled trials involving limited number of patients, and therefore should be viewed still as premature and justified skepticism; the accuracy of such reports must be evaluated in and corroborated by multicenter placebo-controlled trials. To lend to this skepticism, in a number of reports *(99–102)* spiramycin was described as completely lacking in activity against cryptosporidiosis. Some contributing factors to the perceived clinical efficacy of spiramycin may be traced to the observed tendency of the infection to disappear spontaneously *(103)*, or to clinical improvement due to concomitant discontinuation of immunosuppressive medication *(89,90)*, as well as to better control of cryptosporidial diarrhea in the early stage of AIDS as opposed to cryptosporidiosis in advanced stages of AIDS where the state of immune deficiency is much worse *(104)*. In addition, in a report by Weikel et al. *(105)* two of three AIDS patients with cryptosporidiosis receiving high doses of spiramycin developed acute intestinal injury as the likely result of direct damage to the epithelium by the drug.

A multicenter, placebo-controlled, clinical trial of chronic cryptosporidiosis in AIDS patients treated with spiramycin is currently under way and will undoubtedly shed more light on its clinical efficacy; preliminary data from the trial indicated that when administered orally at 1.0 g, 3 times daily, the antibiotic is nontoxic and may reduce the severity of cryptosporidial diarrhea *(106)*.

Dupont et al. *(107)* reported a favorable outcome in an AIDS patient with pulmonary cryptosporidiosis after treatment with azithromycin. What made this particular case unusual was the presence of extracellular invasive forms of the parasite in the bronchoalveolar lavage of the patient. Hicks et al. *(108)* described a successful outcome in 3 of 4 pediatric AIDS patients (a marked decrease in stool volume and frequency within 36 h of initiating therapy, and resolution of diarrhea within 5 d) after treatment with azithromycin for severe diarrheal illness solely due to *C. parvum*; the fourth patient required prolonged therapy with azithromycin to achieve clearance. In another report, Vargas et al. *(109)* described two pediatric patients with cancer who received azithromycin for *Cryptosporidium*-associated diarrhea that was unresponsive to supportive care. One child had choleriform diarrhea requiring daily fluid replacement of up to 65% of his total body weight; the other had protracted diarrhea and wasting. In both cases, administration of azithromycin resulted in prompt clinical improvement.

In a retrospective study, Jordan *(110)* compared the incidence of cryptosporidial enteritis in AIDS patients ($n = 63$) receiving prophylactic clarithromycin (500 mg, b.i.d.) for MAC with patients ($n = 73$) not treated with clarithromycin who served as the control group. None of the patients who received clarithromycin developed cryptosporidial enteritis, compared with 4 patients (all with CD4$^+$ of less than 25 cells/mm^3) from the control group. In a subsequent 2-yr follow-up study of an additional 217 AIDS patients with CD4$^+$ of <50 cells/mm^3 receiving clarithromycin (500 mg, b.i.d.) as MAC prophylaxis, no patient developed cryptosporidial enteritis.

To evaluate the rates of cryptosporidiosis in HIV-infected patients who either received or did not receive MAC chemoprophylaxis, Holmberg et al. *(111)* conducted a nested analysis of data collected prospectively from 1019 patients (seen during 1992–1996 at 10 HIV clinics in 9 U.S. cities) with CD4$^+$ counts of less than 75 cells/mm^3. The results showed a marked decrease in incidence of *C. parvum* enteritis in 312 patients taking clarithromycin and 214 taking rifabutin compared with those not taking these antibiotics, but not among the comparatively few (54) patients taking azithromycin.

In a contradictory report, Fichtenbaum et al. *(112)* retrospectively evaluated the efficacy of macrolide therapy for prevention of cryptosporidiosis in 2291 HIV-positive patients enrolled in two clinical trials for MAC (ACTG 196) and cytomegalovirus (ACTG 204) prophylaxis. There were 60 cases of cryptosporidiosis during the duration of these studies (12/92–6/95). Azithromycin and clarithomycin were given to 1292 patients for more than 1 mo. The results indicated that the incidence of cryptosporidiosis was similar in both who did and did not receive macrolide therapy, and that macrolide therapy had no protective effect in doses prescribed to prevent MAC infections in HIV-infected patients *(112)*.

2.2. Paromomycin

Recently, paromomycin, a poorly absorbed per os aminoglycoside antibiotic known for its activity against *Giardia* and amebic intestinal infections, has been tested for activity against cryptosporidiasis both in experimental animal models and in humans *(113–130)*. The clinical results were inconclusive due to a major degree on the variable nature of the disease, during which some patients may improve without intervention *(131)*.

Gatlie et al. *(132)* have found paromomycin able to control the symptoms of gastrointestinal cryptosporidiosis and to eradicate the parasite in some patients without evidence of serious toxicity. Clezy et al. *(133)* used paromomycin in five HIV-infected patients with gastrointestinal cryptosporidiosis. The drug was administered at 1.5 g daily (divided in 6 equal doses) or 2.0 g daily (divided in 5 equal doses) depending on the patient's weight (over 60 kg or less than 60 kg, respectively). The patients were evaluated on a biweekly basis mainly to monitor symptoms of diarrhea and changes in the weight. Within 24 h of commencing the therapy, four patients had reduction in diarrhea (to 1–3 semiformed bowel actions daily), and in one patient the bowel movements returned to normal after 1 wk of medication. The control of diarrhea was maintained in all patients during the first 4 wk of therapy, but four of five patients continued to have detectable oocysts in stools during the treatment. Paromomycin was tolerated well, with serum levels reaching over 6.2 mg/L (lower limit of detection) *(133)*.

Hoepelman *(56)* and Fichtenbaum et al. *(129)* have recommended for therapy with paromomycin an initial regimen of 500 mg of the drug given 4 times daily for 2–3 wk followed by a maintenance therapy with 500 mg b.i.d. to prevent relapse.

In a prospective, randomized, double-blind trial, the therapeutic efficacy of paromomycin was tested against cryptosporidiosis in 10 AIDS patients *(125)*. Patients were randomized to receive either paromomycin or placebo; after 14 d, they were switched to the other treatment for 14 additional days. During the paromomycin treatment phase, oocyst excretion decreased from 314×10^6 to $10^9 \times 10^6$ per 24 h ($p < 0.02$). The oocyst excretion increased for the four patients initially on placebo as compared with a median decrease of $128 \times 10^6/24$ h for the six patients initially treated with paromomycin ($p < 0.02$). Furthermore, stool frequency also decreased more in those treated with the antibiotic (3.6 fewer vs 1.25 fewer/24 h; $p < 0.05$). The overall trend was in favor of drug over placebo for stool weight, stool character, and the Karnofsky score, leading to improvement in both clinical and parasitologic parameters of cryptosporidiosis in AIDS patients. The results presented by White et al. *(125)* enticed extensive comments from other investigators *(114–116)*.

Mohri et al. *(120)* described an AIDS patient with hemophilia A and intractable diarrhea and fever, who, approx 2 mo after admission, developed respiratory infection and hypoxia due to *Cryptosporidium* but was successfully treated with paromomycin inhalation.

In a randomized, double-blind trial (ACTG 192) involving 35 patients with advanced HIV disease, treatment with paromomycin resulted in no clinical benefit *(131)*. The patients were given paromomycin at 500 mg, q.i.d. for 3 wk or placebo; after that, all patients received open-label paromomycin (500 mg for another 3 wk). Patients without complete response could then receive 1000 g, q.i.d. for an additional 21 d; patients with a partial or complete response after 9 wk were offered an optional 16-wk maintenance therapy. The results showed no significant differences in change from baseline in diarrhea, antidiarrheal pill use, weight, number of oocysts, or other gastrointestinal symptoms *(131)*.

Samson and Brown *(134)* successfully treated cryptosporidiosis in an AIDS patient with a combination of paromomycin and clofazimine.

Smith et al. *(135)* have assessed a 4-wk combination therapy of oral paromomycin (1.0 g, b.i.d.) and oral azithromycin (600 mg, 4 times daily), followed by paromomycin alone for 8 wk in AIDS patients with cryptosporidial chronic diarrhea. The treatment resulted in marked improvement and significant reduction in oocyst excretion. However, not all reports regarding the anticryptosporidium activity of paromomycin-azithromycin combination were positive. Thus, an HIV-positive patient with disseminated cryptosporidiosis failed to respond clinically to repeated treatment with oral paromomycin (1.0 mg/mL) and azithromycin (8.0 mg/L), and then nitazoxanide (10 mg/L) *(136)*.

2.3. Rifaximin

At doses of 600 mg given 3 times daily for 2 wk, rifaximin, a nonabsorbable, locally active antibiotic with a broad antimicrobial activity was found effective in resolving the clinical symptoms and clearing cryptosporidial infections in HIV-1-positive patients with CD4$^+$ of over or 200/mm^3 *(137)*.

2.4. Nitazoxanide (NTZ, Cryptaz)

Nitazoxanide, an anthelmintic agent, has been available for several years in developing countries for treatment of tapeworm and liver fluke infestations *(138,139)*. Initial trials conducted in Mali and Mexico have shown promising results in controlling cryptosporidial diarrhea and lowering the level of parasite in the stool of AIDS patients *(139)*. Side effects, although rare, included decreased liver function, discolored urine, and hives *(138)*. However, a U.S. government-sponsored study (ACTG 336) failed to provide convincing supportive data due to poor enrollment *(140,141)*. Ultimately, a Food and Drug Administration (FDA) Advisory Committee rejected the drug because of insufficient and incomplete evidence (small and not randomized control trial) *(141–145)*.

2.5. Somatostatin and Analogues

Somatostatin (a tetradecapeptide factor inhibiting the release of somatotropin) has been found useful in the treatment of secretory diarrhea related to various diseases, such as Zollinger-Ellison syndrome *(146)*, Verner-Morrison syndrome *(147,148)*, the carcinoid syndrome *(149)*, glucagonomas *(147)*, and ileostomy *(150)*. Somatostatin is known to prolong the intestinal transit time and to induce the net intestinal water and electrolyte reabsorption in patients with diarrhea. Because the native form of somatostatin has a short half-life (3–4 min) necessitating its intravenous administration *(151)*, analogs with longer half-life were subsequently developed *(152)*.

For the past several years attention has focused on one somatostatin analog, octreotide (sandostatin, SMS 201-995), for its activity against cryptosporidial diarrhea in AIDS patients *(153–157)*. Structurally, octreotide is a small peptide comprising of eight amino acid residues that share homology with a four-amino acid sequence present in somatostatin *(158)*. The biological activity of octreotide mimicked to a great extent that of the endogenous somatostatin, especially its potent ability to inhibit the release of vasoactive intestinal peptide, and/or its action on the intestinal mucosal target tissue *(159,160)*. Octreotide has a longer half-life (90–120 min) and duration of activity of up to 8 h *(161,162)*. In an open-label, multicenter, controlled clinical trial involving 49 AIDS patients with profuse diarrhea, octreotide was administered subcutaneously for 14 d (50 µg every 8 h for 3 d, then 100 µg, 250 µg, and 500 µg every 8 h for 3 d each, if no response to prior dose was observed) *(163)*. Four patients responded completely and 13 partially, for an overall rate of 34.7%. After ceasing the therapy, diarrhea recurred in all patients who had initially responded *(163)*.

Fanning et al. *(164)* reported results from a pilot-escalating study of 17 nonconsecutive HIV-positive patients given subcutaneous octreotide for refractory diarrhea. The outcome of the trial was quite modest: of the 11 patients who completed the therapy, only 5 responded and were ultimately maintained on a long-term octreotide medication (dose range of 50–250 µg); although 3 of the patients remained stable on the same dose regimen, the remaining two had worsening of their diarrhea and required further increase in drug dosage.

Moroni et al. *(165)* examined the effect of octeotride on the bowel frequency of 13 patients with AIDS-associated refractory diarrhea. All patients received 100 µg t.i.d. of subcutaneous octeotride for 1 wk; those patients who did not improve were given 250 µg, t.i.d. for an additional 1 wk. The bowel frequency returned to normal in one patient, and decreased by more than 50% in seven others; one patient improve at the higher dose.

In general, octreotide was well-tolerated and its toxicity was limited to mild adverse reactions, such as pain at the injection site, nausea, abdominal pain, and discomfort or bloating *(161,166)*.

In a study conducted by Nousbaum et al. *(153)* the resolution of cryptosporidial infection in one immunosuppressed patient receiving AZT and the somatostatin analog octreotide was not attributed to the prior improvement of immune functions by the effects of AZT, but rather to the efficacy of octreotide—the progressive disappearance of diarrhea, malabsorption, and cryptosporidia in stools coincided with the octreotide medication.

In the broader context of *Cryptosporidium*-induced diarrhea, especially the inability to treat this condition in AIDS patients, the probable mode of action of octreotide deserves special consideration. Severe manifestations of watery diarrhea observed in AIDS patients have been frequently associated with infection by cryptosporidia. This, however, has not always been the case because the immunodeficiency virus itself may cause directly mucosal hypersecretory response *(162)*, which would result in enteropathy *(167–169)* and diarrhea. Furthermore, an HIV invasion into the enterochromaffin cells of the intestinal mucosa (which is known to occur *[167–169]*), may create a local deficiency of somatostatin. Such deficiency, if developed, may explain the beneficial effect of octreotide in ameliorating the cryptosporidial diarrhea in some AIDS patients *(170)*.

Alternatively, the protein coat of HIV was found to contain amino acid sequences that are homologous with the vasoactive intestinal peptide (VIP) *(171)*. Based on the fact that VIP is an effective stimulant of intestinal fluid secretion *(172)*. Gaginella and O'Dorisio *(159)* advanced the hypothesis that HIV may activate the VIP receptors, thereby triggering, at least partially, a diarrheal response.

The mechanism of action of octreotide on the cryptosporidial diarrhea, although still not fully elucidated, may involve a nonspecific effect on the gastrointestinal mucosal fluid and electrolyte secretion *(162)*. The fact, that both somatostatin and octreotide inhibited the effect of VIP on the intestinal secretion may provide one aspect of the mechanism of action of octreotide, namely, its ability to act on the membrane receptor that recognizes VIP. In one report *(173)*, somatostatin itself was also found effective against refractory cryptosporidial diarrhea in a patient with AIDS.

Although it is still possible that octeotride may prove to be useful against some cases of AIDS-associated intestinal cryptosporidiosis, this will require not only stringently conducted placebo-controlled trials, but also the participation of homogeneous patient populations with regard to their probable cause of diarrhea and better compliance with stool collections *(174)*.

2.6. Immunotherapy of Cryptosporidiosis

The lack of effective anticryptosporidial chemotherapy in immunocompromised patients on one hand, and the importance of the immune system in determining the host's response towards invading pathogens on the other, have prompted the evaluation of some immunotherapeutic approaches for prevention and treatment of cryptosporidiosis.

Some of the novel immunotherapeutic approaches towards treatment of cryptosporidiosis include the use of cow's milk globulin *(175)* and hyperimmune bovine colostrums (HBC) *(65,176,177)*.

Initial reports have indicated that bovine colostrum obtained from cows that were naturally infected with *Cryptosporidium*, when administered orally to three patients with cryptosporidiosis failed to exert any beneficial effect *(178)*. However, Tzipori et al. *(65,179)* demonstrated that a specially produced HBC was effective in three patients (one with AIDS) with intestinal cryptosporidiosis. In vitro evaluation *(180)*, as well as controlled experiments in animal models and neonatal calves, confirmed the immunotherapeutic activity of HBC as evidenced by the reduction of parasite load *(181,182)*.

This potentially new anticryptosporidial therapy was tested successfully by Ungar et al. *(183)* in one AIDS patient with fulminant cryptosporidial diarrhea by passively transferring large amounts of immune elements present in HBC to the affected host; the patient showed remission of diarrhea and elimination of *Cryptosporidium* oocysts from stool specimens. Nord et al. *(184)* conducted a randomized, double-blind, controlled pilot study in five AIDS patients with cryptosporidial diarrhea. HBC was administered by continuous nasogastric infusion at 20 mL/h (approx 30 mg total immunoglobulin/ mL) for 10 d. Although the study was hampered by such factors as the small number of patients, significant difference among patients (oocyst load and severity of diarrhea at the onset of the trial), and the inability to obtain adequate baseline information about daily stool volumes before treatment was started, the overall results have demonstrated that HBC may prove to be effective in treating patients with cryptosporidiosis *(184)*.

In a prospective study, Greenberg and Cello *(185)* have evaluated the safety and efficacy of colostrum-derived bovine immunoglobulin concentrate in the treatment of *C. parvum*-induced severe chronic diarrhea in AIDS patients. The treatment lasted for 21 d, with the medication given either in powder or capsule forms. Patients receiving the powder form experienced a significant decrease in mean stool weight, from 1158 ± 114 g/d at baseline, to 595 ± 63 g/d ($p = 0.04$) at the end of treatment, and 749 ± 123 g/d ($p = 0.03$) 1 mo after completion of therapy. The stool frequency also decreased from 6.6 ± 0.6 bowel movements per day at study entry, to 5.4 ± 0.7 during treatment ($p = 0.04$), and 5.4 ± 0.9 during observation ($p = 0.12$). Patients who received the medication in capsule form showed no improvement. Although showing certain benefits, the optimal dosage, duration of therapy and overall efficacy of bovine immunoglobulin concentrate need to be determined in placebo-controlled trials *(185)*.

The active ingredient(s) of HBC are presently unknown. However, it may be possible that the bovine IgG_1 immunoglobulin, which is very closely related to human IgA, may elicit a protective effect similar to the one already postulated for bovine IgG_1 in enteropathogenic and enterotoxigenic *Escherichia coli*-related diarrheas, and enteric infection caused by rotavirus *(186–189)*. It is also plausible that the active ingredient of HBC is a cytokine.

"Colostrum Specific" has been used successfully against cryptospidiosis in regimens that included four times daily administration for 3 wk *(177)*.

Fourteen AIDS patients with symptomatic cryptosporidiosis were treated with either a specific bovine dialyzable leukocyte extract (immune DLE) prepared from lymph node lymphocytes of calves immunized with cryptosporidia, or with a nonspecific (nonimmune) DLE prepared from nonimmunized calves *(190,191)*. Of the seven patients who received immune DLE, six gained weight and had a decrease in bowel movement frequency; eradication of oocysts from stools was observed in five patients. By comparison, six of seven recipients of nonimmune DLE showed no decrease in bowel movements and in four of them no clearing of oocysts from stools was observed; five of the patients continued to lose weight. When five of the nonimmune DLE recipients were treated with immune DLE, four experienced a decrease in bowel movement frequency and considerable weight gain, with eradication of oocysts from stools in two patients *(190)*. Even though sustained symptomatic improvement of patients given immune DLE was evident, the lack of an appropriate cryptosporidial antigen would only allow a postulation that the observed microbiologic and clinical improvements were indeed caused by the immune-DLE-induced augmentation of cellular immunity towards *C. parvum*. In this regard, DLE has been found to contain an antigen-binding product of T-helper lymphocytes that enhanced the cell-mediated immune responses in man *(192,193)*. In several studies, DLE was found beneficial in the treatment of various bacterial, fungal, and viral infections *(194–196)* as well as against parasites such as *Eimeria bovis* in cattle *(197)* and *Eimeria ferrisi* in mice *(198)*.

Because the intestinal cytokine signals involved with eradication of cryptosporidiosis are unknown, Okhuysen et al. *(199)* initiated a study to assess the role of cytokines in human cryptosporidiosis in healthy adult volunteers experimentally infected with *C. parvum* and AIDS patients with naturally acquired chronic cryptosporidiosis using endoscopy and jejunal biopsies for human interferon-γ (IFN-γ) and interleukin-15 (IL-15). The overall data suggested a key roles for intestinal IFN-γ and IL-15 in controlling human cryptosporidiosis. IL-15 seemed to function by initiation of the immune response while IFN-γ functions in the anamnestic response that limits reinfection *(199)*.

Kern et al. *(200)* studied the effects of recombinant interleukin-2 (rIL-2) against cryptosporidiosis in patients having AIDS or persistant lymphadenopathy syndrome (LAS). Increasing doses of rIL-2 (from 10^3 U/m^2 to 10^6 U/m^2) were administered as an intravenous bolus injection. Two of the patients with severe intestinal cryptosporidiosis had their diarrhea ceased under the treatment with rIL-2, and not occuring during the following 2 mo. At the high-dose level, the rIL-2 caused some minor adverse reactions, such as fever, chills, and malaise or vomiting *(200)*. The observed anticryptosporidial effect of rIL-2 was likely due to its ability to enhance immune responses to foreign antigens *(201,202)* by acting as a second messenger of T-lymphocyte activation *(202,203)*. After its release from IL-2-producer lymphocytes (mainly within the T4$^+$ subsets), IL-2 facilitates an adequate reaction by the T-responder lymphocytes against infectious pathogens or allogeneic malignant cells *(201,202,204)*.

Capetti et al. *(205)* studied the therapeutic efficacy of recombinant human granulocyte-macrophage colony-stimulating factor (rHuGM-CSF) in HIV-positive patients (CD4$^+$ counts of <50 cells/mm^3) with paromomycin-resistant cryptosporidiosis. rHuGM-CSF was given subcutaneously at 300 mg daily for 14 d, then at each other day for additional 14 d together with zidovudine (500 mg) and paromomycin. The patients showed prompt clinical response to rHuGM-CSF (cessation of diarrhea in 2 d), but relapsed when therapy was discontinued.

2.7. Antiretroviral Therapies and Cryptosporidiosis

There have been a number of studies aimed at better understanding whether or not potent antiretroviral therapies can modify the natural history of HIV-associated cryptosporidiosis (206–210). Effective antiretroviral therapy has been associated with restoration of the immune response with accompanying resolution of opportunistic infections including cryptosporidiosis. Thus, Maggi et al. (206) collected retrospective data for 50 HIV-positive patients with chronic diarrhea concerning demographics, clinical and microbiological characteristics of cryptosporidial and microsporidial infections, antiretroviral therapies, and prophylaxis against these parasitic infections. The data strongly supported the hypothesis that combination antiretroviral therapy had significantly modified the course of both cryptosporidiosis and microsporidiosis in HIV-1-infected patients. The resolution of diarrhea seemed to be related to an increased $CD4^+$ cell count rather than the viral load (206).

Treatment of HIV-1 infections with protease inhibitors has resulted in dramatic decreases in the HIV-1 viral load with concomitant increases in $CD4^+$ counts. In a case of progressive cryptosporidiosis, an HIV patient with $CD4^+$ count of 33 cells/mm^3 cleared parasite oocysts in stool samples and has the symptoms resolved following treatment with indinavir (207). In another study, there was clearance of *Cryptosporidium* and *Microsporidium* and clinical improvement in 85% of the cases following treatment with indinavir (9 patients) or ritonavir in combination with two nucleoside analogs (6 patients) (208).

2.8. Alternative Therapies for Cryptosporidiosis

In addition to chemotherapy, one important aspect in the management of cryptosporidial infections in immunodeficient patients has been the need to provide supportive care by decreasing the intestinal motility and maintaining a proper fluid and electrolyte balance by giving patients oral rehydration reduced-osmolarity solutions (211) containing glucose, sodium bicarbonate and potassium (94,212), and parenteral feeding (213,214).

Furthermore, in immunocompromised hosts, the reversal of underlying immune deficiencies by discontinuation of immunosuppressive therapy has led to successful recovery from cryptosporidiosis (67,71,79,89,2150). In one case described by Holley and Thiers (216), the patient, with bullous pemphigoid, did not have cryptosporidia in the stools until after the initiation of immunosuppressive therapy with steroids and azathioprine. It was postulated that the patient had reactivation of a latent infection, possibly representing a previously asymptomatic carrier state. The medication, which involved daily doses of 80 mg prednisone was sufficient to cause immunosuppression by eliciting T-cell depletion and dysfunction (217,218) that had not only indirectly affected the humoral responses (219), but also interfered with the antibody binding and monocyte IgG and complement receptor functions (220).

REFERENCES

1. Berkowitz, C. D. AIDS and parasitic infections, including *Pneumocystis carinii* and cryptosporidiosis. *Pediatr. Clin. North Am.*, 32, 933, 1985.
2. Current, W. L. and Blagburn, B. L. *Cryptosporidium* and Microsporidia: some closing comments. *J. Protozool.*, 38, 244S, 1991.
3. Current, W. L. and Garcia, L. S. Cryptosporidiosis. *Clin. Microb. Rev.*, 4, 325, 1991.
4. Garcia, L. S. and Current, W. L. Cryptosporidiosis: clinical features and diagnosis. *Crit. Rev. Clin. Lab. Sci.*, 27, 439, 1989.
5. Current, W. L. and Garcia, L. S., Cryptosporidiosis, *Clin. Lab. Med.*, 11, 873, 1991.
6. Bhan, M. K., Bhandari, N., Bhatnagar, S., and Bahl, R. Epidemiology and management of persistent diarrhoea in children of developing countries. *Indian J. Med. Res.*, 104, 103, 1996.
7. Assefa, T., Mohammed, H., Abebe, A., Abebe, S., and Tafesse, B. Cryptosporidiosis in children seen at the children's clinic of Yakatit 12 Hospital, Addis Ababa. *Ethiop. Med. J.*, 34, 43, 1996.

8. Fraser, D., Naggan, L., El-On, J., Deckelbaum, R. J., and Dagan, R. Risk factors for symptomatic and asymptomatic *Cryptosporidium* (CR) and *Giardia lamblia* (GL) infection in a cohort of Israeli bedouin children. *Proc. 36th Intersci. Conf. Antimicrob. Agents Chemother.*, American Society for Microbiology, Washington, D.C., abstract # K153, 1996.
9. Neill, M. A., Rice, S. K., Ahmad, N. V., and Flanigan, T. P. Cryptosporidiosis: an unrecognized cause of diarrhea in elderly hospitalized patients. *Clin. Infect. Dis.*, 22, 168, 1996.
10. Gerba, C. P., Rose, J. B., and Haas, C. N. Sensitive populations: who is at the greatest risk? *Int. J. Food Microbiol.*, 30, 113, 1996.
11. Poirot, J. L., Deluol, A. M., Antoine, M., et al. Broncho-pulmonary cryptosporidiosis in four HIV- infected patients. *J. Eukaryot. Microbiol.*, 43, 78S, 1996.
12. Farthing, M. J., Kelly, M. P., and Veitch, A. M. Recently recognized microbial enteropathies and HIV infection. *J. Antimicrob. Chemother.*, 37(Suppl. B), 61, 1996.
13. Greenberg, P. D., Koch, J., and Cello, J. P. Diagnosis of *Cryptosporidium parvum* in patients with severe diarrhea and AIDS. *Dig. Dis. Sci.*, 41, 2286, 1996.
14. Manatsathit, S., Tansupasawasdikul, S., Wanachiwanawin, D., et al. Causes of chronic diarrhea in patients with AIDS in Thailand: a prospective clinical and microbiological study. *J. Gastroenterol.*, 31, 533, 1996.
15. Tarimo, D. S., Killewo, J. Z., Minjas, J. N., and Msamanga, G. I. Prevalence of intestinal parasites in adult patients with enteropathic AIDS in north-eastern Tanzania. *East Afr. Med. J.*, 73, 397, 1996.
16. Ghorpade, M. V., Kulkarni, S. A., and Kulkarni, A. G. *Cryptosporidium, Isospora* and *Strongyloides* in AIDS. *Natl. Med. J. India*, 9, 201, 1996.
17. Lanjewar, D. N., Rodrigues, C., Saple, D. G., Hira, S. K., and DuPont, H. L. *Cryptosporidium, Isospora* and *Strongyloides* in AIDS. *Natl. Med. J. India*, 9, 17, 1996.
18. Dieng, T., Ndir, O., Diallo, S., Coll-Seck, A. M., and Dieng, Y. Prevalence of *Cryptosporidium* sp. and *Isospora belli* in patients with acquired immunodeficiency syndrome (AIDS) in Dakar (Senegal). *Dakar Med.*, 39, 121, 1994.
19. Gunthard, M., Meister, T., Luthy, R., and Weber, R. Intestinal cryptosporidiosis in HIV infection: clinical features, course and therapy. *Dtsch. Med. Wochenschr.*, 121, 686, 1996.
20. Moolasart, P., Eampokalap, B., Ratanasrithong, M., Kanthasing, P., Tansupaswaskul, S., and Tanchanpong, C. Cryptosporidiosis in HIV infected patients in Thailand. *Southeast Asian J. Trop. Med. Public Health*, 26, 335, 1995.
21. Esfandiari, A., Jordan, W. C., and Brown, C. P. Prevalence of enteric parasitic infection among HIV-infected attendees of an inner city AIDS clinic. *Cell. Mol. Biol. (Noisy-le- Grand)*, 41(Suppl. 1), S19, 1995.
22. Lopez-Velez, R., Tarazona, R., Garcia Camacho, A., et al. Intestinal and extraintestinal cryptosporidiosis in AIDS patients. *Eur. J. Clin. Microbiol. Infect. Dis.*, 14, 677, 1995.
23. Moon, H. W. and Woodmansee, D. B. Cryptosporidiosis. *J. Am. Vet. Med. Assoc.*, 189, 643, 1986.
24. Angus, K. W. Cryptosporidiosis in man, domestic animals and birds: a review. *J. R. Soc. Med.*, 76, 62, 1983.
25. Forgacs, P., Tarshis, A., Ma, P., et al. Intestinal and bronchial cryptosporidiosis in an immunodeficient homosexual man. *Ann. Intern. Med.*, 99, 793, 1983.
26. Guarda, L. A., Stein, S. A., Cleary, K. A., and Ordonez, N. G. Human cryptosporidiosis in the acquired immune deficiency syndrome. *Arch. Pathol. Lab. Med.*, 107, 562, 1983.
27. Pitlik, S. D., Fainstein, V., Rios, A., Guarda, L., Mansell, P. W. A, and Hersh, E. M. Cryptosporidial cholecystitis. *N. Engl. J. Med.*, 308, 967, 1983.
28. Blumberg, R. S., Kelsey, P., Perrone, T., Dickersin, R., Laguaglia, M., and Ferruci, J. Cytomegalovirus- and *Cryptosporidium*-associated acalculous gangrenous cholecystitis. *Am. J. Med.*, 76, 1118, 1984.
29. French, A. L., Beaudet, L. M., Benator, D. A., Levy, C. S., Kassa, M., and Orenstein, J. M. Cholecystectomy in patients with AIDS: clinicopathologic correlations in 107 cases. *Clin. Infect. Dis.*, 21, 852, 1995.
30. Mifsud, A. J., Bell, D., and Shafi, M. S. Respiratory cryptosporidiosis as a presenting feature of AIDS. *J. Infect.*, 28, 227, 1994.
31. Ito, A. and Kawata, K. Liver cryptosporidiosis, *Ryoikibetsu Shokogun Shirizu*, (7), 75, 1995.
32. Talens, A., Montoya, E., Cubells, M. L., et al., Acute pancreatitis and acquired immunodeficiency syndrome. *Rev. Esp. Enferm. Dig.*, 88, 155, 1996.
33. Rose, J. B. Occurence and significance of *Cryptosporidium* in water. *J. Am. Water Works Assoc.*, 80, 53, 1988.
34. Dworkin, M. S., Goldman, D. P., Wells, T. G., Kobayashi, J. M., and Herwaldt, B. L. Cryptosporidiosis in Washington State: an outbreak associated with well water. *J. Infect. Dis.*, 174, 1372, 1996.
35. Kuroki, T., Watanabe, Y., Asai, Y., et al., An outbreak of waterborne cryptosporidiosis in Kanagawa, Japan. *Kansenshogaku Zasshi*, 70, 132, 1996.
36. Osewe, P., Addiss, D. G., Blair, K. A., Hightower, A., Kamb, M. L., and Davis, J. P. Cryptosporidiosis in Wisconsin: a case-control study of post-outbreak transmission. *Epidemiol. Infect.*, 117, 297, 1996.
37. Addiss, D. G., Pond, R. S., Remshak, M., Juranek, D. D., Stokes, S., and Davis, J. P. Reduction of risk of watery diarrhea with point-of-use water filters during a massive outbreak of waterborne *Cryptosporidium* infection in Milwaukee, Wisconsin, 1993. *Am. J. Trop. Med. Hyg.*, 54, 549, 1996.
38. Goldstein, S. T., Juranek, D. D., Ravenholt, O., et al. Cryptosporidiosis: an outbreak associated with drinking water despite state-of-the-art water treatment. *Ann. Intern. Med.*, 124, 459, 1996.
39. Kramer, M. H., Herwaldt, B. L., Craun, G. F., Calderon, R. L., and Juranek, D. D., Surveillance for waterborne-disease outbreaks - United States, 1993–1994. *Morb. Mortal. Wkly Rep. [CDC Surveill. Summ.]*, 45, 1, 1996.
40. Bridgman, S. A., Robertson, R. M., Syed, O., Speed, N., Andrews, N., and Hunter, P. R. Outbreak of cryptosporidiosis associated with a disinfected groundwater supply. *Epidemiol. Infect.*, 115, 555, 1995.

41. Mackenzie, W. R., Kazmierczak, J. J., and Davis, J. P. An outbreak of cryptosporidiosis associated with a resort swimming pool. *Epidemiol. Infect.*, 115, 545, 1995.
42. Fayer, R. and Nerad, T. Effects of low temperatures on viability of *Cryptosporidium parvum* oocysts. *Appl. Environ. Microbiol.*, 62, 1431, 1996.
43. Fayer, R., Trout, J., and Nerad, T. Effects of a wide range of temperatures on infectivity of *Cryptosporidium parvum* oocysts. *J. Eukaryot. Microbiol.*, 43, 64S, 1996.
44. Shepherd, K. M. and Wyn-Jones, A. P. An evaluation of methods for the simultaneous detection of *Cryptosporidium* oocysts and *Giardia* cysts from water. *Appl. Environ. Microbiol.*, 62, 1317, 1996.
45. Drozd, C. and Schartzbrod, J. Hydrophobic and electrostatic cell surface properties of *Cryptosporidium parvum*. *Appl. Environ. Microbiol.*, 62, 12,227, 1996.
46. Rochelle, P. A., Ferguson, D. M., Handojo, T. J., De Leon, R., Stewart, M. H., and Wolfe, R. L. Development of a rapid detection procedure for *Cryptosporidium*, using in vitro cell culture combined with PCR. *J. Eukaryot. Microbiol.*, 43, 72S, 1996.
47. Anderson, B. C., Donndelinger, T., Wilkins, R. M., and Smith, J. Cryptosporidiosis in a veterinary student. *J. Am. Vet. Med. Assoc.*, 180, 408, 1982.
48. Baxby, D., Hart, C. A., and Blundell, N. Shedding of oocysts by immunocompetent individuals with cryptosporidiosis. *J. Hyg.*, 95, 708,1985.
49. Brasseur, P., Lemeteil, D., and Mallet, E. La cryptosporidiose chez l'enfant immunocompetent. *Presse Med.*, 16, 177, 1987.
50. Current, W. L., Reese, N. .C, Ernest, J. V., Bailey, W. S., Heyman, M. B., and Weinstein, W. M. Human cryptosporidiosis in immunocompetent and immunodeficient persons. *N. Engl. J. Med.*, 308, 1252, 1983.
51. Laurent, F., McCole, D., Eckmann, L., and Kagnoff, M. F. Pathogenesis of *Cryptosporidium parvum* infection. *Microbes Infect.*, 1, 141–148, 1999.
52. Navin, T. R. and Juranek, D. D. Cryptosporidiosis - clinical, epidemiologic and parasitologic review. *Rev. Infect. Dis.*, 6, 313, 1984.
53. Reese, N. C., Current, W. L., Ernest, J. V., and Bailey, W. S. Cryptosporidiosis of man and calf: a case report and results of experimental infections in mice and rats. *Am. J. Trop. Med. Hyg.*, 31, 226, 1982.
54. Casemore, D. P. The epidemiology of human cryptosporidiosis, in *Cryptosporidiosis. Proc. 1st Int. Workshop*, Edinburgh, Angus, K. W. and Blewett, D. A., Eds. 65, 1988.
55. Malla, N., Sehgal, R., Ganguly, N. K., and Mahajan, R. C. Cryptosporidiosis - the Indian scene. *Indian J. Pediatr.*, 56, 6, 1989.
56. Hoepelman, A. I. Current therapeutic approaches to cryptosporidiosis in immunocompromised patients. *J. Antimicrob. Chemother.*, 37, 871, 1996.
57. Colford, J. M. Jr., Tager, I. B., Hirozawa, A. M., Lemp, G. F., Aragon, T., and Petersen, C. Cryptosporidiosis among patients infected with human immunodeficiency virus: factors related to symptomatic infection and survival. *Am. J. Epidemiol.*, 144, 807, 1996.
58. Heyworth, M. F. Parasitic diseases in immunocompromised hosts: cryptosporidiosis, isosporiasis, and strongyloidiasis. *Gastroenterol. Clin. North Am.*, 25, 691, 1996.
59. Ballal, M., Prabhu, T., Chandran, A., and Shivananda, P. G. *Cryptosporidium* and *Isospora belli* diarrhoea in immunocompromised hosts. *Indian J. Cancer*, 36, 38–42, 1999.
60. Issacs, D. *Cryptosporidium* and diarrhea. *Arch. Dis. Child.*, 60, 608, 1985.
61. Malenbranche, R., Arnous, E., Guerin, J. M., et al. Acquired immunodeficiency syndrome with severe gastrointestinal manifestations. *Lancet*, 2, 873, 1983.
62. Vakil, N. B., Schwartz, S. M., Buggy, B. P., et al. Biliary cryptosporidiosis in HIV-infected people after the waterborne outbreak of cryptosporidiosis in Milwaukee. *N. Engl. J. Med.*, 334, 19, 1996.
63. Lasser, K. H., Lewin, K. J., and Ryning, F. W. Cryptosporidial enteritis in a patient with congenital hypogammaglobulinaemia. *Hum. Pathol.*, 10, 234, 1979.
64. Sloper, K. S., Dourmashkin, R. R., Bird, R. B., Slavin, G., and Webster, A. D. B. Chronic malabsorption due to cryptosporidiosis in a child with immunoglobulin deficiency. *Gut*, 23, 80, 1982.
65. Tzipori, S., Robertson, D., and Chapman, C. Remission of diarrhea due to cryptosporidiosis in an immunodeficient child treated with hyperimmune bovine colostrums. *Br. Med. J.*, 293, 1276, 1986.
66. Kocoshis, S. A., Cibull, M. L., Davis, T. E., Hinton, J. T., Seip, M., and Banwell, J. G. Intestinal and pulmonary cryptosporidiosis in an infant with severe combined immunoglobulin deficiency. *J. Pediatr. Gastroenterol. Nutr.*, 3, 149, 1984.
67. Miller, R. A., Holmberg, R. E., and Clausen, C. R. Life-threatening diarrhoea caused by *Cryptosporidium* in a child undergoing therapy for acute lymphocytic leukaemia. *J. Pediatr.*, 103, 256, 1983.
68. Lewis, I. J., Hart, C. A., and Baxby, D. Diarrhoea due to *Cryptosporidium* in acute lymphoblastic leukaemia. *Arch. Dis. Child.*, 60, 60, 1985.
69. Foot, A. B., Oakhill, A., and Mott, M. G. Cryptosporidiosis and acute leukaemia. *Arch. Dis. Child.*, 65, 236, 1990.
70. Gentile, G., Venditti, M., Micozzi, A., et al. Cryptosporidiosis in patients with hematologic malignancies. *Rev. Infect. Dis.*, 13, 842, 1991.
71. Weisburger, W. R., Hutcheson, D. F., Yardley, J. H., Roche, J.C., Hillis, W. D., and Charache, P. Cryptosporidiosis in an immunosuppressed renal-transplant recipient with IgA deficiency. *Am. J. Clin. Pathol.*, 72, 473, 1979.
72. Soave, R. Cryptosporidiosis and isosporiasis in patients with AIDS. *Infect. Dis. Clin. North Am.*, 2, 485, 1988.
73. Connolly, G. M., Dryden, M.S., Shanson, D. C., and Gazzard, B. G. Cryptosporidial diarrhoea in AIDS and its treatment. *Gut*, 29, 593, 1988.
74. Soave, R. and Johnson, W. D. Jr. *Cryptosporidium* and *Isospora belli* infections. *J. Infect. Dis.*, 157, 225, 1988.

75. Hudson, R. No treatment for cryptosporidiosis in AIDS patients. *J. Am. Osteopath. Assoc.*, 89, 716, 1989.
76. Soave, R. Treatment strategies for cryptosporidiosis. *Ann. NY Acad. Sci.*, 616, 442, 1990.
77. Georgiev, V. St. Opportunistic infections: treatment and developmental therapeutics of cryptosporidiosis and isosporiasis. *Drug Dev. Res.*, 28, 445, 1993.
78. Sterling, C. R., Cryptosporidiosis: the treatment dilemma. *J. Med. Microbiol.*, 49, 207–208, 2000.
79. Centers for Disease Control. Cryptosporidiosis: assessment of chemotherapy of males with acquired immunodeficiency syndrome (AIDS). *Morbid. Mortal. Wkly Rep.*, 31, 589, 1982.
80. U. S. Public Health Service (USPHS) and Infectious Diseases Society of America (IDSA), 1999 USPHS/IDSA guidelines for the prevention of opportunistic infections in persons infected with human immunodeficiency virus. *Infect. Dis. Obstet. Gynecol.*, 8, 5–74, 2000.
81. Holmberg, S. D., Moorman, A. C., Von Bargen, J. C., et al. Possible effectiveness of clarithromycin and rifabutin for cryptosporidiosis chemoprophylaxis in HIV disease. *J. Am. Med. Assoc.*, 279, 384–386, 1998.
82. Brasseur, P., Lemeteil, D., and Ballet, J. J. Anti-cryptosporidial activity screened with an immunosuppressed rat model. *J. Protozool.*, 38, 230S, 1991.
83. Gross, T. L., Wheat, J., Bartlett, M., and O'Connor, K. W. AIDS and multiple system involvement with Cryptosporidium. *Am. J. Gastroenterol.*, 8, 456, 1986.
84. Pilla, A. M., Rybak, M. J., and Chandrasekar, P. H. Spiramycin in the treatment of cryptosporidiosis. *Pharmacotherapy*, 7, 188, 1987.
85. Centers for Disease Control. Update: treatment of cryptosporidiosis in patients with acquired immunodeficiency syndrome (AIDS). *Morb. Mortal. Wkly Rep.*, 33, 117, 1984.
86. Portnoy, D., Whiteside, M. E., Buckley, E., and MacLeod, C. L. Treatment of intestinal cryptosporidiosis with spiramycin. *Ann. Intern. Med.*, 101, 202, 1984.
87. Decaux, G. M. and Devroeda, C. Acute colitis related to spiramycin. *Lancet*, 2, 993, 1978.
88. Moskovitz, B. L., Stanton, T. L., and Kusmierek, J. J. Spiramycin therapy for cryptosporidial diarrhoea in immunocompromised patients. *J. Antimicrob. Chemother.*, 22(Suppl B), 189, 1988.
89. Collier, A. C., Miller, P. A., and Meyers, J. D. Cryptosporidiosis after marrow transplantation: person-to-person transmission and treatment with spiramycin. *Ann. Intern. Med.*, 101, 205, 1984.
90. Mead, G. M., Sweetenham, J. W., Ewins, D. L., Furlong, M., and Lowes, J. A. Intestinal cryptosporidiosis: a complication of cancer treatment. *Cancer Treat. Rep.*, 70, 769, 1986.
91. Fafard, J. and Lalonde, R. Long-standing symptomatic cryptosporidiosis in a normal man: clinical response to spiramycin. *J. Clin. Gastroenterol.*, 12, 190, 1990.
92. Galvano, G., Cattaneo, G., and Reverso-Giovantin, E. Chronic diarrhea due to *Cryptosporidium*: the efficacy of spiramycin treatment. *Pediatr. Med. Chir.*, 15, 297, 1993.
93. Wilmsmeyer, B., Dopfer, R., Hoppe, J. E., and Niethammer, D. *Cryptosporidium* enteritis. *Monatsschr. Kinderheilkd.*, 141, 130, 1993.
94. Descotes, J., Vial, T., Delattre, D., and Evreux, J.-C. Spiramycin: safety in man. *J. Antimicrob. Chem.*, 22, 207, 1988.
95. Kotler, D. P., Gaetz, H. P., Lange, M., Klein, E. B., and Holt, P. R. Enteropathy associated with the acquired immunodeficiency syndrome. *Ann. Intern. Med.*, 101, 421, 1984.
96. Saez-Llorens, X., Odio, C. M., Umana, M. A., and Morales, M. V. Spiramycin vs. placebo for treatment of acute diarrhea caused by *Cryptosporidium*. *Pediatr. Infect. Dis. J.*, 8, 136, 1989.
97. Saez-Llorens, X. Spiramycin for treatment of *Cryptosporidium* enteritis. *J. Infect. Dis.*, 160, 342, 1989.
98. Connolly, G. M., Dryden, M. S., Shanson, D. C., and Gazzard, B. G. Cryptosporidial diarrhoea in AIDS and its treatment. *Gut*, 29,593, 1988.
99. Casemore, D.P., Sands, R. L., and Curry, A. *Cryptosporidium* species: a "new" human pathogen. *J. Clin. Pathol.*, 38, 1321, 1985.
100. Woolf, G. M., Townsend, M., and Guyatt, G. Treatment of cryptosoridiosis with spiramycin in AIDS: an "N of 1". *J. Clin. Gastroenterol.*, 9, 632, 1987.
101. Wittenberg, D. F., Miller, N. M., and van den Ende, J. Spiramycin is not effective in treating *Cryptosporidium* diarrhea in infants: results of a double-blind randomized trial. *J. Infect. Dis.*, 159, 131, 1989.
102. Wittenberg, D. F. Spiramycin for treatment of *Cryptosporidium* enteritis. *J. Infect. Dis.*, 160, 342, 1989.
103. Berkowitz, C. D. and Seidel, J. S. Spontaneous resolution of cryptosporidiosis in a child with acquired immunodeficiency syndrome. *Am. J. Dis. Child.*, 139, 967, 1985.
104. Current, W. L. Cryptosporidium: *Its Biology and Potential For Environmental Transmission* [CRC Crit. Rev. Environ. Control, vol. 17], 21, 1986.
105. Weikel, C., Lazenby, A., Belitsos, P., McDewitt, M., Fleming, H. E. Jr., and Barbacci, M. Intestinal injury associated with spiramycin therapy of *Cryptosporidium* infection in AIDS. *J. Protozool.*, 38, 147S, 1991.
106. Soave, R. Cryptosporidiosis and isosporiasis in patients with AIDS. *Infect. Dis. Clin. North Am.*, 2, 485, 1988.
107. Dupont, C., Bougnoux, M. E., Turner, L., Rouveix, E., and Dorra, M. Microbiological findings about pulmonary cryptosporidiosis in two AIDS patients. *J. Clin. Microbiol.*, 34, 227, 1996.
108. Hicks, P., Zwiener, R. J., Squires, J., and Savell, V. Azithromycin therapy for *Cryptosporidium parvum* infection in four children infected with human immunodeficiency virus. *J. Pediatr.*, 129, 297, 1996.
109. Vargas, S. L., Shenep, J. L., Flynn, P. M., Pui, C. H., Santana, V. M., and Hughes, W. T. Azithromycin for treatment of severe *Cryptosporidium* diarrhea in two children with cancer. *J. Pediatr.*, 123, 154, 1993.

110. Jordan, W. C. Clarithromycin prophylaxis against *Cryptosporidium* enteritis in patients with AIDS. *J. Natl. Med. Assoc.*, 88, 425, 1996.
111. Holmberg, S. D., Moorman, A. C., Von Bargen, J. C., Palella, F. J., Loveless, M. O., and Navin, T. R. Apparent chemoprophylaxis of cryptosporidiosis with clarithromycin and rifabutin. *4th Conf. Retroviruses Opportunistic Infect., Jan. 22–26, 1997*, 191, abstract 685.
112. Fichtenbaum, C., Griffiths, J., Zackin, R., Feinberg, J., and Benson, C. Macrolides do not prevent cryptosporidiosis in AIDS. *5th Conf. Retroviruses Opportunistic Infect., Feb. 1–5, 1998*, 169, abstract 479.
113. Tzipori, S., Rand, W., Griffiths, J., Widmer, G., and Crabb, J. Evaluation of an animal model system for cryptosporidiosis: therapeutic efficacy of paromomycin and hyperimmune bovine colostrum-immunoglobulin. *Clin. Diagn. Lab. Immunol.*, 1, 450, 1994.
114. Cirioni, O., Giacometti A., Balducci, M., Drenaggi, D., Del Prete, M. S., and Scallise, G. Anticryptosporidial activity of paromomycin. *J. Infect. Dis.*, 172, 1169, 1995.
115. Verdon, R., Polianski, J., Gaudebout, C., and Pocidalo, J. J. Paromomycin for cryptosporidiosis in AIDS. *J. Infect. Dis.*, 171, 1070, 1071, 1995.
116. Tsipori, S., Griffiths, J., and Theodus, C. Paromomycin treatment against cryptosporidiosis in patients with AIDS. *J. Infect. Dis.*, 171, 1069, 1071, 1995.
117. Mancassola, R., Reperant, J. M., Naciri, M., and Chartier, C. Chemoprophylaxis of *Cryptosporidium parvum* infection with paromomycin in kids and immunological study. *Antimicrob. Agents Chemother.*, 39, 75,1995.
118. Jimenez-Beatty Navarro, M. D., de la Fuente Aguado, J., Sopena Arguelles, B., and Martinez Vazquez, C. Paromomycin in the treatment of cryptosporidiosis. *Rev. Clin. Esp.*, 195, 62, 1995.
119. Healey, M. C., Yang, S., Rasmussen, K. R., Jackson, M. K., and Du, C. Therapeutic efficacy of paromomycin in immunosuppressed adult mice infected with *Cryptosporidium parvum*. *J. Parasitol.*, 81, 114, 1995.
120. Mohri, H., Fujita, H., Asakura, Y., et al. Case report: inhalation therapy of paromomycin is effective for respiratory infection and hypoxia by cryptosporidium with AIDS. *Am. J. Med. Sci.*, 309, 60, 1995.
121. Verdon, R., Polianski, J., Gaudebout, C., Marche, C., Garry, L., and Pocidalo, J.-J. Evaluation of curative anticryptosporidial activity of paromomycin in a dexamethazone- treated rat model. *Antimicrob. Agents Chemother.*, 38, 1681, 1994.
122. Scaglia, M., Atzori, C., Marchetti, G., et al. Effectiveness of aminosidine (paromomycin) sulfate in chronic *Cryptosporidium* diarrhea in AIDS patients: an open, uncontrolled, prospective clinical trial. *J. Infect. Dis.*, 170, 1349, 1994.
123. Rehg, J. E. A comparison of anticryptosporidial activity of paromomycin with that of other aminoglycosides and azithromycin in immunosuppressed rats. *J. Infect. Dis.*, 170, 934, 1994.
124. Youssef, M. M., Hammam, S. M., Abou Samra, L. M., and Khalifa, A. M. Aminosidine sulphate in experimental cryptosporidiosis. *J. Egypt. Soc. Parasitol.*, 24, 239, 1994.
125. White, A. C. Jr., Chappell, C. L., Hayat, C. S., Kimball, K. T., Flanigan, T. P., and Goodgame, R. W. Paromomycin for cryptosporidiosis in AIDS: a prospective, double-blind trial. *J. Infect. Dis.*, 170, 419, 1994.
126. Forester, G., Sidhom, O., Nahass, R., and Andavolu, R. AIDS-associated cryptosporidiosis with gastric structure and a therapeutic response to paromomycin. *Am. J. Gastroenterol.*, 89, 1096, 1994.
127. Wallace, M. R., Nguyen, M. T., and Newton, J. A. Jr. Use of paromomycin for the treatment of cryptosporidiosis in patients with AIDS. *Clin. Infect. Dis.*, 17, 1070, 1993.
128. Anand, A. Cryptosporidiosis in patients with AIDS. *Clin. Infect. Dis.*, 17, 297, 1993.
129. Fichtenbaum, C. J., Ritchie, D. J., and Powderly, W. G. Use of paromomycin for treatment of cryptosporidiosis in patients with AIDS. *Clin. Infect. Dis.*, 16, 298, 1993.
130. Goodgame, R. W., Genta, R. M., White, A. C., and Chappell, C. L. Intensity of infection in AIDS-associated cryptosporidiosis. *J. Infect. Dis.*, 167, 704, 1993.
131. Hewitt, R. G., Yiannoutsos, C. T., Carey, J et al. A double-blind, placebo-controlled trial of paromomycin for the treatment of cryptosporidiosis in patients with advanced HIV disease and CD4 counts under 150 (ACTG 192). *4th Conf. Retroviruses Opportunistic Infect., Jan. 22–26, 1997*, 65, abstract 4.
132. Gatlie, J. Jr., Piot, D., Hawkins, K., Bernal, A., Clemmons, J., and Stool, E. Treatment of gastrointestinal cryptosporidium. *Proc. VIth Int. Conf. AIDS*, San Francisco, 1990, abstract no. 2121.
133. Clezy, K., Gold, J., Blaze, J., and Jones, P. Paromomycin for the treatment of cryptosporidial diarrhoea in AIDS patients. *AIDS*, 5, 1146, 1991.
134. Samson, V. E. and Brown, W. R. Pneumatosis cystoides intestinalis in AIDS-associated cryptosporidiosis: more than incidental finding? *J. Clin. Gastroenterol.*, 22, 311, 1996.
135. Smith, N. S., Cron, S., Chappell, C., Valdez, L., and White, A. C. Combination paromomycin and azithromycin for cryptosporidiosis in AIDS. *5th Conf. Retroviruses Opportunistic Infect., Feb. 1–5, 1998*, 170, abstract 481.
136. Giacometti, A., Burzachhini, F., Cirioni, O., Barchiesi, F., Dini, M., and Scalise, G. Efficacy of treatment with paromomycin, azithromycin, and nitazoxanide in a patient with dissiminated cryptosporidiosis. *Eur. J. Clin. Microbiol. Infect. Dis.*, 18, 885–889, 1999.
137. Amenta, M., Dalle Nogare, E. R., Colomba, C., et al. Intestinal protozoa in HIV-infected patients: effect of rifaximin in *Cryptosporidium parvum* and *Blastocystis hominis* infections. *J. Chemother.*, 11, 391–395, 1999.
138. Bowers, M. Nitazoxanide for cryptosporidial diarrhea. *BETA*, (April), 30-31, 1998.
139. Bornhoeft, M. A. Cryptosporidiosis gets a new treatment. *Body Posit.*, XI(3), 13, 1998.
140. James, J. S. NTZ: advisory committee votes against approval. *AIDS Treat. News*, (No. 295), 7, 1998.
141. James, J. S. Prospective case series in clinical trial design - proposal, and NTZ example. *AIDS Treat. News*, (No. 296), 5-6, 1998.

142. Baker, R. FDA panel rejects drug for cryptosporidial diarrhea. Food and Drug Administration. *BETA*, (July), 7, 1998.
143. Roehr, B. Another failed promise? NTZ gets the nix. *J. Int. Assoc. Phycisians AIDS Care* 4, 26–27, 29, 1998.
144. Learned, J. NTZ - still promising but Unimed walks. *Notes Undergr.*, (No. 37), 10, 1998.
145. Cadman, J. Diarrhea drug rejection raises a ruckus. *GMHC Treat Issues*, 12, 1-3, 1998.
146. Bonfils, S., Ruszniewski, P., Costil, V., et al. Prolonged treatment of Zollinger-Ellison syndrome by long-acting somatostatin. *Lancet*, 1, 554, 1986.
147. Ch'ng, J. L., Anderson, J. V., Williams, S. J., Carr, D.H., and Bloom, S. R. Remission of symptoms during long term treatment of metastatic pancreatic endocrine tumours with long- acting somatostatin analogue. *Br. Med. J.*, 292, 981, 1986.
148. Maton, P. N., O'Dorisio, T. M., Howe, B. A., et al. Effect of a long-acting somatostatin analogue (SMS 201-995) in a patient with pancreatic cholera. *N. Engl. J. Med.*, 312, 17, 1985.
149. Dharmsathaphorn, K., Sherwin, R. S., Cataland, S., Jaffe, B., and Dobbins, J. Somatostatin inhibits diarrhea in the carcinoid syndrome. *Ann. Intern. Med.*, 92, 68, 1980.
150. Williams, N. S., Cooper, J. C., Axon, A. T. R., King, R. F. G. J, and Barker, M. Use of a long-acting somatostatin analogue in controlling life threatening ileostomy diarrhoea. *Br. Med. J.*, 289, 1027, 1984.
151. Sheppard, M., Shapiro, B., Pimstone, B., Kronheim, M. B., and Gregory, M. The metabolic clearance and plasma half disappearance time of exogenous somatostatin in man. *J. Clin. Endocrinol. Metab.*, 49, 50, 1979.
152. Bauer, W., Briner, U., Doepfner, W., et al. SMS 201-995: a very potent and selective octapeptide analogue of somatostatin with prolonged action. *Life Sci.*, 31, 1133, 1982.
153. Nousbaum, J. B., Robaszkiewicz, M., Cauvin, J. M., Garre, M., and Gouerou, H. Treatment of intestinal cryptosporidiosis with zidovudine and SMS 201-995, a somatostatin analog. *Gastroenterology*, 101, 874, 1989.
154. Casals, A., Lorente, L., Jou, B., and Clotet, A. Usefulness of a somatostatin analog in the treatment of chronic severe diarrhea caused by *Cryptosporidium*. *Med. Clin. (Barcelona)*, 92, 358, 1989.
155. Santos, G. I., Mur Gimeno, P., Herreros Fernandez, M., and del Arco Galan, C. The usefulness of somatostatin analog SMS 201-995 in treating *Cryptosporidium*-induced diarrhea associated with the acquired immunodeficiency syndrome. *Med. Clin. (Barcelona)*, 95, 796, 1990.
156. Robinson, E. N. Jr. and Fogel, R. SMS 201-995, a somatostatin analogue, and diarrhea in the acquired immunodeficiency syndrome (AIDS). *Ann. Intern. Med.*, 109, 680, 1988.
157. Oehler, R. and Loos, U. Therapy of severe AIDS-associated diarrhea with the somatostatin analog octreotide. *Med. Klin.*, 88, 45, 1993.
158. Longnecker, S. M. Somatostatin and octreotide: literature review and description of therapeutic activity in pancreatic neoplasia. *Drug Intell. Clin. Pharm.*, 22, 1, 1988.
159. Gaginella, T. S. and O'Dorisio, T. M. Octreotide: entering the new era of peptodomimetic therapy. *Drug Intell. Clin. Pharm.*, 22, 154, 1988.
160. Santangelo, W. C., O'Dorisio, T. M., Kim, J. G., Severino, G., and Krejs, G. VIPoma syndrome: effect of a synthetic somatostatin analogue. *Scand. J. Gastroenterol.*, 21, 187, 1986.
161. Gorden, P. Somatostatin and somatostatin analogue (SMS 201-995) in the treatment of hormone-secreting tumors of the pituitary and gastrointestinal tract and non-neoplastic diseases of the gut. *Ann. Intern. Med.*, 110, 35, 1989.
162. Katz, M. D., Erstad, B. L., and Rose, C. Treatment of severe *Cryptosporidium*-related diarrhea with octreotide in a patient with AIDS. *Drug Intell. Clin. Pharm.*, 22, 134, 1988.
163. Cello, J. P., Grendell, J. H., Basuk, P., et al. Controlled clinical trial of octeotride (sandostatin) for refractory AIDS-associated diarrhea. *Gastroenterology*, 98, A163, 1990.
164. Fanning, M., Monte, M., Sutherland, L. R., Broadhead, M., Murphy, G. F., and Harris, A. G. Pilot study of sandostatin (octreotide) therapy of refractory HIV-associated diarrhea. *Dig. Dis. Sci.*, 36, 476, 1991.
165. Moroni, M., Esposito, R., Cernuschi, M., Franzetti, F., Carosi, G. P., and Fiori, G. P. Treatment of AIDS-related refractory diarrhoea with octreotide. *Digestion*, 54(Suppl. 1), 30, 1993.
166. Crawford, F. G. and Vermund, S. H. Human cryptosporidiosis. *CRC. Crit. Rev. Microbiol.*, 16, 113, 1988.
167. Nelson, J. A., Wiley, C. A., Reynolds-Kohler, C., Reese, C. E., Margaretten, W., and Levy, J. A. Human immunodeficiency virus detected in bowel epithelium from patients with gastrointestinal symptoms. *Lancet*, 1, 259, 1988.
168. Levy, J. A., Margaretten, W., and Nelson, J. Detection of HIV in enterochromaffin cells in the rectal mucosa of an AIDS patient. *Am. J. Gastroenterol.*, 84, 787, 1989.
169. Bigornia, E., Simon, D., Weiss, L., Tanowitz, H., Jones, J., Wittner, M., and Lyman, W. Detection of HIV-1 viral protein and genomic sequences in enterochromaffin cells of HIV-1- seropositive patients. *Am. J. Gastroenterol.*, 85, 1264, 1990.
170. Kreinik, G., Burstein, O., Landor, M., Bernstein, L., Weiss, L. M., and Wittner, M. Successful management of intractable cryptosporidial diarrhea with intravenous octreotide, a somatostatin analogue. *AIDS*, 5, 765, 1991.
171. Ruff, M. R., Martin, B. M., Guins, E. I., Farrar, W. L., and Pert, C.B. CD4 receptor-binding peptides that block HIV infectivity cause human monocyte chemotaxis: relationship to vasoactive intestinal polypeptide. *FEBS Lett.*, 211, 17, 1987.
172. Gaginella, T. S., Hubel, K. A., and O'Dorisio, T. M. Vasoactive intestinal polypeptide and intestinal chloride secretion, in *Vasoactive Intestinal Peptide*, Said, I., Ed. Raven Press, New York, 211, 1982.
173. Cook, D. J., Kelton, J. G., Stanisz, A. M., and Collins, S. M. Somatostatin treatment for cryptosporidial diarrhea in a patient with the acquired immunodeficiency syndrome (AIDS). *Ann. Intern. Med.*, 108, 708, 1988.
174. Friedman, L. S. Somatostatin therapy for AIDS diarrhea: muddy waters. *Gastroenterology*, 101, 1446, 1991.
175. Kotler, D. P. Preliminary observations of the effect of cow's milk globulin upon intestinal cryptosporidiosis in AIDS. *Proc. IIIrd Int. Conf. AIDS*, 1987, Washington DC, abstract.

176. Perryman, L. E., Riggs, M. W., Mason, P. H., and Fayer, R. Kinetics of *Cryptosporidium parvum* sporozoite neutralization by monoclonal antibodies, immune bovine serum, and immune bovine colostral antibodies. *Infect. Immun.*, 58, 257, 1990.
177. Anonymous. Jarrow formulas: "colostrums specific" for cryptosporidiosis. *Posit. Health News*, (17), 22, 1998.
178. Saxon, A. and Weinstein, W. Oral administration of bovine colostrum anti-cryptosporidia antibody fails to alter the course of human cryptosporidiosis. *J. Parasitol.*, 73, 413, 1987.
179. Tzipori, S., Robertson, D., Chapman, C., and White, L. Chronic cryptosporidial diarrhoea and hyperimmune cow colostrum. *Lancet*, 2, 344, 1987.
180. Flanigan, T., Marshall, R., Redman, D., Kaetzel, C., and Ungar, B. In vitro screening of therapeutic agents against *Cryptosporidium*: hyperimmune cow colostrum is highly inhibitory. *J. Protozool.*, 38, 225S, 1991.
181. Fayer, R., Perryman, L. E., and Riggs, M. W. Hyperimmune bovine colostrum neutralizes *Cryptosporidium* sporozoites and protects mice against challenge. *J. Parasitol.*, 75, 151, 1989.
182. Fayer, R., Andrews, B., Ungar, B. L. P., and Blagburn, B. Efficacy of hyperimmune bovine colostrum for prophylaxis of cryptosporidiosis in neonatal calves. *J. Parasitol.*, 75, 393, 1989.
183. Ungar, B. L. P., Ward, D. J., Fayer, R., and Quinn, C. A. Cessation of *Cryptosporidium*- associated diarrhea in an acquired immunodeficiency syndrome patient after treatment with hyperimmune bovine colostrum. *Gastroenterology*, 98, 486, 1990.
184. Nord, J., Ma, P., DiJohn, D., Tzipori, S., and Tacket, C.O. Treatment with bovine hyperimmune colostrum of cryptosporidial diarrhea in AIDS patients. *AIDS*, 4, 581, 1990.
185. Greenberg, P. D. and Cello, J. P. Treatment of severe diarrhea caused by *Cryptosporidium parvum* with oral bovine immunoglobuline concentrate in patients with AIDS. *J. Acquir. Immune Defic. Syndr. Hum. Retrovirol.*, 13, 348, 1996.
186. Mietens, C., Keinhorst, H., Hilpert, H., Gerber, H., Amster, H., and Pahud, J. J. Treatment of infantile *E. coli* gastroenteritis with specific bovine anti-*E. coli* milk immunoglobulins. *Eur. J. Pediatr.*, 132, 239, 1979.
187. Brussow, H., Hilpert, H., Walther, I., Sidoti, J., Mietens, C., and Bachmann, P. Bovine milk immunoglobulin for passive immunity to infantile rotavirus gastroenteritis. *J. Clin. Microbiol.*, 25, 982, 1987.
188. Hilpert, H., Brussow, H., Mietens, C., Sidoti, J., Lerner, L., and Werchau, H. Use of bovine milk concentrate containing antibody to rotavirus to treat rotavirus gastroenteritis in infants. *J. Infect. Dis.*, 156, 158, 1987.
189. Tacket, C. O., Losonsky, G., Link, H., et al. Protection by milk immunoglobulin concentrate against oral challenge with enterotoxigenic *Escherichia coli*. *N. Engl. J. Med.*, 318, 1240, 1988.
190. McMeeking, A., Borkowsky, W., Klesius, P. H., Bonk, S., Holzman, R. S., and Lawrence, S. A controlled trial of bovine dialyzable leukocyte extract for cryptosporidiosis in patients with AIDS. *J. Infect. Dis.*, 161, 108, 1990.
191. Louie, E., Borkowsky, W., Klesius, P. H., et al. Treatment of cryptosporidiosis with oral bovine transfer factor. *Clin. Immunol. Immunopathol.*, 44, 329, 1987.
192. Borkowsky, W. and Lawrence, H. S. Antigen-specific inducer factor in human leukocyte dialysates: a product of T_H cells which binds to anti-V region and anti-Ia region antibodies, in *Immunology of Transfer Factor*, Kirkpatrick, C. H., Burger, D. R., and Lawrence, H. S., Eds. Academic Press, New York, 75, 1983.
193. Jeter, W. S., Kibler, R., Soli, T. C., and Stephens, C. A. Oral administration of bovine and human dyalizable transfer factor to human volunteers, in *Immune Regulators in Transfer Factor*, Kahn, A., Kirkpatrick, C. H., and Hill, N. O., Eds. Academic Press, New York, 451, 1979.
194. Lawrence, H. S. Transfer factor in cellular immunity. *Harvey Lecture Series 68*, Academic Press, New York, 239, 1974.
195. Schulkind, M. L. and Ayoub, E. M. Transfer factor and its clinical applications, in *Advances in Pediatrics, Barness*, L. A., Ed. Year Book Medical Publishers, Chicago, 89, 1980.
196. Jones, J. F., Jeter, W. S., Fulginiti, V. A., Munnich, L. L., Pritchett, R. F., and Wedgwood, R. J. Treatment of childhood combined Epstein-Barr virus/cytomegalovirus infection with oral bovine transfer factor. *Lancet*, 2, 122, 1091.
197. Klesius, P. H. and Kristensen, F. Bovine transfer factor: effect on bovine and rabbit coccidiosis. *Clin. Immunol. Immunopathol.*, 7, 240, 1977.
198. Klesius, P. H., Quals, D. F., Elston, A. L., and Fudenberg, H. H. Effects of bovine transfer factor (TFd) in mouse coccidiosis (*Eimeria ferrisi*). Clin. Immunol. Immunopathol., 10, 214, 1987.
199. Okhuysen, P., Robinson, P., Watson, V., et al. Intestinal IL-15 and interferongamma (Ifgamma) in cryptosporidiosis. *6th Conf. Retroviruses Opportunistic Infect., Jan. 31–Feb. 4, 1999*, 113, abstract 243.
200. Kern, P., Toy, J., and Dietrich, M. Preliminary clinical observations with recombinant interleukin-2 in patients with AIDS or LAS. *Blut*, 50, 1, 1985.
201. Donahue, J. H., Resenstein, M., Chang, A. E., Lotze, M. T., Robb, R. J., and Rosenberg, S. A. The systemic administration of purified interleukin 2 enhances the ability of sensitized murine lymphocytes to cure a disseminated syngeneic lymphoma. *J. Immunol.*, 132, 2123, 1984.
202. Ruscetti, F. W. and Gallo, R. C. Human T-lymphocyte growth factor: regulation of growth and function of T lymphocytes. *Blood*, 57, 379, 1981.
203. Wagner, H., Kronke, M., Solbach, W., Scheurich, P., Rollinghoff, M., and Pfizenmaier, K. Murine T cell subsets and interleukins: relationships between cytotoxic T cells, helper T cells and accessory cells. *Clin. Haematol.*, 11, 607, 1982.
204. Pearlstein, K. T., Palladino, M. A., Welte, K., and Vilcek, J. Purified human interleukin-2 enhances induction of immune interferon. *Cell Immunol.*, 80, 1, 1983.
205. Capetti, A., Bonfanti, P., Rizzardini, G., and Milazzo, F. Can rHuGM-CSF help treating drug-resistant cryptosporidiosis

in AIDS. *Proc. 36th Intersci. Conf. Antimicrob. Agents Chemother.*, American Society for Microbiology, Washington, DC, abstract # G33, 1996.
206. Maggi, P., Larocca, A. M., Quarto, M., et al. Effect of antiretroviral therapy on cryptosporidiosis and microsporidiosis in patients infected with human immunodeficiency virus type 1. *Eur. J. Clin. Microbiol. Infect. Dis.*, 19, 213–217, 2000.
207. Mileno, M. D., Tashima, K., Farrar, D., Elliot, B. C., Rich, J. D., and Flanigan, T. P. Resolution of AIDS-related opportunistic infections with addition of protease inhibitor treatment. *4th Conf. Retroviruses Opportunistic Infect., Jan. 22–26, 1997*, 129, abstract 355.
208. Benhamou, Y., Bochet, M. V., Carriere, J., et al. Effects of triple antiretroviral therapies including a HIV protease inhibitor on chronic intestinal cryptosporidiosis and microsporidiosis in HIV- infected patients. *4th Conf. Retroviruses Opportunistic Infect., Jan. 22–26, 1997*, 130, abstract 357.
209. Landau, A., Aaron, L., Pialoux, G., Eliaszewicz, M., Zylberberg, H., Poncelet, H., and Dupont, B. Impact of antiretroviral therapy (ART) on cryptosporidiosis outcome and factors of clinical resistance. *5th Conf. Retroviruses Opportunistic Infect., Feb. 1–5, 1998*, 169, abstract 480.
210. Moore, R. D., Keruly, J. C., and Chaisson, R. E. Decline in CMV and other opportunistic disease with combination antiretroviral therapy. *5th Conf. Retroviruses Opportunistic Infect., Feb. 1–5, 1998*, 113, abstract 184.
211. Lentidoro, I., Anastasio, E., Pensabene, L., Apollini, M., and Guandalini, S. Oral rehydration in infants with acute diarrhea: using a new preparation of reduced osmolarity. *Pediatr. Med. Chir.*, 18, 67, 1996.
212. Posada, G., Pizarro, D., and Mohs, E. Oral rehydration in children with *Cryptosporidium muris* infection. *Bol. Med. Hosp. Infant Mex.*, 44, 740, 1987.
213. Gerberding, J. L. Diagnosis and management of HIV-infected patients with diarrhoea. *J. Antimicrob. Chemother.*, 23(Suppl A), 83, 1989.
214. Wu, K. Z., Chew, S. K., Oh, H. M., Lin, R. V., Allen, D. M., and Monteiro, E. H. Acquired immunodeficiency syndrome and *Cryptosporidium* infection. *Singapore Med. J.*, 35, 418, 1994.
215. Meisel, J. L., Perera, D. R., Meligro, C., and Rubin, C. E. Overwhelming water diarrhea associated with *Cryptosporidium* in an immunosuppressed patient. *Gastroenterology*, 70, 1156, 1976.
216. Holley, H. P. Jr. and Thiers, B. H. Cryptosporidiosis in a patient receiving immunosuppressive therapy: possible activation of latent infection. *Dig. Dis. Sci.*, 31, 1004, 1986.
217. Katz, P., Immunosuppressive therapy, in *Advances in Internal Medicine*, Stollerman, G. H., Ed. Year Book Medical Publishers, Chicago, 167, 1984.
218. Fauci, A. S. Mechanisms of the immunosuppressive and anti-inflammatory effects of glucocorticosteroids. *J. Immunopharmacol.*, 1, 1, 1978.
219. Fauci, A. S., Haynes, B. F., and Katz, P. Drug-induced T- and B-lymphocyte and monocyte dysfunction, in *Infections in the Abnormal Host*, Grieco, M. H., Ed. Yorke Medical Books, Brooklyn, New York, 163, 1980.
220. Schreiber, A. D., Parsons, J., McDermott, P., and Cooper, R. A. Effect of corticosteroids on the human monocyte IgG and complement receptors. *Clin. J. Invest.*, 56, 1189, 1975.

14
Isospora spp.

1. INTRODUCTION

Isospora spp. are apicomplexan protozoan parasites that are taxonomically related to *Cryptosporidium*, *Toxoplasma*, and *Sarcocystis* spp., all members of the family Eimeriidae (suborder Eimeriina). Two species of *Isospora*, *I. belli*, and *I. hominis*, have been diagnosed in humans *(1)*.

The life cycle of *Isospora* is similar to that of other enteric coccidia. It involves a multistep asexual stage (merogony), followed by sexual reproduction (gamogony) and the subsequent development of oocysts. Both the asexual and sexual stages develop in the intestinal cells of their hosts (several mammal species and humans), and produce an environmentally resistant cyst stage, the oocysts. The latter, when released into the environment, are usually unsporulated and noninfective, requiring maturation to become infective *(1–4)*.

The mechanism of *I. belli*-induced infections is still not well understood *(3)*. The disease is transmitted usually by oocysts through fecal contamination of the environment, food, or water. Unsporulated oocysts, initially noninfective in the large intestine or the perianal area, may become infective within 20–24 h at 25–29°C *(3,5)*.

Immunocompromised hosts, such as patients with HIV/AIDS *(6–13,48)* and malignancies (Hodgkin's disease *[14]*), are particularly at risk to the effect of this parasite *(6)*. A case of HTLV-1-associated ATLL complicated by isosporiasis and strongyloidiasis was described by Peng and Tsai *(15)*.

Isosporiasis is also often associated with traveller's diarrhea in many regions of Africa, South America, and Southeast Asia *(16–19)*.

Using data from a surveillance registry conducted over an 8-yr period, Sorvillo et al. *(20)* found that AIDS patients receiving continuous prophylactic medication of trimethoprim-sulfamethoxazole against *Pneumocystis carinii* pneumonia have been less likely to develop primary isosporiasis infection to express latent isosporiasis because of the anti-isosporidial effect of trimethoprim-sulfamethixazole.

Cases of disseminated isosporiasis (lymph nodes, liver, and spleen) in AIDS patients have been reported *(21,22)*. In order to assess the effect of the HIV epidemic on mortality from opportunistic infections, in 1993 Selik et al. *(23)* examined the national multiple-cause death certificate data. The overall results showed that the HIV epidemic had greatly increased the mortality from opportunistic infections; thus, the percentage of death with HIV as the underlying cause and the ratio of observed to predicted death rate for cryptosporidiosis/isosporiasis were respectively, 90% and infinite (1.61/0.00).

A case of fatal malabsorption syndrome caused by stronyloidiasis complicated with isosporiasis and human cytomegalovirus infection has been reported by Yoon et al. *(24)*.

According to some reports *(25,26)*, *Isospora* infections have been observed in 15–20% of Haiti's AIDS population. By other accounts *(26,27)*, in the United States, only 0.2% of AIDS patients had the infection. Clinical manifestations of isosporiasis may range from acute, but self-limited gastroenteritis in the immunocompetent host to chronic, usually intermittent illness in immunodeficient patients *(2,9,27–35)*. The clinical signs and symptoms of isosporiasis are frequently indistinguishable from those of cryptosporidiosis. Charcot-Leyden crystals and high fat content in stool specimens, as well as peripheral eosinophilia, are among the common signs of the infections *(27)*. In one AIDS patient, *Isospora* parasites were identified in the lymph nodes, in what appeared to be perhaps the only reported case of extraintestinal involvement of this protozoan *(34)*.

Hermier et al. *(36)* reported a case of severe form of isosporiasis caused by *I. hominis*.

2. TREATMENT OF ISOSPORIASIS

Contrary to cryptosporidiosis, isosporiasis is treated rather successfully.Thus, clinical and parasitologic cure has been achieved within 7–10 d after initiation of oral therapy with trimethoprim-sulfamethoxazole (co-trimoxazole) *(10,12,25,27,33–35,37–40)*. One recommended regimen consists of oral trimethoprim (160 mg)-sulfamethoxozale (800 mg) given every 6 h for 10 d *(40)*.

Lumb and Hardiman *(3)* described a rapid response of two AIDS patients with isosporidial diarrhea (one of them also with concurrent cryptosporidiosis) to treatment with co-trimoxazole (960 mg, 4 times daily) for 10 d. However, the diarrhea recurred after cessation of treatment thereby necessitating a maintenance therapy *(3)*.

High risk of adverse reactions in AIDS patients treated with co-trimoxazole has been reported *(41)*.

Deluol et al. *(42)* described somewhat disappointing results from treatment of 11 AIDS patients with isosporiasis. Sulfamethoxazole appeared to be the only drug found effective; however, a prolonged parasitologic surveillance was required in order to detect frequent relapses and to assess the long-term efficacy of the drug.

Verdier et al. *(43)* conducted a randomized, controlled trial in HIV-infected patients comparing trimethoprim-sulfamethoxazole with ciprofloxacin for the treatment and prophylaxis of chronic diarrhea caused by *Isospora belli* (22 patients) and *Cyclospora cayetanensis* (20 patients). Oral co-trimoxazole (160 mg or 800 mg) or ciprofloxacin (500 mg) were administered twice daily for 7 d. Patients who showed clinical and microbiological response received prophylaxis for 10 wk (1 tablet orally, 3 times weekly); prophylaxis was measured by recurrent disease rate. The success rates for co-trimoxazole and ciprofloxacin were 95% and 87%, respectively. All patients receiving prophylaxis with co-trimoxazole remained disease-free, and 15 of 16 patients receiving secondary prophylaxis with ciprofloxacin remained disease-free. Ciprofloxacin may prove useful as an alternative therapy for isosporiasis in patients who do not tolerate sulfa drugs.

Because the recurrence rate of isosporiasis in AIDS patients is approaching 50% *(41)*, patients are required to undergo chronic suppressive therapy with either co-trimoxazole, pyrimethamine-sulfadoxine, or trimethoprim-sulfadoxine *(10,25,44)*. The fact that AIDS patients have shown high-incidence intolerance to these agents has prevented their use in a long-term maintenance therapy *(44,45)*.

In addition to co-trimoxazole, other anti-infective agents have also been used to treat isosporiasis. Among published reports have been treatment of isosporiasis in AIDS patients with combined albendazole and ornidazole *(46)*, therapies consisting of metronidazole and quinacrine *(30–32)*, diclazuril *(44)*, and pyrimethamine *(47)*.

A combination of albendazole (400 mg, t.i.d. for 20 d) and ornidazole (2.0 g single dose on d 1, 10, and 20) may prove to be a useful alternative therapy for isosporiasis in patients allergic to cotrimoxazole; when applied to two AIDS patients, the combination led to resolution of diarrhea and eradication of *I. belli* oocysts at the end of treatment *(46)*.

Limson-Pobre et al. *(44)* have described an AIDS patient with isosporiasis and sulfonamide allergy who showed a dramatic clinical response to diclazuril therapy applied at low-level, steady-state concentration (300 mg, b.i.d.). Because the pharmacokinetics of diclazuril in humans have not been defined fully, appropriate dose regimens should be established in every case.

Pyrimethamine was used in two AIDS patients with sulfonamide allergy: the drug was given at 75 mg daily, and recurrence was prevented with a 25-mg daily dose of pyrimethamine. Treatment with pyrimethamine alone seems to be another reasonable alternative therapy for *I. belli* infection in patients with sulfonamide allergy or intolerance *(47)*.

REFERENCES

1. Levine, N. D. Taxonomy and life cycles, in *The Biology of the Coccidia*, (Long, P. L., ed.) University Park Press, Baltimore, 1, 1982.
2. Faust, E. C., Russell, P. F., Jung, R. C. *Craig and Faust's Clinical Parasitology*, 8th ed., Lea & Fabiger, Philadelphia, 177, 1974.
3. Lumb, R. and Hardiman, R. *Isospora belli* infection: a report of two cases in patients with AIDS. *Med. J. Aust.*, 155, 194–196, 1991.
4. Lindsay, D. S., Dubey, J. P., and Blagburn, B. L. Biology of *Isospora* spp. from humans, nonhuman primates, and domestic animals. *Clin. Microbiol. Rev.*, 10, 19–34, 1997.
5. Morakote, N., Muangimpong, Y., Somboon, P., Khamboonruang, C. Acute human isosporiasis in Thailand: a case report. *S. E. Asian. J. Trop. Med. Pub. Health*, 18, 107–117, 1987.
6. Shein, R. and Gelb, A. *Isospora belli* in a patient with acquired immunodeficiency syndrome. *J. Clin. Gastroenterol.*, 6, 525.
7. Rogowska-Szadkowska, D. Parasitic infectons in AIDS. *Wiad. Parazytol.*, 42, 145, 196.
8. Risse, J. H., Adam, G., Langen, H. J., Biesterfeld, S., and Hoffmann, R. Intestinal strongyloidiasis and isosporiasis in AIDS. *Rofo. Fortschr. Geb. Rontgenstr. Neuen Bildgeb. Verfahr.*, 161, 564, 1994.
9. Chaika, N. A. Isosporiasis and AIDS. *Med. Parazitol. (Mosk.)*, (3), 45–48, 1993.
10. Shekhar, K. C., Ng, K. P., and Rokiah, I. Human isosporiasis in an AIDS patient—report of first case in Malaysia. *Med. J. Malaysia*, 48, 355–360, 1993
11. Wittner, M., Tanowitz, H. B., and Weiss, L. M. Parasitic infections in AIDS patients: cryptosporidiosis, isosporiasis, microsporidiosis, cyclosporiasis. *Infect. Dis. Clin. North Am.*, 7, 569–586.
12. Sakamoto, M., Adachi, T., Sagara, H., and Izeki, M. A case of AIDS complicated with isosporiasis as initial manifestation. *Kansenshogaku Zasshi*, 72, 643–646, 1998
13. Pape, J. W., Verdier, R. I., Boncy, M., Boncy, J., and Johnson, W. D., Jr.*Cyclospora* infection in adults infected with HIV. Clinical manifestations, treatment, and prophylaxis. *Ann. Intern. Med.*, 121, 654–65, 1994..
14. Peng, C. Y. and Tsai, W. *Isospora belli* infection in a patient with Hodgkin's disease: report of a case. *J. Formos. Med. Assoc.*, 90, 260–263, 1991.
15. Massey, A. C., Weinstein, D. L., Petri, W. A., Williams, M. E., and Hess, C. E. ATLL complicated by strongyloidiasis and isosporiasis: case report. *Va. Med. Q.*, 117, 311–316, 1990.
16. Skinner, J. I. Human infection with *Isospora belli* in England: a case report. *J. Med. Microbiol.*, 5, 271, 1972.
17. Sorvillo, F., Lieb, L., Iwakoshi, K., and Waterman, S. H. *Isospora belli* and the acquired immunodeficiency syndrome. *N. Engl. J. Med.*, 322, 131, 1990.
18. Butler, T. and De Boer, W. G.R. M. (1981) *Isospora belli* infection in Australia. *Pathology*, 13, 593, 1981.
19. Shaffer, N. and Moore, L. Chronic traveller's diarrhea in a normal host due to *Isospora belli*. *J. Infect. Dis.*, 159, 596, 1989.
20. Sorvillo, F. J., Lieb, L. E., Seidel, J., Kerndt, P., Turner, J., and Ash, L. R. Epidemiology of isosporiasis among persons with acquired immunodeficiency syndrome in Los Angeles County. *Am. J. Trop. Med. Hyg.*, 53, 656–659, 1995.
21. Bernard, E., Delgiudice, P., Carles, M., et al. Disseminated isosporiasis in an AIDS patient. *Eur. J. Clin. Microbiol. Infect. Dis.*, 16, 699–701, 1997.
22. Michiels, J. F., Hofman, P., Bernard, E., et al. Intestinal and extraintestinal *Isospora belli* infection in an AIDS patient. A second case report. *Pathol. Res. Pract.*, 190, 1089–1093, 1994.
23. Selik, R. M., Karon, J. M., and Ward, J. W. Effect of the human immunodeficiency virus epidemic on mortality from opportunistic infections in the United States in 1993. *J. Infect. Dis.*, 176, 632–636, 1997.
24. Yoon, D. H., Yang, S. J., Kim, J. S., et al.A case of fatal malabsorption syndrome caused by strongyloidiasis complicated with isosporiasis and human cytomegalovirus infection. *Kisaengchunghak Chapchi*, 30, 53–58, 1992.
25. DeHovitz, J. A., Pape, J. W., Boncy, M., and Johnson, W. D. Jr. Clinical manifestations and therapy of *Isospora belli* in patients with acquired immunodeficiency syndrome. *N. Engl. J. Med.*, 315, 87–90, 1986.
26. Soave, R. and Johnson, W. D., Jr. *Cryptosporidium* and *Isospora belli* infections. *J. Infect. Dis.*, 157, 225–229, 1988.
27. Soave, R. Cryptosporidiosis and isosporiasis in patients with AIDS. *Infect. Dis. Clin. North Am.*, 2, 485, 1988.
28. Brandborg, L., Goldberg, S. B., and Briedenbach, W. C. Human coccidiosis: a possible cause of malabsorption: the life cycle in small-bowel mucosal biopsies as a diagnostic feature. *N. Engl. J. Med.*, 283, 1306, 1970.
29. Trier, J. S., Moxey, P. C., Schimmel, E. M., and Robles, E. Chronic intestinal coccidiosis in man: intestinal morphology and response to treatment. *Gastroenterology*, 66, 923, 1974.
30. Faust, E. C., Giraldo, L. E., Caicedo, G., and Bonfante, R. Human isosporiasis in the Western Hemisphere. *Am. J. Trop. Med. Hyg.*, 10, 343, 1961.
31. Forthal, D. N. and Guest, S. S. *Isospora belli* enteritis in three homosexual men. *Am. J. Trop. Med. Hyg.*, 33, 1060, 1984.
32. Liebman, W. M., Thaler, M. M., DeLorimier, A., Brandborg, L. L., and Goodman, J. Intractable diarrhea of infancy due to intestinal coccidiosis. *Gastroenterology*, 78, 579, 1980.
33. Ma, P., Kaufman D., and Montana, J. *Isospora belli* diarrheal infection in homosexual men. *AIDS Res.*, 1, 327–338, 1983.

34. Restrepo, C., Macher, A. M., and Radany, E. H. Disseminated extraintestinal isosporiasis in a patient with acquired immune deficiency syndrome. *Am. J. Clin. Pathol.*, 87, 536, 1987.
35. Westerman, E. L. and Christensen, R. P. Chronic *Isospora belli* infection treated with co- trimoxazole. *Ann. Intern. Med.*, 91, 413, 1979.
36. Hermier, M., Mojon, M., Piens, M. A., Louis, J. J., and Descos, B. Severe form of isosporiasis caused by *Isospora hominis*. *Pediatrie*, 36, 211–216, 1981.
37. Gorricho Mendevil, J., Torres Sopena, L., Paradineiro Somoza, J. C., and Moles Calandre, B. Treatment of recurrent *Isospora belli* diarrhea. *Rev. Esp. Enferm. Dig.*, 87, 612, 1995.
38. Gerberding, J. L. Diagnosis and management of HIV-infected patients with diarrhoea. *J. Antimicrob. Chemother.*, 23(Suppl. A), 83, 1989.
39. Gelb, A. and Miller, S. AIDS and gastroenterology. *Am. J. Gastroenter.*, 81, 619, 1986.
40. Santana Ane, M., Villaverde Ane, B., Morales Landrove, A., and Perez Avila, J. HIV infection and isosporiasis. Presentation of a case. *Rev. Cubana Med. Trop.*, 49, 142–144, 1997.
41. Pape, J. W., Verdier, R. I., and Johnson, W. D. Jr. Treatment and prophylaxis of *Isospora belli* infection in patients with the acquired immunodeficiency syndrome. *N. Engl. J. Med.*, 320, 1044–1047, 1989.
42. Deluol, A. M., Cenac, J., Michon, C., Matheron, S., Coulaud, J. P., and Savel, J. 11 cases of isosporiasis (*Isospora belli*) in patients with AIDS. *Bull. Soc. Pathol. Exot. Filiales*, 81, 164–172, 1988.
43. Verdier, R. I., Fitzgerald, D. W., Johnson, W. D., Jr., and Pape, J. W. Trimethoprim- sulfamethoxazole compared with ciprofloxacin for treatment and prophylaxis of *Isospora belli* and *Cyclospora cayetanensis* infection in HIV-infected patients. A randomized, controlled trial. *Ann. Intern. Med.*, 132, 885–888, 2000.
44. Limson-Pobre, R. N., Merrick, S., Gruen, D., and Soave, R. Use of diclazuril for the treatment of isosporiasis in patients with AIDS. *Clin. Infect. Dis.*, 20, 201–202, 1995.
45. Gordin, F. M., Simon, G. L., Wofsy, C. B., and Mills, J., Adverse reactions to thrimethoprim- sulfamethoxazole in patients with the acquired immunodeficiency syndrome. *Ann. Intern. Med.*, 100, 495–499, 1984.
46. Dionisio, D., Sterrantino, G., Meli, M., Leoncini, F., Orsi, A., and Nicoletti, P., Treatment of isosporiasis with combined albendazole and ornidazole in patients with AIDS. *AIDS*, 10, 1301–1302, 1996.
47. Weiss, L. M., Perlman, D. C., Sherman, J., Tanowitz, H., and Wittner, M.,*Isospora belli* infection: treatment with pyrimethamine. *Ann. Intern. Med.*, 109, 474–475, 1988.
48. Ballal, M., Prabhu, T., Chandran, A., and Shivananda, P. G., *Cryptosporidium* and *Isospora belli* diarrhoea in immunocompromised hosts. *Indian J. Cancer*, 36, 38–42, 1999.

15
Toxoplasma gondii

1. INTRODUCTION

Toxoplasma is a genus of coccidian protozoa classified into the suborder Eimeriina, order Eucoccidiida, comprising intracellular parasites of many organs and tissues of birds and mammals, including humans. The only known complete hosts of these parasites are cats and other Felidae, in which both asexual and sexual developmental cycles occur in the intestinal epithelium, culminating in the passage of oocysts in the feces. The intestinal stages do not occur in other hosts.

Toxoplasma gondii is considered to be the causative agent of toxoplasmosis. It is a widespread intracellular parasite infecting wide range of birds and mammals, including humans. The sexual cycle of the organism takes place in the intestinal epithelium of the cat, which is the definitive host. *T. gondii* exists in three forms: tachyzoite, tissue cysts (pseudocysts), and oocysts.

Although persistence of *Toxoplasma* cysts within host tissues may contribute to maintenance of immunity against reinfection, their presence may also represent, under certain conditions, a potential danger for reactivation of infection, especially in immunocompromised patients and infants with congenital toxoplasmosis (1).

Transmission of infection is caused by ingestion of either parenteral cysts (trophozoites) from raw, uncooked infected meat, or oocysts from feces of domestic pets (cats), by transplantation of infected organs (2,3), tainted blood transfusion (4), or even accidental inoculation in a laboratory setting (5). In immunocompetent hosts, toxoplasmosis is asymptomatic and benign (6,7). The incidence of the disease is most frequent between 16 and 25 yr of age (8).

Human toxoplasmosis is expressed either as congenital or acquired. Congenital toxoplasmosis is present in newborn infants and is characterized by encephalitis, rash, jaundice, and hepatomegally, usually associated with chorioretinitis, hydrocephalus, and microcephaly, and with high mortality rate (9–11). *T. gondii* can be transmitted from mother to fetus during primary maternal infection acquired after, or possibly slightly before, conception (12). The incidence of congenital toxoplasmosis is highest in the third trimester, whereas severity is most pronounced when maternal infection is acquired during the first trimester (12). Studies of congenital toxoplasmosis in twins confirmed the definite role of the placenta in the modalities and mechanism of fetal contamination by *Toxoplamsa* (13).

By and large, acquired (i.e., noncongenital) toxoplasmosis is manifested by lymphadenopathy, fatigue or malaise, fever, sore throat, headache, myocardial disease, chorioretinitis, and seizures (6). The lymphadenopathy is most likely to be cervical (97%) with lymph nodes being usually enlarged, rubbery, and nontender. Lymphadenopathy may be also febrile, nonfebrile, or subclinical (8).

Chorioretinitis associated with toxoplasmosis is believed to be the most often infection of the posterior segment of the eye, which may also lead to blindness (14–16). Encysted *T. gondii* bradyzoites when persisting in ocular tissues may cause recurrence of the disease. Chemotherapeutic eradication of encysted bradyzoites from chronically infected tissues is usually hampered by the structure of the cyst walls, as well as the organism's low metabolism.

From: Opportunistic Infections: Treatment and Prophylaxis
By: Vassil St. Georgiev © Humana Press Inc., Totowa, NJ

Cerebral toxoplasmosis is manifested by fever, encephalitis, convulsions, delirium, lymphadenopathy, and mononuclear pleocytosis, followed by death. In the brain, *T. gondii* multiplies in the neurons and other cells, causing cellular and interstitial necrosis. Occasionally, the infarction necrosis may lead to formation of extensive lesions *(8,17)*.

Until recently, toxoplasmic encephalitis (TE) was diagnosed predominantly in immunocompromised patients with malignancies of the reticuloendothelial system or organ-transplant recipients *(3,18,19)*. However, after the advent of the AIDS epidemic TE has became one of the most common causes of encephalitis in this population *(20–28)*. Whereas toxoplasmosis comprised about 75% of all cases of nonviral infections in AIDS patients *(21)*, the incidence of central nervous system (CNS) toxoplasmosis alone was estimated in various reports to range between 3% and 44% *(20,23,29)*. It is believed that the occurrence of TE in AIDS patients has most likely been the result of reactivation of a latent infection rather than diagnosed as acute acquired infection *(10)*. A study encompassing 31 medical centers and 61 patients with AIDS, concluded that presently the overall prognosis of TE is poor; the median survival time following initiation of therapy was 4 mo *(30)*. Clinically, TE is characterized mainly with neurological disorders such as seizures, mental status change, coma, confusion, psychosis, anemia, as well as focal neurological abnormalities (hemiparesis, hemiplegia, hemisensory loss, cranial nerve palsies, aphasia, ataxia, and alexia), and meningeal symptoms *(22,23,31)*. Computerized axial tomography (CAT) has been of considerable help in diagnosing TE; mild to severe edema is observed on CT scan in almost every patient *(22)*. Lesions were rounded, single or multiple, and isodense or hypodense *(23)*. Furthermore, contrast studies have revealed the presence of ring or nodular enhancement in over 90% of patients *(32)*. Recently, magnetic resonance imaging (MRI) has been used to detect lesions not demonstrated by CAT *(18)*. It is recommended, therefore, that MRI be performed in seropositive AIDS patients with neurological signs or symptoms, even when the CAT scan does not produce evidence of TE *(18)*. In several reports *(33–36)*, the diagnosis and treatment strategies of CNS toxoplasmosis in AIDS patients have been reviewed.

Pulmonary toxoplasmosis in AIDS patients is the second most frequent localization after the brain *(37–39)*. Its frequency is estimated to be between 0.2 and 3.7%, and it is seldom identified prior to autopsy. Clinical manifestations include severe interstitial pneumonitis occurring in profoundly immunodeficient patients *(40)*. Disseminated *T. gondii* infection may also present with fulminant pneumonia *(41)*. In a retrospective and descriptive study of *T. gondii*-induced pneumonia in AIDS patients, Oksenhendler et al. *(42)* discussed the clinical presentation, diagnostic procedures, results of therapy, and hypotheses on the pathophysiology of the infection.

Cardiac *(43,44)* and liver *(45–47)* toxoplasmosis have been described in only a limited number of patients.

Besnier et al. *(48)* described a case of toxoplasmosis disseminated in the bladder of an AIDS patient.

Another rare case of reversible anterior bilateral opercular syndrome (Foix-Chavany-Marie syndrome) secondary to cerebral *Toxoplasma* abscesses has been described in an AIDS patient by Grassi et al. *(49)*.

2. TREATMENT OF TOXOPLASMOSIS

Current therapeutic strategies and future prospects for the treatment of congenital and acquired toxoplasmosis have been extensively reviewed *(50–55)*. One of the major problems confronting the development of successfull anti-*Toxoplasma* agents has been the ability of the parasite to differentiate from the actively growing tachyzoite form, which is susceptible to drug action, into the chronic, almost latent bradyzoite state, which is not susceptible and, therefore, cannot be eradicated by any of the currently known antitoxoplasmic agents. Because the bradyzoites remain as a source of recrudescing infection, drug therapy must be maintained for the life of the patient.

The molecular signals and mechanism(s) involved in the tachyzoite-bradyzoite interconversion are not known *(56)*. Blocking this differentiation process would be a major breakthrough in the cure of toxoplasmosis by preventing reactivation of the latent forms, and thereby attenuating disease progression. Similarly, stimulating bradyzoites to differentiate back to the drug-sensitive tachyzoites would facilitate chemotherapy that may completely clear the body of the protozoan *(56)*.

Therapy of congenital toxoplasmosis, in general, is based on spiramycin, which is capable of achieving high concentrations in the placenta; if the fetus is uninfected, pyrimethamine and sulfonamides are administered from the fourth month of pregnancy *(12)*. Lambotte *(57)* found prenatal therapy of congenital toxoplasmosis to be beneficial in reducing the frequency of infant infection. Derouin et al. *(58)* considered the potential of co-timoxazole for the prenatal prevention and treatment of toxoplasmic fetal death. Various options for prevention of ocular toxoplasmosis associated with congenital toxoplasmosis were discussed by Bloch-Michel *(59)*.

For primary therapy of toxoplasmosis in immunocompromised patients, in severe cases of the disease, and in congenital toxoplasmosis, treatment with synergistic combinations of either trimethoprim or pyrimethamine and sulfonamide (e.g., co-trimoxazole) have been widespread *(60)*.

Spiramycin, alone or in combination with pyrimethamine-sulfonamide, is used often in pregnant women with acute infection to prevent congenital toxoplasmosis *(51)*.

Clindamycin is utilized frequently for the management of acute flares of toxoplasmic chorioretinitis and as second-line therapy for toxoplasmic encephalitis in AIDS patients *(25,51)*. Holliman *(61)* discussed the effect of folate supplements in the therapy of cerebral toxoplasmosis, and Grange et al. *(62)* surveyed the therapy of *T. gondii*-induced myocarditis in AIDS patients.

Immunomodulating drugs such as interferon-γ (IFN-γ), alone or in combination with roxithromycin, were found effective in murine models of toxoplasmosis; interleukin (IL)-2 was also found to be effective in a murine model *(51)*.

When treating toxoplasmosis in immunocompromised patients, it is important to take into consideration the tendency of such patients to develop simultaneously other opportunistic diseases, such as cytomegalovirus (CMV) infection and *Pneumocystis carinii* pneumonia *(63)*. If it occurs, the management of such conditions would, undoubtedly, be very difficult. In this regard, gross alterations of the host microbial flora, as a result of excessive antimicrobial medication and unduly prolonged treatment, must be avoided in order to prevent undesired superinfections.

2.1. Pyrimethamine-Sulfonamide Combinations

Leport et al. *(31)* have treated 35 AIDS patients with TE with combination of pyrimethamine-sulfadiazine over a 30-mo period. The initial use of higher daily dose of pyrimethamine (50–100 mg instead of the conventional 25-mg dose) was justified because of the poor prognosis of cerebral toxoplasmosis. In spite of the higher dose regimen, only two of the patients experienced hematologic toxicity that warranted discontinuation of pyrimethamine therapy, whereas 31 patients showed improvement. Furthermore, of the 24 patients who were evaluable for long-term therapy, 14 (58%) achieved complete resolution and 10 had late clinical and/or CT scan sequelae. Reintroduction of the combination therapy resulted in complete resolution of relapse in 8 of 10 cases *(31)*. Gonzalez-Clemente et al. *(64)* also recommended the use of combination pyrimethamine-sulfadiazine for 3–6 wk to treat acute episodes of toxoplasmic encephalitis.

In an open randomized, multicenter trial, Podzamczer et al. *(65,66)* found no difference in the survival rate of HIV-infected patients with toxoplasmic encephalitis following a three times per wk regimen of pyrimethamine-sulfadiazine combination (consisting of 1.0 g of sulfadiazine given twice daily, 50 mg of pyrimethamine daily, and 15 mg of folinic acid) vs the same regimen administered daily (containing 25 mg of pyrimethamine instead).

Holliman *(67)* reported satisfactory response to sulfonamide-pyrimethamine medication of 20 AIDS patients with toxoplasmosis, although a high incidence of toxicity has been present. Wanke et al. *(68)* found that 11 of 13 AIDS patients with CNS toxoplasmosis receiving pyrimethamine-sulfadiazine combination showed clinical and radiologic improvement; toxic side effects included neutropenia, fever, and rash. Autopsies performed in five patients revealed evidence of *T. gondii* *(68)*. In one report *(69)*, treatment of AIDS patients having toxoplasmosis with pyrimethamine-sulfadiazine was found to produce complications in 29%, and serious complications in 8% of treated cases.

Pyrimethamine-sulfadiazine (1.0 g, q.i.d. and 25 mg, q.i.d, respectively)-resistant cerebral toxoplasmosis in AIDS patients has been reported *(70,71)*.

Contrary to previous reports *(72)*, which described successful therapy of cerebral toxoplasmosis using pyrimethamine and clindamycin in place of sulfadiazine, Bell et al. *(73)* observed progression of cerebral lesions in one patient receiving the pyrimethamine-clindamycin combination. It was this latter finding that necessitated sulfadiazine desensitization as a useful alternative. The sulfadiazine desensitization was carried out in three AIDS patients with cerebral toxoplasmosis and prior severe sulfonamide reactions (diffused maculopapular rash) *(73)*. The achieved maximum tolerated daily doses were 2.0 g of the drug in one patient and 4.0 g for the remaining two patients. Side effects comprised of transient fever, mild pruritis, and hyperglycemia (presumably exacerbated by the steroid given before desensitization) *(73)*. Tenant-Flowers et al. *(74)* conducted a study to assess the efficacy of a sulfadiazine desensitization protocol to treat patients with AIDS and cerebral toxoplasmosis and known sulfonamide allergy, and to ensure that an adequate dose of sulfadiazine (2.0–4.0 g daily) was achieved rapidly (within 4–5 d). Moreover, the effect of concurrent corticosteroid therapy on the success rate of the sulfadiazine regimen was also evaluated. The proposed desensitization protocol employed the oral administration of gradually increasing increments of sulfadiazine every 3 h over a 5-d period. The overall success rate of desensitization was reported to be 62%; seven patients achieved a final dose of 4.0 g daily, and for three patients the dose was 2.0 g daily. The concurrent corticosteroid administration did not appear to affect the outcome in the number of patients studied (total of 16) *(74)*. Gilquin et al. *(75)* also described an efficient protocol to induce tolerance towards sulfadiazine in an AIDS patient using betamethasone and dexchlorpheniramine.

Leport et al. *(76)* have assessed results from potential interactions of multiple drug regimens (pyrimethamine-clindamycin, pyrimethamine-sulfadiazine, and pyrimethamine alone) administered to 35 AIDS patients receiving maintenance therapy for toxoplasmosis. Adverse side effects were associated to pyrimethamine in 10 cases, to clindamycin in 7, and to sulfadiazine in 8 patients *(76)*. Pedrol et al. *(77)* concluded that an intermittent (2 d/wk) maintenance therapy for CNS toxoplasmosis with pyrimethamine-sulfadiazine combination was effective in preventing relapses in AIDS patients, although prospective randomized studies still remain to be done. The application of low-dose, alternate-day pyrimethamine medication as a maintenance therapy for cerebral toxoplasmosis in AIDS was also discussed *(78)*.

A Swiss HIV cohort study *(79)* had the objective of determining whether a long-term maintenance therapy for cerebral toxoplasmosis may be protective also against *Pneumocystis carinii* pneumonia in patients with AIDS. The medication applied consisted of either pyrimethamine-sulfonamides (in 50% of patients), pyrimethamine-clindamycin (in 25%), or pyrimethamine alone (in 9% of patients). Overall, patients with cerebral toxoplasmosis showed a low risk of subsequently developing *P. carinii* pneumonia, most likely due to the chronic suppressive effects of pyrimethamine and sulfonamides.

Twelve patients with toxoplasmic chorioretinitis were treated with fansidar (pyrimethamine and sulfadoxine at 25 and 500 mg/kg, respectively), starting with a loading zone of two tablets of fansidar, followed by one tablet daily; prednisone (0.5 mg/kg daily) was added and gradually tapered off. The duration of treatment was 21–50 d (median, 28 d). In 83% of patients, the scar was considerably smaller than the original lesion (on average 25% of original lesion), with no side effects observed *(80)*.

A case of severe dermatomyositis in association with high serum *Toxoplasma* antibody titers responded to treatment with pyrimethamine and sulfadiazine *(81)*.

In utero treatment of congenital toxoplasmosis with pyrimethamine-sulfadiazine has also been reported *(82,83)*. Mothers in 52 cases of toxoplasmic fetopathy (group 1) were treated in utero with combination of pyrimethamine and sulfadiazine (or sulfisoxazole), and with spiramycin *(83)*. The results were compared with those obtained from 51 other infants with congenital toxoplasmosis whose mothers (group 2) had received spiramycin alone. Furthermore, patients of both groups received the same medication of pyrimethamine-sulfadiazine and spiramycin after birth. Parasitologic examination of the placenta was positive in 42% for group 1, and 76.6% for group 2, while specific IgM titers in newborns were detected in 17.4% and 69.2% of cases, respectively; these findings indicated that prenatal treatment with pyrimethamine-sulfonamides resulted in less progressing infection at birth *(83)*. The limitations of prenatal therapy of congenital toxoplasmosis with pyrimethamine-sulfadiazine combination *(84)* and its passage through the placenta *(85)* have also been explored.

Cottrell *(86)* described the successful treatment of a 4-yr-old child with acquired toxoplasmic encephalitis using combination of pyrimethamine and sulfamidine for a period of 6 mo. Acquired toxoplasmic encephalitis in children, although not common, was first reported in 1941 *(87)*.

One case of toxoplasmosis complicated with myeloblastic leukemia was treated with pyrimethamine (50 mg daily) and sulfadimidine (1.0 g, 3 times daily); the therapy against myeloblastic leukemia was started prior to that and consisted of cytosine arabinoside and daunorubicine *(88)*. After two and half weeks of treatment (and still with leukemia in no relapse), the patient suffered profound thrombocytopenia and neutropenia (due to bone-marrow aplasia) from which the patient did not recover. The fatal outcome was attributed to the cumulative effect of antileukemia drugs and the combination pyrimethamine-sulfadimidine *(88)*. Commenting on this case, Price et al. *(89)* strongly suggested that pyrimethamine not only acted, as expected, as antagonist to dihydrofolate reductase, but also destroyed both normal and malignant stem cells during the DNA synthesis S-phase of the cell cycle. It is believed that prolonged administration of S-phase-active drugs will draw normal marrow stem cells out of their resting stage (G_0) and into the reproductive cycle. Such action will abolish the selective advantage of normal stem cells over malignant cells in response to chemotherapeutic drugs, thereby allowing the normally resting marrow cells to become vulnerable to antitumor agents (such as cytosine arabinoside and daunomycin) as they are being drawn into the cell cycle *(90–92)*.

Studying the mechanism of increased serum creatinine levels after administration of pyrimethamine and dapsone in healthy volunteers and HIV-infected patients, Opravil et al. *(93)* found that pyrimethamine inhibited the renal secretion of creatinine by what appeared to be a reversible inhibition of the renal tubular secretion of creatinine without affecting the glomerular filtration rate.

2.1.1. Acute Renal Failure to Sulfadiazine Therapy in AIDS Patients

Acute renal failure due to crystal deposition of sulfadiazine in the urinary tract should be of growing concern if appropriate prophylactic measures had not been taken promptly *(94–106)*.

Carbone et al. *(107)* have observed the presence of sulfadiazine-associated obstructive nephropathy in one patient with AIDS. According to Becker et al. *(97)*, due to the high prevalence of potential risk factors, the incidence of sulfadiazine-associated renal impairment was 1.9–7.5% in patients with AIDS compared with 1–4% in HIV-seronegative controls. Furthermore, its occurence appeared to be delayed in HIV-infected individuals with a median of 3 wk of medication compared with about 10 d in HIV-negative subjects; in conformance, the cumulative sulfadiazine dose at time of manifestation has doubled in AIDS patients (median of 84 g vs 40 g in controls).

Molina et al. *(108)* reported four cases of AIDS patients with toxoplasmic encephalitis who developed sulfadiazine-induced crystalluria after receiving combination of sulfadiazine and pyrimethamine. The crystalluria can rapidly reverse by rehydration and urine alkalinization *(97,101,108,109)*. It was recommended that after high doses of sulfadiazine, patients be adequately hydrated and their urinary pH maintained above 7.5 *(108)*. Diaz et al. *(95)* treated an AIDS patient with sulfadiazine-induced urolithiasis acute renal failure (acute lumbar pain, dysuria, urinary frequency, and hematuria) with intravenous fluids and alkalinization of the urine.

2.1.2. Adverse Cutaneous Reactions to Pyrimethamine Combinations in AIDS Patients

The value of various clinical and laboratory parameters in predicting the occurence of skin reactions in AIDS patients with toxoplasmic encephalitis induced by pyrimethamine combinations with either sulfadiazine or clindamycin, and the effects of continued therapy for patients with these reactions, have been studied retrospectively by Caumes et al. *(110)*. Seventy-five percent of patients (18 of 25) treated pyrimethamine-sulfadiazine developed cutaneous reactions after a mean of 11 d, whereas 58% (15 of 26) of patients who received pyrimethamine-clindamycin had cutaneous reactions after a mean of 13 d ($p = 0.56$). Nine (50%) of the 18 patients continued to receive pyrimethamine-sulfadiazine throughout the duration of hypersensitivity, compared with all 15 patients who were treated with pyrimethamine-clindamycin ($p = 0.002$). Thus, treatment throughout the duration of hypersensitivity is more likely to succeed for patients receiving the pyrimethamine-clindamycin combination, whereas therapy with pyrimetamine-sulfadiazine has been associated with more pronounced cutaneous side effects and a high risk of developing Lyell's syndrome and Stevens-Johnson syndrome *(110)*.

2.2. Trimethoprim-Sulfonamide Combinations

In patients with toxoplasmosis, therapy with trimethoprim (160 mg) and sulfamethoxazole (800 mg) daily for 10 d, resulted in a significant remission of symptoms *(111)*. Norrby et al. *(112)* treated five patients with lymphadenopathy due to toxoplasmosis with good therapeutic results by using co-trimoxazole for a period of 4 wk. No adverse effects on the bone marrow were observed during a 3-mo trial; however, a transient stomatitis was present, as well as allergic exanthema *(112)*. In another study, Norrby and Eilard *(113)* described one case of recurrent toxoplasmosis that required repeated (on three different occasions) treatment with co-trimoxazole. This and other reports *(114,115)* of recurrent toxoplasmosis (which seemed to be independent of the type of drug-combination therapy), would necessitate the need for long-term monitoring of patients, especially in those cases where an immune deficiency is present (or might be developed) resulting in increased virulence of the *Toxoplasma* pathogen.

Williams and Savage *(116)* have described as dramatic the recovery of a child with generalized toxoplasmosis following therapy with co-trimoxazole (400 mg sulfamethoxazole and 80 mg trimethoprim, twice daily for 1 mo). This result led to the recommendation that co-trimoxazole be used as the treatment of choice for acquired toxoplasmosis, especially in immunocompromised patients and cases of congenital toxoplasmosis. However, Remington *(117)* seriously questioned the recommendation of Williams and Savage.

Esposito et al. *(118)* described the use of co-trimoxazole in the management of cerebral encephalitis in AIDS patients showing severe hematologic damage caused by pyrimethamine and concurrent zidovudine therapy; the lesions completely resolved after 3 wk of therapy. Solbreux et al. *(119)* conducted a retrospective study on the use of co-trimoxazole as diagnostic support and treatment of suspected cerebral toxoplasmosis in AIDS patients. The drug was reported to be effective as evidenced by the improved clinical and radiological status. However, further prospective randomized therapeutic trials seem to be in order to confirm these observations.

Data by Jick *(120)* demonstrated that of 1,121 hospitalized patients receiving trimethoprim-sulfamethoxazole, only 91 (8%) experienced side effects attributed to this combination; the most common adverse reactions were gastrointestinal upset (nausea, vomiting, anorexia, and diarrhea) (3.9%) and skin reactions (erythema, urticaria, and itch) (3.3%).

2.3. Antibiotic Therapy of Toxoplasmosis

2.3.1. Spiramycin

Over the years, spiramycin has been used extensively in the treatment of human congenital toxoplasmosis *(121–126)*. Fetuses infected with *T. gondii* often developed impaired vision or neurologic disorders, even after 5 yr post-partum *(127)*. The risk of congenital infections due to acute toxoplasmosis acquired during the first trimester of pregnancy has been estimated at 15% *(122)*. Although such a risk is usually higher during the second (30%) and third (60%) trimesters, only acute toxoplasmosis acquired in the first trimester has been associated with severe congenital infections *(122)*. Alternating 3 wk of therapy with oral spiramycin with 2 wk of no treatment resulted in a diminished incidence of congenital toxoplasmosis from 61% to 23% *(121)*.

Hohfeld et al. *(128)* reported their experience in treating 98 cases of fetal *Toxoplasma* infection with spiramycin during pregnancy. Of the 52 pregnancies allowed to proceed, 43 were treated additionally with pyrimethamine and sulfonamides. After a mean follow-up period of 19 mo, 41 infants showed evidence of subclinical toxoplasmosis. The therapeutic efficacy of the additional treatment with pyrimethamine and sulfonamides was evidenced by a marked reduction of severe congenital toxoplasmosis and the relative decrease in the ratio of benign to subclinical forms *(128)*.

In a clinical trial involving 67 patients, Chodos and Habegger-Chodos *(129)* described spiramycin to be effective in treating posterior uveitis caused by *Toxoplasma*. However, Fajardo et al. *(130)* found that in 87 patients with posterior uveitis, therapy with combination pyrimethamine-sulfadiazine was superior to that of spiramycin (and/or steroids). In two other studies *(131,132)*, spiramycin was reported to be ineffective in treating toxoplasmic uveitis.

Timsit and Bloch-Michel *(133)* have studied 54 patients with active toxoplasmic chorioretinitis and found the therapy with pyrimethamine-sulfadiazine to be statistically more effective than a corresponding treatment with systemic steroids either given alone or in combination with spiramycin.

As reported by Descotes et al. *(134)*, there has been little serious toxicity associated with spiramycin. Contrary to other macrolide antibiotics, spiramycin was not damaging to the liver. It caused mild gastrointestinal disturbance, and allergic reactions were confined to transient skin eruptions *(134)*. Ostlere et al. *(135)* reported the development of allergy towards spiramycin during prophylactic treatment of fetal toxoplasmosis.

Kawakami et al. *(136)* described a case of dermatomyositis in a patient with toxoplasmosis, which was successfully cured with prednisolone for the dermatomyositis and acetylspiramycin for toxoplasmosis. Facial erythema and cervical lymphadenopathy preceded myalgia and muscle weakness of the extremities.

2.3.2. Clindamycin and Clindamycin-Pyrimethamine Combinations

Burke and Mills *(137)* described one case of acute toxoplasmic lymphadenitis treated with 600 mg daily of oral clindamycin. The therapy was continued for 28 d after which the patient was apyrexial and clinically well.

Dannemann et al. *(138)* have used clindamycin with promising results to treat 15 AIDS patients with toxoplasmic encephalitis *(139,140)* as part of either primary or alternative therapy. Eleven of the patients responded by clinical or radiologic improvement after receiving the antibiotic either alone or in combination with pyrimethamine. Twelve patients continued to receive oral clindamycin as suppressive therapy on outpatient basis. The adverse reactions of clindamycin were mainly diarrhea, reversible granulocytopenia, and skin reaction *(138)*. Westblom and Belshe *(141)* described as successful the treatment of cerebral toxoplasmosis in one AIDS patient using combination of intravenous clindamycin (600 mg, every 6 h) and pyrimethamine (25 mg daily) for 37 d. There was clinical improvement and complete resolution of CT scan abnormalities.

One side effect often associated with the use of clindamycin (as much as 80% of recorded cases) has been the development of colitis of pseudomembranous type *(142)*. Marcos et al. *(143)* have provided a protocol for clindamycin desensitization in an AIDS patient.

Rolston *(144,145)* reported treatment of four AIDS patients with clindamycin (1200–1800 mg daily) and pyrimethamine (25 mg daily); only oral clindamycin was used in the initial therapy (in an earlier study, Podzamczer and Gudiol *(146)* have used the antibiotic intravenously). Three of four patients who responded to the initial 8-wk regimen, also remained symptom-free through a maintenance therapy with oral clindamycin (600 mg daily) and pyrimethamine (25 mg daily), three times weekly for a period of 6–8 mo *(144)*. Previously, Kaplan et al. *(147)* recommended a dose regimen of 3,600 mg clindamycin daily, whereas Rolston and Hoy *(148)* applied 1200–2400 mg of the drug daily to treat three AIDS patients with TE.

Ruf and Pohle *(149)* found that in the treatment of AIDS patients with cerebral toxoplasmosis, combination regimens consisting of pyrimethamine, clindamycin, and spiramycin, and pyrimethamine-clindamycin proved to be equally effective, and that the addition of spiramycin did not provide additional benefit. Myelosuppressive side effects due to pyrimethamine prevented the addition of folinic acid at the start of the antitoxoplasmic therapy.

Dannemann et al. *(150)* reported interim results from an ongoing large-scale, prospective, randomized study to determine the potential role of clindamycin in the management of toxoplasmic encephalitis. Data were presented on 33 patients, 15 of whom received oral pyrimethamine and clindamycin (intravenously, then orally), and 18 of whom received pyrimethamine and sulfadiazine (both drugs given orally). The interim evaluation did not reveal any significant differences between the two regimens in the clinical and radiologic response. Both regimens caused similar adverse side effects; however, patients on pyrimethamine-clindamycin medication had more pronounced gastrointestinal side effects and more adverse hematologic reactions than those receiving pyrimethamine-sulfadiazine *(150)*. In a further report by Dannemann et al. *(151)*, a randomized unblinded phase II, multicenter clinical trial was conducted in California to compare the therapeutic efficacy of combination of pyrimethamine and clindamycin to that of pyrimethamine and sulfadiazine. The study allowed for crossover in the event of failure or intolerance of the assigned regimen. The patients were treated for 6 wk with pyrimethamine and folinic acid plus either sulfadiazine or clindamycin (the latter injected intravenously during the first 3 wk). The results of several end points for efficacy, when taken together, indicated that the relative efficacies of clindamycin and sulfadiazine appeared to be approximately the same. Hence, the use of clindamycin should be considered as an acceptable alternative to sulfadiazine in patients unable to tolerate sulfadiazine *(151)*.

Through the European Network for the Treatment of AIDS, a multicenter trial was conducted to compare, again, the potency and safety of pyrimethamine (50 mg daily)-clindamycin (2.4 mg daily) and pyrimethamine (50 mg daily)-sulfadiazine (4.0 mg daily) for treatment and maintenance therapy of toxoplasmic encephalitis *(152)*. The preliminary results have demonstrated that 77% of the 148 patients evaluated, responded completely or showed improvement with minor sequelae during therapy; 20% of the patients deteriorated. The adverse side effects consisted primarily of rash (52 patients), fever (31 patients), diarrhea (17 patients), and nausea (12 patients).

Fourteen AIDS patients with toxoplasmic encephalitis who were not treated with the standard regimen of pyrimethamine and sulfonamide because of previous history of bone-marrow suppression and severe allergic reactions to sulfonamide, were given instead pyrimethamine-clindamycin combination (both drugs were administered orally) *(153)*. The therapy comprised of pyrimethamine (first, a 100-mg loading dose, followed by 50 mg daily) and clindamycin (600–900 mg every 8 h); the duration of treatment was between 6 and 8 wk. All patients received oral folinic acid (15 mg daily). Complete or partial response was evident in all 14 patients at the end of 2 mo of primary therapy (10 of 14 patients showed complete resolution of clinical signs, and 8 of 14 patients showed complete resolution of neuroradiologic signs). All patients continued on a maintenance therapy of 25 mg daily of pyrimethamine, and 300 mg (every 6 h) or 450 mg (every 8 h) of clindamycin. Although no relapses were observed, symptoms that did not resolve at the end of the 2-mo period of acute therapy tended to remain unchanged *(153)*.

Leport et al. *(154)* have also conducted an open study in AIDS patients with brain toxoplasmosis using pyrimethamine-clindamycin combination. Cohn et al. *(155)* reported no difference in the survival of AIDS patients with toxoplasmic encephalitis who were treated continuously with either pyrimethamine-sulfadiazine or pyrimethamine-clindamycin (median therapy of 311 and 422 d, respectively; $p = 0.25$).

A combination of 5-fluorouracil and clindamycin was also used to treat a case of cerebral toxoplasmosis in AIDS *(156)*.

2.3.3. Clarithromycin

Clarithromycin (1.5–2.0 g) combined with pyrimetamine (25 mg) was used successfully (regression of neurologic signs and encephalitic abnormalities) to treat cerebral toxoplasmosis in two AIDS patients *(157)*. The use of clarithromycin-pyrimetamine was suggested as an alternative treatment of toxoplasmosis in AIDS patients who cannot receive or tolerate sulfonamides.

The role of clarithromycin-minocycline combination treatment *(158)* and in maintenance *(159)* therapies of toxoplasmosis in AIDS patients was also examined.

Alba et al. *(160)* have also reviewed the use of clarithromycin for the treatment of cerebral toxoplasmosis associated with HIV infection.

2.3.4. Azithromycin

A prospective study was conducted to evaluate azithromycin in combination with pyrimethamine for treatment of acute toxoplasmic encephalitis in AIDS patients *(161)*. Fourteen patients were given 75 mg of pyrimethamine and 500 mg azithromycin daily for 4 wk. Of the eight patients who were evaluable for clinical response, five responded favorably, one had an intermediate response, and two patients did not respond. Based on the adverse effects observed (rash, abnormal liver function, vomiting, and hypoacousia), it seemed that the azithromycin dosage used in the combination was not optimal.

Godofsky *(162)* has also described the use of azithromycin in the treatment of cerebral toxoplasmosis.

2.3.5. Doxycycline

Two reports of treating cerebral toxoplasmosis with combination of doxycycline and pyrimethamine have appeared *(163,164)*. Clinical improvement was described in a patient with AIDS and toxoplasmic encephalitis after daily treatment with doxycycline (400 mg) and pyrimethamine (25 mg)—CT scanning of the brain showed complete resolution of two ring-enhanced lesions within 5 wk of therapy *(164)*.

2.4. Atovaquone

So far, atovaquone has been studied in small number of patients ($n = 5-24$) with cerebral toxoplasmosis who were mostly unresponsive to conventional chemotherapy *(165–168)*. When given at doses of 750 mg, q.i.d., atovaquone produced a complete or partial radiologic response in 37–87.5% of patients. In the largest trial involving 87 patients after 6 wk of treatment, 35% of the patients had a partial clinical response and 12% had the disease stabilized, although the mortality rate associated with the disease reached 40%, 18 wk after initiation of therapy *(169)*.

Bouboulis et al. *(170)* used atovaquone to resolve successfully cerebral toxoplasmic lesions in a child and in an adult HIV-positive patient who failed to respond to conventional therapy with high-dose (3.0 mg/kg daily) pyrimethamine, as well as clindamycin, and azithromycin. A rapid oral desensitization was initiated in the adult patient because of maculopapular rash developed during the attempted treatment with pyrimetamine.

Schimkat et al. *(171)* described the successful treatment of bifocal ocular toxoplasmosis in an AIDS patient using 750 mg, t.i.d. of the drug; the infiltrates healed within 8 d leaving retinochoroidal scars. During maintenance therapy (atovaquone at 750 mg 3 times daily) two relapses had occured, but were successfully treated by increasing the dosage of atovaquone to 750 mg, q.i.d. and the addition of trimethoprim-sulfamethoxazole and clindamycin-pyrimethamine, respectively.

Durand et al. *(172)* reported a treatment failure of atovaquone in one patient with cerebral toxoplamosis.

In an uncontrolled, open-label study, Katlama et al. *(173)* have evaluated the efficacy and tolerance of atovaquone as a long-term maintenance therapy in patients with toxoplasmic encephalitis and intolerant to conventional anti-*Toxoplasma* drugs. The patients, who received 750 mg, q.i.d. of the drug were followed up for a mean period of 1 year. While 17 patients (26%) experienced a toxoplasmic encephalitis relapse, the survival probability was 70% at 1 yr after the episode of TE. The overall results suggested that atovaquone has been well-tolerated and effective maintenance therapy in patients who were intolerant to conventional anti-*Toxoplasma* drugs.

2.5. Trimetrexate

The therapeutic efficacy of trimetrexate has been evaluated in nine sulfonamide-intolerant AIDS patients and biopsy-proven cerebral toxoplasmosis *(174)*. Patients received trimetrexate (30–280 mg/m^2 daily) plus leucovorin (20–90 mg/m^2, every 6 h) for 28–149 d. Radiographic responses were documented in eight patients, and clinical responses in five patients. Despite the improvement, however, all patients showed both clinical and radiographic deterioration within 12–109 d of their initial improvement. The activity of trimetrexate administered alone, although dramatic in sulfonamide-intolerant patients, has been transient in nature, thereby making this drug inappropriate as a single-agent therapy for AIDS-associated toxoplasmosis *(174)*.

2.6. Management of Ocular Toxoplasmosis

The frequency of ocular toxoplasmosis in AIDS patients has been on the increase *(175)*. As reported by Chakroun et al. *(176)*, the incidence rose from 3.3% in 1983, to 6.1% in 1988, and 5.9% during the first trimester of 1989.

Blanc-Jouvan et al. *(177)* have described a case of *T. gondii*-associated chorioretinitis following liver transplantation. Peacock et al. *(178)* have identified bone-marrow transplant recipients who are seropositive for antibody to *T. gondii* and have findings consistent with previous *Toxoplasma* retinochoroiditis on pre-transplant ophthalmologic examination, as yet another high-risk population for reactivation of ocular toxoplasmosis in the early post-transplant period.

In 1991, Engstrom et al. *(179)* conducted a survey on the current practices for management of ocular toxoplasmosis. The results have shown the use of systemic corticosteroids as part of the initial treatment regimen in 95% of cases. Systemic corticosteroids are usually administered to patients having their vision threatened *(5)*. Patients with unilateral focal chorioretinitis (without associated old scars in the posterior pole) presumably caused by acquired toxoplasmosis, when treated with systemic or periocular corticosteroids not accompanied by antiparasitic medication showed rapid increase of inflamation *(180)*.

The most often used therapy for ocular toxoplasmosis *(181–184)* consisted of combination of pyrimethamine, sulfadiazine, and corticosteroids (32% of cases) *(185–187)*; or pyrimethamine, sulfadiazine, clindamycin and corticosteroids (27%) *(188)*; adjunct therapies involving photocoagulation, cryotherapy, or vitrectomy have been used in 33% of the cases *(188)*. In a typical example, Psilas et al. *(185)* reported positive response of patients with acute toxoplasmic chorioretinitis following treatment with sulfonamides, pyrimethamine, and corticosteroids for a period of 4 wk.

Rothova et al. *(189)* conducted a perspective multicenter study to evaluate the efficacy of therapeutic strategies for treatment of ocular toxoplasmosis in 106 patients. Medication was given for at least 4 wk and consisted of three combinations, namely, pyrimethamine, sulfadiazine and corticosteroids (group 1; 29 patients), clindamycin, sulfadiazine and corticosteroids (group 2; 37 patients), and co-trimoxazole (trimethoprim-sulfamethoxazole) and corticosteroids (group 3; 8 patients); patients with peripheral retinal lesions remained without systemic therapy (group 4; 32 patients). Patients from group 1 received leucovorin (5.0 mg twice weekly). No difference in the duration of inflammatory activity was noticed between the separate groups of patients. The investigators concluded that independently of the therapy given, the size of the retinal focus was the most important factor in predicting the duration of inflammatory activity ($p < 0.05$). There was a 52% reduction in the size of the retinal inflammatory focus in the pyrimethamine-treated patients, as compared with only 25% of untreated cases. The most frequently observed side effects of pyrimethamine treatment included hematologic complications (thrombocytopenia and leukopenia, despite the leucovorin medication) *(189)*.

Colin and Harie *(190)* conducted a prospective, randomized study in 29 patients with presumed toxoplasmic retinochoroiditis to compare the efficacy of oral pyrimethamine-sulfadiazine with subconjunctival injections of clindamycin. Results from both treatments showed no difference in the mean visual acuity after completion of therapy, with mean healing times being similar (1.80 mo for clindamycin, and 1.88 mo for pyrimethamine-sulfadiazine). At the 14 mo follow-up examination, recurrence of ocular toxoplasmosis developed in both groups: 21% (clindamycin) and 36% (pyrimethamine-sulfadiazine) of patients. In general, other than discomfort, the subconjunctival injection of clindamycin did not produce any significant adverse side effects, thus providing an useful alternative in the choice of anti-*Toxoplasma* ocular therapy *(190)*. A report by Hansen et al. *(191)* discussed the successful therapy of toxoplasmic retinochoroiditis following specific treatment with pyrimethamine, sulfamethoxydiazine, clindamycin, and spiramycin, in double or triple combinations.

After evaluating the data of 33 patients with active toxoplasmic retinochoroiditis that were followed up for 2–9 yr, Theodossiadis et al. *(192)* found no real differences between treatment with argon laser and medication in terms of success rate, time of regression of lesion recurrences, and complications. The regression of the active lesion in the laser-treated group was accomplished in 25–50 d, whereas in the medication-treated group it took 50–150 d.

Atovaquone at oral doses of 750 mg, q.i.d. resolved vitreal inflammation and improved visual acuity from 20/200 to 20/40 in a pediatric AIDS patient with toxoplasmic retinochoroiditis; there was no evidence of recurrence at 5 mo follow-up examination *(193)*.

Tassignon et al. *(194)* examined the intraocular penetration of anti-toxoplasmic drugs administered either by subconjunctival, retrobulbar, or intramuscular routes. Drug measurements were performed in the anterior chamber, the vitreous, and the retina-choroid of a healthy rabbit eye; the best results were obtained for spiramycin, trimethoprim-sulfamethoxazole, and clindamycin. The therapeutic efficacy on *Toxoplasma*-infected rabbit eye was investigated using indirect method; pyrimethamine, and especially doxycycline have shown the best results *(194)*.

Neuroretinitis is a distinct clinical entity consisting of moderate to severe visual loss, optic nerve head edema, macular exudate in a stellate pattern, and variable vitreous inflammation. Several cases of neuroretinitis associated with *T. gondii* infection have been described by Fish et al. *(195)*. Treatment with systemic antibiotics and corticosteroides resulted in restoration of visual acuity to 20/25 or better, thereby suggesting that although rare, toxoplasmic neuroretinitis is a potentially treatable ocular disorder.

Falcone et al. *(196)* described a case in which toxoplasmic papillitis was the initial manifestation of AIDS.

3. PROPHYLAXIS OF CEREBRAL TOXOPLASMOSIS

Immunocompromised patients (e.g., HIV-infected) with $CD4^+$ counts of less than 100 cells/μL should be given prophylaxis against toxoplamic encephalitis (Table 1).

In a comparative study to evaluate the efficacy and safety of three regimens for primary prophylaxis of toxoplasmic encephalitis, Antinori et al. *(198)* have found co-trimoxazole (160 mg trimethoprim and 800 mg sulfamethoxazole every other day) significantly reducing the risk of TE. The double-strength tablet daily dose of TMP-SMZ, which is recommended as the preferred regimen for *P. carinii* pneumonia prophylaxis, appeared to be effective against TE and has been recommended for this infection as well *(26)*.

If patients cannot tolerate TMP-SMZ, the combination dapsone-pyrimethamine (100 mg weekly dapsone and 25 mg biweekly pyrimethamine) was equally effective *(197)*. Aerozolized pentamidine (300 mg monthly) was found efficacious only against *Pneumocystis carinii* pneumonia. A similar finding was also reported by Nielsen et al. *(199)*.

Klinker et al. *(200)* used pyrimethamine alone (50 mg daily) as prophylaxis for toxoplasmic encephalitis in 56 patients with advanced HIV infection (38 patients with $CD4^+$ counts of <200 cells/μL) and presence of serum IgG antibodies to *T. gondii*. All patients received folinic acid (7.5 mg daily) as supplement. During prophylaxis (697 mo; mean, 12.5 ± 12.1) only one patient developed TE, and four patients had their treatment discontinued because of adverse side effects.

However, based on the results of a randomized trial in patients with advanced AIDS disease (absolute $CD4^+$ counts of <200 cells/μL) who had been treated with trimethoprim-sulfamethoxazole for

Table 1
Prophylaxis against Toxoplasmosis[a]

Patients	Indication	Prophylactic drug regimens	
		First line	Alternative line
Adults and adolescents	First episode: IgG antibody to *Toxoplasma* and CD4+ count <100 cells/μL	TMP-SMZ, one double-strength tablet, p.o., daily	TMP-SMZ, one single-strength tablet, p.o., daily; or Dapsone 50 mg, p.o., daily + pyrimethamine 50 mg, p.o., daily + leucovorine 25 mg, p.o., daily; or Atovaquone 1.5 g, p.o., daily (with or without pyrimethamine 25 mg, daily + leukovorin 10 p.o., daily;
	Prior toxoplasmic encephalitis	Sulfadiazine 0.5–1.0 g, p.o., daily + pyrimethamine 25–75 mg, p.o., daily + leucovorin 10–25 mg, p.o., daily	Clindamycin 0.3–0.45 g, p.o., every 6–8 h + pyrimethamine 25–75 mg, p.o., daily + leucovorin 10–25 mg p.o., daily; or Atovaquone 0.75 g, every 6–8 h (with or without pyrimethamine 25 mg, p.o., daily + leucovorin 10 mg, p.o., daily
Infants and children	First episode (IgG antibody to *Toxoplasma* and severe immunosuppression[b]	TMP-SMZ 150/750 mg/m²/d in 2 divided doses, p.o., daily	Dapsone[c] 2 mg/kg or 15 mg/m² (max. 25 mg), p.o. +pyrimethamine 1 mg/kg, p.o., daily + leucovorin 5 mg, p.o., every 3 d; or Atovaquone 30 mg/kg, p.o., daily[d]; or 45 mg/kg, p.o., daily[e]
	Prior toxoplasmic encephalitis	Sulfadiazine 85–120 mg/kg/d in 2–4 divided doses, p.o., daily + pyrimethamine 1 mg/kg or 15 mg/m² (max 25 mg), p.o., daily + leucovorin 5 mg, p.o., every 3 d	Clindamycin 20–30 mg/kg/d in 4 divided doses, p.o., daily + pyrimethamine 1 mg/kg, p.o., daily + leucovorin 5 mg, p.o. every 3 d

[a]Data taken from the U.S. Public Health Service and the Infectious Diseases Society of America guidelines for the prevention of opportunistic infections in persons infected with human immunodeficiency virus *(197)*.
[b]Generally recommended prophylactic drug regimens for infants and children.
[c]For children aged ≥1 mo.
[d]Recommended for infants aged 1–3 mo and >24 mo.
[e]Recommended for children aged 14–24 mo.

toxoplasmic encephalitis, additional prophylaxis for TE with pyrimethamine appeared unnecessary *(201)*. Still, Van Delden et al. *(202)* attributed the continuing occurence of toxoplasmic encephalitis among AIDS patients to the lack of prophylaxis; according to data obtained from a Swiss HIV cohort study, at least one-half of the cases of TE could have been prevented with a combination of prophylaxis, better motivation of physicians, and increased compliance of patients. High doses of co-trimoxazole prophylaxis appeared to be more effective than low doses in decreasing the risk of toxoplasmic encephalitis in HIV-infected patients *(203)*.

Meta-analysis of data from 16 trials by Saillourglenisson et al. *(204)* suggested that dapsone may be used safely as a primary prophylactic regimen for toxoplasmosis. In a randomized trial of HIV-infected patients, the combination of dapsone (50 mg, daily) and pyrimethamine (50 mg, weekly) plus leucovorin (25 mg, weekly) was found superior to co-trimoxazole as primary prophylaxis against toxoplasmosis as well as *P. carinii* pneumonia *(205)*.

The use of pyrimethamine in combination with folinic acid was found to be beneficial as secondary prophylaxis for ocular toxoplasmosis, and may be helpful in preventing recurrence of sight-threatening and/or frequent ocular toxoplasmosis *(206)*.

4. PROPHYLAXIS AGAINST TOXOPLASMOSIS AND HAART IN HIV-INFECTED PATIENTS

Recent reports have suggested that interruption of primary prophylaxis against toxoplasmosis in HIV patients receiving highly active antiretroviral therapy (HAART), may be possible when the $CD4^+$ counts surpass the 200 cells/µL treshhold *(197,207–214)*. However, data on the feasibility of discontinuing secondary prophylaxis are more scarce and involve a limited number of patients *(215)*.

Although reported results have lent credence to the efficiency of immune restoration following HAART and have been beneficial to patients *(216)*, because of the potential for reinfection *(207)* caution must be applied before making a decision based on immunologic and virologic consideration, especially shortly after instituting HAART *(217)*.

5. IMMUNOTHERAPY OF TOXOPLASMOSIS

Ultimately, the control of severe *Toxoplasma* infections will rest with the ability of the host to develop an adequate cell-mediated immune response. With the advance of recombinant lymphokines, as well as drugs capable of enhancing the cell-mediated immunity, immunotherapy alone or in conjunction with specific chemotherapy will play an increasing role in the management of toxoplasmosis, especially in immunocompromised patients *(18,218)*.

IFN-γ, with its pleiotropic adjuvant effects on host defenses, plays an active role in the development of appropriate cell-mediated immune responses by the host *(219)*. It is thought that endogenous IL-12 is required for the development and long-term maintenance of IFN-γ-dependent resistance against *T. gondii (220)*. The activation of microglia and astrocytes by IFN-γ or its combination with tumor-necrosis factor-α (TNF-α) appears to be an important effector mechanism in the host immunity. GM-CSF, IL-1β, and IL-6 may participate in this activation. Alternatively, IL-10 may play a pathogenic role by downregulating IFN-γ production *(221)*.

Administration of IFN-γ can enhance the antibody production and survival time of mice infected with *Toxoplasma (222)*. Furthermore, IFN-γ also augments the activity of natural killer (NK) cells and activates the macrophages, making these cells important factors in the development of viable host resistance against *Toxoplasma (18)*.

Fegies and Guerrero *(223)* used levamisole to boost the immune response in five patients with toxoplasmosis. The drug, when given alone (at 150 mg daily for 3 d, every 14 d during a 2-mo period), or in combination with trimethoprim-sulfamethoxazole (300 mg daily for 30 d) induced significant increase and normalization of the T-lymphocyte counts, and consequently, an enhancement of the cellular immune response with suppression of antitoxoplasmic antibody titers. The lower

T-lymphocyte counts in *T. gondii*-infected patients correlated with the depressed thymus activity found in *T. gondii*-infected animals *(223)*. Later, however, the results of Fegies and Guerrero were contradicted by Zastera et al. *(224)*, who did not find any activity of levamisole against experimental toxoplasmosis in mice; the drug was administered in the stomach at the same doses and schedule (2.5 mg/kg for 3 consecutive days, every 2 wk for a 2-mo period), as described in ref. *(223)*. The effect of levamisole on toxoplasmosis during pregnancy in guinea pigs was also investigated *(225)*.

REFERENCES

1. Nguyen, B. T. and Stadtsbaeder, S. Comparative effects of cotrimoxazole (trimethoprim- sulfamethoxazole), pyrimethamine-sulfadiazine and spiramycin during avirulent infection with *Toxoplasma gondii* (Beverley strain) in mice. *Br. J. Pharmacol.*, 79, 923, 1983.
2. Renoult, E., Biava, M. F., Hulin, C., Frimat, L., Hestin, D., and Kessler, M. Transmission of toxoplasmosis by renal transplant: a report of four cases. *Transplant. Proc.*, 28, 181, 1996.
3. Gallino, A., Maggiorini, M., Kiowski, W., et al. Toxoplasmosis in heart transplant recipients. *Eur. J. Clin. Microbiol. Infect. Dis.*, 15, 389, 1996.
4. Kimball, A. C., Kean, B. H., and Kellner, A. The risk of transmitting toxoplasmosis by blood transfusion. *Transfusion*, 5, 447, 1965.
5. Feldman, H. A. Toxoplasmosis. *N. Engl. J. Med.*, 279, 1370, 1968.
6. Jones, T. C., Kean, B. H., and Kimball, A. C. Acquired toxoplasmosis. *NY State J. Med.*, 69, 2237, 1969.
7. Bamford, C. R. Toxoplasmosis mimicking a brain abscess in an adult with treated scleroderma. *Neurology*, 25, 343, 1975.
8. Levine, N. D. *Protozoan Parasites of Domestic Animals and of Man*. Burgess Publishing Co., Minneapolis, 294, 1973.
9. Feldman, H. A. The clinical manifestations and laboratory diagnosis of toxoplasmosis. *J. Trop. Med. Hyg.*, 2, 420, 1953.
10. Feldman, H. A. and Miller, L. T. Congenital human toxoplasmosis. *Ann. NY Acad. Sci.*, 64, 180, 1956.
11. Conyn-van Spaendonck, M. A., van Knapen, F., and de Jong, P. T. Congenital toxoplasmosis. *Tijdschr. Kindergeneeskd.*, 58, 227, 1990.
12. Russo, M. and Calanti, B. Prevention of congenital toxoplasmosis. *Clin. Ter.*, 134, 383, 1990.
13. Couvreur, J., Thulliez, T., Daffos, F., et al. 6 cases of toxoplasmosis in twins. *Ann. Pediatr. (Paris)*, 38, 63, 1991.
14. Woods, A.C. Modern concepts of the etiology of uveitis. *Am. J. Ophthalmol.*, 50, 1170, 1960.
15. O'Connor, G. R. Ocular toxoplasmosis. *Jpn. J. Ophthalmol.*, 19, 1, 1975.
16. Pivetti-Pezzi, P., Accorinti, M., Tamburi, S., Ciapparoni, V., and Abdulaziz, M. A. Clinical features of toxoplasmic retinochoroiditis in patients with acquired immunodeficiency syndrome. *Ann. Ophthalmol.*, 26, 73, 1994.
17. Martin-Duverneuil, N., Cordoliani, Y. S., Sola-Martinez, M. T., Miaux, Y., Weill, A., and Chiras, J. Cerebral toxoplasmosis: neuroradiologic diagnosis and prognostic monitoring. *J. Neuroradiol.*, 22, 196, 1995.
18. Luft, B. J. and Remington, J. S. Toxoplasmic encephalitis. *J. Infect. Dis.*, 157, 1, 1988.
19. Rostaing, L., Baron, E., Fillola, O., et al. Toxoplasmosis in two renal transplant recipients: diagnosis by bone marrow aspiration. *Transplant. Proc.*, 27, 1733, 1995.
20. Luft, B. J. and Remington, J. S. Toxoplasmosis of the central nervous system, in *Current Clinical Topics in Infectious Diseases*, vol. 6, Remington, J. S. and Swartz, M. N., Eds. McGraw-Hill, New York, 315, 1985.
21. Levy, R. M., Bredersen, D. E., and Rosenblum, M. L. Neurobiological manifestations of the acquired immunodeficiency syndrome (AIDS): experience of UCSF and review of the literature. *J. Neurosurg.*, 621, 475, 1985.
22. Tuazon, C. U. Toxoplasmosis in AIDS patients. *J. Antimicrob. Chemother.*, 23(Suppl. A), 77, 1989.
23. Ferrer, S., Fuentes, I., Domingo, P., et al., Cerebral toxoplasmosis in patients with human immunodeficiency virus (HIV) infection: clinico-radiological and therapeutic aspects in 63 patients. *Ann. Med. Intl.*, 13, 4, 1996.
24. Winstanley, P. Drug treatment of toxoplasmic encephalitis in acquired immunodeficiency syndrome. *Postgrad. Med. J.*, 71, 404, 1995.
25. Luft, B. J., Hafner, R., Korzun, A. H., et al. Toxoplasmic encephalitis in patients with the acquired immunodeficiency syndrome. *N. Engl. J. Med.*, 329, 995, 1993.
26. Carr, A., Tindall, B., Brew, B. J., et al. Low-dose trimethoprim-sulfamethoxazole prophylaxis for toxoplasmic encephalitis in patients with AIDS, *Ann. Intern. Med.*, 117, 106- 111, 1992.
27. Alappat, J. P., Mathew, C. F., Jayakumar, K., Suresh, I. C., and Kumar, S. A case of cerebral toxoplasmosis. *Neurol. India*, 48, 185–187, 2000.
28. Schlager, S. I., Management of opportunistic infections in acquired immunodeficiency syndrome. I. Treatment. *Am. J. Ther.*, 5, 45–49, 1998.
29. Wilson, C. B., Remington, J. S., Stagno, S., and Reynolds, D. W. Development of adverse sequelae in children born with subclinical congenital *Toxoplasma* infection. *Pediatrics*, 66, 767, 1980.
30. Haverkos, H. W. (coordinator), Assessment of therapy for *Toxoplasma* encephalitis. The TE Study Group. *Am. J. Med.*, 82, 907, 1987.
31. Leport, C., Raffi, F., Metherton, S., et al. Treatment of central nervous system toxoplasmosis with pyrimethamine/ sulfadiazine combination in 35 patients with acquired immunodeficiency syndrome: efficacy of long-term continuous therapy. *Am. J. Med.*, 84, 94, 1988.

32. Post, M. J. D., Kusunoglu, S. J., Hensley, C. T., Chan, J. C., Moskowitz, L. B., and Hoffman, T. A. Cranial CT in acquired immunodeficiency syndrome: spectrum of diseases and optimal contrast enhancement technique. *Am. J. Radiol.*, 145, 929, 1985.
33. Tuazon, C. U. Toxoplasmosis in AIDS patients. *J. Antimicrob. Chemother.*, 23(Suppl. A), 77, 1989.
34. Altes, J., Salas, A., Ricart, C., Villalonga, C., Riera, M., and Casquero, P. Cerebral toxoplasmosis in patients with AIDS. *Arch. Neurobiol. (Madr.)*, 52(Suppl. 1), 121, 1989.
35. Carrazana, E. J., Rossitch, E. Jr., and Samuels, M. A. Cerebral toxoplasmosis in the acquired immune deficiency syndrome. *Clin. Neurol. Neurosurg.*, 91, 291, 1989.
36. Artigas, J., Grosse, G., Niedobitek, F., Kassner, M., Risch, W., and Heise, W., Severe toxoplasmic ventriculomeningoencephalomyelitis in two AIDS patients following treatment of cerebral toxoplasmic granuloma. *Clin. Neuropathol.*, 13, 120, 1994.
37. Mortier, E., Poirot, J. L., Marteau, M., et al. Pulmonary toxoplasmosis in patients with human immunodeficiency virus infection: 21 cases. *Presse Med.*, 25, 485, 1996.
38. Halme, M., Jokipil, L., Jokipil, A. M., Ristola, M., and Lahdevirta, J. *Toxoplasma* pneumonia in a patient with AIDS. *J. Infect.*, 31, 252, 1995.
39. Gadea, I., Cuenca, M., Benito, N., Pereda, J. M., and Soriano, F. Bronchoalveolar lavage for the diagnosis of disseminated toxoplasmosis in AIDS patients. *Diagn. Microbiol. Infect. Dis.*, 22, 339, 1995.
40. Knani, L., Bouslama, K., Varette, C., et al. Pulmonary toxoplasmosis in AIDS: report of 3 cases. *Ann. Med. Interne (Paris)*, 141, 469, 1990.
41. Miller, R. F., Lucas, S. B., and Bateman, N. T. Disseminated *Toxoplasma gondii* infection presenting with a fulminant pneumonia. *Genitourin. Med.*, 72, 139, 1996.
42. Oksenhendler, E., Cadranel, J., Sarfati, C., et al. *Toxoplasma gondii* pneumonia in patients with the acquired immunodeficiency syndrome. *Am. J. Med.*, 88(5N), 18N, 1990.
43. Albrecht, H., Stellbrink, H. J., Fenske, S., Schafer, H., and Greten, H. Successfull treatment of *Toxoplasma gondii* myocarditis in an AIDS patient. *Eur. J. Clin. Microbiol. Infect. Dis.*, 13, 500, 1994.
44. Duffield, J. S., Jacob, A. J., and Miller, H. C. Recurrent, life-threatening atrioventricular dissociation associated with *Toxoplasma* myocarditis. *Heart*, 76, 453, 1996.
45. Mastroianni, A., Coronado, O., Scarani, P., Manfredi, R., and Chiodo, F. Liver toxoplasmosis and acquired immunodeficiency syndrome. *Recenti Prog. Med.*, 87, 353, 1996.
46. Bonacini, M., Kanel, G., and Alamy, M. Duodenal and hepatic toxoplasmosis in a patient with HIV infection: review of the literature. *Am. J. Gastroenterol.*, 91, 1838, 1996.
47. Kume, H. and Takai, T. Toxoplasmosis of the liver. *Ryoikibetsu Shokogun Shirizu*, (7), 93, 1995.
48. Besnier, J. M., Verdier, M., Cotty, F., Fétisof, F., Besancenez, A., and Choutet, P. Toxoplasmosis of the bladder in a patient with AIDS. *Clin. Infect. Dis.*, 21, 452, 1995.
49. Grassi, M. P., Borella, M., Clerici, F., Perin, C., Bini, M. T., and Mongoni, A. Reversible bilateral opercular syndrome secondary to AIDS-associated cerebral toxoplasmosis. *Ital. J. Neurol. Sci.*, 15, 115, 1994.
50. Piens, M. A. and Garir, J. P. New perspectives in the chemoprophylaxis of toxoplasmosis. *J. Chemother.*, 1, 46, 1989.
51. McCabe, R. E. and Oster, S. Current recommendations and future prospects in the treatment of *Toxoplasma*. *Drugs*, 38, 973, 1989.
52. Georgiev, V. St. Opportunistic/nosocomial infections: treatment and developmental therapeutics. Toxoplasmosis, *Med. Res. Rev.*, 13, 529, 1993.
53. Georgiev, V. St. Management of toxoplasmosis. *Drugs*, 48, 179, 1994.
54. Boyer, K. M. Diagnosis and treatment of congenital toxoplasmosis, *Adv. Pediatr. Infect. Dis.*, 11, 449, 1996.
55. Behbahani, R., Moshfeghi, M., and Baxter, J. D. Therapeutic approaches for AIDS-related toxoplasmosis. *Ann. Pharmacother.*, 29, 960, 1995 [see comment in *Ann. Pharmacother.*, 29, 1303, 1995].
56. Tomavo, S. and Boothroyd, J. C. (1995) Interconnection between organellar functions, development and drug resistance in the protozoan parasite. *Toxoplasma gondii. Int. J. Parasitol.*, 25, 1293.
57. Lambotte, R. Toxoplasmose congenitale: evaluation du benefice therapeutique prenatal. *J. Gynecol. Obstet. Biol. Reprod. (Paris)*, 5, 265, 1976.
58. Derouin, F., Jacqz-Aigrain, E., Thulliez, P., Couvreur, J., and Leport, C. Cotrimoxazole for prenatal treatment of congenital toxoplasmosis? *Parasitol. Today*, 16, 254–256, 2000.
59. Bloch-Michel, E. Ocular toxoplasmosis in 1989. *Bull. Soc. Belge Ophthalmol.*, 230, 53, 1989.
60. Finielz, P., Chuet, C., Ramdane, M., and Guiserix, J. Treatment of cerebral toxoplasmosis in AIDS with cotrimoxazole. *Presse Med.*, 24, 917, 1995.
61. Holliman, R. E. Folate supplements and the treatment of cerebral toxoplasmosis. *Scand. J. Infect. Dis.*, 21, 475, 1989.
62. Grange, F., Kinney, E. L., Monsuez, J. J., et al. Successful therapy for *Toxoplasma gondii* myocarditis in acquired immunodeficiency syndrome. *Am. Heart J.*, 120, 443, 1990.
63. McNamara, J. J. Antibiotic therapy in compromised hosts. *Calif. Med.*, 119, 49, 1973.
64. Gonzalez-Clemente, J. M., Miró, J. M., Pedrol, E., et al. Encephalic toxoplasmosis in patients with acquired immunodeficiency syndrome. A clinico-radiological study and the therapeutic results in 78 cases. *Med. Clin. (Barcelona)*, 95, 441, 1990.
65. Podamczer, D., Miró, J. M., Ferrer, E., et al. Thrice-weekly sulfadiazine-pyrimethamine for maintenance therapy of toxoplasmic encephalitis in HIV-infected patients. Spanish Toxoplasmosis Study Group. *Eur. J. Clin. Microbiol. Infect. Dis.*, 19, 89–95, 2000.
66. Podzamczer, D., Miró, J. M., Ferrer, E., and Gatell, J. M. Thrice-weekly vs. daily sulfadiazine-pyrimethamine (SP) for

maintenance therapy of toxoplasmic encephalitis (TE). *5th Conf. Retroviral Opportunistic Infect.*, Feb. 1–5, 167, abstract 468, 1998.
67. Holliman, R. E. Clinical and diagnostic findings in 20 patients with toxoplasmosis and acquired immune deficiency syndrome. *J. Med. Microbiol.*, 35, 1, 1991.
68. Wanke, C., Tuazon, C. U., Kovacs, A., et al. *Toxoplasma* encephalitis in patients with acquired immune deficiency syndrome: diagnosis and response to therapy. *Am. J. Trop. Med. Hyg.*, 36, 509, 1987.
69. Cimino, C., Lipton, R. B., Williams, A., Feraru, E., Harris, C., and Hirschfeld, A. The evaluation of patients with human immunodeficiency virus-related disorders and brain mass lesions. *Arch. Intern. Med.*, 151, 138l, 1991.
70. Langmann, P., Klinker, H., and Richter, E. Pyrimethamine-sulphadiazine resistant cerebral toxoplasmosis in AIDS. *Dtsch. Med. Wochenschr.*, 120, 780, 1995.
71. Huber, W., Bautz, W., Classen, M., and Schepp, W. Pyrimethamine-sulfadiazine resistant cerebral toxoplasmosis in AIDS. *Dtsch. Med. Wochenschr.*, 120, 60, 1995.
72. Luft, B. J., Brooks, R. G., Conley, P. K., McCabe, R. E., and Remington, J. S. Toxoplasmic encephalitis in patients with acquired immune deficiency syndrome. *J. Am. Med. Assoc.*, 252, 913, 1984.
73. Bell, E. T., Tapper, M. L., and Pollock, A. A. Sulphadiazine desensitization in AIDS patients. *Lancet*, 1, 163, 1985.
74. Tenant-Flowers, M., Boyle, M. J., Carey, D., et al. Sulphadiazine desensitization in patients with AIDS and cerebral toxoplasmosis. *AIDS*, 5, 311, 1991.
75. Gilquin, J., Magar, Y., Acar, J. F., and Blamontier, J. Induction de tolerance a la sulfadiazine chez un malade atteint de syndrome d'immunodeficit acquit. *Presse Med.*, 17, 2306, 1988.
76. Leport, C., Tournerie, C., Raguin, G., Fernandez-Martin, J., Niyongabo, T., and Vildé, J.-L. Long-term follow-up of patients with AIDS on maintenance therapy for toxoplasmosis. *Eur. J. Clin. Microbiol. Infect. Dis.*, 10, 191, 1991.
77. Pedrol, E., Gonzalez-Clemente, J. M., Gatell, J. M., et al. Central nervous system toxoplasmosis in AIDS patients: efficacy of an intermittent maintenance therapy. *AIDS*, 4, 511, 1990.
78. Bhatti, N. and Larson, E. Low-dose alternate-day pyrimethamine for maintenance therapy in cerebral toxoplasmosis complicating AIDS. *J. Infect.*, 21, 119, 1990.
79. Heald, A., Flepp, J. M., Chave, J. P., et al. Treatment for cerebral toxoplasmosis protects against *Pneumocystis carinii* pneumonia in patients with AIDS. *Ann. Intern. Med.*, 115, 760, 1991.
80. Michalova, K., Rihova, E., and Havlikova, M. Fansidar in the treatment of toxoplasmosis. *Cesk. Slov. Oftalmol.*, 52, 173, 1996.
81. Harland, C. C., Marsden, J.R., Vernon, S. A., and Allen, B. R. Dermatomyositis responding to treatment of associated toxoplasmosis. *Br. J. Dermatol.*, 125, 76, 1991.
82. Couvreur, J., In utero treatment of congenital toxoplasmosis with a pyrimethamine-sulfadiazine combination. *Presse Med.*, 20, 1136, 1991.
83. Couvreur, J., Thulliez, P., Daffos, F., et al. Fetal toxoplasmosis: in utero treatment with pyrimethamine sulfamides. *Arch. Fr. Pediatr.*, 48, 397, 1991.
84. Boulot, P., Pratlong, F., Sarda, P., et al. Limitations of prenatal treatment of congenital toxoplasmosis with a sulfadiazine-pyrimethamine combination. *Presse Med.*, 31, 570, 1990.
85. Dorangeon, P., Fay, R., Marx-Chemba, C., et al. Transplacental passage of the pyrimethamine-sulfadoxine combination in the prenatal treatment of congenital toxoplasmosis. *Presse Med.*, 19, 2036, 1990.
86. Cottrell, A. J. Acquired *Toxoplasma* encephalitis. *Arch. Dis. Child.*, 61, 84, 1986.
87. Sabin, A. B. Toxoplasmic encephalitis in children. *J. Am. Med. Assoc.*, 116, 801, 1941.
88. Rose, M. S., Black, P. J., and Barkhan, P. Fatal outcome after combined therapy for myeloblastic leukaemia and toxoplasmosis. *Lancet*, 1, 600, 1973.
89. Price, I. A., Bondy, P. K., and Ferench, G. E. Fatal outcome after combined therapy for myeloblastic leukaemia and toxoplasmosis. *Lancet*, 1, 727, 1973.
90. Bruce, W. R., Meeker, B. E., and Valeriote, F. A. Comparison of the sensitivity of normal hematopoietic and transplanted lymphoma colony-forming cells to chemotherapeutic agents administered in vivo. *J. Natl. Cancer Inst.*, 37, 233, 1966.
91. Valeriote, F. A. and Bruce, W. R. Comparison of the sensitivity of hematopoietic colony-forming cells in different proliferative states to vinblastine. *J. Natl. Cancer Inst.*, 38, 393, 1967.
92. Bruce, W. R. and Meeker, B. E. Comparison of the sensitivity of hematopoietic colony-forming cells in different proliferative states to 5-fluorouracil. *J. Natl. Cancer Inst.*, 38, 401, 1967.
93. Opravil, M., Keusch, G., and Luthy, R. Pyrimethamine inhibits renal secretion of creatinine. *Antimicrob. Agents Chemother.*, 37, 1056, 1993.
94. Simon, D. I., Brosius III, F. C., and Rothstein, D. M. Sulfadiazine crystalluria revisited: the treatment of *Toxoplasma* encephalitis in patients with acquired immunodeficiency syndrome. *Arch. Intern. Med.*, 150, 2379, 1990.
95. Diaz, F., Collazos, J., Mayo, J., and Martinez, E., Sulfadiazine-induced multiple urolithiasis and acute renal failure in a patient with AIDS and *Toxoplasma* encephalitis. *Ann. Pharmacother.*, 30, 41, 1996.
96. Rodriguez-Carballeira, M., Casagran, A., More, J., Argilaga, R., and Garcia, M. Acute renal insufficiency caused by sulfadiazine in a patient with cerebral toxoplasmosis and AIDS. *Enferm. Infecc. Microbiol. Clin.*, 14, 125, 1996.
97. Becker, K., Jablonowski, H., and Haussinger, D. Sulfadiazine-associated nephrotoxicity in patients with the acquired immunodeficiency syndrome. *Medicine (Baltimore)*, 75, 185, 1996.
98. Peh, C. A., Kimber, T. E., Shaw, D. R., and Clarkson, A. R. Acute renal failure due to sulphadiazine in a patient with acquired immunodeficiency syndrome (AIDS). *Aust. N. Z. J. Med.*, 25, 58, 1995.
99. Potter, J. L. and Kofron, W. G. Sulfadiazine/N^4-acetylsulfadiazine crystalluria in a patient with the acquired immune deficiency syndrome (AIDS). *Clin. Chim. Acta*, 230, 221, 1994.

100. Bressollette, L., Carlhant, D., Bellein, V., Morand, C., Mottier, D., and Riche, C. Crystalluria induced by sulfadiazine in an AIDS patient. *Therapy*, 49, 154, 1994.
101. Furrer, H., von Overbeck, J., Jaeger, P., and Hess, B. Sulfadiazine nephrolithiasis and nephropathy. *Schweiz. Med. Wochenschr.*, 124, 2100, 1994.
102. Marques, L. P., Madeira, E. P., and Santos, O. R. Renal alterations induced by sulfadiazine therapy in an AIDS patient. *Clin. Nephrol.*, 42, 68, 1994 [see comments in *Clin. Nephrol.*, 39, 254, 1993].
103. Kronawitter, U., Jacob, K., Zoller, W. G., Rauh, G., and Goebel, F. D. Acute kidney failure caused by sulfadiazine stones: a complication of the therapy of toxoplasmosis in AIDS. *Dtsch. Med. Wochenschr.*, 118, 1683, 1993.
104. Hein, R., Brunkhorst, R., Thon, W. F., Schedel, I., and Schmidt, R. E. Symptomatic sulfadiazine crystalluria in AIDS patients: a report of two cases. *Clin. Nephrol.*, 39, 254, 1993 [see comments in *Clin. Nephrol.*, 42, 68, 1994].
105. Farinas, M. C., Echevarria, S., Sampedro, I., et al. Renal failure due to sulphadiazine in AIDS patients with cerebral toxoplasmosis. *J. Intern. Med.*, 233, 365, 1993.
106. Diaz, F., Collazos, J., Mayo, J., and Martinez, E. Sulfadiazine-induced multiple urolithiasis and acute renal failure in a patient with AIDS and *Toxoplasma* encephalitis. *Ann. Pharmacother.*, 30, 41, 1996.
107. Carbone, L. G., Bendixen, B., and Appel, G. B. Sulfadiazine-associated obstructive nephropathy occuring in a patient with the acquired immunodeficiency syndrome. *Am. J. Kidney Dis.*, 12, 72, 1988.
108. Molina, J. M., Belefant, X., Doco-Lacompte, T., Idatte, J. M., and Modai, J., Sulfadiazine induced crystalluria in AIDS patients with *Toxoplasma* encephalitis. *AIDS*, 5, 587, 1991.
109. Oster, S., Hutchinson, F., and McCabe, R. Resolution of acute renal failure in toxoplasmic encephalitis despite continuance of sulfadiazine. *Rev. Infect. Dis.*, 12, 618, 1990.
110. Caumes, E., Bocquet, H., Guermonprez, G., et al. Adverse cutaneous reactions to pyrimethamine/sulfadiazine and pyrimethamine/clindamycin in patients with AIDS and toxoplasmic encephalitis. *Clin. Infect. Dis.*, 21, 656, 1995.
111. Lafrenz, M., Ziegler, K., Saender, R., Budde, E., and Naumann, G. Treatment of toxoplasmosis. *Muenchen. Med. Wochenschr.*, 115, 2057, 1973.
112. Norrby, R., Eilard, T., Svedhen, A., and Lycke, E. Treatment of toxoplasmosis with trimethoprim-sulphamethoxazole. *Scand. J. Infect. Dis.*, 7, 72, 1975.
113. Norrby, R. and Eilard, T. Recurrent toxoplasmosis. *Scand. J. Infect. Dis.*, 8, 275, 1976.
114. Burchall, J. J. Mechanism of action of trimethoprim-sulfamethoxazole. II. *J. Infect. Dis.*, 128(suppl.-Nov), S473, 1973.
115. Greenlee, J. E., Johnson, W. D. Jr., Campa, J. F., Adelman, L. S., and Sande, M. A. Adult cerebellar ataxia. *Ann. Intern. Med.*, 82, 367, 1975.
116. Williams, M. and Savage, D. C.L. Acquired toxoplasmosis in children. *Arch. Dis. Child.*, 53, 829, 1978.
117. Remington, J. S. Acquired toxoplasmosis in children. *Arch. Dis. Child.*, 55, 80, 1980.
118. Esposito, R., Lazzarin, A., Orlando, G., Gallo, M., and Foppa, C. U. ABC of AIDS: treatment of infections and antiviral agents. *Br. Med. J. (Clin. Res.)*, 295, 668, 1987.
119. Solbreux, P., Sonnet, J., and Zech, F. A retrospective study about the use of cotrimoxazole as diagnostic support and treatment of suspected cerebral toxoplasmosis in AIDS. *Acta Clin. Belg.*, 45, 85, 1990.
120. Jick, H. Adverse reactions to trimethoprim-sulfamethoxazole in hospitalized patients. *Rev. Infect. Dis.*, 4, 426, 1982.
121. Desmonts, G. and Couvreur, J. Congenital toxoplasmosis: a prospective study of the offspring of 542 women who acquired toxoplasmosis during pregnancy. Pathophysiology of congenital disease, in *Proc. 6th European Congr. Perinat. Med., Vienna*, Thalhammer, O., Baumgarten, K., and Polak, A., Eds. Georg Thieme, Stuttgart, 51, 1979.
122. Chang, H. R. and Pechère, J. C. Activity of spiramycin against *Toxoplasma gondii* in vitro, in experimental infections and in human infection. *J. Antimicrob. Chemother.*, 22(Suppl.), 87, 1988.
123. Martin, C. and Mahon, R. Traitment de la toxoplasmose. *Nouv. Presse Med.*, 2, 2202, 1974.
124. Desmonts, G. and Couvreur, J. Congenital toxoplasmosis: a prospective study of 378 pregnancies. *N. Engl. J. Med.*, 290, 1110, 1974.
125. Desmonts, G., Couvreur, J., and Thulliez, P. Prophylaxis of congenital toxoplasmosis: effects of spiramycin on placental injection. *J. Antimicrob. Chemother.*, 22(Suppl.), 193, 1988.
126. Fortier, B., Ajana, F., Pinto de Sousa, M. I., Aissi, E., and Camus, D. Prevention and treatment of materno-fetal toxoplasmosis. *Presse Med.*, 20, 1374, 1991.
127. Koppe, J. G., Loewer-Siegler, D. H., and De Roever-Bonnet, H. Results of 20-year follow-up of congenital toxoplasmosis. *Lancet*, 1, 254, 1986.
128. Hohfeld, P., Daffos, F., Thilliez, P., et al. Fetal toxoplasmosis: outcome of pregnancy and infant follow-up after in utero treatment. *J. Pediatr.*, 115, 765, 1989.
129. Chodos, J. B. and Habegger-Chodos, H. E. The treatment of ocular toxoplasmosis with spiramycin. *Arch. Ophthalmol.*, 65, 401, 1961.
130. Fajardo, R. V., Furguiele, F. P., and Leopold, J. M. Treatment of toxoplasmosis uveitis. *Arch. Ophthalmol.*, 67, 712, 1962.
131. Cassidy, J. V., Bahler, J. W., and Minken, M. V. Spiramycin for toxoplasmosis. *Am. J. Ophthalmol.*, 57, 227, 1964.
132. Canamucio, C. J., Hallet, J. W., and Leopold, J. M. Recurrence of treated toxoplasmic uveitis. *Am. J. Ophthalmol.*, 55, 1035, 1963.
133. Timsit, J. C. and Bloch-Michel, E. Efficacite de la chimiotherapie specifique dans la prevention des recidives des chorioretinitis toxoplasmiques dans les quatre annees qui suivent la traitment. *J. Fr. Ophthalmol.*, 10, 15, 1987.
134. Descotes, J., Vial, T., Delattre, D., and Evreux, J. C. Spiramycin: safety in man. *Antimicrob. Agents Chemother.*, 22(Suppl. B), 207, 1988.
135. Ostlere, L. S., Langtry, J. A., and Staughton, R. C. Allergy to spiramycin during prophylactic treatment of fetal toxoplasmosis. *Br. Med. J.*, 302, 970, 1991.

136. Kawakami, Y., Hayashi, J., Fujisaki, T., et al., A case of toxoplasmosis with dermatomyositis. *Kansenshogaku Zasshi*, 69, 1312, 1995.
137. Burke, G. J. and Mills, A. F. Toxoplasmosis and clindamycin. *S. Afr. Med. J.*, 55, 156, 1979.
138. Dannemann, B. R., Israelski, D. M., and Remington, J. S. Treatment of toxoplasmic encephalitis with intravenous clindamycin. *Arch. Intern. Med.*, 148, 2477, 1988.
139. Remington, J. S. and Vildé, J.-L., Clindamycin for *Toxoplasma* encephalitis in AIDS. *Lancet*, 338, 1142, 1991.
140. Santos Gil, I., Noguerado Asensio, A., del Arco Galan, C., and Garcia Polo, I. Clindamycin in the treatment of cerebral toxoplasmosis in a patient with AIDS. *Rev. Clin. Esp.*, 185, 47, 1989.
141. Westblom, T. U. and Belshe, R. B. Clindamycin therapy of cerebral toxoplasmosis in an AIDS patient. *Scand. J. Infect. Dis.*, 20, 561, 1988.
142. Goldsmith, J. M. Toxoplasmosis and clindamycin. *S. Afr. Med. J.*, 57, 37, 1980.
143. Marcos, C., Sopena, B., Luna, I., Gonzalez, R., de la Fuente, J., and Martinez-Vazquez, C. Clindamycin desensitization in an AIDS patient. *AIDS*, 9, 1201, 1995.
144. Rolston, K. V. I., Clindamycin in cerebral toxoplasmosis, *Am. J. Med.*, 85, 254, 1988.
145. Rolston, K. V. Treatment of acute toxoplasmosis with oral clindamycin. *Eur. J. Clin. Microbiol. Infect. Dis.*, 10, 181, 1991.
146. Podzamczer, D. and Gudiol, F. Clindamycin in cerebral toxoplasmosis. *Am. J. Med.*, 84, 800, 1988.
147. Kaplan, L., Wofsy, C., and Volberding, P. Treatment of patients with acquired immune deficiency syndrome and associated manifestations. *J. Am. Med. Assoc.*, 257, 1374, 1987.
148. Rolston, K. V. I. and Hoy, J. Role of clindamycin in the treatment of central nervous system toxoplasmosis. *Am. J. Med.*, 83, 551, 1987.
149. Ruf, B. and Pohle, H. D. Role of clindamycin in the treatment of acute toxoplasmosis of the central nervous system. *Eur. J. Clin. Microbiol. Infect. Dis.*, 10, 183, 1991.
150. Dannemann, B. R., McCutchan. J. A., Israelski, D. M., et al. Treatment of acute toxoplasmosis with intravenous clindamycin, *Eur. J. Clin. Microbiol. Infect. Dis.*, 10, 193, 1991.
151. Dannemann, B., MacCutchan, J. A., Israelski, D., et al. Treatment of toxoplasmic encephalitis in patients with AIDS: a randomized trial comparing pyrimethamine plus clindamycin to pyrimethamine plus sulfadiazine. *Ann. Intern. Med.*, 116, 33, 1992.
152. Katlama, C. Evaluation of the efficacy and safety of clindamycin plus pyrimethamine for induction and maintenance therapy of toxoplasmic encephalitis in AIDS. *Eur. J. Clin. Microbiol. Infect. Dis.*, 10, 189, 1991.
153. Foppa, C. U., Bini, T., Gregis, G., Lazzarin, A., Esposito, R., and Moroni, M. A retrospective study of primary and maintenance therapy of toxoplasmic encephalitis with oral clindamycin and pyrimethamine. *Eur. J. Clin. Microbiol. Infect. Dis.*, 10, 187, 1991.
154. Leport, C., Bastuji-Garin, S., Perronne, C., et al. An open study of the pyrimethamine-clindamycin combination in AIDS patients with brain toxoplasmosis. *J. Infect. Dis.*, 160, 557, 1989.
155. Cohn, J. A., McMeeking, A., Cohen, W., Jacobs, J., and Holzman, R. S., Evaluation of the policy of empiric treatment of suspected *Toxoplasma* encephalitis in patients with acquired immunodeficiency syndrome. *Am. J. Med.*, 86, 521, 1989.
156. Dhiver, C., Milandre, C., Poizot-Martin, I., Drogoul, M. P., Gastaut, J. L., and Gastaut, J. A., 5-Fluorouracil-clindamycin for treatment of cerebral toxoplasmosis. *AIDS*, 7, 143, 1993.
157. Dalston, M. O., Tavares, W., Bazin, A. R., Hahn, et al., Clarithromycin combined with pyrimethamine in cerebral toxoplasmosis: a report of 2 cases. *Rev. Soc. Bras. Med. Trop.*, 28, 409, 1995.
158. Lacassin, F., Schaffo, D., Perronne, C., Longuet, P., Leport, C., and Vildé, J.-L. Clarithromycin-minocycline combination as salvage therapy for toxoplasmosis in patients infected with human immunodeficiency virus. *Antimicrob. Agents Chemother.*, 39, 276, 1995.
159. Sellal, A., Rabaud, C., Amiel, C., Hoen, B., May, T., and Canton, Ph. Maintenance treatment of cerebral toxoplasmosis in AIDS: role of clarithromycin-minocycline combination. *Presse Med.*, 25, 509, 1996.
160. Alba, D., Molina, F., Ripoli, M. M., and del Arco, A. Clarithromycin in the treatment of cerebral toxoplasmosis associated with HIV infection. *Rev. Clin. Esp.*, 192, 458, 1993.
161. Saba, J., Morlat, P., Raffi, F., et al. Pyrimethamine plus azithromycin for treatment of acute toxoplasmic encephalitis in patients with AIDS. *Eur. J. Clin. Microbiol. Infect. Dis.*, 12, 853, 1993.
162. Godofsky, E. W. Treatment of presumed cerebral toxoplasmosis with azithromycin. *N. Engl. J. Med.*, 330, 575, 1994.
163. Valencia, M. E., Laguna, F., Soriano, V., and Gonzalez Lahoz, J. Favorable course of cerebral toxoplasmosis treated with doxycycline and pyrimetamine. *Rev. Clin. Esp.*, 192, 197, 1993.
164. Hagberg, L., Palmertz, B., and Lindberg, J. Doxycycline and pyrimethamine for toxoplasmic encephalitis. *Scand. J. Infect. Dis.*, 25, 157, 1993.
165. Clumeck, N., Katlama, C., Ferrero, T., et al., Atovaquone (1,4-hydroxynaphthoquinone, 566C80) in the treatment of acute cerebral toxoplasmosis (CT) in AIDS patients. *32nd Intersci. Conf. Antimicrob. Agents Chemother.*, American Society for Microbiology, Washington, DC, abstract 1217, 1992.
166. Grundman, M., Torres, R. A., Thorn, M., Hriso, and Britton, D. Neuroradiologic response to 566C80 salvage therapy for CNS toxoplasmosis. *Proc. VIIth Int. Conf. AIDS*, Amsterdam, 1992, abstract PoB 3185.
167. Kovacs, J. A. NIAID-Clinical CIAIDSP: efficacy of atovaquone in treatment of toxoplasmosis in patients with AIDS. *Lancet*, 340, 637, 1992.
168. Lafeuillade, A., Pellegrino, P., Poggi, C., et al. Efficacité de l'atovaquone dans les toxoplasmoses résistantes du SIDA. *Presse Med.*, 22, 1708, 1993.

169. Spencer, C. M. and Goa, K. L. Atovaquone: a review of its pharmacological properties and therapeutic efficacy in opportunistic infections. *Drugs*, 50, 176, 1995.
170. Bouboulis, D. A., Rubinstein, A., Shliozberg, J., Madden, J., and Frieri, M. Cerebral toxoplasmosis in childhood and adult HIV infection treated with 1,4-hydroxynaphthoquinone and rapid desensitization with pyrimethamine. *Ann. Allergy Asthma Immunol.*, 74, 491, 1995.
171. Schimkat, M., Althaus, C., Armbrecht, C., Jablonowski, H., and Sundmacher, R. Treatment of toxoplasmosis retinochoroiditis with atovaquone in an AIDS patient. *Klin. Monatsbl. Augenheilkd.*, 206, 173, 1995.
172. Durand, J. M., Cretel, E., Bagneres, D., Guillemot, E., Kaplanski, G., and Soubeyrand, J. Failure of atovaquone in the treatment of cerebral toxoplasmosis. *AIDS*, 9, 812, 1995.
173. Katlama, C., Mouthon, B., Gourdon, D., Lapierre, D., and Rousseau, F. Atovaquone as long-term suppressive therapy for toxoplasmic encephalitis in patients with AIDS and multiple drug intolerance. *AIDS*, 10, 1107, 1996.
174. Masur, H., Polis, M. A., Tuazon, C. U., et al. Salvage trial of trimetrexate-leucovorin for the treatment of cerebral toxoplasmosis in patients with AIDS. *J. Infect. Dis.*, 167, 1422, 1993.
175. Tabbara, K. F. Ocular toxoplasmosis: toxoplasmic retinochoroiditis. *Int. Ophthalmol. Clin.*, 35, 15, 1995.
176. Chakroun, M., Meyohas, M. C., Pelosse, B., et al. Ocular toxoplasmosis in AIDS. *Ann. Med. Interne (Paris)*, 141, 472, 1990.
177. Blanc-Jouvan M., Boibieux, A., Fleury, J., et al. Chorioretinitis following liver transplantation: detection of *Toxoplasma gondii* in aqueous humor. *Clin. Infect. Dis.*, 22, 184, 1996.
178. Peacock, J. E. Jr., Greven, C. M., Cruz, J. M., and Hurd, D. D. Reactivation of toxoplasmic retinochoroiditis in patients undergoing bone marrow transplantation: is there a role for chemoprophylaxis? *Bone Marrow Transplant.*, 15, 983, 1995.
179. Engstrom, R. E. Jr., Holland, G. N., Nussenblatt, R. B., and Jabs, D. A. Current practices in the management of ocular toxoplasmosis. *Am. J. Ophthalmol.*, 111, 601, 1991.
180. Ronday, M. J., Luyendijk, L., Baarsma, G. S., Bollemeijer, J. G., Van der Lelij, A., and Rothova, A. Presumed acquired ocular toxoplasmosis. *Arch. Ophthalmol.*, 113, 1524, 1995.
181. Mittelviefhaus, H. Treatment of ocular toxoplasmosis. Part 2: therapeutic approaches. *Kinderarztl. Prax.*, 61, 154, 1993.
182. Mittelviefhaus, H. Treatment of ocular toxoplasmosis. Part 1: basic principles and diagnosis. *Kinderarztl. Prax.*, 61, 90, 1993.
183. Rothova, A. Ocular involvement in toxoplasmosis. *Br. J. Ophthalmol.*, 77, 371, 1993 [correction in *Br. J. Ophthalmol.*, 77, 683, 1993].
184. Rothova, A., Meenken, C., Buitenhuis, H. J., et al. Therapy of ocular toxoplasmosis. *Am. J. Ophthalmol.*, 115, 517, 1993.
185. Psilas, K., Petroutsos, G., and Aspiotis, M. Treatment of toxoplasmosis. *J. Fr. Ophthalmol.*, 13, 551, 1990.
186. Lebech, A. M., Lebech, M., Borme, K. K., and Mathiesen, L. R. Toxoplasmosis- chorioretinitis: clinical course and treatment of seven patients. *Ugeskr. Laeger*, 158, 3935, 1996.
187. Holland, G. N. and Lewis, K. G. An update on current practices in the management of ocular toxoplasmosis. *Am. J. Opthamol.*, 134, 102–114, 2002.
188. Lam, S. and Tessler, H. H. Quadruple therapy for ocular toxoplasmosis. *Can. J. Ophthalmol.*, 28, 58, 1993.
189. Rothova, A., Buitenhuis, H. J., Meenken, C., et al. Therapy of ocular toxoplasmosis. *Int. Ophthalmol.*, 13, 415, 1989.
190. Colin, J. and Harie, J. C. Presumed toxoplasmic chorioretinitis: comparative study of treatment with pyrimethamine and sulfadiazine or clindamycin. *J. Fr. Ophthalmol.*, 12, 161, 1989.
191. Hansen, L. L., Nieuwenhuis, I., Hoeffken, G., and Heise, W. Retinitis in AIDS patients: diagnosis, follow-up and treatment. *Fortschr. Ophthalmol.*, 86, 232, 1988.
192. Theodossiadis, G. P., Koutsandrea C., and Tzonou, A. A comparative study concerning the treatment of active toxoplasmic retinochoroiditis with argon laser and medication (follow-up 2-9 years). *Ophthalmologica*, 199, 77, 1989.
193. Lopez, J. S., de Smet, M. D., Masur, H., Mueller, B. U., Pizzo, P. A., and Nessenblatt, R. B. Orally administered 566C80 for treatment of ocular toxoplasmosis in a patient with the acquired immunodeficiency syndrome. *Am. J. Ophthalmol.*, 113, 331, 1992.
194. Tassignon, M. J., Brihaye, M., De Meuter, F., Vercruysse, A., Van Hoof, F., and De Wilde, F. Efficacy of treatments in experimental toxoplasmosis. *Bull. Soc. Belge Ophthalmol.*, 230, 59, 1989.
195. Fish, R. H., Hoskins, J. C., and Kline, L. B. Toxoplasmosis neuroretinitis. *Ophthalmology*, 100, 1177, 1993.
196. Falcone, P. M., Notis, C., and Merhige, K. Toxoplasmic papillitis as the initial manifestation of acquired immunodeficiency syndrome. *Ann. Ophthalmol.*, 25, 56, 1993.
197. U.S. Public Health Service and Infectious Diseases Society of America. 1999 USPHS/IDSA guidelines for prevention of opportunistic infections in persons infected with human immunodeficiency virus. *Infect. Dis. Obstet. Gynecol.*, 8, 5–74, 2000.
198. Antinori, A., Murri, R., Ammassari, A., et al. Aerosolized pentamidine, cotrimoxazole and dapsone-pyrimethamine for primary prophylaxis of *Pneumocystis carinii* pneumonia and toxoplasmic encephalitis. *AIDS*, 9, 1343, 1995.
199. Nielsen, T. L., Jensen, B. N., Nelsing, S., Mathiesen, L. R., Skinhoj, P., and Nielsen, J. O. Randomized study of sulfamethoxazole-trimethoprim versus aerosolized pentamidine for secondary prophylaxis of *Pneumocystis carinii* pneumonia in patients with AIDS. *Scand. J. Infect. Dis.*, 27, 217, 1995.
200. Klinker, H., Langmann, P., and Richter, E. Pyrimethamine alone as prophylaxis for cerebral toxoplasmosis in patients with advanced HIV infection. *Infection*, 24, 324, 1996.

201. Jacobson, M. A., Besch, C. L., Child, C., et al. Primary prophylaxis with pyrimethamine for toxoplasmic encephalitis in patients with advanced human immunodeficiency virus disease: results of a randomized trial. *J. Infect. Dis.*, 169, 384, 1994.
202. Van Delden, C., Gabriel, V., Sudre, P., Flepp, M., von Overbeck, J., Hirschel, B., and the Swiss HIV Cohort Study. Reasons for failure of prevention of *Toxoplasma* encephalitis. *AIDS*, 10, 509, 1996.
203. Ribera, E., Fernandez-Sola, A., Juste, C., et al. Comparison of high and low doses of trimethoprim- sulfamethoxazole for primary prevention of toxoplasmic encephalitis in human immunodeficiency virus-infected patients. *Clin. Infect. Dis.*, 29, 1461–1466, 1999.
204. Saillourglenisson, F., Chene, G., Salmi, L. R., Hafner, R., and Salamon, R. Effet de la dapsone sur la survie des patients infectes par le VIH: une metanalyse des essais termines. *Rev. Epidemiol. Sante Publique*, 48, 17–30, 2000.
205. Antinori, A., Murri, R., Ammassari, A., et al. Risk of bacterial infections in a cohort of HIV-positive patients receiving anti *P. carinii/T. gondii* prophylaxis. *38th Intersci. Conf. Antimicrob. Agents Chemother.*, American Society of Microbiology, Washington DC, 549, abstract L-9, 1998.
206. Gourdon, F., Laurichesse, H., Dalens, H., et al. Ocular toxoplasmosis: clinical experience using pyrimethamine as secondary prophylaxis. *38th Intersci. Conf. Antimicrob. Agents Chemother.*, American Society of Microbiology, Washington DC, 566, abstract L-66, 1998.
207. Jubault, V., Pacanowski, J., Rabian, C., and Viard, J. P. Interruption of prophylaxis for major opportunistic infections in HIV-infected patients receiving triple combination antiretroviral therapy. *Ann. Med. Interne (Paris)*, 151, 163–168, 2000.
208. Maenza, J. Discontinuation of prophylaxis in HAART-responders. *Hopkins HIV Rep.*, 11, 2–3, 1999.
209. Furrer, H., Opravil, M., Bernasconi, E., Telenti, A., and Egger, M. Stopping primary prophylaxis in HIV-1-infected patients at high risk of *Toxoplasma* encephalitis. Swiss HIV Cohort Study. *Lancet*, 355(9222), 2217–2218, 2000.
210. Mussini, C., Pezotti, P., Govoni, A., et al. Discontinuation of primary prophylaxis for *Pneumocistis carinii* pneumonia and toxoplasmic encephalitis in human immunodeficiency virus type I-infected patients: the changes in opportunistic prophylaxis study. *J. Infect. Dis.*, 181, 1635–1642, 2000.
211. Guex, A. C., Radziwill, A. J., and Bucher, H. C. Discontinuation of secondary prophylaxis for toxoplasmic encephalitis in human immunodeficiency virus infection after immune restoration with highly active antiretroviral therapy. *Clin. Infect. Dis.*, 30, 602–603, 2000.
212. Antinori, A., Cingolani, A., Ammassari, A., Pezzotti, P., Murri, R., de Luca, A., Larocca, L. M., and Ortona, L. AIDS-related focal brain lesions in the era of HAART. *6th Conf. Retroviral Opportunistic Infect.*, Jan. 31–Feb. 4, 145, abstract 413, 1999.
213. Ravaux, I., Quinson, A. M., Chadapaud, S., and Gallais, H. Discontinue primary and secondary prophylaxis regimens in selected HIV-infected patients treated with HAART. *38th Intersci. Conf. Antimicrob. Agents Chemother.*, American Society of Microbiology, Washington DC, 429, abstract I-203, 1998.
214. Moore, R. D., Keruly, J. C., and Chaisson, R. E. Decline in CMV and other opportunistic diseases with combination antiretroviral therapy. *5th Conf. Retroviral Opportunistic Infect.*, Feb. 1–5, 113, abstract 184, 1998.
215. Soriano, V., Dona, C., Rodriguez-Rosado, R., Barreiro, P., and Gonzalez-Lahoz, J. Discontinuation of secondary prophylaxis for opportunistic infections in HIV-infected patients receiving highly active retroviral therapy. *AIDS*, 14, 383–386, 2000.
216. Michaels, S., Clark, R., and Kissinger, P. Differences in the incidence rates of opportunistic processes before and after the availability of protease inhibitors. *5th Conf. Retroviral Opportunistic Infect.*, Feb. 1–5, 112, abstract 180, 1998.
217. Rodriguez-Rosado, R., Soriano, V., Dona, C., and Gonzalez-Lahoz, J. Opportunistic infections shortly after beginning highly active retroactive antiretroviral therapy. *Antiviral Ther.*, 3, 229–231, 1998.
218. Krahenbuhl, J. L. and Remington, J. S. The immunology of toxoplasma and toxoplasmosis, in *Immunology of Parasitic Infections*, Cohen, S. and Warren, K. S., Eds. Blackwell, Oxford, 356, 1982.
219. Gallin, J. I., Farber, J. M., Holland, S. M., and Nitman, T. B. Interferon-gamma in the management of infectious diseases [clinical conference]. *Ann. Intern. Med.*, 123, 216, 1995 [see comments in *Ann. Intern. Med.*, 124, 1095, 1996].
220. Yap, G., Pesin, M., and Sher, A. Cutting edge: IL-12 is required for the maintenance of IFN-gamma production in T cells mediating chronic resistance to the intracellular pathogen. *Toxoplasma gondii. J. Immunol.*, 165, 628–631, 2000.
221. Suzuki, Y. Genes, cells and cytokines in resistance against development of toxoplasmic encephalitis. *Immunobiology*, 201, 255–271, 1999.
222. McCabe, R. E., Luft, B. J., and Remington, J. S. Effect of murine interferon gamma on murine toxoplasmosis. *J. Infect. Dis.*, 150, 961,1984.
223. Fegies, M. and Guerrero, J. Treatment of toxoplasmosis with levamisole. *Trans. R. Soc. Trop. Med. Hyg.*, 71, 178, 1977.
224. Zastera, M., Fruehbauer, Z., and Pokorny, J. Levamisole therapy of experimental toxoplasmosis in white mice. *Cesk. Epidemiol. Mikrobiol. Immunol.*, 31, 94, 1982.
225. Youssef, M. Y., el-Ridi, A. M., Arafa, M. S., el-Sawy, M. T., and el-Sayed, W. M. Effect of levamisole on toxoplasmosis during pregnancy in guinea pigs. *J. Egypt. Soc. Parasitol.*, 15, 41, 1985.

16
Microsporidia

1. INTRODUCTION

Microsporidia is a nontaxonomic designation used to commonly describe a group of obligate, intracellular, single-cell protozoa sharing a unique organelle, the polar filament, and classified under the order Microsporida, phylum Microspora, class Microsporea. Identified in a wide range of vertebrate and invertebrate hosts, their primary habitat is invertebrates, especially arthropods, although they were also found in lower and very rarely in higher vertebrates. Microsporida comprises of two suborders: Pansporoblastina and Apansporoblastina.

In 1957, Matsubayashi et al. *(1)* diagnosed the first case of microsporidiosis in humans, followed by several more cases *(2–5)*. The particular microsporidial species and the competence of the immune response may lead to different host-parasite interactions *(2)*. In otherwise healthy persons, usually microsporidial infections will develop into acute intestinal, self-limiting disease *(6)*. So far, systemic microsporidiosis has not been clearly documented in previously healthy patients. By comparison, patients with severe immunodeficiency are at highest risk for developing microsporidial disease. What is not well-understood in such cases was whether the disease represent reactivation of latent infection acquired prior to the state of suppressed immunity, or whether microsporidiosis has been associated with recently acquired infection *(2)*.

Initially, microsporidia species pathogenic to humans have been classified in five genera: *Enterocytozoon* spp. (*Enterocytozoon. bieneusi*), *Encephalitozoon* spp. (*Encephalitozoon cuniculi, E. hellem*), *Septata* spp. (*Septata intestinalis*), *Nosema* spp. (*Nosema connori, N. corneum, N. ocularum*), and *Pleistophora* sp., as well as a number of unclassified microsporidial organisms collectively referred to as *Microsporidium* sp. (*Microsporidium ceylonensis*, and *M. africanum*). However, based on genetic and immunologic studies, recently, *Septata intestinalis* has been reclassified as *Encephalitozoon intestinalis (7)*.

The potential sources and means of transmission of human microsporidial infections are still not very clear *(2)*. It is likely that parasites may be ingested via food contaminated with spores, which are resistant to environmental extremes and can survive for months, or via insect stings *(8,9)*. Inside the host, ingested spores travel to the intestine where the polar tubules of the parasite evert, penetrate the intestinal epithelial cells, and inject their cellular contents, or sporoplasm into these host cells *(10)*. The latter eventually rupture and release spores that infect other nearby cells or travel hematogenously or via infected macrophages to other organs, such as liver, brain, heart, and kidney *(4,11,12)*.

In humans, some microsporidial species may develop in particular host cells of a single organ system, whereas others may cause systemic infections involving different organ systems *(2,13,14)*. *E. bieneusi* appears to exhibit a strong preference for small intestinal epithelium *(15)*. Its development occurs predominantly in the apical cytoplasm, especially in the Golgi region immediately above the nucleus *(16–18)*. It seem likely that this may be the preferred site of morphogenesis; because microsporidians lack mitochondria they must rely on those of the host cells, which are particularly

From: Opportunistic Infections: Treatment and Prophylaxis
By: Vassil St. Georgiev © Humana Press Inc., Totowa, NJ

rich in this region of the cytoplasma *(19)*. It is of interest to note that *E. bieneusi* displays strong preference for infecting absorptive cells; only rarely it is seen in goblet or enterochromatin cells *(16)*. Belcher et al. *(20)* even reported a rare case of mandibular microsporidiosis.

Microsporidia have been recognized as opportunistic pathogens *(21,22)* in immunocompromised patients *(3,5,11,23–26)* with impaired cell immunity especially patients with hematologic neoplasia, solid transplant and bone-marrow recipients, patients receiving high-dose corticosteroids, and those with HIV *(3,5,12,23,27–38)*. Three microsporidial species, *E. intestinalis (33,39–45)*, *E. hellem (8,46)*, and *E. bieneusi (8,33,47)* were first diagnosed in intestinal and disseminated infections in AIDS patients *(41–43,48–53)*. In addition, *E. bieneusi* has also been isolated from immunocompetent patients *(6,54)* and from immunocompromised patients secondary to organ transplantation *(2,55,56)*. Guerard et al. *(57)* have reported the onset of intestinal *E. bieneusi* infection in two renal transplant recipients believed to be secondary to an increase in immunosuppression after azathioprine replacement by mycophenolate mofetil.

It should be noted that any imbalance of host-parasite interactions may result in proliferation and dissemination of the parasites, causing distruction of the host cells *(2)*. One unexpected occurence during a case of dissemination of *E. hellem* has been the parasitic infestation of respiratory epithelial-lining cells extending from the proximal trachea distally into small-order conducting airways *(46)*.

Disease manifestations may vary depending on the infecting species, mode of infection, age of the host at the time of infection, and the competence of the host's immune response *(3,5,58)*. They include intestinal, ocular, muscular, and systemic disease *(59)*. The number of sufficiently documented cases of microsporidiosis among non-HIV-infected patients is rather limited *(3–5,23,60)* including a case of *Microsporidium ceylonensis* being identified as a cause of corneal microsporidiosis *(61)*. However, the number of cases of microsporidiosis in HIV-infected individuals has been in the hundredths *(23)*. Chronic diarrhea coupled with wasting syndrome *(62–65)*, and disseminated infections *(41,46,50,66–68)* (particularly in patients with CD4+ cell counts below 50/mm^3) have been observed most frequently, whereas ocular microsporidiosis has been limited to the superficial epithelium of the cornea and conjuctiva.

2. ENTEROCYTOZOON BIENEUSI

Enterocytozoon bieneusi is currently the most commonly recognized microsporidian species in humans *(69)*. With very few exceptions, it has been found predominantly in HIV-positive patients *(18,43,70–72)*. An HIV-seronegative heart-lung transplant recipient presented with chronic diarrhea due to *E. bieneusi*; the clinical symptoms and evolution of the disease ware identical to those usually observed in AIDS patients *(73)*.

E. bieneusi has been associated with diarrhea and wasting syndrome *(47,74,75)*, cholecystitis and cholangitis *(76,77)*, bronchitis and pneumonia *(72,78,79)*, and sinusitis and rhinitis *(48,80)*.

Thus, in 7–50% of severely immunodeficient patients (CD4+ cell counts below 100/mm^3), *E. bieneusi* has been associated with chronic diarrhea which has been difficult to treat *(16,43,49,81–86)*. In HIV-infected patients with less severe cellular immunodeficiency (CD4+ cell counts above 100–200/mm^3), *E. bieneusi* may cause a self-limiting diarrhea *(2)*. Overall, intestinal microsporidiasis likely accounts for approx 15–30% of all cases of chronic diarrhea in AIDS patients *(9)*. The infection is localized to the small intestine with the jujenum (or ileum) seemingly more heavily infested than the duodenum *(87)*. Both electron and light microscopic studies suggested that the pathogenic mechanism involved in intestinal microsporidiasis involved the shedding of infected enterocytes containing large numbers of spores *(88)*. HIV-associated infections with other microsporidia are relatively less frequent *(28)*.

Blanshard et al. *(89)* recorded the first case in an AIDS patient of intestinal microsporidiosis involving simultaneous infection with two different types of microsporidia: *E. bieneusi* and a non *E. bieneusi* microsporidian. In another case of co-infection, an endoscopic biopsy from an AIDS patient with chronic diarrhea showed the presence of both *Giardia lamblia* and *E. bieneusi (90)*.

3. ENCEPHALITOZOON SPP.

Encephalitozoon spp. have been isolated from corneal and conjunctival specimens of patients with keratoconjunctivitis *(8,23,91–99)*. In addition, *Encephalitozoon* infections *(3,23)* have been associated with bronchiolitis *(67)*, sinusitis *(48,92)*, nephritis *(100)*, cystitis or ureteritis *(46,68,100)*, hepatitis *(101)*, peritonitis *(102)*, and disseminated infection *(66,68)*. *Encephalitozoon* microsporidia develop and mature within parasitophorous vacuoles, enlarging the vacuole over time until it occupies most of the cytoplasm of the host cells subsequently blocking multiple points of the cell cycle *(103)*.

E. cuniculi was recently confirmed to infect both AIDS *(66,100–102,104,105)* as well as HIV-seronegative patients *(1,106)*. In HIV-positive patients, *E. cuniculi* has been associated with fulminant hepatitis *(101)*, peritonitis *(102)*, sinusitis and keratoconjunctivitis *(107)*, and disseminated infection *(66)* reaching even the brain *(108)*.

Encephalitozoon hellem (109) has been most often identified as the causative agent of ocular microsporidiasis (keratoconjunctivitis and conjunctivitis) *(8,94,96,99,110)*. It was isolated from conjunctival scrappings and corneal tissue of several male homosexual AIDS patients with keratoconjunctivitis where it develops within parasitophorous vacuoles located in the most superficial layers of epithelial cells.

Although keratitis may be severe, it rarely, if ever, led to corneal ulceration *(99)*. A typical pattern of systemic *E. hellem* infection involves concomitant keratoconjunctival, urinary tract, and bronchial infection *(46,67,68)*. Associated clinical manifestations may include keratoconjunctival inflammation, cystitis, nephritis, renal failure, bronchtis, pneumonia, and possibly, progressive respiratory failure *(2)*.

Also, *E. hellem* has been identified as the causative agents of disseminated infection (tubulointerstitial nephritis, ureteritis, cystitis, colonization of bronchial epithelium) *(46,111)*, prostatic abscess *(112)*, and bronchiolitis and pneumonia *(67)*. *E. hellem* respiratory tract infection may also be asymptomatic *(113)*.

In a recent case of dual microsporidial infection, an AIDS patient has been diagnosed with sinunasal *Encephalitozoon hellem* infection and urinary tract infection due to *Vittaforma corneae (114)*.

E. intestinalis was associated with diarrhea, and disseminated infection (tubulointerstitial nephritis, diarrhea, enteritis, cystitis, and cholecystitis) *(39–42,115)*, keratoconjunctivitis *(116)*, and cholangiopathy *(117,118)*.

4. PLEISTOPHORA SPP.

Myositis associated with *Pleistophora* sp. has been described in immunocompromised patients *(10,119–121)*. In addition, some non-designated *Encephalitozoon* species have been found to cause keratoconjunctivitis *(91)*, and sinusitis and nasal polyps *(92,122)*.

5. TRACHIPLEISTOPHORA HOMINIS

Trachipleistophora hominis, a *Pleistophora*-like microsporidian caused myositis in a patient with AIDS *(123)*. The infection presented with progressive and severe disease with fever and weight loss.

6. NOSEMA SPP.

In an earlier report, Margileth et al. *(124)* described an infant with severe immunodeficiency to be heavily infected with *Nosema connori* with extensive involvement of the renal tubular epithelium. *Nosema* has since been identified as the causative agent of corneal infections *(125–128)*. *Nosema corneum*, the first human microsporidium isolated, has been recovered from the corneal stroma of an HIV-seronegative patient with keratitis and iritis *(125,126)*, and high *Nosema algerae* antibody titers were observed in humans with ocular microsporidiasis *(129)*.

7. BRACHIOLA VESICULARUM

Brachiola vesicularum is a recently identified microsporidium genus placed in the family Nosematidae that was associated with myositis in AIDS *(130)*.

8. TREATMENT OF MICROSPORIDIOSIS

The viability of the host cellular immune responses represents one critical aspect for preventing symptomatic microsporidiosis, which is predominantly associated with $CD4^+$ cellular deficiency. Results from an in vitro study by Khan et al. *(131)* have shown that host $CD8^+$ T-cells were essential for providing protective immunity against *E. cuniculi* infection.

It is suggested *(5)* that some species as *E. bieneusi* may be natural parasites of humans possibly causing transient diarrhea but normally remaining below the threshold of detection. However, with progression of cellular immunodeficiency, reactivation of latent microsporidial infection may occur.

The role of humoral immune responses is yet to be understood fully, but similarly to other human opportunistic protozoal infections, microsporidian-specific antibodies alone may not be protective *(2)*.

At present, there is no established and effective therapy for microsporidiosis. Patients are often treated empirically, usually with several drugs. Accepted therapy, such as diet alterations and antidiarrheal medications, have often been ineffective in alleviating the diarrhea and malabsorption associated with intestinal microsporidiosis *(132)*. In a clinical trial, a medium-chain triglyceride-based diet in HIV-positive patients with chronic microsporidial diarrhea reduced diarrhea and malabsorption *(133)*.

Different agents, such as metronidazole, itraconazole, albendazole, octreotide, primaquine, lomotil, sulfalazine, paromomycin, trimethoprim-sulfamethoxazole, sulfisoxazole, and loperamide, have been used to patients with variable results. In several reports, the incidence of microsporidia-associated diarrheal illness in HIV-positive patients has been decreased since the introduction of the HAART. It is thought that patients that successfully responded to HAART may have the microsporidial organisms eradicated *(134,135)*. To this end, clinical data *(136–138)* suggested that some protease inhibitors (indinavir, saquinavir) may be capable of eradicating microsporidial (and/or cryptosporidial) infection refractory to other treatments. (The relapse of cryptosporidiosis in two patients who discontinued antiretroviral therapy suggest that the infection may have remained in a latent stage) *(135)*.

In patients with *E. bieneusi*-elicited diarrhea, symptomatic management is carried out usually with standard nonspecific antidiarrheal drugs *(63)*. In cases of failure to respond, subcutaneous octeotride (a somatostatin analog) has been recommended at 100–500 µg, t.i.d. *(139)*. For patients on parenteral nutrition, octreotide up to 500 µg (not to exceed 50 µg/h) may be added directly to the total parenteral nutrition *(140)*.

Matsubayashi et al. *(1)* have used sulfisoxazole to treat successfully *E. cuniculi* infection of the CNS. Although trimethoprim-sulfamethoxazole and octreotide relieved diarrhea in a few cases *(63,139)*, neither drug was successful in eliminating the parasite from the gastrointestinal tract. On the other hand, therapy with trimethoprim-sulfamethoxazole followed by sulfadiazine was found to be effective against *Pleistophora*-associated myositis *(119,120)*.

Eeftinck Schattenkerk et al. *(82)* have observed pronounced improvement in six patients or disappearance of diarrhea in four patients in 10 of 13 patients treated empirically with metronidazole. With one exception (250 mg, b.i.d.), the drug was given at 500 mg, t.i.d. In four of the patients, the response was prolonged; however, repeat biopsies showed continued presence of microsporidia regardless of the response to metronidazole *(82)*. In another case, one patient with microsporidiosis treated similarly also showed transient improvement *(141)*. In an appatrent contradiction, a study by Blanshard and Gazzard *(142)* showed no improvement in four patients following metronidazole therapy.

A 4-wk course with 400 mg of albendazole orally, twice daily, in six HIV-infected patients with intestinal *E. bieneusi* resulted in cessation of diarrhea and either weight gain or cessation of weight loss; three patients who relapsed after treatment received a 6-wk course *(132)*. Molina et al. *(86)* have observed transient improvement in five AIDS patients treated with metronidazole (given at 1.5 mg daily), but a longer response in three patients treated with albendazole (at 800 mg daily). However, in all patients, the diarrhea recurred after the end of therapy, and spores of *E. bieneusi*, were recovered from the stools of all patients *(86)*. At low concentrations albendazole may bind reversibly to its tubulin target in *E. bieneusi* which, in turn, may provide a partial explanation why diarrhea may return to pretreatment levels when the low-dose treatment had been discontinued *(132)*.

Dieterich et al. *(143)* studied the effect of albendazole on 29 severely immunocompromised AIDS patients (peripheral blood CD4+ lymphocyte counts ranging from 1–60 cells/mm^3) with intestinal microsporidiosis (persistent watery diarrhea, and a slow but progressive weight loss). At doses of 400 mg, b.i.d., albendazole was effective in substantially reducing diarrhea. In another study, Aarons et al. *(144)* described a case of *Encephalitozoon*-associated renal failure in an HIV-positive patient. Treatment with albendazole (400 mg, b.i.d.) led to disappearance of spores from the urine, clinical improvement, and return of renal function virtually to normal. One case of an AIDS patient with *Encephalitozoon*-associated disseminated microsporidiosis (intestinal, urinary, nasal, and ocular involvement) has been successfully treated with albendazole given at 400 mg, b.i.d. *(145)*.

In the experience of Leder et al. *(33)* treatment with albendazole resulted in a better clinical response against *Encephalitozoon intestinalis* infection *(146)* but not *Enterocytozoon bieneusi* infection. To this end, eighteen patients with *E. bieneusi* chronic diarrhea that did not respond symptomatically to albendazole received 100-mg daily of thalidomide for 1 mo; seven subjects had a complete response, and three showed a partial response *(147)*.

Weber et al. *(148)* described two patients with HIV-associated chronic diarrhea caused by *Encephalitozoon (Septata) intestinalis* who after receiving a 2-wk course of 400 mg (b.i.d.) of albendazole became asymptomatic with no parasites detected in stool specimens.

A double-blind, placebo-controlled trial was conducted to evaluate the safety and efficacy of albendazole (given at 400 mg twice daily for 3 wk) for the treatment of *E. intestinalis* in AIDS patients *(149)*. All patients cleared microsporidia from the intestinal tract. To assess the effect of albendazole in preventing relapse, patients were randomly assigned to receive for the next 12 mo either albendazole (400 mg b.i.d.) or no treatment; albendazole significantly delayed the occurrence of relapse ($p = .04$, one-sided log-rank test).

In a case of *E. intestinalis*-induced sclerosing cholangitis in an AIDS patient, albendazole therapy was successful in eradicating the microsporidia with clinical improvement and increased CD4 count. However, the cholangiographic picture did not improve and repeated cholangiography revealed progressive bile duct injury *(117)*.

A 15-d regimen of albendazole and metronidazole resolved *E. bieneusi* diarrheal disease in a HIV-negative renal transplant recipient; 2 mo later, the patient recovered completely *(55)*.

Dionisio et al. *(150)* after investigating the morphological changes in *E. bieneusi* and the duration of symptomatic relief after combination treatment with albendazole and furazolidone (800 and 500 mg daily, respectively) in AIDS patients, concluded that this drug regimen may result in lasting remission even in severely immunocompromised patients. In another study by the same group *(151)* conducted in six AIDS patients with symptomatic *E. bieneusi* infection of the small intestine, treatment with furazolidone alone resulted in both clinical and parasitologic response with transient clearance or decrease of spore shedding in stools.

Itraconazole has been used to treat *Nosema* infections in invertebrates *(152)*. Yee et al. *(96)* found itraconazole (200 mg orally, twice daily) found effective in the treatment of *E. cuniculi*-associated epithelial keratopathy in an AIDS patient. After 6 wk of treatment, there was improvement of vision and reduction of foreign body sensation and punctuate staining; topical application of coltrin (intravenous trimethoprim-sulfisoxazole formulation) resulted in no significant improvement *(96)*. Rossi et al. *(107)* reported complete resolution of sinusitis and keratoconjunctivitis in an AIDS patient after treatment with itraconazole at 200 mg daily for 8 wk; previous albendazole therapy (400 mg daily for 6 wk) was unsuccessful.

Brachiola vesicularum myositis in AIDS was successfully cleared both clinically and histologically) by treatment with albendazole and itraconazole *(130).*

However, Albrecht et al. *(153)* reported failure of itraconazole to prevent *E. bieneusi* infection in an AIDS patient who developed intestinal microsporidiosis while on a high-dose itraconazole therapy (200 mg, b.i.d.) for secondary prophylaxis against histoplasmosis; the serum level of itraconazole was determined at 7.9 µg/mL (levels above 2.0 µg/mL are considered to be therapeutic).

While fumagillin, a naturally secreted water-soluble antibiotic has been used successfully in the treatment of superficial keratitis in AIDS patients *(116,154,155).* Systemic therapy has been somewhat limited because of the toxicity of the currently available fumagillin salt *(156,157).* Thus, treatment of bilateral microsporidial keratitis in an AIDS patient with local fumagillin-eye-drops (0.07 mg/mL seven times daily) led to significant improvement *(158).*

French studies have been designed to assess the safety and efficacy of oral fumagillin against *E. bieneusi* chronic diarrhea in HIV-positive patients *(159,160).* The drug was given to four groups of patients for 14 d at daily doses of 10, 20, 40, and 60 mg. The safety and efficacy was assessed at wk 1, 2, 4, and 6; during the study, 21 patients (out of 29) transiently cleared the pathogen from their stools. By wk 6, however, all patients taking 10, 20, and 40 mg daily fumagillin had parasitic relapse; by comparison, 8 out of 11 (72%) patients receiving 60 mg daily of the drug apparently had cleared microsporidia from gastrointestinal tract and gained weight without parasitic relapse during a mean follow-up of 11.5 mo *(159).*

TNP-470, a semisynthetic analog of fumagillin was found highly effective in vitro and in vivo *(156,157).* Against *E. cuniculi,* treatment with TNP-470 resulted in prolonged survival and prevention of the development of ascites in infected athymic mice *(156).*

An AIDS patient with *E. bieneusi*-induced chronic diarrhea was successfully treated with nitazoxanide (a 5-nitrothiazole benzamide antiparasitic drug used primarily against cryptosporidiosis) producing a complete clinical and parasitologic response while off of antiviral therapy *(161).*

Anwar-Bruni et al. *(162)* reported a promising clinical response of HIV-1-positive patients with symptomatic intestinal microsporidiosis to a minimum of 1 mo of atovaquone therapy.

A long-term therapy with oral clindamycin cured dissiminated nodular cutaneous *Encephalitozoon* microsporidiosis in an AIDS patient *(163).*

Metcalfe et al. *(98)* used propamidine isethionate (4,4'-diamidino-α,ω-diphenoxypropane isethionate) 0.1% eye drops (6 times daily) to treat successfully *E. cuniculi*-associated keratoconjunctivitis in an AIDS patient.

REFERENCES

1. Matsubayashi, H., Koike, T., Mikata, T., and Hagiwara, S. A case of *Encephalitozoon*-like body infection in man. *Arch. Pathol.,* 67, 181, 1959.
2. Weber, R., Bryan, R. T., Schwartz, D. A., and Owen, R. L. Human microsporidial infections. *Clin. Microbiol. Rev.,* 7, 426, 1994.
3. Bryan, R. T. Microsporidia, in *Principles and Practice of Infectious Diseases,* Mandell, G. L., Douglas, R. G., and Bennett, J. E., Eds., 3rd ed., Churchill Livingston, New York, 2130, 1990.
4. Bryan, R. T., Cali, A., Owen, R. L., and Spencer, H. C. Microsporidia: opportunistic pathogens in patients with AIDS, in *Progress in Clinical Parasitology,* vol. 2, Sun, T., Ed., Field and Wood, Philadelphia, 1, 1991.
5. Canning, E. U. and Hollister, W. S. Human infections with microsporidia. *Rev. Med. Microbiol.,* 3, 35, 1992.
6. Sandfort, J., Hannemann, A., Gelderblom, H., Stark, K., Owen, R. L., and Ruf, B. *Enterocytozoon bieneusi* infection in an immunocompetent patient who had acute diarrhea and who was not infected with the human immunodeficiency virus. *Clin. Infect. Dis.,* 19, 514, 1994.
7. Hartskeerl, R. A., van Gool, T., Schuitema, A. R. J., Didier, E. S., and Terpstra, W. J. Genetic and immunological characterization of the microsporidian *Septata intestinalis* Cali, Kotler and Orenstein, 1993; reclassification to *Encephalitozoon intestinalis*. *Parasitology,* 110, 277, 1995.
8. Didier, AE. S., Didier, P. J., Friedberg, D. N., et al. Isolation and characterization of a new human microsporidian, *Encephalitozoon hellem* (n. sp.), from three AIDS patients with keratoconjunctivitis. *J. Infect. Dis.,* 163, 617, 1991.
9. Weber, R., Bryan, R. T., Owen, R. L., Wilcox, C. M., Gorelkin, L., and Visvesvara, G. S. Improved light-microscopical detection of microsporidia spores in stool and duodenal aspirates. *N. Engl. J. Med.,* 326, 161, 1992.

10. Chupp, G. L., Alroy, J., Adelman, L. S., Breen, J. C., and Skolnik, P. R. Myositis due to *Pleistophora* (Microsporidia) in a patient with AIDS. *Clin. Infect. Dis.*, 16, 15, 1993.
11. Canning, E. U., Lom, J., and Dykova, I. *The Microsporidia of Vertebrates*, Academic Press, New York, 1986.
12. Shadduck, J. A. Human microsporidiosis and AIDS. *Rev. Infect. Dis.*, 11, 203, 1989.
13. Georges, E., Rabaud, C., Amiel, C., et al. *Enterocytozoon bieneusi* multiorgan microsporidiosis in a HIV-infected patient. *J. Infect.*, 36, 223–225, 1998.
14. Corcoran, G. D., Isaacson, J. R., Daniels, C., and Chiodini, P. L. Urethritis associated with disseminated microsporidiosis: clinical response to albendazole. *Clin. Infect. Dis.*, 22, 592–593, 1996.
15. Orenstein, J. M., Tenner, M., and Kotler, D. P. Localization of infection by the microsporidian *Enterocytozoon bieneusi* in the gastrointestinal tract of AIDS patients with diarrhea. *AIDS*, 6, 195, 1992.
16. Orenstein, J. M. Microsporidiosis in the acquired immunodeficiency syndrome. *J. Parasitol.*, 77, 843, 1991.
17. Cali, A. and Owen, R. I. Intracellular development of *Enterocytozoon*, a unique microsporidian found in the intestine of AIDS patients. *J. Protozool.*, 37, 145, 1990.
18. Orenstein, J. M., Chiang, J., Steinberg, W., Smith, P. D., Rotterdam, H., and Kotler, D. P. Intestinal microsporidiosis as a cause of diarrhea in human immunodeficiency virus-infected patients: a report of 20 cases. *Human Pathol.*, 21, 475, 1990.
19. Gourley, W. K. and Swedo, J. L. Intestinal infection by microsporidia *Enterocytozoon bieneusi* of patients with AIDS: an ultrastructural study of the use of human mitochondria by a protozoan. *Lab. Invest.*, 58, 35A, 1988.
20. Belcher, J. W., Jr., Guttenberg, S. A., and Schmooker, B. M. Microsporidiosis of the mandible in a patient with acquired immunodeficiency syndrome. *J. Oral Maxillofac. Surg.*, 55, 424–426, 1997.
21. Canning, E. U. and Hollister, W. S. Microsporidia of mammals - widespread pathogens or opportunistic curiosities? *Parasitol. Today*, 3, 267, 1987.
22. Canning, E. U. and Hollister, W. S. In vitro and in vivo investigations of human microsporidia. *J. Parasitol.*, 38, 631, 1991
23. Bryan, R. T. and Weber, R. Microsporidia: emerging pathogens in immunodeficient persons. *Arch. Pathol. Lab. Med.*, 117, 1243, 1993.
24. Canning, E. U. Microsporidia, in *Parasitic Protozoa*, 2nd ed., vol. 6, Kreier, J. P. and Baker, J. R., Eds. Academic Press, New York, 299, 1993.
25. Ferreira, M. S. Infections by protozoa in immunocompromised hosts. *Mem. Inst. Oswaldo Cruz*, 95(Suppl. 1), 159–162, 2000.
26. Wasson, K. and Peper, R. L. Mammalian microsporidiosis. *Vet. Pathol.*, 37, 113–128, 2000.
27. Shadduck, J. A. and Greeley, E. Microsporidia and human infections. *Clin. Microbiol. Rev.*, 2, 158, 1989.
28. Orenstein, J. M., Tenner, M., Cali, A., and Kotler, D. P. A second species of microsporidia that causes intestinal disease in AIDS. *Immunol. Microbiol.*, 98, A467, 1990.
29. Kotler, D. P., Francisco, A., Clayton, F., Scholes, J. V., and Orenstein, J. M. Small intestinal injury and parasitic diseases in AIDS. *Ann. Intern. Med.*, 113, 444, 1990.
30. Wittner, M., Tanowitz, H. B., and Weiss, L. M. Parasitic infections in AIDS patients: cryptosporidiosis, isosporiasis, microsporidiosis, cyclosporiasis. *Infect. Dis. Clin. North Am.*, 7, 569, 1993.
31. Schottelius, J. and da Costa, S. C. Microsporidia and acquired immunodeficiency syndrome. *Mem. Inst. Oswaldo Cruz*, 95(Suppl. 1), 133–139, 2000.
32. Brasil, P., Lima, D. B., Paiva, D. D., et al. Clinical and diagnostic aspects of intestinal microsporidiosis in HIV-infected patients with chronic diarrhea in Rio de Janeiro, Brazil. *Rev. Inst. Med. Trop. Sao Paulo*, 42, 299–304, 2000.
33. Leder, K., Ryan, N., Spelman, D., and Crowe, S. M. Microsporidial disease in HIV-infected patients: a report of 42 patients and review of the literature. *Scand. J. Infect. Dis.*, 30, 331–338, 1998.
34. Kopicko, J. J., Frazer, T., Dascomb, K., Clark, R., Didier, E. S., and Kissinger, P. Influence of seasonal variation with enteric microsporidiosis among HIV-infected individuals. *J. Acquir. Immune Defic. Syndr.*, 22, 408-409, 1999.
35. Gamboa Dominguez, A., Bencosme Vinas, C., and Kato Maeda, M. Microsporidiasis in AIDS patients with chronic diarrhea. Experiences at the National Institute of Nutrition "Salvador Zubriran." *Rev. Gastroenterol. Mex.*, 64, 70-74, 1999.
36. Dascomb, K., Clark, R., Aberg, J., et al. Natural history of intestinal microsporidiosis among patients infected with human immunodeficiency virus. *J. Clin. Microbiol.*, 37, 3421-3422, 1999.
37. Goodgame, R., Stager, C., Marcantel, B., Alcocer, E., and Segura, A. M. Intensity of infection in AIDS-related intestinal microsporidiosis. *J. Infect. Dis.*, 180, 929-932, 1999.
38. Kelkar, R., Sastry, P. S., Kulkarni, S. S., Saikia, T. K., Parikh, P. M., and Advani, S. H. Pulmonary microsporidial infection in a patient with CML undergoing allogeneic marrow transplant. *Bone Marrow Transplant.*, 19, 179-182, 1997.
39. Cali, A., Kotler, D. P., and Orenstein, J. M. *Septata intestinalis* n.g., n.sp., an intestinal microsporidian associated with chronic diarrhea and dissemination in AIDS patients. *J. Protozool.*, 40, 101, 1993.
40. Cali, A., Orenstein, J. M., Kotler, D. P., and Owen, R. L. A comparison of two microsporidian parasites in enterocytes of AIDS patients with chronic diarrhea. *J. Protozool.*, 38, S96, 1991.
41. Orenstein, J. M., Dieterich, D. T., and Kotler, D. P. Systemic dissemination by a newly recognized intestinal microsporidia species in AIDS. *AIDS*, 6, 1143, 1992.
42. Orenstein, J. M., Tenner, M., Cali, A., and Kotler, D. P. A microsporidian previously undescribed in humans, infecting enterocytes and macrophages, and associated with diarrhea in an acquired immunodeficiency syndrome patient. *Human Pathol.*, 23, 722, 1992.

43. Field, A., Hing, M., Milliken, S., and Marriott, D. Microsporidia in the small intestine of HIV infected patients: a new diagnostic technique and a new species. *Med. J. Aust.*, 158, 390, 1993.
44. Didier, E. S., Rogers, L. B., Orenstein, J. M., et al. Characterization of *Encephalitozoon* (*Septata*) *intestinalis* isolates cultured from nasal mucosa and bronchoalveolar lavage fluids of two AIDS patients. *J. Eukariot. Microbiol.*, 43, 34, 1996.
45. Kelly, P., McPhail, P., Ngwenya, B., et al. *Septata intestinalis*: a new microsporidian in Africa. *Lancet*, 344, 271, 1995.
46. Schwartz, D. A., Bryan, R. T., Hewan-Lowe, K. O., et al. Disseminated microsporidiosis (*Encephalitozoon hellem*) and acquired immunodeficiency syndrome: autopsy evidence for respiratory acquisition. *Arch. Pathol. Lab. Med.*, 116, 660, 1992.
47. Desportes, I., Le Charpantier, Y., Galian, A., et al. Occurence of a new microsporidian, *Enterocytozoon bieneusi* n.g., n.sp. in the enterocytes of a human patient with AIDS. *J. Protozool.*, 32, 250, 1985.
48. Eeftinck Schattenkerk, J. K. M., van Gool, T., Schot, L. S., van den Bergh Weerman, M., and Dankert, J. Chronic rhinosinusitis, a new clinical syndrome in HIV-infected patients with microsporidiosis. *Workshop on Intestinal Microsporidia in HIV Infection*, Paris, abstract, 1992.
49. van Gool, T., Snijders, F., Reiss, P. et al. Diagnosis of intestinal and disseminated microsporidial infections in patients with HIV by a new rapid fluorescence technique. *J. Clin. Pathol.*, 46, 694, 1993.
50. Asmuth, D. M., DeGirolami, P. C., Federman, M., et al. Clinical features of microsporidiosis in patients with AIDS. *Clin. Infect. Dis.*, 18, 819, 1993.
51. Wanke, C. A. and Mattia, A. R. A 36-year-old man with AIDS, increase in chronic diarrhea, and intermittent fever and chills. *N. Engl. J. Med.*, 329, 1946, 1993.
52. Canning, E. U. and Hollister, W. S. *Enterocytozoon bieneusi* (Microspora): prevalence and pathogenicity in AIDS patients. *Trans. R. Soc. Trop. Med. Hyg.*, 84, 181, 1990.
53. Leitch, G. J., Scanlon, M., Shaw, A., and Visvesvara, G. S. Role of P glycoprotein in the course and treatment of *Encephalitozoon* microsporidiosis. *Antimicrob. Agents Chemother.*, 45, 73–78, 2001.
54. Deluol, A.-M., Poirot, J.-L., Heyer, F., Roux, P., and Levy, D. Intestinal microsporidiosis: about clinical characteristics and laboratory diagnosis. *J. Eukariot. Microbiol.*, 41, 33S, 1994.
55. Metge, S., Van Nhieu, J. T., Dahmane, D., et al. A case of *Enterocytozoon bieneusi* infection in an HIV-negative renal transplant recipient. *Eur. J. Clin. Microbiol. Infect. Dis.*, 19, 221–223, 2000.
56. Gumbo, T., Hobbs, R. E., Carlyn, C., Hall, G., and Isada, C. M. Microsporidia infection in transplant patients. *Transplantation*, 67, 482–484, 1999.
57. Guerard, A., Rabodonirina, M., Cotte, L., et al. Intestinal microsporidiosis occurring in two renal transplant recipients treated with mycophenolate mofetil. *Transplantation*, 68, 699–707, 1999.
58. Font, R. L., Samaha, A. N., Keener, M. J., Chevez-Barrios, P., and Goosey, J. D. Corneal microsporidiosis. Report of case, including electron microscopic observations. *Ophthalmology*, 107, 1769–1775, 2000.
59. Kotler, D. P. and Orenstein, J. M. Clinical syndromes associated with microsporidiosis. *Adv. Parasitol.*, 40, 321–349, 1998.
60. Silverstein, B. E., Cunningham, E. T., Jr., Margolis, T. P., Cevallos, V., Wong, I. G. Microsporidial keratoconjunctivitis in a patient without human immunodeficiency virus infection. *Am. J. Ophthalmol.*, 124, 395–396, 1997.
61. Canning, E. U., Curry, A., Vavra, J., and Bonshek, R. E. Some ultrastructural data on *Microsporidium ceylonensis*, a cause of corneal microsporidiosis. *Parasite*, 5, 247–254, 1998.
62. Bartlett, J. G., Belitsos, P. C., and Sears, C. L. AIDS enteropathy. *Clin. Infect. Dis.*, 15, 726, 1992.
63. Current, W. L. and Owen, R. L. Cryptosporidiosis and microsporidiosis, in *Enteric Infection: Mechanism, Manifestations, and Management*, Farthing, J. M. C. and Keusch, G. T., Eds. Chapman and Hall, London, 223, 1989.
64. Guerrant, R. L. and Bobak, D. A. Medical progress: bacterial and protozoal gastroenteritis. *N. Engl. J. Med.*, 325, 327, 1991.
65. Smith, P. D., Quinn, T. C., Strober, W., Janoff, E. M., and Masur, H. Gastriintestinal infections in AIDS. *Ann. Intern. Med.*, 116, 63, 1992.
66. De Groote, M. A., Visvesvara, G. S., Wilson, M. L., et al. Polymerase chain reaction and culture confirmation of disseminated *Encephalitozoon cuniculi* infection in a patient with AIDS: successful therapy with albendazole. *J. Infect. Dis.*, 171, 1375, 1995.
67. Schwartz, D. A., Visvesvara, G. S., Leitch, G. J., et al. Pathology of symptomatic microsporidial (*Encephalitozoon hellem*) bronchiolitis in AIDS: a new respiratory pathogen diagnosed from lung biopsy, bronchoalveolar lavage, sputum, and tissue culture. *Human Pathol.*, 24, 937, 1993.
68. Weber, R., Kuster, H., Visvesvara, G. S., Bryan, R. T., Schwartz, D. A., and Lüthy, R. Disseminated microsporidiosis due to *Encephalitozoon hellem*: pulmonary colonization, microhematuria and mild conjunctivitis in a patient with AIDS. *Clin. Infect. Dis.*, 17, 415, 1993.
69. Cali, A. General microsporidian features and recent findings on AIDS isolates. *J. Protozool.*, 38, 625, 1991.
70. Orenstein, J. M., Zierdt, W., Zierdt, C., and Kotler, D. P. Identification of spores of *Enterocytozoon bieneusi* in stool and duodenal fluid from AIDS patients. *Lancet*, 336, 1127, 1990.
71. Ditrich, O., Lom, J., Dykova, I., and Vavra, J. First case of *Enterocytozoon bieneusi* in the Czech Republic: comments on the ultrastructure and teratoid sporogenesis of the parasite. *J. Eukariot. Microbiol.*, 41, 35S, 1994.
72. del Aguila, C., Lopez-Velz, R., Fenoy, S., et al. Identification of *Enterocytozoon bieneusi* spores in respiratory samples from an AIDS patient with a 2-year history of intestinal microsporidiosis. *J. Clin. Microbiol.*, 35, 1862–1866, 1997.
73. Rabodonirina, M., Bertocchi, M., Desportes-Livage, I., et al. *Enterocytozoon bieneusi* as a cause of chronic diarrhea in

a heart-lung transplant recipient who was seronegative for human immunodeficiency virus. *Clin. Infect. Dis.*, 23, 114–117, 1996 [see also: *Clin. Infect. Dis.*, 24, 534–535, 1997].
74. Dobbins, W. O. III and Weinstein, W. M. Electron microscopy of the intestine and rectum in acquired immunodeficiency syndrome. *Gastroenterology*, 88, 738, 1985.
75. Modigliani, R., Bories, C., Le Charpentier, Y., et al. Diarrhoea and malabsorption in acquired immune deficiency syndrome: a study of four cases with special emphasis on opportunistic protozoan infections. *Gut*, 26, 179, 1985.
76. McWhinney, P. H. M., Nathwani, D., Green, S. T., Boyd, J. F., and Forrest, J. A. H. Microsporidiosis detected in association with AIDS-related sclerosing cholangitis. *AIDS*, 5, 1394, 1991.
77. Pol, S., Romana, C., Richard, S., et al. *Enterocytozoon bieneusi* infection in acquired immunodeficiency syndrome-related sclerosing cholangitis. *Gastroenterology*, 102, 1778, 1992.
78. Weber, R., Kuster, H., Keller, R., et al. Pulmonary and intestinal microsporidiosis in a patient with the acquired immunodeficiency syndrome. *Am. Rev. Respir. Dis.*, 146, 1603, 1992.
79. Lores, B., Arias, C., Fenoy, S., et al. *Enterocytozoon bieneusi*: a common opportunistic parasite in lungs of HIV-positive patients? *J. Eukariot. Microbiol.*, 46, 6S-7S, 1999.
80. Hartskeerl, R. A., Schuitema, A. R. J., van Gool, T., and Terpstra, J. Genetic evidence for the occurence of extraintestinal *Enterocytozoon bieneusi* infections. *Nucleic Acids Res.*, 21, 4150, 1993.
81. Cello, J. P., Grendell, J. H., Basuk, P., et al. Effect of octreotide on refractory AIDS-associated diarrhea. *Ann. Intern. Med.*, 115, 705, 1991.
82. Eeftinck Schattenkerk, J. K. M., van Gool, T., van Ketel, R. J., et al. Clinical significance of small-intestinal microsporidiosis in HIV-1-infected individuals. *Lancet*, 337, 895, 1991.
83. Greenson, J. K., Belitsos, P. C., Yardley, J. H., and Bartlett, J. G. AIDS enteropathy: occult enteric infections and duodenal mucosal alterations in chronic diarrhea. *Ann. Intern. Med.*, 114, 366, 1991.
84. Lucas, S. B., Papadaki, L., Conlon, C., Sewankambo, N., Goodgame, R., and Serwadda, D. Diagnosis of intestinal microsporidiosis in patients with AIDS. *J. Clin. Pathol.*, 42, 885, 1989.
85. Michiels, J. F., Hofman, P., Saint Paul, M. C., and Loubière, R. Pathological features of intestinal microsporidiosis in HIV positive patients. *Pathol. Res. Pract.*, 189, 377, 1993.
86. Molina, J. M., Sarfati, C., Beauvais, B., et al. Intestinal microsporidiosis in human immunodeficiency virus-infected patients with chronic unexplained diarrhea: prevalence and clinical and biologic features. *J. Infect. Dis.*, 167, 217, 1993.
87. Orenstein, J. M., Tenner, M., and Kotler, D. P. Localization of infection by microsporidia *Enterocytozoon bieneusi* in the gastrointestinal tracts of AIDS patients. *Immunol. Microbiol.*, 98, A467, 1990.
88. Peacock, C. S., Blanshard, C., Tovey, D. G., Ellis, D. S., and Gazzard, B. G. Histological diagnosis of intestinal microsporidiosis in patients with AIDS. *J. Clin. Pathol.*, 44, 558, 1991.
89. Blanshard, C., Hollister, W. S., Peacock, C. S., et al. Simultaneous infection with two types of intestinal microsporidia in a patient with AIDS. *Gut*, 33, 418, 1992.
90. Hewan-Lowe, K., Furlong, B., Sims, M., and Schwartz, D. A. Coinfection with *Giardia lamblia* and *Enterocytozoon bieneusi* in a patient with acquired immunodeficiency syndrome and chronic diarrhea. *Arch. Pathol. Lab. Med.*, 121, 417-422, 1997.
91. Centers for Disease Control. Microsporidial keratoconjunctivitis in patients with AIDS. *Morb. Mortal. Wkly Rep.*, 39, 188, 1990.
92. Lacey, C. J. N., Clark, A., Frazer, P., Metcalfe, T., and Curry, A. Chronic microsporidian infection in the nasal mucosae, sinuses and conjunctivae in HIV disease. *Genitourin. Med.*, 68, 179, 1992.
93. Lowder, C. Y., Meisler, D. M., McMahon, J. T., Longworth, D. L., and Rutherford, I. Microsporidia infection of the cornea in a man seropositive for human immunodeficiency virus. *Am. J. Ophthalmol.*, 109, 242, 1990.
94. Friedberg, D. N., Stenson, S. M., Orenstein, J. M., Tierno, P. M., and Charles, N. C. Microsporidial keratoconjunctivitis in acquired immunodeficiency syndrome. *Arch. Ophthalmol.*, 108, 504, 1990.
95. Cali, A., Meisler, D. M., Rutherford, I., et al. Corneal microsporidiosis in a patient with AIDS. *Am. J. Trop. Med. Hyg.*, 44, 463, 1991.
96. Yee, R. W., Tio, F. O., Martinez, J. A., Held, K. S., Shadduck, J. A., and Didier, E. S. Resolution of microsporidial epithelial keratopathy in a patient with AIDS. *Ophthalmology*, 98, 196, 1991.
97. Desser, S. S., Hong, H., and Yang, J. Ultrastructure of the development of a species of *Encephalitozoon* cultured from the eye of an AIDS patient. *Parasitol. Rev.*, 78, 677, 1992.
98. Metcalfe, T. W., Doran, R. M. L., Rowlands, P. L., Curry, A., and Lacey, C. J. M. Microsporidial keratoconjunctivitis in a patient with AIDS. *Br. J. Ophthalmol.*, 76, 177, 1992.
99. Schwartz, D. A., Visvesvara, G. S., Diesenhouse, M. D., et al. Pathologic features and immunofluorescent antibody demonstration of ocular microsporidiosis (*Encephalitozoon hellem*) in seven patients with acquired immunodeficiency syndrome. *Am. J. Ophthalmol.*, 115, 285, 1993.
100. Hollister, W. S., Canning, E. U., and Colbourn, N. I. A species of *Encephalitozoon* isolated from an AIDS patient: criteria for species differentiation. *Folia Parasitol.*, 40, 293, 1993.
101. Terada, S., Reddy, K. R., Jeffers, L. J., Cali, A., and Schiff, E. R. Microsporidian hepatitis in the acquired immunodeficiency syndrome. *Ann. Intern. Med.*, 107, 61, 1987.
102. Zender, H. O., Arrigoni, E., Eckert, J., and Kapanci, Y. A case of *Encephalitozoon cuniculi* peritonitis in a patient with AIDS. *Vet. Pathol.*, 92, 352, 1989.
103. Scanlon, M., Shaw, A. P., Zhou, C. J., Visvesvara, G. S., and Leitch, G. J. Infection by microsporidia disrupts the host cell cycle. *J. Eukariot. Microbiol.*, 47, 525–531, 2000.

104. Bergquist, R., Morfeldt-Mansson, Pehrson, P. O., Petrini, B., and Wasserman, J. Antibody against *Encephalitozoon cuniculi* in Swedish homosexual men. *Scand. J. Infect. Dis.*, 16, 389, 1984.
105. Didier, E. S., Vossbrinck, C. R., Baker, M. D., Rogers, L. B., Bertucci, D. C., and Shadduck, J. A. Identification and characterization of three *Encephalitozoon cuniculi* strains. *Parasitology*, 111, 4121, 1995.
106. Bergquist, N. R., Stinzing, G., Smedman, L., Waller, T., and Andersson, T. Diagnosis of encephalitozoonosis in man by serological studies. *Br. Med. J.*, 288, 902, 1984.
107. Rossi, P., Urbani, C., Donelli, G., and Pozio, E. Resolution of microsporidial sinusitis and keratoconjunctivitis by itraconazole treatment. *Am. J. Ophthalmol.*, 127, 210–212, 1999.
108. Weber, R., Deplazes, P., Flepp, M., et al. Cerebral microsporidiosis due to *Encephalitozoon cuniculi* in a patient with human immunodeficiency virus infection. *N. Engl. J. Med.*, 336, 474–478, 1997 [see also: *N. Engl. J. Med.*, 337, 640–641, 1997].
109. Didier, P. J., Didier, E. S., Orenstein, J. M., and Shadduck, J. A. Fine structure of a new human microsporidian, *Encephalitozoon hellem*, in culture. *J. Protozool.*, 38, 502, 1991.
110. Friedberg, D. N., Didier, E. S., and Yee, R. W. Microsporidial keratoconjunctivitis. *Am. J. Ophthalmol.*, 116, 380, 1993.
111. Hollister, W. S., Canning, E. U., Colbourn, N. I., Curry, A., and Lacey, C. J. N. Characterization of *Encephalitozoon hellem* (Microspora) isolated from the nasal mucosa of a patient with AIDS. *Parasitology*, 107, 351, 1993.
112. Schwartz, D. A., Visvesvara, G., Weber, R., and Bryan, R. T. Male genital microsporidiosis and AIDS: prostatic abscess due to *Encephalitozoon hellem.*, *J. Eukariot. Microbiol.*, 41, 61S, 1994.
113. Scaglia, M., Gatti, S., Sacchi, L., et al. Asymptomatic respiratory tract microsporidiosis due to *Encephalitozoon hellem* in three patients with AIDS. *Clin. Infect. Dis.*, 26, 174–176, 1998.
114. Deplazes, P., Mathis, A., van Saanen, M., et al. Dual microsporidial infection due to *Vittaforma corneae* and *Encephalitozoon hellem* in a patient with AIDS. *Clin. Infect. Dis.*, 27, 1521–1524, 1998.
115. Soule, J. B., Halverson, A. L., Becker, R. B., Pistole, M. C., and Orenstein, J. M. A patient with acquired immunodeficiency syndrome and untreated *Encephalitozoon (Septata) intestinalis* microsporidiosis leading to small bowel perforation. Response to albendazole. *Arch. Pathol. Lab. Med.*, 121, 880–887, 1997.
116. Lowder, C. Y., McMahon, J. T., Meisler, D. M., et al. Microsporidial keratoconjunctivitis caused by *Septata intestinalis* in a patient with acquired immunodeficiency syndrome. *Am. J. Ophthalmol.*, 121, 715–717, 1996.
117. Sheikh, R. A., Prindiville, T. P., Yenamandra, S., Munn, R. J., and Ruebner, B. H. Microsporidial AIDS cholangiopathy due to *Encephalitozoon intestinalis*: case report and review. *Am. J. Gastroenterol.*, 95, 2364–2371, 2000.
118. Liberman, E. and Yen, T. S. Foamy macrophages in acquired immunodeficiency syndrome cholangiopathy with *Encephalitozoon intestinalis*. *Arch. Pathol. Lab. Med.*, 121, 985–988, 1997.
119. Ledford, D. K., Overman, M. D., Gonzalvo, A., Cali, A., Mester, S. W., and Lockey, R. F. Microsporidiosis myositis in a patient with the acquired immunodeficiency syndrome. *Ann. Intern. Med.*, 102, 628, 1985.
120. Macher, A. M., Neafie, R., Angritt, P., and Tuur, S. M. Microsporidial myositis and the acquired immunodeficiency syndrome (AIDS): a four-year follow-up. *Ann. Intern. Med.*, 109, 343, 1988.
121. Grau, A., Valls, M. E., Williams, J. E., Ellis, D. S., Muntane, M. J., and Nadal, C. Myositis caused by *Pleistophora* in a patient with AIDS. *Med. Clin. (Barc.)*, 107, 779–781, 1996.
122. Canning, E. U., Curry, A., Lacey, C. J., and Fenwick, D. Ultrastructure of *Encephalitozoon* sp. infecting the conjunctival, corneal, and nasal epithelia of a patient with AIDS. *Eur. J. Parasitol.*, 28, 226, 1992.
123. Field, A. S., Marriott, D. J., Milliken, S. T., et al. Myositis associated with a newly described microsporidian, *Trachipleistophora hominis*, in a patient with AIDS. *J. Clin. Microbiol.*, 34, 2803–2811, 1996.
124. Margileth, A. M., Strano, A. J., Chandra, R., Neafie, R., Blum, M., and McCully, R. M. Disseminated nosematosis in an immunologically compromised infant. *Arch. Pathol.*, 95, 145, 1973.
125. Shadduck, J. A., Meccoli, R. A., Davis, R., and Font, R. L. First isolation of a microsporidian from a human patient. *J. Infect. Dis.*, 162, 773, 1990.
126. Davis, R. M., Font, R. L., Keisler, M. S., and Shadduck, J. A. Corneal microsporidiosis: a case report including ultrastructural observations. *Ophthalmology*, 97, 953, 1990.
127. Ashton, N. and Wirasinha, P. A. Encephalitozoonosis (Nosematosis) of the cornea. *Br. J. Ophthalmol.*, 57, 669, 1973.
128. Pinnolis, M., Egbert, P. R., Font, R. L., and Winter, F. C. Nosematosis of the cornea. *Arch. Ophthalmol.*, 99, 1044, 1981.
129. Didier, E. S., Shadduck, J. A., Didier, P. J., Millichamp, N., and Vossbrinck, C. R. Studies on ocular microsporidia. *J. Protozool.*, 38, 635, 1991.
130. Cali, A., Takvorian, P. M., Lewin, S., et al. *Brachiola vesicularum*, n.g., n. sp., a new microsporidium associated with AIDS and myositis. *J. Eukaryot. Microbiol.*, 45, 240–251, 1998.
131. Khan, I. A., Schwartzman, J. D., Kasper, L. H., and Moretto, M. CD+ CTLs are essential for protective immunity against *Encephalitozoon cuniculi* infection. *J. Immunol.*, 162, 6086–6091, 1999.
132. Blanshard, C., Ellis, D. S., Tovey, D. G., Dowell, S., and Gazzard, B. G. Treatment of intestinal microsporidiosis with albendazole in patients with AIDS. *AIDS*, 6, 311, 1992.
133. Wanke, C. A., Pleskow, D., Degirolami, P. C., Lambl, B. B., Merkel, K., and Akrabawi, S. A medium chain triglyceride-based diet in patients with HIV and chronic diarrhea reduces diarrhea and malabsorption: a prospective controlled trial. *Nutrition*, 12, 766–771, 1996.
134. Miao, Y. M., Awad-El-Kariem, F. M., Franzen, C., et al. Eradication of cryptosporidia and microsporidia following successful antiretroviral therapy. *J. Aquir. Immun. Defic. Syndr.*, 25, 124–129, 2000.

135. Maggi, P., Larocca, A. M., Quarto, M., et al. Effect of antiretroviral therapy on cryptosporidiosis and microsporidiosis in patients infected with human immunodeficiency virus type 1. *Eur. J. Clin. Microbiol. Infect. Dis.*, 19, 213–217, 2000.
136. Bobin, S., Bouhour, D., Durupt, S., Boibieux, A., Girault, V., and Peyramond, D. Importance of antiproteases in the treatment of microsporidia and/or cryptosporidia infections in HIV-seropositive patients. *Pathol. Biol. (Paris)*, 46, 418–419, 1998.
137. Contes, C. N., Berlin, O. G., Speck, C. E., Pandhumas, S. S., Lariviere, M. J., and Fu, C. Modification of the clinical course of intestinal microsporidiasis in acquired immunodeficiency syndrome patients by immune status and anti-human immunodeficiency virus therapy. *Am. J. Trop. Med. Hyg.*, 58, 555–558, 1998.
138. Goguel, J., Katlama, C., Sarfati, C., Maslo, C., Leport, C., and Molina, J. M. Remission of AIDS-associated intestinal microsporidiosis with highly active antiretroviral therapy. *AIDS*, 11, 1658–1659, 1997.
139. Simon, D., Weiss, L. M., Tanowitz, H. B., Cali, A., Jones, J., and Wittner, M. Light microscopic diagnosis of human microsporidiosis and variable response to octreotide. *Gastroenterology*, 100, 271, 1991.
140. Kreinik, G., Burstein, O., Landor, E. W., Burnstein, L., Weiss, L. M., and Wittner, M. Successful treatment of intractable cryptosporidial diarrhea with intravenous octreotide (sandostatin), a somatostatin analogue. *AIDS*, 5, 765, 1991.
141. Bernard, E., Michiels, J. F., Durant, J., et al. Intestinal microsporidiosis due to *Enterocytozoon bieneusi*: a new case report in an AIDS patient. *Lancet*, 5, 606, 1991.
142. Blanshard, C. and Gazzard, B. G. Microsporidiosis in HIV-1-infected individuals. *Lancet*, 337, 1488, 1991.
143. Dieterich, D. T., Lew, E. A., Kotler, D. P., Poles, M. A., and Orenstein, J. M. Treatment with albendazole for intestinal disease due to *Enterocytozoon bieneusi* in patients with AIDS. *J. Infect. Dis.*, 169, 178, 1994.
144. Aarons, E. J., Woodrow, D., Hollister, W. S., Canning, E. U., Francis, N., and Gazzard, B. G. Reversible renal failure caused by a microsporidian infection. *AIDS*, 8, 1119, 1994.
145. Lecuit, M., Oksenhendler, E., and Sarfati, C. Use of albendazole for disseminated microsporidian infection in a patient with AIDS. *Clin. Infect. Dis.*, 19, 332, 1994.
146. Joste, N. E., Rich, J. D., Busam, K. J., and Schwartz, D. A. Autopsy verification of *Encephalitozoon intestinalis* (microsporidiosis) eradication following albendazole therapy. *Arch. Pathol. Lab. Med.*, 120, 199–203, 1996.
147. Sharpstone, D., Rowbottom, A., Francis, N., et al. Thalidomide: a novel therapy for microsporidiosis. *Gastroenterology*, 112, 1823–1829, 1997 [published erratum in *Gastroenterology*, 113, 1054, 1997].
148. Weber, R., Sauer, B., Spycher, M. A., et al. Detection of *Septata intestinalis* in stool specimens and coprodiagnostic monitoring of successful treatment with albendazole. *Clin. Infect. Dis.*, 19, 342, 1994.
149. Molina, J. M., Chastang, C., Goguel, J., et al. Albendazole for treatment and prophylaxis of microsporidiosis due to *Encephalitozoon intestinalis* in patients with AIDS: a randomized double-blind controlled trial. *J. Infect. Dis.*, 177, 1373–1377, 1998.
150. Dionisio, D., Manneschi, L. I., Di Lollo, S., et al. Persistent damage to *Enterocytozoon bieneusi*, with persistent symptomatic relief, after combined furazolidone and albendazole in AIDS patients. *J. Clin. Pathol.*, 51, 731–736, 1998.
151. Dionisio, D., Manneschi, L. I., Di Lollo, S., et al. *Enterocytozoon bieneusi* in AIDS: symptomatic relief and parasite changes after furazolidone. *J. Clin. Pathol.*, 50, 472–476, 1997.
152. Liu, T. P. and Myrick, G. R., Deformities in the spore of *Nosema apis* as induced by itraconazole. *Parasitol. Res.*, 75, 498, 1989.
153. Albrecht, H., Stellbrink, H.-J., and Sobottka, I. Failure of itraconazole to prevent *Enterocytozoon bieneusi* infection. *Genitourin. Med.*, 71, 325, 1995.
154. Gritz, D. C., Holsclaw, D. S., Neger, R. E., Whitcher, J. P., Jr., and Margolis, T. P. Ocular and sinus microsporidial infection cured with systemic albendazole. *Am. J. Ophthalmol.*, 124, 241–243, 1997.
155. Didier, E. S., Rogers, L. B., Brush, A. D., Wong, S., Traina-Dorge, V., and Bertucci, D. Diagnosis of disseminated microsporidian *Encephatlitozoon hellem* infection by PCR- Southern analysis and successful treatment with albendazole and fumagillin. *J. Clin. Microbiol.*, 34, 947–952, 1996.
156. Coyle, C., Kent, M., Tanowitz, H. B., Wittner, M., and Weiss, L. M. TNP-470 is an effective antimicrosporidial agent. *J. Infect. Dis.*, 177, 515–518, 1998.
157. Didier, E. S. Effects of albendazole, fumagillin, and TNP-470 on microsporidial replication in vitro. *Antimicrob. Agents Chemother.*, 41, 1541–1546, 1997.
158. Kersten, A., Althaus, C., Seitz, H. M., Pfahl, H. G., and Sundmacher, R. Bilateral microsporidial keratitis in an HIV-positive patient with AIDS stage infection. *Klin. Monatsbl. Augenheilkd.*, 212, 476–479, 1998.
159. Molina, J. M., Goguel, J., Sarfati, C., et al. Trial of oral fumagillin for the treatment of intestinal microsporidiosis in patients with HIV. ANRS 054 Study Group. Agence Nationale de Recherche sur le SIDA. *AIDS*, 14, 1341–1318, 2000.
160. Molina, J. M., Goguel, J., Sarfati, C., et al. Potential efficacy of fumagillin in intestinal microsporidiosis due to *Enterocytozoon bieneusi* in patients with HIV infection: results of a drug screening study. The French Microsporidiosis Study Group. *AIDS*, 11, 1603–1610, 1997.
161. Bicart-See, A., Massip, P., Linas, M. D., and Datry, A. Successful treatment with nitazoxanide of *Enterocytozoon bieneusi* microsporidiosis in a patient with AIDS. *Antimicrob. Agents Chemother.*, 44, 167–168, 2000.
162. Anwar-Bruni, D. M., Hogan, S. E., Schwartz, D. A., Wilcox, C. M., Bryan, R. T., and Lennox, J. L. Atovaquone is effective treatment for symptoms of gastrointestinal microsporidiosis in HIV-1-infective patients. *AIDS*, 10, 619–623, 1996.
163. Kester, K. E., Turiansky, G. W., and McEvoy, P. L., Nodular cutaneous microsporidiosis in a patient with AIDS and successful treatment with long-term oral clindamycin therapy. *Ann. Intern. Med.*, 128, 911–914, 1998.

17
Strongyloides stercoralis

1. INTRODUCTION

Strongyloides stercoralis, the causative agent of strongyloidiasis, is an intestinal nematod classified in the genus Strongyloides. The latter are plasmids widely distributed as intestinal parasites in mammals. *S. stercoralis* (known also as *S. intestinalis*, *Anguillula intestinalis*, *A. stercoralis*) is a roundworm occuring mainly in tropical and subtropical countries *(1)*. In the U. S., strongyloidiasis is endemic in certain southern regions (eastern Kentucky, Tennessee, Lousiana, and southern Appalachia) *(2–4)*, although cases have been reported in all major geographic areas of the country *(2,3,5–18)*, with fatal outcomes being reported in malnourished children from socioeconomically deprived circumstances *(13,19,20)*.

S. stercoralis is uniquely capable of perpetuating itself both in the soil and within the human host *(21,22)*. Strongyloidiasis may be characterized with overwhelming proliferation of worms in the gastrointestinal tract and by maturation of noninfective rhabtidiform larvae into the infective filariform larvae before the latter are excreted into the stool. In addition, the worms can cause damage directly by invading tissues or by carrying with them intestinal microorganisms that cause secondary infections *(5,6,23–31)*.

S. stercoralis, which inhabits the gastrointestinal tract of a substantial proportion of the human population, can cause a chronic and essentially asymptomatic infection showing little if any symptoms in the immunocompetent host *(18,32–37)*. However, in the presence of abnormalities in the immune responses *(38,39)* (mainly cellular *[5,6,40,41]* but also humoral immunity), hyperinfection may develop *(8,23,27,42–47)*.

Clinically, strongyloidiasis is often asymptomatic but may be manifested by abdominal pain, distention, or ileus, and by secondary infections due to enteric (bacterial or fungal) microorganisms.

2. STRONGYLOIDIASIS AS OPPORTUNISTIC INFECTION IN IMMUNOCOMPROMISED HOSTS

Because the parasite is uniquely able to carry out its entire life cycle inside the human body, in immunocompromised patients strongyloidiasis can lead to a hyperinfection syndrome with high morbiduty and mortality due to the accelerated endogenous autoinfection *(1,6,45–47)*.

Patients on corticosteroid therapy *(5,6,48–54)* renal-transplant recipients *(55–60)* or renal deficiency *(23,27,61–63)*, patients with systemic lupus erythematosus (SLE) *(38)*, diabetes *(64–66)*, asthma *(25,29,50)*, chronic dermatosis *(10,23,27,61)*, chronic infections (lepromatous leprosy *[23,38]*, tuberculoid leprosy *[38]*, and tuberculosis *[23,27,67]*) as well as those with neoplastic conditions (lymphoma, leukemia, and solid tumors) *(6–9,23,24,28,38,61,68–74)*, protein-calorie malnutrition *(10,19,23,32,75,76)* (shown to compromise cell-mediated immunity *[23,77]*), chronic alcoholism *(11,78,79)*, and achlorhydria *(12,80,81)*, are all at higher risk and may develop systemic

From: Opportunistic Infections: Treatment and Prophylaxis
By: Vassil St. Georgiev © Humana Press Inc., Totowa, NJ

strongyloidiasis. Parana et al. *(82)* described two cases of severe strongyloidiasis coincident with ribavirin plus interferon therapy for treating hepatitis C virus infection pointing to a possible role of ribavirin in modifying the immune response to *S. stercoralis*.

Patients infected with HIV *(83–85)* and the human T-lymphotropic virus type 1 (HTLV-1) *(86–90)* may be also at high risk for strongyloidiasis. High prevalence of HTLV-1-directed antibodies has been found in carriers of *S. stercoralis (91,92)*. Occurrence of strongyloidiosis always progresses to hyperinfestation or dissemination with severe clinical carriers of HTLV-1 *(93)*. This phenomenon may be linked to selective immunosuppression by the retrovirus (as evidenced by the very low total serum levels of IgE) creating a favorable environment for nematode proliferation *(94)*. Furthermore, it has been also suggested that the *Strongyloides* infection may, in turn, contribute to the leukemogenesis by HTLV-1 in cases of adult T-cell leukemia lymphoma *(87,95)*.

Disseminated strongyloidiasis and the hyperinfection syndrome are among the opportunistic infections that would be considered indicative for underlying cell-mediated immunodeficiency such as in patients with AIDS *(83,96,97)*. Sexually active homosexual men are at increased risk for *S. stercoralis* infection, which can be acquired as a sexually transmitted disease.

The underrepresentation of the hyperinfection among the opportunistic infections linked to AIDS may be explained, at least partially, with the specific immunodeficiency state of AIDS, which may be more conducive to reactivation of infection with unicellular protozoa (e.g., *Toxoplasma gondii*) rather than to proliferation of infections involving complex, multicellular worms *(96)*. Other factors, such as underdiagnosis and underreporting may also account for the small number of strongyloidiasis cases in AIDS patients.

According to Gompels et al. *(83)*, there was compelling evidence to suggest that the development of hypeinfection occurred only in a subset of doubly infected patients because of the greater severity of HIV-induced immunodeficiency and the presence of an additional defect of the host defense, such as granulocytopenia. That is, that cell-mediated immunodeficiency due to HIV alone will not predispose to *Strongyloides* hyperinfection, but will also require a reduced numbers or function of granulocytes.

In cases reported in the literature *(84,98–104)*, the disease has been localized mainly in the intestines. Peripheral blood eosinophilia is common. Spillover infection to the colon did occur *(105)*.

Because *S. stercoralis* can pass through the lungs it can induce also chronic obstructive pulmonary disease *(106)* and extensive intra-alveolar hemorrhage *(107,108)*. Pulmonary signs and symptoms include cough, shortness of breath, wheezing, and hepoptysis, adult respiratory distress syndrome (ARDS), and pulmonary infiltrates *(108)*.

Severe disseminated strongyloidiasis can often be fatal *(52,64,66,71,106,109)*. Kiyuna et al. *(110)* have reported a case of periarteritis nodosa associated with disseminated strongyloidiasis. In addition to gastrointestinal and pulmonary disease, cutaneous manifestations (urticaria, maculopapular exanthema, localized or generalized pruritus, and prurigo) may also arise from the migration of the larvae in the skin *(47)*. Strongyloidiasis presenting as generalized prurigo nodularis and lichen simplex chronicus was described by Jacob and Patten *(111)*.

Cases associated with nephrotic syndrome brought on by infection of *S. stercoralis* have also been reported *(112,113)*. The remission of the nephrotic syndrome after treatment of the infection suggested the possibility of *Strongyloides*-associated glomerulonephtitis *(113)*. Cases of reactive arthritis induced by *S. stercoralis* are exceedingly rare *(114)*.

The eosinophil count is typically elevated in immunocompetent patients *(115,120)*, but is usually absent in immunosuppressed patients with the hyperinfection syndrome *(52,115–117)*. As reported by Aziz et al. *(32)* as many as 94% of patients with strongyloidiasis showed peripheral blood eosinophilia as a symptom of the disease. Savage et al. *(121)* reported an unusual case of an immunosuppressed patient with strongyloidiasis who was minimally symptomatic but with a dramatic increase in his eosinophil count. Although the mechanism of this phenomenon was unclear some synergistic association between the eosinophilopoietic effects of helminth infection *(117,122)* and chemotherapy *(123)* seemed plausible. In several other reports *(115,124–126)*, cases of immunosuppressed patients with mild strongyloidiasis and higher eosinophilic counts, have also been described. Because there is no eosinophilia in AIDS patients, it may be the lack of eosinophils that is the most relevant factor to predisposition *(83)*.

Although individuals with asymptomatic infection do not have raised IgE titers, it is often a feature in immunocompromised patients, such as AIDS *(83)*. It has been suggested that greater survival may be associated with higher IgE levels *(1)*.

3. CORTICOSTEROID THERAPY AS A PREDISPOSING FACTOR FOR STRONGYLOIDIASIS

One of the major stages of the development cycle of *S. stercoralis* within the human body is the transformation of rhabdiform larvae into invasive filariform larvae in the gut *(5)*. On average, it takes between 24–48 h for this process to complete. There is evidence that the conversion of rhabdiform larve into the filariform could be altered by corticosteroid administration *(22)*. It has been established by several groups *(127–129)*, that during corticosteroid administration in animals infected with *Nippostrongylus brasiliensis* or *S. ratti*, there have been an absolute rise in worm numbers and a fractional increase in invasive filariform larve relative to rhabdiform larvae in the intestinal tracts. However, the mechanism of this augmentation of metamorphosis is poorly understood. Moreover, the corticosteroids may also reduce the local inflammation which, in turn, may further impair the containment of the parasites allowing increased number of invasive filiform larvae to penetrate the gut wall and complete the endogenous autoinfection cycle. Finally, the immunosuppression activity of corticosteroids (or any other immunosuppressive drug, such as azathioprine and cyclophosphamide) will also help enhance the predisposition of the host to hyperinfection *(5,50,51,53)*.

4. TREATMENT OF STRONGYLOIDIASIS

Even though the morbidity and mortality rates are relatively high, especially in immunocompromised hosts with hyperinfection syndrome, those patients who receive prompt and adequate treatment have a reasonably favorable prognosis to survive.

Thiabendazole, a 2-(4-thiazolyl)benzimidazole anthelmintic agent, has been the drug of choice in the treatment of strongyloidiosis especially in cases of refractory infections *(10)*. Thiabendazole, however, is not available for parenteral administration. Thiabendazole has been especially effective in immunocompetent patients *(130,131)*. For uncomplicated gastrointestinal infections, the usual recommended dose has been 25 mg/kg b.i.d. for 2 or more d *(5,6,11,38,62,83,96)*. However, in immunocompromised patients, the therapy may take longer than that *(132)*, as well as the necessity of higher doses *(5,6,109,133,134)*. According to Levi et al. *(109)*, in cases of prolonged therapy, daily administration of 3 g of thiabendazole may be adequate. Adam et al. *(24)* have used courses of 15–40 g of thiabendazole for over 10–15 d in order to achieve favorable response.

Because of its adverse side effects (dizziness, hypotension, neurotoxicity, leukopenia *[135]*, elevated hepatic enzymes *[135,136]*, and often severe cholestatic hepatitis *[137,138]*) in some patients, at least the prophylatic use of thiabendazole is controversial and did not receive wide acceptance *(139)*. Levi et al. *(109)* suggested cambendazole as an useful alternative for disseminated strongyloidiasis in cases of intolerance (high incidence of liver dysfunction) to thiabendazole. Persistent infection despite of adequate antiparasitic therapy with thiabendazole has been associated with the development of lung abscesses *(14)* harboring the parasite. The lesions are refractory to oral medication and may result in death. To this end, surgical resection or drainage may be helpful *(5)*.

Scowden et al. *(5)* treated a number of immunocompromised patients with strongyloidiasis using combination of thiabendazole (15–25 mg/kg, b.i.d., orally or via a nasogastric tube) and metronidazole.

In spite of thiabendazole therapy, in two cases *(140,141)* of ARDS associated with *S. stercoralis,* the outcome was fatal. In one of the reported cases *(141)*, ARDS had developed after successful therapy of the parasitic disease and coincided with the rapid taper of the immunosuppressive corticosteroid therapy. In two previous reports by the same group *(142,143)*, treatment of pulmonary strongyloidiasis has been successful despite continued therapy with high-dose systemic corticosteroids. One recommended treatment regimen for patients with ARDS involved thiabendazole (25 mg/kg, b.i.d.) given for 7 d rather than the 3-d treatment with the same dose applied to patients without ARDS *(108)*.

Savage et al. *(121)* treated strongyloidiasis in an immunosuppressed patient with albendazole (also a benzimidazole derivative) at daily doses of 400 mg given in four 3-d cycles. Other reports *(144–146)* have corroborated the efficacy of this dose regimen. In another treatment regimen, albendazole was administered at 400 mg given twice daily for 6 d, followed by a maintenance dose of 400 mg once daily *(73)*. Hanck and Holzer *(48)* also reported the use of oral albendazole to treat an immunosuppressed patient on corticosteroid therapy, and severe diarrhea and dehydration because of strongyloidiasis. Significant improvement has been reported in a case of fulminating strongyloidiasis complicating kala-azar after treatment with albendazole *(147)*.

Recent reports have indicated that ivermectin, a macrolide antibiotic primarily known for its activity against onchocerciasis, was also efficacious in the treatment of strongyloidiasis in immunocompetent patients with cure rates averaging 94% *(92,148)*. Ivermectin has been used in HIV-infected patients with *S. stercoralis*-associated hyperinfection *(84,85)*. Two regimens have been applied: a single 200-μg/kg daily oral dose *(84,149)*, or the same dose given on a multiple schedule (on d 1, 2, 15, and 16) *(84)*. All seven patients who received multiple doses showed sustained clinical and parasitological cure, whereas one of two patients who were given the single dose relapsed promptly and fatally. Ashraf et al. *(150)* also reported a case of strongyloidiasis in a patient with hypogammaglobulinemia in which ivermectin failed to clear the nematode larvae from stool, despite repeated courses of treatment throughout 14 mo. Nevertheless, because of its different pharmacokinetic profile and lesser toxicity, ivermectin may become an attractive alternative to thiabendazole.

Other drugs that have been used in the treatment of strongyloidiasis were pyrvinium pamoate and mebendazole. Giannoulis et al. *(151)* used in a patient with disseminated strongyloidiasis mebendazole (200 mg b.i.d., over a 3-d period) with dramatic clinical improvement; the dose regimen was repeated in 2 and 5 wk to completely eliminate the nematode from feces. As the case with thiabendazole, mebendazole has also been associated with high incidence of liver dysfunction *(152)*. In addition, relapse of pulmonary strongyloidiasis after medication with mebendazole (100 mg b.i.d.) was ceased, has been reported *(106)*. To this end, it is important to note that because of the high relapse rate of pulmonary strongyloidiasis (15%), serial follow-up of stool and sputum should be carried out.

Whereas in some studies pyrvinium pamoate and mebendazole were found to be effective against hookworms (*Necator Americana*, *Ancylostoma duodenale*, *A. caninum*, *A. brasiliensis*), their efficacy against strongyloidiasis was questionable *(119,152)*.

4.1. Comparative Studies

Toma et al. *(153)* have undertaken a study to compare the efficacy of ivermectin (6 mg in a single dose), albendazole (400 mg daily for 3 d), and pyrvinium pamoate (5 mg/kg daily for 3 d) in 211 patients with strongyloidiasis. For each treatment, the same regimen was repeated once 2 wk later, and the efficacy was assessed at wk 2, 6 mo, and 12 mo after the second course of treatment. The coprological cure rates were 97.0% (65 out of 67 patients), 77.4% (65 out of 84), and 23.3% (14 out of 60 patients) for ivermectin, albendazole and pyrvinium pamoate, respectively. In general, the cure rates were lower in males and patients with concurrent HTLV-1 infection.

A comparative randomized trial of a single dose ivermectin (200 μg/kg) vs albendazole (400 mg daily for 3 d) for treatment of 301 children with strongyloidiasis showed ivermectin to be superior with cure rates of 83% and 45%, respectively *(154)*. No severe side effects were observed and mild side effects were of transient nature for both treatments.

An open randomized study for comparing the efficacy of albendazole (400 mg, b.i.d. for 5 d; group A) and thiabendazole (1.0 g, b.i.d. for 5 d; group B) in chronic strongyloidiasis was conducted in 1990–1992 *(155)*. The cure rates for group A (23 patients) and group B (12 patients) were 95% and 100%, respectively.

REFERENCES

1. Genta, R. M. Global prevalence of strongyloidiasis: critical review with epidemiologic insights into the prevention of disseminated disease. *Rev. Infect. Dis.*, 11, 755, 1989.
2. Fulmer, H. S. and Huempfner, H. R. Intestinal helminths in eastern Kentucky: a survey in rural counties. *Am. J. Trop. Med. Hyg.*, 14, 269, 1965.
3. Ophüs, W. A fatal case of strongyloidiasis in man, with autopsy. *Arch. Pathol.*, 8, 1, 1929.
4. Berk, S. L., Verghese, A., Alvarez, S., Hall, K., and Smith, B. Clinical and epidemiologic features of strongyloidiasis: a prospective study in rural Tennessee. *Arch. Intern. Med.*, 147, 1257, 1987.
5. Scowden, E. B., Schaffner, W., and Stone, W. J. Overwhelming strongyloidiasis: an unappreciated opportunistic infection. *Medicine (Baltimore)*, 57, 527, 1978.
6. Igra-Siegman, Y., Kapila, R., Sen, P., Kaminski, Z. C., and Louria, D. B. Syndrome of hyperinfection with *Strongyliodes stercoralis*. *Rev. Infect. Dis.*, 3, 397, 1981.
7. Pollock, T. W. and Perencevich, E. N. Hyperinfection with *Strongyloides stercoralis* in a patient with Hodgkin's disease. *J. Am. Ostheopath. Assoc.*, 76, 171, 1976.
8. Rogers, W. A. Jr. and Nelson, B. Strongyloidiasis and malignant lymphoma:"opportunistic infection" by a nematode. *J. Am. Med. Assoc.*, 195, 685, 1966.
9. Buss, D. H. *Strongyliodes stercoralis* infection complicating granulocytic leukemia. *N. C. Med. J.*, 32, 269, 1971.
10. Civantos, F. and Robinson, M. J. Fatal strongyloidiasis following corticosteroid therapy. *Am. J. Dig. Dis.*, 14, 643, 1969.
11. Cahill, K. M. Thiabendazole in massive strongyloidiasis. *Am. J. Trop. Med. Hyg.*, 16, 451, 1967.
12. Amir-Ahmadi, H., Braun, P., Neva, F. A., Gottlieb. L. S., and Zamcheck, N. Strongyloidiasis at the Boston City Hospital. *Am. J. Dig. Dis.*, 13, 959, 1968.
13. Smith, S. B., Schwartzman, M., Mencia, L. F., et al. Fatal disseminated strongyloidiasis presenting as acute abdominal distress in an urban child. *J. Pediatr.*, 91, 607, 1977.
14. Seabury, J. H., Abadie, S., and Savoy, F. Jr. Pulmonary strongyloidiasis with lung abscess: ineffectiveness of thiabendazole therapy. *Am. J. Trop. Med. Hyg.*, 20, 209, 1971.
15. Cuni, L., Rosner, F., and Chawla, S. K. Fatal strongyloidiasis in immunosuppressed patients. *NY State J. Med.*, 77, 2109, 1977.
16. Cummins, R. O., Suratt, P. M., and Horwitz, D. A. Disseminated *Strongyloides stercoralis* infection. *Arch. Intern. Med.*, 138, 1005, 1978.
17. Berger, R., Kraman, S., and Paciotti, M. Pulmonary strongyloidiasis complicating therapy with corticosteroids. *Am. J. Trop. Med. Hyg.*, 29, 31, 1980.
18. Milder, J. E., Walzer, P. D., Kilgore, G., Rutherford, I., and Klein, M. Clinical features of *Strongyloides stercoralis* infection in an endemic area of the United States. *Gastroenterology*, 80, 1481, 1981.
19. Cookson, J. B., Montgomery, R. D., Morgan, H. V., and Tudor, R. W. Fatal paralytic ileus due to strongyloidiasis. *Br. Med. J.*, 4, 771, 1972.
20. Huchton, P. and Horn, R. Strongyloidiasis. *J. Pediatr.*, 55, 602, 1959.
21. Faust, E. C. and DeGroat, A. Internal autoinfection in human strongyloidiasis. *Am. J. Trop. Med.*, 20, 359, 1940.
22. Galliard, H. Pathogenesis of *Strongyloides*. *Helminthol. Abstr.*, 36, 247, 1967.
23. Purtilo, D. T., Meyers, W. M., and Connor, D. H. Fatal strongyloidiasis in immunosuppressed patients. *Am. J. Med.*, 56, 488, 1974.
24. Adam, M., Morgan, O., Persaud, C., and Gibbs, W. N. Hyperinfection syndrome, with *Strongyloides stercoralis* in malignant lymphoma. *Br. Med. J.*, 1, 264, 1973.
25. Ali-Khan, Z. and Seemayer, T. A. Fatal bowel infaction and sepsis: an unusual complication of systemic strongyloidiasis. *Trans. R. Soc. Trop. Med. Hyg.*, 69, 473, 1975.
26. Brown, H. W. and Perna, V. P., An overwhelming *Strongyloides* infection. *J. Am. Med. Assoc.*, 168, 1648, 1958.
27. Cruz, T., Reboucas, G., and Rocha, H. Fatal strongyloidiasis in patients receiving corticosteroids. *N. Engl. J. Med.*, 275, 1093, 1966.
28. Kuberski, T. T., Gabor, E. P., and Boudreaux, D. Disseminated strongyloidiasis: a complication of the immunosuppressed host. *West. J. Med.*, 122, 504, 1975.
29. Higenbottam, T. W. and Heard, B. E. Opportunistic pulmonary strongyloidiasis complicating asthma treated with steroids. *Thorax*, 31, 226, 1976.
30. Liepman, M. Disseminated *Strongyloides stercoralis*, a complication of immunosuppression. *J. Am. Med. Assoc.*, 231, 287, 1975.
31. Cadham, F. T. Infestation with *Strongyloides stercoralis* associated with severe symptoms. *Can. Med. Assoc. J.*, 29, 18, 1933.
32. Aziz, E. M. *Strongyloides stercoralis* infestation: review of the literature and report of 33 cases. *South. Med. J.*, 62, 806, 1969.
33. Rojas, R. A. M. *Pathology of Protozoal and Helminthic Diseases*. Williams & Wilkins, Baltimore, 713, 1971.
34. Scaglia, M., Brustia, R., Gatti, S., et al. Autochthonous strongyloidiasis in Italy: an epidemiological and clinical review of 150 cases. *Bull. Soc. Pathol. Exot. Filiales*, 77, 328, 1984.

35. Genta, R. M., Gatti, S., Linke, M. J., Cevini, C., and Scaglia, M. Endemic strongyloidiasis in northern Italy: clinical and immunological aspects. *Q. J. Med.*, 258, 679, 1988.
36. Davidson, R. A. Strongyloidiasis: a presentation of 63 cases. *N. C. Med. J.*, 43, 23, 1982.
37. Davidson, R. A., Fletcher, R. H., and Chapman, L. E. Risk factros for strongyloidiasis: a case-control study. *Arch. Intern. Med.*, 144, 321, 1984.
38. Rivera, E., Maldonado, N., Velez-Garcia, E., Grillo, A. J., and Malaret, G. Hyperinfection syndrome with *Strongyloides stercoralis*. *Ann. Intern. Med.*, 72, 199, 1970.
39. Keller, R. and Keist, R. Protective immunity to *Nippostrongylus brasiliensis* in the rat: central role of the lymphocyte in worm expulsion. *Immunology*, 22, 767, 1972.
40. Neva, F. A. Biology and immunology of human strongyloidiasis. *J. Infect. Dis.*, 153, 397, 1986.
41. Genta, R. M. *Strongylodes stercoralis*: immunobiological considerations on an unusual worm. *Parasitology Today*, 2, 241, 1986.
42. Wong, B. Parasitic diseases in immunocompromised hosts. *Am. J. Med.*, 76, 479, 1984.
43. Longworth, D. L. and Weller, P. F. Hyperinfection syndrome with strongyloidiasis, in *Current Clinical Topics in Infectious Diseases*, Remington, J. S. and Swartz, M. N., Eds., McGraw-Hill, New York, 1, 1986.
44. Willis, A. J., P. and Nwokolo, C. Steroid therapy and strongyloidiasis. *Lancet*, 1, 1396, 1966.
45. Smith, J. W. Strongyloidiasis. *Clin. Microbiol. Newsletter*, 13, 33, 1991.
46. Armstrong, D. and Paredes, J. Strongyloidiasis, in *Respiratory Disease in the Immunocompromised Host*, Shalamer, J., Pizzo, P. A., Parrillo, J. E., and Masur, H., Eds. J. B. Lippincott, Philadelphia, 428, 1991.
47. Karolyi, Z., Eros, N., and Kriston, R. Cutaneous manifestations of strongyloidosis. *Orv. Hetil.* 140, 191–194, 1999.
48. Hanck, Ch. and Holzer, B. R. Strongyloidiasis unter immunosuppressiver therapy. *Schweiz. Med. Wcshr.*, 122, 899, 1992.
49. Stewart, J. B. and Heap, B. J. Fatal disseminated strongyloidiasis in an immunocompromised former war prisoner of the Japanese. *J. R. Army Med. Corps*, 131, 47, 1985,
50. Rivals, A., Rouquet, R. M., Recco, P., Linas, M. D., Leophonte, P., and Didier, A. A rare cause of asthma exacerbation: systemic anguilluliasis. *Rev. Mal. Respir.*, 17, 99–102, 2000.
51. Thomas, M. C. and Costello, S. A. Disseminated strongyloidiasis arising from a single dose of dexamethasone before stereotactic radiosurgery. *Int. J. Clin. Pract.*, 52, 520–521, 1998.
52. Suvajdzic, N., Kranjcic-Zec, I., Jovanovic, V., Popovic, D., and Colovic, M. Fatal strongyloidosis following corticosteroid therapy in a patient with chronic idiopathic thrombocytopenia. *Haematologia (Budap.)*, 29, 323–326, 1999.
53. Link, K. and Orenstein, R. Bacterial complications of strongyloidiasis: *Streptococcus bovis* meningitis. *South Med. J.*, 92, 728–731, 1999.
54. Suvajdzic, N., Kranjcic-Zec, I., Jovanovic, V., Popovic, D., and Colovic, M. Fatal strongyloidosis following corticosteroid therapy in a patient with chronic idiopathic thrombocytopenia. *Haematologia (Budap)*, 29, 323–326, 1999.
55. Batoni, F. L., Ianhez, L. E., Saldanha, L. B., and Sabbaga, E. Acute respiratory insufficiency caused by disseminated strongyloidiasis in a renal transplant. *Rev. Inst. Ned. Trop. Sao Paulo*, 18, 283, 1976.
56. Fagundes, L. A., Busato, O., and Brentano, L. Strongyloidiasis: fatal complication of renal transplantation. *Lancet*, 2, 439, 1971.
57. Meyers, A. M., Shapiro, D. J., Milne, F. J., Myburgh, J. A., and Rabkin, R. *Strongyloides stercoralis* hyperinfection in a renal allograft recipient. *S. Afr. Med. J.*, 50, 1301, 1976.
58. Scoggin, C. H. and Call, N. B. Acute respiratory failure due to disseminated strongyloidiasis in a renal transplant recipient. *Ann. Intern. Med.*, 87, 456, 1977.
59. DeVault, G. A., King, J. W., Rohr, M. S., Landreneau, M. D., Brown, S.T. III, and McDonald, J. C., Opportunistic infections with *Strongyloides stercoralis* in renal transplantation. *Rev. Infect. Dis.*, 12, 653, 1990.
60. Palau, L. A. and Pankey, G. A. *Strongyloides* hyperinfection in a renal transplant recipient receiving cyclosporine: possible *Strongyloides stercoralis* transmission by kidney transplant. *Am. J. Trop. Med. Hyg.*, 57, 413–415, 1997.
61. Dwork, K. G., Jaffe, J. R., and Lieberman, H. D. Strongyloidiasis with massive hyperinfection. *NY State J. Med.*, 75, 1230, 1975.
62. Neefe, L. I., Pinilla, O., Garagusi, V. F., and Bauer, H. Disseminated strongyloidiasis with cerebral involvement. *Am. J. Med.*, 55, 832, 1973.
63. Said, S., Nevez, G., Moriniere, P., Fournier, A., and Raccurt, C. P. Hemodialyse et strongyloidose: une cause presumee d'hypereosinophilie peut en cacher une autre. *Nephrologie*, 20, 343–346, 1999.
64. Ho, P. L., Luk, W. K., Chan, A. C., and Yuen, K. Y. Two cases of fatal stroingyloidiasis in Hong Kong. *Pathology*, 29, 324–326, 1997.
65. Emad, A. Exudative eosinophilic pleural effusion due to *Strongyloides stercoralis* in a diabetic man. *South. Med. J.*, 92, 58–60, 1999.
66. Bozikov, V., Dzebro, S., Seidle, K., Dominis, M., Zambal, Z., and Skrabalo, Z. Fatal "overwhelming" strongyloidiasis in an immunosuppressed patient. *Lijec Vjesn.*, 118, 23–26, 1996.
67. Nagalotimath, S. J., Ramaprasad, A. V., and Chandrashekhar, N. K. Fatal strongyloidiasis in a patient receiving corticosteroids. *Indian J. Pathol. Bacteriol.*, 17, 190, 1974.
68. Yim, Y., Kikkawa, Y., Tanowitz, H., and Wittner, M. Fatal strongyloidiasis in Hodgkin's disease after immunosuppressive therapy. *J. Trop. Med. Hyg.*, 73, 245, 1970.
69. Rassiga, A. L., Lowry, J. L., and Forman, W. B. Diffuse pulmonary due to *Strongyloides stercoralis*. *J. Am. Med. Assoc.*, 230, 426, 1974.

70. Suzuki, T., Nara, N., Miyake, S., Eishi, Y., Sugiyama, E., and Aoki, N. Fatal strongyloidiasis latent over 42 years in the antineoplastic chemotherapy of a case with malignant lymphoma. *Jpn. J. Med.*, 28, 96, 1989.
71. Patil, P., Jayshree, R. S., Acharya, R. S., Sridhar, H., Babu, G., and Suresh, T. M. Fulminant fatal *Strongylides stercoralis* infection in a post-chemotherapy immunosuppressed cancer patient. *Med. Pediatr. Oncol.*, 33, 504–555, 1999.
72. Daubenton, J. D., Buys, H. A., and Hartley, P. S. Disseminated strongyloidiasis in a child with lymphoblastic lymphoma. *J. Pediatr. Hematol. Oncol.*, 20, 260–263, 1998.
73. Muller, A., Fatkenheuer, G., Salzberger, B., Schrappe, M., and Diehl, V. *Strongyloides stercoralis* infection in a patient with AIDS and non-Hodgkin lymphoma. *Dtsch. Med. Wochenschr.*, 123, 381–385, 1998.
74. Graeff-Teixeira, C., Leite, C. S., Sperhacke, C. L., et al. Prospective study of strongyloidosis in patients with hematologic malignancies. *Rev. Soc. Bras. Med. Trop.*, 30, 355-357, 1997.
75. Hartz, P. H. Human strongyloidiasis with internal autoinfection. *Arch. Pathol.*, 41, 601, 1946.
76. Yoeli, M., Most, H., Berman, H. H., and Scheinesson, G. P., II. The clinical picture and pathology of a massive *Strongyloides* infection in a child. *Trans. R. Soc. Trop. Med. Hyg.*, 57, 346, 1963.
77. Bistrian B. R., Sherman, M., Blackburn, G. L., Marshall, R., and Shaw, C. Cellular immunity in adult marasmus. *Arch. Intern. Med.*, 137, 1408, 1977.
78. Gage, J. G. A case of *Strongyloides intestinalis* with larvae in the sputum. *Arch. Intern. Med.*, 7, 561, 1911.
79. Tullis, D. C. H. Bronchial asthma associated with intestinal parasites. *N. Engl. J. Med.*, 282, 370, 1970.
80. Giannella, R. A., Broitman, S. A., and Zamcheck, N. Influence of gastric acidity on bacterial and parasitic enteric infections. *Ann. Intern. Med.*, 78, 271, 1973.
81. Shikhobalova, N. P. and Semenova, N. E. On the problem of the clinical study and treatment of strongyloidiasis. *Trop. Dis. Bull.*, 41, 411, 1944.
82. Parana, R., Portugal, M., Vitvitski, L., Cotrim, H., Lyra, L., and Trepo, C. Severe strongyloidiasis during interferon plus ribavirin therapy for chronic HCV infection. *Eur. J. Gastroenterol. Hepatol.*, 12, 245-246, 2000.
83. Gompels, M., Todd, J., Peters, B., Main, J., and Pinching, A. J. Disseminated strongyloidiasis in AIDS: uncommon but important. *AIDS*, 5, 329, 1991.
84. Torres, J. R., Isturiz, R., Murillo, J., Guzman M., and Contreras, R. Efficacy of ivermectin in the treatment of strongyloidiasis complicating AIDS. *Clin. Infect. Dis.*, 17, 900, 1993.
85. Heath, T., Riminton, S., Garsia, R., and Macleod, C. Systemic strongyloidiasis complicating HIV: a promising response to ivermectin. *Int. J. STD AIDS*, 7, 294–296, 1996.
86. Chieffi, P. P., Chiattone, C. S., Feltrim, E. N., Alves, R. C., and Paschoalotti, M. A. Coinfection by *Strongyloides stercoralis* in blood donors infected with human T-cell leukemia/lymphoma virus type 1 in Sao Paulo City, Brazil. *Mem. Inst. Oswaldom Cruz*, 95, 711–712, 2000.
87. Sorensen, M., Andersen, O., Friis-Moller, A., and Kvinesdal, B. B. Fatal outcome of *Strongyloides stercoralis* infection in a patient with no previously known immunosuppression. *Ugeskr. Laeger*, 162, 2894–2895, 2000.
88. Oya, H., Mori, S., Tsuchihashi, H., et al. A case of pleuritis caused by strongyloides in a carrier of T-cell lymphoma virus type I (HTLV-I). *Nihon Kokyuki Gakkai Zasshi*, 36, 262–267, 1998.
89. Bonnet, C., Vergne, P., Bertin, P., and Treves, R. Anguillulose associee a une infection par HTLV1. *Presse Med.*, 28, 788, 1999.
90. Gotuzzo, E., Terashima, A., Alvarez, H., et al. *Strongyloides stercoralis* hyperinfection associated with human T cell lymphotropic virus type-1 infection in Peru. *Am. Trop. Med. Hyg.*, 60, 146–149, 1999.
91. Nakada, K., Kohakura, M., Komoda, H., and Hinuma, Y. High incidence of HTLV-I antibody in carriers of *Strongyloides stercoralis*. *Lancet*, 1, 633, 1984.
92. Higashiyama, Y., Sakata, H., Obase, Y., et al. A case of bacterial emningitis induced by strongyloidiasis. *Kansenshogaku Zasshi*, 71, 680–683, 1997.
93. Foucan, L., Genevier, I., Lamaury, I., and Strobel, M. Meningite purulente aseptique chez deux patients co-infectes par HTLV-1 et *Strongyloides stercoralis*. *Med. Trop. (Mars.)*, 57, 262–264, 1997.
94. Newton, R. C., Limpuangthip, P., Greenberg, S., Gam, A., and Neva, F. A. *Strongyloides stercoralis* hyperinfection in a carrier of HTLV-1 virus with evidence of selective immunosuppression. *Am. J. Med.*, 92, 202, 1992.
95. Yamaguchi, K., Matutes, E., Catovsky, D., Galton D. A. G., Nakada, K., and Takatsuki, K. *Strongyloides stercoralis* as candidate co-factor for HTLV-1-induced leukaegenesis. *Lancet*, 2, 94, 1987.
96. Maayan, S., Wormser, G. P., Widerhorn, J., Sy, E. R., Kim, Y. H., and Ernst, J. A. *Strongyloides stercoralis* hyperinfection in a patient with the acquired immune deficiency syndrome. *Am. J. Med.*, 83, 945, 1987.
97. Vieyra-Herrera, G., Becerril-Carmona, G., Padua-Gabriel, A., Jessurun, J., and Alonso-de Ruiz, P. *Strongyloides stercoralis* hyperinfection in a patient with the acquired immune deficiency syndrome. *Acta Cytologica*, 32, 277, 1988.
98. Pialoux, G., Beriel, P., Caudron, J., Chousterman, M., and Meyrignac, C. Syndrome d'imminodépression acquise associé a une anduillulose sévere. *Presse Med.*, 13, 1960, 1984.
99. René, E., Marche, C., Régnier, B., et al. Manifestations digestives du syndrome d'immunodéficience acquise (SIDA): étude chez 26 patients. *Gastroenterol. Clin. Biol.*, 9, 327, 1985.
100. Baird, J. K., De Vinatea, M. L., Macher, A. M., Sierra, J. A. R., and Lasala, G. AIDS: case for diagnosis series. *Milit. Med.*, 152, M17, 1987.
101. Hillyer, G. V. and Climent, C. Acquired immunodeficiency syndrome (AIDS) and parasitic disease in Puerto Rico. *Bol. Asoc. Med. PR*, 80, 312, 1988.

102. Petithory, J. C. and Derouin, F. AIDS and strongyloidiasis in Africa. *Lancet*, 1, 921, 1987.
103. Gachot, B., Bouvet, E., Bure, A., et al. HIV infection and malignant strongyloidiasis. *Rev. Prat.*, 40, 2129, 1990.
104. Goyal, S. B. Intestinal strongyloidiasis as eosinophilic pleural effusion. *South. Med. J.*, 91, 768–769, 1998.
105. Weight, S. C. and Barrie, W. W. Colonic *Strongyloides stercoralis* infection masquerading as ulcerative colitis. *J. R. Coll. Surg. Edinb.*, 42, 202–203, 1997.
106. Ting, Y. M. Pulmonary strongyloidiasis; case report of 2 cases. *Kaohsiung J. Med. Sci.*, 16, 269–274, 2000.
107. Kinjo, T., Tsuhako, K., Nakazato, I., et al. Extensive intra-alveolar haemorrhage caused by disseminated strongyloidiasis. *Int. J. Parasitol.*, 28, 323–330, 1998.
108. Woodring, J. H., Halfhill, H. 2nd, Berger, R., Reed, J. C., and Moser, N. Clinical and imaging features of pulmonary strongyloidiasis. *South. Med. J.*, 89, 10–19, 1996.
109. Levy, G. C., Kallas, E. G., and Ramos Moreira Leite, K. Disseminated *Strongyloides stercoralis* infection in an AIDS patient: the role of suppressive therapy. *Braz. J. Infect. Dis.*, 1, 48–51, 1997.
110. Kiyuna, M., Toda, T., Tamamoto, T., et al. An autopsy case of periarteritis nodosa associated with disseminated strongyloidiasis. *Rinsho Byori*, 42, 883, 1994.
111. Jacob, C. I. and Patten, S. F. *Strongyloides stercoralis* infection presenting as generalized prurigo nodularis and lichen simplex chronicus. *J. Am. Acad. Dermatol.*, 41(2 Pt. 2), 357–361, 1999.
112. Mori, S., Konishi, T., Matsuoka, K., et al. Strongyloidiasis associated with nephritic syndrome. *Intern. Med.*, 37, 606–610, 1998.
113. Wong, T. Y., Szeto, C. C., Lai, F. F., Mak, C. K., and Li, P. K. Nephrotic syndrome in strongyloidiasis: remission after eradication with anthelmintic agents. *Nephron*, 79, 333–336, 1998.
114. Brocq, O., Breul, V., Agopian, V., et al. Reactive arthritis induced by *Strongyloides stercoralis*. *Rev. Rhum. Engl. Ed.*, 63, 217–219, 1996.
115. Genta, R. M., Douce, R. W., and Walzer, P. D. Diagnostic implications of parasite-specific immune responses in immunocompromised patients with strongyloidiasis. *J. Clin. Microbiol.*, 23, 1099, 1986.
116. Pearson, R. D. and Guerrant, R. L. *Strongyloides* infections, in *Hunter's Tropical Medicine*, 7th ed., Strickland, G. T., Ed. W. B. Saunders, Philadelphia, 706, 1991.
117. Spry, C. J. F. *Eosinophils: A Comprehensive Review, and Guide to the Scientific and Medical Literature*. Oxford University Press, Oxford, 1988.
118. Moro-Furlani, A. M. and Krieger, H. Familial analysis of eosinophilia caused by helminthic parasites. *Genet. Epidemiol.*, 9, 185, 1992.
119. Fisher, D., McCary, F., and Currie, B. Strongyloidiasis in the Northern Territory. *Med. J. Aust.*, 159, 88, 1993.
120. Prociv, P. Strongyloidiasis in the Northern Territory. *Med. J. Aust.*, 159, 636, 1993.
121. Savage, D., Foadi, M. Haworth, C., and Grant, A. Marked eosinophilia in an immunosuppressed patient with strongyloidiasis. *J. Intern. Med.*, 236, 473, 1994.
122. Sher, A. and Coffman, R. L. Regulation of immunity to parasites by T cells and T cell-derived cytokines. *Annu. Rev. Immunol.*, 10, 385, 1992.
123. Thomson, A. W., Mathie, I. H., and Sewell, H. F. Cyclophosphamide-induced eosinophilia in the rat: concomitant changes in T-cell subsets, B cell and large granular lymphocytes within lymphoid tissues. *Immunology*, 60, 383, 1987.
124. Gherman, I., Oproiu, A., Aposteneau, G., et al. Observations on 35 cases of strongyloidiasis hospitalized at a clinical digestive disease unit. *Rev. Med. Interna*, 41, 169, 1989.
125. Stey, C., Jost, J., and Lüthy, R. Extraintestinale strongyloidiasis bei erworbenem immunmangelsyndrom. *Dtsch. Med. Wschr.*, 115, 1716, 1990.
126. Azab, M. E., Mohamed, N. H., Salem, S. A., et al. Parasitic infections associated with malignancy and leprosy. *J. Egypt. Soc. Parasitol.*, 22, 59, 1992.
127. Harley, J. P. and Gallicchio, V. Effect of cortisone on the establishment of *Nippostrongylus brasiliensis* in the rabbit. *J. Parasitol.*, 56, 271, 1970.
128. Moqbel, R. Effect of corticosteroids on experimental strongyloidiasis. Proc. Br. Soc. Parasitology. *Parasitology*, 69, xviii, 1974.
129. Ogilvie, B. M. Use of cortisone derivatives to inhibit resistance to *Nippostrongylus brasiliensis* and to study the fate of parasites in resistant hosts. *Parasitology*, 55, 723, 1965.
130. Franz, K. H. Clinical trials with thiabendazole against human strongyloidiasis. *Am. J. Trop. Med. Hyg.*, 12, 211, 1963.
131. Most, H. Treatment of common parasitic infections of man encountered in the United States (first of two parts). *N. Engl. J. Med.*, 287, 495, 1972.
132. Wehner, J. H. and Kirsch, C. M. Pulmonary manifestations of strongyloidiasis. *Semir. Respir. Infect.*, 12, 122–129, 1997.
133. Gordon, S. M., Gal, A. A., Solomon, A. R., and Bryan, J. A. Disseminated strongyloidiasis with cutaneous manifestations in an immunocompromised host. *J. Am. Acad. Dermatol.*, 31, 255, 1994.
134. Kramer, M. R., Gregg, P., Goldstein, M., Llamas, R., and Krieger, B. P. Disseminated strongyloidiasis in AIDS and non-AIDS immunocompromised hosts: diagnosis by sputum and bronchoalveolar lavage. *South. Med. J.*, 83, 1226, 1990.
135. Schumaker, J. D., Band, J. D., Lensmeyer, G. L., and Craig, W. A. Thiabendazole treatment of severe strongyloidiasis in a hemodialyzed patient. *Ann. Intern. Med.*, 89, 644, 1978.
136. Royle, G., Fraser-Moodie, A., and Jones, M. W. Hyperinfection with *Strongyloides stercoralis* in Great Britain. *Br. J. Surg.*, 61, 498, 1974.
137. Eland, I. A., Kerkhof, S. C., Overbosch, D., Wismans, P. J., and Stricker, B. H. Cholestatic hepatis ascribed to the use of thiabendazole. *Ned. Tijdschr. Geneeskd.*, 142, 1331–1334, 1998.

138. Skandrani, K., Richardet, J. P., Duvoux, C., Cherqui, D., and Zafrani, E. S. Hepatic transplantaion for severe ductopenia related to ingestion of thiabendazole. *Gastroenterol. Clin. Biol.*, 21, 623–625, 1997.
139. Bush, A., Gabriel, R., Gatus, S. J., and Thornton, J. G. Recurrent hyperinfestation with *Strongyloides stercoralis* in a renal allograft patient. *Br. Med. J.*, 286, 52, 1983.
140. Cook, G. A., Rodriguez, A., Silva, H., Rodriguez-Iturbe, B., and Bohorquez de Rodriguez, H. Adult respiratory distress secondary to strongyloidiasis. *Chest*, 92, 1115, 1987.
141. Thomson, J. R. and Berger, R. Fatal adult respiratory distress syndrome following successfull treatment of pulmonary strongyloidiasis. *Chest*, 99, 772, 1991.
142. Berger, R., Kramm, S., and Paciotti, M. Pulmonary strongyloidiasis complicating therapy with corticosteroids. *Am. J. Trop. Med. Hyg.*, 29, 31, 1980.
143. Thomson, J. R. and Berger, R. *Strongyloides stercoralis* infection: a review of 66 cases. *South. Med. J.*, 82(Suppl.), 7, 1989.
144. Bidulph, J. Mebendazole and albendazole for infants. *Pediatr. Infect. Dis. J.*, 5, 373, 1990.
145. Currie, B. Why does Australia have no national drug policy? *Med. J. Aust.*, 157, 210, 1992.
146. Sreenivas, D. V., Kumar, A., Kumar, Y. R., Bharavi, C., Sundaram, C., and Gayathri, K., Intestinal strongyloidiasis; a rare opportunistic infection. *Indian J. Gastroenterol.*, 16, 105–106, 1997.
147. Nandy, A., Addy, M., Patra, P., and Bandyopashyay, A. K. Fulminating strongyloidiasis complicating Indian kala-azar. *Trop. Geogr. Med.*, 47, 139, 1995.
148. Naquira, C., Jimenez, G., Guerra, J. G., et al. Ivermectin for human strongyloidiasis and other intestinal helminthes. *Am. J. Trop. Med. Hyg.*, 40, 304, 1989.
149. Adenusi, A. A. Cure by ivermectin of a chronic, persistent intestinal strongyloidosis. *Acta Trop.*, 66, 163–167, 1997.
150. Ashraf, M., Gue, C. L., and Baddour, L. M., Case report: strongyloidiasis refractory to treatment with ivermectin. *Am. J. Med. Sci.*, 311, 178–179, 1996.
151. Giannoulis, E., Arvanitakis, C., Zaphirolopoulos, A., Nakos, V., Karkavelas, G., and Haralambidis, S. Disseminated strongyloidiasis with uncommon manifestations in Greece. *J. Trop. Med. Hyg.*, 89, 171, 1986.
152. Zaha, O., Hirata, T., Kinjo, F., and Saito, A. Strongyloidiasis - progress in diagnosis and treatment. *Intern. Med.*, 39, 695–700, 2000.
153. Toma, H., Sato, Y., Siroma, Y., Kobayashi, J., Shimabukuro, I., and Takara, M. Comparative studies on the efiicacy of three anthelminthics on treatment of human strongyloidiasis in Okinawa, Japan. *Southeast Asian J. Trop. Med. Public Health*, 31, 147–151, 2000.
154. Marti, H., Haji, H. J., Savioli, L., et al. A comparative trial of a single-dose ivermectin versus theree days of albendazole for treatment of *Strongyloides stercoralis* and other soil-transmitted helminth infections in children. *Am. J. Trop. Med. Hyg.*, 55, 477–481, 1996.
155. Pitisuttithum, P., Supanaranond, W., and Chindanond, D. A randomized comparative study of albendazole and thiabendazole in chronic strongyloidiasis. *Southeast Asian J. Trop. Med. Public Health*, 26, 735–738, 1995.

18
Cyclospora spp.

1. INTRODUCTION

Cyclospora infections in humans have been documented since at least 1977. However, in the past 10 years or so, this pathogen has come into attention as the result of several major foodborne outbreaks in USA and Canada, cases of prolonged gastrointestinal disease in travelers and expatriates associated with southeast Asia (Nepal, Pakistan), and the rise of the immunocompromised population *(1–7)*. In addition to southeast Asia, *Cyclospora*-induced gastroenteritis has been diagnosed in an increasing number of regions throughout the world (the Americas and the Caribbean, Africa, Australia, Indonesia, England, and eastern Europe).

Sporulation characteristics combined with light and electron microscopic *(8–10)* identification of the life cycle stages of *Cyclospora* sp. (Coccidia, Apicomplexa) provided evidence that these organisms require only a single host to complete their entire life cycle. Although not fully known, the life cycle of *Cyclospora* is believed to involve both asexual and sexual stages of proliferation. Recent phylogenetic analysis based on rRNA sequences suggested that *Cyclospora* was closely related to the *Eimeria* genus *(11)*. In humans, the habitat of *Cyclospora* is the enterocyte of the small intestine *(10–12)*. All four asexual stages of *Cyclospora* (sporozoite, trophozoite, schizont, and merozoite) were observed within the parasitophorous vacuoles located in the apical supranuclear region of the enterocytes *(10)*. The term *Cyclospora cayetanensis* was first suggested in 1993 to define the infectious species in tropical and subtropical regions.

Various modes of transmission of the parasite to humans have been suggested *(13–15)*. However, it appears clear that cyclosporiasis can be contracted through consumption of fecally contaminated water supplies or food *(16–21)*. Some patients have been infected from accidental ingestion of aquarium water and from swimming in Lake Michigan *(22)*. It seems likely that water supplies may be contaminated by bird droppings *(16,23)*. Person-to-person transmission is unlikely because excreted oocysts require days to weeks, under favorable environmental conditions, to sporulate and become infectious *(24)*.

Cyclosporiasis has been diagnosed in immunocompetent adults *(22,25,26)*, in children *(25,27,28)*, immunocompromised patients (especially those with HIV infection) *(2,14,15,22,29–32)*, patients with malignancies such as leukemia *(33)*, and on rare occasions in asymptomatic carriers *(17,25,27,31,34,35)*.

The most typical signs of *C. cayetenensis* disease include persistent, acute or protracted, relapsing watery, nonbloody diarrhea that begins days or weeks after infection *(1,17,24,25)*. The onset may be abrupt or gradual *(25)*, with such symptoms as nausea, vomiting, anorexia, bloating, abdominal cramping, increased gas, watery diarrhea, fatigue, and malaise *(13,17,18,22,25,36–38)*. In immunocompetent hosts, the diarrhea appeared to be prolonged but self-limited, lasting on average between 3 and 6 wk, according to the various reports *(16,17,22,25,27,36)*. Although *Cyclospora*-associated diarrhea may be acute or chronic, the latter appeared to occur more frequently *(12,17,22,34,39)*. The resolution of symptoms seemed to correlate with the disappearance of the organisms from the stool, although diarrhea may persist after parasites are no longer detected *(40)*.

In immunocompromised patients, such as those with AIDS or diabetes *(39)*, the diarrhea tends to be persistent, unremitting, and more prolonged (for up to 15 wk) *(17,22)* with higher morbidity (profound loss of weight and fatigue) *(39)* and recurrence after therapy is completed *(38,41)*. According to data by Pape et al. *(41)*, *Cyclospora*-induced diarrhea may be considered an opportunistic infection in HIV-infected individuals because it preceded the development of AIDS in 37% of patients. Coinfection with *Cryptosporidium* sp. and *Cyclospora* sp. in an AIDS patient has also been reported *(42)*.

After studying the difference in the clinical course of cyclosporiasis in patients with and without AIDS, Sifuentes-Osornio et al. *(39)* suggested a possible extraintestinal involvement (acalculous cholecystitis) of *Cyclospora* in AIDS patients. Although these investigators did not provide a direct evidence of biliary infection due to *C. cayetanensis*, other *Cyclospora* spp. have been found in the biliary tract of moles *(43)*, which is an indirect proof of tissue tropism by these parasites.

The mechanism by which *Cyclospora* causes diarrhea has not been fully defined. Currently, cyclosporiasis is known to be associated with an inflammatory process in the small bowel *(44)* resulting in villus fusion and atrophy, which may reduce the surface area available for absorption and thus cause diarrhea *(39)*. This hypothesis has been supported by findings of impaired xylose absorption in patients with *Cyclospora* infection *(44,45)*.

Little is known about the host immune response to *C. cayetanensis (46)*. Its oocysts do not react with monoclonal antibody (MAb) specific for *Cryptosporidium parvum (25,27)*. Although Long et al. *(47)* found that patients passing *Cyclospora* in the stool have produced antibodies against these organisms, recurrent disease has been reported, indicating that infection did not provide lasting immunity *(17)*.

Richarson et al. *(48)* presented a case of a patient who developed Guillain-Barré syndrome after a *Cyclospora*-induced diarrheal illness, raising the possibility of *Cyclospora* being an infectious trigger for this syndrome.

2. TREATMENT OF CYCLOSPORIASIS

Treatment of cyclosporiasis consists of supportive care, maintenance of fluid and electrolyte status, symptomatic relief, and antibiotic therapy *(3)*.

A number of antibiotics have been used in the treatment of cyclosporiasis, including metronidazole, norfloxacin, ciprofloxacin, quinacrine, nalidixic acid, tinidazole, diloxanide, spiramycin, and azithromycin, but without apparent benefit *(13,22,25,36,49,50)*.

Orally administered trimethoprim-sulfamethoxazole (TMP-SMX, co-trimoxazole) has been clearly efficacious and is currently the drug of choice *(3,24,51,53)*. The recommended dosage regimens have been for adults, 160 mg of TMP and 800 mg of SMX, twice daily; and for children, daily oral doses of 5.0 and 25 mg/kg of TMP and SMX, respectively, twice daily *(52–54)*. In a randomized, double-blind, placebo-controlled trial recently completed in Nepal *(55)*, 960 mg of co-trimoxazole (160 mg of TMP, and 800 mg of SMX) when administered twice-daily for 7 d, eradicated the parasites in approx 90% of immunocompetent adults, with no signs of relapse among treated patients followed for an additional 7 d. Usually, the treatment lasts for 7 d, although in immunosuppressed patients greater dose regimens may be necessary as well as duration of medication for several weeks; in such cases, individual treatment planning is required. A 31-d course of co-trimoxazole has also been recommended *(56)*, although uncontrolled data collected for treatment of *Isospora belli* infections have suggested that as little as 2 d of treatment may be sufficient for immunocompetent patients *(57,58)*. Treatment regimens for patients who cannot tolerate sulfa drugs (part of the co-trimoxazole combination) have not yet been identified *(24)*.

In the largest trial so far of HIV-infected patients with cyslosporiasis, co-trimoxazole (160 mg of TMP, and 800 mg of SMX) was given orally 4 times daily for 10 d—both clinical improvement (cessation of symptoms in mean of 2.5 d) and parasitologic efficacy have been reported *(41)*. Secondary prophylaxis was successful with only a single relapse in a group of 12 patients taking co-trimoxazole prophylaxis for a mean of 7 mo.

Verdier et al. *(51)* conducted a randomized, controlled trial in HIV-infected patients comparing trimethoprim-sulfamethoxazole with ciprofloxacin for the treatment and prophylaxis of chronic diarrhea caused by *Isospora belli* (22 patients) and *Cyclospora cayetanensis* (20 patients). Oral co-trimoxazole (160 mg or 800 mg) or ciprofloxacin (500 mg) were administered twice daily for 7 d. Patients who showed clinical and microbiological response received prophylaxis for 10 wk (1 tablet orally, 3 times weekly); prophylaxis was measured by recurrent disease rate. The success rates for co-trimoxazole and ciprofloxacin were 95% and 87%, respectively. All patients receiving prophylaxis with co-trimoxazole remained disease-free, and 15 of 16 patients receiving secondary prophylaxis with ciprofloxacin remained disease-free.

Because patients with known allergies to sulfa drugs cannot take co-trimoxazole, a number of antibiotics (azithromycin, norfloxacin, tinidazole, diloxanide furoate, and quinacrine hydrochloride) have been tried against *Cyclospora* but without much success. To this end, trimethoprim, the nonsulfa component of co-trimoxazole, was used in an open trial in Nepal involving non-Nepalese subjects *(59)*. A dose of 200 mg trimethoprim was given b.i.d. for 7 d. The results have shown no benefits using trimethoprim alone for cyclosporiasis. Moreover, two of three sulfa-allergic patients appeared to have an allergic reaction to trimethoprim alone.

REFERENCES

1. Herwaldt, B. L. *Cyclospora cayetanensis*: a review, focusing on the outbreaks of cyclosporiasis in the 1990s. *Clin. Infect. Dis.*, 31, 1040–1057, 2000.
2. Mossimann, M., Nguyen, X. M., and Furrer, H. Excessive watery diarrhea and pronounced fatigue due to *Cyclospora cayetanensis* infection in an HIV infected traveler returning from the tropics. *Schweiz. Med. Wochenschr.*, 129, 1158–1161, 1999.
3. Brown, G. H. and Rotschafer, J. C. *Cyclospora*: review of emerging parasite. *Pharmacotherapy*, 19, 70–75, 1999.
4. Soave, R., Herwaldt, B. L., and Relman, D. A. *Cyclospora. Infect. Dis. Clin. North Am.*, 12, 1–12, 1998.
5. Connor, B. A. *Cyclospora* infection: a review. *Ann. Acad. Med. Singapore*, 26, 632–636, 1997.
6. Ortega, Y. R., Sterling, C. R., and Gilman, R. H. *Cyclospora cayetanensis. Adv. Parasitol.*, 40, 399–418, 1998.
7. Crowley, B., Path, C., Moloney, C., and Keane, C. T. *Cyclospora* species: a cause of diarrhoea among Irish travelers to Asia. *Ir. Med. J.*, 89, 110–112, 1996.
8. Nhieu, J. T. V., Nin, F., Fleury-Feith, J., Chaumette, M.-T., Schaeffer, A., and Bretagne, S. Identification of intracellular stages of *Cyclospora* species by light microscopy of thick sections using hematoxylin. *Hum. Pathol.*, 27, 1107, 1996.
9. Deluol, A.-M., Teilhac, M. F., Poirot, J.-L., Heyer, F., Beaugerie, L., and Chatelet, F.-P. *Cyclospora* sp.: life cycle studies in a patient by electron microscopy. *J. Eukar. Microbiol.*, 43, 128S, 1996.
10. Sun, T., Ilardi, C., Asnis, D., et al. Light and electron microscopic identification of *Cyclospora* species in the small intestine. *Clin. Microbiol. Infect. Dis.*, 195, 216, 1996.
11. Colombia Rodriguez, J. and Villar Serrano, J. Morphological, clinical and therapeutic characteristics of *Cyclospora cayetanensis. Bol. Chil. Parasitol.*, 52, 26–32, 1997.
12. Bendall, R. P., Lucas, S., Moody, A., Tovey, G., and Chiodini, P. L. Diarrhoea associated with cyanobacterium-like bodies: a new coccidian enteritis in man. *Lancet*, 341, 590, 1993.
13. Ashford, R. W. Occurence of an undescribed coccidian in man in Papua New Guinea. *Ann. Trop. Med. Parasitol.*, 73, 497, 1979.
14. Hart, A. S., Ridinger, M. T., Soundarajan, R., Peters, C. S., Swiatlo, A. L., and Kocka, F. E. Novel organism associated with chronic diarrhea in AIDS. *Lancet*, 335, 169, 1990.
15. Long, E. G., Ebrahimzadeh, A., White, E. H., Swisher, B., and Callaway, C. S. Alga associated with diarrhea in patients with acquired immunodeficiency syndrome and in travelers. *J. Clin. Microbiol.*, 28, 1101, 1990.
16. Centers for Disease Control. Outbreaks of diarrheal illness associated with cyanobacteria (blue-green algae)-like bodies, Chicago and Nepal, 1989 and 1990. *Morb. Mortal. Wkly Rep.*, 40, 325, 1991.
17. Hoge, C. W., Shlim, D. R., Rajah, R., et al. Epidemiology of diarrhoeal illness associated with coccidian-like organism among travelers and foreign residents in Nepal. *Lancet*, 341, 1175, 1993.
18. Brennan, M. K., MacPherson, D. W., Palmer, J., and Keystone, J. S. Cyclosporiasis: a new cause of diarrhea, *Can. Med. Assoc. J.*, 155, 1293, 1996.
19. Huang, P., Weber, J. T., Sosin, D. M., et al. The first reported outbreak of diarrheal illness associated with *Cyclospora* in the United States. *Ann. Intern. Med.*, 123, 409, 1995.
20. Rabold, J. G., Hoge, C. W., Shlim, D. R., Kefford, C., Rajah, R., and Echeverria, P. *Cyclospora* outbreak associated with chlorinated drinking water. *Lancet*, 344, 1360, 1994.

21. Connor, B. A. and Shlim, D. R., Foodborne transmission of *Cyclospora*. *Lancet*, 346, 1634, 1995.
22. Wurtz, R. M., Kocka, F. E., Peters, C. S., Weldon-Linne, C. M., Kuritza, A., and Yungbluth, P. Clinical characteristics of seven cases of diarrhea associated with a novel acid-fast organism in the stool. *Clin. Infect. Dis.*, 16, 136, 1993.
23. Wurtz, R. M., Kocka, F. E., Kallick, C., Peters, C., and Dacumos, E., Blue green algae associated with a diarrheal outbreak. *Proc. 91st Meet. Am. Soc. Microbiol.*, American Society for Microbiology, Washington, DC, abstract # C-21, 1991.
24. Chambers, J., Somerfeldt, S., Mackey, L., et al. Outbreaks of *Cyclospora cayetanensis* infection - United States, 1996. *Morb. Mortal. Wkly Rep.*, 276, 183, 1996.
25. Shlim, D. R., Cohen, M. T., Eaton, M., Rajah, R., Long, E. G., and Ungar, B. L. P. An alga-like organism associated with an outbreak of prolonged diarrhea among foreigners in Nepal. *Am. J. Trop. Med. Hyg.*, 45, 383, 1991.
26. Ooi, W. W., Zimmerman, S. K., and Needham, C. A. *Cyclospora* species as a gastrointestinal pathogen in immunocompetent hosts. *J. Clin. Microbiol.*, 33, 1267, 1995.
27. Ortega, Y. R., Sterling, C. R., Gilman, R. H., Cama, V. A., and Diaz, F. *Cyclospora* species: a new protozoan pathogen in humans. *N. Engl. J. Med.*, 328, 1308, 1993.
28. Hoge, C. W., Echeverria, P., Rajah, R., et al. Prevalence of *Cyclospora* species and other enteric pathogens among children less than 5 years of age in Nepal. *J. Clin. MIcrobiol.*, 33, 3058, 1995.
29. Robinson, R. D. Parasitic infections associated with HIV/AIDS in the Carribean. *Bull. Pan. Am. Health Organ.*, 29, 129, 1995.
30. Raguin, C., Heyer, F., Rousseau, C., Aerts, J., Desplaces, N., and Deluol, A. *Cyclospora* infection in an HIV infected patient. *Presse Med.*, 24, 1134, 1995.
31. Maggi, P., Brandonisio, O., Larocca, A. M., et al., *Cyclospora* in AIDS patients: not always an agent of diarrhoic syndrome. *New Microbiol.*, 18, 73, 1995.
32. O'Mahony, C. and Mannion, P. T. *Cyclospora cayetanensis* and HIV-related diarrhoea. *Int. J. STD AIDS*, 9, 59, 1998.
33. Jayshree, R. S., Acharya, R. S., and Sridhar, H. *Cyclospora cayetanensis*-associate diarrhoea in a patients with acute myeloid leukaemia. *J. Diarrhoeal Dis. Res.*, 16, 254–255, 1998.
34. Pollock, R. C., Bendall, R. P., Moody, A., Chiodini, P. L., and Churchill, D. R. Traveller's diarrhoea associated with a cyanobacterium-like bodies: a new coccidium enteritis in man. *Lancet*, 340, 556, 1992
35. Goodgame, R. W. Understanding intestinal spore-forming protozoa: Cryptosporidia, Microsporidia, Isospora, and *Cyclospora*. *Ann. Intern. Med.*, 124, 429–441, 1996.
36. Soave, R., Dubey, J. P., Ramos, L. J., and Tummings, M. A new intestinal pathogen? *Clin. Res.*, 34, 533A, 1986.
37. McDougall, R. J., and Tandy, M. Coccidian/cyanobacterium-like bodies as a cause of diarrhea in Australia. *Pathology*, 25, 375, 1993.
38. Farthing, M. J. G., Kelly, M. P., and Veitch, A. M. Recently recognized microbial enteropathies and HIV infection. *J. Antimicrob. Chemother.*, 37(Suppl. B), 61–70, 1996.
39. Sifuentes-Osornio, J., Porras-Cortés, G., Bendall, R. P., Morales-Villareal, F., Reyes-Teran, G., and Ruiz-Palacios, G. M. *Cyclospora cayetanensis* infection in patients with and without AIDS: biliary disease as another clinical manifestation. *Clin. Infect. Dis.*, 21, 1092, 1995.
40. Wurtz, R. *Cyclospora*: a newly identified intestinal pathogen in humans. *Clin. Infect. Dis.*, 18, 620, 1994.
41. Pape, J. W., Verdier, R.-I., Boncy, M., Boncy, J., and Johnson, W. D. Jr. *Cyclospora* infection in adults infected with HIV. *Ann. Intern. Med.*, 121, 654–657, 1994.
42. Belagra, N., Ajana, F., Coignard, C., Caillaux, M., and Mouton, Y. Co-infection with *Cryptosporidium* sp. and *Cyclospora* sp. in an AIDS stage HIV patient. *Ann. Biol. Clin. (Paris)*, 56, 476–478, 1998.
43. Mohamed, H. A. and Molyneux, D. H. Developmental stages of *Cyclospora talpae* in the liver and bile duct of the mole (Talpa europeae). *Parasitology*, 101, 345, 1990.
44. Connor, B. A., Shlim, D. R., Scholes, J. V., Rayburn, J. L., Reidy, J., and Rajah, R. Pathologic changes in the small bowel in nine patients with diarrhea associated with a coccidia-like body. *Ann. Intern. Med.*, 119, 377, 1993.
45. Bendall, R. P. and Chiodini, P. L. Intestinal malabsorption associated with human *Cyclospora* infection. *Proc. 1st Biannual Conf. Federation Infectious Societies (London)*, Federation of Infectious Societies, Manchester, U.K., abstract # 817, 1994.
46. Clarke, S. C. and McIntyre, M. An attempt to demonstrate a serological immune response in patients infected with *Cyclospora cayetanensis*. *Br. J. Biomed. Sci.*, 54, 73–74, 1997.
47. Long, E. G., White, E. H., Carmichael, W. W., et al. Morphologic and staining characteristics of a cyanobacterium-like organism associated with diarrhea. *J. Infect. Dis.*, 164, 199, 1991.
48. Richardson, R. F., Jr., Remler, B. F., Katirij, B., and Murad, M. H. Guillain-Barré syndrome after *Cyclospora* infection. *Muscle Nerve*, 21, 669–671, 1998.
49. Gascon, J., Corachan, M., Bombi, J. A., Valls, M. E., and Bordes, J. M. *Cyclospora* in patients with traveller's diarrhea. *Scand. J. Infect. Dis.*, 27, 511, 1995.
50. Shear, M., Connor, B. A., Shlim, D. R., Taylor, D. N., and Rabold, J. G. Azithromycin treatment of *Cyclospora* infections. *Gastroenterology*, 106(Suppl. 4), 772A, 1994.
51. Verdier, R. I., Fitzgerald, D. W., Johnson, W. D., Jr., and Pape, J. W. Trimethoprim- sulfamethoxazole compared with ciprofloxacin for treatment and prophylaxis of *Isosporra belli* and *Cyclospora cayetanensis* infection in HIV-infected patients. A randomized, controlled trial. *Ann. Intern. Med.*, 132, 885–888, 2000.

52. Lepes, T. Newly established causes of diarrhea: the protozoan *Cyclospora cayetanensis* (Coccidia, Apicomplexa). *Med. Pregl.*, 51, 242–244, 1998.
53. Fryauff, D. J., Krippner, R., Purnomo, Ewald, C., and Echeverria, P. Short report: case report of *Cyclospora* infection acquired in Indonesia and treated with cotrimoxazole. *Am. J. Trop. Med. Hyg.*, 55, 584–585, 1996.
54. Madico, G., Gilman, R. H., Miranda, E., Cabrera, L., and Sterling, C. R. Treatment of *Cyclospora* infections with co-trimoxazole. *Lancet*, 342, 122–123, 1993.
55. Hoge, C. W., Shlim, D. R., Ghimire, M., et al. Placebo-controlled trial of co-trimoxazole for *Cyclospora* infections among travellers and foreign residents in Nepal. *Lancet*, 345, 691–693, 1995.
56. Anonymous. Drugs for parasitic infections. *Med. Lett.*, 35, 111, 1993.
57. Westerman, E. L. and Christensen, R. P. Chronic *Isospora belli* infection treated with co-trimoxazole. *Ann. Intern. Med.*, 91, 413, 1979.
58. DeHovitz, J. A., Pape, J. W., Bongy, M., and Johnson, W. D. Jr. Clinical manifestations and therapy of *Isospora belli* infection in patients with the acquired immunodeficiency syndrome. *N. Engl. J. Med.*, 315, 87, 1986.
59. Shlim, D. R., Pandey, P., Rabold, J. G., Walch, A., and Rajah, R. An open trial of trimethoprim alone against *Cyclospora* infections. *J. Travel Med.*, 4, 44–45, 1997.

PART IV
FUNGAL INFECTIONS

During the last two decades or so, the incidence of fungal infections has increased dramatically. Deep-seated mycoses are creating serious problems for clinicians working with certain populations of patients, such as those with cancer, the immunocompromised, and physiologically compromised patients *(1,2)*.

With the ever-expanding application of immunosuppressive therapy, the role host factors (the T-lymphocyte system) in the defense against systemic fungal infections is currently the subject of intensive studies, and new approaches for antifungal therapy are being investigated.

The need for effective antifungal drugs has been felt more and more acutely with the emergence of the AIDS pandemic and the AIDS-related complex (ARC), which are nearly always associated with opportunistic fungal infections.

Another factor facilitating the spread of opportunistic mycoses has been the significant improvement achieved in the management of bacterial infections.

At present, the majority of antifungal agents available to clinicians, in addition of having some unacceptable side effects are, by mechanism of action, fungistatic. Such a mode of action, for the most part, requires prolonged periods of treatment, and relapses after treatment is ceased are frequent. Because both human and fungal cells are eukaryotic by nature, prolonged antifungal chemotherapy would be damaging to host cells too. Overcoming an obstacle such as this should present a fundamental challenge to scientists in their quest for safer, more selective, and effective antifungal agents *(1,2)*.

REFERENCES

1. Georgiev, V. St. *Antifungal Drugs*. Ann. NY Acad. Sci., vol. 544, The New York Academy of Sciences, New York, 1988.
2. Georgiev, V. St. Fungal infections and the search for novel antifungal agents. *Ann. NY Acad. Sci.*, 544, 1, 1988.

19
Cryptococcus neoformans

1. INTRODUCTION

Cryptococcus neoformans is a yeast-like fungus that is pathogenic to both animals and man. It was first isolated in 1894 by Busse *(1)* from a patient with osteomyelitis of the tibia. The fungus is a saprophitic organism that can be found in soil, on a variety of fruits, as well as in close association with pigeon nests *(2,3)*. There are two varieties of *C. neoformans*: *C. neoformans* var. *neoformans* and *C. neoformans* var. *gattii*. Each of these varieties, in turn, has two serotypes: A and D for var. *neoformans*, and B and C for var. *gattii*. In addition, there have been reports of human infections caused by two other *Cryptococcus* species: *C. albidus* and *C. laurentii*.

Infection with *C. neoformans* is usually acquired by its inhalation. Although the fungus is common in pigeon feces, the birds are not clinically infected *(4)*. There is no observation of human-to-human transmission of the disease *(5)*.

Cell-mediated immunity seems to provide the major defense against cryptococcal infections, leaving patients with compromised cell-mediated responses (lymphoma, leukemia, sarcoidosis, and those patients receiving corticosteroid therapy) more vulnerable and, therefore, more likely to develop a cryptococcal infection *(6–15)*. The alveolar macrophages represent the initial host's defense against the cryptococcal pathogen and may arrest infection before dissemination occurs. To this end, experiments by Ieong et al. *(16)* have shown that the innate fungicidal activity of primary human alveolar macrophages against *C. neoformans* was impaired after HIV-1 infection in vitro by a mechanism that might have involved a defect of intracellular antimicrobial processing. Also, human neutrophils are known to inhibit and kill *C. neoformans* in vitro and are thought to play an important role in the host's defense against cryptococcosis through both oxidative and nonoxidative mechanisms *(17)*.

Aguirre et al. *(18)* have demonstrated that both interferon-γ (IFN-γ) and tumor necrosis factor-α (TNF-α) were important factors in mediating acquired resistance to cryptococcal meningoencephalitis. To this end, Kawakami et al. *(19)* found that in mice with defective IL-12 production, IL-18 contributed to the hosts's resistance to cryptococcal infection through the induction of IFN-γ production by natural killer (NK) cells, but not through the development of Th1 cells, under the condition in which IL-12 synthesis was deficient.

Cryptococcosis may develop as an acute, subacute or chronic pulmonary, systemic or meningeal mycosis. Although the pulmonary form is usually transitory, mild and often asymptomatic, the involvement of the central nervous system (CNS) is manifested by subacute or chronic meningitis that in immunocompromised hosts could be life-treatening. Cases of patients with idiopathic $CD4^+$ T-lymphocytopenia accosiated with CNS cryptococcosis have also been reported *(20)*.

During dissemination of the disease, skeletal and visceral lesions may occur. Nearly all of the immunocompromised patients are likely to develop disseminated cryptococcosis *(21,22)* with susceptibility to infection being reported for the skin *(23–27)*, bone *(28)*, prostate *(29)*, kidney *(30)*, eyes

From: Opportunistic Infections: Treatment and Prophylaxis
By: Vassil St. Georgiev © Humana Press Inc., Totowa, NJ

(31,32), liver *(33–35)*, spleen *(36)*, adrenals *(36,37)* lymph nodes *(24,35,38,39)*, and the gastrointestinal tract *(40)*. Although infrequently, deep cryptococcal infections of the breast have been reported *(41)*. Hypereosinophilia in disseminated disease has also been observed *(42)*.

Larsen et al. *(43)* reported a persistent cryptococcal infection of the prostate in AIDS patients even after an adequate therapy with amphotericin B alone or in combination with flucytosine; this observation suggest the possibility of the prostate serving as a sequestered reservoir of infection from which systemic relapse may occur. To this end, cryptococcal prostatitis in a patient with Behcet's disease was also described *(44)*.

The co-existence of different diseases within the same lesion could be a distinct possibility in patients with HIV infection. In this context, there have been several reports of simultaneous Kaposi's sarcoma and cutaneous cryptococcosis occuring at the same site in a patient with AIDS *(45)*. Limbal nodules and multifocal choroidal lesions due to *C. neoformans* may also occur in AIDS patients *(46)*. Benard et al. *(47)* have presented case reports of two patients with immunodeficiency secondary to paracoccidiodomycosis and opportunistic cryptococcosis. Secondary immunodeficiency likely occured as a consequence of the intestinal loss of proteins and lymphocytes associated with malabsorption syndrome due to obstructed lymphatic drainage; both patients had severe abdominal involvement during the acute paracoccidiodomycosis disease *(47)*.

Molnar-Nadasdy et al. *(48)* have described a unique case of placental cryptococcosis in a pregnant mother with systemic lupus erythematosus (SLE) and steroid treatment. Although there were no clinical or placental signs of transplacental infection, immunohistochemical labeling of villous stromal cells showed a conspicuously increased number of fetal macrophages.

In patients with AIDS, cryptococcal infections are often associated with high relapse rate and poor response to treatment *(49–53)*. Currently, cryptococcosis is considered to be the one of the most life-threatening mycoses in patients with AIDS *(54–60)*. Munoz-Perez et al. *(61)* have described disseminated cryptococcosis presenting as molluscum-like lesions as the first manifestation of AIDS.

Although a common opportunistic mycosis in adults, cryptococcosis complicating pediatric AIDS have also been well-documented *(62)*.

In the majority of patients with normal immunity, cryptococcosis is confined to the lung or the hilar nodes *(21,63–68)* and will hardly require any antifungal therapy *(21,69,70)*. Occasionally, cryptococcal osteomyelitis has also been described in normal hosts *(71)*. Cutaneous cryptococcosis in the nonimmunocompromised host is also a rare entity, and when it does occur, it presents with protean manifestations making clinical diagnosis difficult *(72,73)*. One unusual case of progressive pulmonary disease in an immunocompetent patient presenting as a discrete endobronchial cryptococcoma has been reported by Emmons et al. *(60)*. Mahida et al. *(71)* also reported a patient with endobronchial cryptococcal obstruction. Cryptococcal meningitis with severe visual and hearing loss and radiculopathy was described in an immunocompetent patient *(75)*, as well as CNS cryptococcosis with multiple intraventricular cysts *(76)*. The development of adult respiratory distress syndrome (ARDS) caused by pulmonary cryptococcosis in an immunocompetent host has been reported *(77)*.

By far, cryptococcal meningitis is the most dangerous form of the disease. Because some of the patients with cryptococcal meningitis may be asymptomatic *(6,8,78–80)* it is important that the cerebrospinal fluid (CSF) be examined whenever *C. neoformans* is isolated or detected from any site. The onset of cryptococcal meningitis would most likely be insidious, but often it is acute in cases of severely immunocompromised hosts. In the latter case, if untreated, the infection is always fatal *(6,81–84)*.

2. TREATMENT OF CRYPTOCOCCOSIS

The choice of therapy for cryptococcal disease largely dependent on both the anatomic site of infection and the patient's immune status *(88)*.

Presently, there are no clinical trials to evaluate the outcome of therapy for AIDS-related cryptococcal pneumonia. The optimal therapeutic approaches for management of cryptococcal meningitis,

Table 1
Treatment of Cryptococcosis in Immunocompromised Patients

Patients	Site of infection	Drug Regimens
HIV-negative	Pulmonary and non-CNS involvement	Amphotericin B 0.7–1.0 mg/kg, daily + flucytosine 100 mg/kg, daily for 2 wk, then fluconazole 400 mg, daily for at least 10 weeks[a,b,c]
	CNS involvement	Amphotericin B 0.7–1.0 mg/kg, daily for 2 wk, then fluconazole 400-800 mg, daily for 8–10 wk, followed by lower dose fluconazole (200 mg, daily) for 6–12 mo[b,c]
HIV-positive	Pulmonary[d]	Fluconazole 200–400 mg, daily for life; Itraconazole 200–400 mg, daily for life; Fluconazole 400 mg, daily + flucytosine 100–150 mg/kg, daily for 10 wk[a]
	CNS involvement	Amphotericin B 0.7–1.0 mg/kg, daily + flucytosine 100 mg/kg, daily for 2 wk, then fluconazole 400 mg, daily for at least 10 wk[e]

[a]Patients receiving flucytosine for over 2 wk should be monitored for renal toxicity.

[b]For patients with significant renal disease, lipid formulation of amphotericin B may be used. Intrathecal or intraventricular amphotericin B may be used in refractory cases where systemic administration of antifungal therapy had failed.

[c]For patients who cannot tolerate fluconazole, itraconazole (200 mg, b.i.d.) may be taken instead.

[d]Mild-to-moderate symptoms. In patients with more severe disease, amphotericin B should be used initially until symptoms are controlled, and then substituted with an oral azole antimycotic (preferably fluconazole).

[e]Induction/consolidation therapy. In cases where flucytosine is not tolerated, amphotericin B (at the same doses) alone is an acceptable alternative. Lipid amphotericin B may also be used in patients with renal insufficiency.

especially in AIDS patients with underlying T-cell dysfunction, and those with neoplasia or on corticosteroid therapy, are also not completely defined and still subject to discussion (Table 1) *(85–88)*.

Currently, the most recommended therapy for cryptococcosis in HIV-negative immunocompromised patients with pulmonary disease and non-CNS involvement, consists of amphothericin B alone or in combination with flucytosine for the first 2 wk, followed by fluconazole both to complete initial treatment and provide a lifelong maintenance therapy *(88)*.

Although fluconazole and itraconazole have been associated with response rates of 50–60%, amphotericin B is still the drug of choice for inducing a rapid clearance of the fungus, and therefore, a preferable option for initial therapy. Results from a recently completed large clinical trial (MSG 17/ACTG 159) *(85)* have indicated that initial treatment for 2 wk with amphotericin B (0.7 mg/kg once daily), followed by triazole (fluconazole at 400 mg daily, or itraconazole at 400 mg daily) therapy for further 8 wk resulted in mortality rate of less than 8%, which is substantially lower than that of previous studies *(89)*.

Based on the results of a retrospective review of 30 consecutive AIDS patients with cryptococcal infection (median CD4+ count of 0.042×10^9 cells/L) given fluconazole at 400 mg daily, Nightingale *(90)* supported the use fluconazole as initial therapy for AIDS-associated cryptococcosis in these patients. In fact, in the largest comparative study *(91)* there was no difference in the response rates associated with amphotericin B and fluconazole.

Studies by Haubrich et al. *(92)* have also shown that a high-dose (800 mg daily) of fluconazole was well-tolerated by HIV-infected patients and appeared effective primary therapy for cryptococcal disease in AIDS patients.

First-line fluconazole therapy (200–400 mg daily) has also been found effective and well-tolerated in patients with AIDS-associated nonmeningeal cryptococcosis *(93)*.

The standard therapy of disseminated cryptococcosis, particularly of cerebral manifestations, is still amphotericin B-flucytosine combination *(59,86)*. The use of high-dose oral fluconazole for treatment of disseminated cryptococcosis has also been recommended *(94)*.

Disease relapses are frequent in AIDS patients (20–60%) if a long-term maintenance therapy is not applied promptly. In this regard, fluconazole at 200 mg daily has shown to be superior than itraconazole at the same dosage level *(85)*.

Fluconazole has also been used prophylactically *(95–97)*. At 200–400 mg daily, it reduced significantly the incidence of cryptococcosis (and mucosal candidiasis), especially in AIDS patients with CD4$^+$ counts of less than 50 cells/mm^3.

2.1. Amphotericin B

Before the introduction of chemotherapy, 86% of all cases of cryptococcal infections associated with neurological involvement were fatal within one year of onset *(84)*, with death usually resulting from raised intracranial pressure producing cerebral compression. Amphotericin B, which has been in use for treatment of cryptococcosis since the 1950s, is still one of the most frequently applied therapeutic agents against this infection *(98,99)*. Thus, following the introduction of amphotericin B, cure rates as high as 85% have been reported *(100)*.

When given intravenously at daily doses of up to 1.0–1.5 mg/kg (or every other day), amphotericin B accounted for as high as 64% cure rate of patients with cryptococcal meningitis *(5)*. In AIDS patients with cryptococcal meningitis, continuing weekly infusions of amphotericin B after the standard course of therapy has been completed, apparently offered some degree of protection against relapse *(101)*.

A typical primary course of therapy may consist of amphothericin B given daily for at least 4 wk with a total dose ranging from 1.60 to 2.76 g (mean 2.11 g), whereas a maintenance therapy would include treatment with 40–100 mg/wk of amphotericin B ranging from 0.7–1.5 mg/kg body weight *(101)*. It should be emphasized that although a maintenance therapy with this antibiotic will not necessarily provide a total protection against relapse of cryptococcosis in patients with AIDS, the weekly maintenance regimen with amphotericin B is still a recommended current practice that may be carried out indefinitely with AIDS patients who had survived their primary course of antifungal therapy *(102,103)*. However, the continued infusion of amphotericin B is not without a danger and may cause toxicity making it unacceptable to many patients *(101)*.

The total dose of the antibiotic administered during primary therapy may be highly variable; this, in addition to the requirement for maintenance therapy (which may become a life-long treatment) will make the end point of amphothericin B therapy not well defined. Thus, in one study *(103)* involving 48 cases of cryptococcosis complicating AIDS, the cumulative amphotericin B dosage administered to the time of clinical response (defervescence and resolution of symptoms in 48% of the patients) varied between 0.1 and 1.76 g; in the majority of patients, the clinical response was noted early in the treatment when the average cumulative dose was 0.4 g *(103)*.

In a study involving 31 consecutive AIDS patients with cryptococcal disease (28 with meningitis, and 3 with disseminated extrameningeal cryptococcosis), investigators *(104–106)* have examined the efficacy and safety of a short-course primary treatment with relatively high dose of amphotericin B at 1.0 mg/kg daily for 14 d (26 patients also received flucytosine at 100–150 mg/kg daily, given either intravenously or orally), followed by maintenance therapy with fluconazole or itraconazole. Successful therapy was defined as the resolution of symptoms and negative cultures of CSF and/or blood 2 mo after the initial diagnosis. The therapeutic regimen was successful in 29 (93.5%) of all 31 cases, and in 26 (92.8%) of the 28 cases of culture-proven or presumed cryptococcal meningitis; treatment failed in two patients.

A therapy comprising amphotericin B and flucytosine, if maintained over a period of 6 wk, although showing a high rate of success, had also required a permanent relapse prevention *(56)*. With regard to prevention therapy, oral fluconazole could be very effective and is considered by some investigators to be the drug of choice *(56)*.

As reported by Zugar et al. *(49)* and Kovacs et al. *(50)*, in spite of antifungal medication, the mortality rate resulting from cryptococcal meningitis in AIDS patients has ranged from 17–35%, and was 25% in patients having persistently positive cultures *(50)*. By comparison, the relapse rate in non-AIDS patients was between 0% and 35% *(6,10,107)*.

Polsky et al. *(108)* have conducted a retrospective study evaluating the use of intraventricular application of amphotericin B in cases of cryptococcal meningitis in non-AIDS patients. Death during therapy occured in only one of the six patients who had received intraventricular and systemic therapy, and in six of the seven patients on systemic therapy alone. No major adverse effects were reported with the intraventricular administration of the drug. However, the preliminary information in AIDS patients did not provide much encouragment because those patients who received intraventricular amphotericin B did not show any therapeutic benefits *(48,49)*. In addition, the treatment was often complicated by infection of the ventricular shunt and chemical arachnoiditis (consisting of fever, headache, and CSF pleocytosis) forcing the premature discontinuation of the intraventricular therapy *(49,50)*.

An earlier long-term study involving 31 patients with cryptococcal meningitis receiving intravenous amphotericin B (with half of the patients on intrathecal therapy as well) had shown an overall mortality rate of 45% of which 39% was due to cryptococcal meningitis *(8)*. Roberts and Douglas *(109)* reported a successful amphotericin B therapy (with a total dose of 3.0 g) in one case of cryptococcal meningitis accompanied by cryptococcemia. In another study, Sapico *(110)* described the disappearance of focal cryptococcal brain lesion following intravenous infusion of amphotericin B at gradually increasing doses (a total of 3.0 g), whereas Bastin et al. *(111)* applied the drug to cure a case of cryptococcal meningitis associated with polyradiculitis.

Although amphotericin B therapy greatly improved the prognosis of patients with cryptococcal meningitis, overall, there are still important clinical limitations associated with its use, including modest efficacy, nephrotoxicity, and the inconvenience of intravenous application *(112)*.

Ambisome®, an unilamellar liposomal formulation of amphotericin B, was used in the treatment of cryptococcal meningitis in three patients; clinical and mycological remission were observed in two of the patients, with the remaining one showing improvement *(113)*. Coker et al. *(114)* described a successful treatment of cryptococcal meningitis with liposomal amphotericin B after failure of treatment with fluconazole and conventional amphotericin B. Schurmann et al. *(115)* investigated the safety and efficacy of liposomal amphotericin B in treating AIDS-associated disseminated cryptococcosis.

Japanese scientists *(116,117)* have described an unusual therapy of cryptococcal meningitis consisting of small doses of amphotericin B, a large dose of prednisolone, and a continuous removal of CSF.

An individual case of a patient with a solid intracranial cryptococcal granuloma in the motor cortex area was treated initially with intrathecal and intravenous amphotericin B; because no regression of the granuloma was observed, a subsequent gross total surgical excision was successfully performed *(118)*. There are several other reports of combined treatment of intracranial cryptococcal infection with surgery and systemic amphotericin B *(119–122)*.

Intrathecal administration of amphotericin B has been routinely performed by usage of subcutaneous CSF reservoir. The latter comprised a subcutaneous dome of siliconized rubber that can fit into a cranial burr hole with a catheter extending from the dome into a lateral cerebral ventricle *(107,123,124)*. Schonheyder et al. *(125)* observed some complications following intrathecal infusion of amphotericin B using the Rickham reservoir; mainly a persistent infection resulting from the presence of the reservoir.

A renal-transplant recipient who was on immunosuppressive medication (prednisone, azathioprine) and with developed pulmonary cryptococcosis was successfully treated with intravenous amphotericin B *(126)*. In this regard, a Japanese study *(127)* indicated a poor prognosis of antifungal therapies for cryptococcal infections in renal transplant recipients; thus, only one of six patients survived following the graft. Although amphotericin B was found most effective, its nephrotoxicity has always been of prime concern in graft survival.

Shindo *(128)* has found amphotericin B superior to fluconazole, itraconazole, miconazole, and flucytosine (given in various combinations) in the treatment of one patient with cryptococcal meningitis and slight azotemia caused by hypertensive nephrosclerosis.

A diabetic patient with isolated adrenal cryptococcosis (characterized with fungal granuloma and poorly encapsulated pathogen) was treated successfully with surgery and medication with amphotericin B; after a 7-mo follow-up period, there was no evidence of recurrence or dissemination *(129)*.

The use of intravenous amphotericin B in nine cases involving pulmonary cryptococcosis was also reported *(130)*.

Amphotericin B when used at cumulative doses of 189–551 mg, effectively decreased the systemic infections in patients with lymphocytic lymphoma and progranulocytic leukemia *(131)*. Fajardo *(132)* has reported the failure of topical amphotericin B to cure cutaneous cryptococcosis in a patient who previously had Hodgkin's disease in a cervical lymph node; the topical treatment comprised 3% amphotericin B ointment in a polyethylene and mineral oil gel base applied four times daily. In another case report, Kojima et al. *(133)* described a successful treatment by amphotericin B of acute lymphocytic leukemia (ALL) complicated with a generalized cryptococcosis.

Mycotic endocarditis is a rare fungal infection *(134,135)*. Colmers et al. *(2)* described a successful therapy of *C. neoformans*-induced endocarditis manifesting fungemia with intravenous amphotericin B (total dose of 1.58 g).

2.1.1. Toxicity of Amphotericin B

Toxicity studies included a follow-up evaluation of 53 patients treated with amphotericin B. The patients showed an increase in the blood urea nitrogen, acute and permanent nephrotoxicity (age- but not dose-dependent), and a transient reduction of the creatinine clearance during therapy *(136)*. The antibiotic has also been used in cases of pregnancy complicated with cryptococcosis and showing no clinical damage to the fetus *(137,138)*. Li and Lai *(139)* observed acute visual loss in a patient with SLE and cryptococcal meningitis who was receiving a test dose (1.0 mg) of intravenous amphotericin B; caution was recommended in using the anibiotic in cases of cryptococcal meningitis when a desease of the optic nerve is strongly suspected.

2.2. Combinations of Amphotericin B with 5-Fluorocytosine and Other Drugs

Currently, the combination of amphotericin B and 5-fluorocytosine is one of the most frequently used for the treatment of cryptococcosis *(140)*. According to Armstrong *(141)*, therapy of invasive cryptococcosis should include daily doses of amphotericin B (1.0 mg/kg, intravenously) and oral flucytosine (100 mg/kg daily, divided in 4 doses) for a duration (or total dose) depending on the patient's response; maintenance therapy of fluconazole (200 mg daily) is often required and can be administered indefinitely.

Concerning the mechanism of combined amphotericin B/5-FC treatment, it is thought that amphotericin B at low doses would potentiate *(142,143)* the uptake of the flucytosine, thus facilitating a synergistic effect *(144)*.

In 1978, Jimbow et al. *(145)* reported an evaluation of the therapeutic effectiveness of amphotericin B and flucytosine, alone and in combination, in 28 patients with cryptococcal meningitis. The combined regimen (at 0.35 mg/kg amphotericin B daily, i.v., and 150 mg/kg daily of oral flucytosine) was significantly more effective than either drug given alone, both in terms of toxicity and shorter duration of treatment.

Bennett et al. *(146)* conducted a prospective, uncontrolled trial of 15 patients with cryptococcal meningitis to compare a combined therapy of intravenous amphotericin B and oral flucytosine (a 6-wk trial) with amphotericin B given alone (a 10-wk trial). Results showed that as compared to monotherapy with amphotericin B, the combination cured more patients with fewer failures or relapses, more rapid sterilization of CSF ($p < 0.001$), and less nephrotoxicity ($p < 0.05$). The applied regimens were as follows: (1) combination therapy: 0.3 mg/kg of amphotericin B daily, i.v., and 150 mg/kg of 5-FC daily, divided in 6 hourly oral doses; and (2) amphotericin B alone: 0.4 mg/kg daily, i.v. for 42 d, followed by 0.8 mg/kg every other day for 28 d *(146)*.

In order to reduce potential toxicity without compromising the efficacy, Dismukes et al. *(51)* conducted a multicenter, prospective, randomized clinical trial of 194 patients having cryptococcal meningitis. The trial was designed to compare the efficacy and toxicity of 4- vs 6-wk regimens (identical with those applied by Bennett et al. *[146]*) of combined amphotericin B/5-fluorocytosine therapy. Cure or improvement was observed in 75% of those patients who were treated for 4 wk, and in 85% of those treated for 6 wk, with relapse rates of 27% and 16%, respectively, and a similar incidence of toxicity (44 and 43%, respectively). Based on the results of the trial, the investigators recommended that the 4-wk regimen be applied to patients having no neurological complications, underlying disease or immunosuppressive therapy; patients who do not meet these criteria should be receiving for at least 6 wk the combined amphotericin B/5-fluorocytosine treatment *(51)*. Alternatively, MacGregor *(147)* suggested a modified therapy involving a relatively short course of amphotericin B treatment (3–4 wk) combined with a longer course of 5-fluorocytosine medication. It was assumed that the period necessary for the pathogen to develop a resistance towards 5-FC is early in the treatment when the cryptococcal population is in its peak; therefore, a short initial period of combined therapy (involving the use of amphotericin B) would be sufficient to reduce the cryptococcal population and thereby, the possibility of developing a resistance towards flucytosine. In turn, such therapeutic regimen will allow for a more extended course of single 5-FC therapy and less of amphotericin B-induced toxicity *(147)*.

In an earlier study, Utz et al. *(10)* described the treatment of 15 patients with cryptococcal meningitis with a combination of low-dose intravenous amphotericin B (20 mg daily) and oral flucytosine (150 mg/kg daily); 53% of the patients were reported cured with no relapse. Other reports have indicated that increasing the doses of the antibiotic to conventional levels (0.6–1.0 mg/kg daily) improved the cure rate of patients on a single amphotericin B therapy to 47–58%; repeated courses of amphotericin B treatment increased the cure rate even further (61–67%) *(6,8,9)*.

Schmutzhard and Vejajjiva *(148)* conducted a trial of 24 patients with cryptococcal meningitis using as therapy amphotericin B (1.0 mg/kg daily, i.v.) and oral flucytosine (150 mg/kg daily). None of the patients received corticosteroid therapy. The duration of treatment ranged from 56–104 d. Upon completion, none of the patients died. However, four patients had a relapse within 6 mo; an overall relapse rate of 17% was observed in spite of the higher total dosage of amphotericin B and 5-FC and longer duration of therapy.

In addition to data already discussed, there have been reports from various groups that indicate that, in general, the difference between amphotericin B administered alone, or as part of combined therapy with flucytosine, has not been statistically significant *(49,50,149)*. Furthermore, 5-FC would be difficult to consider for AIDS patients because of its adverse bone marrow-suppressive *(149,150)* and gastrointestinal *(51)* effects, which often are superimposed on symptoms caused by the human immunodeficiency virus (HIV) *(151,152)*. After reviewing the records of 106 patients with cryptococcal infections and AIDS (criteria considered included: efficacy of treatment with amphotericin B alone or in combination with flucytosine, efficacy of suppressive therapy, prognostic clinical characteristics, and the course of nonmeningeal cryptococcosis), Chuck and Sande *(153)* concluded that addition of flucytosine to amphotericin B neither enhanced survival nor prevented relapse, but long-term suppressive therapy appeared to be beneficial. Nevertheless, in a significant number of patients, the flucytosine medication had to be stopped because of cytopenia *(153,154)*.

Cryptococcal infections associated with the CNS can be manifested as focal granulomatous lesions that may contribute to increased mortality (often exceeding 50%). A case report of cerebral cryptococcoma linked to cryptococcal meningitis was treated successfully with a short course of intravenous amphotericin B and oral flucytosine *(155)*. The combined therapy consisted of 20 mg daily of amphotericin B and 150 mg/kg daily of 5-FC for a period of 6 wk, after which the antibiotic was administered alone at a dose of 50 mg given every other day until a total dose of 2.16 g of the antibiotic had been dispensed. The observed side effects (parasthesia of the hands, edema of the ankles, increased serum creatinine level [168 mol/L], and a lowered serum potassium level [to 3.0 mmol/L]) were transitory *(155)*. One case of cryptococcal meningoencephalitis, which developed after 9 yr of corticosteroid therapy, was resolved successfully with amphotericin B and flucytosine (for 6 wk) and with itraconazole (for another 8 wk) *(156)*.

Systemic treatment with amphotericin B and flucytosine led to resolution of choroidal infiltrates in two AIDS patients with optic edema and cryptococcal choroiditis *(157)*. Picon et al. *(158)* successfully treated with amphotericin B and flucytosine an AIDS patient with cutaneous cryptococcosis manifecting as molluscum contagiosum-like skin lesions.

Tobias et al. *(159)* reported the treatment of two patients with Hodgkin's disease and cryptococcal meningitis with amphotericin B and oral flucytosine; amphotericin B was administered intrathecally as well as by a rapid low-dose intravenous injection.

Watson et al. *(160)* described a long-term study (spanning over 11 yr) that involved treatment of cryptococcal infection in renal-transplant recipients on continued immunosuppressive therapy (prednisolone). The treatment of cryptococcosis, which consisted of combination amphotericin B (0.3–0.5 mg/kg daily, i.v.) and/or oral flucytosine (150 mg/kg daily) led to cure in 10 of 11 patients. In order to preserve graft viability in those patients with stable renal function at the time of diagnosis, maintenance immunosuppressive therapy was continued throughout the antifungal medication *(160)*. Previous reports *(12,161,162)* suggested the need to reduce or even to discontinue the immunosuppressive therapy in order to achieve a cure of cryptococcal infection in cases of renal transplantation. Kong et al. *(163)* treated cryptococcal meningitis in eight cases of renal transplant recipients with SLE. The therapy comprised amphotericin B and flucytosine; at the time of medication all patients were also receiving immunosuppressive therapy (steroids in association with either azathioprine or cyclosporine) *(163)*. Kimura et al. *(164)* described the successful treatment of a case of SLE complicated with cryptococcal meningitis using combination of amphotericin B and 5-FC.

Pulmonary cryptococcosis with an early systemic spread was managed with combination amphotericin B, and flucytosine; following that, a rapid 1-h intravenous infusion of amphotericin B (30 mg) on alternative days was instituted as an outpatient maintenance therapy for a period of approx 6 wk *(165)*.

Cryptococcal osteomyelitis (manifested either as a single bone lesion or a systemic illness in addition to osteomyelitis), has been described on several occasions *(166–169)*. Poliner et al. *(40)* discussed a case of cryptococcal cervical vertebral osteomyelitis that was cured with oral 5-FC (150 mg/kg daily) and amphotericin B (0.3 mg/kg daily, i.v.) for 6 wk with no evidence of systemic toxicity or relapse. In another case *(170)*, a patient who developed osteomyelitis of the skull due to cryptococcosis was successfully treated with amphotericin B and flucytosine.

An AIDS patient who presented with oral lesion of cryptococcosis (gingival ulceration) was successfully cured with amphotericin and flucytosine given over a 4-wk period *(171)*.

Iida et al. *(172)* described the successful treatment of cryptococcal meningitis with combined amphotericin B-ketoconazole therapy.

Echevarria et al. *(173)* reported a case of pulmonary cryptococcosis that was treated successfully with combination of amphotericin B and ketoconazole.

A "fungus ball," which developed in an inactive tuberculosis cavity, was treated with infusion of amphotericin B (total dose of 2.4 g) and sodium iodide (total of 56 g over a 30-d period) directly into the cavity through an indwelling percutaneously inserted endobronchial catheter for a period of 3 mo. A marked improvement was observed without any complications caused by the use of the catheter *(174)*.

2.2.1. Toxicity of Amphotericin B-5-Fluorocytosine Combinations

In view of the existing toxicity of both amphotericin B and flucytosine (especially the negative effect of the latter on the bone marrow), medication of cryptococcal infections with combination of these two drugs should be considered very carefully when severely immunocompromised patients (advanced state of AIDS) are involved. Thus, in a multicenter, prospective randomized trial *(175)* that lasted for either 4 or 6 wk, the treatment with intravenous amphotericin B (0.3 mg/kg daily) and oral 5-FC (150 mg/kg daily) of 194 patients with cryptococcal meningitis led to the development of one or more adverse side effects in 103 patients. The toxicity included azotemia (51 patients), renal tubular necrosis (2 patients), leukopenia (30 patients), thrombocytopenia (22 patients), diarrhea (26 patients), nausea/vomiting (10 patients), and hepatitis (13 patients). Overall, both the 4- and 6-wk regimens were complicated by toxicity in 44 and 43% of the patients, respectively. In general, the observed side effects appeared during the first 2 wk of therapy in 56%, and during the first 4 wk in 87% of the patients (175).

Shindo et al. (176) observed, alongside improvement, the presence of granulocytopenia and thrombocytopenia in one patient given concomitantly amphotericin B and low-dose flucytosine (50 mg/kg daily); it was suggested that both side effects might have been the result of toxic reactions by flucytosine in the azotemic state caused by amphotericin B. In another example, Bryan and McFarland (177) reported a fatal bone-marrow aplasia in one patient with multiple myeloma and cryptococcal meningitis, following medication of the infection with combined amphotericin B and flucytosine (a total of 151 mg and 30.5 g, respectively). Although amphotericin B is considered beneficial in reducing the flucytosine toxicity on the bone marrow, again, caution should be in order with patients having hematologic malignancies and where a reduced marrow reserve is suspected (178).

2.3. 5-Fluorocytosine (5-FC)

In 1965, flucytosine was first introduced in the therapy of cryptococcosis (178,179). The drug is effective orally and also readily absorbed. Over 90% of it is excreted in the urine within the first 48 h; the observed levels in the CSF were half those present in the plasma (180,181).

Although encouraging, earlier studies on the clinical usefulness of 5-FC against cryptococcal infections were carried out only with a limited number of patients. For example, when 5-FC (100 mg/kg daily, given in 4 oral doses for 20 wk) was applied to one patient following excision of multiple intracerebral supperative cryptococcal granulomas, the drug was well-tolerated and the patient was apparently free of cryptococcal infection 1 yr after the end of medication (182). However, a rapid development of resistance towards 5-FC by *C. neoformans* is commonly observed (183). This has been especially true for patients receiving less than 150 mg/kg daily of the drug at the onset of the infection when the cryptococcal population is at its peak (183).

Consequently, in the therapy of either cryptococcal meningitis or pulmonary cryptococcosis, 5-FC alone was found often inadequate for a successful treatment because of the development of resistance. According to one study (184), only 30% cure rate was observed while relapses and failures resulting from development of drug resistance were common (185–187). For this reason, the use of flucytosine alone limits its use in cryptococcosis. Currently, the combination of amphotericin B and 5-FC is recommended whenever cryptococcal infection (especially with neurological involvement) is diagnosed.

Flucytosine-associated toxicity included liver damage, transient thrombocytopenia, neutropenia, anemia, and eosinophilia (188). In addition, pancytopenia and severe agranulocytosis were also reported (189–191). The damage on bone marrow (185,192) (including a fatal marrow aplasia [192,193]) is by far the most severe adverse effect of 5-FC and should be addressed properly. Philpot and Lo (194) reported the use of flucytosine in the treatment of cryptococcal meningitis in pregnancy without damage to the fetus.

2.4. Azole Derivatives

2.4.1. Miconazole

One general regimen for miconazole therapy of cryptococcal meningitis that has been recommended (195), required an initial intravenous infusion of 30 mg/kg of the drug daily for 3 wk; following that period, if the patient was still unresponsive, miconazole was applied into the CSF space at a dosage of 20 mg twice daily, then going to 20 mg every other day.

In one Japanese study *(196)*, deep-seated mycoses were treated with miconazole at an initial dose of 200 mg (dissolved in at least 200 mL of solvent medium) injected intravenously (by drip-infusion) over a 30–60 min period. If no side effects were observed, 200–400 mg of the drug were administered intravenously over 30 min, 1–3 times daily.

On a negative note, Sung et al. *(197)* reported the failure of miconazole (administered both intravenously and intrathecally) to cure one patient with cryptococcal meningitis and suffering from multiple other complications; a previous combined amphotericin B-flucytosine therapy had also been unsuccessful *(197)*. Deresinsky et al. *(195)* applied miconazole intravenously to two patients with cryptococcosis with inconclusive results and a clinical response that could not be evaluated.

Because of many contradicting reports, the efficacy of miconazole in the therapy of cryptococcal meningitis is still very much in doubt. Since miconazole penetrates poorly into CSF when given systemically, the therapy of most cryptococcal infections associated with CNS involvement will eventually require intrathecal administration of flucytosine *(195,198–200)*. Controlled, randomized trials will be necessary to define unambiguously the usefulness of miconazole in the management of cryptococcal meningitis. In the treatment of pulmonary cryptococcosis, the efficacy of miconazole has also been very much in doubt.

2.4.2. Ketoconazole

Although ketoconazole has shown potent in vitro activity against *C. neoformans*, it is generally ineffective in treating cryptococcal meningitis *(88)*. Perfect et al. *(201)* found ketoconazole ineffective in the treatment of cryptococcal meningitis following therapy with high doses. In a contradicting report *(202)*, a case of cryptococcal meningitis showed improvement after high doses of the drug were applied.

Karaffa et al. *(203)* initiated a ketoconazole therapy in a patient with AIDS and disseminated cryptococcosis; the drug was applied at 400 mg daily but the patient, who continued to do well 5 mo after the diagnosis, still had extremely high serum levels of cryptococcal antigen.

Granier et al. *(204)* reported a successful therapy of localized cutaneous cryptococcosis in a renal allograft recipient receiving ketoconazole in conjunction with systemic steroids and azathioprine; ketoconazole was given orally at 400 mg daily for 6 mo with no relapse or dissemination observed.

2.4.3. Fluconazole

Fluconazole has been extensively studied for its therapeutic efficacy against cryptococcosis *(27,205–210)* especially against cryptococcal meningitis *(211–218)*.

Jones et al. *(219)* conducted a clinical trial using oral fluconazole to treat 32 AIDS patients with cryptococcal meningitis. Of the 11 patients who received a daily primary therapy of 200–400 mg/kg of fluconazole, 67% had a favorable clinical response; in 87% of these cases, the CSF cultures were negative. In addition, fluconazole was used as a secondary therapy in 15 patients who were not responsive to amphotericin B (or amphotericin B-fluconazole combination); positive clinical and mycological responses were obtained in over 60% of the patients. As maintenance therapy, 26 patients received 100–200 mg/kg fluconazole daily; the relapse rate of cryptococcal meningitis was 3.2 cases per 1,000 patient weeks (mean duration of 22 wk of maintenance therapy) *(219)*.

Dupont *(220)* reported a study involving 16 patients with AIDS and cryptococcal meningitis treated with oral fluconazole. The majority of patients received an initial loading dose of 400 mg, followed by 200 mg daily for 2 mo, then maintenance therapy of 100 mg daily. Eleven of 16 patients were clinically cured, concurrent with mycological clearance of all infected sites as well; 4 of 16 patients had clinical improvement but still showed positive CSF cultures; and 1 of 16 patients had clinical deterioration and died with positive CSF culture in spite of being switched to standard treatment *(220)*. This study, however, was not an open one, and the obtained results were not compared to standard therapy with amphotericin B-flucytosine.

Byrne and Wajszczuk *(221)* also described a successful use of 150 mg daily of fluconazole against cryptococcal meningitis in one patient with AIDS who had not responded well to an initial therapy with amphotericin B.

In more extensive clinical trials, the therapeutic efficacy of fluconazole was compared to that of amphotericin B. In a randomized, multicenter study *(92)* lasting for 10 wk, intravenously injected amphotericin B was compared with oral fluconazole (200 mg daily) as primary therapies in AIDS patients with acute cryptococcal meningitis; amphotericin B was given either at a mean daily dose of 0.4 mg/kg, or at 0.5 mg/kg depending on patients' response ($p = 0.34$). The treatment was successful in 25 of 63 patients receiving amphotericin B (40%; 95% confidence interval, 26–53%) and in 44 of the 131 fluconazole recipients (34%; 95% confidence interval, 25–42%) ($p = 0.40$). There was no significant difference in the overall mortality rate between the two groups (amphotericin B vs fluconazole, 14 and 18%, respectively; $p = 0.48$); however, during the first 2 wk of treatment, the mortality in the fluconazole group was higher (15 vs 8%; $p = 0.25$). Treatment was considered successful when the patients had two consecutive negative CSF cultures by the end of the 10-wk trial period. The median length of time to the first negative CSF culture was 42 d (95 confidence interval, 28–71%) for the amphotericin B group, and 64 d (95% confidence interval, 53–67%) for the fluconazole group ($p = 0.25$) *(92)*.

In a recently completed retrospective clinical study, the efficacies of amphotericin B and fluconazole were evaluated in HIV-negative patients (organ-transplant recipients, patients with neoplastic disease) and with meningeal and extrameningeal cryptococcosis *(222)*. Patients with more severe infections (i.e., meningitis, neurological disorders, or higher level of antigen in CSF) were more frequently treated with amphotericin B; a cure rate of less than 70% was achieved regardless of the initial treatment and severity of infection. In general, a Cox regression analysis has shown that in patients older than 60 yr, neoplastic disease, abnormal mental status, disseminated infection at the time of diagnosis, and therapeutic failure were independent predictors of death. Although fluconazole appeared to be equipotent to amphotericin B, only a prospective multicenter study would be sufficient to determine the best treatment regimen for cryptococcal infections in HIV-negative patients *(222)*.

In another randomized clinical trial of AIDS patients with cryptococcal meningitis, Larsen et al. *(223)* compared the therapeutic efficacies of fluconazole with a combination of amphotericin B and flucytosine. The all-male group was randomly assigned to either oral fluconazole (400 mg daily) for 10 wk, or to amphotericin B (0.7 mg/kg daily) for 1 wk, then 3 times weekly for 9 wk combined with flucytosine (150 mg/kg daily, in 4 divided doses). Eight of 14 patients (57%) assigned to fluconazole failed to respond, compared to none of 6 patients assigned to amphotericin B plus flucytosine therapy. The mean duration of positive CSF cultures was 40.6 ± 5.4 d in patients receiving fluconazole, and 15.6 ± 6.6 d in those receiving amphotericin B plus flucytosine. Although such results show that combined amphotericin B-flucytosine medication may be superior to fluconazole in the treatment of cryptococcal meningitis in AIDS patients, the intravenous therapy of amphotericin B has been associated with frequent and often severe side effects compared to oral fluconazole given once daily. Further studies should provide the necessary information to determine the feasibility of the amphotericin B-flucytosine combination and the contribution of flucytosine *(224)*. According to a cost-minimization analysis conducted by Buxton et al. *(225)*, costs associated with the use of fluconazole as primary therapy will likely be significantly lower than those for amphotericin B, but similar (or slightly less) for a maintenance therapy.

A case of cryptococcal meningoencephalitis in a patient with Hodgkin's disease at third-stage B became asymptomatic after 1 wk of therapy with intravenous fluconazole (400 mg daily); 2 mo later, all laboratory tests of CSF and blood specimens were negative *(226)*. Combination of amphotericin B (20 mg daily, i.v.) and flucytosine (2.5 g daily, i.v.) did not lead to any improvement *(226)*. Iacopino et al. *(227)* also used fluconazole to treat disseminated cryptococcosis in a patient with Hodgkin's disease.

Oral fluconazole (once daily at doses of 50–200 mg/kg) was applied to 20 AIDS patients having disseminated cryptococcosis *(228)*. All patients received amphotericin B as primary therapy before entry. Fluconazole medication was successfully maintained in nine patients for a median of 11 mo; seven patients died (five of them did not have evidence of active cryptococcosis at the time of death), and two patients experienced a relapse. Fluconazole had to be discontinued in only one patient when thrombocytopenia developed, and then resolved when the drug was stopped *(228)*.

Bozzette et al. *(229)* also evaluated maintenance therapy with fluconazole in a placebo-controlled, double-blind, clinical trial of AIDS patients with cryptococcal meningitis. The drug was given at 100 mg daily in the first phase of the study, and 200 mg daily in the second phase. Following a clinically successful therapy with flucytosine, 19% of the enrolled patients presented a silent, persistent cryptococcal infection. However, there was no recurrent meningeal infection observed in those patients taking fluconazole (mean duration of follow-up, 164 d; $p = 0.03$), suggesting it as an effective alternative for maintenance therapy against cryptococcal infections *(229)*.

The suppressive efficacy of fluconazole in preventing relapse from cryptococcal meningitis in AIDS patients was corroborated by findings from a larger trial *(230)*. Two suppressive regimens were compared: fluconazole at daily oral doses of 200 mg (11 patients; 59%) vs amphotericin B at 1.0 mg/kg per week (78 patients; 41%). The failure rate of the amphotericin B-treated group was markedly higher (33%; 26 of 78 patients) compared to only 8% of the fluconazole-receiving patients (9 of 11 patients) *(230)*. A successful maintenance therapy of cryptococcosis with fluconazole was also described for 80 AIDS patients from Burundi *(231)*.

In an uncontrolled, open trial with a small number of AIDS patients with cryptococcosis, fluconazole was found to be effective in preventing relapses after the active disease was controlled with amphotericin B *(232)*; however, the drug was found not very effective at conventional doses (50–100 mg daily) usually applied for treatment of active cryptococcosis. Observed side effects of fluconazole included an increase in hepatic function test values in one patient, and seisures in another; in both cases fluconazole had to be discontinued.

C. neoformans-induced pleural empyema secondary to liver cirrhosis due to hepatitis C virus infection responded well to oral fluconazole *(233)*.

Retinitis resulting from disseminated cryptococcosis in a renal allograft recipient showed remarkable improvement following therapy with oral fluconazole *(234)*. Cryptococcal endophthalmitis is a rare disorder, nearly always diagnosed after enucleation or at postmortem examination. Custis et al. *(235)* have described a culture-positive cryptococcal endophthalmitis in a patient with chronic uveitis diagnosed by vitreous biopsy at the time of retinal detachment repair. The fungus, *Cryptococcus laurentii* is a previously unreported non-*neoformans* ocular pathogen. After a 5-mo course of oral fluconazole, the patient was culture-negative; however, the visual declined to hand motions because of hyphema and hypotony.

Although cutaneous cryptococcosis is frequently diagnosed in AIDS patients, it has only seldom been observed in other immunocompromised patients *(27,236–238)*. In one such case, Abraham et al. *(27)* described a renal allograft recipient with necrotic cryptococcal granulomata on the dorsum of the hand but no clinical evidence of systemic infection; the infection was successfully cured after a 6-mo treatment with oral fluconazole (400 mg, daily). Vandersmissen et al. *(236)* described the successful use of a 6-wk course of oral fluconazole in two corticosteroid-treated HIV-negative patients who developed cutaneous cryptococcosis. In a relevant case *(239)*, cryptoccocal whitlow in an HIV-positive patient (unusual clinical presentation of cutaneous cryptococcosis never seen before in this population) was cured with fluconazole at 400 mg daily for 2 mo, and 200 mg daily thereafter. Contrary to AIDS patients who need life-long antifungal maintenance therapy to prevent relapses, suppressive treatment may not be indicated for immunocompromised non-AIDS patients *(236)*.

Other reports describing successful use of oral fluconazole against cryptococcal infections, included laryngeal cryptococcosis *(240)*, neck mass resulting in lytic destruction of portion of the cervical vertebrae *(241)*, and pulmonary cryptococcosis in non-AIDS patients (400 mg daily, for 10–12 wk) *(242)*.

After evaluation of 4,048 patients who received fluconazole for at least 7 d, some of the undesirable side effects included: nausea (3.7%), headache (1.9%), skin rash (1.8%), vomiting (1.7%), abdominal pain (1.7%), and diarrhea (1.5%) *(243)*. Although adverse effects are more likely to occur in HIV-positive patients, their pattern remained essentually the same, with only 1.5% of patients having their medication discontinued because of side effects *(244)*. Fluconazole may also induce multiple hepatic abnormalities usually characterized by asymptomatic and reversible mild hepatic necrosis. However, Guillaume et al. *(245)* described severe subacute liver damage occuring in an AIDS patient that may be related to prolonged fluconazole maintenance therapy for cryptococcsis; electron microscopic studies revealed the presence of a unusual giant mitochondria with paracrystalline inclusions and enlarged smooth endoplasmic reticulum. All microscopic abnormalities were reversed after discontinuation of fluconazole. Alopecia appeared to be a common adverse effect associated with higher-dose (400 mg daily) of fluconazole given for 2 mo or longer; although sometimes severe, the effect is reversed by discontinuing fluconazole therapy or substantially reducing the daily dose *(246,247)*.

Drug-interaction studies demonstrated that when fluconazole was administered in multiple daily doses of up to 400 mg, it did not produce noticeable effects on testosterone, estrogen, or the ACTH-stimulated cortisol concentrations *(243)*. Furthermore, no drug interaction has been observed when fluconazole was administered (at daily doses of 100 mg or more) concomitantly with cyclosporin A to bone-marrow transplant recipients (but not renal-transplant patients) *(243)*.

Failures of fluconazole in treatment of cryptococcal meningitis *(248)* and prostate cryptococcosis *(249)* have also been reported. For example, a 10-wk regimen of fluconazole, if first given intravenously then orally, resulted in failure in 62% of patients (8 of 13) *(250)*. However, when the drug was administered entirely by oral route, the failure rate was only 10% (5 of 17 patients) *(251)*. To this end, Aller et al. *(252)* have found that MIC valued determined by a modified microdilution method could serve as potential predictors of the clinical response to fluconazole therapy and may help in the identification of patients who will not respond to fluconazole therapy.

Cases of fluconazole-resistant *C. neoformans* have also been reported *(253,254)*.

2.4.4. Itraconazole

Itraconazole, another recently developed triazole-containing antimycotic *(255)*, has been used in the treatment of AIDS patients with meningeal and/or additional neurological cryptococcosis at daily oral doses of 200–400 mg *(220)*. There was no report on the success rate of the treatment, but a maintenance therapy with the drug (200–400 mg daily) was recommended to prevent relapses.

According to Van Cutsem and Cauwenbergh *(256)*, in patients with meningeal or pulmonary cryptococcosis, daily treatment with 200 mg itraconazole for 88 (median) or 139 (median) d produced global responses of 57 and 83% of patients, respectively, and negative mycological response in 51 and 50%, respectively; a similar study involving daily administration of 400 mg of itraconazole to both groups for 160–216 d (median; meningeal) and 160 d (median; pulmonary) resulted in global responses of 86 and 89%, respectively *(256)*.

Data from itraconazole treatment (200 mg daily) of three AIDS patients with disseminated cryptococcosis were reported by Viviani et al. *(257)*. All patients received conventional therapy with amphotericin B prior to itraconazole. Within 1 mo of treatment, suppression of clinical symptoms in two of the patients, and further improvement in the third, were observed. Although cultures became negative, two of the patients still had encapsulated yeast present in the CSF *(381)*. A long-term maintenance therapy with the drug (3.0 mg/kg) has been recommended *(258)*.

The therapeutic efficacy of itraconazole has been examined in 33 patients with various manifestations of cryptococcosis (meningitis, cryptococcemia, cryptococcuria, osteomyelitis, pulmonary cryptococcosis, and soft-tissue cryptococcosis) *(259)*. Thirty-two of the patients were immunocompromised, including 4 transplant recipients and 26 with AIDS. The treatment consisted of 200 mg oral itraconazole, two times daily. Results showed that cryptococcemia was abolished 100%. Furthermore, 65% of the patients with cryptococcal meningitis showed complete response (as manifested by clinical resolution and negative cultures), whereas 25% had partial response, and in 10% the treatment had failed. In 71% of patients with AIDS who had meningitis and were treated with itraconazole as their sole therapy, the response was complete, whereas 21% responded partially, and the therapy failed in 7%. All patients who had pulmonary cryptococcosis, soft-tissue cryptococcosis, or osteomyelitis responded 100% to itraconazole therapy, compared to only 60% of patients with cryptococcuria. Because itraconazole hardly penetrated the CSF, the results for cryptococcal meningitis suggested that meningeal and parenchymal penetration was important in lowering the therapeutic efficacy *(259)*.

In another report *(260)*, oral itraconazole was successful in 28 patients with cryptococcal meningitis; 18 of them have achieved complete response, including 16 of 24 patients with AIDS.

A clinical trial of five AIDS patients conducted by de Gans et al. *(261)*, demonstrated a promise for itraconazole as maintenance therapy for cryptococcal meningitis. Each patient received initial treatment with amphotericin B (0.3 mg/kg daily, intravenously) and oral 5-FC (150 mg/kg daily, every 6 h) for 6–8 wk. In four of the patients, the titer of cryptococcal antigen in CSF declined. Two of the patients were still alive, respectively, 10 and 12 mo after a maintenance therapy with itraconazole had began with no toxic side effects from the drug *(261)*.

Batungwanayo et al. *(262)* found itraconazole to be highly effective in the prevention of disseminated cryptococcal disease among HIV-positive Rwandan patients with primary pulmonary cryptococcosis.

Oral itraconazole at 100 *(263)*, 200 *(264)*, or 400 mg *(265)* once daily was also used successfully in treatment of localized cutaneous cryptococcosis *(263)*. In another case of cutaneous cryptococcosis in a patient receiving immunosuppressive therapy, medication with itraconazole resulted in lesion improvement after topical treatment proved ineffective *(238)*.

Among the interactions of itraconazole with other drugs, it should be mentioned that its levels were decreased by rifampicin, phenytoin, and phenobarbital, while itraconazole increased the levels of cyclosporin A. Caution should be applied in patients receiving concomitant anticoagulants.

3. PROPHYLAXIS AND MAINTENANCE THERAPY OF CRYPTOCOCCOSIS

Based on results from prospective controlled trials, fluconazole and itraconazole were both able to reduce the frequency of cryptococcosis in patients with advanced HIV disease *(266)*. Although not routinely recommended, the prophylaxis of cryptococcal disease is usually carried out in patients with $CD4^{4+}$ T-lymphocyte counts of less than 50 cells/µL using daily doses of 100–200 mg fluconazole (Table 2) *(266–269)*. After a documented first episode of cryptococcosis, patients should receive lifelong maintenace therapy (secondary prophylaxis) *(266)*.

4. *CRYPTOCOCCUS NEOFORMANS* VAR. *GATTII*

Before the rise of the AIDS epidemic, cryptococcal meningitis in the tropical and subtropical regions usually affected apparently immunocompetent persons, in contrast to those presenting in temperate climates, where infection was most often associated with immunosuppression *(270,271)*. Biotyping of clinical isolates showed that, serotypes B and C characteristic for *C. neoformans* var. *gattii* were commonly identified in patients from the tropical and subtropical areas *(272–276)* whereas serotypes A, D, and A/D of *C. neoformans* var. *neoformans* were found in predominantly temperate regions *(277)*. It seemed that the human disease caused by var. *gattii* had predilection for the respiratory and central nervous systems, and has been endemic for Australia *(278,279)*, Papua New Guinea *(271–275)*, Southern California, and parts of Africa, India, Southeast Asia, and Central and South America (Mexico, Brasil, and Paraguay) *(277)*. Based on results of searches conducted in Australia, the eucalypt species *Eucalyptus camaldulensis* and *E. tereticornis* constituted, although circumstantially, the only known environmental niche of *C. neoformans* var. *gattii (273,280–282)*. Comparison of a single Californian environmental isolate with three environmental isolates from Australia by karyotyping revealed that although genetically different the four isolates were related *(283,284)*.

The course of meningitis caused by the two different varieties of *C. neoformans* may differ *(285,286)*, with mortality rate in the tropics remaining particularly high *(271,275,287)*.

Treatment of *C. neoformans* var. *gattii*-associated meningitis has been most successful with amphotericin B (0.3–1.0 mg/kg daily, parenterally) and flucytosine (150 mg/kg daily, orally) *(275)*.

Table 2
Prophylaxis Against Cryptococcosis

Patients	Indication	Prophylactic drug regimens	
		First line	Alternative line
Adults and adolescents	First episode: CD^{4+} counts of >50 µL	Fluconazole 100–200 mg, p.o., daily	Itraconazole 200 mg, p.o., daily
	Documented disease	Fluconazole 200 mg, p.o., daily	Amphotericin B 0.6–1.0 mg/kg, i.v., 3 times weekly; or Itraconazole 200 mg, p.o., daily
Infants and children[a]	Severe immunosuppression	luconazole 3–6 mg/kg, p.o., daily	Itraconazole 2–5 mg/kg, p.o., every 12–24 h
	Documented disease	Fluconazole 3–6 mg/kg, p.o., daily	Amphotericin B 0.5–1.0 mg/kg, i.v., 1–3 times weekly; or Itraconazole 2–5 mg/kg, p.o., every 12–24 h

[a]Prophylaxis not recommended for most children but only in cases of severe immunosuppression.

Treatment of an AIDS patient with *C. neoformans* var. *gattii*-induced meningitis resulted in poor clinical and mycological response; in vitro sensitivity testing revealed high MIC value suggesting fluconazole resistance *(288)*. Kamei et al. *(289)* have found voriconazole, a new triazole antimycotic, to be more effective than fluconazole when tested in vitro in two different systems.

5. *CRYPTOCOCCUS ALBIDUS*

C. albidus, is commonly isolated yeast from skin of healthy persons, as well as in indoor or outdoor air *(290)*. The organism has also been isolated from blood specimens *(291,292)*. Although rarely, this yeast has been the cause of meningitis *(293–295)*, lung abscess *(291,296)*, and empyema *(297)* in immunocompromised patients. Studying the distribution of yeast isolates from the oral mucosa of HIV-positive patients, Mckee et al. *(298)* found among non-*Candida* yeasts also *C. albidus*.

Loison et al. *(299)* described what appeared to be the first case of septicemia due to *C. albidus* in an HIV-positive patient. The yeast was sensitive in vitro to amphotericin B, fluconazole, miconazole, itraconazole, and 5-FC. Although the infection was resolved initially with a 2-wk treatment with oral fluconazole at 600 mg daily, followed by fluconazole prophylaxis, a relapse did occur prompting change of the antifungal treatment to oral itraconazole (400 mg daily); the patient died shortly thereafter from cardiovascular arrest. In another fatal case, an AIDS patient with *C. albidus* cryptococcemia died on the 14th day of treatment with amphotericin B-flucytosine combination therapy *(300)*.

6. *CRYPTOCOCCUS LAURENTII*

The natural habitat of *C. laurentii* and its prevalence in the environment have not yet been established. There has been no data about its isolation from normal respiratory flora either, although it would appear to be extraordinarily rare *(301,302)*.

Lynch et al. *(301)* reported the first case of pulmonary infection caused by *C. laurentii* manifested as a lung abscess in a patient with dermatomyositis receiving corticosteroid therapy. The isolation of the yeast appeared to be consistent with an opportunistic infection (pulmonary infiltration with cavity formation developed in association with corticosteroid therapy), rather than saprophytic colonization. Treatment has been carried out successfully with a 6-wk course of amphotericin B (total dose, 2.0 g). In vitro, the antibiotic showed a MIC value of 0.1 μg/mL against a clinical isolate. The latter was not susceptible to 5-FC (MIC = 500 μg/mL), and there has been no synergism between amphotericin B and 5-FC.

C. laurentii has been diagnosed as the etiologic pathogen in a rare case of cryptococcal endophthalmitis cured successfully with oral fluconazole *(303)*.

Kordossis et al. *(300)* described the first case of *C. laurentii* meningitis in an AIDS patient; the condition was controlled after 2 wk of treatment with amphotericin B and flucytosine and no evidence of infection 20 mo later.

REFERENCES

1. Busse, O. Über Parasitare zelleinschlusse und ihre Zuchtung. *Centralbl. Bakt.*, 16, 175, 1894.
2. Colmers, R. A,, Irniger, W., and Steinberg, D. H. *Cryptococcus neoformans* endocarditis cured by amphotericin. *J. Am. Med. Assoc.*, 199, 762, 1967.
3. Arasteh, K., Staib, F., Grosse, G., Futh, U., and L'Age, M. Cryptococcosis in HIV infection of man: an epidemiological and immunological indicator? *Zentralbl. Bakteriol.*, 284, 153, 1996.
4. Littman, M. C. and Walter, J. E. Cryptococcosis: current status. *Am. J. Med.*, 45, 922, 1968.
5. Sabetta, J. R., and Andriole, V. T. Cryptococcal infection of the central nervous system. *Med. Clin. North Am.*, 69, 333, 1985.
6. Butler, W. T., Alling, D. W., Spickard, A., and Utz, J. P. Diagnostic and prognostic value of clinical and laboratory findings in cryptococcal meningitis. *N. Engl. J. Med.*, 270, 59, 1964.
7. De Wytt, C. N., Dickson, P. L., and Holt, G. W. Cryptococcal meningitis: a review of 32 years' experience. *J. Neurol. Sci.*, 53, 283, 1982.
8. Sarosi, G. A., Parker, J. D., Doto, I. L., and Tosh, F. E. Amphotericin B in cryptococcal meningitis: long-term results of treatment. *Ann. Intern. Med.*, 71, 1079, 1969.
9. Spickard, A., Butler, W. T., Andriole, V., and Utz, J. P. The improved prognosis of cryptococcal meningitis with amphotericin B therapy. *Ann. Intern. Med.*, 58, 66, 1963.
10. Utz, J. P., Garriques, I. L., Sande, M. A., et al. Therapy of cryptococcosis with a combination of flucytosine and amphotericin B. *J. Infect. Dis.*, 132, 368, 1975.
11. Zimmerman, L. E. and Rappaport, H. Occurence of cryptococcosis in patients with malignant disease of the reticuloendothelial system. *Am. J. Clin. Pathol.*, 24, 1050, 1954.
12. Perfect, J. R., Durack, D. T., and Gallis, H. A. Cryptococcemia. *Medicine (Baltimore)*, 62, 98, 1983.
13. Graybill, J. R. and Alford, R. H. Cell-mediated immunity in cryptococcosis. *Cell. Immunol.*, 14, 12, 1974.
14. Schimpff, S. C. and Bennett, J. E. Abnormalities in cell-mediated immunity in patients with *C. neoformans* infections. *J. Allergy Clin. Immunol.*, 55, 430, 1975.
15. Krick, J. A. Familial cryptococcal meningitis. *J. Infect. Dis*, 143, 133, 1981.
16. Ieong, M. H., Reardon, C. C., Levitz, S. M., and Kornfeld, H. Human immunodeficiency virus type 1 infection of alveolar macrophages impairs their innate fungicidal activity. *Am. J. Respir. Crit. Care Med.*, 162(3 Pt. 1), 966–970, 2000.
17. Mambula, S. S., Simons, E. R., Hastey, R. P., and Levitz, S. M. Human neutrophil-mediated nonoxidative antifungal activity against *Cryptococcus neoformans*. *Abstr. 99th Abstr. Gen. Meet. Am. Soc. Microbiol.*, May 30–June 3, 303, abstract F-42, 1999.
18. Aguirre, K., Havell, E. A., Gibson, G. W., and Johnson, L. L. Role of tumor necrosis factor and gamma interferon in acquired resistance to *Cryptococcus neoformans* in the central nervous system of mice. *Infect. Immun.*, 63, 1725, 1995.
19. Kawakami, K., Koguchi, Y., Qureshi, M. H., et al. IL-18 contributes to host resistance against infection with *Cryptococcus neoformans* in mice with defective IL-12 synthesis through induction of IFN-gamma production by NK cells. *J. Immunnol.*, 165, 941–947, 2000.
20. Watanabe, H., Inukai, A., Doyu, M., and Sobue, G. CNS cryptococcosis with idiopathic CD4+ T lymphocytopenia. *Rinsho Shinkeigaku*, 40, 249–253, 2000.
21. Kerkering, T. M., Duma, R. J., and Shadomy, S. The evolution of pulmonary cryptococcosis. *Ann. Intern. Med.*, 94, 611, 1981.
22. Reblin, T., Meyer, A., Albrecht, H., and Greten, H. Disseminated cryptococcosis in a patient with AIDS. *Mycoses*, 37, 275, 1994.
23. Sarosi, G. A., Silberfarb, P. M., and Tosh, F. E. Cutaneous cryptococcosis: a sentinel of disseminated disease. *Arch. Dermatol.*, 104, 1, 1971.
24. Srur, E., Misad, C., and Henriquez, A. Extrameningeal cryptococcosis in a patient with AIDS. *Rev. Med. Chil.*, 123, 1009, 1995.
25. Houston, S., Lipp, K., Cobian, L., and Sinnott, J. T. Skin rash in a renal transplant recipients. *Hosp. Pract. (Off. Ed.)*, 30, 89, 1995.
26. Haight, D. O., Esperanza, L. E., Greene, J. N., et al., Case report: cutaneous manifestations of cryptococcosis. *Am. J. Med. Sci.*, 308, 192, 1994.

27. Abraham, K. A., Little, M. A., Casey, R., Smyth, E., and Walshe, J. J. A novel presentation of cryptococcal infection in a renal allograft recipient. *Ir. Med. J.*, 93, 82-84, 2000.
28. Gosling, H. R. and Gilmer, W. S. Skeletal cryptococcosis: report of a case and review of the literature. *J. Bone Joint Surg.*, 38A, 660, 1956.
29. Hinchey, W. W. and Someren, A. Cryptococcal prostatis. *Am. J. Clin. Pathol.*, 75, 257, 1981.
30. Randal, R. E. Jr., Stacy, W. K., Prout, G. R. Jr., et al. Cryptococcal pyelonephritis. *N. Engl. J. Med.*, 279, 60, 1968.
31. Okun, E. and Butler, W. T. Ophthalmologic complications of cryptococcal meningitis. *Arch. Ophthalmol.*, 71, 52, 1964.
32. Weiss, C., Perry, I. H., and Shevky, M. C. Infections of the human eye with *Cryptococcus neoformans* (*Torula histolytica*). *Arch. Ophthalmol.*, 39, 739, 1948.
33. Procknow, J. J., Benfield, J. R., Ripon, J. W., Diener, C. F., and Archer, F. L. Cryptococcal hepatitis presenting as a surgical emergency. *J. Am. Med. Assoc.*, 191, 269, 1965.
34. Sabesin, S. M., Fallon, H. J., and Andriole, V. T. Hepatic failure as a manifestation of cryptococcosis. *Arch. Intern. Med.*, 111, 661, 1963.
35. Goenka, M. K., Mehta, S., Yachha, S., Nagi, B., Chakraborty, A., Malik, A. K. Hepatic involvement culminating in cirrhosis in a child with disseminated cryptococcosis. *J. Clin. Gastroenterol.*, 20, 57, 1995.
36. Baker, R. D. and Haugen, R. K. Tissue damages and tissue diagnosis in cryptococcosis. *Am. J. Clin. Pathol.*, 25, 14, 1955.
37. Bowman, H. E. and Ritchey, J. O. Cryptococcosis (torulosis) involving brain, adrenal, and prostate. *J. Urol.*, 71, 373, 1954.
38. Voyles, G. O. and Beck, E. M. Systemic infection due to *Torula histolytica* (*C. hominis*): report of four cases and review of the literature. *Arch. Intern. Med.*, 77, 504, 1946.
39. Zelman, S., O'Neil, H., and Plaut, A. Disseminated visceral torulosis without nervous system involvement with clinical appearance of granulocytic leukemia. *Am. J. Med.*, 11, 568, 1951.
40. Poliner, J. R., Wilkins, E. B., and Fernald, G. W. Localized osseous cryptococcosis. *J. Pediatr.*, 94, 597, 1979.
41. Goldman, M. and Pottage, J. C. Jr. Cryptococcal infection of the breast. *Clin. Infect. Dis.*, 21, 1166, 1995.
42. Merwaha, R. K., Trehan, A., Jayashree, K., and Vasishta, R. K. Hypereosinophilia in disseminated cryptococcal disease. *Pediatr. Infect. Dis. J.*, 14, 1103, 1995.
43. Larsen, R. A., Bozzette, S., McCutchan, J. A., et al. Persistent *Cryptococcus neoformans* infection of the prostate after successful treatment of meningitis. *Ann. Intern. Med.*, 111, 125, 1989.
44. Fuse, H., Ohkawa, M., Yamaguchi, K., Hirata, A., and Matsubara, F. Cryptococcal prostatitis in a patient with Behcet's disease treated with fluconazole. *Mycopathologia*, 130, 147, 1995.
45. Glassman, S. J. and Hale, M. J. Cutaneous cryptococcosis and Kaposi's sarcoma occuring in the same lesions in a patient with the acquired immunodeficiency syndrome. *Clin. Exp. Dermatol.*, 20, 480, 1995.
46. Muccioli, C., Belfort Junior, R., Neves, R., and Rao, N. Limbal and choroidal *Cryptococcus* infection in the acquired immunodeficiency syndrome. *Am. J. Ophthalmol.*, 120, 539, 1995.
47. Benard, G., Gryschek, R. C., Duarte, A. J., and Shakanai-Yasuda, M. A. Cryptococcosis as an opportunistic infection in immunodeficiency secondary to paracoccidioidomycosis. *Mycopathologia*, 133, 65, 1996.
48. Molnar-Nadasdy, G., Haesly, I., Reed, J., and Altshuler, G. Placental cryptococcosis in a mother with systemic lupus erythematosus. *Arch. Pathol. Lab. Med.*, 118, 757, 1994.
49. Zuger, A., Louie, E., Holzman, R. S., Simberkoff, M. S., and Rahal, J. J. Cryptococcal disease in patients with acquired immunodeficiency syndrome: diagnostic features and outcome of treatment. *Ann. Intern. Med.*, 104, 234, 1986.
50. Kovacs, J. A., Kovacs, A. A., Polis. M., et al. Cryptococcosis in the acquired immunodeficiency syndrome. *Ann. Intern. Med.*, 103, 533, 1985.
51. Dismukes, W. E., Cloud, G., Gallis, H. A., et al. Treatment of cryptococcal meningitis with combination amphotericin B and flucytosine for four as compared with six weeks. *N. Engl. J. Med.*, 317, 334, 1987.
52. Eng, R. H.K., Bishburg, E., Smith, S. M., and Kapila, R. Cryptococcal infections in patients with acquired immune deficiency syndrome. *Am. J. Med.*, 81, 19, 1986.
53. Theunissen, A. W. J. and Zanen, H. C. Dertig petienten net een "verborgen" ziekte: cryptococcen-meningitis. *Ned. Tijdschr. Geneeskd.*, 131, 1123, 1987.
54. Castro Guardiola, A., Ocana Rivera, I., Gasser Laguna, I., et al. 16 cases of infections by *Cryptococcus neoformans* in patients with AIDS. *Enferm. Infec. Microbiol. Clin.*, 9, 90, 1991.
55. Sugar, A. M. Overview: cryptococcosis in the treatment of AIDS. *Mycopathologia*, 114, 153, 1991.
56. Fur, B. Cryptococcosis in AIDS: therapeutic concepts. *Mycoses*, 33(Suppl.1), 55, 1990.
57. Kirchner, J. T. Opportunistic fungal infections in patients with HIV disease: combating cryptococcosis and histoplasmosis. *Postgrad. Med.*, 99, 209, 1996.
58. Mitchell, T. G. and Perfect, J. R. Cryptococcosis in the era of AIDS: 100 years after the discovery of *Cryptococcus neoformans*. *Clin. Microbiol. Rev.*, 8, 515, 1995.
59. Just-Nübling, G. Therapy of candidiasis and cryptococcosis in AIDS. *Mycoses*, 37(Suppl. 2), 56, 1994.
60. Emmons III, W. W., Luchsinger, S., and Miller, L. Progressive pulmonary cryptococcosis in a patient who is immunocompetent. *South. Med. J.*, 88, 657, 1995.
61. Munoz-Peréz, M. A., Colmenero, M. A., Rodriguez-Pichardo, A., Rodriguez-Pinero, F. J., Rios, J. J., and Camacho, F. Disseminated cryptococcosis presenting as moluscum-like lesions as the first manifestation of AIDS. *Int. J. Dermatol.*, 35, 646, 1996.
62. Gonzalez, C. E., Shetty, D., Lewis, L. L., Mueller, B. U., Pizzo, P. A., and Walsh, T. J. Cryptococcosis in human immunodeficiency virus-infected children. *Pediatr. Infect. Dis. J.*, 15, 796, 1996.

63. Littman, M. L. and Zimmerman, L. E. *Cryptococcosis.* Grune & Stratton, New York, 1956.
64. Haugen, R. K. and Baker, R. D. The pulmonary lesions in cryptococcosis with special reference to subpleural nodules. *Am. J. Clin. Pathol.,* 24, 1381, 1954.
65. Talerman, A., Bradley, J. M., and Woodland, B. Cryptococcal lymphadenitis. *J. Med. Microbiol.,* 3, 633, 1970.
66. Salyer, W. R., Salyer, D. C., and Baker, R. D. Primary complex of *Cryptococcus* and pulmonary lymph nodes. *J. Infect. Dis.,* 130, 74, 1974.
67. Houk, V. N. and Moser, K. M. Pulmonary cryptococcosis: must all receive amphotericin B. *Ann. Intern. Med.,* 63, 583, 1965.
68. Campbell, G. D. Primary pulmonary cryptococcosis. *Am. Rev. Respir. Dis.,* 94, 236, 1966.
69. Duperval, R., Hermans, P. E., Brewer, N. S., and Roberts, G. D. Cryptococcosis with emphasis on the significance of isolation of *C. neoformans* from the respiratory tract. *Chest,* 72, 13, 1977.
70. Hammerman, K. J., Powell, K. E., and Christianson, C. S. Pulmonary cryptococcosis: clinical forms and treatment - CDC cooperative mycoses study. *Am. Rev. Respir. Dis.,* 108, 1116, 1973.
71. Gurevitz, O., Goldschmiedt-Reuven, A., Block, C., Kopolovic, J., Farfel, Z., and Hassin, D. *Cryptococcus neoformans* vertebral osteomyelitis. *J. Med. Vet. Mycol.,* 32, 315, 1994.
72. Anthony, S. A. and Anthony, S. J. Primary cutaneous cryptococcosis in nonimmunocompromised patients. *Cutis,* 56, 96, 1995.
73. Gordon, P. M., Ormerod, A. D., Harvey, G., Atkinson, P., and Best, P. V. Cutaneous cryptococcal infection without immunodeficiency. *Clin. Exp. Dermatol.,* 19, 181, 1994.
74. Mahida, P., Morar, R., Goolam Mohamed, A., Song, E., Tissandie, J. P., and Feldman, C. Cryptococcosis: an unusual cause of endobronchial obstruction. *Eur. Respir. J.,* 9, 837, 1996.
75. Schepelmann, K., Muller, F., and Dichgans, J. Cryptococcal meningitis with severe visual and hearing loss and radiculopathy in a patient without immunodeficiency. *Mycoses,* 36, 429, 1993.
76. Vender, J. R., Miller, D. M., Roth, T., Nair, S., and Reboli, A. C. Intraventricular cryptococcal cysts. *AJNR Am. J. Neuroradiol.,* 17, 110, 1996.
77. Yu, F. C., Perng, W. C., Wu, C. P., Shen, C. Y., and Lee, H. S. Adult respiratory distress syndrome caused by pulmonary cryptococcosis in an immunocompetent host: a case report. *Chung Hua I Hsueh Tsa Chih (Taipei),* 52, 120, 1993.
78. Hellman, R. N., Hinrichs, J., Sicard, G., Hoover, R., Golden, P., and Hoffsten, P. Cryptococcal pyelonephritis and disseminated cryptococcosis in a renal transplant recipient. *Arch. Intern. Med.,* 141, 128, 1984.
79. Liss, H. P. and Rimland, D. Asymptomatic cryptococcal meningitis. *Am. Rev. Respir. Dis.,* 124, 88, 1981.
80. Tarala, R. A. and Smith, J. D. Cryptococcosis treated by rapid infusion of amphotericin B. *Br. Med. J.,* 281, 28, 1980.
81. Mosberg, W. H. and Arnold, J. G. Torulosis of the central nervous system: review of the literature and report of five cases. *Ann. Intern. Med.,* 32, 1153, 1950.
82. Beeson, P. B. Cryptococcal meningitis of nearly sixteen years' duration. *Arch. Intern. Med.,* 89, 797, 1952.
83. Campbell, G. D., Carrier, R. D., and Busey, J. F. Survival in untreated cryptococcal meningitis. *Neurology,* 31, 1154, 1981.
84. Carton, C. A. and Mount, L. A. Neurosurgical aspects of cryptococcosis. *J. Neurosurg.,* 8, 143, 1951.
85. Powderly, W. G. Recent advances in the management of cryptococcal meningitis in patients with AIDS. *Clin. Infect. Dis.,* 22(suppl. 2), S119, 1996.
86. Dismukes, W. E. Management of cryptococcosis. *Clin. Infect. Dis.,* 17(Suppl. 2), S507, 1993 [see also: *Clin. Infect. Dis.,* 19, 975, 1994].
87. Powderly, W. G. Current approach to the acute management of cryptococcal infections. *J. Infect.,* 41, 18–22, 2000.
88. Saag, M. S., Graybill, R. J., Larsen, R. A., et al. Practice guidelines for the management of cryptococcal disease. Infectious Diseases Society of America. *Clin. Infect. Dis.,* 30, 710–718, 2000.
89. Van der Horst, C., Saag, M., Cloud, G., et al. Randomized double blind comparison of amphotericin B (AMB) plus flucytosine to AMB alone (step 1) followed by a comparison of fluconazole to itraconazole (step 2) in the treatment of acute cryptococcal meningitis in patients with AIDS. Part I, *35th Intersci. Conf. Antimicrob. Agents Chemother.,* American Society for Microbiology, Washington, DC, abstract I-216, 1995.
90. Nightingale, S. D. Initial therapy for acquired immunodeficiency syndrome-associated cryptococcosis with fluconazole. *Arch. Intern. Med.,* 13, 538, 1995.
91. Saag, M. S., Powderly, W. G., Cloud, G. A., et al. Comparison of amphotericin B with fluconazole in the treatment of acute AIDS-associated cryptococcal meningitis. *N. Engl. J. Med.,* 326, 83, 1992.
92. Haubrich, R. H., Haghighat, D., Bozzette, S. A., Tilles, J., and McCutchan, J. A. High-dose fluconazole for treatment of cryptococcal disease in patients with human immunodeficiency virus infection. *J. Infect. Dis.,* 170, 238, 1994.
93. Meyohas, M. C., Meynard, J. L., Bollens, D., et al. Treatment of non-meningeal cryptococcosis in patients with AIDS. *J. Infect.,* 33, 7, 1996.
94. Sitbon, O., Fourme, T., Bouree, P., Du Pasquier, L., and Salmeron, S. Successful treatment of disseminated *Cryptococcus*is with high-dose oral fluconazole. *AIDS,* 7, 1685, 1993.
95. Ammassari, A., Linzalone, A., Murri, R., Marasca, G., Morace, G., and Antinori, A. Fluconazole for primary prophylaxis of AIDS-associated cryptococcosis: a case controlled study. *Scand. J. Infect. Dis.,* 27, 235, 1995.
96. Nelson, M. R., Fisher, M., Cartledge, J., Rogers, T., and Gazzard, B. G. The role of azoles in the treatment and prophylaxis of cryptococcal disease in HIV infection. *AIDS,* 8, 651, 1994 [see also: *AIDS,* 9, 300, 1995].
97. Manfredi, R., Mastroianni, A., Coronado, O. V., and Chiodo, F. Fluconazole as prophylaxis against fungal infection in patients with advanced HIV infection. *Arch. Intern. Med.,* 157, 64, 1997

98. Georgiev, V. St. Opportunistic/nosocomial infections: treatment and developmental therapeutics. I. Cryptococcosis. *Med. Res. Rev.*, 13, 493–506, 1993.
99. Fernandez-Concepcion, O., Ariosa-Acuna, M. C., Giroud-Benitez, J. L., Pando-Cabrera, A., Garcia-Fidalgo, J. A., and Mestre-Miguelez, R. Cryptococcosis of the central nervous system. A report of five cases. *Rev. Neurol.*, 30, 935–938, 2000.
100. Emmons, C. W., Binford, C. H., and Utz, J. P. *Medical Mycology*, 2nd ed. Lea & Fabiger, Philadelphia, 190, 1970.
101. Zuger, A., Schuster, M., Simberkoff, M. S., Rahal, J. J., and Holzman, R. S. Maintenance amphotericin B for cryptococcal meningitis in the acquired immunodeficiency syndrome (AIDS). *Ann. Intern. Med.*, 109, 592, 1988.
102. Holmberg, K. and Meyer, R. D. Fungal infections in patients with AIDS and AIDS-related complex. *Scand. J. Infect. Dis.*, 18, 179, 1986.
103. Chechani, V. and Kamholz, S. L. Optimal therapy of cryptococcosis in patients with the acquired immunodeficiency syndrome. *NY State J. Med.*, 91, 292, 1991.
104. de Lalla, F., Pellizzer, G., Vaglia, A., et al., Amphotericin B as primary therapy for cryptococcosis in patients with AIDS: reliability of relatively high doses administered over a relatively short period. *Clin. Infect. Dis.*, 20, 263, 1995.
105. Churchill, D. and Coker, R. Amphotericin B as primary therapy for cryptococcosis in patients with AIDS: reliability of relatively high doses over a relatively short period. *Clin. Infect. Dis.*, 21, 1352, 1995.
106. de Lalla, F., Pellizzer, G., Vaglia, A., et al. Amphotericin B as primary therapy for cryptococcosis in patients with AIDS: reliability of relatively high doses over a relatively short period: a reply. *Clin. Infect. Dis.*, 21, 1353, 1995.
107. Diamond, R. D. and Bennett, J. E. A subcutaneous reservoir for intrathecal therapy of fungal meningitis. *N. Engl. J. Med.*, 288, 186, 1973.
108. Polsky, B., Depman, M. R., Gold, J. W. M., Galicich, J. H., and Armstrong, D. Intraventricular therapy of cryptococcal meningitis via a subcutaneous reservoir. *Am. J. Med.*, 81, 24, 1986.
109. Roberts, N. J. and Douglas, R. G. Cryptococcal meningitis: cure despite cryptococcemia. *Arch. Neurol.*, 35, 179, 1978.
110. Sapico, F. L. Disappearance of focal cryptococcal brain lesion on chemotherapy alone. *Lancet*, 1, 560, 1979.
111. Bastin, R., Vildé, J. L., Drouhet, E., and Carbon, C. Primary meningitis due to *Cryptococcus neoformans* associated with polyradiculitis: cure by amphotericin B. *Sem. Hop. Paris.*, 50, 337, 1974.
112. Sugar, A. M., Stern, J. J., and Dupont, B. Overview: treatment of cryptococcal meningitis. *Rev. Infect. Dis.*, 12(Suppl 3), S338, 1990.
113. Hay, R. J. Use of ambisome, liposomal amphotericin B in systemic fungal infections: preliminary findings of a European multicenter study, in *Recent Progress in Antifungal Chemotherapy*, Yamaguchi, H., Kobayashi, G. S., and Takeuchi, H., Eds. Marcel Dekker, New York, 323, 1992.
114. Coker, R., Tomlinson, D., and Harris, J. Successful treatment of cryptococcal meningitis with liposomal amphotericin B after failure of treatment with fluconazole and conventional amphotericin B. *AIDS*, 5, 231, 1991.
115. Schurmann, D., de Matos Marques, B., Grunewald, T., Pohle, H. D., Hahn, H., and Ruf, B. Safety and efficacy of liposomal amphotericin B in treating AIDS-associated disseminated cryptococcosis. *J. Infect. Dis.*, 164, 620, 1991.
116. Ikemoto, H., Yashiro, M., Furugori, T., and Kudo, Y. Unusual treatment of cryptococcal meningitis successfully treated with a small amount of amphotericin B, a large amount of prednisolone, and continued removal of cerebrospinal fluid. *J. Antibiot.*, 20, 374, 1967.
117. Yashiro, M., Furugori, T., Kudo, Y., and Ikemoto, H. Cryptococcal meningitis successfully treated with amphotericin B, adrenal corticosteroid, and continuous removal of the cerebrospinal fluid. *Naika*, 20, 1155, 1967.
118. Brisman, R., Reid, R., and Harrington, G. Intracranial cryptococcal granuloma - amphotericin B and surgical excision. *Surg. Neurol.*, 1, 43, 1973.
119. Dillon, M. C. and Sealy, W. C. Surgical aspects of opportunistic fungus infection. *Lab. Invest.*, 11, 1231, 1962.
120. Reeves, D. C. Cryptococcic (*Torula*) granuloma of the scull. *J. Neurol.*, 27, 70, 1967.
121. Rish, B. L. and Meacham, W. F. Intracerebral cystic toruloma. *J. Neurosurg.*, 28, 603, 1968.
122. Vijayan, N., Bhatt, G. P., and Dreyfus, P. M. Intraventricular cryptococcal granuloma. *Neurology*, 21, 728, 1971.
123. Einstein, H. E., Brown, J. F., and Holmes, C. W. Some treatment aspects of coccidioidal meningitis, in *Progress Report of the VA-Armed Forces Coccidioidomycosis Study Group No 7*, Salkin, D. and Huppert, M., Eds. California VA Hospital, San Francisco, 17, 1969.
124. Pappagianis, D. Meningitis in children, in *Progress Report of the VA- Armed Forces Coccidioidomycosis Study Group No 8*, Salkin, D. and Hupper, M., Eds. California VA Hospital, San Francisco, 16, 1969.
125. Schonheyder, H., Thestrup-Pedersen, K., Esmann, V., and Stenderup, A. Cryptococcal meningitis: complications due to intrathecal treatment. *J. Infect. Dis.*, 12, 155, 1980.
126. Swenson, R. S., Kountz, S. L., Blank, N., and Merigan, T. C. Successful renal allograft in a patient with pulmonary cryptococcosis. *Arch. Intern. Med.*, 124, 502, 1969.
127. Oka, S., Sugimoto, H., and Shimada, K. Problems in the treatment of fungal infections after renal transplantation in Japan, in *Recent Progress in Antifungal Chemotherapy*, Yamaguchi, H., Kobayashi, G. S., and Takeuchi, H., Eds. Marcel Dekker, New York, 239, 1992.
128. Shindo, K. Treatment of cryptococcal meningitis with five antifungal drugs: the role of amphotericin B. *Drugs Exp. Clin. Res.*, 16, 327, 1991.
129. Liu, Y. C., Cheng, D. L., Liu, C. Y., Yen, M. Y., and Wang, R. S. Isolated cryptococcosis of the adrenal gland. *J. Intern. Med.*, 230, 285, 1991.
130. Perkins, W. Pulmonary cryptococcosis: report on the treatment of nine cases. *Dis. Chest*, 56, 398, 1969.
131. Lopez-Berestein, G., Fainstein, V., Hersh, E. M., et al. Treatment of disseminated fungal infections in mammals with liposome- encapsulated amphotericin B. *U.S. Patent 4,663,167*, 1987.

132. Fajardo, L. F. Failure of topical amphotericin B in cryptococcosis. *Ann. Intern. Med.*, 78, 777, 1973.
133. Kojima, T., Matsuzaki, M., Sano, M., et al. Acute lymphocytic leukemia, complicated with generalized cryptococcosis successfully treated by amphotericin B: a case report. *Rinsho Ketsueki*, 26, 217, 1985.
134. Lerner, P. I. and Weinstein, L. Infective endocarditis in the antibiotic era. *N. Engl. J. Med.*, 274, 388, 1966.
135. Lombardo, T. A., Rabson, A. D., and Dodge, H. T. Mycotic endocarditis: report of a case due to *Cryptococcus neoformans*. *Am. J. Med.*, 22, 664, 1957.
136. Miller, R. P. and Bates, J. H. Amphotericin B toxicity: a follow-up report of 53 patients. *Ann. Intern. Med.*, 71, 1089, 1969.
137. Ellincy, B. R. Amphotericin B usage in pregnancy complicated by cryptococcosis. *Am. J. Obstet. Gynecol.*, 115, 285, 1973.
138. Silberfarb, P. M., Sarosi, G. A., and Tosh, F. E. Cryptococcosis and pregnancy. *Am. J. Obstet. Gynecol.*, 112, 714, 1972.
139. Li, P. K. and Lai, K. N. Amphotericin B induced ocular toxicity in cryptococcal meningitis. *Br. J. Ophthalmol.*, 73, 397, 1989.
140. Kaminaga, Y., Shindo, K., Ito, A., and Iizuma, H. Mycological and clinical study of cryptococcosis in Yokohama City University Hospital during the period from 1965 to 1989. *Kansenshogaku Zasshi*, 65, 374, 1991.
141. Armstrong, D. Treatment of fungal infections in the immunocompromised host, in *Recent Progress in Antifungal Chemotherapy*, Yamaguchi, H., Kobayashi, S. G., and Takeuchi, H., Eds. Marcel Dekker, New York, 251, 1992.
142. Hackett, A. J., Sylvester, S. S., Joss, U. R., and Calvin, M. Synergistic effect of rifamycin derivatives and amphotericin B on viral transformation of a murine cell line. *Proc. Natl. Acad. Sci. USA*, 69, 3653, 1972.
143. Kuwano, M., Akiyama, S., Endo, H., and Kohga, M. Potentiation of fusidic acid and lentinan effects upon normal and transformed fibroblastic cells by amphotericin B. *Biochem. Biophys. Res. Commun.*, 49, 1241, 1972.
144. Medoff, G. and Kobayashi, G. S. Amphotericin B and 5-fluorocytosine. *J. Infect. Dis.*, 132, 489, 1975.
145. Jimbow, T., Tejima, Y., and Ikemoto, H. Comparison between 5-fluorocytosine, amphotericin B and the combined administration of these agents in the therapeutic effectiveness for cryptococcal meningitis. *Chemotherapy*, 24, 374, 1978.
146. Bennett, J. E., Dismukes, W. E., Duma, R. J., et al. A comparison of amphotericin B alone and combined with flucytosine in the treatment of cryptococcal meningitis. *N. Engl. J. Med.*, 301, 127, 1979.
147. MacGregor, R. R. Treatment of cryptococcal meningitis. *N. Engl. J. Med.*, 318, 380, 1988.
148. Schmutzhard, E. and Vejajjiva, A. Treatment of cryptococcal meningitis with high-dose, long-term combination amphotericin B and flucytosine. *Am. J. Med.*, 85, 737, 1988.
149. Sahai, J. Management of cryptococcal meningitis in patients with AIDS. *Clin. Pharmacy*, 7, 528, 1988.
150. Kauffman, C. A. and Frame, P. T. Bone marrow toxicity associated with 5-fluorocytosine therapy. *Antimicrob. Agents Chemother.*, 11, 244, 1977.
151. Donahue, R. E., Johnson, M. M., Zon, L. I., Clark, S. C., and Groopman, J. E. Suppression of in vitro haematopoiesis following human immunodeficiency virus infection. *Nature*, 326, 200, 1987.
152. Kotler, D. P., Gaetz, H. P., Lange, M., Klein, E. B., and Holt, P. R. Enteropathy associated with acquired immunodeficiency syndrome. *Ann. Intern. Med.*, 101, 421, 1984.
153. Chuck, S. L. and Sande, M. A. Infections with *Cryptococcus neoformans* in the acquired immunodeficiency syndrome. *N. Engl. J. Med.*, 321, 794, 1989.
154. Dismukes, W. E. Treatment of systemic fungal diseases in patients with AIDS, in *Recent Progress in Antifungal Chemotherapy*, Yamaguchi, H., Kobayashi, G. S., and Takeuchi, H., Eds. Marcel Dekker, New York, 227, 1992.
155. Bayardelle, P., Giard, N., Maltais, R., Delorme, J., and Brazean, M. Success with amphotericin B and 5-fluorocytosine in treating cerebral cryptococcoma accompanying cryptococcal meningitis. *Can. Med. Assoc. J.*, 127, 732, 1982.
156. Koeleman, J. G., Rustemejer, C., Wijermans, P. W., and MacLaren, D. M. Cryptococcal meningo-encephalitis after prolonged corticosteroid therapy. *Neth. J. Med.*, 36, 242, 1990.
157. Carney, M. D., Combs, J. L., and Waschler, W. Cryptococcal choroiditis. *Retina*, 10, 27, 1990.
158. Picon, L., Vaillant, L., Duong, T., et al. Cutaneous cryptococcosis resembling molluscum contagiosum: a first manifestation of AIDS. *Acta Derm. Venereol. (Stockholm)*, 69, 365, 1989.
159. Tobias, J. S., Wrigley, P. F. M., and Shaw, E. Combination antifungal therapy for cryptococcal meningitis. *Postgrad. Med. J.*, 52, 305, 1976.
160. Watson, A. J., Russell, R. P., Cabreja, R. F., Braverman, R., and Whelton, A. Cure of cryptococcal infection during continued immunosuppressive therapy. *Q. J. Med.*, 55, 169, 1985.
161. Gallis, H. A., Berman, R. A., Cate, T. R., Hamilton, J. D., Gunnels, J.C., and Stickel, D. L. Fungal infection following renal transplantation. *Arch. Intern. Med.*, 135, 1163, 1975.
162. Mills, S. A., Seigler, H. F., and Wolfe, W. G. The incidence and management of pulmonary mycosis in renal allograft patients. *Ann. Surg.*, 182, 617, 1975.
163. Kong, N. C., Sharriah, W., Morad, Z., Suleiman, A. B., and Wong, Y. H. Cryptococcosis in a renal unit. *Aust. N. Z. J. Med.*, 20, 645, 1990.
164. Kimura, K., Hatekayama, M., Miyagi, J., et al. A case of systemic lupus erythematosus with cryptococcal meningitis successfully treated with amphotericin B and 5-FC. *Nipon Naika Gakkai Zasshi*, 75, 406, 1986.
165. Butler, W. P. and Kaufer, G. I. Primary cutaneous cryptococcosis successfully treated with outpatient amphotericin B and 5-fluorocytosine. *Nita*, 8, 295, 1985.
166. Woolfitt, R., Park, H. M., and Greene, M. Localized cryptococcal osteomyelitis. *Radiology*, 120, 290, 1976.

167. Nottebart, H. C., McGehee, R. F., and Utz, J. P. *Cryptococcus neoformans* osteomyelitis: case report of two patients. *Sabouraudia*, 12, 127, 1974.
168. Chand, K. and Lall, K. S. Cryptococcosis of the knee joint. *Acta Orthop. Scand.*, 47, 432, 1976.
169. Nathan, C. F. Cryptococcal osteomyelitis treated with 5-fluorocytosine. *Am. Rev. Respir. Dis.*, 110, 78, 1974.
170. Luhr, H. and Svane, S. Pulmonary pseudomotor caused by *Cryptococcus neoformans*. *Tidsskr. Nor. Laegeforen.*, 111, 3288, 1991.
171. Schmidt-Westhausen, A., Grunewald, T., Reihart, P. A., and Pohle, H. D. Oral cryptococcosis in a patient with AIDS: a case report. *Oral. Dis.*, 1, 77, 1995 [see also: *Oral Dis.*, 1, 61, 1995].
172. Iida, Y., Maehara, K., Okamoto, Y., et al. A case of cryptococcal meningitis treated by ketoconazole and amphotericin B combination therapy. *Kansenshogaku Zasshi*, 60, 189, 1986.
173. Echevarria, A., Pinzon, V., Toro, J., and Diaz Issacs, M. Pulmonary cryptococcosis. *Rev. Med. Panama*, 16, 50, 1991.
174. Aslam, P. A., Larkin, J., Eastridge, C. E., and Hughes, F. A. Endocavitary infusion through percutaneous endobronchial catheter. *Chest*, 57, 94, 1970.
175. Stamm, A. M., Diasio, R. B., Dismukes, W. E., et al. Toxicity of amphotericin B plus flucytosine in 194 patients with cryptococcal meningitis. *Am. J. Med.*, 83, 236, 1987.
176. Shindo, K., Mizuno, T., Matsumoto, Y., et al. Granulocytopenia and thrombocytopenia associated with combination therapy of amphotericin B and low-dose flucytosine in a patient with cryptococcal meningitis. *DICP*, 23, 672, 1989.
177. Bryan, C. S. and McFarland, J. A. Cryptococcal meningitis: fatal marrow applasia from combined therapy. *J. Am. Med. Assoc.*, 239, 1068, 1978.
178. Tassel, D. and Madoff, M. A., Treatment of *Candida* sepsis and *Cryptococcus* meningitis with 5-fluorocytosine: a new antifungal agent. *J. Am. Med. Assoc.*, 260, 830, 1968.
179. Sanati, H., Messer, S. A., Pfaller, M., et al. Multicenter evaluation of broth microdilution method for susceptibility testing of *Cryptococcus neoformans* against fluconazole. *J. Clin. Microbiol.*, 34, 1280, 1996.
180. Koechlin, B. A., Rubio, S., Palmer, S., Gabriel, T., and Duschinsky, R. The metabolism of 5-fluorocytosine-2[^{14}C] and cytosine[^{14}C] in the rat and the disposition of 5-fluorocytosine- 2[^{14}C] in man. *Biochem. Pharmacol.*, 15, 435, 1966.
181. Shadomy, S. Further in vitro studies with 5-fluorocytosine. *Infect. Immun.*, 2, 484, 1970.
182. Roberts, M., Rinaudo, P. A., Tilton, R. C., and Vilinskas, J. Treatment of multiple intracerebral cryptococcal granulomas with 5-fluorocytosine. *J. Neurosurg.*, 37, 229, 1972.
183. Editorial. Cryptococcosis and 5-fluorocytosine. *Aust. N. Z. J. Med.*, 4, 296, 1974.
184. Sabetta, J. R. and Andriole, V. T. Cryptococcal infections in the central nervous system. *Med. Clin. North Am.*, 69, 334, 1985.
185. Block, E. R. and Bennett, J. E. Clinical and pharmacological studies with 5-fluorocytosine (5-FC). *Clin. Res.*, 20, 525, 1972.
186. Utz, J. P., Shadomy, S., McGehee, R. F., and Tynes, B. S. 5-Fluorocytosine: experience in patients with pulmonary and other forms of cryptococcosis. *Am. Rev. Respir. Dis.*, 99, 975, 1969.
187. Zylstra, W. Cryptococcosis and 5-fluorocytosine: comment. *Aust. N. Z. J. Med.*, 4, 296, 1974.
188. Vandevelle, A. G., Nauceri, A. A., and Johnson III, J. E. 5-Fluorocytosine in the treatment of mycotic infections. *Ann. Intern. Med.*, 77, 43, 1972.
189. Fass, R. J. and Perkins, R. L. 5-Fluorocytosine in the treatment of cryptococcal and *Candida* mycoses. *Ann. Intern. Med.*, 74, 535, 1971.
190. Schlegel, R. J., Bernier, G. M., Bellanti, J. A., et al. Severe candidiasis asociated with thymic displasia, IgA deficiency and plasma antilymphocyte effects. *Pediatrics*, 45, 926, 1970.
191. McDonnell, F. I., Clunie, G. J. A., Petrie, J. J. G., and Rao, A. Experience with 5- fluorocytosine in a dialysis-transplant unit. *Aust. N. Z. J. Med.*, 3, 438, 1973.
192. Kauffman, C. A. and Frame, P. T. Bone marrow toxicity associated with 5-fluorocytosine therapy. *Antimicrob. Agents Chemother.*, 11, 244, 1977.
193. Bryan, C. S. and McFarland, J. A. Cryptococcal meningitis: fatal marrow aplasia from combined therapy. *J. Am. Med. Assoc.*, 239, 1068, 1978.
194. Philpot, C. R. and Lo, D. Cryptococcal meningitis in pregnancy. *Med. J. Aust.*, 2, 1005, 1972.
195. Deresinski, S. C., Lilly, R. B., Levine, H. B., Galgiani, J. N., and Stevens, D. A. Treatment of fungal meningitis with miconazole. *Arch. Intern. Med.*, 137, 1180, 1977.
196. Ito, A., Therapeutic results with miconazole in Japan, in Recent Progress in *Antifungal Chemotherapy*, Yamaguchi, H., Kobayashi, G. S., and Takeuchi, H., Eds. Marcel Dekker, New York, 183, 1991.
197. Sung, J. P., Grendale, J. G., and Levine, H. B., Intravenous and intrathecal miconazole therapy for systemic mycosis. *West. J. Med.*, 126, 5, 1977.
198. Weinstein, L. and Jacoby, I., Successful treatment of cerebral cryptococcoma and meningitis with miconazole. *Ann. Intern. Med.*, 93, 569, 1980.
199. Belle, W. E., Treatment of fungal infections of the central nervous system. *Ann. Neurol.*, 9, 417, 1981.
200. Sung, J. P., Campbell, G. D., and Grendahl, J. C., Miconazole therapy for fungal meningitis. *Arch. Neurol.*, 35, 443, 1978.
201. Perfect, J. R., Durack, D. T., Hamilton, J. D., and Gallis, H. A., Failure of ketoconazole in cryptococcal meningitis. *J. Am. Med. Assoc.*, 247, 3349, 1982.
202. Ogushi, F., Tamura, M., Ozaki, T., et al. A case of cryptococcal meningitis improved in the treatment of high dose ketoconazole. *Kansenshogaku Zasshi*, 59, 405, 1985.

203. Karaffa, C. A., Rehm, S. J., and Keys, T. F. The acquired immunodeficiency syndrome and cryptococcosis. *Ann. Intern. Med.*, 104, 891, 1986.
204. Granier, F., Kamitakis, J., Hermier, C., Zhu, Y. Y., and Thivolet, J. Localized cutaneous cryptococcosis successfully treated with ketoconazole. *J. Am. Acad. Dermatol.*, 16, 243, 1987.
205. Bernard, E., Carles, M., Toussaint-Gari, M., Fournier, J. P., and Dellamonica, P. Value of fluconazole in the treatment of systemic yeast infection. *Pathol. Biol. (Paris)*, 37, 690, 1989.
206. Shuttleworth, D., Philpot, C. M., and Knight, A. G. Cutaneous cryptococcosis: treatment with oral fluconazole. *Br. J. Dermatol.*, 120, 683, 1989.
207. Nakashima, M. The clinical study of fluconazole against pulmonary cryptococcosis and aspergillosis, and its pharmacokinetics in patients. *Jpn. J. Antibiot.*, 42, 127, 1989.
208. Mares, M., Sartori, M. T., Carretta, M., Bertaggia, A., and Girolami, A. Rhinophyma-like cryptococcal infection as an early manifestation of AIDS in a hemophilia B patient. *Acta Haematol.*, 84, 101, 1990.
209. Zalcman, G., Lechapt, E., Milleron, B., Denis, M., Mayaud, C., and Akoun, G. Pleuropulmonary cryptococcosis disclosing AIDS. *Rev. Pneumol. Clin.*, 47, 133, 1991.
210. Bozzette, S. A., Larsen, R. A., Chiu, J., et al. Fluconazole treatment of persistent *Cryptococcus neoformans* prostatic infection in AIDS. *Ann. Intern. Med.*, 115, 285, 1991.
211. Sugar, A. M. Overview: cryptococcosis in the treatment of AIDS. *Mycopathologia*, 114, 153, 1991.
212. Levesque, H., Alie-Legrand, M. C., Omnient, Y., et al. *Cryptococcus neoformans* meningitis and cirrhosis: value of fluconazole. *Clin. Biol.*, 13, 942, 1989.
213. Michelone, G., Tacconi, F., Maccabruni, A., Lanzarini, P., Tinelli, M., and Dei Cas, A. Clinical and therapeutic profile of 3 cases of cryptococcal meningitis in patients with AIDS. *G. Ital. Chemoter.*, 36, 95, 1989.
214. Krisch, H. and Sarnow, E. Collection of cases in relation to clinical trials of fluconazole in Germany. *Mycoses*, 33(Suppl. 1), 14S, 1990.
215. Reents, S. B. and Powell, G. Fluconazole success after amphotericin B and flucytosine failure in cryptococcal meningitis. *DICP*, 24, 885, 1990.
216. Lindberg, J. and Edebo, L. Successful treatment of cryptococcal meningitis with fluconazole. *Lakartidningen*, 88, 2245, 1991.
217. Good, C. B. and Leeper, H. F. Profound papilledema due to cryptococcal meningitis in acquired immunodeficiency syndrome: successful treatment with fluconazole. *South. Med. J.*, 84, 394, 1991.
218. Dismukes, W. E. Treatment of systemic fungal diseases in patients with AIDS, in *Recent Progress in Antifungal Chemotherapy*, Yamaguchi, H., Kobayashi, G. S., and Takahashi, H., Eds. Marcel Dekker, New York, 227, 1992.
219. Jones, P. D., Marriott, D., and Speed, B. R. Efficacy of fluconazole in cryptoccocal meningitis. *Diagn. Microbiol. Infect. Dis.*, 12(Suppl. 4), 235S, 1989.
220. Dupont, B. Treatment of cryptococcal meningitis, in *Proc. Xth Congr. Int. Soc. Human Animal Mycol., Barcelona*, Torres-Rodriguez, J. M., Ed. J. R. Prous, 197, 1988.
221. Byrne, W. R. and Wajszczuk, C. P. Cryptococcal meningitis in the acquired immunodeficiency syndrome (AIDS): successful treatment with fluconazole after failure of amphotericin B. *Ann. Intern. Med.*, 108, 384, 1988.
222. Dromer, F., Mathoulin, S., Dupont, B., Brugiere, O., and Letenneur, L., Comparison of the efficacy of amphotericin B and fluconazole in the treatment of cryptococcosis in human immunodeficiency virus-negative patients: retrospective analysis of 83 cases. *Clin. Infect. Dis.*, 22(Suppl. 2), S154, 1996.
223. Larsen, R. A., Leal, M. A., and Chan, L. S. Fluconazole compared with amphotericin B plus flucytosine for cryptococcal meningitis in AIDS: a randomized trial. *Ann. Intern. Med.*, 113, 183, 1990.
224. Wong, R. D. and Goetz, M. B., Treatment of cryptococcal meningitis in AIDS. *J. Infect. Dis.*, 113, 992, 1990.
225. Buxton, M. J., Dubois, D. J., Turner, R. R., Sculpher, M. J., Robinson, P. A., and Searcy, C., Cost implications of alternative treatments for AIDS patients with cryptococcal meningitis: comparison of fluconazole and amphotericin-based therapies. *J. Infect.*, 23, 17, 1991.
226. Bolignano, G., Chindemi, G., and Criseo, G., Cryptococcal meningoencephalitis in a patient with Hodgkin's lymphoma: successful treatment with fluconazole. *Mycoses*, 34, 63, 1991.
227. Iacopino, P., Morabito, F., Martino, B., Bolignano, G., and Nobile, F., Fluconazole for disseminated cryptococcosis in a patient with Hodgkin's disease. *Haematologica*, 76, 260, 1991.
228. Sugar, A. M. and Saunders, C. Oral fluconazole as suppressive therapy of disseminated cryptococcosis in patients with acquired immunodeficiency syndrome. *Am. J. Med.*, 85, 481, 1988.
229. Bozzette, S. A., Larsen, R. A., Chiu, J., et al. A placebo-controlled trial of maintenance therapy with fluconazole after treatment of cryptococcal meningitis in the acquired immunodeficiency syndrome. *N. Engl. J. Med.*, 324, 580, 1991.
230. Powderly, W., Saag, M., Cloud, G., et al., Fluconazole versus amphotericin B as maintenance therapy for prevention of relapse of AIDS-associated cryptococcal meningitis. *30th Intersci. Conf. Antimicrob. Agents Chemother*. American Society for Microbiology, Washington, DC, abstract 1162, 1990.
231. Laroche, R., Deppner, M., Floch, J. J., et al. Cryptococcosis in Bujumbura, Burundi: apropos of 80 observed cases in 42 months. *Bull. Soc. Pathol. Exot. Fil.*, 83, 159, 1990.
232. Stern, J. J., Hartman, B. J., Sharkey, K., et al. Oral fluconazole therapy for patients with acquired immunodeficiency syndrome and cryptococcosis: experience with 22 patients. *Am. J. Med.*, 85, 477, 1988.
233. Sort, P., Morales, M., Gomez, J., Pares, A., and Rodes, J. Pleural empyema caused by *Cryptococcus neoformans* in a patient with liver cirrhosis. *Gastroenterol. Hepatol.*, 19, 302, 1996.
234. Agarwal, A., Gupta, A., Sakhuja, V., Talwar, P., Joshi, K., and Chugh, K. S. Retinitis following disseminated

cryptococcosis in a renal allograft recipient: efficacy of oral fluconazole. *Acta Ophthalmol (Copenhagen)*, 69, 402, 1991.
235. Custis, P. H., Haller, J. A., and de Juan, E. Jr. An unusual case of cryptococcal endophthalmitis. *Reina*, 15, 300, 1995.
236. Vandersmissen, G., Meuleman, L., Tits, G., Verhaeghe, A., and Peetermans, W. E. Cutaneous cryptococcosis in corticosteroid-treated patients without AIDS. *Acta Clin. Belg.*, 51, 111, 1996.
237. Halweg, H., Korzeniewska-Kosela, M., Podsiadlo, B., and Krakowka, P. A case of skin cryptococcosis in systemic lupus erythematosus. *Pneumonol. Pol.*, 58, 544, 1990.
238. Pineski, R., Mathurin, S. A., Ruffinengo, O., Alonso, H. O., and Corallini de Bracelenti, B. Cutaneous cryptococcosis in a patient receiving chronic immunosuppressive therapy. *Cutis*, 57, 229, 1996.
239. Verneuil, L., Dompmartin, A., Duhamel, C., et al. Cryptococcal whitlow in a HIV-positive patient. *Ann. Dermatol. Venereol.*, 122, 688, 1995.
240. Kerchner, J. E., Ridley, M. B., and Greene, J. N. Laryngeal *Cryptococcus*: treatment with oral fluconazole. *Arch. Otolaryngol. Head Neck Surg.*, 121, 1193, 1995.
241. Schmidt, D. M., Sercarz, J. A., Kevorkian, K. F., and Canalis, R. F. *Cryptococcus* presenting as a neck mass. *Ann. Otol. Rhinol. Laryngol.*, 104, 711, 1995.
242. Yew, W. W., Wong, P. C., Wong, C. F., Lee, J., and Chau, C. H. Oral fluconazole in the treatment of pulmonary cryptococcosis in non-AIDS patients. *Drugs Exp. Clin. Res.*, 22, 25, 1996.
243. Feczko, J. M. Overview of fluconazole in *Recent Progress in Antifungal Chemotherapy*, Yamaguchi, H., Kobayashi, G. S., and Takahashi, H., Eds. Marcel Dekker, New York, 191, 1992.
244. Troke, P. F., Marriott, M. S., Richardson, K., and Tarbit, M. H. In vitro potency and in vivo activity of azoles. *Ann. NY Acad. Sci.*, 544, 284, 1988.
245. Guillaume, M. P., De Prez, C., and Cogan, E. Subacute mitochondroal liver disease in a patient with AIDS: possible relationship to prolonged fluconazole administration. *Am. J. Gastroenterol.*, 91, 165, 1996.
246. Pappas, P. G., Kauffman, C. A., Perfect, J., et al. Alopecia associated with fluconazole therapy. *Ann. Intern. Med.*, 123, 354, 1995 [see comment in *Ann. Intern. Med.*, 125, 153, 1996].
247. Weinroth, S. E., and Tuazon, C. U. Alopecia associated with fluconazole treatment. *Ann. Intern. Med.*, 119, 637, 1993.
248. Coker, R. J. and Harris, J. R. Failure of fluconazole treatment in cryptococcal meningitis despite adequate CSF levels. *J. Infect.*, 123, 101, 1991.
249. Bailly, M. P., Boibieux, A., Biron, F., et al. Persistence of *Cryptococcus neoformans* in prostate: failure of fluconazole despite high doses. *J. Infect. Dis.*, 164, 435, 1991.
250. Pietroski, N., Buckley, R. M., Braffman, M. N., and Stern, J. J. Intravenous and oral fluconazole in treatment of acute cryptococcal meningitis in AIDS. *30th Intersci. Conf. Antimicrob. Agents Chemother.*, American Society for Microbiology, Washington, DC, abstract 576, 1990.
251. Squires, K., Rowland, V., Gassyuk, E., et al. Fluconazole as therapy for acute cryptococcal meningitis. *30th Intersci. Conf. Antimicrob. Agents Chemother.*, American Society for Microbiology, Washington, DC, abstract 573, 1990.
252. Aller, A. I., Martin-Mazuelos, E., Lozano, F., et al. Correlation of fluconazole MICs with clinical outcome in cryptococcal infection. *Antimicrob. Agents Chemother.*, 44, 1544-1548, 2000.
253. Orni-Wasserlauf, R., Siegman-Igra, Y., Izkhakov, E., Bash, E., Polacheck, I., and Giladi, M. Fluconazole-resistant *Cryptococcus neoformans* isolated from an immunocompetent patient without prior exposure to fluconazole. *38th Intersci. Conf. Antimicrob. Agents Chemother.*, American Society of Microbiology, Washington, DC, 458, abstract J-24, 1998.
254. Abi-Hanna, P., Marichal, P., Vandenbossche, H., and Williamson, P. R. Study of fluconazole resistance in *Cryptococcus neoformans* by insertional mutagenesis. *99th Abstr. Gen. Meet. Am. Soc. Microbiol.*, May 30–June 3, 6, abstract A-29, 1999.
255. Georgiev, V. St. Opportunistic/nosocomial infections: treatment and developmental therapeutics. II. Cryptococcosis. *Med. Res. Rev.*, 13, 507–527, 1993.
256. Van Cutsem, J. and Cauwenbergh, G. Results of itraconazole treatment in systemic mycoses in animals and man, in *Recent Progress in Antifungal Chemotherapy*, Yamaguchi, H., Kobayashi, G. S., and Takahashi, H., Eds. Marcel Dekker, New York, 203, 1992.
257. Viviani, M. A., Tortorano, A. M., Giani, P. C., et al. Itraconazole for cryptococcal infection in the acquired immunodeficiency syndrome. *Ann. Intern. Med.*, 106, 106,1987.
258. Viviani, M. A., Tortorano, A. M., Langer, M., et al. Experience with itraconazole in cryptococcosis and aspergillosis. *J. Infect.*, 18, 151, 1989.
259. Denning, D. W., Tucker, R. M., Hanson, L. H., Hamilton, J. R., and Stevens, D. A. Itraconazole therapy for cryptococcal meningitis and cryptococcosis. *Arch. Intern. Med.*, 149, 2301, 1989.
260. Denning, D. W., Tucker, R. M., Hanson, L. H., and Stevens, D. A. Itraconazole in opportunistic mycoses: cryptococcosis and aspergillosis. *J. Am. Acad. Dermatol.*, 3, 602, 1990.
261. de Gans, J., Eeftinck Schattenkerk, J. K. M., and van Ketel, R. J. Itraconazole as maintenance treatment for cryptococcal meningitis in the acquired immunodeficiency syndrome. *Br. Med. J.*, 296, 339, 1988.
262. Batungwanayo, J., Taelman, H., Bogaerts, J., et al. Pulmonary cryptococcosis associated with HIV-1 infection in Rwanda: a retrospective study of 37 cases. *AIDS*, 8, 1271, 1994.
263. Sato, T., Koseki, S., Takahashi, S., and Maie, O., Localized cutaneous cryptococcosis successfully treated with itraconazole: review of medication in 18 cases reported in Japan. *Mycoses*, 33, 455, 1990.
264. Goh, C. L., Cutaneous cryptococcosis successfully treated with itraconazole. *Cutis*, 51, 377, 1993.

265. Bettoli, V., Virgili, A., Zampino, M. R., Bedetti, A., and Montanari, P., Cutaneous cryptococcosis in AIDS: successful treatment with itraconazole. *Mycoses*, 36, 433, 1993.
266. 1999 USPHS/IDSA guidelines for the prevention of opportunistic infections on persons infected with human immunodeficient virus. *Infect. Dis. Obstetr. Gynecol.*, 8, 5–74, 2000 & *Clin. Infect. Dis.*, 30(Suppl. 1), S29–S65, 2000.
267. Powderly, W. G., Finkelstein, D. M., Feinberg, J., et al. A randomized trial comparing fluconazole with clotrimazole troches for the prevention of fungal infections in patients with advanced human immunodeficiency virus infection. *N. Engl. J. Med.*, 332, 700–705, 1995.
268. Schuman, P., Capps, L., Peng, G., et al. Weekly fluconazole for the prevention of mucosal candidiasis in women with HIV infection: a randomized, double-blind, placebo-controlled trial. *Ann. Intern. Med.*, 126, 689–696, 1997.
269. Havlir, D. V., Dube, M. P., McCutchan, J. A., et al. Prophylaxis with weekly versus daily fluconazole for fungal infections in patients with AIDS. *Clin. Infect. Dis.*, 27, 1369–1375, 1998.
270. Lewis, J. L. and Rabinovich, S. The wide spectrum of cryptococcal infections. *Am. J. Med.*, 53, 315, 1972.
271. Lalloo, D., Fisher, D., Naraqi, S., et al. Cryptococcal meningitis (*C. neoformans* var.*gattii*) leading to blindness in previously healthy Melanesian adults in Papua New Guinea. *Q. J. Med.*, 87, 343, 1994.
272. Currie, B., Vigus, T., Leach, G., and Dwyer, B. *Cryptococcus neoformans* var. *gattii*. *Lancet*, 336, 1442, 1990.
273. Laurenson, I. F., Naraqi, S., Howcroft, N., Burrows, I., and Saulei, S. Cryptococcal meningitis in Papua New Guinea: ecology and the role of eucalypts. *Med. J. Aust.*, 158, 213, 1993.
274. Laurenson, I. F., Naraqi, S., Trevett, A., et al. Cryptococcal investigations in Papua New Guinea. *Proc. 2nd Int. Conf. Cryptococcus & Cryptococcosis*, Milan, 114, 1993.
275. Laurenson, I. F., Trevett, A. J., Lalloo, D. G., et al. Meningitis caused by *Cryptococcus neoformans* var. *gattii* and var. *neoformans* in Papua New Guinea. *Trans. R. Soc. Trop. Med. Hyg.*, 90, 57, 1996.
276. Castanon-Olivares, L. R., Arreguin-Espinosa, R., Ruiz-Palacios y Santos, G., and Lopez-Martinez, R. Frequency of *Cryptococcus* species and varieties in Mexico and their comparison with some Latin American countries. *Rev. Latinoam. Microbiol.*, 42, 35–40, 2000.
277. Kwon-Chung, K. J. and Bennett, J. E. Epidemiologic differences between the two varieties of *Cryptococcus neoformans*. *Am. J. Epidemiol.*, 120, 123, 1984.
278. Ellis, D. H. *Cryptococcus neoformans* var. *gattii* in Australia. *J. Clin. Microbiol.*, 25, 430, 1987.
279. Marriott, D. J., Speed, B. R., Spelman, D., Shaw, D., French, M., and Harkness, J. L. *Cryptococcus neoformans* var. *gattii* infections in Australian HIV-infected patients: a review of seven cases. *8th Annu. Conf. Australs. Soc. HIV Med.*, Nov. 14–17, 86, abstract 88, 1996.
280. Sorrell, T. C., Brownlee, A. G., Ruma, P., Malik, R., Pfeiffer, T. J., and Ellis, D. H. Natural environmental sources of *Cryptococcus neoformans* var. *gattii*. *J. Clin. Microbiol.*, 34, 1261, 1996.
281. Pfeiffer, T. J. and Ellis, D. H. Environmental isolation of *Cryptococcus neoformans* var. *gattii* from *Eucalyptus tereticornis*. *J. Med. Vet. Mycol.*, 30, 407, 1992.
282. Sorrell, T. C., Chen, S. C. A., Ruma, P., et al. Concordance of clinical and environmental isolates of *Cryptococcus neoformans* var. *gattii* by random amplification of polymorphic DNA analysis and PCR fingerprinting. *J. Clin. Microbiol.*, 34, 1253, 1996.
283. Kwon-Chung, K. J., Wickes, B. L., Stockman, L., Roberts, G. D., Ellis, D., and Howard, D. H. Virulence, serotype, and molecular characteristics of environmental strains of *Cryptococcus neoformans* var. *gattii*. *Infect. Immun.*, 60, 1869, 1992.
284. Varma, A., Swinne, D., Staib, F., Bennett, J. E., and Kwon-Chung, K. J. Diversity of DNA fingerprints in *Cryptococcus neoformans*. *J. Clin. Microbiol.*, 33, 1807, 1995.
285. Mitchell, D. H., Sorrell, T. C., Allworth, A. M., et al. Cryptococcal disease of the CNS in immunocompetent hosts: influence of cryptococcal variety on clinical manifestations and outcome. *Clin. Infect. Dis.*, 20, 611, 1995.
286. Speed, R. and Dunt, D. Clinical and host differences between the two varieties of *Cryptococcus neoformans*. *Clin. Infect. Dis.*, 21, 28, 1995.
287. Slobodnik, R. and Naraqi, S. Cryptococcal meningitis, in the Central Province of Papua New Guinea. *Papua New Guinea Med. J.*, 23, 111, 1980.
288. Peetermans, W., Bobbaers, H., Verhaegen, J., and Vandepitte, J. Fluconazole-resistant *Cryptococcus neoformans* var. *gattii* in an AIDS patient. *Acta Clin. Belg.*, 48, 405-409, 1993.
289. Kamei, K., Brummer, E., Nishimura, K., and Miyaji, M. Activity of voriconazole against *Cryptococcus neoformans* var. *gattii* vs. var. *neoformans*: effect of human serum. *Abstr. 98th Gen. Meet. Am. Soc. Microbiol.*, May 17–21, 270, abstract F-100, 1998.
290. Gluck, J. L., Myers, J. P., and Pass, L. M. Cryptococcemia due to *Cryptococcus albidus*. *South. Med. J.*, 80, 511, 1987.
291. Gordon, M. A. Pulmonary cryptococcosis: a case due to *Cryptococcus albidus*. *Am. Rev. Respir. Dis.*, 106, 786, 1972.
292. Lin, S. R., Peng, C. E., Yung, S. A., and Yu, H. S. Isolation of *Cryptococcus albidus* var. *albidus* in patient with pemphigus foliaceous. *Kao-Hsiung I Hsueh Ko Hsueh Tsa Chih*, 5, 126, 1989.
293. Weiser, H. G. Zur frage der pathogenität der *Cryptococcus albidus*. *Schweiz. Med. Wochenschr.*, 103, 475, 1973.
294. da Cunha, T. and Lusins, J. *Cryptococcus albidus* meningitis. *South. Med. J.*, 66, 1230, 1973.
295. Mello, J. C., Srinivasan, S., Scott, M. L., and Raff, M. J. *Cryptococcus albidus* meningitis. *J. Infect.*, 2, 79, 1980.
296. Krumholz, R. A. Pulmonary cryptococcosis: a case due to *Cryptococcus albidus*. *Am. Rev. Respir. Dis.*, 105, 421, 1972.
297. Horowitz, I. D., Blumberg, E. A., and Krevolin, L. *Cryptococcus albidus* and mucormycosis empyema in a patient receiving hemodialysis. *South. Med. J.*, 86, 1070, 1993.

298. Mckee, M., Arthington-Skaggs, B. A., Motley, M., et al. Distribution of yeast isolates recovered from the oral mucosa of HIV+ patients: relationship to antifungal drug use. *Abstr. 99th Gen. Meet. Am. Soc. Microbiol., May 30–June 3*, 137, abstract C-161, 1999.
299. Loison, J., Bouchara, J. P., Gueho, E., et al. First report of *Cryptococcus albidus* septicemia in an HIV patient. *J. Infect.*, 33, 139, 1996.
300. Kordossis, T., Avlami, A., Velegraki, A., et al. First report of *Cryptococcus laurentii* meningitis and a fatal case of *Cryptococcus albidus* cryptococcaemia in AIDS patients. *Med. Mycol.*, 36, 335-339, 1998.
301. Lynch III, J. P., Schaberg, D. R., Kissner, D. G., and Kauffman, C. A. *Cryptococcus laurentii* lung abscess. *Am. Rev. Respir. Dis.*, 123, 135, 1981.
302. Chander, J., Sapra, R. K., and Talwar, P. Incidence of cryptococcosis in and around Chandigarch, India during the period 1982–1991. *Mycoses*, 37, 23, 1994.
303. Custis, P. H., Haller, J. A., and de Juan, E. Jr. An unusual case of cryptococcal endophthalmitis. *Reina*, 15, 300, 1995.

20
Candida albicans

1. INTRODUCTION

Candidiasis is an acute or chronic, superficial or disseminated mycosis caused by species of the genus *Candida*. The latter is a genus of nearly 200 yeast-like anamorphic (sexual imperfect) fungi (form-order Cryptococcales, form-class Blastomycetes), characterized by a polymorphic nature because of their ability to produce budding yeast cells (blastoconidia), mycelia, pseudomycelia, and blastospores *(1–3)*. Some *Candida* spp. have been found capable of mating producing teleomorphic (sexual perfect) form.

Although commonly part of the normal flora of the skin, mouth, intestinal tract, and vagina, *Candida* spp. are the etiologic agents of variety of infections, including candidiasis, onychomycosis, tinea corporis, tinea pedis, vaginitis, and thrush. The fungus appears to have receptors (known as adhesins) for human fluid-phase glycoproteins, such as fibronectin and immobilized basement-membrane glycoproteins in order to establish itself in mucus-lined cavities. The *Candida* adhesins may be analogous or perhaps homologous to the human integrin receptors *(4)*. Adherence of *C. albicans* to host tissue is an essential virulence factor in the early stages of colonization and tissue invasion. It is achieved by a combination of specific (ligand-receptor interactions) and nonspecific (electrostatic charge, van der Waals forces) mechanisms that allow the yeast to attach to a wide range of tissue types and inanimate surfaces *(5)*.

Several conditions have been identified to favor the predominance of *Candida* spp. over normal microbial flora, namely, elimination of bacterial competition following oral or parenteral antibacterial therapy, the use of cimetidine or histamine-2 blockers, as well as the significant elevation of extracellular glucose concentrations in diabetic patients *(6–12)*. The reason histamine antagonists promote candidal growth is because of their ability to elevate the local pH, thereby creating an environment more conducive to fungal growth.

C. albicans is the most frequent etiologic agent of candidiasis capable of causing any of the clinical types of mycosis, and the leading cause of oropharyngeal and cutaneous fungal disease. In addition to *C. albicans*, *C. albicans* var. *stellatoidea*, *C. tropicalis*, *C. parapsilosis*, *C. krusei*, *C. lusitaniae*, *C. dubliniensis*, and *C. guilliermondii* have been increasingly identified as causative agents of opportunistic infections in the immunocompromised host *(13,14)*. The advent of the AIDS pandemic and the widespread use of azole antimycotics (fluconazole) has contributed to a significant increase in *C. krusei* infections (even though this species is less virulent than *C. albicans*), particularly because of the high incidence of resistance of this yeast to fluconazole *(15)*.

2. HUMAN CANDIDIASIS

By some accounts *(16)*, *Candida* spp. are the seventh most common pathogens to cause nosocomial infections *(17)*, and the fifth most common cause of primary blood-stream infections *(18)*.

Based on pathologic studies, three distinct forms of human candidiasis have been distinguished: supeficial, locally invasive, and deep (systemic) mycoses.

From: Opportunistic Infections: Treatment and Prophylaxis
By: Vassil St. Georgiev © Humana Press Inc., Totowa, NJ

Cases of superficial candidiasis are most commonly observed in lining surfaces (skin, oropharynx, gastrointestinal tract, and upper and lower respiratory tracts). Characteristic features include velvety appearance of the lesions, whereas the adjacent mucosal membrane appears dark red and moderately swollen; ulcerative or necrotic lesions indicate deeper tissue invasion *(19)*.

Among immunosuppressed patients, locally invasive candidiasis may present as pneumonia, cystitis, esophagitis, or pyelonephritis. Typically, it is characterized by fairly sharply defined ulcerations of the intestinal, respiratory, or genitourinary tract *(19)*.

Systemic candidiasis is the most serious manifestation of the disease that can affect any organ, but most frequently it involves the heart, kidneys, liver, spleen, lung, and the brain. Usually, dissemination is defined as an invasive infection striking the parenchyma of two or more visceral organs, excluding the mucosa of the gastrointestinal, respiratory, or the genitourinary tract *(19–21)*. The most likely organ combination involved has been the gastrointestinal tract, liver, kidney, and the lung *(20)*.

Because of their decreased resistance to infection, patients at high risk of developing systemic candidiasis include immunocompromised patients, those with hematologic and solid malignancies, or on immunosuppressive therapy, and postoperative patients *(20,22–25)*. The most severe form of systemic candidiasis has been observed in leukemic patients and organ-transplant recipients receiving immunosuppressive therapy (irradiation, corticosteroids, antineoplastic and antibacterial drugs) *(26–31)*. The gastrointestinal tract is the most frequent source of systemic candidiasis in patients with hematologic malignancies and neutropenia *(27)*. Ocular candidiasis, although very infrequent has also been diagnosed *(20,22,32)*. Derkinderen et al. *(33)* described the first case of documented epidural involvement in *C. albicans*-associated candidal spondylodiscitis.

Using genotyping of *C. albicans* isolates obtained from hospitalized patients and healthcare workers in a geriatric unit, Fanello et al. *(34)* demonstrated person-to-person transmission of candidal infection.

Prostatic abscess due to *Candida* is generally secondary to systemic disease in immunosuppressed patients and usually takes place with affection of other organs in a septic patient. Only in exceptional cases it will occur alone with no systemic manifestations *(35)*.

2.1. Candidal Infections in HIV-Infected Patients

Oral candidiasis is the most common and usually the earliest opportunistic infection affecting HIV-positive patients *(36)*. It has been used as an initial manifestation of AIDS in all high-risk population *(37)*, although by some accounts it is considered more prevalent in the homosexual HIV-infected population *(38,39)*. Risk factors for esophageal candidiasis in HIV-infected populations include initial low CD4$^+$ T-cell count and plasma viremia. In addition, that risk may also be influenced by such factors as homosexual/bisexual behavior, prior zidovudine therapy, recent antibacterial therapy, and oral candidiasis *(39)*.

Moreover, low levels of serum testosterone may have negative implications on the morbidity of esophageal candidiasis in HIV-infected men *(40)*. In this regard, early detection of low serum testosterone would allow for expedient testosterone supplementation therapy to improve the morbidity of the disease.

If oral candidiasis is not treated, it may progress to candidal esophagitis *(41,42)*. In the HIV-infected persons, the latter may be presented with similar manifestations as herpes virus or cytomegalovirus disease necessitating the use of esophagoscopy and biopsy to establish the diagnosis.

Hairy leukoplakia, which is a more imminent sign of impending AIDS, should be differentiated from candidal infection by its reticulate, smooth plaque, typically found on the lateral side of the tongue and that will not come off by scraping. Hairy leukoplakia is caused by the Epstein-Barr virus and will often carry herpes virus, papillomavirus, and *Candida* as secondary invaders *(43)*.

Virtually all HIV-infected individuals with cutaneous candidiasis will harbor *C. albicans* as the pathogen, with *C. tropicalis* only rarely being diagnosed *(43)*. In patients with the AIDS-related complex (ARC), the observed perirectal pain and ulceration has often been associated with *C. albicans*. In female patients with HIV infection, candidal vaginitis is a recurring problem.

As the CD4+ T-helper cell population is progressively depleted, the development of systemic candidiasis in AIDS patients becomes increasingly likely *(43)*.

3. TREATMENT OF CANDIDIASIS

C. albicans is usually susceptible to all major antifungal drugs (fluconazole, itraconazole, flucytosine, and amphotericin B). However, although consensus exists about the necessity of treating all candidemic patients with antifungal agents, presently little is known about the optimal duration of treatment. To this end, Oude Lashof et al. *(44)* conducted a retrospective study to define whether there were any correlations between the length of treatment and the development of delayed complications such as metastatic foci. The findings have suggested that whereas the early failure rate of treatment for candidemia was high, there were few instances of delayed complications due to hematologic dissemination. Further, there were no correlation between the duration of treatment and the development of late complications, suggesting that treatment of 2 wk or less may be sufficient provided that the initial response to therapy has been favorable *(44)*.

Despite continuing efforts *(45,46)* so far there are no effective prophylactic and/or therapeutic vaccines developed against *C. albicans (47)*.

Lopez et al. *(48)* undertook a study to identify prescribing policies likely to potentiate or limit *Candida* resistance to fluconazole in a clinical environment. The fluconazole utilization was determined by the number of fluconazole treatrment-days per 100 hospitalization days (penetration index) after prescription of either low-dose fluconazole (50 mg; prescribed as intermittent or prolonged treatment) or higher-dose fluconazole regimens (200 mg). The data suggested that prolonged or repeated exposure to low-dose fluconazole, rather than total cumulative use, was associated with fluconazole resistance. Moreover, restoration of a normal ecology was observed when low-dose prolonged or intermittent prescriptions were reduced.

3.1. Cutaneous Candidiasis

The therapy of cutaneous candidiasis is best determined after evaluation of the location, the extent of involvement, and the immune status of the patient *(49)*. It could involve both topical and/or oral therapy. In case of immunocompromised patients, especially in extensive fungal involvement, systemic antimycotic therapy may be required. Both oral ketoconazole and fluconazole have been used, with the latter being preferred when treating resistant organisms.

In a double-blind, randomized study of 40 patients with culturally proven dermatophytosis (pityriasis versicolor) or cutaneous candidiasis, del Palacio et al. *(50)* compared the efficacy and tolerance of flutrimazole and bifonazole (both as 1% solutions applied once daily for 4 wk). At the end of therapy, negative microscopy and cultures were recorded in 85% of the flutrimazole group and 65% in the bifonazole group. However, there was significant difference in the efficacy: 80% of the flutrimazole-treated patients received effective treatment, as compared to only 40% in the bifonazole group.

Topical antifungal therapy may be added in conjunction with systemic medication, or used alone in less extensive disease *(49)*. Topical nystatin and amphotericin B are not effective against cutaneous candidiasis and have been largely supplanted by the more effective azole (ketoconazole, miconazole, clotrimazole, econazole) antimycotics.

In a multicenter, randomized, double-blind, double-dummy trial, Stengel et al. *(51)* compared the therapeutic activities of fluconazole and ketoconazole in the treatment of cutaneous candidiasis and dermatophytoses (tinea corporis, tinea cruris) lasting for 2–4 wk. The patients received either fluconazole (150 mg once weekly, plus daily placebo), or ketoconazole (200 mg once daily plus weekly placebo for 2–6 wk). The results have shown that both drug regimens were equally effective in terms of clinical and mycological cure rates, with fluconazole having the advantage of once-weekly oral administration, which is not only more cost-effective, but also may improve patient compliance *(52)*.

Nesseem *(53)* has used tertiary polyoxyethylene stearyl ether/oil and water to form a liquid crystalline system cream as a dosage form for 1% itraconazole for topical dermal drug delivery. The incorporation of itraconazole in liquid crystal increased its efficacy against *C. albicans*.

Ibuprofen, a nonsteroidal anti-inflammatory drug (NSAID), was found to exert activity against both *C. albicans* and non-*albicans* strains. Thus, at 10 mg/mL, ibuprofen showed a rapid cidal activity against exponential growth-phase *C. albicans*, accompanied by rapid and extensive leakage of intracellular K^+, permeation to propidium iodide, lysis of spheroplasts, and severe membrane ultrastructural alteration *(54)*. Moreover, the combination of ibuprofen with fluconazole resulted in synergistic activity in 8 of 12 *Candida* strains studied, including 4 of the 5 fluconazole-resistant strains. In view of ibuprofen's antifungal and anti-inflammatory properties, its use has been suggested together with fluconazole in the topical treatment of candidosis.

3.2. Chronic Mucocutaneous Candidiasis

Amphotericin B, which at one time was used exclusively in the treatment of chronic mucocutaneous candidiasis *(55)*, is being substituted by oral systemic azole antifungals. Polizzi et al. *(56)* evaluated the clinical efficacy of a 16-mo course of cimetidine (400 mg t.i.d.) and zinc sulfate (200 mg daily) in a patient with chronic mucocutaneous candidiasis. The favorable response was attributed to the immunopotentiating effect of the combined treatment.

3.3. Candidal Onychomycosis

Candidal onychomycosis does not occur very often, and therapy with itraconazole appears to be effective (200 mg, b.i.d. for 1 wk); the therapy is most effective when repeated monthly for 3–4 mo *(57,58)*.

3.4. Oropharyngeal and Esophageal Candidiasis

In addition to oral systemic therapy, topical antimycotics, such as clotrimazole buccal troches, have been effective in the treatment of chronic oral candidiasis without developing evidence of drug resistance *(59,60)*. However, if no maintenance suppressive antifungal therapy is applied, nearly all patients with HIV and successfully treated esophageal candidiasis develop a recurrence, usually within 2–3 mo *(61)*. Little is known about the epidemiology and clinical features of esophageal candidiasis in pediatric AIDS. In this regard, Chiou et al. *(62)* investigated the clinical manifestations and risk factors of esophageal candidiasis in a prospectively monitored population of HIV-infected children. Concurrent oropharyngeal candidiasis was the most common clinical presentation (94%), followed by odynophagia (80%), retrosternal pain (57%), and nausea/vomiting (24%), with *C. albicans* being the causative organism.

Initial treatment of oral and esophageal candidiasis should focus on minimizing predisposing factors. Subsequent therapy would consist of either topical or systemic agents according to the clinical status of the patient (Table 1) *(43,63,64)*.

One recommended regimen in HIV-infected patients consists of nystatin suspension (usually 5.0 mL of nystatin, q.i.d.) or clotrimazole troches (q.i.d.), or both *(43)*. Although in the early stages of HIV infection this regimen is usually effective, *Candida* recurrence is nearly a certainty and patients may have to be on this regimen continuously *(43)*. Encarnacion and Chin *(65)* have determined the salivary nystatin concentrations after administration of an osmotic-controlled release tablet for oral cavity therapy. The tablet was designed to deliver approx 200,000 U of nystatin over 2-h dosing; the mean salivary drug concentrations, which consistently exceeded those produced by a pastille at the same time points, were 279 µg/mL, 654 µg/mL, and 532 µg/mL at 30, 60, and 120 min, respectively.

Although clotrimazole troches are widely used in the treatment of mucosal candidiasis, little is known about the potential contribution of resistance to clotrimazole to the development of refractory mucosal candidiasis. In this regard, Pelletier et al. *(66)* investigated the potential emergence of resis-

Table 1
Treatment of Oropharyngeal and Esophageal Candidiasis (43,63,64)

Drug	Dose
Topical:	
Nystatin	0–30 mL (1,000,000–3,000,000 U), 4–5 times daily (swish and swallow)
Clotrimazole	1 Troche (10 mg), 4–5 times daily
Systemic:	
Ketoconazole	200–400 mg daily, orally[a]
Fluconazole	50–200 mg daily, orally
Itraconazole	100–200 mg daily, orally[b]
Amphotericin B	0.4–0.6 mg/kg daily, i.v.

[a]Proper gastric acidity is required for adequate absorption.
[b]Taken with food and proper gastric acidity to ensure adequate absorption.

tance to clotrimazole in a prospectively monitored HIV-infected pediatric population receiving clotrimazole. The corresponding MICs were compared in macro- and microdilution assays and the results correlated with the clinical response to antifungal therapy. The observed resistance to clotrimazole was highly associated with the clinically overt failure af the azole therapy. Furthermore, the findings suggested that an interpretive breakpoint of 0.5 µg/mL may be useful in defining clotrimazole resistance in *C. albicans*.

In comparison with other drugs used to treat mucosal candidiasis in HIV-infected patients, fluconazole was found to be superior to nystatin, similar to itraconazole, and at least as effective as clotrimazole and ketoconazole (67). Furthermore, in a study of AIDS patients with candidal esophagitis, fluconazole was shown to elicit a rapid clinical response that may necessitate only a 1-wk course of empiric treatment for newly developed esophageal symptoms (68).

Pagani et al. (69) evaluated treatment of oropharyngeal candidiasis clinically resistant to oral fluconazole (400 mg daily for 7 d) with daily escalating doses, and measured the tolerance and safety of these higher doses in HIV-infected patients. The patients received a 7-d course of oral fluconazole at 800 mg daily; in cases of no response, a 7-d dose regimen of 1.2 g of the drug was initiated, and if no response, 1.6 g of fluconazole. No significant adverse effects were observed except one episode of skin allergy.

In a multicenter, prospective, randomized trial of 334 HIV-infected patients with oropharyngeal candidiasis, Pons et al. (70) found a 2-wk course of oral fluconazole (100 mg daily) and clotrimazole troches (10 mg orally 5 times daily) to be equally effective; the clinical response was statistically equivalent in both groups (98 and 94% of fluconazole and clotrimazole recipients, respectively, were cured or improved). However, fluconazole was more effective in eliminating *C. albicans* from the oral flora (65 vs 48%) and maintaining an asymptomatic state through 2 wk of follow-up examination (82.3 vs 50%) (70).

Systemic therapy is usually considered for immunocompromised patients (with granulocytopenia, or receiving immunosuppressive therapy) who are at high risk for dissemination, or for patients unresponsive to topical therapy (63). In a prospective study in AIDS patients with esophageal candidiasis, Laine and Rabeneck (64) examined the clinical efficacy of fluconazole suspensions (200 mg loading dose followed by 100 mg, q.d.s.). The therapy, which was implemented for 2 wk after symptom resolution, was successful in all 41 evaluable patients.

Newton et al. (71) implemented weekly fluconazole therapy for the suppression of recurrent thrush in HIV-infected patients. However, Azon-Masoliver and Vilaplana (72) reported a case of an HIV-infected patient who developed a toxic epidermal necrolysis affecting over 70% of the body surface area and severe mucosal involvement after starting fluconazole for a recurrent oral trush with dysphagia.

In an open Phase III clinical trial of 103 HIV-infected patients with oral candidiasis, therapy with oral fluconazole at 100 mg daily for 7–21 d, achieved clinical cure in 71% of patients and improvement in another 16%; mycological tests revealed elimination in 57% and reduction in colony counts in 23% of patients *(73)*.

In a double-blind, randomized study of 102 HIV-infected patients with endoscopically diagnosed esophageal candidiasis, Barbaro and Di Lorenzo *(74)* compared the therapeutic efficacies of orally given fluconazole and itraconazole. Two groups of 60 patients each, received a 3-wk course of either fluconazole (100 mg b.i.d.) or itraconazole (100 mg, b.i.d.), and were monitored for another 2 mo post-therapy. The results showed complete remission of endoscopic lesions in 45 patients (75%) from the fluconazole group and in 23 patients (38%) from the itraconazole group ($p < 0.001$); partial remission was achieved in 25 and 47% of patients from the fluconazole and itraconazole groups, respectively. In each group, the number of nonresponders was the same (9 patients; 15%). Complete clinical remission was observed in 47 patients (78%) in the fluconazole group and in 44 patients (73%) in the itraconazole group. Partial clinical remission was shown in 22 and 20% of the fluconazole and itraconazole groups, respectively, and no clinical response was observed in four patients (7%) from the itraconazole group. No apparent side effects were seen in patients of either treatment group. Overall, the results of this study demonstrated that fluconazole was significantly better than itraconazole in resolving endoscopic lesions, with both drugs nearly equipotent in eliciting complete clinical remission of esophageal candidiasis *(74)*. The same investigators *(75)* also compared the efficacies of fluconazole and flucytosine in a double-blind, placebo-controlled trial of 60 AIDS patients with endoscopically diagnosed esophageal candidiasis. Three randomly selected groups of 20 patients each, received orally either fluconazole (3.0 mg/kg daily), flucytosine (100 mg/kg daily), or placebo. After 2 wk of treatment, the placebo-receiving patients were double-blindly randomized to receive fluconazole (8 patients) or flucytosine (9 patients). The results at the end of 2 wk showed that endoscopic cure was achieved in 13 patients (65%) of the fluconazole group versus only 3 patients (15%) in the flucytosine group, whereas partial endoscopic cure was evident in 2 patients (10%) in the placebo-receiving group. Complete clinical remission was observed in 16 patients (80%) from the fluconazole group and 12 patients (60%) from the flucytosine group, while 6 patients from the placebo group presented with partial clinical remission. At the end of the follow-up period (5 wk post-treatment) the number of patients showing endoscopic cure were 19 (70%) and 9 (33%) from the fluconazole- and flucytosine-treated groups, respectively; the corresponding number of patients achieving complete clinical remission was 21 (77.7%) in the fluconazole group, and 17 (63%) in the flucytosine group. Overall, although both fluconazole and flucytosine were safe and well-tolerated by AIDS patients with esophageal candidiasis, fluconazole exhibited greater therapeutic efficacy than flucytosine, especially in the rate of endoscopic cure *(75)*.

The efficacy of amphotericin B oral suspension (ABOS) for fluconazole-refractory oral candidiasis in HIV-infected patients was evaluated in a prospective, multicenter, open-label trial at 25 study centers within the AIDS Clinical Trial Group *(76)*. Treatment with ABOS (100 mg/mL, 5 mL swish and swallow, 4 times daily for 14 d) was commenced after patients with diffuse oral candidiasis were treated daily with 200 mg of fluconazole for 14 d. The results showed that although ABOS was well-tolerated, it has limited efficacy for the treatment of fluconazole-refractory oral candidiasis. In the same vein, a randomized study was conducted to compare the safety and efficacy of amphotericin B oral solution with fluconazole oral solution in head and neck cancer patients following radiotherapy *(77)*. The patients were divided in three regimen groups receiving for up to 4 wk: (1) amphotericin B at 4.0 g, q.i.d.; (2) fluconazole at 50 mg o.d.; or (3) fluconazole at 100 mg o.d. The three drug regimens were found equally efficacious and well-tolerated.

Smith et al. *(78)* randomized HIV-infected patients with oral or esophageal candidosis to 4 wk of treatment with itraconazole (200 mg daily), followed by itraconazole or matching placebo for a prophylaxis phase of 24 wk. Seventy-four percent of the patients were clinically cured and 40% were also mycologically cured. In the 44 patients enrolled in the prophylactic stage, there were significantly more relapses of candidosis, with time to candidosis also significantly shorter in the placebo group as compared with the itraconazole-treated group ($p = 0.0001$) *(78)*.

In liquid formulation, itraconazole increased the absorption by 30% as compared to its solid form; nearly 99% success rate of yeast lesions clearance was observed during a 14-d treatment course *(79)*. In an open-label, multicenter trial, Saag et al. *(80)* evaluated the efficacy and safety of an oral solution in HIV-infected/AIDS patients with fluconazole-refractory oropharyngeal candidiasis. After failing fluconazole therapy at 200 mg daily, the patients were treated with 100 mg of oral itraconazole solution administered twice daily for 14 d. Additional treatment for another 14 d (28 d total) was given to patients with incomplete response. Clinical response by d 28 was achieved in 55% of the patients.

An open-label, sequential dose escalation Phase I/II clinical trial was conducted to evaluate the safety, pharmacokinetics, and efficacy of cyclodextrin itraconazole (2.5 mg/kg given either once or twice daily) in the treatment of oropharyngeal candidiasis on HIV-positive pediatric patients *(81)*. On d 15 of therapy, 22 of 26 children showed improvement of their condition. The drug was well tolerated with no associated hepatotoxicity.

In a double-blind trial in HIV-positive patients with oral and esophageal candidiasis, Smith et al. *(82)* compared the efficacies of oral itraconazole (200 mg once daily) and oral ketoconazole (200 mg b.i.d.). The clinical responses at the end of the 4-wk trial were equal for both drug regimens. In another study, de Repentigny et al. *(83)* also compared the potencies of itraconazole and ketoconazole in 128 HIV-infected patients. Both drugs were administered orally once daily at doses of 200 mg to 76 patients with oropharyngeal, and 16 patients with endoscopically proven esophageal candidiasis for 14 and 28 d, respectively. Although no significant differences in time to clearing infection was observed between the two regimens, time to relapse was greater and cumulative relapse rates were lower in patients treated with itraconazole as compared to ketoconazole *(83)*.

Capetti et al. *(84)* treated resistant esophageal candidiasis in AIDS patients with GM-CSF. The latter was given consecutively for 10 d at 150 µg daily. Three of the four patients treated showed complete resolution of colonization within 7 d and one patient only partial regression over the treatment period. Scadden *(85)* has suggested that GM-CSF might play an important role in the treatment of HIV-positive patients by its ability to correct HIV-correlated or drug-induced neutropenia, and potentiating the monocyte-macrophage response *(86)* to fungal and mycobacterial infections.

Vazquez et al. *(87)* have used GM-CSF as an adjuvant to fluconazole in the treatment of refractory oropharyngeal candidiasis in three advanced AIDS patients. The latter received subcutaneously 300 µg daily of GM-CSF for 14 d along with 400 mg daily of fluconazole; all had complete resolution of the disease.

The adjunctive use of chlorhexidine (a broad-spectrum antimicrobial agent) in the therapy of oral candidoses, has been reviewed by Ellepola and Samaranayake *(88)*.

3.5. Systemic Candidiasis

The clinical status of the patients, the nature of the *Candida* spp., and the susceptibility of the infecting isolate to antifungal drugs usually will determine the choice of therapy against disseminated candidiasis (Table 2) *(89)*. Although empirical therapy for suspected disseminated candidiasis in febrile non-neutropenic patients is not well-defined, treatment options include intravenous amphotericin B or either oral or intravenous fluconazole. For neutropenic patients with prolonged and persistent fever (in spite of antimicrobial therapy), the recommended treatment is amphotericin B at 0.5–0.7 mg/kg daily until resolution of neutropenia. The use of liposomal amphotericin B (AmBisome) in the same setting has the added advantages of a smaller daily dose (3.0 mg/kg) and less toxicity *(89)*. In patients with disseminated (hepatosplenic) candidiasis, therapy should proceed until calcification or resolution of lesions, especially in patients receiving chemotherapy or immuno-

Table 2
Recommended Treatment of Systemic Candidiasis (89)

Condition	Drug regimens
Candidemia[a] and acute hematogenously disseminated candidiasis	Fluconazole, ≥6.0 mg/kg, orally, daily[b,c] Amphotericin B, ≥0.7 mg/kg, i.v., daily[b,d,e]
Chronic disseminated (hepatosplenic) candidiasis	Fluconazole, 6.0 mg/kg, orally, daily[f] Amphotericin B, 0.6–0.7 mg/kg, daily, i.v.[f]
Disseminated cutaneous neonatal (congenital) candidiasis[g]	Amphotericin B, 0.5–1.0 mg/kg daily (total: 10–25 mg/kg[g])
Candidal endophthalmitis	Amphotericn B alone (≥200 mg) or in combination with flucytosine[h]
Candidal meningitis	Amphotericin B, 0.7–1.0 mg/kg, daily + flucytosine, q.i.d.[i]
Candidal endocarditis	Amphotericin B, 1.0–2.0 g, i.v. (after surgery)[j] Fluconazole, 200–400 mg, daily, orally or i.v.[k]
Urinary candidiasis	Fluconazole, 200 mg, daily, orally for 1–2 wk Amphotericin B, 0.3–1.0 mg/kg, daily for 1–7 d Flucytosine, 2.5 mg/kg, q.i.d., orally[l]
Candidal peritonitis	Fluconazole, 400 mg, daily
Candidal arthritis and osteomyelitis	Amphotericin B, 0.5–1.0 mg/kg, i.v., daily for 6–10 wk[m] Flucytosine, 6.0 mg/kg, daily, orally for 6–12 mo[m]
Laryngeal candidiasis	Amphotericin B, 0.7–1.0 mg/kg, daily, i.v.

[a]For candidemia, therapy should be continued for 2 wk after the last positive blood culture and resolution of signs and symptoms of infection have been observed.

[b]It is recommended that *C. albicans*, *C. tropicalis*, and *C. parapsilosis* are treated daily with either amphotericin B at 0.6 mg/kg or fluconazole at 6.0 mg/kg.

[c]Because *C. lusitaniae* is resistant to amphotericin B, daily fluconazole at 6.0 mg/kg is the preferred therapy.

[d]Because *C. glabrata* often is less susceptible to both azoles and amphotericin B, the latter is the mostly recommended initial therapy at ≥0.7 mg/kg, daily. Fluconazole, at 12 mg/kg, daily may also be beneficial, especially in less critically ill patients.

[e]For *C. krusei*, the regimen of choice is amphotericin B at 1.0 mg/kg, daily.

[f]The use of fluconazole is recommended for patients in stable condition, whereas amphotericin B is preferred in acutely ill patients or those with refractory disease.

[g]Treatment of infants with congenital candidiasis with amphotericin B is usually considered when there is a high risk for developing acute disseminated candidiasis. Fluconazole may also be used as a second-line agent.

[h]Dose regimens of 1.0–1.5 g of amphotericin B, if tolerated by the patient) have been recommended in severe cases of vitreous abscess formation *(92)*.

[i]Recommended as an initial therapy; the flucytosine dose should be adjusted to produce serum levels of 40–60 μg/mL.

[j]In patients with no severe heart failure, a course of parenteral amphotericin B (500 mg) may be implemented, followed by additional treatment after valvular replacement *(145)*.

[k]If valve replacement is not possible, a life-long suppressive therapy with fluconazole has been recommended *(93,94)*.

[l]Recommended in the absence of renal insufficiency, especially in patients with urologic infections caused by non-*albicans Candida* species.

[m]Initially, a course of amphotericin B for 2–3 wk, followed by fluconazole for a total duration of therapy of 6–12 mo has also been recommended *(89)*.

suppressive drugs. To this end, an initial 1–2-wk course of amphotericin B for all patients followed by a prolonged course of fluconazole, has also been recommended *(89)*.

Amphotericin B is the most often used in the treatment of candidal endophthalmitis either alone or in combination with flucytosine. Therapy should last until complete resolution of visible disease; vitrectomy may also be carried out to save the eyesight *(89)*.

Because in candidal meningitis sterilization of the cerebrospinal fluid (CSF) often may precede eradication of the parenchymal infection, treatment should continue until achieving both the normalization of all CSF analyses and radiological findings, and the stabilization of the neurologic function *(89)*.

Combination of antifungal therapy and surgical intervention is most beneficial in the treatment of candidal endocarditis, pericarditis, and supporative phlebitis *(90,91)*. Thus, in cases of pericarditis, surgical debridement and/or resection, depending on the extent of the disease, has often been performed *(91)*. Considering the antifungal treatment, intravenous amphotericin B and oral and intravenous fluconazole have been the preferential choice, with oral flucytosine used in combination with amphotericin B *(89)*.

Depending on its severity, frequency, and organism involved, vulvovaginal candidiasis may be classified as either uncomplicated or complicated. Although uncomplicated vaginitis is diagnosed in about 90% of patients and often requires a short-course of oral or topical treatment with over-the-counter azole antimycotics (clotrimazole, butoconazole, miconazole, and tioconazole), nystatin, oral azoles (ketoconazole, itraconazole, and fluconazole), and boric acid, the complicated form of vulvovaginal candidiasis (seen in approx 10% of patients) requires antimycotic therapy of at least 7 d. In this regard, azole therapy is often unreliable in non-*albicans* vaginitis. *C. glabrata* and other non-*albicans* infections respond to a 2-wk course of daily treatment with topical boric acid, or topical flucytosine *(89)*.

Amphotericin B has been used extensively in the therapy of life-threatening systemic candidiasis *(95)*. The antibiotic is given intravenously at 0.5–1.0 mg/kg *(96)*. Nevertheless, the use of the drug in the traditional deoxycholate formulation (d-AmB) has been limited by severe toxicity. Its drawbacks include extensive toxicity (renal toxicity, nausea, headache, neutropenia, as well as a general flu-like illness [43]) and prolonged hospitalization. In this regard, several relatively new formulations have received regulatory approval, including amphotericin B colloidal dispersion (ABCD), amphotericin B lipid complex (ABLC), and liposomal amphotericin B (AmBisome). Jensen et al. *(97)* quantitated the level of reduction of intrinsic toxicity of these new formulations over d-AmB using a red blood cell potassium release assay and found the physicochemical component of therapeutic index improvement to follow the order AmBisome >> ABLC = ABCD > d-AmB.

Miyata et al. *(98)* successfully applied intrahepatic arterial infusion of amphotericin B (5.0–20 mg daily) using an inplantable drug-delivery system (reservoir) to treat patients with acute myelocytic leukemia (AML) who developed intractable *Candida*-associated multiple liver abscesses. Following orthotopic liver transplantation, there was increased mortality and morbidity of associated invasive fungal infections *(99)*.

Bowden et al. *(100)* applied a colloidal dispersion of amphotericin B (amphocil) in a Phase I dose-escalation study of 75 marrow-transplant recipients with invasive fungal infections (primarily *Aspergillus* or *Candida* spp.) to evaluate its toxicity, maximum tolerated dose, and clinical response. Escalating doses of 0.5–8.0 mg/kg in 0.5-mg/kg per patient increments were given up to 6 wk. No infusion-related toxicity was observed in 32% of the patients, and no appreciable renal toxicity was observed at any dose level. The estimated maximum tolerated dose was 7.5 mg/kg as defined by rigors and chills, and hypotension. The complete or partial response rate across dose levels and infection types was 52% *(100)*. Caillot et al. *(101)* also determined the efficacy and tolerance of a new amphotericin B lipid emulsion (Amb-OL) in 14 neutropenic patients with candidemia. The formulation, consisting of the antibiotic diluted in a lipid solution for parenteral nutrition, was applied at a mean daily dosage of 1.18 mg/kg (range 0.73–1.55) for 22 d (range 6–62). Seven patients were cured, and six showed improvement *(101)*.

Studies on the tolerance of high doses of amphotericin B by infusion of a liposomal formulation in children with cancer showed that daily doses ranging from 1.0–6.0 mg/kg (median 3.0 mg/kg) and cumulative doses of 13–311 mg/kg (median 75 mg/kg) were tolerated well in terms of acute toxicity and duration of treatment *(102)*.

In a multicenter, prospective, observational study involving 427 consecutive patients with candidemia, Nguyen et al. *(103)* assessed the efficacy of low- vs high-dose amphotericin B, and fluconazole vs amphotericin B, as well as the morbidity and mortality of *Candida* fungemia. The results showed a 34% mortality rate for patients with candidemia. The mortality rate for patients with catheter-related candidemia in whom the catheters were retained was significantly higher than that of patients having their catheters removed (41 vs 21%, $p < 0.001$). Furthermore, there was no overall difference in mortality in patients treated with low-dose (total amphotericin B dose of 500 mg or less) (13%) as compared to those receiving high-dose amphotericin B (total dose of >500 mg) (15%); however, patients who received the low-dose regimen experienced fewer side effects (40 vs 55%, $p = 0.03$). In addition to being as effective as amphotericin B, fluconazole also elicited fewer side effects than amphotericin B (12 and 44%, respectively, $p < 0.001$) *(103)*.

In an open label trial, 60% of non-neutropenic patients with refractory invasive candidiasis (positive blood cultures for *Candida* spp.) showed mycological success and clinical improvement after treatment with liposomal nystatin (Nyotran) *(104)*. The latter was well-tolerated with no serious nephrotoxicity observed.

Results from a randomized trial comparing fluconazole (400 mg daily, i.v. infusion for the first 7 d, then oral administration) with intravenous amphotericin B (0.5–0.6 mg/kg daily for the first week, then three times weekly) for the treatment of candidemia in 206 patients with neutropenia and no major immunodeficiency (most common diagnoses were renal failure, nonhematologic cancer, and gastrointestinal disease) revealed that the therapeutic efficacies of both drugs were not significantly different *(105)*. Even though fluconazole may be considered a safe alternative to amphotericin B in treating candidemia in non-neutropenic patients, a high risk of death is still present *(106,107)*, as well as some uncertainties with regard to duration of treatment, the need to initiate the therapy intravenously, the optimal timing to remove intravenous catheters, and the most proper medication of children *(108–110)*.

Kullberg et al. *(111)* conducted a double-blind, randomized, placebo-controlled, Phase II trial to evaluate the safety, feasibility, and preliminary efficacy of filgrastim in combination with fluconazole in 51 non-neutropenic patients with invasive candidiasis and candidemia. Filgrastim (recombinant granulocyte colony-stimulating factor, rG-CSF), which stimulates the production, numbers, and augments the biological function of circulating phagocytes and thereby increases the host defense against candidiasis, appeared to be potentially beneficial in the treatment of systemic candidiasis in non-neutropenic patients.

5-Fluorocytosine (5-FC) was also found to be beneficial in the treatment of systemic candidiasis *(112,113)*, although there may be a problem with drug resistance *(114)* and adverse myelosuppressive toxicity. In vitro and in vivo experiments showed that amphotericin B and 5-FC acted synergistically *(115,116)*.

Two azole derivatives, miconazole and ketoconazole, have also been shown to be effective in some cancer patients with disseminated candidiasis *(117,118)*.

3.5.1. Endogenous (Hematogenous) Candidal Endophthalmitis (HCE)

The recommended therapy for HCE is intravenous amphotericin B either alone or in combination with 5-FC. The latter combination should be considered in cases of either lesions threatening the macula, the presence of extensive intraocular inflammation, and/or when the inflammatory response is rapidly progressive *(119)*. Despite the low eye levels of amphotericin B *(101)*, its use apparently facilitated healing of HCE. Thus, Edwards et al. *(92)* reported that in a group of 76 patients with HCE, the 7 patients who received 200 mg or more of intravenous amphotericin B had the highest rate of healing. The recommended minimal therapeutic dose of amphotericin B should be at least 200 mg. However, dose regimens of 1.0–1.5 g (if tolerated by the patient) should be used in cases of severe vitrous abscess formation, and if resolution did not occur rapidly *(119)*.

Combination of amphotericin B and rifampin has been used successfully in one patient (the two drugs acted synergistically in an in vitro system) *(120)*.

The use of 5-FC alone has been rather limited and with marginal success (two of four patients responded, and two did not) *(121,122)*.

Miconazole failed to elicit favorable response in one patient with HCE *(123)* whereas the clinical experience with fluconazole in human HCE has been rather limited *(124)*. Its effect in a rabbit model of *C. albicans*-associated disseminated candidiasis and endophthalmitis was short-lived (24 d) and there was evidence that endophthalmitis actually worsened during the later stages of treatment with fluconazole *(125)*. Nomura and Ruskin *(126)* reported failure of fluconazole to prevent blinding from endophthalmitis secondary to candidal sepsis despite aggressive and lengthy therapy. According to Abbasoglu et al. *(127)*, upon single and multiple drop application, topical fluconazole 0.2% penetrated into the aqueous humor in concentrations that satisfied the MICs of most *Candida* strains.

Intravitreal injection of antifungal agents as potential therapy for HCE has not been adequately supported either experimentally *(122)* or clinically *(128,129)*. Moreover, the potential toxicity of intravitreal amphotericin B has raised concern *(130)* although in some studies *(122)*, 5.0- and 10-μg doses of intravitreal amphotericin B were reported safe in a rabbit model of exogenous candidal endophthalmitis. Furthermore, while intravitreally administered therapeutical dose of liposome-bound amphotericin B successfully eradicated *Candida* infection in rabbits with endophthalmitis, the treatment resulted in retinal damage to the eyes of all rabbits *(131)*.

Other therapeutic approaches for HCE include vitrectomy *(122,132,133)* and laser therapy *(134)*. In this regard, Bagnoud et al. *(135)* recommended that for treatment of endogenous candidal endophthalmitis a rapid antifungal therapy associated with or without a vitrectomy would represent a favorable therapeutic option when fungal infection is suspected.

3.5.2. Candidal Meningitis

For treatment of candidal meningitis, the recommended therapy consists of amphotericin B and 5-FC *(136–138)*. In one clinical trial *(137)*, 15 of 17 patients receiving this combination for 4–8 wk improved or were cured, with median time to sterilization of CSF cultures being 7 d. The addition of intrathecal amphotericin B facilitated the sterilization of CSF fluid *(139)*.

Candida meningitis, although rare in children, has been on the increase recently *(140)*.

Fungal infections of ventriculoperitoneal shunts, although occasional, may create significant difficulties in their clinical management. The treatment, with or without the shunt removal and the correct dosage and route of administration of the antifungal agents, is still not well-documented *(141)*. In a case report by Soto-Hernandez et al. *(142)*, cerebral granuloma associated with a nonfunctional CSF shunt caused by *Candida albicans* was resolved by shunt removal and 1.1 g of intravenously administered amphotericin B and oral ketoconazole.

3.5.3. Candidal Endocarditis

Candida endocarditis was nearly always fatal before the introduction of open heart surgery and amphotericin B therapy *(143–146)*. Currently, the recommended treatment of candidal endocarditis uniformly consists of combined medical and surgical interventions with systemic amphotericin B given before and after surgery *(90,147–159)*. However, neither the dose nor the duration of treatment with amphotericin B have been clearly established; rather, both are usually determined by the patient's tolerance of the drug *(90)*. Hallum and Williams *(90)* have recommended that in patients with no severe heart failure, a course of parenteral amphotericin B be implemented at approx 500 mg before surgery and an additional 1.0–1.5 g after valvular replacement. In cases where the patient is in severe heart failure and fails to improve dramatically within 36–48 h after a full medical treatment for the heart failure, emergency valvular replacement may have to be carried out; in such cases, a dose regimen of 1.5–2.0 g of amphotericin B should be given after the cardiac surgery *(90)*.

5-Fluorocytosine has been used adjunctively in several patients with candidal endocarditis with inconclusive results *(148,160)*.

At daily doses of 100–200 mg (3 mg/kg daily), fluconazole has also been used to treat *Candida* endocarditis *(161,162)*. In one of these studies *(161)*, the patient with *C. parapsilosis* complicating treatment for non-Hodgkin's lymphoma received a 3-mo course of intravenous and oral fluconazole in addition to granulocyte-macrophage colony-stimulating factor (GM-CSF) for persistent neutropenia. Furthermore, the therapeutic efficacy of fluconazole has been tested in a rabbit model of candidal endocarditis; at much higher doses (20–50 mg/kg given intraperitoneally), it successfully sterilized all *Candida* vegetations *(163)*.

Nishida et al. *(164)* described a case of active valve infective endocarditis due to *C. glabrata* that was successfully treated by systemic administration of fluconazole. The drug was administered intravenously or orally at doses of 400 mg daily for 46 d.

3.5.4. Vulvovaginal Candidiasis

Vulvovaginal candidiasis is a common mucosal fungal infection in women of child-bearing age. In spite of the role cell-mediated immunity and T cells play in host protection against mucosal *C. albicans* infections, it is still not well defined whether immunosuppression by HIV infection enhances the susceptibility to vaginal candidiasis. In this regard, current data suggest that the role of local mucosal immunity is more important than that in the systemic circulation for host defense against vaginitis *(165)*.

A number of agents have been used to treat acute candidal vaginitis. Among the polyene antifungals, nystatin cream and vaginal suppositories have been used for nearly three decades with approx 75–80% rate of success *(166)*. Other polyenes, such as amphotericin B, meparteicin, and trichomycin, appeared at least as effective as nystatin *(167)*. Several azole derivatives (butoconazole, clotrimazole, miconazole, econazole, fenticonazole, tioconazole, terconazole) when compared to the polyenes seemed to be more effective by achieving clinical and mycological cure rates in the range of 85–90% *(168,169)*.

In several clinical trials, shorter treatment courses or higher single-dose regimens have proven effective for most of the azole antimycotics against acute candidal vaginitis *(170,171)*. The higher dose resulted in the persistence of inhibitory drug concentrations for several days; for example, clotrimazole when given as 500-mg suppositories maintained measurable therapeutic concentrations for at least 2–3 days *(172)*; similar data is now available for miconazole *(173)*. In addition, single high-dosage therapy with clotrimazole was reported beneficial in pregnant women *(174)*.

Of the orally active azole derivatives, ketoconazole (at 400 mg daily, for 5 d), itraconazole (at either 200 mg daily for 3 d, or 400 mg on 1 d), and fluconazole (150 mg single daily dose, or 150 mg once weekly for 3 wk) have been shown to be highly effective in achieving clinical and mycological cure of acute candidal vaginitis *(175–178)*.

In an open, non-comparative study, Kukner et al. *(179)* evaluated the efficacy of neo-penotran, a combination of metronidazole (500 mg) and miconazole nitrate (100 mg), in patients with candidal vaginitis. Each patients was inserted a neo-penotran pessary twice daily for 2 wk; vaginitis was resolved in 84.4% of the cases.

A comparison of oral metronidazole (500 mg b.i.d. for 1 wk), 0.75% metronidazole vaginal gel (5 g b.i.d. for 5 d), and 2% clindamycin vaginal cream (5 g once daily for 1 wk), have shown equivalent cure rates of vulvovaginal candidiasis *(180)*.

In a prospective, randomized, double-blind study of patients with complicated *Candida* vaginitis, Sobel et al. *(181)* compared the efficacy of a single (150 mg) and sequential (2 × 150-mg) doses of fluconazole given 3 d apart. Overall, while treatment of candidal vaginitis still requires individualized therapy, patients with severe vaginitis achieved superior clinical and mycologic eradication when given the two-dose fluconazole regimen.

In a single-blind, randomized, controlled trial, the clinical efficacy of fluconazole (a single daily oral dose of 150 mg) was compared with that of clotrimazole (100-mg suppository given twice daily in the morning and at bedtime) in the treatment of vulvovaginal candidiasis over a 3-d period *(182)*. There was no significant difference between the two drugs regarding mycological cure 1 week after treatment (79.2% for fluconazole- and 80% for clotrimazole-treated groups); approx 4 wk after treatment, the corresponding cure rates were 60.4 and 66%, respectively. The toxic side effects were minimal.

Sobel et al. *(183)* conducted a randomized study of 151 patients with a history of recurrent vulvovaginal candidiasis to compare the efficacy of oral ketoconazole (400 mg daily for 2 wk) with that of topical clotrimazole (100 mg daily as vaginal suppositories for 1 wk). One week after the completion of therapy, clinical cure or improvement was observed in 86.4% of the ketoconazole- and 81.7% of clotrimazole-treated groups, with mycological response of 80.3 and 81.7%, respectively. However, in the absence of maintenance suppressive antifungal therapy, the clinical and mycologic failures in both groups were very high, reaching 52.5 and 62.6% for the ketoconazole and clotrimazole groups, respectively, thus necessitating the need for immediate initiation of maintenance therapy following the initial clinical improvement *(183)*.

Azzena and Vasoin *(184)* successfully treated candidal vulvovaginitis with itraconazole with a single daily oral dose of 200 mg for 3 d.

The management of recurrent and chronic vulvovaginal infections is more problematic especially in immunocompromised hosts *(167)*, especially when there is underlying conditions (e.g., diabetes) and/or predisposing factors (corticosteroid or other immunosuppressive, or estrogen therapies). In general, recalcitrant candidal infection will require long-term maintenance suppressive prophylactic therapy *(185–187)*. Treatment with low-dose oral ketoconalzole (100 mg daily for 6 mo) has been described as maintenance therapy *(185)*.

Orungal (Janssen-Cilag) (an extremely lipophilic and keratophilic antifungal triazole agent) was found to be highly effective in alleviating vaginal candidiasis after 1-d treatment with 2 × 200 mg of the drug; 91% of patients showed no clinical signs and negative cultures after control examination 1 mo after treatment *(188)*.

C. albicans is known to be a potent allergen in some situations, and it has been suggested that local hypersensitivity to this yeast can be a factor in the prolongation of infection. In a prospective cohort study of women with recurrent vaginal candidiasis, Moraes et al. *(189)* evaluated the efficacy of a 24-mo *C. albicans* allergen immunotherapy in women with immediate skin test positive for this species that were unresponsive to other modes of treatment. The results showed a decrease in the number and intensity of episodes following the allergen immunotherapy.

3.5.5. Urinary and Peritoneal Candidiasis

One of the recommended therapies of *Candida*-associated cystitis and candiduria is treatment with intravenous amphotericin B. Doses as high as 200 µg/mL have been reported to cause minimal toxicity *(190,191)*. The usual amphotericin B concentrations are in the 50–60 µg/mL range added to 1.0 L of 5% dextrose and water and infused at a rate of 40 mL/h *(191)*. Other drugs used to treat candidal cystitis include 5-FC and azole (fluconazole *[192]*) antimycotics *(193)*. Because fungal resistance against 5-FC is likely to develop, combined therapy with amphotericin B may be beneficial *(194)*.

Strassner and Friesen *(195)* showed that alkalinization of the urine (to adjust the pH to 7.0–7.5) with oral potassium-sodium-hydrogen citrate may provide a simple and effective method to treat candiduria in patients with an indwelling catheter. An additional advantage was the metaphylaxis and prophylaxis of renal stone formation in immobilized patients.

Because candiduria has emerged as major therapeutic problem over the past 40 yr, treatment by means of bladder irrigation with amphotericin B solutions has been widely used in clinical practice.

However, some specific aspects of this procedures, such as drug concentrations and duration of treatment, and the benefit of continuous washing over instillation with cross-clamping (to allow "dwell-times,") have not been clearly defined by prospective, randomized, double-blind trials. In view of the current knowledge (based exclusively on anecdotal experiences), Sanford *(196)* recommended that 200–300 mL of amphotericin B solution at optimal concentrations of 5.0–10 mg/L, should be administered by triple-lumen urethral catheter with cross-clamping for 60–90 min; because of potential uroepithelial damage, irrigation for no more than 2 d should be sufficient. However, some aspects of the Sanford's recommended procedure have drawn criticism from a number of investigators *(197–200)*.

Treatment of catheter-associated candiduria with fluconazole irrigation (prepared as 1.0 mg/mL solution with normal saline) was effective and safe in eliminating the candiduria without changing the catheter *(201)*. In this regard, the use of fluconazole may also prove to be cost-effective because in patients with candiduria there is often the dilemma of deciding whether a patient's candiduria is the result of colonization or an infectious agent. Although repeated catheterized urinalysis is helpful in selecting those patients with true candiduria, this procedure is expensive. While catheter change alone rarely results in elimination of candiduria (in less than 20% of cases), discontinuation of the catheter alone may result in eradication of candiduria in nearly 40% of patients *(89)*. In terms of duration, 1–2 wk therapy is more likely to succeed.

Candidal pyelonephritis, which is one of the most common manifestations of upper urinary tract infections, may be life-threatening, and intravenous amphotericin B is the recommended therapy *(202–204)*. The recommended regimen usually commences with 10 mg of the antibiotic on the first day, and 25 mg daily on the subsequent 4 d *(205)*. Instillation of amphotericin B directly into the renal pelvis has been successful in several cases *(204,206)*.

The incidence of *Candida*-associated peritoneal infections have increased, with *C. albicans* and *C. tropicalis* being the most frequent etiologic agents *(207)*. In addition to peritoneal dialysis *(208–215)*, imunosuppression and broad-spectrum antibiotic therapies are risk factors for the development of candidal peritonitis *(205)*.

In patients on peritoneal dialysis in whom the infection has been localized to the peritoneum, treatment with either intraperitoneal 5-FC or miconazole plus oral ketoconazole was reported to be well-tolerated and effective *(207)*. In two other reports, treatment of patients on chronic ambulatory peritoneal dialysis (CAPD) included intraperitoneal lavage with 5-FC alone *(216,217)* or low-dose amphotericin B (2.0–4.0 µg/mL final concentration in dialysate fluid); in the latter case, although effective this treatment may not only cause abdominal pain during instillation *(215,218)*, but may also preclude patients of continuing peritoneal dialysis *(205)*. The amphotericin B-associated abdominal pain may be dose-related because it occurs at doses of 4.0 µg/mL or higher. In addition, intraperitoneal amphotericin B has been linked with peritoneal fibrosis and adhesion *(208)*. Two patients who developed fungal peritonitis after receiving CAPD were successfully treated with intracatheter retention of amphotericin B (1.0–2.0 mg) and oral flucytosine or fluconazole (50 mg b.i.d.) for 5 wk; the catheter was not removed and efficient peritoneal permeability was maintained *(219)*.

The peritoneal penetration of amphotericin B lipid complex and fluconazole in a pediatric patient with *C. albicans* peritonitis receiving continuous cyclic peritoneal dialysis was studied. While fluconazole rapidly and efficiently penetrated the peritoneal fluid, achieving concentrations that exceeded the MIC for most *Candida* species, the amount of amphotericin B in the dialysate was below the limit of quantification despite measurable blood concentrations *(220)*. Montenegro et al. *(221)* treated candidal peritonitis with fluconazole with delayed removal of the peritoneal dialysis catheter. Because of its ability to penetrate into the peritoneal fluid after oral administration *(222,223)* fluconazole was found effective (100–200 mg daily, for 2–6 wk) in the treatment of candidal peritonitis *(224,225)*.

Voss et al. *(226)* reviewed the efficacy of fluconazole in the management of candidal urinary tract infections in several small studies (a total of 99 patients). The drug appeared to be of value in the treatment of both uncomplicated and complicated infections.

Corbella et al. *(227)* reported a case of *C. glabrata* upper urinary tract infection causing urethral obstruction that was successfully treated with intravenous fluconazole (200 mg daily) combined with urethral catheterization; oral fluconazole at 200 mg daily was instituted as preventive maintenance therapy for 1 mo post-treatment. However, Ansari et al. *(228)* cautioned about the possibility of failing to eradicate fluconazole in such settings due either to inheritant resistance of *C. glabrata* to fluconazole *(229,230)* or to development of resistance after prolonged therapy with the drug *(231,232)*.

In another therapeutic strategy *(233)*, a combination of intravenous or intraperitoneal administration of 5-fluorocytosine and oral fluconazole was also used.

In a recent randomized, double-blind study, Sobel et al. *(234)* compared fungal eradication rates among 316 consecutive caniduric (asymptomatic or minimally symptomatic) hospitalized patients treated with fluconazole (200 gm) or placebo daily for 14 d. Findings have shown that in an intent-to-treat analysis, candiduria cleared by d 14 in 79 (50%) of 159 receiving fluconazole and 46 (29%) of 157 patients receiving placebo, including 33 (52%) of 64 catheterized and 42 (78%) of 54 non-catheterized patients. Overall, although oral fluconazole was safe and effective for short-term eradication, especially following catheter removal, the long-term eradication rates were disappointing and not associated with clinical benefit.

3.5.6. Candidal Arthritis and Osteomyelitis

Amphotericin B has been the drug of choice for therapy of candidal arthritis *(31)*. In cases of no response, the therapy was supplemented with either flucytosine or ketoconazole. Local candidal arthritis healed in all cases. However, candidal arthritis in an artificial joint resulted in all cases in removal of the prostheses *(235)*.

Lafont et al. *(236)* described three patients with a history of intravenous heroin addiction who presented with indolent persistant lumbar pain, revealing septic spondilodiscitis and vertebral osteomyelitis caused by *C. albicans*. Two of the patients were treated with intravenous amphotericin B, and the other with fluconazole, with excellent results. Fluconazole alone was also found effective in the treatment of *C. albicans* prosthetic arthritis *(237)*.

Treatment of arthritis and osteomyelitis secondary to disseminated *C. tropicalis* infection in a premature infant with amphotericin B and oral flucytosine (25 mg/kg q.i.d.) resulted in sterilization of the synovial fluid within 4 d. The intraarticular level of flucytosine (synovial fluid) was 39.6 µg/mL; corresponding serum level was 47.5 µg/mL *(238)*. In another case *(239)*, *C. lusitaniae* osteomyelitis in premature infant was successful following therapy with flucytosine and fluconazole.

The use of amphotericin B-loaded bone cement to treat a case of *C. albicans*-associated osteomyelitis was reported by Marra et al. *(240)*.

Tang *(241)* reported a case of patient with candidal osteomyelitis who, because of renal impairment, was treated with fluconazole rather than amphotericin B; the patient made a full recovery. However, fluconazole therapy failed to cure sternal osteomyelitis due to *C. albicans (242)*.

3.5.7. Neonatal Candidiasis

By producing systemic disease in vulnerable low birth-weight infants, *C. albicans* represents a serious opportunistic threat to critically ill infants that is difficult to manage and is associated with high morbidity and mortality. Moreover, because such infections have an insidious and rapid course, it is critically important that key prevention and early treatment measures are provided *(243)*.

A disseminated neonatal candidiasis would necessitate the use of amphotericin B *(244,245)*. However, its toxicity may be a serious problem. Baley et al. *(246)*, found 7 of 10 infants receiving amphotericin B with severe renal abnormalities manifested by oliguria or anuria and significant increase in blood urea nitrogen and creatinine at an average cumulative dose of 6.5 mg/kg; six infant deaths were attributed to amphotericin B-associated nephrotoxicity. In two neonatal studies *(247,248)*, after 1 wk of amphotericin B treatment, the creatinine levels rose an average of 0.299 µg/dL but reversed to baseline levels after the end of therapy. It is recommended that therapy with amphotericin B in infants is started with 0.25 mg/kg diluted in 5 or 10% dextrose and infused over 2–4 h (test dose is usually not necessary), followed by daily increases of 0.25 mg/kg to achieve a daily dose from 0.5 mg/kg to 1.0 mg/kg *(244)*. In severe cases, dose increases have been carried out every 12 h; to this end, daily doses of up to 1.5 mg/kg in cases of persistent fungemia were safely given *(249)*.

Endogenous *Candida* endophthalmitis resulting from candidemia in low birth-weight infants is well-recognized complication. It usually occurs as a retinochondroitis, which is effectively resolved with systemic antifungal therapy. However, in recurrent candidal infections, it is the iris and lens that are affected primarily, rather than the retina and choroids *(250)*. A case of *C. albicans* cataract was found to be unresponsive to systemic and intracameral antifungal therapy and necessitated lensectomy with vitrectomy *(251)*.

Although uncommon complication of invasive candidiasis, a fatal case of *C. albicans* endocarditis in a very low birth-weight (780 g) infant and the failure of fluconazole treatment, have been reported *(252)*.

Aydin et al. *(253)* described three cases of candidal meningitis of low birth-weight infants treated with amphotericin B. *C. albicans* was isolated from CSF cultures and treatment was instituted 1–4 wk before the onset of candidiasis. Amphotericin B was administered intravenously at an initial daily dose of 0.25 mg/kg, which was later increased to 2.0 mg/kg daily. The side effects included a transient and mild elevation in hepatic enzyme concentration, and transient thrombocytopenia *(253)*. Delaplane et al. *(247)* found that in five infants the amphotericin B levels in the CSF were 40–50% of those in the serum; by comparison, in adults, the CSF concentrations were between 2 and 4% that of serum *(254)*.

The management of obstructive uropathy in neonates and infants has been successfully carried out by treatment with intravenous amphotericin B and oral 5-FC *(255)*. Stocker et al. *(256)* successfully treated nonobstructing bilateral renal *C. albicans* balls in an extremely low birth-weight (750 g) infant using combination therapy of intravenous amphotericin B and oral fluconazole for 6 wk, followed by monotherapy with fluconazole until complete resolution.

A case of widespread cutaneous candidiasis in an infant with methylmalonic acidemia was treated successfully with liposomal amphotericin B (AmBisome) *(188)*. Results from other studies *(257,258)* have shown high cure rate of invasive candidiasis in immunocompromised and very low birth-weight infants following AmBisome therapy.

Lackner et al. *(259)* reported the use of liposomal amphotericin B (AmBisome) in the treatment of one low birth-weight infant (1,020 g) with disseminated candidiasis. The liposomal formulation was given intravenously at an initial daily dose of 1.5 mg/kg, which was later increased to 5.0 mg/kg daily with no severe side effects observed. After 1 wk, no fungal contamination was detected, and treatment was stopped after 26 d. However, based on their clinical experience with disseminated candidiasis in low birth-weight infants, Pereira da Silva et al. *(260)* recommended increasing the initial 1.0-mg/kg dose of AmBisome (given for 1 wk) to a lower dose (1.25 mg/kg); after 1 wk at a dose regimen of 1.25 mg/kg AmBisome, clinical improvement was evident.

5-FC usually is used as an adjunctive therapy with amphotericin B *(244)*. However, the need for it has been questioned *(261)*. Dose regimens may vary from 25–50 mg/kg (q.i.d.) to a single daily dosing of 50 or 100 mg/kg *(244)*.

Clarke and Davies *(262)* have found miconazole effective in the treatment of neonatal disseminated candidiasis at 4.0 mg/kg daily. Miconazole antagonism with amphotericin B has been reported *(263)*.

Fluconazole at daily doses of 1.0–16 mg/kg (mean 5.3 mg/kg daily) eliminated *Candida* colonization in a low birth-weight infants with no apparent toxicity *(264,265)*. The clinical and mycological responses reached 97% of the patients *(265)*, and the recommended daily dose of fluconazole is 5.0 mg/kg *(266)*.

Marr et al. *(267)* reported successful treatment of candidal sepsis and meningitis in a very low birth-weight infant using fluconazole and flucytosine. While fluconazole given alone failed in a case of an infant with candidal meningitis *(268)*, it was reported to be effective in resolving *C.*

albicans septicemia when given orally to a premature low birth-weight infant (5.0 mg/kg daily for 20 d) *(269)*.

The therapeutic efficacy of oral itraconazole for disseminated candidiasis in low birth-weight infants was discussed by Bhandari and Narang *(270)*.

Michel et al. *(271)* reported a case of major eosinophilia in a very low birth-weight induced by transcutaneous resorption of topical ketoconazole to treat diaper *C. albicans* dermatitis.

4. AZOLE DRUG RESISTANCE AND REFRACTORY CANDIDIASIS

Although *C. albicans* is usually susceptible to major antifungal drugs (fluconazole, itraconazole, flucytosine, and amphotericin B), there have been numerous reports of resistance to azole agents in HIV-infected patients with relapsing oropharyngeal candidiasis as well as invasive candidiasis *(272)*. For example, daily or every-other-day use of fluconazole was associated with the development of refractory candidal infection *(273)*. Therefore, susceptibility testing for azole derivatives has become increasingly important in establishing an effective therapy *(274)*. Even though most *Candida* isolates still remain susceptible to amphotericin B *(89)*, the emergence of resistance and cross-resistance to antifungal drugs would necessitate in vitro and clinical correlations.

Using MIC values, Schuman et al. *(275)* evaluated in vitro the fluconazole susceptibility patterns of *C. albicans* and non-*albicans Candida* species from oral and vaginal isolates in HIV-positive and at risk HIV-negative women. The results have shown that while reduced susceptibility to fluconazole among the *C. albicans* isolates were rare, in non-*albicans Candida* isolates it occurred frequently and increased during follow-up. Furthermore, recent history of candidiasis and lower CD4 counts were not significantly related to reduced susceptibility. Rodriguez-Tudela et al. *(276)* demonstrated the presence of correlation between in vitro susceptibility (as determined in RPMI-2% glucose broth) and the clinical response to fluconazole and ketoconazole in AIDS patients with oropharyngeal or esophageal candidiasis.

The genotypes and susceptibilities to fluconazole of two sets of samples of *C. albicans* (a total of 78 strains); one from HIV-infected patients and one from a healthy volunteers, were compared in an attempt to define the clonal and spontaneous origins of fluconazole resistance *(277)*. While the analysis revealed little evidence for genotypic clustering according to HIV status or body site, a small group of fluconazole-resistant strains from HIV-infected patients formed a distinct cluster. The overall results suggested both clonal and spontaneous origins of fluconazole resistance in *C. albicans*.

To study the molecular epidemiology of fluconazole-refractory oral candidiasis (FROC) and determine whether patients are colonized with genetically similar or distinct strains of *C. albicans* prior to the development of FROC, Fichtenbaum et al. *(273,278)* conducted a prospective, observational study of 832 patients with advanced HIV. The results confirmed that the pathogenesis of FROC is characterized with two patterns for *C. albicans*, with the majority of patients having genetically distinct isolates emerging when compared to pre-FROC asymptomatic colonization. The observed phenomenon may represent a mutation within an existing strain or acquisition of a new strain.

The phospholipid and sterol composition of plasma membranes of five fluconazole-resistant clinical *C. albicans* isolates was compared to that of three fluconazole-sensitive ones *(279)*. While the three azole-sensitive strains tested and four of the five resistant strains did not exhibit any major difference in their phospholipid and sterol composition, the remaining strain showed a decreased amount of ergosterol and a lower phosphatidylcholine:phosphatidylethanolamine ratio in the plasma membrane. It has been postulated that these changes in the plasma membrane lipid and sterol composition may be responsible for an altered uptake of drugs and thus for a reduced intracellular accumulation of fluconazole thereby providing a possible mechanism for azole resistance.

C. albicans resistance to azole antimycotics is thought to be initiated by multiple mechanisms, including alterations in the target enzyme and increased efflux of drugs *(280)*. For example, overexpression of the ABC-transporter genes CDR1 and CDR2 were found in 20 azole-resistant *C. albicans* clinical isolates from seven HIV-infected patients, and overexpression of the Major Facilitator gene MDR1 was found in nine azole-resitant isolates from six patients *(281)*. The overall results suggested the existence of multiple combinations of mechanisms for the development of azole resistance in *C. albicans*. In another study *(280)*, the expression of ERG11, MDR1, and CDR2 genes involved in *C. albicans* resistance to fluconazole was monitored using Northern-blot technique. The obtained results demonstrated the complexity of the epidemiology of the molecular mechanisms of antifungal resistance and indicated that different subpopulations of yeast may coexist at a given time in the same patient and may develop resistance through different mechanisms.

Although clotrimazole troches are widely used in the treatment of mucosal candidiasis, little is known about clotrimazole resistance and its effect on the development of refractory mucosal candidiasis. Findings from a prospectively monitored HIV-infected pediatric population receiving clotrimazole concentrations ranging from 0.03–16 µg/mL have suggested that clotrimazole resistance had developed in isolates of *C. albicans*, that a concomitant cross-resistance to other azoles may also develop, and that this resistance correlated with refractory candidiasis. To this end, interpretive breakpoint of 0.5 µg/mL may be useful in defining clotrimazole resistance in *C. albicans (66)*.

5. HAART THERAPY AND CANDIDIASIS

Initiation of highly active antretroviral therapy (HAART) in HIV-infected populations has exerted a positive impact on the immunological recovery of such patients, thereby leading to decreased frequency of symptomatic *Candida* infections and an overall decline of some opportunistic infections *(282)*. Thus, in patients receiving HAART, there has been a significant increase in the functional measures of innate immunity, such as fungicidal activity, chemotaxis, and oxidative metabolism of PMNL and monocytes from HIV-positive naive patients *(283)*. However, in a longitudinal study of the relationship between HAART therapy and recurrent oropharyngeal candidiasis in advanced HIV-infected patients, Revankar et al. *(284)* demonstrated that unless HAART is accompanied by significant decrease in the viral load and increase in the $CD4^+$ T-cell count, HAART alone may not lead to reduced recurrence rate of oropharyngeal candidiasis.

Zingman *(285)* reported resolution of refractory (fluconazole-resistant) AIDS-related mucosal candidiasis after initiation of retroviral therapy consisting of didanosine (125 mg, b.i.d.) and sequinavir (600 mg, t.i.d.). Arribas et al. *(286,287)* also noticed continuous improvement of oral *Candida* colonization and skin-test reactivity after 1 yr of treatment with anti-HIV protease inhibitors (ritonavir) of a cohort of advanced HIV-infected patients. Proteinase inhibitors inhibit the *Candida* aspartyl proteinase resulting in reduced fungal growth, as well as having a direct inhibitory activity of *Candida* virulence *(288,289)*.

Connick et al. *(290)* evaluated the effects of a 1-yr zidovudine, lamivudine, and ritonavir treatment on the immune reconstitution of 34 HIV-infected patients and its relationship to virulogic response. The magnitude of virulogic suppression, which was correlated with numeric increases in the $CD4^+$ T-cells but not with measures of functional immune reconstitution, has shown that plasma virus suppression of less than 100 copies/mL was not significantly correlated with increases in $CD4^+$ T-cells or functional immune reconstitution.

6. DRUG ACTIVITIES AND *CANDIDA* VIRULENCE

When given to sensitive surgical patients, cefepime and meropenem did not significantly increase the risk of gastrointestinal colonization by *C. albicans* originating in the gastrointestinal (GI) tract *(291)*. Likewise, with the exception of ciprofloxacin (which caused a slight, statistically insignificant increase in *C. albicans* GI colonization), the quinolone antibiotics (norfloxacine, ciprofloxacin, and ofloxacin) had no effect either *(292)*.

Using *C. albicans* strains, Ueta et al. *(293)* examined the influence of anticancer drugs and irradiation on *Candida* cell virulence (proliferation, adherence to HeLa cells, and the susceptibility toantifungal agents, and neutrophils). After treatment with 5-FC (25–250 µg/mL), *cis*-diamminedichloroplatinum (10–100 µg/mL), peplomycin (0.5–5.0 µg/mL), or ^{137}Cs (20–40 Gy) for 3 d or more, surviving *Candida* cells proliferated more rapidly than did untreated control cells. In addition, they showed an increased adhesion to HeLa cells (indicating increased binding to lectins), decreased susceptibility to amphotericin B and miconazole (except after treatment with peplomycin), and greater resistance towards neutrophils. The results indicated that anticancer drugs and irradiation potentiated the virulence of *Candida* cells, or, by eliminating the cells with low virulence, enhanced the risk of oral and systemic candidiasis.

Willis et al. *(294)* studied the influence of nystatin and fluconazole on the virulence of *C. albicans* in oral candidosis in diabetic patients. Drug therapy was given at 6-h intervals for nystatin or daily with fluconazole for a maximum of 2 wk. Unlike nystatin, treatment with fluconazole reduced the ability of *C. albicans* to colonize the buccal mucosa for up to 8 wk after treatment. In addition of being antifungal, fluconazole reduced the production of phospholipase, modified the buccal epithelial cells, and reduced *C. albicans* adhesion to these cells for up to 8 wk post-treatment in diabetic patients with oral candidosis.

7. PROPHYLAXIS OF *CANDIDA* INFECTIONS

Even though data from prospective controlled trials have indicated that fluconazole can reduce the risk for mucosal (oropharyngeal, esophageal, and vaginal) candidiasis, routine primary prophylaxis is not recommended because of the effectiveness of therapy for acute disease, the low mortality associated with mucosal candidiasis, the potential for developing resistance to *Candida* spp., the possibility of drug interactions, and the cost of prophylaxis *(295)*. In addition, immune reconstitution following the introduction of HAART has led to a remarkable reduction in the incidence of opportunistic infections (and candidiasis, in particular) in patients with advanced AIDS. One of the benefits of HAART had been that in patients experiencing a favorable response to HAART, discontinuation of primary and secondary prophylaxis for candidiasis can be attempted with a decreased risk of recurrent infection *(284,296)*. Nevertheless, if recurrences are frequent or severe, prophylaxis with oral fluconazole or itraconazole solution ought to be considered (Table 3) *(295)*.

Just-Nubling et al. *(297)* conducted a randomized, open-label, clinical trial of fluconazole as a prophylactic treatment for recurrent oral candidiasis in AIDS patients with CD4$^+$ of less than 100 cells/mm^3. As compared to untreated controls, of the 58 evaluable patients who received fluconazole at either 50 or 100 mg daily (observation time: 137–215 d) prophylaxis significantly reduced the frequency of candidiasis relapse. The two fluconazole regimens were equally effective.

In patients undergoing chemotherapy, or bone-marrow transplant recipients, fluconazole as primary prophylaxis has shown greater clinical benefit than clotrimazole. In liver-transplant recipients, prophylaxis with amphotericin B, liposomal amphotericin B (AmBisome), and fluconazole have reduced both fungal colonization and the risk of serious *Candida* infections *(298,299)*. The risk of candidiasis following pancreatic transplantation is similar to that of liver transplantation. Fluconazole prophylaxis at 400 mg, daily for 1 wk after surgery reduced the frequency of intra-abdominal candidiasis from 10% to 7% *(300)*.

Data from a prospective, randomized, and placebo-controlled study of very low birth weight infants (less than 1500 g) have shown that prophylaxis with fluconazole (6.0 mg/kg, given either i.v. or by feeding tube) significantly reduced candidal rectal colonization from day-of-life (DOL) 14 through DOL 56 in all infants with a birth weight of <1250 g, and from DOL 14 through DOL 56 in all infants with a birth weight of 1250 to 1500 g *(301)*. There was no statistical difference between the fluconazole ($n = 53$) and placebo ($n = 50$) groups in the major risk factors known to increase the chances of candidal septicemia.

Table 3
Prophylaxis of Candidiasis in HIV-Infected Patients

Condition	Indication	Drug regimens	
		First line	Second line
Adults and adolescents			
Oropharyngeal, esophageal, or vaginal	Frequent/severe recurrences[a]	Fluconazole, 100–200 mg, orally, daily	Itraconazole solution, 200 mg, orally, daily; Ketoconazole, 200 mg, orally, daily
Hematologic malignancies		Fluconazole, 150 mg/kg, orally, every other day	
Infants and children			
Oropharyngeal	Frequent/severe recurrences[a]	Fluconazole, 3–6 mg/kg, orally, daily	
Esophageal	Frequent/severe recurrences[a]	Fluconazole, 3–6 mg/kg, orally, daily	Itraconazole solution, 5 mg/kg, orally, daily Ketoconazole, 5–10 mk/kg, orally, every 12–24 h
Organ transplantation, neutropenia		Amphotericin B, 10–20 mg, daily, i.v. AmBisome, 1.0 mg/kg, daily Fluconazole, 400 mg, daily, orally	

[a]After chemotherapy for acute disease had been applied.

Studying the impact of oral fluconazole (400 mg daily) prophylaxis in neutropenic patients receiving intensive cytotoxic therapy for acute leukemia or for autologous marrow transplantation, Laverdiere et al. *(302)* found that *C. albicans* colonization decreased from 30 to 10% whereas it increased from 32 to 57% in the placebo-receiving group ($p < 0.001$). Goranov et al. *(303)* have recommended fluconazole prophylaxis of 150 mg of the drug every other day in patients with hematological malignancies; the drug was discontinued when neutrophil count of less than $1.5 \times 10(9)/L$ was maintained.

Harousseau et al. *(304)* conducted a large multicenter, double-blind trial comparing the efficacy of oral itraconazole solution 2.5 mg/kg, b.i.d.) with amphotericin B capsules (500 mg, q.i.d.) in *Candida* prophylaxis. No colonization of the oropharynx was observed in the itraconazole group vs six (with three subsequent fungal infections) in the amphotericin B group. From the latter group, only 2 out of 20 patients showed colonization of the lower alimentary tract. In the itraconazole group, no fungal infections were observed. While the significance of yeast colonization of the lower alimentary tract remains unclear, the result of the trial indicated that itraconazole solution seemed to be an effective drug formulation for preventing candidal infections.

In a recent placebo-controlled study of long-term itraconazole antifungal prophylaxis of AIDS patients, Goldman et al. *(305)* found that it was associated with,

A targeted prophylaxis with three different daily dosages of amphotericin B complex (5.0, 2.5, and 1.0 mg/kg) in liver-transplant recipients requiring prolonged intensive care unit (ICU) treatment and at high risk for the development of invasive candidiasis, was well-tolerated and likely to prevent invasive fungal infections; 1.0-mg/kg daily was the recommended dose for this high-risk group *(306)*.

REFERENCES

1. Bodey, G. P., Ed. Candidiasis: Pathogenesis, Diagnosis, and Treatment, 2nd ed. Raven Press, New York, 1993.
2. Emmons, C. W., Binford, C. H., and Utz, J. P. *Medical Mycology*, 2nd ed. Lea & Fabiger, Philadelphia, 167, 1970.
3. Barnett, J. A., Payne, R. W., and Yarrow, D. *Yeasts - Characteristics and Identification*, 2nd ed. Cambridge University Press, New York, 1991.
4. Klotz, S. A. Plasma and extracellular matrix proteins mediate in the fate of *Candida albicans* in the human host. *Med. Hypotheses*, 42, 328, 1994.
5. Cotter, G. and Kavanagh, K. Adherence mechanisms of *Candida albicans*. *Br. J. Biomed. Sci.*, 57, 241–249, 2000.
6. Nicholls, P. E. and Henry, K. Gastritis and cimetidine: a possible explanation. *Lancet*, 1, 1095, 1978.
7. Ruddell, W. S. J., Azon, A. T. R., Findlay, J. M., Bartholomew, B. A., and Hill, M. J. Effect of cimetidine on the gastric bacterial flora. *Lancet*, 1, 672, 1980.
8. Seelig, M. S. The role of antibiotics in the pathogenesis of *Candida* infections. *Am. J. Med.*, 40, 887, 1966.
9. Stark, F. R., Ninos, N., Hutton, J., Katz, R., and Butler, M. *Candida* peritonitis and cimetidine. *Lancet*, 2, 744, 1978.
10. Triger, D. R., Goepel, J. R., Slater, D. N., and Underwood, J. C. W., Systemic candidiasis complicating acute hepatic failure in patients treated with cimetidine, *Lancet*, 2, 837, 1981.
11. McVay, L. V. Jr. and Sprunt, D. H. A study of moniliasis in aureomycin therapy. *Proc. Soc. Exp. Biol. Med.*, 78, 759, 1951.
12. Hughes, W. T., Kuhn, S., Chaudhary, S., et al. Successful chemoprophylaxis for *Pneumocystis carinii* pneumonia. *N. Engl. J. Med.*, 297, 1419, 1977.
13. Goldman, M., Pottage, J. C. Jr., and Weaver, D. C. *Candida krusei* fungemia: report of 4 cases and review of the literature. *Medicine (Baltimore)*, 72, 143, 1993.
14. Sandin, R. L., Meier, C. S., Crowder, M. L., and Greene, J. N. Concurrent isolation of *Candida krusei* and *Candida tropicalis* from multiple blood cultures in a patient with acute leukemia. *Arch. Pathol. Lab. Med.*, 117, 521, 1993.
15. Smaranayake, Y. H. and Samaranayake, L. P. *Candida krusei*: biology, epidemiology, pathogenicity and clinical manifestations of an emerging pathogen. *J. Med. Microbiol.*, 41, 295, 1994.
16. Wade, J. C. Epidemiology of *Candida* infections, in *Candidiasis: Pathogenesis, Diagnosis, and Treatment*, 2nd ed., Bodey, G. P., Ed. Raven Press, New York, 85, 1993.
17. Schaberg, D. R., Culver, D. H., and Gaines, R. P. Major trends in the microbial etiology of nosocomial infection. *Am. J. Med.*, 91(S3B), 72S, 1991.
18. Banerjee, S. N., Emori, T. G., Culver, D. H., et al. Secular trends in nosocomial primary blood-stream infections in the United States, 1980–1989. *Am. J. Med.*, 91(S3), 86S, 1991.
19. Rinaldi, M., Biology and pathogenicity of *Candida* species, in *Candidiasis: Pathogenesis, Diagnosis, and Treatment*, 2nd ed., Bodey, G. P., Ed. Raven Press, New York, 1, 1993.
20. Maksymiuk, A. W., Thongprasert, S., Hopfer, R., Luna, M. A., Fainstein, V., and Bodey, G. P. Systemic candidiasis in cancer patients. *Am. J. Med.*, 77, 20, 1984.
21. Myerowitz, R. L. Localized and disseminated candidiasis, in *The Pathology of Opportunistic Infections*, Myerowitz, R. L., Ed. Raven Press, New York, 95, 1983.
22. Myerowitz, R. L., Pazin, G. J., and Allen, C. M. Disseminated candidiasis: changes in incidence, underlying disease, and pathology. *Am. J. Clin. Pathol.*, 68, 29, 1977.
23. Gaines, J. D. and Remington, J. S. Disseminated candidiasis in the surgical patient. *Surgery*, 72, 730, 1972.
24. Vartivarian, S. and Smith, C. B. Pathogenesis, host resistance, and predisposing factors, in *Candidiasis: Pathogenesis, Diagnosis, and Treatment*, 2nd ed., Bodey, G. P., Ed. Raven Press, New York, 59, 1993.
25. Badrul, B. and Ruslan, G. *Candida albicans* infection of a prosthetic knee replacement: a case report. *Med. J. Malaysia*, 55(Suppl. C), 93-96, 2000.
26. Stein, D. K. and Sugar, A. M. Fungal infections in the immunocompromised host. *Diagn. Microbiol. Infect. Dis.*, 12, 221S, 1989.
27. Luna, M. A. and Tortoledo, M. E. Histologic identification and pathologic patterns of disease caused by *Candida*, in *Candidiasis: Pathogenicity, Diagnosis, and Treatment*, 2nd ed., Bodey, G. P., Ed. Raven Press, New York, 21, 1993.
28. Mancher, A. M., De Vinatea, M., Tuur, S. M., and Amgritt, P. AIDS and the mycosis. *Infect. Dis. Clin. North Am.*, 2, 827, 1988.
29. Warnock, D. W. Fungal complications of transplantation: diagnosis, treatment and prevention. *J. Antimicrob. Chemother.*, 36(Suppl. B), 73, 1995.
30. Wai, P. H., Ewing, C. A., Johnson, L. B., Lu, A. D., Attinger, C., and Kuo, P. C. *Candida* fascitis following renal transplantation. *Transplantation*, 72, 477–479, 2001.
31. Choi, I. S., Kim, S. J., Kim, B. Y., et al. *Candida* polyarthritis in a renal transplant patient: case report of a patient sussessfully treated with amphotericin B. *Transplant. Proc.*, 32, 1963–1964, 2000.
32. Edwards, J. E., Foos, R. Y., Montgomerie, J. Z., and Guze, J. B. Ocular manifestations of *Candida* septicemia: review of 76 cases of hematogenous *Candida* endophthalmitis. *Medicine (Baltimore)*, 53, 47, 1974.
33. Derkinderen, P., Bruneel, F., Bouchaud, O., and Regnier, B. Spondylodiscitis and epidural abscess due to *Candida albicans*. *Eur. Spine J.*, 9, 72–74, 2000.
34. Fanello, S., Bouchara, J. P., Jousset, N., Delbos, V., and LeFlohic, A. M. Nosocomial *Candida albicans* acquisition in a geriatric unit: epidemiology and evidence for person-to-person transmission. *J. Hosp. Infect.*, 47, 46–52, 2001.
35. Collado, A., Ponce De Leon, J., Salinas, D., Salvador, J., and Vicente, J. Prostatic abscess due to *Candida* with no systemic manifestation. *Urol. Int.*, 67, 186–188, 2001.

36. Wilcox, C. M. and Karowe, M. W. Esophageal infections: etiology, diagnosis, and management. *Gastroenterologist*, 2, 188, 1994.
37. Selik, R. M., Starcher, E. T., and Curran, J. W. Opportunistic diseases reported in AIDS patients: frequencies, associations, and trends. *AIDS*, 1, 175, 1987.
38. Torssander, J., Morfeldt-Manson, L., Biberfeld, G., Karlsson, A., Putkonen, P. O., and Wasserman, J. Oral *Candida albicans* in HIV infection. *Scand. J. Infect. Dis.*, 19, 291, 1987.
39. Abgrall, S., Charreau, I., Bloch, J., et al. Risk factors for esophageal candidiasis in HIV infection. *5th Conf. Retroviruses Opportunistic Infect.*, 172, abstract no. 492, 1998.
40. Kopicko, J. J., Momodu, I., Adedokun, A., Hoffman, M., Clark, R. A., and Kissinger, P. Characteristics of HIV-infected men with low serum testosterone levels. *Int. J. STD AIDS*, 10, 817–820, 1999.
41. Tavitian, A., Raufman, J. P., and Rosenthal, L. E. Oral candidiasis as a marker for esophageal candidiasis in the acquired immunodeficiency syndrome. *Ann. Intern. Med.*, 104, 54, 1986.
42. Pedersen, C., Gerstoft, J., Lindhardt, B. O., and Sindrup, J. *Candida* esophagits associated with acute human immunodeficiency virus infection. *J. Infect. Dis.*, 156, 529, 1987.
43. Green, B. I. Treatment of fungal infections in the human immunodeficiency virus-infected individual in *Antifungal Drug Therapy: A Complete Guide For the Practitioner*, Jacobs, P. H., and Nall, L., Eds. Marcel Dekker, New York, 237, 1990.
44. Oude Lashof, A. M., Donnelly, J. P., Meis, J. F., Van der Meer, J. W., and Kullberg, B. J. Duration of antifungal treatment and development of delayed complications in patients with candidemia. *38th Intersci. Conf. Antimicrob. Agents Chemother.*, 478, abstract no. J-97, 1998.
45. Palma-Carlos, A. G. and Palma-Carlos, M. L. Chronic mucocutaneous candidiasis revisited. *Allerg. Immunol. (Paris)*, 33, 229-232, 2001.
46. Mulero-Marchese, R. D., Blank, K. J., and Sieck, T. G. Genetic basis for protection against experimental vaginal candidiasis by peripheral immunozation. *J. Infect. Dis.*, 178, 227–234, 1998.
47. Elahi, S. Clancy, R., and Pang, G. A therapeutic vaccine for mucosal candidiasis. *Vaccine*, 19, 2516–2521, 2001.
48. Lopez, J., Pernot, C., Aho, S., et al. Decrease in *Candida albicans* strains with reduced susceptibility to fluconazole following changes in prescribing policies. *J. Hosp. Infect.*, 48, 122–123, 2001.
49. Hymes, S. R. and Duvic, M. Cutaneous candidiasis, in *Candidiasis: Pathogenesis, Diagnosis, and Treatment*, 2nd ed. Bodey, G. P., Ed., Raven Press, New York, 159, 1993.
50. del Palacio, A., Cuetara, S., Izquierdo, I., et al. A double-blind, randomized comparative trial: flutrimazole 1% solution versus bifonazole 1% solution once daily in dermatomycoses. *Mycoses*, 38, 395, 1995.
51. Stengel, F., Robles-Soto, M., Galimberti, R., and Suchil, P. Fluconazole versus ketoconazole in the treatment of dermatophytoses and cutaneous candidiasis. *Int. J. Dermatol.*, 33, 726, 1994.
52. Millikan, L. E. and Shrum, J. P. Systemic therapy for mycoses: changing targets and changing agents. *Int.J. Dermatol.*, 33, 701, 1994.
53. Nesseem, D. I. Formulation and evaluation of itraconazole via liquid crystal for topical delivery system. *J. Pharm. Biomed. Anal.*, 26, 387–399, 2001.
54. Pina-Vaz, C., Sansonetty, F., Rodriguez, A. G., Martinez-De-Oliveira, J., Fonseca, A. F., and Mardh, P. A. Antifungal activity of ibuprofen alone and in combination with fluconazole against *Candida* species. *J. Med. Microbiol.*, 49, 831–840, 2000.
55. Kirkpatrick, C. H. and Smith, T. K. Chronic mucocutaneous candidiasis: immunologic and antibiotic therapy. *Ann. Intern. Med.*, 80, 310, 1974.
56. Polizzi, B., Origgi, L., Zuccaro, G., Matti, P., and Scorza, R. Case report: successful treatment with cimetidine and zinc sulphate in chronic mucocutaneous candidiasis. *Am. J. Med. Sci.*, 311, 189, 1996.
57. de Doncker, P., van Lint, J., Dockx, P., and Roseeuw, D. Pulse therapy with one-week itraconazole monthly for three or four months in the treatment of onychomycosis. *Cutis*, 56, 180-183, 1995.
58. Roseeuw, D. and de Doncker, P. New approaches to the treatment of onychomycosis. *J. Am. Acad. Dermatol.*, 29, S45-S50, 1993.
59. Kirkpatrick, C. H. Chronic mucocutaneous candidiasis, in *Candidiasis: Pathogenesis, Diagnosis, and Treatment*, 2nd ed., Bodey, G. P., Ed. Raven Press, New York, 167, 1993.
60. Powderly, W. G., Gallant, J. E., Ghannoum, M. A., Mayer, K. H., Navarro, E. E., and Perfect, J. R. Oropharyngeal candidiasis in patients with HIV: suggested guidelines for therapy. *AIDS Res. Hum. Retroviruse*, 15, 1619-1623, 1999.
61. Laine, L. The natural history of esophageal candidiasis after successful treatment in patients with AIDS. *Gastroenterology*, 107, 744, 1994.
62. Chiou, C. C., Groll, A. H., Gonzalez, C. E., et al. Esophageal candidiasis in pediatric acquired immunodeficiency syndrome: clinical manifestation and risk factors. *Pediatr. Infect. Dis.*, 19, 729-734, 2000.
63. Roseff, S. A. and Sugar, A. M. Oral and esophageal candidiasis, in *Candidiasis: Pathogenesis, Diagnosis, and Treatment*, 2nd ed., Bodey, G. P. Ed. Raven Press, New York, 185, 1993.
64. Laine, L. and Rabeneck, L. Prospective study of fluconazole suspension for the treatment of esophageal candidiasis in patients with AIDS. *Aliment Pharmacol. Ther.*, 9, 553, 1995.
65. Encarnacion, M. and Chin, I. Salivary nystatin concentrations after administration of an osmotic controlled release tablet and a pastille. *Eur. J. Clin. Pharmacol.*, 46, 533, 1994.
66. Pelletier, R., Peter, J., Antin, C., Gonzalez, C., Wood, L., and Walsh, T. J. Emergence of resistance of *Candida albicans* to clotrimazole in human immunodeficiency virus-infected children: in vitro and clinical correlations. *J. Clin. Microbiol.*, 38, 1563-1568, 2000.

67. Goa, K. L. and Barradell, L. B. Fluconazole: an update of its pharmacodynamic and pharmacokinetic properties and therapeutic use in major supeficial and systemic mycoses in immunocompromised patients. *Drugs*, 50, 658, 1995.
68. Wilcox, C. M. Short report: time course of clinical response with fluconazole for *Candida* oesophagitis in patients with AIDS. *Aliment. Pharmacol. Ther.*, 8, 347, 1994.
69. Pagani, J. L., Chave, J. P., Iten, A., Durussel, C., Bille, J., and Glause, M. P. Treatment of oropharyngeal candidiasis (OPC) resistant to fluconazole (F) with escalating doses. *3rd Conf. Retroviruses Opportunistic Infect.*, 158, 1996.
70. Pons, V., Greenspan, D., and Debruin, M. Therapy for oropharyngeal candidiasis in HIV- infected patients: a randomized, prospective multicenter study of oral fluconazole versus clotrimazole troches. *J. Acquir. Immun. Defic. Syndr.*, 6, 1311, 1993.
71. Newton, J. A. Jr., Tasker, S. A., Bone, W. D., et al. Weekly fluconazole for the suppression of recurrent thrush in HIV-seropositive patients: impact on the incidence of disseminated cryptococcal infection. *AIDS*, 9, 1286, 1995.
72. Azon-Masoliver, A. and Vilaplana, J. Fluconazole-induced toxic epidermal necrolysis in a patient with human immunodeficiency virus infection. *Dermatology*, 187, 268, 1993.
73. Plettenberg, A., Stoehr, A., Höffken, G., et al. Fluconazole therapy of oral candidiasis in HIV-infected patients: results of a multicentre study. *Infection*, 22, 118, 1994.
74. Barbaro, G. and Di Lorenzo, G. Comparison of therapeutic activity of fluconazole and itraconazole in the treatment of oesophageal candidiasis in AIDS patients: a double-blind, randomized, controlled clinical study. *Ital. J. Gastroenterol.*, 27, 175, 1995.
75. Barbaro, G., Barbarini, G., and Di Lorenzo, G. Fluconazole vs. flucytosine in the treatment of esophageal candidiasis in AIDS patients: a double-blind, placebo-controlled study. *Endoscopy*, 27, 377, 1995.
76. Fichtenbaum, C. J., Zackin, R., Rajicic, N., Powderly, W. G., Wheat, L. J., and Zingman, B. S. Amphotericin B oral suspension for fluconazole-refractory oral candidiasis in persons with HIV infection. Adult AIDS Clinical Trials Group Study Team 295. *AIDS*, 14, 845–852, 2000.
77. Domenge, C., Wibault, P., Tancrede, C., et al. Randomized study of fluconazole (FCA) oral solution (OS) versus amphotericin B (AB) oral solution in oropharyngeal candidiasis (OPC) in head and neck cancer patients (HNCP) after radiotherapy. *38th Intersci. Conf. Antimicrob. Agents Chemother.*, 488, abstract no. J-131, 1998.
78. Smith, D., Midgley, J., and Gazzard, B. A randomized, double-blind study of itraconazole versus placebo in the treatment and prevention of fluconazole-resistant oral or oesophageal candidosis in patients with HIV infection. *Int. J. Clin. Pract.*, 53, 349–352, 1999.
79. Annonymous. Itraconazole solution for oral yeast infections. *Treat Update*, 10, 2–3, 1998.
80. Saag, M. S., Fessel, W. J., Kaufman, C. A., et al. Treatment of fluconazole-refractory oropharyngeal candidiasis with itraconazole oral solution in HIV-positive patients. *AIDS Res. Hum. Retroviruses*, 15, 1413–1417, 1999.
81. Walsh, T. J., McEvoy, M., Rishforth, B., et al. Cyclodextrin itraconazole in the treatment of oropharyngeal candidiasis (OPC) in pediatric patients with HIV infection: a phase I–II clinical trial. *38th Intersci. Conf. Antimicrob. Agents Chemother.*, 492, abstract no. J-145, 1998.
82. Smith, D. E., Midgley, J., Allan, M., Connolly, G. M., and Gazzard, B. G. Itraconazole versus ketoconazole in the treatment of oral and oesophageal candidiasis in patients infected with HIV. *AIDS*, 5, 1367, 1991.
83. de Repentigny, L., Ratelle, J., and the HIVIK Project group. Itraconazole vs. ketoconazole in HIV-positive patients with oropharyngeal and/or esophageal candidiasis. *Proc. 32nd Intersci. Conf. Antimicrob. Agents Chemother.*, American Society of Microbiology, Washington DC, abstract 1117, 1992.
84. Capetti, A., Bonfanti, P., Magni, C., and Milazzo, F. Employment of recombinant human granulocyte-macrophage colony stimulating factor in oesophageal candidiasis in AIDS patients. *AIDS*, 9, 1378, 1995.
85. Scadden, D. T. The use of GM-CSF in AIDS. *Infection*, 20(Suppl. 2), S103, 1992.
86. Jones, T. C. The effects of rHuGM-CSF on macrophage function. *Eur. J. Cancer*, 29A(Suppl. 3), S10, 1993.
87. Vazquez, J. A., Gupta, S., and Villanueva, A. Use of granulocyte-macrophage colony stimulating factor (GM-CSF) as an adjuvant to fluconazole in antifungal refractory oropharyngeal candidiasis in advanced AIDS patients. *5th Conf. Retroviruses Opportunistic Infect.*, 171, abstract no. 491, 1998.
88. Ellepola, A. N. and Samaranayake, L. P. Adjunctive use of chlorhexidine in oral candidoses: a review. *Oral Dis.*, 7, 11–17, 2001.
89. Rex, J. H., Walsh, T. J., Sobel, J. D., et al. Practice guidelines for the treatment of candidiasis. Infectious Diseases Society of America. *Clin. Infect. Dis.*, 30, 662–678, 2000.
90. Hallum, J. L. and Williams, T. W. Jr. *Candida* endocarditis, in *Candidiasis: Pathogenesis, Diagnosis, and Treatment*, 2nd ed., Bodey, G. P., Ed. Raven Press, New York, 357, 1993.
91. Rabinovici, R., Szewczyk, D., Ovadia, P., Greenspan, J. R., and Sivalingam, J. J. *Candida* pericarditis: clinical profile and treatment. *Ann. Thorac. Surg.*, 63, 1200–1204, 1997.
92. Edwards, J. E. Jr., Foos, R. Y., Montgomerie, J. Z., and Guze, L. B. Ocular manifestations of *Candida* septicemia: review of seventy-six cases of hematogenous *Candida* endophthalmitis. *Medicine (Baltimore)*, 53, 47, 1974.
93. Baddour, L. M. Long-term suppressive therapy for *Candida parapsilosis*-induced prosthetic valve endocarditis. *Mayo Clin. Proc.*, 70, 773–775, 1995.
94. Castiglia, M., Smego, R. A., and Sames, E. L. *Candida* endocarditis and amphotericin B intolerance: potential role of fluconazole. *Infect. Dis. Clin. Pract.*, 3, 248–253, 1994.
95. Bennett, J. E. Chemotherapy of systemic mycoses. *N. Engl. J. Med.*, 290, 30, 1974.
96. Borgers, M., vanden Bossche, H., and Cauwenbergh, G., The pharmacology of agents used in the treatment of pulmonary mycoses. *Clin. Chest Med.*, 7, 439, 1986.
97. Jensen, G. M., Skenes, C. R., Bunch, T. H., et al. Determination of the relative toxicity and efficacy of amphotericin B formulations: potassium release from red blood cells and *Candida albicans* cells. *38th Intersci. Conf. Antimicrob. Agents Chemother.*, 477, abstract no. J-94, 1998.

98. Miyata, A., Honda, K., Fujita, M., and Kikuchi, T. Multiple *Candida* liver abscesses successfully treated by continuous intrahepatic arterial infusion of amphotericin B using a reservoir in a case with acute myelocytic leukemia (M2). *Rinsho Ketsueki*, 36, 1217, 1995.
99. Rabkin, J. M., Orloff, S. L., Corless, C. L., et al. Association of fungal infection and increased mortality in liver transplant recipients. *Am. J. Surg.*, 179, 426–430, 2000.
100. Bowden, R. A., Cays, M., Gooley, T., Mamelok, R. D., and van Burik, J. A. Phase I study of amphotericin B colloidal dispersion for the treatment of invasive fungal infections after marrow transplant. *J. Infect. Dis.*, 173, 1208, 1996.
101. Caillot, D., Casasnovas, O., Solary, E., et al. Efficacy and tolerance of an amphotericin B lipid (intralipid) emulsion in the treatment of *Candidaemia* in neutropenic patients. *J. Antimicrob. Chemother.*, 31, 161, 1993.
102. Emminger, W., Graninger, W., Emminger-Schmidmeier, W., et al. Tolerance of high doses of amphotericin B by infusion of a liposomal formulation in children with cancer. *Ann. Hematol.*, 68, 27, 1994.
103. Nguyen, M. H., Peacock, J. E. Jr., Tanner, D. C., et al. Therapeutic approaches in patients with candidemia: evaluation of a multicenter, prospective, observational study. *Arch. Intern. Med.*, 155, 2429, 1995.
104. Rolston, K., Baird, I., Graham, D. R., and Jauregui, L. Treatment of refractory candemia in non-neutropenic patients with liposomal nystatin (NYOTRAN(tm)). *38th Intersci. Conf. Antimicrob. Agents Chemother.*, 24, abstract no. LB-1, 1998.
105. Rex, J. H., Bennett, J. E., Sugar, A. M., et al. A randomized trial comparing fluconazole with amphotericin B for the treatment of candidemia in patients without neutropenia. *N. Engl. J. Med.*, 331, 1325, 1994.
106. Wey, S. B., Mori, M., Pfaller, M. A., Woolson, R. F., and Wenzel, R. P. Hospital-acquired candidemia: the attributable mortality and excess length of stay. *Arch. Intern. Med.*, 148, 2642, 1988.
107. Fraser, V. J., Jones, M., Dunkel, J., Storfer, S., Medoff, G., and Dunagan, W. C. Candidemia in a tertiary care hospital: epidemiology, risk factors, and predictors of mortality. *Clin. Infect. Dis.*, 15, 414, 1992.
108. Raad, I. I. and Bodey, G. P. Infectious complications of indwelling vascular catheters. *Clin. Infect. Dis.*, 15, 197, 1992.
109. Lecciones, J. A., Lee, J. W., Navarro, E. E., et al. Vascular catheter-associated fungemia in patients with cancer analysis of 155 episodes. *Clin. Infect. Dis.*, 14, 875, 1992.
110. Meunier, F., Management of candidemia. *N. Engl. J. Med.*, 331, 1371, 1994.
111. Kullberg, B. J., Vandewoude, K., Aoun, M., Jacobs, F., Herbrecht, R., and Kujath, P. A double-blind, randomized, placebo-controlled phase II study of filgrastim (recombinant granulocyte colony-stimulating factor) in combination with fluconazole for treatment of invasive candidiasis and candidemia in nonneutropenic patients. *38th Intersci. Conf. Antimicrob. Agents Chemother.*, 479, abstract no. J-100, 1998.
112. Eilard, T., Alestig, K., and Wahlen, P. Treatment of disseminated candidiasis with 5- fluorocytosine. *J. Infect. Dis.*, 130, 155, 1974.
113. Vandevelde, A. G., Mauceri, A. A., and Johnson, J. E. III. 5-Fluorocytosine in the treatment of mycotic infections. *Ann. Intern. Med.*, 77, 1972.
114. Hoeprich, P. D., Ingraham, J. L., Kleker, E., and Winship, M. J. Development of resistance to 5-fluorocytosine in *Candida parapsilosis* during therapy. *J. Infect. Dis.*, 130, 112, 1974.
115. Montgomerie, J. Z., Edwards, J. E., and Guze, L. B. Synergism of amphotericin B and 5-fluorocytosine for *Candida* species. *J. Infect. Dis.*, 132, 82, 1975.
116. Rabinovich, S., Shaw, B. D., Bryant, T., and Donta, S. T. Effect of 5-fluorocytosine and amphotericin B on *Candida albicans* infection in mice. *J. Infect. Dis.*, 130, 28, 1974.
117. Fainstein, V., Bodey, G. P., Elting, L., Maksymiuk, A., Keating, M., and McCredie, K. B. Amphotericin B or ketoconazole therapy of fungal infections in neutropenic cancer patients. *Antimicrob. Agents Chemother.*, 31, 11, 1987.
118. Jordan, W. M., Bodey, G. P., Rodriguez, V., Ketchel, S. J., and Henney, J. Miconazole therapy for treatment of fungal infections in cancer patients. *Antimicrob. Agents Chemother.*, 16, 792, 1979.
119. Moyer, D. V. and Edwards, J. E. Jr. *Candida* endophthalmitis and central nervous system infection, in *Candidiasis: Pathogenesis, Diagnosis, and Treatment,* 2nd. ed., Bodey, G. P., Ed. Raven Press, New York, 331, 1993.
120. Lou, P., Kazdan, J., Bannatyne, R. M., and Cheung, R., Successful treatment of *Candida* endophthalmitis with a synergistic combination of amphotericin B and rifampin. *Am. J. Ophthalmol.*, 83, 12, 1977.
121. Peyman, G. A., Vastine, D. W., and Meisels, H. I., The experimental and clinical use of intravitreal antibiotics to treat bacterial and fungal endophthalmitis. *Doc. Ophthalmol.*, 39, 183, 1975.
122. Huang, K., Peyman, G. A., and McGetrick, J. Vitrectomy in experimental endophthalmitis. Part I. Fungal infection. *Ophthalmic Surg.*, 10, 84, 1979.
123. Blumenkranz, M. S. and Stevens, D. A. Therapy of endogenous fungal endophthalmitis: miconazole or amphotericin B for coccidioidal and candidal infection. *Arch. Ophthalmol.*, 98, 1216, 1980.
124. Venditti, M., De Bernardis, F., Micozzi, A., et al. Fluconazole treatment of catheter-related right-sided endocarditis caused by *Candida albicans* and associated with endophthalmitis and folliculitis. *Clin. Infect. Dis.*, 14, 422, 1992.
125. Filler, S. G., Crislip, M. A., Mayer, C. L., and Edwards, J. E. Jr. Comparison of fluconazole and amphotericin B for treatment of disseminated candidiasis and endophthalmitis in rabbits. *Antimicrob. Agents Chemother.*, 35, 288, 1991.
126. Nomura, J. and Ruskin, J. Failure of therapy with fluconazole for candidal endophthalmitis. *Clin. Infect. Dis.*, 17, 888, 1993.
127. Abbasoglu, O. E., Hosal, B. M., Sener, B., Erdemoglu, N., and Gursel, E. Penetration of topical fluconazole into human aqueous humor. *Exp. Eye Res.*, 72, 147-151, 2001.
128. Stern, G. A., Fetkenhour, C. L., and O'Grady, R. B. Intravitreal amphotericin B treatment of *Candida* endophthalmitis. *Arch. Ophthalmol.*, 95, 89, 1977.

129. Perraut, L. E. Jr., Perraut, E., Bleiman, B., and Lyons, J. Successful treatment of *Candida albicans* endophthalmitis with intravitreal amphotericin B. *Arch. Ophthalmol.*, 99, 1565, 1981.
130. Souri, E. N. and Green, W. R. Intravitreal amphotericin B toxicity. *Am. J. Ophthalmol.*, 78, 77, 1974.
131. Liu, K. R., Peyman, G. A., and Khoobehi, B. Efficacy of liposome-bound amphotericin B for the treatment of experimental fungal endophthalmitis in rabbits. *Invest. Ophthalmol. Vis. Sci.*, 30, 1527, 1989.
132. Aguilar, G. L., Blumenkrantz, M. S., Egbert, P. R., and McCulley, J. P. *Candida* endophthalmitis after intravenous drug abuse. *Arch. Ophthalmol.*, 97, 96, 1979.
133. Snip, R. C. and Michels, R. G. Pars plana vitrectomy in the management of endogenous *Candida* endophthalmitis. *Am. J. Ophthalmol.*, 82, 699, 1976.
134. Santos, R., de Buen, S., and Juarez, P. Experimental *Candida albicans* chorioretinitis treated by laser. *Am. J. Ophthalmol.*, 63, 440, 1967.
135. Bagnoud, M., Baglivo, E., Hengstler, J., Safran, A. B., Pournaris, C. J., and Leuenberger, P. Endogenous fungal endophthalmitis: results of antifungal treatment with and without vitrectomy. *Klin. Monatsbl. Augenheilkd.*, 218, 398-400, 2001.
136. Chesney, P. J., Justman, R. A., and Bogdanowicz, W. M. *Candida* meningitis in newborn infants: a review and report of combined amphotericin B-flucytosine therapy. *Johns Hopkins Med. J.*, 142, 155,1978.
137. Smego, R. A. Jr., Perfect, J. R., and Durack, D. T. Combined therapy with amphotericin B and 5-fluorocytosine for *Candida* meningitis. *Rev. Infect. Dis.*, 6, 791, 1984.
138. Sanchez-Portocarrero, J., Perez-Cecilia, E., Corral, O., Romero-Vivas, J., and Picazo, J. J. The central nervous system and infection by *Candida* species. *Diagn. Microbiol. Infect. Dis.*, 37, 169–179, 2000.
139. Mohan Rao, H. K. and Myers, G. J. *Candida* meningitis in the newborn. *South. Med. J.*, 72, 1468, 1979.
140. Aldress, K., Al Shaalan, M., Memish, Z., Alola, S., and Bannatyne, R. *Candida* meningitis in children: two cases report. *J. Chemother.*,12, 339-344, 2000.
141. Murphy, K., Bradley, J., and James, H. E. The treatment of *Candida albicans* shunt infections. *Childs. Nerv. Syst.*, 16, 4–7, 2000.
142. Soto-Hernandez, J. L., Ramirez-Crescencio, M. A., Moreno Estrada, V. M., and del Valle Robles, R. *Candida albicans* cerebral granulomas associated with a nonfunctional cerebrospinal fluid shunt: case report. *Neurosurgery*, 47, 973-976, 2000.
143. Rubinstein, E., Noriega, E. R., Simberkoff, M. S., Holzman, R., and Rahal, J. J. Fungal endocarditis: analysis of 24 cases and review of the literature. *Medicine (Baltimore)*, 54, 331, 1975.
144. Merchant, R. K., Louria, D. B., Geiseler, P. H., Edgcomb, J. H., and Utz, J. P. Fungal endocarditis: review of the literature and report of three cases. *Ann. Intern. Med.*, 48, 242, 1958.
145. Kay, J. H., Bernstein, S., Feinstein, D., and Biddle, M. Surgical cure of *Candida albicans* endocarditis with open heart surgery. *N. Engl. J. Med.*, 264, 907, 1961.
146. Kay, J. H., Bernstein, S., Tsuji, H. K., Redington, J. V., Milgram, M., and Brem, T. Surgical treatment of *Candida* endocarditis. *J. Am. Med. Assoc.*, 203, 105, 1968.
147. Lerner, P. I. Infective endocarditis: a review of selected topics. *Med. Clin. North Am.*, 58, 605, 1974.
148. Record, C. O., Skinner, J. M., Speight, P., and Speller, D. C. E. *Candida* endocarditis treated with 5-fluorocytosine. *Br. Med. J.*, 1, 262, 1971.
149. McRae, A. T., Pate, J. W., and Richardson, R. L. Aortic valve replacement for *Candida* endocarditis. *Chest*, 62, 757, 1972.
150. Fass, R. J. and Perkins, R. L. 5-Fluorocytosine in the treatment of cryptococcal and *Candida* mycoses. *Ann. Intern. Med.*, 74, 535, 1971.
151. Utley, J. R., Mills, J., Hutchinson, J. C., Edmunds, L. H., Sanderson, R. G., and Roe, B. B. Valve replacement for bacterial and fungal endocarditis. *Circulation*, 42–43(Suppl. 3), 42, 1973.
152. Utley, R. J., Mills, J., and Roe, B. B. Role of valve replacement in the treatment of fungal endocarditis. *J. Thorac. Cardiovasc. Surg.*, 69, 255, 1974.
153. Rubinstein, E., Noriega, E. R., Simberkoff, M. S., and Rahal, J. T. Tissue penetration of amphotericin B in *Candida* endocarditis. *Chest*, 66, 376, 1974.
154. Stinson, E. B., Griepp, R. B., Vostik, K., Copeland, J. G., and Shumway, N. E. Operative treatment of active endocarditis. *J. Thorac. Cardiovasc. Surg.*, 71, 659, 1975.
155. Rotheman, E. B. and Magovern, G. J. Two year cure of *Candida* infection of prosthetic mitral valve. *Postgrad. Med. J.*, 61, 237, 1977.
156. Richardson, J. V., Karp, R. B., Kirklin, J. W., and Dismukes, W. E. Treatment of infective endocarditis: a ten year comparative analysis. *Circulation*, 58, 589, 1978.
157. Stinson, E. B. Surgical treatment of infective endocarditis. *Prog. Cardiovasc. Res.*, 22, 145, 1979.
158. Brown, L. A., Baddley, J. W., Sanchez, J. E., and Bachmann, L. H. Implantable cardioverter-defibrilator endocarditis secondary to *Candida albicans*. *Am. J. Med. Sci.*, 322, 160-162, 2001.
159. Liang, J. D., Fang, C. T., Chen, Y. C., Chang, S. C., and Luh, K. T. *Candida albicans* spinal epidural abscess secondary to prosthetic valve endocarditis. *Diagn. Microbiol. Infect. Dis.*, 40, 121-123, 2001.
160. Montague, N. T. and Sugg, W. L. *Candida* endocarditis with femoral emboli. *J. Thorac. Cardiovasc. Surg.*, 67, 322, 1973.
161. Martino, P., Meloni, G., and Cassone, A. Candidal endocarditis and treatment with fluconazole and granulocyte-macrophage colony-stimulating factor. *Ann. Intern. Med.*, 112, 966, 1990.

162. Wells, C. J., Leech, G. J., Lever, A. M., and Wansbrough-Jones, M. H. Treatment of native valve *Candida* endocarditis with fluconazole. *J. Infect.*, 31, 233, 1995.
163. Longman, L. P., Hibbert, S. A., and Martin, M. V. Efficacy of fluconazole in prophylaxis and treatment of experimental *Candida* endocarditis. *Rev. Infect. Dis.*, 12(Suppl. 3), S294, 1990.
164. Nishida, T., Mayumi, H., Kawachi, Y., et al. The efficacy of fluconazole in treating prosthetic valve endocarditis caused by *Candida glabratal*: repeat of a case. *Surg. Today*, 24, 651–654, 1994.
165. Fidel, P. L., Jr. Vaginal candidiasis: review and role of local mucosal immunity. *AIDS Patient Care STDS*, 12, 359-366, 1998.
166. Isaacs, J. H. Nystatin vaginal cream in monilial vaginitis. *Int. Med. J.*, 143, 240, 1973.
167. Sobel, J. D. Genital candidiasis, in *Candidiasis: Pathogenesis, Diagnosis, and Treatment*, 2nd ed., Bodey, G. P., Ed. Raven Press, New York, 225, 1993.
168. Droegemueller, W., Adamson, D. G., Brown, D., et al. Three day treatment with butoconazole nitrate for vulvovaginal candididasis. *Obstet. Gynecol.*, 64, 530, 1984.
169. Corson, S. L., Kapikian, R. R., and Nehring, R. Terconazole and miconazole cream for treating vulvovaginal candidiasis: a comparison. *J. Reprod. Med.*, 36, 561, 1991.
170. Breuker, G., Jurczok, F., Naerts, M., Weinhold, E., and Krause, U. Single-dose therapy of vaginal mycoses with clotrimazole vaginal cream 10%. *Mykosen*, 29, 427, 1986.
171. Van der Meijden, W. I., Van der Hoek, J. C. S., Staal, H. J. M., Van Joost, T., and Stolz, E. Double-blind comparison of 200 mg ketoconazole oral tablets and 1200 mg miconazole vaginal capsule in the treatment of vaginal candidosis. *Eur. J. Obstet. Gynecol. Reprod. Biol.*, 22, 133, 1986.
172. Ritter, W. Pharmacokinetic fundamentals of vaginal treatment with clotrimazole. *Am. J. Obstet. Gynecol.*, 152, 945, 1985.
173. Odds, F. C. and MacDonald, F. Persistence of miconazole in vaginal secretions after single application of the antifungal: implications for the treatment of vaginal candidosis. *Br. J. Vener. Dis.*, 57, 400, 1981.
174. Lindeque, B. G. and Van Niekerk, W. A. Treatment of vaginal candidiasis in pregnancy with a single clotrimazole 500 mg vaginal pessary. *S. Afr. Med. J.*, 65, 123, 1984.
175. Bingham, J. S. Single blind comparison of ketoconazole 200 mg oral tablets and clotrimazole 100 mg vaginal tablets and 1% cream in treating acute candidosis. *Br. J. Vener. Dis.*, 60, 175, 1984.
176. Cauwenbergh, G. Itraconazole: the first orally active antifungal for single-day treatment of vaginal candidosis. *Curr. Ther. Res.*, 41, 210, 1987.
177. Brammer, K. W. Treatment of vaginal candidiasis with a single oral dose of fluconazole. *Eur. J. Clin. Microbiol. Infect. Dis.*, 7, 364, 1988.
178. Frega, A., Gallo, G., Di Renzi, F., Stolfi, G., and Stentella, P. Persistent vulvovaginal candidiasis: systemic treatment with oral fluconazole. *Clin. Exp. Obstet. Gynecol.*, 21, 259, 1994.
179. Kukner, S., Ergin, T., Cicek, N., Ugur, M., Yesilyurt, H., and Gokmen, O. Treatment of vaginitis. *Int. J. Gynaecol. Obstet.*, 52, 43, 1996.
180. Ferris, D. G., Litaker, M. S., Woodward, L., Mathis, D., and Hendrich, J. Treatment of bacterial vaginosis: a comparison of oral metronidazole, metronidazole vaginal gel, and clindamycin vaginal cream. *J. Fam. Pract.*, 41, 443, 1995.
181. Sobel, J. D., Kapernick, P. S., Zervos, M., et al. Treatment of complicated *Candida* vaginitis: comparison of single and sequential doses of fluconazole. *Am. J. Obstet. Gynecol.*, 185, 363–369, 2001.
182. O-Prasertsawat, P. and Bourlert, A. Comparative study of fluconazole and clotrimazole for the treatment of vulvovaginal candidiasis. *Sex. Transm. Dis.*, 22, 228, 1995.
183. Sobel, J. D., Schmitt, C., Stein, G., Mummaw, N., Christensen, S., and Meriwether, C. Initial management of recurrent vulvovaginal candidiasis with oral ketoconazole and topical clotrimazole. *J. Reprod. Med.*, 39, 517, 1994.
184. Azzena, A. and Vasoin, F. Systemic treatment of recurrent candidal vulvovaginitis by itraconazole. *Clin. Exp. Obstet. Gynecol.*, 21, 59, 1994.
185. Sobel, J. D. Recurrent vulvovaginal candidiasis: a perspective study of the efficacy of maintenance ketoconazole therapy. *N. Engl. J. Med.*, 315, 1455, 1986.
186. Sobel, J. D. Management of recurrent vulvovaginal candidiasis with intermittent ketoconazole prophylaxis. *Obstet. Gynecol.*, 65, 123, 1985.
187. Davidson, F. and Mould, R. F. Recurrent genital candidosis in women and the effect of intermittent prophylactic treatment. *Br. J. Vener. Dis.*, 54, 176, 1978.
188. Pekhlivanov, B. and Markova, R. The treatment of vaginal mycosis with Orungal. *Akush. Ginekol. (Sofia)*, 38, 56–58, 1999.
189. Moraes, P. S., de Lima Goiaba, S., and Taketomi, E. A. *Candida albicans* allergen immunotherapy in recurrent vaginal candidiasis. *J. Investig. Allergol. Clin. Immunol.*, 10, 305–309, 2000.
190. Nix, D. E., Durrence, C. W., and May, J. R. Amphotericin B bladder irrigation. *Drug Intell. Clin. Pharm.*, 19, 299, 1985.
191. Wise, G. J., Kozinn, P. J., and Goldberg, P. Amphotericin B as a urologic irrigant in the management of noninvasive candiduria. *J. Urol.*, 128, 82, 1982.
192. Nito, H. Clinical efficacy of fluconazole in urinary tract fungal infections. *Jpn. J. Antibiot.*, 42, 171, 1989.
193. Edwards, J. E. Jr. *Candida* species, in *Principles and Practice of Infectious Diseases*, Mandell, G. L., Douglas, R. G. Jr., and Bennett, J. E., Eds. Churchill Livingston, New York, 1954, 1990.
194. Dreetz, D. J. and Fetchick, R. Fungal infections of the urinary tract and kidney, in *Diseases of the Kidney*, vol. 1, Schrier, R. W. and Gottschalk, C. W., Eds. Little, Brown & Co., 1015, 1988.

195. Strassner, C. and Friesen, A. Therapy of candiduria by alkalinization of urine: oral treatment with potassium-sodium-hydrogen citrate. *Fortschr. Med.*, 113, 359, 1995.
196. Sanford, J. P. The enigma of candiduria: evolution of bladder irrigation with amphotericin B for management - from anecdote to dogma and a lesson from Machiavelli. *Clin. Infect. Dis.*, 16, 145, 1993.
197. Occhipinti, D. J., Schoonover, L. L., and Danziger, L. H. Bladder irrigation with amphotericin B for treatment of patients with candiduria. *Clin. Infect. Dis.*, 17, 812, 1993.
198. Sanford, J. P. Bladder irrigation with amphotericin B for treatment of patients with candiduria: a reply. *Clin. Infect. Dis.*, 17, 813, 1993.
199. Johnson, J. R. Should all catheterized patients with candiduria be treated? *Clin. Infect. Dis.*, 17, 814, 1993.
200. Sanford, J. P. Should all catheterized patients with candiduria be treated?: a reply. *Clin. Infect. Dis.*, 17, 814, 1993.
201. Simsek, U., Akinci, H., Oktay, B., Kavrama, I., and Ozyurt, M. Treatment of catheter-associated candiduria with fluconazole irrigation. *Br. J. Urol.*, 75, 75, 1995.
202. Cartwright, R. Y., Shaldon, C., and Hall, G. H. Urinary candidiasis after renal transplantation. *Br. Med. J.*, 2, 351, 1972.
203. Price, E., Webb, E. A., and Smith, B. A. Urinary tract candidiasis treated with amphotericin B. *Br. J. Urol.*, 98, 523, 1967.
204. Blum, J. A. Acute monilial pyohydronephrosis: report of a case successfully treated with amphotericin B. *J. Urol.*, 96, 614, 1966.
205. Gentry, L. O. and Price, M. F. Urinary and peritoneal *Candida* infections, in *Candidiasis: Pathogenesis, Diagnosis, and Treatment*, 2nd ed., Bodey, G. P., Ed. Raven Press, New York, 249, 1993.
206. Gerle, R. D. Roentgenographic features of primary renal candidiasis: fungus ball of the renal pelvis and ureter. *Am. J. Roentgenol. Radium Ther. Nucl. Med.*, 119, 731, 1973.
207. Bayer, A. S., Blumenkranta, M. J., Mongomerie, J. Z., Galpin, J. E., Coburn, J. W., and Guze, L. B. *Candida* peritonitis: report of 22 cases and review of the English literature. *Am. J. Med.*, 61, 832, 1976.
208. Eisenberg, E. S., Leviton, I., and Soerio, R. Fungal peritonitis in patients receiving peritoneal dialysis: experience with 11 patients and review of the literature. *Rev. Infect. Dis.*, 8, 309, 1986.
209. Fabris, A., Biasioli, S., Borin, D., et al. Fungal peritonitis in peritoneal dialysis: our experience and review of treatments. *Perit. Dial. Bull.*, 4, 75, 1984.
210. Johnson, R. J., Ramsey, P., Gallagher, N., and Ahmad, S. Fungal peritonitis in patients on peritoneal dialysis: incidence, clinical features and prognosis. *Am. J. Nephrol.*, 5, 169, 1985.
211. Benevent, D., Peyronnet, P., Lagarde, C., and Leroux-Robert, C. Fungal peritonitis in patients on continuous ambulatory peritoneal dialysis: three recoveries in 5 cases without catheter removal. *Nephron*, 41, 203, 1985.
212. Vergemezis, V., Papadopoulou, Z. L., Liamos, H., et al. Management of fungal peritonitis during continuous ambulatory peritoneal dialysis (CAPD). *Perit. Dial. Bull.*, 6, 17, 1986.
213. Tapson, J. S., Mansy, H., Freeman, R., and Wilkinson, R. The high morbidity of CAPD fungal peritonitis - description of 10 cases and review of treatment strategies. *Q. J. Med.*, 61, 1047, 1986.
214. Rubin, J., Kirchner, K., Walsh, D., Green, M., and Bower, J. Fungal peritonitis during continuous ambulatory peritoneal dialysis: a report of 17 cases. *Am. J. Kidney Dis.*, 10, 361, 1987.
215. Struijk, D. G., Krediet, R. T., Boeschoten, E. W., Rietra, P. J., and Arisz, L. Antifungal treatment of *Candida* peritonitis in continuous ambulatory peritoneal dialysis patients. *Am. J. Kidney Dis.*, 9, 66, 1987.
216. Pocheville, M., Charpentier, B., Brocard, J. F., Benarbia, S., Hammouche, M., and Fries, D. Successful in situ treatment of fungal peritonitis during CAPD. *Nephron*, 37, 66, 1984.
217. Cecchin, E., De Marchi, S., Panarello, G., and Tesio, F. Chemotherapy and/or removal of the peritoneal catheter in the management of fungal peritonitis complicating CAPD? *Nephron*, 40, 251, 1985.
218. Arfania, D., Everett, E. D., Nolph, K. D., and Rubin, J. Uncommon causes of peritoneal dialysis. *Arch. Intern. Med.*, 141, 61, 1981.
219. Lee, S. H., Chiang, S. S., Hsieh, S. J., and Shen, H. M. Successful treatment of fungal peritonitis with intracatheter antifungal retention. *Adv. Perit. Dial.*, 11, 172, 1995.
220. Blowey, D. L., Garg, U. C., Kearns, G. L., and Warady, B. A. Peritoneal penetration of amphotericin B lipid complex and fluconazole in a pediatric patient with fungal peritonitis. *Adv. Perit. Dial.*, 14, 247–250, 1998.
221. Montenegro, J., Aguirre, R., Gonzalez, O., Martinez, I., and Saracho, R. Fluconazole treatment of *Candida* peritonitis with delayed removal of the peritoneal dialysis catheter. *Clin. Nephrol.*, 44, 60, 1995.
222. Dismukes, W. E. Azole antifungal drugs: old and new. *Ann. Intern. Med.*, 109, 177, 1988.
223. Saag, M. S. and Dismukes, W. E. Azole antifungal agents: emphasis on new triazoles. *Antimicrob. Agents Chemother.*, 32, 1, 1988.
224. Levin, J., Bernard, D. B., Idelson, B. A., Farnham, H., Saunders, C., and Sugar, A. M. Fungal peritonitis complicating continuous ambulatory peritoneal dialysis: successful treatment with fluconazole, a new orally active antifungal agent. *Am. J. Med.*, 86, 825, 1989.
225. Corbella, X., Sirvent, J. M., and Carratala, J. Fluconazole treatment without catheter removal in *Candida albicans* peritonitis complicating peritoneal dialysis. *Am. J. Med.*, 90, 227, 1991.
226. Voss, A., Meis, J. F., and Hoogkamp-Korstanje, J. A. Fluconazole in the management of fungal urinary tract infections. *Infection*, 22, 247, 1994.
227. Corbella, X., Carratala, J., Castells, M., and Berlanga, B. Fluconazole treatment in *Torulopsis glabrata* upper urinary tract infection causing ureteral obstruction. *J. Urol.*, 147, 1116, 1992.
228. Ansari, S. H., Levin, M. H., and Lipshitz, S. Re: fluconazole treatment in Toluropsis glabrata upper urinary tract infection causing ureteral obstruction. *J. Urol.*, 154, 1870, 1995.

229. Dermoumi, H. In vitro susceptibility of yeast isolates from the blood to fluconazole and amphotericin B. *Chemotherapy*, 38, 112, 1992.
230. Morace, G., Manzara, S., and Dettori, G. In vitro susceptibility of 119 yeast isolates to fluconazole, 5-fluorocytosine, amphotericin B and ketoconazole. *Chemotherapy*, 37, 23, 1991.
231. Hitchcock, C. A., Pye, G. W., Troke, P. F., Johnson, E. M., and Warnock, D. W. Fluconazole resistance in *Candida glabrata*. *Antimicrob. Agents Chemother.*, 37, 1962, 1993.
232. Warnock, D. W., Burke, J., Cope, N. J., Johnson, E. M. von Fraunhofer, N. A., and Williams, E. W., Fluconazole resistance in *Candida glabrata*. *Lancet*, 2, 1310, 1988.
233. Michel, C., Courdavault, L., al Khayat, R., Viron, B., Roux, P., and Mignon, F. Fungal peritonitis in patients on peritoneal dialysis. *Am. J. Nephrol.*, 14, 113, 1994.
234. Sobel, J. D., Kaufmann, C. A., McKinsey, D., et al. Candiduria: a randomized, double-blind study of treatment with fluconazole and placebo. The National Institute of Allergy and Infectious Diseases (NIAID) Mycoses Study Group. *Clin. Infect. Dis.*, 30, 19–24, 2000 [see also: *Clin. Infect. Dis.*, 31, 209–210, 2000].
235. Hansen, B. L. and Andersen, K. Fungal arthritis. *Scand. J. Rheumatol.*, 24, 248, 1995.
236. Lafont, A., Olivé, A., Gelman, M., Roca-Burniols, J., Cots, R., and Carbonell, J. *Candida albicans* spondylodiscitis and vertebral osteomyelitis in patients with intravenous heroin drug addiction: report of 3 new cases. *J. Rheumatol.*, 21, 953, 1994.
237. Merrer, J., Dupont, B., Nieszkowska, A., De Jonghe, B., and Outin, H. *Candida albicans* prosthetic arthritis treated with fluconazole alone. *J. Infect.*, 42, 208–209, 2001.
238. Weisse, M. E., Person, D. A., and Berkenbaugh, J. T. Jr. Treatment of *Candida* arthritis with fluconazole and amphotericin B. *J. Perinatol.*, 13, 402, 1993.
239. Oleinik, E. M., Della-Latta, P., Rinaldi, M. G., and Saiman, L. *Candida lusitaniae* osteomyelitis in a premature infant. *Am. J. Perinatol.*, 10, 313, 1993.
240. Marra, F., Robbins, G. M., Masri, B. A., et al. Amphotericin B-loaded bone cement to treat osteomyelitis caused *Candida albicans*. *Can. J. Surg.*, 44, 383–386, 2001.
241. Tang, C. Successful treatment of *Candida albicans* osteomyelitis with fluconazole. *J. Infect.*, 26, 89, 1993.
242. Dan, M. and Priel, I. Failure of fluconazole therapy for sternal osteomyelitis. *Clin. Infect. Dis.*, 18, 126, 1994.
243. Witek-Janusek, L., Cusack, C., and Mathews, H. L. *Candida albicans*: an opportunistic threat to critically ill low birth weight infants. *Dimens. Crit. Care Nurs.*, 17, 243-255, 1998.
244. Hughes, P. A., Lepow, M. L., and Hill, H. R. Neonatal candidiasis, in *Candidiasis: Pathogenesis, Diagnosis, and Treatment*, 2nd ed., Bodey, G. P., Ed. Raven Press, New York, 261, 1993.
245. Glick, C., Graves, G. R., and Feldman, S. Neonatal fungemia and amphotericin B. *South. Med. J.*, 86, 1368, 1993.
246. Baley, J. E., Kliegman, R. M., and Faranoff, A. A. Disseminated fungal infections in very low birth weight infants: therapeutic toxicity. *Pediatrics*, 73, 153, 1984.
247. Delaplane, D., Wiringa, K. S., Shulman, S. F., and Yogev, R. Congenital mucocutaneous candidiasis following diagnostic amniocentesis. *Am. J. Obstet. Gynecol.*, 147, 342, 1983.
248. Starke, J. R., Mason, E., Kraner, W. G., and Kaplan, S. L. Pharmacokinetics of amphotericin B in infants and children. *J. Infect. Dis.*, 155, 766, 1987.
249. Butler, K. M. and Baker, C. J. *Candida*: an increasingly important pathogen in nursery. *Pediatr. Clin. North Am.*, 35, 543, 1988.
250. Stern, J. H., Calvano, C., and Simon, J. W. Recurrent endogenous candidal endophthalmitis in a premature infant. *J. AAPOS*, 5, 50–51, 2001.
251. Todd Johnston, W. and Cogen, M. S. Systemic candidiasis with cataract formation in a premature infant. *J. AAPOS*, 4, 386–388, 2000.
252. Mogyorosy, G., Soos, G., and Nagy, A. *Candida* endocarditis in a premature infant. *J. Perinat. Med.*, 28, 407–411, 2000.
253. Aydin, M., Kucukoduk, S., Yalin, T., Cetinkaya, F., and Gurses, N. Amphotericin B in the treatment of *Candida* meningitis in three neonates. *Turk. J. Pediatr.*, 37, 247, 1995.
254. Plak, A. Pharmacokinetics of amphotericin B and flucytosine. *Postgrad. Med. J.*, 55, 667, 1979.
255. al-Rasheed, S. A. The management of fungal obstructive uropathy in neonates and infants. *Ann. Trop. Paediatr.*, 14, 169, 1994.
256. Stocker, M., Caduff, J. H., Spalinger, J., and Berger, T. M. Successful treatment of bilateral renal fungal balls with liposomal amphotericin B and fluconazole in an extremely low birth weight infant. *Eur. J. Pediatr.*, 159, 676–678, 2000.
257. Ringdén, O., Tollemar, J., Dahllof, G., and Tyden, G. High cure rate of invasive fungal infections in immunocompromised children using ambisome. *Transplant. Proc.*, 26, 175, 1994.
258. Juster-Reicher, A., Leibovitz, E., Linder, N., et al. Liposomal amphotericin B (AmBisome) in the treatment of neonatal candidiasis in very low birth weight infants. *Infection*, 28, 223–226, 2000.
259. Lackner, H., Schwinger, W., Urban, C., et al. Liposomal amphotericin B (AmBisome) for treatment of disseminated fungal infections in two infants of very low birth weight. *Pediatrics*, 89, 1259, 1992.
260. Pereira da Silva, L., Videira Amaral, J. M., and Cordeiro Ferreira, N. Which is the most appropriate dosage of liposomal amphotericin B (AmBisome) for the treatment of fungal infections in infants of very low birth weight? *Pediatrics*, 91, 1217, 1993.
261. Butler, K. M., Rench, M. A., and Baker, C. J. Amphotericin B as a single agent in the treatment of systemic candidiasis in neonates. *Pediatr. Infect. Dis. J.*, 9, 51, 1990.
262. Clarke, M. and Davies, D. P. Neonatal systemic candidiasis treated with miconazole. *Br. Med. J.*, 281, 354, 1980.

263. Dupont, B. and Drouet, E. In vitro synergy and antagonism of antifungal agents against yeast-like fungi. *Postgrad. Med. J.*, 55, 683, 1979.
264. Viscolli, C., Castagnola, E., Fioredda, F., Ciravegna, B., Barigone, G., and Terragna, A. Fluconazole in the treatment of candidiasis in immunocompromised children. *Antimicrob. Agents Chemother.*, 35, 365, 1991.
265. Fasano, C., O'Keeffe, J., and Gibbs, D. Fluconazole treatment of neonates and infants with severe fungal infections not treatable with conventional agents. *Eur. J. Clin. Microbiol. Infect. Dis.*, 13, 351, 1994.
266. Scwarze, R., Penk, A., and Pittrow, L. Treatment of candidal infections with fluconazole in neonates and infants. *Eur. J. Med. Res.*, 5, 203–208, 2000.
267. Marr, B., Gross, S., Cunningham, C., and Weiner, L. Candidal sepsis and meningitis in a very-low-birth-weight infant successfully treated with fluconazole and flucytosine. *Clin. Infect. Dis.*, 19, 795, 1994.
268. Epelbaum, S., Laurent, C., Morin, G., Berquin, P., and Piussan, C. Failure of fluconazole treatment in *Candida* meningitis. *J. Pediatr.*, 123, 168, 1993.
269. Bode, S., Pedersen-Bjergaard, L., and Hjelt, K. *Candida albicans* septicemia in a premature infant successfully treated with oral fluconazole. *Scand. J. Infect. Dis.*, 24, 673, 1992.
270. Bhandari, V. and Narang, A. Oral itraconazole therapy for disseminated candidiasis in low birth weight infants. *J. Pediatr.*, 120(2 Part 1), 330, 1992.
271. Michel, J. L., Coinde, E., Chalencon, V., and Stephan, J. L. Major eosinophilia in a premature infant induced by topical ketoconazole. *Ann. Dermatol. Venereol.*, 127, 405–407, 2000.
272. Vazquez, J. A., Boikov, D., and Sobel, J. D. Antifungal cross-resistance among *Candida* spp. recovered from fluconazole-refractory thrush in AIDS patients. *5th Conf. Retroviruses Opportunistic Infect.*, abstract no. 490, 1998.
273. Fichtenbaum, C. J., Koletar, S., Yiannoutsos, C., et al. Refractory mucosal candidiasis in advanced human immunodeficiency virus infection. *Clin. Infect. Dis.*, 30, 749–756, 2000.
274. McNeil, M. M., Reiss, E., Elie, C. M., et al. Molecular analysis of serial *Candida albicans* isolates from HIV-infected patients with oropharyngeal candidiasis (OPC) demonstrating clinical resistance to fluconazole. *99th Gen. Meet. Am. Soc. Microbiol.*, 316, abstract no. F-104, 1999.
275. Schuman, P., Vazquez, J., Klein, R. S., Mayer, K., Rompalo, A., and Sobel, J. D. Evolution of fluconazole susceptibility among *Candida* isolates. *6th Conf. Retroviruses Opportunistic Infect.*, 103, abstract no. 186, 1999.
276. Rodriguez-Tudela, J. L., Martinez-Suarez, J. V., Dronda, F., Laguna, F., Chaves, F., and Valencia, E. Correlation of invitro susceptibility test results with clinical response: a study of azole therapy in AIDS patients. *J. Antimicrob. Chemother.*, 35, 793, 1995.
277. Xu, J., Ramos, A. R., Vilgalys, R., and Mitchell, T. G. Clonal and spontaneous origins of fluconazole resistance in *Candida albicans*. *J. Clin. Microbiol.*, 38, 1214–1220, 2000.
278. Fichtenbaum, C., Ignatov, A., Mersman, D., Keath, E., Koletar, S., and Powderly, W. The molecular epidemiology of fluconazole refractory oral candidiasis. *6th Conf. Retroviruses Opportunistic Infect.*, 103, abstract no. 187, 1999.
279. Loffler, J., Einsele, H., Hebart, H., Schumacher, U., Hrastnik, C., and Daum, G. Phospholipid and sterol analysis of plasma membranes of azole-resistant *Candida albicans* strains. *FEMS Microbiol. Lett.*, 185, 59–63, 2000.
280. Vennwald, I., Seebacher, C., and Roitzsch, E. Post-mortem findings in patients with repeatedly mycological demonstration of *Candida glabrata*. *Mycoses*, 41, 125–132, 1998.
281. Calabrese, D. C., Bille, J., Barchiesi, F., and Sanglard, D. Incidence of resistance mechanisms to azole antifungal agents in *Candida* species from HIV+ patients with oropharyngeal candidosis (OPC). *38th Intersci. Conf. Antimicrob. Agents Chemother.*, 112, abstract no. C-152, 1998.
282. Bini, E. J., Micale, P. L., and Weinshel, E. H. Natural history of HIV-associated esophageal disease in the era of protease inhibitor therapy. *Dig. Dis. Sci.*, 45, 1301–1307, 2000.
283. Vullo, V., Mastroianni, C. M., Mengoni, F., et al. Restoration of the innate immunity in HIV-infected patients after protease-inhibitor therapy. *38th Intersci. Conf. Antimicrob. Agents Chemother.*, 422, abstract no. I-182, 1998.
284. Revankar, S. G., Sanche, S. E., Dib, O. P., Caceres, M., and Patterson, T. F. Effect of highly active anti-retroviral therapy (HAART) on recurrent oropharyngeal candidiasis in HIV- infected patients: a complex relationship. *5th Conf. Retroviruses Opportunistic Infect.*, 171, abstract no. 488, 1998.
285. Zingman, B. S. Resolution of refractory AIDS-related mucosal candidiasis after initiation of didanosine plus sequinavir. *N. Engl. J. Med.*, 334, 1674, 1996.
286. Arribas, J. R., Hernandez-Albujar, S., Gonzalez-Garcia, J., et al. Continuous improvement of oral *Candida* colonization and skin test reactivity after one year of treatment with protease inhibitors. *6th Conf. Retroviruses Opportunistic Infect.*, 103, abstract no. 185, 1999.
287. Arribas, J. R., Hernandez-Albujar, S., Gonzalez-Garcia, J., et al. Prospective study of oral *Candida* colonization in advanced AIDS patients treated with ritonavir. *5th Conf. Retroviruses Opportunistic Infect.*, 170, abstract no. 485, 1998.
288. Tacconelli, E., De Bernardis, F., Tumbarello, M., Torosantucci, A., and Cauda, R. A direct effect of HIV protease inhibitors on *Candida albicans*: prevention of oral candidiasis through inhibition of fungal proteinase. *6th Conf. Retroviruses Opportunistic Infect.*, 103, abstract no. 184, 1999.
289. Cassone, A., Adriani, D., Tacconelli, E., Cauda, R., and De Bernardis, F. HIV protease inhibitors have a direct anti-*Candida* effect by inhibition of *Candida* aspartyl proteinase. *12th Int. Conf. AIDS*, 537, abstract no. 31211, 1998.
290. Connick, E., Lederman, M. M., Kotzin, B. L., et al. Immune reconstitution in the first year of potent antiretroviral therapy and its relationship to virulogic response. *J. Infect. Dis.*, 181, 358–363, 2000.
291. Samonis, G., Thomakos, N., Liakakos, T., et al. Effects of cefepime and meropenem on the gastrointestinal colonization of surgical patients by *Candida albicans*. *Chemotherapy*, 47, 350–353, 2001.

292. Mavromanolakis, E., Maraki, S., Cranidis, A., Tselentis, Y., Kontoyiannis, D. P., and Samonis, G. The impact of norfloxacin, ciprofloxacin and ofloxacin on human gut colonization by *Candida albicans*. *Scand. J. Infect. Dis.*, 33, 477–478, 2001.
293. Ueta, E., Tanida, T., Yoneda, K., Yamamoto, T., and Osaki, T. Increase of *Candida* cell virulence by anticancer drugs and irradiation. *Oral Microbiol. Immunol.*, 16, 243–249, 2001.
294. Willis, A. M., Coulter, W. A., Fulton, C. R., Hayes, J. R., Bell, P. M., and Lamey, P. J. The influence of antifungal drugs on virulence properties of *Candida albicans* in patients with diabetes mellitus. *Oral Surg. Oral Med. Oral Pathol. Oral Radiol.*, 91, 317–321, 2001.
295. U.S. Public Health Service (USPHS) and Infectious Diseases Society of America (IDSA). 1999 USPHS/IDSA guidelines for the prevention of opportunistic infections in persons infected with human immunodeficiency virus. *Infect. Dis. Obstet. Gynecol.*, 8, 5–74, 2000.
296. Soriano, V., Dona, C., Rodriguez-Rosado, R., Barreiro, P., and Gonzalez-Lahoz, J. Discontinuation of secondary prophylaxis for opportunistic infections in HIV-infected patients receiving highly active antiretroviral therapy. *AIDS*, 14, 383–386, 2000.
297. Just-Nübling, G., Gentschew, G., Meissner, K., et al. Fluconazole prophylaxis or recurrent oral candidiasis in HIV-positive patients. *Eur. J. Clin. Microbiol. Infect. Dis.*, 10, 917, 1991.
298. Kung, N., Fisher, N., Gunson, B., Hastings, M., and Mutimer, D. Fluconazole prophylaxis for high-risk liver transplant recipients. *Lancet*, 349, 1234–1235, 1995.
299. Tollemar, J., Hockerstedt, K., Ericzon, B. G., Jalanko, H., and Ringdén, O. Liposomal amphotericin B prevents invasive fungal infections in liver transplant recipients: a randomized, placebo-controlled study. *Transplantation*, 59, 45–50, 1995.
300. Benedetti, E., Gruessner, A. C., Troppmann, C., et al., Intra-abdominal fungal infections after pancreatic transplantation: incidence, treatment, and outcome. *J. Am. Coll. Surg.*, 183, 307–316, 1996.
301. Kicklighter, S. D., Springer, S. C., Cox, T., Hulsey, T. C., and Turner, R. B. Fluconazole for prophylaxis against candidal rectal colonization in the very low birth weight infant. *Pediatrics*, 107, 293–298, 2001 [see also: *Pediatrics*, 107, 404–405, 2001].
302. Laverdiere, M., Rotstein, C., Bow, E. J., et al. Impact of fluconazole prophylaxis on fungal colonization and infection rates in neutropenic patients. The Canadian Fluconazole Study. *J. Antimicrob. Chemother.*, 46, 1001–1008, 2000.
303. Goranov, S., Spasov, E., Grudeva-Popova, J., and Vakrilov, V., Antifungal prophylaxis with low doses fluconazole in patients with hematological malignancies. *Folia Med. (Plovdiv)*, 41, 68–72, 1999.
304. Harousseau, J. L., Dekker, W., Stamatoullas-Bastard, A., Fassas, A., et al. Itaconazole oral solution for primary prophylaxis of fungal infections in patients with hematological malignancy and profound neutropenia: a randomized, double-blind, double-placebo, multicenter trial comparing itraconazole and amphotericin B. *Antimicrob. Agents Chemother.*, 44, 1887–193, 2000.
305. Goldman M., Cloud, G. A., Smedema, M., et al. Does long-term itraconazole prophylaxis results in in vitro azole resistance in mucosal *Candida albicans* isolates from persons with advanced human immunodeficiency virus infection? The National Institute of Allergy and Infectious Diseases Mycoses study group. *Antimicrob. Agents Chemother.*, 44, 1585–1587, 2000.
306. Singhal, S., Ellis, R. W., Jones, S. G., et al. Targeted prophylaxis with amphotericin B lipid complex in liver transplantation. *Liver Transpl.*, 6, 588–595, 2000.

21
Emerging *Candida* spp. Infections

1. INTRODUCTION

More than 150 species of *Candida* have been idenfified, but only a dosen or so have been regarded as important pathogens in humans. Although *C. albicans* remains the most common fungal pathogen, over the past decade or so, there has been an increasing number of reports implicating non-*albicans* species causing opportunistic mycoses *(1)*.

Although single reports describing one or more cases of infection caused by unusual *Candida* species do not necessarily mark the emergence of a new yeast infection, at least some of these species may arise as potential human opportunistic pathogens, especially among immunocompromised hosts *(2–4)*. Thus, in one prospective, clinical multicenter study, non-*albicans* candidemia was diagnosed in 77% of the 73 episodes of candidemia with an overall mortalily rate of 49% *(5)*.

Among the various emerging *Candida* spp. pathogenic to humans, *C. glabrata (6,7)*, *C. guilliermondii (8–10)*, *C. krusei (11,12)*, and *C. parapsilosis (13)* are the most frequently isolated. Other emerging pathogenic yeasts include *C. stellatoidea (14,15)*, *C. famata (16,17)*, *C. kefyr (C. pseudotropicalis) (18)*, *C. lusitaniae (19–21)*, *C. norvegensis (22)*, *C. lipolytica (23,24)*, *C. rugosa (25–27)*, *C. utilis (28,29)*, *C. zeylanoides (30,31)*, *C. haemulonii (32)*, *C. humicola (33) C. pintolopesii (34,35)*, *C. pulcherrima (36)*, *C. viswanathii (37) C. tropicalis (38)*, and lately *C. dubliniensis (39–46)*.

Concurrent isolation of more than one non-*albicans* species of *Candida* from blood cultures of patients with disseminated candidiasis, although rare, has been reported *(47)*. Given the increased clinical significance of these yeasts in immunocompromised hosts and the difference in virulence, maximum caution should be applied to properly identifying the emerging non-*C. albicans* species. To this end, in vitro susceptibility testing will be most helpful in deciding on the treatment regimens of non-*albicans Candida* infections, especially in cases where patients have already been treated with azole antimycotics and the development of drug resistance.

Some of the particular clinical and/or microbiological aspects of these less frequently encountered but emerging non-*albicans Candida* infections are reviewed in this section.

2. *CANDIDA GLABRATA*

C. glabrata (also known as *Torulopsis glabrata* and *Cryptococcus glabratus*) is a small, round yeast thought to be saprophytic in humans. Most commonly, *C. glabrata* is found as a commensal of the gastrointestinal (GI) tract, and incidently has been isolated from the oral cavity, skin, and urine cultures of healthy individuals *(48–52)*.

Until recently, *C. glabrata* was considered a relatively nonpathogenic commensal of human mucosal tissues such as the vagina *(53)*. However, with the increased use of immunosuppressive drugs, mucosal and systemic infections caused by this yeast have increased significantly, especially in the HIV-infected population. Currently, *C. glabrata* ranks second or third as the causative agent of superficial (oral, esophageal, vaginal, or urinary) or systemic candidal infections, which are often nosocomial *(53,54)*, and overall, the non-*albicans* species now surpass *C. albicans* as the cause of nosocomial bloodstream infections in hospitalized patients *(55)*. Sfameny et al. *(56)* reported two severe cases of *C. glabrata* chorioamnionitis occurring in pregnancies achieved by in vitro fertilization techniques that resulted in preterm delivery and pregnancy loss.

As it increasingly becomes an opportunistic pathogen, *C. glabrata* is associated with high mortality rates ranging from 38–83% *(52,57–59)*. It has been frequently isolated from various secretions of hospitalized patients *(48,60–62)*. Blot et al. *(63)* conducted a retrospective study to determine population characteristics and outcome in critically ill patients with fungemia due to *C. albicans* ($n = 41$) and *C. glabrata* ($n = 15$). Patients with *C. glabrata* fungemia were significantly older as compared with the *C. albicans* group with no other differences in population characteristics or severity of illness. Because age was an independent predictor of mortality, the observed trend towards a higher mortality in patients with *C. glabrata* was explained by this population being significantly older *(63)*. Using univariate analysis, Viscoli et al. *(64)* associated *C. glabrata* with the highest mortality rate in a prospective, multicenter surveillance study of candidemia in cancer patients.

The underlying conditions most often associated with fungemia, bronchopneumonia, salpingitis, and urinary tract infections caused by *C. glabrata* included malignancies *(64,65)*, diabetes mellitus *(52)*, transplantation *(66)*, and alcoholism *(48,67)*. This yeast could also become pathogenic under other conditions leading to altered host immune defenses, such as therapies with corticosteroids, immunosuppressive drugs, and broad-spectrum antibiotics or major surgery *(6,57,68,69)*. A fatal case of spontaneous *C. glabrata*-associated peritonitis was reported in a patient with cirrhosis secondary to autoimmune hepatitis *(70)*. Recently, the first case of a ventriculoperitoneal shunt infection by *C. glabrata* was also reported *(71)*. Presentation of *C. glabrata* spinal osteomyelitis 25 mo after documented candidemia was discussed by Dwyer et al. *(72)*.

Among the risk factors commonly associated with *C. glabrata* fungemia in neonates have been extreme prematurity, indwelling central lines (in the umbilical vessels or the vena cava), prolonged intubation, and excessive use of broad-spectrum antibiotics *(7,58,73,74)*.

The most common clinical manifestations of *C. glabrata* fungemia have been high fever and hypotension, resembling bacterial endotoxic shock *(75)*. However, *C. glabrata* urinary infections have become more prevalent over the last decade in immunocompromised patients *(76–78)*.

2.1. Treatment of C. glabrata Infections

A major obstacle in the treatment of *C. glabrata* is the innate resistance of this species to azole antimycotics that are usually very effective in treating infections caused by other *Candida* infections *(53,79–81)*. There are few recognized virulence factors of *C. glabrata* and scarce information about the host defense mechanisms to protect against this yeast infection *(53)*. Therapy of *C. glabrata* most often includes the use of amphotericin B alone or in combination with flucytosine. Because of increased resistance, the use of azole antimycotics such as fluconazole would require higher doses to achieve clinical cure *(81)*. Rather, fluconazole is used frequently in prophylactic treatment.

Treatment with amphotericin B has been the most preferred treatment modality for *C. glabrata* fungemia *(6,57,82)*. Multiple tests evaluating the sensitivity of the yeast to amphotericin B furnished MIC values ranging from 0.1 to 1.0 µg/mL *(57)*. In the presence of disseminated infection, the use of higher doses of amphotericin B (30 mg/kg) has been recommended *(74)*. Glick et al. *(7)* reported a successful outcome of *C. glabrata* fungemia in a neonate patient following treatment with amphotericin B at 0.5 mg/kg daily for 5 d and then every other day for 5 more doses. Yet, Komshian et al. *(83)* found no statistical difference in mortality whether antifungal therapy was administered or not (55 and 69% mortality rates, respectively), although an early initiation of therapy may improve the response rate *(7)*. High mortality rates among neonates have also been reported *(58,84–86)*.

Khemakhem et al. *(76)* successfully used surgical drainage and amphotericin B therapy to treat a perinephric abscess caused by *C. glabrata* in a diabetic patient who underwent ureteropelvic surgery for lithiasic urinary tract obstruction.

AmBisome, a liposomal amphotericin B was evaluated at 2.5–7 mg/kg/daily (as a continuous 1-h infusion) in very low birth-weight infants with systemic candidiasis *(87)*. Fungal eradication was achieved in 92% of the episodes; mean duration of AmBisome therapy until achieving eradication was 9 d.

A synergistic combination of amphotericin B and flucytosine was used successfully to treat a *C. glabrata* periprosthetic infection after total hip replacement *(70)*. In another case, a combination of intravenous amphotericin B lipid complex and flucytosine resolved a case of *C. glabrata* endophthalmitis *(88)* which occurred 2 mo after urologic surgery *(68)*.

Rolston et al. *(89)* reported the treatment of refractory candidemia in non-neutropenic patients with liposomal nystatin (Nyotran). Patients with positive blood culture for *Candida* species (including *C. glabrata*) were given Nyotran at 2.0 or 4.0 mg/kg daily within 96 h of obtaining a positive culture. Nyotran was found effective in at least 60% of episodes of refractory candidemia, including those treated with amphotericin B.

Reporting on four episodes of *C. glabrata*-associated peritonitis in three patients on continuous ambulatory peritoneal dialysis (CAPD), Kleinpeter and Butt *(90)* suggested that treatment should include removal of the peritoneal dialysis catheter with appropriate antifungal therapy.

2.1.1. Fluconazole in the Treatment of C. glabrata Infections

While fluconazole was found effective in the treatment of non-*albicans* pelvic candidal gynecological infections *(91)*, developing resistance of *C. glabrata* to fluconazole has often been the case *(79,92–94)*. To this end, fluconazole-susceptible colonies were replaced by resistant colonies that exhibited both increased fluconazole efflux and increased transcrips of a gene that codes for a protein with 72.5% identity to Pdr5p, an ABC multidrug transporter in *Saccharomyces cerevisiae*. When the earliest and most azole-susceptible isolate of *C. glabrata* was exposed to fluconazole, increased transcripts of the PDR5 homolog appeared linking azole exposure to regulation of this gene *(95)*. Further evidence was provided when the ATP-binding cassette transporter gene CgCDR1 from *C. glabrata* was also found involved in the resistance to fluconazole as well as other azoles *(80)*. Thus, the deletion of CgCDR1 in an azole-resistant *C. glabrata* clinical isolates rendered the resulting mutant (DSY1041) susceptible to azole derivatives, thereby providing genetic evidence that a specific mechanism was involved in the azole resistance of a clinical isolate.

In addition, shortly after commencing oral fluconazole, fluconazole-induced torsade de pointes (TDP) has been reported in a patient with *C. glabrata*-associated presacral abscess *(96)*. The condition resolved after treatment was discontinued. One possible mechanism of the observed use of fluconazole and the development of TDP might have been the depression of rapidly activating delayed rectifier potassium currents.

Comparison of critically ill patient populations with and without fluconazole treatment found increased mortality and longer hospital and intensive care unit (ICU) lengths of stay in the fluconazole-treated group. The latter also showed higher bacterial pathogen resistance to antibiotics after fluconazole administration compared with bacterial resistance of patients without fluconazole treatment *(97)*. Moreover, the use of fluconazole was specifically associated with *C. glabrata* catheter-associated candiduria (but not with *C. albicans* candiduria) *(78)*.

2.1.2. C. glabrata-Induced Vulvovaginal Candidiasis

Chronically recidivist vulvovaginal candidiasis is one of the most stubborn problematic diagnosis in the dermatology and gynecology ward. Prognosis and therapy are essentially determined by the causative yeast and its interaction with the antifungal agent *(98–100)*. An Italian study of women with symptomatic *Candida* infection of the low genital tract has shown differences in the epidemiological characteristics of women with *albicans* and non-*albicans Candida* infections; of the causative non-*albicans* yeasts, *C. glabrata* was by far the most frequently isolated pathogen *(101)*. Using 55 clinical yeast isolates from 40 patients, Czaika et al. *(98)* found that *C. glabrata* was the predominant causative agent of recidivist vaginal candidiasis. Further, these investigators have identified the initial dose adaptation of the drug used, which in the case of oral fluconazole was 800 mg daily when *C. glabrata* was the causative agent of vulvovaginal candidiasis. Low-dose fluconazole therapy has always been unsussessful in recurrent vaginal candidiasis and induced secondary resistance *(98)*. Cross et al. *(102)* provided evidence that spontaneous mutants of *C. glabrata* selected for resistance to clotrimazole were cross-resistant to fluconazole and other azole-based antifungals as well.

Patients with vaginitis due to highly azole-resistant *C. glabrata* can be particularly difficult to treat *(102)*. White et al. *(103)* reported the once-daily use of combination of flucytosine (1.0 g) and amphotericin B (100 mg) formulated in lubricating jelly base for a total of 8.0 g delivered dose per vagina. After a 14-d treatment, there was a significant clinical and microbiological improvement.

A double-blind, randomized, placebo-controlled, comparative Phase II study of flutrimazole site-release vaginal cream (1, 2, and 4%) was undertaken over a 10-mo period in patients ($n = 124$) with acute vulvovaginal candidiasis *(104)*. There was a significant association between *C. glabrata* and treatment failure, and *C. glabrata* and carrier state in vagina and vulvovagina. Although there were no significant differences in the clinical and mycological activities between the three concentrations applied, overall, the flutrimazole 2% site-release vaginal cream was chosen for clinical use due to its tolerance profile *(104)*.

Polish investigators have found nystatin effective in the treatment of vulvovaginal candidiasis by defining the drug resistance of 93 *Candida* isolates (81.97% *C. albicans*, and 11.06% *C. glabrata* being the major isolates). Thus, nystatin was found effective in 81.72% of the sensitive strains *(105)*. Although mucocutaneous adverse side effects have rarely been reported with nystatin despite its long years of use, severe vulvovaginitis associated with intravaginal nystatin therapy for *C. glabrata* recently has been reported *(106)*.

In postmenopausal women, long-term tamoxifen (a breast cancer cell estrogen antagonist) medication may be complicated by recurrent vulvovaginal candidiasis due to *C. glabrata*; tamoxifen has not previously been reported to predispose to vulvovaginal candidiasis *(107)*.

2.2. Candida glabrata *Prophylaxis*

The impact of fluconazole prophylaxis on fungal colonization and infection rates in neutropenic cancer patients receiving intensive cytotoxic therapy for acute leukemia or for autologous marrow transplantation was investigated in a Canadian study *(108)*. Oral fluconazole (400 mg daily) or an identical placebo was applied until prophylaxis failure or marrow recovery. By the end of prophylaxis, colonization with non-*albicans Candida* species increased from 7 to 21% and 8 to 18% in the fluconazole and placebo groups, respectively. Although *C. glabrata* was isolated more frequently at the end of the prophylactic period in the fluconazole patients than in the placebo patients (16 vs 7%), only one definite invasive *C. glabrata* infection was observed. By comparison, *C. albicans* colonization was reduced from 30 to 10% in the fluconazole recipients while it increased from 32 to 57% in the placebo patients *(108)*.

Following a low-dose (100–200 mg, daily) fluconazole prophylaxis given to 14 patients after high-risk allogeneic marrow transplantation (all carrying a central venous catheter), Safdar et al. *(109)* reported no adverse effects on incidence and outcome of *C. glabrata* fungemia as compared with high-dose fluconazole (400 mg, daily) prophylaxis.

The effect of fluconazole prophylaxis on the vaginal flora of 323 HIV-infected women was evaluated in a multicenter, randomized, double-blind, placebo-controlled trial in which patients with CD4 cell counts of $300/mm^3$ or less received either 200 mg of the drug or placebo *(110)*. The results showed that fluconazole was associated with a 50% reduction in the odds of being colonized with *C. albicans* but with higher rates for non-*albicans Candida* species. The effect of fluconazole prophylaxis was attributed to the reduction in vaginal *C. albicans* colonization; however, in the case of *C. glabrata*, colonization rapidly supervened.

3. CANDIDA KRUSEI

Previously, *C. krusei* was characterized as a less virulent pathogen in humans. This assumption was based on experimental data stemming from its decreased abilities to adhere to human mucosal epithelial cells in vitro *(111)*, and to elicit cell death in mouse kidney tissue culture *(112)*. In addition, Edwards et al. *(113)* showed that higher inocula of *C. krusei*, compared to other *Candida* species, were required to establish infections in animal models.

Recently, however, there have been an increasing number of reports describing substantial virulence of this yeast in immunocompromised hosts *(12,114–119)*. Thus, in a retrospective study by Abbas et al. *(120)*, *C. krusei* fungemia in cancer patients led to a mortality rate of 49% as compared to 28% for *C. albicans* with persistant neutropenia ($p = 0.02$) and septic shock ($p = 0.002$) being the predictors of poor prognosis. The overall mortality in patients with *C. krusei* fungemia may approach 50%, and if left untreated, the outcome has been nearly always fatal *(11)*. The increase of *C. krusei* infections in recent years may be the result of its intrinsic resistance to fluconazole, which has been widely used in immunocompromised patients to suppress the infections due to azole-susceptible *C. albicans (81,94,120–125)*.

In a study by Goldman et al. *(11)*, at the onset of *C. krusei* fungemia 85% of patients were neutropenic with neutrophil counts below 1,000 cells/mm^3. This prevalence of neutropenia was significantly higher than the 40% previously reported for cancer patients with *C. albicans* fungemia and only slightly higher than the 70% prevalence of neutropenia reported for patients with *C. tropicalis* fungemia *(116)*. Furthermore, over 75% of the patients studied by Goldman et al. *(11)* showed evidence of gastrointestinal mucosal barrier damage, mostly the result of cytotoxic chemotherapy or radiation. The GI tract is believed to be an important portal of entry for *Candida* spp. into the bloodstream *(126)*, and GI mucosal breakdown has been reported to be a risk factor for both nosocomially acquired candidemia in nonleukemic patients *(127)*, and cancer patients sustaining damage to the GI mucosa from the presence of tumor infiltrates or directly from cytotoxic antitumor agents themselves *(128–130)*.

Goldman et al. *(11)* found 69% of the evaluable patients with evidence of *C. krusei* colonization, which was in agreement with the results of Wey et al. *(131)* who described colonization by *Candida* spp. to be a risk factor for candidemia. Merz et al. *(115)* reported that *C. krusei* colonized 12.4% of granulocytopenic patients undergoing chemotherapy for hematologic malignancies or bone-marrow transplantation.

A common risk factor of patients with *C. krusei*-induced endophthalmitis was prolonged intravenous catheterization *(132)*.

Clinical manifestations of *C. krusei* most often include the development of cutaneous lesions (diffuse erythematous maculopapular eruption, erythematous macronodular skin lesions, skin nodules), myalgias, endophthalmitis *(11,132,133)*, and disseminated disease *(11,115,116,126,132,134–136)*. Gordon et al. *(137)* described a case of an immunocompromised leukemic patient with well-localized intra-abdominal abscess caused by *C. krusei*, which disseminated when treated by surgical drainage. In another unusual case, Diggs et al. *(138)* reported on a fatal *C. krusei* muscle granulomata in a patient with acute lymphoblastic leukemia (ALL) and granylocytopenia. Other rarely diagnosed *C. krusei* infections include infectious arthritis *(139,140)*, ureteral obstruction *(141)*, ocular infections (blepharoconjunctivitis without retinitis) *(142,143)*, sinusitis *(144)*, and esophagitis *(145)*.

Recommended treatment of *C. krusei* fungemia included amphotericin B alone (0.5–1.0 mg/kg daily) or in combination with flucytosine (at doses adequate to achieve levels of 30–60 µg/mL), as well as liposomal amphotericin B (2.6 mg/kg daily); adjunctive leukocyte transfusion has also been applied *(11,132,137)*.

3.1. Prophylaxis Against C. krusei Infections and Azole Resistance

Although the prophylactic use of fluconazole has contributed significantly to the decline in the number of disseminated infections caused by the more virulent *C. albicans* and *C. tropicalis*, recent reports of another disturbing trend, have focused attention on the emergence of fungemia caused by the less virulent but drug-resistant *C. krusei* in immunocompromised patients (such as bone-marrow transplant recipients) treated prophylactically with fluconazole *(12,17,114,124,146–152)*. However, in several reports of controlled trials *(109, 115,151,153–155)*, the use of prophylactic fluconazole was not associated with increased incidence of *C. krusei* fungemia. There may be a host of other epidemiologic factors *(151)* that need to be considered in order to explain the different results seen at various centers. As compared to amphotericin B (MIC = 1.25 µg/mL *[146]*), fluconazole was consistently much less susceptible *(17,156,157)* (e.g., MIC = 25 µg/mL *[146]* or 32 µg/mL *[147]*). However, the MIC values themselves cannot imply resistance because the clinical efficacy of fluconazole is thought to be greater than that predicted by its minimum inhibitory concentration *(158)*. On the other hand, the use of animal models have suggested that *C. krusei* indeed displayed a high degree of resistance to fluconazole *(26)*. Moreover, a patient with acute monocytic leukemia and typhlitis (neutropenic enterocolitis) has developed *C. krusei* fungemia while receiving intravenous fluconazole given at 400 mg loading dose followed by 200 mg every 24 h *(158)*.

One established mechanism for azole resistance has been the drug efflux by ATP-binding cassette (ABC) transporters. Because these transporters recognize structurally diverse drugs, their overexpression may result in multidrug resistance. To this end, Katiyar and Edlind *(159)* have identified two *C. krusei* genes, ABC1 and ABC2, as potentially involved in azole resistance by having one or two related gene copies in the *C. krusei* genome. Furthermore, ABC1 was upregulated following brief treatment of *C. krusei* with miconazole and clotrimazole (but not other azoles), and the unrelated albendazole and cycloheximide. The latter two compounds antagonized the fluconazole activity against *C. krusei*, thereby supporting a role for the ABC1 transporter in azole efflux. Moreover, miconazole-resistant mutants selected in vitro demonstrated increase in constitutive expression of ABC1 *(159)*.

4. *CANDIDA LUSITANIAE*

Candida lusitaniae was first described by van Uden and Buckley *(160)* as common commensal of the GI tract of warm-blooded animals. In humans, it was recovered from a variety of clinical specimens, but most often from blood, urine, and the respiratory tract *(19,161–171)*. In view of these findings, the most likely portals of entry appeared to be the genitourinary and respiratory tracts or colonized indwelling intravascular catheters.

The identification of *C. lusitaniae*, especially in earlier reports *(18,164,172)* has proven difficult because of misidentification with *C. parapsilosis*, *C. tropicalis (20,162,164,169,172)*, or even *Saccharomyces* spp. *(19,161)*. The major differential characteristics of *C. lusitaniae* relate to the assimilation of cellobiose and fermentation of trehalose (both negative for *C. parapsilosis*) *(164,169)*. In addition, the lack of growth on cycloheximide-containing medium, pink-appearing colonies on triphenyltetrazolium chloride agar, the assimilation of rhamnose, and the absence of maltose and sucrose fermentation serve to distinguish *C. lusitaniae* from *C. tropicalis (164,173)*.

Pappagianis et al. *(20)* and Holzschu et al. *(169)* reported the first documented case of opportunistic infection associated with *C. lusitaniae* in a patient with acute leukemia.

Although so far *C. lusitaniae* seems to be a rare opportunistic pathogen, it has been associated with serious and often fatal disease *(19,21,161,162,164–168,172–174)*. From the reported cases, immunocompromised patients with hematologic malignancies *(175,176)*, solid tumors *(175)*, bone-marrow transplant recipients *(175)*, patients on CAPD *(177–179)*, and patients with central venous catheters *(180,181)* or receiving immunosuppressive therapies (corticosteroids, broad-spectrum antibiotics) *(182)* were at high risk of developing infection *(19,161,164–167,172)*. In addition, *C. lusitaniae* has emerged as an opportunistic pathogen in premature infants *(21,183,184)*. This yeast has also become an increasingly important nosocomial bloodstream pathogen *(60,176,183,185)*.

In vitro susceptibility testing of *C. lusitaniae* isolates conducted in several laboratories *(21,162,168,174)* have shown mean inhibitory concentrations of 0.1–0.4, 0.03–0.2/>160, and <0.03

μg/mL for amphotericin B, flucytosine, and ketoconazole, respectively. Ahearn and McGlohn *(186)* while reviewing the susceptibilities of several *M. lusitaniae* isolates, found that although the MIC values of amphotericin B fell within attainable serum levels, the minimal fungicidal concentrations were more than two dilutions greater. Based on their overall results, Ahearn and McGlohn concluded that flucytosine might be the drug of choice for *C. lusitaniae* infections. To this end, Oleinik et al. *(184)* used a combination of flucytosine and fluconazole to treat *C. lusitaniae* osteomyelitis in a premature infant.

Treatment of *C. lusitaniae* infections is challenging because of its frequent resistance to antifungal agents and the lack of standardized susceptibility testing for fungi.

In 1985, Pensler et al. *(171)* reported the first successful therapy of *C. lusitaniae*. Later, Blinkhorn et al. *(19)* also described two leukemic patients with *C. lusitaniae* fungemia who responded to treatment with amphotericin B.

However, developing resistance to amphotericin B seemed to be a major problem with *C. lusitaniae (20,167,172,187–190)*. Guinet et al. *(164)* have described the first case of a *C. lusitaniae* isolate resistant to amphotericin B before therapy. Of all of the reported fatal cases of *C. lusitaniae*, fungemia was associated with such resistance *(164,166,167,169,172,191)*, suggesting that amphotericin B should not be used as a single therapeutic modality in the management of *C. lusitaniae*, especially with the possibility of developing drug resistance during treatment *(20,162,168)*. Despite their widespread use, *Candida* spp. resistance to polyene antibiotics (e.g., amphotericin B, nystatin) has been relatively rare *(20,171,172,192–196)*. For this reason, the clearly observed resistance to amphotericin B by *C. lusitaniae*, although unusual (see also, *C. rugosa* and *C. guilliermondii* below), has not been entirely unexpected. It is well-documented that resistance to polyenes is associated with alterations in fungal cell-membrane sterols *(8,172,193–195,197,198)*.

The efficacy and tolerance of an amphotericin B lipid emulsion (AmB-IL), in which amphotericin B was diluted in a lipid solution for parenteral nutrition (Intralipid), was assessed in 14 neutropenic patients (one of them with *C. lusitaniae* candidemia) *(199)*. The AmB-IL, which was administered at a mean dosage of 1.18 mg/kg/d (range 0.73–1.55) for 22 d, was well-tolerated in most patients.

Flucytosine-ketoconazole was one combination that was successfully used by Yinnon et al. *(21)* to eradicate the yeast from the urinary tract of an infant; both drugs were given at daily oral doses of 75 mg/kg and 9.0 mg/kg (divided every 6 h), respectively. Thomas et al. *(200)* reported that the addition of flucytosine to a therapeutic regimen consisting of amphotericin B, resulted in sterilization of the blood in what appeared to be a persistent *C. lusitaniae* fungemia. In contrast, Baker et al. *(170)* described a failure of flucytosine to control *C. lusitaniae* urinary tract infection, which was eradicated with amphotericin B bladder irrigation.

After examining 1,372 yeast isolates collected from 308 patients, Dick et al. *(194)* found the emergence of polyene resistance only in patients undergoing treatment for acute leukemia or in aplastic patients following bone-marrow transplantation. In general, these patients experienced prolonged periods of hospitalization, granulocytopenia, therapy with cytotoxic drugs, and extended treatment with antibiotics. Both Pappagianis et al. *(20)* and Dick et al. *(194)* concluded that the use of cytotoxic drugs should be considered a contributing factor in the development of resistance to polyene antibiotics.

5. CANDIDA DUBLINIENSIS

Although *C. albicans* remains the most common fungal pathogen, over the past decade or so, there has been an increasing number of reports implicating "atypical" *C. albicans* strains as the causative agents of opportunistic mycoses *(41)*. Two such groups of isolates recovered from cases of oral candidiasis in Irish and Australian HIV-infected and AIDS patients have been defined to constitute a novel species termed *Candida dubliniensis (201,202)*. The classification of *C. dubliniensis* as a separate species was confirmed by phylogenetic analysis, whereby the comparison of ribosomal RNA sequences demonstrated that *C. dubliniensis* isolates formed a cluster clearly distinct from other *Candida* species, including *C. albicans (202,203)*. The latter could be readily discriminated from *C.*

dubliniensis isolates on chromogenic medium CHROMagar *Candida*, and by their inability to grow at 42°C *(41,43,45)*.

A number of findings *(42,44,204–209)* have demonstrated that the geographical distribution of *C. dubliniensis* is widespread, and likely to be a significant constituent of the normal oral flora with the potential to cause oral candidiasis, especially in immunocompromised individuals.

At present, isolates of *C. dubliniensis* have been recovered mainly from oral cavities of HIV-infected patients causing recurrent oropharyngeal candidiasis *(39–46,210,211)*. In a small sample, Meiller et al. *(44)* found that *C. dubliniensis* represented 25% of yeast-positive cultures isolated from HIV-positive patients in United States. Velegraki et al. *(211)* implicated *C. dubliniensis* as the possible causative agent of linear gingival erythema in vertically HIV-infected children. In insulin-using diabetes mellitus patients, Willis et al. *(212)* found *C. dubliniensis* in the oral cavity of 15.4% of the population, second only to *C. albicans* (77%).

In general, the binding of microorganisms to each other and oral surfaces contributes to the progression of microbial infections in the oral cavity. To this end, Jabra-Rizk et al. *(213)* found *Fusobacterium nucleatum* to be a coaggregation partner of *C. dubliniensis* at 37°C; by comparison, *C. albicans* did not coaggregate with *F. nucleatum* at that temperature, thereby providing a rapid, specific, and inexpensive assay to differentiate between the two species in the clinical laboratory *(39)*.

Meis et al. *(214)* described invasive *C. dubliniensis* in two immunocompomised patients: one of them becoming candidemic during treatment for graft-vs-host disease after receiving an allogenic bone-marrow transplant for chronic myeloid leukemia (CML); the other patient received cytotoxic chemotherapy for nasopharyngeal rhabdomyosarcoma. In another case, a patient with oral cancer receiving head and neck radiation, has also been diagnosed with oropharyngeal *C. dubliniensis* infection *(215)*.

5.1. Molecular and Phenotypic Characterization of C. dubliniensis

Phenotypically, *C. dubliniensis* isolates are similar to *C. albicans* and *C. stellatoidea* in that they produce germ tubes and chlamydospores, but possess unusual carbohydrate assimilation patterns and grow poorly or not at all at 42°C *(43,201,203,208,216)*. In contrast to the other two species, *C. dubliniensis* produce large number of chlamidospores often arranged in contiguous pairs, triplets and other multiples suspended from a single suspensor cell *(216)*. Further, using a variety of DNA fingerprinting techniques and karyotype analysis, the genomic organization of *C. dubliniensis* was shown to be distinctly different from that of *C. albicans (43,201–203,208,216,217)*.

In view of the increase of both reports of the isolation of *C. dubliniensis* from immunocompromised individuals and the number of unusual genotypic groups of *C. albicans* (C and D), McCullough et al. *(218)* have used molecular tools to characterize further these strains and to compare them with authentic strains of *C. dubliniensis* and type I *C. stellatoidea*. The results have shown that all *C. albicans* genotype D isolates were identical to *C. dubliniensis*, that no difference were found between *C. stellatoidea* and *C. albicans* genotype B straines, and that the *C. albicans* genotype C straines appeared to contained the transposable intron incompletely inserted throughout the ribosomal repeats of their genome.

5.2. Treatment of C. dubliniensis Candidiasis

In general, treatment of *C. dubliniensis*-associated candidiasis follows the same pattern as that of *C. albicans*, with fluconazole being the drug of choice. To this end, the in vitro susceptibilities of *C. dubliniensis* to current and new (such as the echinocandins, BMS-2071147, Sch 56592, and voriconazole) antifungal agents have been the subject of recent studies *(41,219)*. Most of *C. dubliniensis* isolates were susceptible to ketoconazole (75.9%), fluconazole (86.2%), and itraconazole (86.2%); however, some isolates were found resistant to fluconazole (MIC = 64 µg/mL and higher), itraconazole (MIC = 1.0 µg/mL or higher) and ketoconazole *(219)*. In addition, the new liposomal and lipid formulations of amphotericin B, and the liposomal nystatin may also provide new alternatives to fluconazole.

5.2.1. C. dubliniensis Resistance to Fluconazole

Fluconazole-resistant *C. dubliniensis* clinical isolates have been recovered *(220)*. In a case of an AIDS patient, from the appearance of the first episode of oral candidiasis until the patient became unresponsive 18 mo later, the treatment consisted of fluconazole at 400 mg daily *(221)*. In this regard, findings by Moran et al. *(220)* suggested that *C. dubliniensis* might have encoded multidrug transporters similar to those encoded by the *C. albicans* MDR1, CDR1, and CDR2 genes (CaMDR1, CaCDR1, and CaCDR2, respectively). Indeed, a *C. dubliniensis* homolog of CaMDR1, termed CdMDR1 was cloned, and by polymerase chain reaction (PCR), *C. dubliniensis* was also found to encode CdCDR1 and CdCDR2 (homologues of CDR1 and CDR2, respectively). Furthermore, overexpression of CaCDR1 was associated with fluconazole resistance in *C. albicans*; increased levels of the CdMdr1p protein were also detected in fluconazole-resistant isolates. These and other results obtained with fluconazole-resistant *C. dubliniensis* generated in vitro (increased levels of CdCDR1 mRNA and CdCdr1p protein) have demonstrated that *C. dubliniensis* is able to encode multidrug transporters that mediate fluconazole resistance in clinical isolates *(220)*. Molecular typing confirmed the persistence of the same *C. albicans* and *C. dubliniensis* strains that developed resistance to fluconazole after up to 3 yr of asymptomatic colonization *(221)*.

6. CANDIDA RUGOSA

Candida rugosa was originally isolated from human feces in 1917 by Anderson and named *Mycoderma rugosa (222)*. Later, it was found in bovine droppings, stale butter, seawater *(222)*, and implicated as a causative agent of bovine mastitis *(223,224)*.

In humans, *C. rugosa* has been reported to cause opportunistic infections predominantly in immunocompromised patients *(25,27,225–228)*. In one case *(226)* the patient was suffering from acute myelocytic leukemia (ALL) and had disseminated infection with cutaneous lesions that yielded *C. rugosa*. Another patient had alcoholic cirrhosis and an intravenous catheter-associated fungemia *(227)*. Guymon et al. *(228)* and Dubé et al. *(225)* reported frequent colonization by *C. rugosa* of seriously burned patients.

Cases of intravenous catheter-associated *C. rugosa* fungemia have been reported *(25,229)*. In one case, the patient after being treated with intravenous amphotericin B (total dose, 500 mg) made an uneventful recovery *(25)*. Another case of invasive *C. rugosa* disease in a pediatric cystic fibrosis (CF) patient with central venous catheter also responded completely to amphotericin B (at 10 mg/kg) and removal of the catheter *(27)*.

Susceptibility testing of one clinical *C. rugosa* isolate revealed inhibition of growth by 0.156, 0.39, and 0.4 µg/mL of amphotericin B, 5-fluorocytosine (5-FC), and ketoconazole, respectively *(25)*. In a recent study *(225)*, *C. rugosa* isolates from patients in a burn unit showed resistance to nystatin (MIC = 18.5 µg/mL or higher at 24 h) and only moderate susceptibility to amphotericin B (MIC = 0.58 µg/mL at 24 h) and fluconazole (mean MIC = 4.44 µg/mL); ketoconazole uniformly inhibited all isolates at low to moderate concentrations (range, 0.012–0.2 µg/mL at 24 h). While yeast resistance to nystatin and amphotericin B has been linked *(194)*, subtle differences in the mechanism of action of these two polyene antibiotics may not always produce cross-resistance (see also *C. lusitaniae* and *C. guilliermondii*) *(198,225)*.

By comparison, of 18 yeast species isolated from infected bovine mammary glands, *C. rugosa* was the least susceptible of all species evaluated *(223)*. In another study, although none of 13 bovine mammary gland isolates was susceptible to a 9.6-µg amphotericin B disk and 45-µg fluorocytosine disk, and only 25% were inhibited by a 4.8-µg miconazole disk, 100% of the isolates were inhibited by a 1.0-µg ketoconazole disk *(230)*.

7. CANDIDA ZEYLANOIDES

In nature, *Candida zeylanoides* has been isolated from fish *(231)*, as well as a spoilage in poultry *(232–234)* and artisanal Portuguese ewes' cheese *(235)*. Bialasiewicz et al. *(236)* recovered *C. zeylanoides* from the oral cavity of children with retrogenic and other defects. The organism persisted despite the use of disinfectants and treatment with nystatin.

Meyer et al. *(237)* indicated that *C. zeylanoides* did not grow at 37°C, an observation that has also been substantiated by the behavior of the American Type Culture Collection (ATCC) strains.

In several reports, *C. zeylanoides* has been isolated and identified as the causative agent of human disease. Liao et al. *(238)* reported four cases of superficial *C. zeylanoides* mycosis presenting as tinea cruris, which responded to treatment with ketoconazole. In addition, on several occasions, this yeast has been identified as the causative agent of onychomycosis *(239,240)*.

After Roberts *(241)* described the first case of *C. zeylanoides*-induced fungemia, two other accounts followed *(30,31)*. Bisbe et al. *(30)* reported on an insulin-dependent diabetic who underwent kidney and pancreas transplantation and subsequently developed septic arthritis of the knee due to *C. zeylanoides*. The fungemia, which resulted from hematogenous spread of the organism to the synovium, responded to intravenous amphotericin B (total dose 1.0 g). *C. zeylanoides* strain obtained by arthrocentesis was sensitive in vitro to amphotericin B, 5-FC, miconazole, econazole, clotrimazole, and ketoconazole *(30)*. Next, Levenson et al. *(31)* described a patient with a long history of scleroderma and gastrointestinal malabsorption requiring total parenteral nutrition who was diagnosed with *C. zeylanoides* fungemia. While the patient responded to therapy with amphotericin B (total dose, 716 mg), on two subsequent admissions for episodes of fever, blood cultures yielded the same yeast that necessitated further treatment with amphotericin B.

Antimicrobial susceptibility testing performed on three clinical isolates and one control strain of *C. zeylanoides* has shown MIC values, at 48 h, of <0.13, 1.0/2.0, 4.0/8.0, and 0.173–0.5 µg/mL for 5-FC, amphotericin B, fluconazole, and ketoconazole, respectively; in contrast, a fourth clinical isolate was resistant to 5-FC and fluconazole with corresponding MIC values of >128 and 16 µg/mL, respectively *(31)*. Furthermore, the clinical isolates also differed from the description of Meyer et al. *(237)* by exhibiting luxuriant growth at 35°C and 37°C; however, the control strains did not grow at the elevated temperatures, but grew only at 30°C.

Recently, Whitby et al. *(242)* reported a case of *C. zeylanoides* endocarditis in an HIV-positive patient, which developed in the absence of the usual risk factors for systemic candidiasis.

8. CANDIDA FAMATA

Candida famata (formerly known as *Torulopsis candida*) is a saprophytic yeast that has been previously isolated from human skin *(243–245)* and mucosa *(245,246)* but regarded as a contaminant *(243)*. On Sabouraud dextrose agar, the yeast produced smooth, cream-colored colonies after 24 h of incubation at 30°C, which under microscopic examination revealed round-to-oval cells ranging in size from 3.7–5.0 by 2.7–4.7 µm *(16)*.

The first report of human *C. famata*-induced fungemia by Albaret et al. *(247)* did not provide any clinical or mycological description. Later, St.-Germain and Laverdière *(16)* described the first documented case of intravenous-catheter-associated fungemia due to *C. famata* in leukemic patient following allogeneic bone-marrow transplantation. Both the intravascular cannula and the immunosuppressed status of the patient were believed to have played major role as predisposing factors. To this end, Khan et al. *(248)* demonstrated the ability of *C. famata* to produce systemic disease in cortisone-treated mice, thus emphasizing the potential of this yeast to cause disease in immunosuppressed individuals such as cancer patients *(249)*. Removal of the catheter and treatment with intravenous amphotericin B rapidly resolved the fungemia *(16)*.

Quindos et al. *(249)* reported a fatal case of *C. famata*-induced peritonitis in a patient undergoing continuous ambulatory peritoneal dialysis who failed to respond to fluconazole therapy. However in a report by Carrega et al. *(250)*, *C. famata* fungemia in a surgical patient was successfully treated with fluconazole.

In another report *(251)*, *C. famata* was associated with endophthalmitis following extracapsular cataract extraction with implantation of a posterior chamber intraocular lens. The localized intraocular inflammation presented with symptoms virtually identical to *Propionibacterium acnes* infection. The infection was cured with oral flucytosine (2.0 g, q.i.d. for 6 wk; then reduced to 1.0 g, q.i.d. daily because of toxicity).

When tested for antimicrobial susceptibility, a clinical isolate of *C. famata* showed MIC values of 0.08, 0.2, and 0.78 µg/mL for amphotericin B, flucytosine, and ketoconazole, respectively *(16)*.

9. CANDIDA GUILLIERMONDII

Candida guilliermondii is part of the normal fungal flora of the skin. Although, within the genus *Candida*, it appeared to be the least pathogenic in experimental animal models *(252) C. guilliermondii* has been occasionally associated with cases of endocarditis and septic arthritis *(253)*, as well as non-*albicans* nosocomial candidemia in cancer patients *(3)*.

A case of chronic eosinophilic meningoencephalitis due to *C. guilliermondii* has been reported *(254)*. The condition, which is characterized by a meningeal syndrome and an eosinophilic reaction of the cerebrospinal fluid (CSF), is thought to have multiple etiologies including fungal. The neurological disorder was successfully resolved after treatment with amphotericin B.

Dick et al. *(8)* have described a rare case of fatal disseminated candidiasis due to amphotericin B-resistant *C. guilliermondii*. The drug was given daily on d 11 through 24 and every other day on d 24 through 37 (total dose, 883 mg). The patient, with aplastic anemia, died after developing a progressive resistance to amphotericin B. The most disturbing aspect of this case was the emergence of resistance to amphotericin B during therapy by seemingly weakly pathogenic yeast. Yet in another report *(190)*, *C. guilliermondii* resistance to amphotericin B has been reported in a pediatric patient after previous neurosurgery for brain tumor. The decrease and eventual loss of ergosterol with increasing amphotericin B resistance supported previous descriptions of the mechanism of resistance by *Candida* spp. to polyene antibiotics *(172,193–195)* (see also *C. lusitaniae* and *C. rugosa* above).

Resistance to fluconazole was also reported; the drug was given at 5 mg/kg daily to neonates with systemic candidiasis *(255)*.

10. CANDIDA NORVEGENSIS

The occurence in nature of *Candida norvegensis* is largely unknown. This yeast was found to contaminate nonheat-sterilizable food, such as soft cheese *(256)*. On several occasions, however, this yeast has been isolated from clinical specimens *(186)*. A yeast species, *Pichia norvegensis* Leask et Yarrow, isolated on three occasions from human vaginas, has been described as the perfect state of *C. norvegensis (257)*.

C. norvegensis formed yellowish gray colonies when cultured on Sabouraud maltose agar, pH 4.0; at 25°C and 37°C after 2 d, but produced no filaments in the serum tube test *(22)*.

C. norvegensis has been an unusual cause of infections in humans. In Norway, this yeast has been isolated from eight patients from 1990–1996, with all isolates showing resistance to fluconazole *(258)*. This and a previous report of resistance to fluconazole led to the assumption that the fluconazole resistance of *C. norvegensis* is inherent. Polymerase chain reaction (PCR) amplification of the region containing the internally transcribed spacers and 5.8S rRNA gene of *C. norvegensis* yielded a 500 bp fragment *(259)*.

Nielsen et al. *(22)* have reported a fatal case of invasive *C. norvegensis* fungemia related to CAPD peritonitis in a renal-transplant recipient receiving immunosuppressive therapy with prednisone, cyclosporine, and azathioprine. Treatment with flucytosine and amphotericin B (in the peritoneal dialysis fluid) and intravenous amphotericin B failed to control the infection.

Nolla-Salas et al. *(260)* reported the successful treatment of an intra-abdominal abscess due to *C. norvegensis* associated with a Gore-Tex mesh infection using liposomal amphotericin B and mesh removal.

Results from susceptibility antifungal testing of one clinical isolate of *C. norvegensis* revealed sensitivity to amphotericin B and ketoconazole (MIC = 0.2 and 0.4 µg/mL, respectively) but not to flucytosine (MIC = 3.2 µg/mL). After 10 and 4 d, respectively, of flucytosine and amphotericin B therapy, another clinical isolate showed an increase in the MIC values to 0.8 µg/mL for amphotericin B, 12.5 µg/mL for flucytosine, and 1.0 µg/mL for ketoconazole *(22)*.

11. *CANDIDA LIPOLYTICA*

On Sabouraud glucose agar, *C. lipolytica* formed distinctive cerebriform, convoluted, and whiter firm colonies. Blastoconidia, which generally developed only after several days of incubation, were found at the apices and less commonly along the length of the hyphae *(24)*.

C. lipolytica (Harrison) Diddens et Lodder is another yeast that has emerged as pathogenic to humans. Initially included in several large-case series *(261–264)*, only very few well-documented cases of *C. lipolytica*-induced fungemia have been published *(24,265)*. In general, the yeast was weakly pathogenic to humans, and most clearly associated with vascular catheter fungemia *(266)*. There was no evidence of deep visceral infection, such as endophthalmitis, osteomyelitis, arthritis, or hepatic infection *(24,265)*. Catheter removal or empirical amphotericin B treatment was reported to be successful *(266)*. However, even after the removal of infected catheters, fungemia may still persists *(24)*. A treatment regimen of amphotericin B at 0.5 mg/kg daily has been recommended *(24)*.

In vitro susceptibility testing of nine *C. lipolytica* isolates have rendered mean MIC values after 24 h of incubation of 0.660 (range, 0.313–1.25) and 0.22 (0.078–0.313) µg/mL for amphotericin B and ketoconazole, respectively *(24)*.

12. *CANDIDA VISWANATHII*

The major morphologic and biochemical characteristics of *Candida viswanathii* include the absence of chlamydospore formation, and the ability to hydrolyze β-glucosides *(37)*. Although a preliminary study have demonstrated low pathogenicity in laboratory animals *(267)*, *C. viswanathii* was shown to be very pathogenic in cortisone-treated mice, where 5 of 10 animals died during 1 wk, and 3 during the second week following intravenous challenge *(37)*.

In humans, *C. viswanathii* was first isolated in 1959 from the CSF of a fatal case of meningitis in a pediatric patient *(268)*. Later, Sandhu and Rahdhawa *(269)* recovered the yeast in routine sputum cultures.

In a second report of human infection *(37)*, *C. viswanathii* was again isolated from the CSF of a patient with meningitis who also died.

In addition to humans, *C. viswanathii* has also been isolated from gill of fish caught in the Indian Ocean *(270)* and from soil in South Africa *(160)*, which suggested a wide geographic distribution for this fungal species.

13. *CANDIDA HAEMULONII*

Candida haemulonii (van Uden et Kolipinski) Meyer et Yarrow was isolated initially from the scales of the common grunt (*Haemulon scirius*) in the Atlantic Ocean *(271)*. In humans, Lavarde et al. *(272)* reported the first clinical isolation of *C. haemulonii* from the blood of patient with indwelling catheter who died from renal failure, after failing to respond to antifungal therapy with flucytosine and amphotericin B. Marjolet *(273)* has described an additional case of fungemia due to *C. haemulonii* in a cancer patient.

Results from a study by Gargeya et al. *(32)* confirmed the occurence of *C. haemulonii* among clinical specimens, particularly isolates from feet and nails. All of the clinical isolates demonstrated extracellular proteolysis on casein agar but no hydrolysis of keratin (suspended in yeast carbon base agar), and no structures resembling conjugation tubes or ascospores were observed. The major phenotypic difference between *C. famata* and *C. haemulonii* was the absence of "capped cells" and the generally negative assimilation of raffinose by the latter *(32)*.

14. *PICHIA JADINII (CANDIDA UTILIS)*

When grown on Sabouraud dextrose agar medium, the colonies of *Candida utilis* were smooth and cream colored. On cornmeal agar, the yeast produced the typically branched chains of cylindrical blastoconidia *(231)*.

Although still commonly referred to as *Candida utilis*, in 1979, this anamorphic yeast has been determined by Kurtzman et al. *(274)* to be conspecific with the teleomorhic yeast *Hansenula jadinii* based on DNA reasssociation. Subsequently, *H. jadinii* was transferred to the genus *Pichia* by Kurtzman et al. *(275)* who considered the two genera to be synonymous through comparisons of deoxyribonucleic acid and relatedness. Later, the conspecificity of *C. utilis* and *H. jadinii* was corroborated by genomic studies carried out by Bougnoux et al. *(29)* as well as philogenetic relationships based on identical partial sequenses of their 18S and 26S ribosomes *(276)*.

Furthermore, Kogan et al. *(277)* have investigated the structure of a cell-wall glucomannan from *C. utilis* and found that it differed from the cellular mannans of other *Candida* species in that the longer tetra- and pentasaccharide side-chains were terminated with a glucosyl residue. This presence of nonreducing glucosyl groups at the ends of the side chains prevented *C. utilis* from cross-reacting in a double immunodiffusion test with other *Candida* species that possessed mannan antigens and to cross-react with *Hansenula* species with glucomannan antigens.

Only rarely, *C. utilis* has been isolated as a contaminant from clinical specimens (e.g., sputum, digestive tract, vaginal discharge) *(278,279)*. When tested in immunosuppressed mice, *C. utilis* showed low pathogenicity *(280)*. Yet, the first case of opportunistic fungemia due to *C. utilis* was reported by Alsina et al. *(28)* in an AIDS patient with indwelling catheter. Removal of the catheter and treatment with amphotericin B (0.5 mg/kg daily) and flucytosine cleared the infection.

Bougnoux et al. *(29)* have described a case fungemia caused by *C. utilis* in a nonneutropenic, immunocompetent host. Treatment with intravenous amphotericin B (0.5 mg/kg every 2 d) for 26 d resolved the fungemia. Recently, a chronic urinary tract infection due to *C. utilis* was diagnosed in an elderly male patient who developed benign prostatic hypertrophy and chronic obstructive pulmonary disease during a 3-yr course *(281)*.

15. *CANDIDA CIFERRII*

Gunsilius et al. *(282)* have reported the first case of invasive systemic mycosis caused by a fluconazole-resistant *Candida ciferrii* in a patient with acute myeloid leukemia who suffered a relapse after autologous periferal blood progenitor-cell transplantation. Erythematous skin papulae and spotted pulmonary infiltrations were present. Until now, *C. ciferrii* has not been known to cause invasive fungal infections in humans.

REFERENCES

1. Meis, J. F., Ruhnke, M., De Pauw, B. E., Odds, F. C., Siegert, W., and Verweij, P. E. *Candida dubliniensis* candidemia in patients with chemotherapy-induced neutropenia and bone marrow transplantation. *Emerg. Infect. Dis.*, 5, 150-153, 1999.
2. Hazen, K. C. New and emerging yeast pathogens. *Clin. Microbiol. Rev.*, 8, 462, 1995.
3. Krcmery, V., Jr., Mrazova, M., Kunova, A., et al. Nosocomial candidaemias due to species other than *Candida albicans* in cancer patients. Aetiology, risk factors, and outcome of 45 episodes within 10 years in a single cancer institution. *Support Care Cancer*, 7, 428–431, 1999.
4. Hazen, K. C. New and emerging yeast pathogens. *Clin. Microbiol. Rev.*, 8, 462–478, 1995.
5. Colombo, A. L., Nucci, M., Caiuby, M. J., et al. High incidence of non-*albicans* candidemia despite rare use of azoles. *36th Intersci. Conf. Antimicrob. Agents Chemother.*, 226, abstract no. J45, 1996.

6. Morris, J. T. and McAllister, C. K. Fungemia due to *Torulopsis glabrata*. *South. Med. J.*, 86, 356, 1993.
7. Glick, C., Graves, G. R., and Feldman, S. Neonatal fungemia and amphotericin B. *South. Med. J.*, 86, 1368, 1993.
8. Dick, J. D., Rosengard, B. R., Merz, W. G., Stuart, R. K., Hutchins, G. M., and Saral, R., Fatal disseminated candidiasis due to amphotericin B-resistant *Candida guilliermondii*. *Ann. Intern. Med.*, 102, 67, 1985.
9. Booth, L. V., Collins, A. L., Lowes, J. A., and Radford, M. Skin rash associated with *Candida guilliermondii*. *Med. Pediatr. Oncol.*, 16, 295, 1988.
10. Gugnani, H. C., Okafor, B. C., Nzelibe, F., and Njoku-Obi, A. N. Etiological agents of otomycosis in Nigeria. *Mycoses*, 32, 224, 1989.
11. Goldman, M., Pottage, J. C. Jr., and Weaver, D. C. *Candida krusei* fungemia: report of 4 cases and review of the literature. *Medicine (Baltimore)*, 72, 143, 1993.
12. Winegard, J. R., Merz, W. G., Rinaldi, M. G., Johnson, T. H., Karp, J. E., and Saral, R. Increase in *Candida krusei* infection among patients with bone marrow transplantation and neutropenia treated prophylactically with fluconazole. *N. Engl. J. Med.*, 325, 1274, 1991.
13. Piper, J. P., Rinaldi, M. G., and Winn, R. E. *Candida parapsilosis*: an emerging problem. *Infect. Dis. Newsl.*, 7, 49, 55, 1988.
14. Myerowitz, R. L., Pazin, G. L., and Allen, C. M. Disseminated candidiasis: changes in incidence, underlying disease, and pathology. *Am. J. Clin. Pathol.*, 68, 29, 1977.
15. Myers, B. R., Lieberman, T. W., and Ferry, A. P. *Candida* endophthalmitis complicating candidemia. *Ann. Intern. Med.*, 79, 647, 1973.
16. St.-Germain, G. and M. Laverdière, M. *Torulopsis candida*, a new opportunistic pathogen. *J. Clin. Microbiol.*, 24, 884, 1986.
17. Price, M. F., LaRocco, M. T., and Gentry, L. O. Fluconazole susceptibilities of *Candida* species and distribution of species recovered from blood cultures over a 5-year period. *Antimicrob. Agents Chemother.*, 38, 1422, 1994.
18. Morgan, M. A., Wilkowske, C. J., and Roberts, G. D. *Candida pseudotropicalis* fungemia and invasive disease in an immunocompromised patient. *J. Clin. Microbiol.*, 20, 1006, 1984.
19. Blinkhorn, R. J., Adelstein, A., and Spagnuolo, P. J. Emergence of a new opportunistic pathogen, *Candida lusitaniae*. *J. Clin. Microbiol.*, 27, 236, 1989.
20. Pappagianis, D., Collins, M. S., Hector, R., and Remington, J. Development of resistance to amphotericin B in *Candida lusitaniae* infecting a human. *Antimicrob. Agents Chemother.*, 16, 123, 1979.
21. Yinnon, A. M., Woodin, K. A., and Powell, K. R. *Candida lusitaniae* infection in the newborn: case report and review of the literature. *Pediatr. Infect. Dis. J.*, 11, 878–880, 1992.
22. Nielsen, H., Stenderup, J., Bruun, B., and Ladefoged, J. *Candida norvegensis* peritonitis and invasive disease in a patient on continuous ambulatory peritoneal dialysis. *J. Clin. Microbiol.*, 28, 1664–1665, 1990.
23. Rajagopalan, B., Mathews, M. S., and Jacob, M. Vaginal colonization by *Candida lypolitica*. *Genitourin. Med.*, 72, 146–147, 1996.
24. Walsh, T. J., Salkin, I. F., Dixon, D. M., and Hurd, N. J. Clinical, microbiological, and experimental animal studies of *Candida lipolytica*. *J. Clin. Microbiol.*, 27, 927, 1989.
25. Reinhardt, J. F., Ruane, P. J., Walker, L. J., and George, W. L. Intravenous catheter-associated fungemia due to *Candida rugosa*. *J. Clin. Microbiol.*, 22, 1056, 1985.
26. Fisher, M. A., Shueh-Hui, S., Haddad, J., and Tarry, W. F. Comparison of in vivo activity of fluconazole with that of amphotericin B against *Candida tropicalis*, *Candida glabrata*, and *Candida krusei*. *Antimicrob. Agents Chemother.*, 33, 1443, 1989.
27. Arisoy, E. S., Correa, A., Seilheimer, D. K., and Kaplan, S. L. *Candida rugosa* central venous catheter infection in a child. *Pediatr. Infect. Dis. J.*, 12, 961, 1993.
28. Alsina, A., Mason, M., Uphoff, R. A., Riggsby, W. S., Becker, J. M., and Murphy, D. Catheter-associated *Candida utilis* fungemia in a patient with acquired immunodeficiency syndrome: species verification with a molecular probe. *J. Clin. Microbiol.*, 26, 621, 1986.
29. Bougnoux, M.-E., Gueho, E., and Potocka, A.-C. Resolutive *Candida utilis* fungemia in a nonneutropenic patient. *J. Clin. Microbiol.*, 31, 1644, 1993.
30. Bisbe, J., Vilardell, J., Valls, M., Moreno, A., Brancos, M., and Andreu, J. Transient fungemia and candida arthritis due to *Candida zeylanoides*, *Eur. J. Clin. Microbiol.*, 6, 668, 1987.
31. Levenson, D., Pfaller, M. A., Smith, M. A., Hollis, R., Gerarden, T., Tucci, C. B., and Isenberg, H. D., *Candida zeylanoides*: another opportunistic yeast, *J. Clin. Microbiol.*, 29, 1689, 1991.
32. Gargeya, I. B., Pruitt, W. R., Meyer, S. A., and Ahearn, D. G. *Candida haemulonii* from clinical specimens in the USA. *J. Med. Vet. Mycol.*, 29, 335, 1991.
33. Al-Hedaithy, S. S. A. The medically important yeasts present in clinical specimens. *Ann. Saudi Med.*, 12, 57, 1992.
34. Anaissie, E., Bodey, G. P., Kantarjian, H., et al. New spectrum of fungal infections in patients with cancer. *Rev. Infect. Dis.*, 11, 369, 1989.
35. Krogh, P., Holmstrup, P., Thorn, J. J., Vedtofte, P., and Pindborg, J. J. Yeast species and biotypes associated with oral leukoplakia and lichen planus. *Oral Surg. Oral Med. Oral Pathol.*, 63, 48, 1987.
36. Pospisil, L. The significance of *Candida pulcherrima* findings in human clinical specimens. *Mycoses*, 32, 581, 1989.
37. Sandhu, D. K., Sandhu, R. S., and Misra, V. C. Isolation of *Candida viswanathii* from cerebrospinal fluid. *Sabouraudia*, 14, 251, 1976.
38. Aldress, K., Al Shaalan, M., Memish, Z., Alola, S., and Bannatyne, R. *Candida* meningitis in children: two cases report. *J. Chemother.*, 12, 339–344, 2000.

39. Brown, D. M., Jabra-Rizk, M. A., Falkler, W. A., Jr., Baqui, A. A., and Meiller, T. F. Identification of *Candida dubliniensis* in a study of HIV-seropositive pediatric dental patients. *Pediatr. Dent.*, 22, 234–238, 2000.
40. Jabra-Rizk, M. A., Falkler, W. A., Jr., Merz, W. G., Baqui, A. A., Kelley, J. I., and Meiller, T. F. Retrospective identification and characterization of *Candida dubliniensis* isolates among *Candida albicans* clinical laboratory isolates from human immunodeficiency virus (HIV)-infected and non-HIV-infected individuals. *J. Clin. Microbiol.*, 38, 2423–2426, 2000.
41. Kirkpatrick, W. R., Revenkar, S. G., McAtee, R. K., et al. Detection of *Candida dubliniensis* in oropharyngeal samples from human immunodeficiency virus- infected patients in North America by primary CHROMagar candida screening and susceptibility testing of isolates. *J. Clin. Microbiol.*, 36, 3007–3012, 1998.
42. Kirkpatrick, W. R., McAtee, R. K., Lopez-Ribot, J. L., et al. Identification of *Candida dubliniensis* isolates in oropharyngeal samples from HIV-infected patients in North America. *98th Gen. Meet. Am. Soc. Microbiol.*, 261, abstract no. F-48, 1998.
43. Sullivan, D., Harrington, B. J., McCreary, C., Moran, G., and Coleman, D. *Candida dubliniensis*: a new species associated with oral candidiasis in HIV-infected individuals. *11th Int. Conf. AIDS*, 263, abstract no. Th.A.4057, 1996.
44. Meiller, T. F., Jabra-Rizk, M. A., Baqui, A. A., et al. Oral *Candida dubliniensis* as a clinically important species in HIV-seropositive patients in the United States. *Oral Surg. Oral Med. Oral Pathol. Oral Radiol. Endod.*, 88, 573–580, 1999.
45. Jabra-Rizk, M. A., Baqui, A. A., Kelley, J. I., Falkler, W. A. Jr., Merz, W. G., Meiller, T. F. Identification of *Candida dubliniensis* in a prospective study of patients in the United States. *J. Clin. Microbiol.*, 37, 321–326, 1999.
46. Schorling, S. R., Kortunga, H. C., Froschb, M., and Muhlschlegel, F. A. The role of *Candida dubliniensis* in oral candidiasis in human immunodeficiency virus-infected individuals. *Crit. Rev. Microbiol.*, 26, 59–68, 2000.
47. Sandin, R. L., Meier, C. S., Crowder, M. L., and Greene, J. N. Concurrent isolation of *Candida krusei* and *Candida tropicalis* from multiple blood cultures in a patient with acute leukemia. *Arch. Pathol. Lab. Med.*, 117, 521, 1993.
48. Valdivieso, M., Luna, M., Bodey, G. P., Rodriguez, V., and Groschell, D. Fungemia due to *Torulopsis glabrata* in the compromised host. *Cancer*, 38, 1750, 1976.
49. Marks, M., Langston, C., and Eickhoff, T. *Torulopsis glabrata*: an opportunistic pathogen in man. *N. Engl. J. Med.*, 283, 1131, 1970.
50. Hahn, H., Condie, F., and Bulger, R. Diagnosis of *Torulopsis glabrata* infection. *J. Am. Med. Assoc.*, 203, 835, 1968.
51. Friedman, E., Blahut, R., and Bender, M. Hepatic abscesses and fungemia from *Torulopsis glabrata*. *J. Clin. Gastroenterol.*, 9, 711, 1987.
52. Connolly, J. and Mitas, J. *Torulopsis glabrata* fungemia in a diabetic patient. *South. Med. J.*, 83, 352, 1990.
53. Fidel, P. L., Jr., Vazquez, J. A., and Sobel, J. D. *Candida glabrata*: review of epidemiology, pathogenesis, and clinical disease with comparison to *C. albicans*. *Clin. Microbiol. Rev.*, 12, 80-96, 1999.
54. Vazquez, J. A., Dembry, L. M., Sanchez, V., et al. Nosocomial *Candida glabrata* colonization: an epidemiologic study. *J. Clin. Microbiol.*, 36, 421-426, 1998.
55. Gumbo, T., Isada, C. M., Hall, G., Karafa, M. T., and Gordon, S. M. *Candida glabrata* fungemia. Clinical features of 139 patients. *Medicine (Baltimore)*, 78, 220-227, 1999.
56. Sfameni, S. F., Talbot, J. M., Chow, S. L., Brenton, L. A., and Scurry, J. P. *Candida glabrata* chorioamnionitis following in vitro fertilization and embryo transfer. *Aust. N. Z. J. Obstet. Gynecol.*, 37, 88-91, 1997.
57. Sandford, G. R., Merz, W. G., Winegard, J. R., Charache, P., and Saral, R. The value of fungal surveillance cultures as predictors of systemic fungal infections. *J. Infect. Dis.*, 142, 503, 1980.
58. Walter, E., Gingras, J., and McKinney, R. Systemic *Torulopsis glabrata* in a neonate. *South. Med. J.*, 83, 837, 1990.
59. Roger, P. M., Boissy, C., Gari-Toussaint, M., et al. Medical treatment of a pacemaker endocarditis due to *Candida albicans* and to *Candida glabrata*. *J. Infect.*, 41, 176–178, 2000.
60. Luzzati, R., Amalfitano, G., Lazzarini, L., et al. Nosocomial candidemia in non-neutropenic patients at an Italian tertiary care hospital. *Eur. J. Clin. Microbiol. Infect. Dis.*, 19, 602–607, 2000.
61. Vennwald, I., Seebacher, C., and Roitzsch, E. Post-mortem findings in patients with repeatedly mycological demonstration of *Candida glabrata*. *Mycoses*, 41, 125–132, 1998.
62. Maruyama, H., Nakamaru, T., Oya, M., et al. Posthysteroscopy *Candida glabrata* peritonitis in a patient on CAPD. *Perit. Dial. Int.*, 17, 404–405, 1997.
63. Blot, S., Vandewoude, K., Hoste, E., Poelaert, J., and Colardyn, F. Outcome in critically ill patients with candidal fungaemia: *Candida albicans* vs. *Candida glabrata*. *J. Hosp. Infect.*, 47, 308–313, 2001.
64. Viscoli, C., Girmenia, C., Marinus, A., et al. Candidemia in cancer patients: a prospective, multicenter surveillance study by the Invasive Fungal Infection Group (IFIG) of the European Organization for Research and Treatment of Cancer (EORTC). *Clin. Infect. Dis.*, 28, 1071–1079, 1999.
65. Aisner, J., Schimpff, S., Sutherland, J., Young, V. M., and Wiernick, P. H. *Torulopsis glabrata* infections in patients with cancer. *Am. J. Med.*, 61, 23, 1976.
66. Hughes, D. A., Davies, D. R., Young, R., et al. Fine needle aspiration cytology (FNAC) detection of early renal allograft infection with *Candida glabrata* - a case report. *Cytopathology*, 10, 349–353, 1999.
67. Zmierczak, H., Goemaere, S., Mielants, H., Verbruggen, G., and Veys, E. M. *Candida glabrata* arthritis: case report and review of the literature of *Candida* arthritis. *Clin. Rheumatol.*, 18, 406–409, 1999.
68. Darling, K., Singh, J., and Wilks, D., Successful treatment of *Candida glabrata* endophthalmitis with amphotericin B lipid complex (ABLC). *J. Infect.*, 40, 92–94, 2000.
69. Nayeri, F., Cameron, R., Chryssanthou, E., Johansson, L., and Soderstrom, C. *Candida glabrata* prosthesis infection following pyelonephritis and septicaemia. *Scand. J. Infect. Dis.*, 29, 635–638, 1997.

70. Nair, S., Kumar, K. S., Sachan, P., and Corpuz, M. Spontaneous fungal peritonitis (*Candida glabrata*) in a patient with cirrhosis. *J. Clin. Gastroenterol.*, 32, 362–364, 2001.
71. Angel-Moreno, A., Frances, A., Granado, J. M., and Perez-Arellano, J. L. Ventriculoperitoneal shunt infection by *Candida grabrata* in an adult. *J. Infect.*, 41, 178–179, 2000.
72. Dwyer, K., McDonald, M., and Fitzpatrick, T. Presentation of *Candida glabrata* spinal osteomyelitis 25 months after documented candidaemia. *Aust. N. Z. Med.*, 29, 571–572, 1999.
73. Faix, R. G., Kovarik, S. M., Shaw, T. R., and Johnson, R. V. Mucocutaneous and invasive candidiasis among very low birth weight (<1500 grams) infants in intensive care nurseries: a prospective study. *Pediatrics*, 83, 101, 1989.
74. Weese-Mayer, D. E., Fondriest, D. W., Brouillette, R. T., and Schulman, S. T. Risk factors associated with candidemia in the neonatal intensive care unit: a case-control study. *Pediatr. Infect. Dis. J.*, 6, 190, 1987.
75. Pankey, G. and Daloviso, J. Fungemia caused by *Torulopsis glabrata*. *Medicine (Baltimore)*, 52, 395, 1973.
76. Khemakhem, B., Kanoun, F., Ben Jemaa, M., et al. *Candida glabrata* perinephric abscess. A case report. *Ann. Med. Interne (Paris)*, 152, 134–136, 2001.
77. Kauffman, C. A., Vazquez, J. A., Sobel, J. D., et al. Prospective multicenter surveillance study of funguria in hospitalized patients. The National Institute of Allergy and Infectious Diseases (NIAID) Mycoses Study Group. *Clin. Infect. Dis.*, 30, 14–18, 2000.
78. Harris, A. D., Castro, J., Sheppard, D. C., Carmeli, Y., and Samore, M. H. Risk factors for nosocomial candiduria due to *Candida glabrata* and *Candida albicans*. *Clin. Infect. Dis.*, 29, 926-928, 1999.
79. Hoegl, L., Thoma-Greber, E., Rocken, M., and Korting, H. C. Persistent oral candidosis by non-*albicans Candida* strains including *Candida glabrata* in a human immunodeficiency virus-infected patient observed over a period of 6 years. *Mycoses*, 41, 335-338, 1998.
80. Sanglard, D., Ischer, F., Calabrese, D., Majcherczyk, P. A., and Bille, J. The ATP binding cassette transporter gene CgCDR1 from *Candida glabrata* is involved in the resistance of clinical isolates to azole antifungal agents. *Antimicrob. Agents Chemother.*, 43, 2753–2765, 1999.
81. Redding, S. W., Kirkpatrick, W. R., Dib, O., Fothergill, A. W., Rinaldi, M. G., and Patterson, T. F. The epidemiology of non-*albicans Candida* in oropharyngeal candidiasis in HIV patients. *Spec. Care Dentist.*, 20, 178–181, 2000.
82. Phillips, P., Shafran, S., Garber, G., et al. Multicenter randomized trial of fluconazole versus amphotericin B for treatment of candidemia in non-neutropenic patients. Canadian Candidemia Study Group. *Eur. J. Clin. Microbiol. Infect. Dis.*, 16, 337–345, 1997.
83. Komshian, S. V., Uwaydah, A. K., Sobel, J. D., and Crane, L. R. Fungemia caused by *Candida* species and *Torulopsis glabrata* in the hospitalized patient: frequency, characteristics and evaluation of factors influencing outcome. *Rev. Respir. Dis.*, 11, 379, 1989.
84. Baley, J. E., Kliegman, R. M., Annable, W. L., Dahms, B. B., and Fanaroff, A. A., *Torulopsis glabrata* sepsis appearing as necrotizing enterocolitis and endophthalmitis. *Am. J. Dis. Child.*, 138, 965, 1984.
85. Sander, C. H., Martin, J. N., Rogers, A. L., Barr, M. Jr., and Heidelberger, K. P. Perinatal infection with *Torulopsis glabrata*: a case associated with maternal sickle cell anemia. *Obstet. Gynecol.*, 61, 21S, 1983.
86. Quirke, P., Hwang, W. S., and Validen, C. C. Congenital *Torulopsis glabrata* infection in man. *Am. J. Cin. Pathol.*, 73, 137, 1980.
87. Juster-Reicher, A., Leibovitz, E., Linder, N., et al. Liposomal amphotericin B (AmBisome) in the treatment of neonatal candidiasis in very low birth weight infants. *Infection*, 28, 223-226, 2000.
88. Chapman, F. M., Orr, K. E., Armitage, W. J., Easty, D. L., and Cottrell, D. G. *Candida glabrata* endophthalmitis following penetrating keratoplasty. *Br. J. Ophthalmol.*, 82, 712- 713, 1998.
89. Rolston, K., Baird, I., Graham, D. R., and Jauregui, L. Treatment of refractory candemia in non-neutropenic patients with liposomal nystatin (NYOTRAN(tm)). *38th Intersci. Conf. Antimicrob. Agents Chemother.*, 24, abstract no. LB-1, 1998.
90. Kleinpeter, M. A. and Butt, A. A. Non-*Candida albicans* fungal peritonitis in continuous ambulatory peritoneal dialysis patients. *Adv. Perit. Dial.*, 17, 176-179, 2001.
91. Mikamo, H., Sato, Y., Hayasaki, Y., and Tamaya, T. Current status and fluconazole treatment of pelvic fungal gynecological infections. *Chemotherapy*, 46, 209-212, 2000.
92. Fortun, J., Lopez-San Roman, A., Velasco, J. J., et al. Selection of *Candida glabrata* strains with reduced susceptibility to azoles in four liver transplant patients with invasive candidiasis. *Eur. J. Clin. Microbiol. Infect. Dis.*, 16, 314–318, 1997.
93. Piemonte, P., Conte, G., Flores, C., et al. Emergency of fluconazole-resistant infections by *Candida krusei* and *Candida glabrata* in neutropenic patients. *Rev. Med. Chil.*, 124, 1149, 1996.
94. Raffalli, J., Falvo, C., Seiter, K., et al. Risk factors for non-*albicans Candida* bloodstream infections in a university hospital. *38th Intersci. Conf. Antimicrob. Agents Chemother.*, 458, abstract no. J-25, 1998.
95. Miyazaki, H., Miyazaki, Y., Geber, A., et al. Fluconazole resistance associated with drug efflux and increased transcription of a drug transporter gene, PDH1, in *Canida glabrata*. *Antimicrob. Agents Chemother.*, 42, 1695–16701, 1998.
96. Tholakanahalli, V. N., Potti, A., Hanley, J. F., and Merliss, A. D. Fluconazole-induced torsade de pointes. *Ann. Pharmacother.*, 35, 432–434, 2001.
97. Rocco, T. R., Reinert, S. E., and Simms, H. H. Effects of fluconazole administration in critically ill patients: analysis of bacterial and fungal resistance. *Arch. Surg.*, 135, 160–165, 2000.
98. Czaika, V., Titz, H. J., Schmalreck, A., Sterry, W., and Schultze, W. Antifungal susceptibility testing in chronically recurrent vaginal candidosis as basis for effective therapy. *Mycoses*, 43(Suppl. 2), 45–50, 2000.

99. Otero, L., Fleites, A., Mendez, F. J., Palacio, V., and Vazquez, F. Susceptibility of *Candida* species isolated from female prostitutes with vulvovaginitis to antifungal agents and boric acid. *Eur. J. Clin. Microbiol. Infect. Dis.*, 18, 59–61, 1999.
100. Sobel, J. D. Vulvovaginitis due to *Candida glabrata*. An emerging problem. *Mycoses*, 41(Suppl. 2), 18–22, 1998.
101. Parazzini, F., Di Cintio, E., Chiantera, V., and Guaschino, S. Determinants of different *Candida* species infections of the genital tract in women. Sporachrom Study Group. *Eur. J. Obstet. Gynecol. Reprod. Biol.*, 93, 141–145, 2000.
102. Cross, E. W., Park, S., and Perlin, D. S. Cross-resistance of clinical isolates of *Candida albicans* and *Candida glabrata* to over-the-counter azoles used in the treatment of vaginitis. *Microb. Drug Resist.*, 6, 155–161, 2000.
103. White, D. J., Habib, A. R., Vanthyne, A., Langford, S., and Symonds, M. Combined topical flucytosine and amphotericin B for refractory vaginal *Candida glabrata* infections. *Sex. Transm. Infect.*, 77, 212–213, 2001.
104. del Palacio, A., Sanz, F., Sanchez-Alor, G., et al. Double-blind randomized dose-finding study in acute vulvovaginal candidosis. Comparison of flutrimazole site-release cream (1, 2 and 4%) with placebo site-release vaginal cream. *Mycoses*, 43, 355–365, 2000.
105. Lisiak, M., Klyszejko, C., Marcinkowski, Z., and Gwiezdzinski, Z. Yeast species identification in vulvovaginal candidiasis: susceptibility to nystatin. *Ginekol. Pol.*, 71, 959–963, 2000.
106. Dan, M. Severe vulvovaginitis associated with intravaginal nystatin. *Am. J. Obstet. Gynecol.*, 185, 254–255, 2000.
107. Sobel, J. D., Chaim, W., and Leaman, D. Recurrent vulvovaginal candidiasis associated with long-term tamoxifen treatment in postmenopausal women. *Obstet. Gynecol.*, 88(4 Part 2), 704–706, 1996.
108. Laverdiere, M., Rotstein, C., Bow, E. J., et al. Impact of fluconazole prophylaxis on fungal colonization and infection rates in neutropenic patients. The Canadian Fluconazole Study. *J. Antimicrob. Chemother.*, 46, 1001–1008, 2000.
109. Safdar, A., van Rgee, F., Henslee-Downey, J. P., Singhal, S., and Mehta, J. *Candida glabrata* and *Candida krusei* fungemia after high-risk allogeneic marrow transplantation: no adverse effect of low-dose fluconazole prophylaxis on incidence and outcome. *Bone Marrow Transplant.*, 28, 873–878, 2001.
110. Vazquez, J. A., Sobel, J. D., Peng, G., et al. Evolution of vaginal *Candida* species recovered from human immunodeficiency virus-infected women receiving fluconazole prophylaxis: the emergence of *Candida glabrata*? Terry Beirn Community Programs for Clinical Research in AIDS (CPCRA). *Clin. Infect. Dis.*, 28, 1025–1031, 1999.
111. King, R. D., Lee, J. C., and Morris, A. L. Adherence of *Candida albicans* and other *Candida* species to mucosal epithelial cells. *Infect. Immun.*, 27, 667, 1980.
112. Stanley, V. C. and Hurley, R. Growth of *Candida* species in cultures of mouse epithelial cells. *J. Pathol. Bacteriol.*, 94, 301, 1967.
113. Edwards, J. E. Jr., Montgomerie, J. Z., Ishida, K., Morrison, J. O., and Guze, L. B. Experimental hematogenous endophthalmitis due to *Candida*: species variation in ocular pathogenicity. *J. Infect. Dis.*, 135, 294, 1977.
114. Casasnovas, R.-O., Caillot, D., Solary, E., et al. Prophylactic fluconazole and *Candida krusei* infection. *N. Engl. J. Med.*, 326, 891, 1992.
115. Merz, W. G., Karp, J. E., Schron, D., and Saral, R. Increased incidence of fungemia caused by *Candida krusei*. *J. Clin. Microbiol.*, 24, 581, 1986.
116. Horn, R., Wong, B., Kiehn, T. E., and Armstrong, D. Fungemia in a cancer hospital: changing frequency, earlier onset, and results of therapy. *Rev. Infect. Dis.*, 7, 646, 1985.
117. Meunier, F., Aoun, M., and Bitar, N. Candidemia in immunocompromised patients. *Clin. Infect. Dis.*, 14, S120, 1992.
118. Krcméry, V., Jr., Spanik, S., Kunova, A., et al. Nosocomial *Candida krusei* fungemia in cancer patients: report of 10 cases and review. *J. Chemother.*, 11, 131–136, 1999.
119. Launay, O., Lortholary, O., Bouges-Michel, C., Jarrousse, B., Bentata, M., and Guillevin, L. Candidemia: a nosocomial complication in adults with late-stage AIDS. *Clin. Infect. Dis.*, 26, 1134–1141, 1998.
120. Abbas, J., Bodey, G. P., Hanna, H. A., et al. *Candida krusei* fungemia. An escalating serious infection in immunocompromised patients. *Arch. Intern. Med.*, 160, 2659–2664, 2000.
121. Revankar, S. G., Kirkpatrick, W. R., McAtee, R. K., et al. Prevalence of fluconazole resistance in oropharyngeal candidiasis in HIV infected patients using chromogenic media. *3rd Conf. Retroviruses Opportunistic Infect.*, 158, 1996.
122. Vazquez, J. A., Boikov, D., and Sobel, J. D. Antifungal cross-resistance among *Candida* spp. recovered from fluconazole-refractory thrush in AIDS patients. *5th Conf. Retroviruses Opportunistic Infect.*, abstract no. 490, 1998.
123. Calabrese, D. C., Bille, J., Barchiesi, F., and Sanglard, D. Incidence of resistance mechanisms to azole antifungal agents in *Candida* species from HIV+ patients with oropharyngeal candidosis (OPC). *38th Intersci. Conf. Antimicrob. Agents Chemother.*, 112, abstract no. C-152, 1998.
124. Jarque, I., Saavedra, S., Martin, G., Peman, J., Perez Belles, C., and Sanz, M. A. Delay of onset of candidemia and emergence of *Candida krusei* fungemia in hematologic patients receiving prophylactic fluconazole. *Haematologica*, 85, 441–443, 2000
125. Graybill, J. R. Changing strategies for treatment of systemic mycoses. *Braz. J. Infect. Dis.*, 4, 47–54, 2000.
126. Meunier-Carpentier, F., Kiehn, T. E., and Armstrong, D. Fungemia in the immunocompromised host. *Am. J. Med.*, 71, 363, 1981.
127. Bross, J., Talbot, G. H., Maislin, G., Hurvitz, S., and Strom, B. L. Risk factors for nosocomial candidemia: a case-control study in adults without leukemia. *Am. J. Med.*, 87, 614, 1989.
128. Slavin, R. E., Dias, M. A., and Saral, R. Cytosine arabinoside induced gastrointestinal toxic alterations in sequential chemotherapeutic protocols: a clinical-pathologic study of 33 patients. *Cancer*, 42, 1747, 1978.
129. Burke, P. J., Karp, J. E., Braine, H. G., and Vaughan, W. P. Timed sequential therapy of human leukemia based upon the response of leukemic cells to humoral growth factors. *Cancer Res.*, 37, 2138, 1977.
130. Burke, B. J., Vaughan, W. P., Karp, J. E., and Saylor, P. L. The correlation of maximal drug dose, tumor recruitment,

and sequence timing with therapeutic advantage: schedule-dependent toxicity of cytosine arabinoside. *Med. Pediatr. Oncol.*, 1(Suppl.), 201, 1982.
131. Wey, S. B., Mori, M., Pfaller, M. A., Woolson, R. F., and Wenzel, R. P. Risk factors for hospital acquired candidemia: a matched case-control study. *Arch. Intern. Med.*, 149, 2349, 1989.
132. McQuillen, D. P., Zingman, B. S., Meunier, F., and Levitz, S. M. Invasive infections due to *Candida krusei*: report of ten cases of fungemia that include three cases of endophthalmitis. *Clin. Infect. Dis.*, 14, 472, 1992.
133. Rubinstein, E., Noriega, E. R., Simberkoff, M. S., Holzman, R., and Rahal, J. J. Jr. Fungal endocarditis: analysis of 24 cases and review of the literature. *Medicine (Baltimore)*, 54, 331, 1974.
134. Young, R. C., Bennett, J. E., Geelhoed, G. W., and Levine, A. S. Fungemia with compromised host resistance. *Ann. Intern. Med.*, 80, 605, 1974.
135. Jacobs, M. I., Magid, M. S., and Jarowski, C. I. Disseminated candidiasis: newer approaches to early recognition and treatment. *Arch. Dermatol.*, 116, 1277, 1980.
136. Rose, H. D. and Varkey, B. Deep mycotic infection in the hospitalized adult: a study of 132 patients. *Medicine (Baltimore)*, 54, 499, 1975.
137. Gordon, R. A., Simmons, B. P., Appelbaum, P. C., and Aber, R. C. Intra-abdominal abscess and fungemia caused by *Candida krusei*. *Arch. Intern. Med.*, 140, 1239, 1980.
138. Diggs, C. H., Eskenasy, G. M., Sutherland, J. C., and Wiernik, P. H. Fungal infection of muscle in acute leukemia. *Cancer*, 38, 1771, 1976.
139. Nguyen, V. Q. and Penn, R. L. *Candida krusei* infectious arhtritis - a rare complication of neutropenia. *Am. J. Med.*, 83, 963, 1987.
140. Carcassi, A., Saletti, M., and Boschi, S. Artrite acuta da *Candida*: isolamento di *Candida krusei* in un eroinomane. *Minerva Med.*, 73, 2905, 1982.
141. Thomalla, J. V., Steidle, C. P., Leapman, S. B., and Filo, R. S. Ureteral obstruction of a renal allograft secondary to *Candida krusei*. *Transplant. Proc.*, 20, 551, 1988.
142. Segal, E., Romano, A., Eylan, E., et al., Isolation of *Candida tropicalis* from an orbital infection as a complication of maxillary osteomyelitis. *Infection*, 2, 111, 1974.
143. Segal, E., Romano, A., Eylin, E., and Stein, R. Experimental and clinical studies of 5- fluorocytosine activity in *Candida* ocular infections. *Chemotherapy*, 21, 358, 1975.
144. Alva, E. M. and Khayr, W. *Candida krusei* sinusitis. *Am. J. Ther.*, 5, 121–123, 1998.
145. Mathieson, R. and Dutta, S. K. *Candida* esophagitis. *Dig. Dis. Sci.*, 28, 365, 1983.
146. Bugnardi, G. E., Savage, M. A., Coker, R., and Davis, S. G. Fluconazole and *Candida krusei* infections. *J. Hosp. Infect.*, 18, 326, 1991.
147. Case, C. P., MacGowan, A. P., Brown, N. M., Reeves, D. S., Whitehead, P., and Felmingham, D. Prophylactic oral fluconazole and *Candida* fungemia. *Lancet*, 337, 790, 1991.
148. NcIlroy, M. A. Failure of fluconazole to suppress fungemia in a patient with fever, neutropenia, and typhlitis. *J. Infect. Dis.*, 163, 420, 1991.
149. Persons, D. A., Laughlin, M., Tanner, D., Perfect, J., Gockerman, J. P., and Hathorn, J. W. Fluconazole and *Candida krusei* fungemia. *N. Engl. J. Med.*, 325, 1315, 1991.
150. Tam, J. Y., Blume, K. G., and Prober, C. G. Prophylactic fluconazole and *Candida krusei* infections: a reply. *N. Engl. J. Med.*, 326, 891, 1992.
151. Schuler, U. and Ehninger, G. Prophylactic fluconazole and *Candida krusei* infections: a reply. *N. Engl. J. Med.*, 326, 892, 1992.
152. Winston, D. J., Islam, Z., and Buell, D. N. for the Acute Leukemia Study Group. Fluconazole prophylaxis of fungal infections in acute leukemia patients: results of a placebo- controlled, double-blind, multicenter trial. *Proc. 31st Intersci. Conf. Antimicrob. Agents Chemother.*, American Society for Microbiology, Washington, DC, 99, 1991.
153. Chandrasekar, P. H. and Gathy, C. for the Bone Marrow Transplantation Team. Reduction of candidal colonization with fluconazole in neutropenic cancer patients. *Proc. 31st Intersci. Conf. Antimicrob. Agents Chemother.*, American Society for Microbiology, Washington, DC, 292, 1991.
154. Goodman, J., Beull, D., Gilbert, G., et al., Fluconazole prevents fungal infections in bone marrow transplantations: results of a placebo-controlled, double-blind, randomized, multi-center trial. *Proc. 31st Intersci. Conf. Antimicrob. Agents Chemother.*, American Society for Microbiology, Washington, DC, 149, 1991.
155. Samonis, G., Rolston, K., Karl, C., Miller, P., and Bodey, G. P. Prophylaxis of oropharyngeal candidiasis with fluconazole. *Rev. Infect. Dis.*, 12(Suppl. 3), S369, 1990.
156. Morace, G., Manzara, S., and Dettori, G. In vitro susceptibility of 119 yeast isolates to fluconazole, 5-fluorocytosine, amphotericin B and ketoconazole. *Chemotherapy*, 37, 23, 1991.
157. Galgiani, J. N., Susceptibility of *Candida albicans* and other yeast to fluconazole: relation between in vitro and in vivo studies. *Rev. Infect. Dis.*, 12, S272, 1990.
158. Hay, R. J. Fluconazole, *J. Infect.*, 21, 1, 1990.
159. Katiyar, S. K. and Edlind, T. D. Identification and expression of multidrug resistance-related transporter genes in *Candida krusei*. *Med. Mycol.*, 109–116, 2001.
160. van Uden, N. and Buckley, H. *Candida* Berkhout, in *The Yeasts - A Taxonomic Study*, Lodder, J., Ed. North-Holland Publishing Co., Amsterdam, 893, 1970.
161. Hadfield, T. L., Smith, M. B., Winn, R. E., Rinaldi, M. G., and Guerra, C. Mycoses caused by *Candida lusitaniae*. *Rev. Infect. Dis.*, 9, 1006, 1987.
162. Sanchez, P. J. and Cooper, B. H. *Candida lusitaniae*: sepsis and meningitis in a neonate. *Pediatr. Infect. Dis. J.*, 6, 758, 1987.

163. Kauffman, C. A., Shea, M. J., and Frame, P. T. Invasive fungal infections in patients with chronic mucocutaneous candidiasis. *Arch. Intern. Med.*, 141, 1076, 1981.
164. Guinet, R., Chanas, J., Goullier, A., Bonnefoy, G., and Ambroise-Thomas, P. Fatal septicemia due to amphotericin B-resistant *Candida lusitaniae*. *J. Clin. Microbiol.*, 18, 443, 1983.
165. Bradsher, R. W. Transient fungemia due to *Candida lusitaniae*. *South. Med. J.*, 78, 626, 1985.
166. Libertin, C. R., Wilson, W. R., and Roberts, G. D. *Candida lusitaniae*: an opportunistic pathogen. *Diagn. Infect. Dis. J.*, 3, 69, 1985.
167. Merz, W. G. *Candida lusitaniae*: frequency of recovery, colonization, infection and amphotericin resistance. *J. Clin. Microbiol.*, 20, 1194, 1984.
168. Christenson, J. C., Guruswamy, A., Mukwaya, G., and Rettig, P. J. *Candida lusitaniae*: an emerging human pathogen. *Pediatr. Infect. Dis. J.*, 6, 755, 1987.
169. Holzschu, D. L., Presley, H. L., Miranda, M., and Phaff, H. J. Identification of *Candida lusitaniae* as an opportunistic yeast in humans. *J. Clin. Microbiol.*, 10, 202, 1979.
170. Baker, J. G., Nadler, H. L., Forgacs, P., and Kurtz, S. R. *Candida lusitaniae*: a new opportunistic pathogen of the urinary tract. *Diagn. Microbiol. Infect. Dis.*, 2, 145, 1984.
171. Pensler, M. I., Krawczyk, P., and LeBar, W. D. *Candida lusitaniae*. *Clin. Microbiol. Newsl.*, 7, 86, 1985.
172. Merz, W. G. and Sanford, G. R. Isolation and characteristics of a polyene-resistant variant of *Candida tropicalis*. *J. Clin. Microbiol.*, 9, 677, 1979.
173. Schlitzer, R. L. and Ahearn, D. G. Characterization of atypical *Candida tropicalis* and other uncommon clinical yeast isolates. *J. Clin. Microbiol.*, 15, 511, 1982.
174. Leggiadro, R. J. and Collins, T. Postneurosurgical *Candida lusitaniae* meningitis. *Pediatr. Infect. Dis. J.*, 7, 368, 1988.
175. Minari, A., Hachem, R., and Raad, I. *Candida lusitaniae*: a cause of breakthrough fungemia in cancer patients. *Clin. Infect. Dis.*, 32, 186–190, 2001.
176. Krcmery, V. Jr., Oravcova, E., Spanik, S., et al. Nosocomial breakthrough fungemia during antifungal prophylaxis or empirical antifungal therapy in 41 cancer patients receiving antineoplastic chemotherapy: analysis of aetiology risk factors and outcome. *J. Antimicrob. Chemother.*, 41, 373–380, 1998.
177. Bren, A. Fungal peritonitis in patients on continuous ambulatory peritoneal dialysis. *Eur. J. Clin. Microbiol. Infect. Dis.*, 17, 839–843, 1998.
178. Garcia-Martos, P., Diaz, J., Castano, M., Perez, M., and Marin, P. Peritonitis caused by *Candida lusitaniae* in patient on continuous ambulatory peritoneal dialysis (CAPD). *Clin. Nephrol.*, 36, 50, 1991.
179. Garcia-Martos, P., Diaz Portillo, J., Perez Ruilopez, M. A., Castano Lopez, M. A., Fernandez Gutierez del Alamo, C., Fungal peritonitis during continuous ambulatory peritoneal dialysis (CAPD). *Enferm. Infecc. Microbiol. Clin.*, 9, 30–32, 1991.
180. Wendt, B., Haglund, L., Razavi, A., and Rath, R. *Candida lusitaniae*: an uncommon cause of prosthetic valve endocarditis. *Clin. Infect. Dis.*, 26, 769–770, 1998.
181. Kjaeldgaard, P., Schultz, K. S., Nielsen, K., and Stenderup, J. Fatal catheter septicemia with finding of *Candida lusitaniae*. *Ugeskr. Laeger*, 152, 611–612, 1990.
182. Behar, S. M. and Chertow, G. M. Olecranon bursitis caused by infection with *Candida lusitaniae*. *J. Rheumatol.*, 25, 598–600, 1998.
183. Fowler, S. L., Rhoton, B., Springer, S. C., Messer, S. A., Hollis, R. J., and Pfaller, M. A. Evidence for person-to-person transmission of *Candida lusitaniae* in a neonatal intensive care unit. *Infect. Control Hosp. Epidemiol.*, 19, 343–345, 1998.
184. Oleinik, E. M., Della-Latta, P., Rinaldi, M. G., and Saiman, L. *Candida lusitaniae* osteomyelitis in a premature infant. *Am. J. Perinatol.*, 10, 313–315, 1993.
185. Sanchez, V., Vazquez, J. A., Barth-Jones, D., Dembry, L., Sobel, J. D., and Zervos, M. J. Epidemiology of nosocomial acquisition of *Candida lusitaniae*. *J. Clin. Microbiol.*, 30, 3005–3008, 1992.
186. Ahearn, D. G. and McGlohn, M. S. In vitro susceptibilities of sucrose-negative *Candida tropicalis*, *Candida lusitaniae*, and *Candida norvegensis* to amphotericin B, 5- fluorocytosine, miconazole, and ketoconazole. *J. Clin. Microbiol.*, 19, 412, 1984.
187. Abuhammour, W. and Habte-Gabr, E. Systemic antifungal agents. *Indian J. Pediatr.*, 68, 655–668, 2001.
188. Collin, B., Clancy, C. J., and Nguyen, M. H., Antifungal resistance in non-*albicans Candida* species. *Drug Resist. Updat.*, 2, 9–14, 1999.
189. Vanden Bosshe, H., Dromer, F., Improvisi, I., Lozano-Chiu, M., Rex, J. H., and Sanglard, D. Antifungal drug resistance in pathogenic fungi. *Med. Mycol.*, 1, 119–128, 1998.
190. Kovacicova, G., Hanzen, J., Pisarcikova, M., et al. Nosocomial fungemia due to amphotericin B-resistant *Candida* spp. in three pediatric patients after previous neurosurgery for brain tumors. *J. Infect. Chemother.*, 7, 45–48, 2001.
191. Bründel, K.-H. Zum problem der dermatomykosen bei bergleuten der grube. *Anna. Berufs.- Dermatosen*, 25, 181, 1977.
192. Hamilton-Miller, J. Non-emergence of polyene-resistant yeasts: a hypothesis. *Microbios*, 10(Suppl. A), 91, 1974.
193. Safe, L., Safe, S., Subden, R., and Morris, D. Sterol content and polyene antibiotic resistance in isolates of *Candida krusei*, *Candida parakrusei*, and *Candida tropicalis*. *Can. J. Microbiol.*, 23, 398, 1977.
194. Dick, J. D., Merz, W. G., and Saral, R. Incidence of polyene-resistant yeasts recovered from clinical specimens. *Antimicrob. Agents Chemother.*, 18, 158, 1980.
195. Drutz, D. J. and Lehrer, R. I. Development of amphotericin B-resistant *Candida tropicalis* in a patient with defective leukocyte function. *Am. J. Med. Sci.*, 276, 77, 1978.

196. Bodenhoff, J. Resistance studies of *Candida albicans*, with special reference to two patients subjected to prolonged antibiotic treatment. *Odontol. Tidskr.*, 76, 279, 1968.
197. Hamilton-Miller, J. M. T. Chemistry and biology of the polyene macrolide antibiotics. *Bacteriol. Rev.*, 37, 166, 1973.
198. Woods, R. A. Nystatin-resistant mutants of yeast: alterations in sterol content. *J. Bacteriol.*, 108, 69, 1971.
199. Caillot, D., Casanovas, O., Solary, E., et al. Efficacy and tolerance of an amphotericin B lipid (Intralipid) emulsion in the treatment of candidaemia in neutropenic patients. *J. Antimicrob. Chemother.*, 31, 161–169, 1993.
200. Thomas, M. G., Parr, D. H., di Menna, M., and Lang, S. D. R. *Candida lusitaniae* septicemia: successful combination therapy. *Clin. Microbiol. Newsl.*, 7, 142, 1985.
201. Sullivan, D. and Coleman, D. *Candida dubliniensis*: characteristics and identification. *J. Clin. Microbiol.*, 36, 329–334, 1998.
202. Sullivan, D. and Coleman, D. *Candida dubliniensis*: an emerging pathogen. *Curr. Top. Med. Mycol.*, 8, 15–25, 1997.
203. Sullivan, D. J., Westerneng, T. J., Haynes, K. A., Bennett, D. E., and Coleman, D. C. *Candida dubliniensis* sp. nov.: phenotypic and molecular characterization of a novel species associated with oral candidosis in HIV-infected individuals. *Microbiology*, 141(Part 7), 1507–1521, 1995.
204. Milan, E. P., de Laet Sant' Ana, P., de Azevedo Melo, A. S., et al. Multicenter prospective surveillance of oral *Candida dubliniensis* among adult Brazilian human immunodeficiency virus-positive and AIDS patients. *Diagn. Microbiol. Infect. Dis.*, 41, 29–35, 2001.
205. Marriott, D., Laxton, M., and Harkess, J. *Candida dubliniensis* candidemia in Australia. *Emerg. Infect. Dis.*, 7, 479, 2001.
206. Sullivan, D., Haynes, K., Bille, J., et al. Widespread geographic distribution of oral *Candida dubliniensis* strains in human immunodeficiency virus-infected individuals. *J. Clin. Microbiol.*, 35, 960–964, 1997.
207. Meis, J. F., Lunel, F. M., Verweij, P. E., and Voss, A. One-year prevalence of *Candida dubliniensis* in a Dutch university hospital. *J. Clin. Microbiol.*, 38, 3139–3140, 2000 [see also: *J. Clin. Microbiol.*, 38, 170–174, 2000].
208. Diaz-Guerra, T. M., Laguna, F., and Rodriguez-Tudela, J. L. Molecular characterization by PCR fingerprinting of isolates of *C. dubliniensis* from two HIV-positive patients in Spain. *38th Intersci. Conf.Antimicrob. Agents Chemother.*, 457, abstract no. J-21, 1998.
209. Polacheck, I., Strahilevitz, J., Sullivan, D., Donnelly, S., Salkin, I. F., and Coleman, D. C. Recovery of *Candida dubliniensis* from non-human immunodeficiency virus-infected patients in Israel. *J. Clin. Microbiol.*, 38, 170–174, 2000 [see also: *J. Clin. Microbiol.*, 38, 3139–3140, 2000].
210. Patterson, T. F., Kirkpatrick, W. R., McAtee, R. K., et al. Detection of *Candida dubliniensis* isolates in oropharyngeal candidiasis in HIV-infected patients. *10th Int. Symp. Infect. Immunocompromised Host*, abstract no. 048, 1998.
211. Velegraki, A., Nicolatou, O., Theodoridou, M., Mostrou, G., and Legakis, N. J. Paediatric AIDS-related linear gingival erythema: a form of erythematous candidiasis? *J. Oral. Pathol. Med.*, 28, 178-182, 1999.
212. Willis, A. M., Coultier, W. A., Sullivan, D. J., et al. Isolation of *C. dubliniensis* from insulin-using diabetes mellitus patients. *J. Oral. Pathol. Med.*, 29, 86-90, 2000.
213. Jabra-Rizk, M. A., Falkler, W. A., Jr., Merz, W. G., Kelley, J. I., Baqui, A. A., and Meiller, T. F. Coaggregation of *Candida dubliniensis* with *Fusobacterium nucleatum*. *J. Clin. Microbiol.*, 37, 1464, 1468, 1999.
214. Meis, J. F., Van Belkum, A., Odds, F., et al. Invasive candidiasis due to the new species *Candida dubliniensis*. *38th Intersci. Conf. Antimicrob. Agents Chemother.*, 460, abstract no. J-34, 1998.
215. Redding, S. W., Bailey, C. W., Lopez-Ribot, J. L., et al. *Candida dubliniensis* in radiation-induced oropharyngeal candidiasis. *Oral Surg. Oral Med. Oral Pathol. Oral Radiol. Endod.*, 91, 659–662, 2001.
216. Sullivan, D., Coleman, D., Harrington, B., et al. Molecular and phenotypic analysis of *Candida dubliniensis*: a recently identified species linked with oral candidosis in HIV- infected and AIDS patients. *Oral Dis.*, Suppl. 1, S96–S101, 1997.
217. Sullivan, D. C. and Coleman, D. J. Candidiasis: the emergence of a novel species, *Candida dubliniensis*. *AIDS*, 11, 557–567, 1997.
218. McCullough, M. J., Clemons, K. V., and Stevens, D. A. Molecular and phenotypic characterization of the three genotypic subgroups of *Candida albicans*, *Candida dubliniensis* and *Candida stellatoidea*. *98th Gen. Meet. Am. Soc. Microbiol.*, 260, abstract no. F-44, 1998.
219. Quindos, G., Carrillo-Munoz, A. J., Arevalo, M. P., et al. In vitro susceptibility of *Candida dubliniensis* to current and new antifungal agents. *Chemotherapy*, 46, 395–401, 2000.
220. Moran, G. P., Sanglard, D., Donnelly, S. M., Shanley, D. B., Sullivan, D. J., and Coleman, D. C. Identification and expression of multidrug transporters responsible for fluconazole resistance in *Candida dubliniensis*. *Antimicrob. Agents Chemother.*, 42, 1819–1830, 1998.
221. Ruhnke, M., Schmidt-Westhausen, A., and Morschhauser, J. Development of simultaneous resistance to fluconazole in *Candida albicans* and *Candida dubliniensis* in a patient with AIDS. *J. Antimicrob. Chemother.*, 46, 291–295, 2000.
222. van Uden, N. and Buckley, H., *Candida rugosa* (Anderson) Duddens et Lodder, in *The Yeasts - A Taxonomic Study*, Lodder, J., Ed. North-Holland Publishing Co., Amsterdam, 1032, 1970.
223. Richard, J. L., McDonald, J. S., Fichtner, R. E., and Anderson, A. J. Identification of yeasts from infected bovine mammary glands and their experimental infectivity in cattle. *Am. J. Vet. Res.*, 41, 1991, 1980.
224. Dion, W. M. and Dukes, T. W. *Candida rugosa*: experimental mastitis in a diary cow. *Sabouraudia*, 20, 95, 1982.
225. Dubé, M. P., Heseltine, P. N., Rinaldi, M. G., Evans, S., and Zawacki, B. Fungemia and colonization with nystatin-resistant *Candida rugosa* in a burn unit. *Clin. Infect. Dis.*, 18, 77, 1994.
226. Sugar, A. M. and Stevens, D. A. *Candida rugosa* in immunocompromised infection: case reports, drug susceptibility and review of the literature. *Cancer*, 56, 318, 1985.

227. Reinhardt, J. F., Ruane, P. J., Walker, L. J., and George, W. L. Intravenous catheter- associated fungemia due to *Candida rugosa*. *J. Clin. Microbiol.*, 22, 1056, 1985.
228. Guymon, C. H., McManus, A. T., Mason, A. D., and McManus, W. F. Yeast colonization and infection in seriously burned patients, in *Proc. 91st Gen. Meet. Am. Soc. Microbiol.*, American Society for Microbiology, Washington, DC, 429(abstract # L-38), 1991.
229. Shenoy, S., Samuga, M., Urs, S., et al. Intravenous catheter-related *Candida rugosa* fungaemia. *Trop. Doct.*, 26, 31, 1996.
230. McDonald, J. S., Richard, J. L., Anderson, A. J., and Fichtner, R. E. In vitro antimycotic sensitivity of yeasts isolated from infected bovine mammary glands. *Am. J. Vet. Res.*, 41, 1987, 1980.
231. Vazquez-Juarez, R., Ascencio, F., Andlid, T., Gustafson, L., and Wadstrom, T. The expression of potential colonization factors of yeasts isolated from fish during different growth conditions. *Can. J. Microbiol.*, 39, 1135, 1993.
232. Deak, T. Identification of yeast isolated from poultry meat. *Acta Biol. Hung.*, 52, 195–200, 2001.
233. Ismail, S. A., Deak, T., El-Rahman, H. A., Yassien, M. A., and Beuchat, L. R. Presence and changes in population of yeasts on raw and processed poultry products stored at refrigeration temperature. *Int. J. Food Microbiol.*, 62, 113–121, 2000.
234. Deak, T., Chen, J., and Beuchat, L. R. Molecular characterization of *Yarrowia lipolytica* and *Candida zeylanoides* isolated from poultry. *Appl. Environ. Microbiol.*, 66, 4340–4344, 2000.
235. Pereira-Dias, S., Potes, M. E., Marinho, A., Malfeito-Ferreira, M., and Loureiro, V. Characterization of yeast flora isolated from an artisanal Portuguese ewes' cheese. *Int. J. Food Microbiol.*, 60, 55–63, 2000.
236. Bialasiewicz, D., Kurnatowska, A., and Smiech-Slomkowska, G. Characteristics of fungi and attempts of their elimination from the oral cavity in children treated with orthodontic appliances. *Med. Dosw. Mikrobiol.*, 45, 389, 1993.
237. Meyer, S. A., Ahearn, D. G., and Yarrow, D., in *The Yeasts: A Taxonomic Study*, 3rd ed., Kreeger-van Rij, N. J. W., Ed. Elsevier Science, Amsterdam, 839, 1984.
238. Liao, W. Q., Li, Z. G., Guo, M., and Zhang, J. Z. *Candida zeylanoides* causing candidiasis as tinea cruris. *Chin. Med. J.*, 106, 542, 1993.
239. Rippon, J. W. Candidiasis and the pathogenic yeasts, in *Medical Mycology*, Rippon, J. W., Ed. W. B. Saunders, Philadelphia, 484, 1982.
240. Crosier, W. J. Two cases of onychomycosis due to *Candida zeylanoides*. *Australas. J. Dermatol.*, 34, 23, 1993.
241. Roberts, G. Detection of fungemia. *Infect. Dis. Newsl.*, 4, 18, 1985.
242. Whitby, S., Madu, E. C., and Bronze, M. S. Case report: *Candida zeylanoides*, infective endocarditis complicating infection with the human immunodeficiency virus. *Am. J. Med. Sci.*, 312, 138–139, 1996.
243. Cooper, B. H. and Silva-Hutner, M. Yeast of medical importance, in *Manual of Clinical Microbiology*, 4th ed., Lennette, E. H., Balows, A., Hausler, W. J. Jr., and Shadomy, J., Eds. American Society for Microbiology, Washington, DC, 526, 1985.
244. Badillet, G., Sené, S., Barnel, C., and Jung, C. Les levures du genre *Torulopsis* en dermatologie. *Bull. Soc. Fr. Mycol. Méd.*, 14, 235, 1985.
245. Barthe, J. and Barthe, M.-F. The ecology of *Torulopsis* in man. *Sabouraudia*, 11, 192, 1973.
246. De Closets, F. and Combescot, C. Étude de levures isolées de prélèvements pathologiques. *Bull. Soc. Fr. Mycol. Méd.*, 9, 9, 1980.
247. Albaret, S., Hoquet, P., Cavellat, J.-F., Delhumean, A., and Cavellat, M. Le traitement des septicémies a levures: ses limites. *Anasth. Analg. Reanim.*, 36, 13, 1979.
248. Khan, Z. V., Misra, V. C., Randhawa, H. S., and Damodaran, V. N. Pathogenicity of some ordinarily harmless yeast for cortisone-treated mice. *Sabouraudia*, 18, 319, 1980.
249. Quindos, G., Cabrera, F., Arilla, M. C., et al. Fatal *Candida famata* peritonitis in a patient undergoing continuous ambulatory peritoneal dialysis who was treated with fluconazole. *Clin. Infect. Dis.*, 18, 658, 1994.
249. Krcméry, V. and Kunova, A. *Candida fumata* fungemia in a cancer patient: case report. *J. Chemother.*, 12, 189–190, 2000.
250. Carrega, G., Riccio, G., Santoriello, L., Pasqualini, M., and Pellucci, R. *Candida fumata* fungemia in a surgical patient successfully treated with fluconazole. *Eur. J. Clin. Microbiol. Infect. Dis.*, 16, 698–699, 1997.
251. Rao, N. A., Nerenberg, A. V., and Forster, D. J. *Torulopsis candida* (*Candida famata*) endophthalmitis simulating *Propionibacterium acnes* syndrome. *Arch. Ophthalmol.*, 109, 1718–1721, 1991.
252. Hurley, R. and Winner, H. I., Pathogenicity in the genus *Candida*. *Mycopathologia*, 24, 337, 1964.
253. Rippon, J. W. Candidiasis and the pathogenic yeasts, in *Medical Mycology: The Pathogenic Fungi and the Pathogenic Actinomycetes*, Rippon, J. W., Ed. W. B. Saunders, Philadelphia, 565, 1982.
254. Paz-Sendin, L., Gonzalez-Torres, R., Gomez-Morales, L., Hernandez-Gonzalez, G. Chronic eosinophylic meningoencephalitis due to *Candida guilliermondii*. *Rev. Neurol.*, 29, 817–818, 1999.
255. Narang, A., Agrawal, P., Chakraborti, A., and Kumar, P. Fluconazole in the management of neonatal systemic candidiasis. *Indian Pediatr.*, 33, 823–826, 1996.
256. Bouakline, A., Lacroix, C., Roux, N., Gangneux, J. P., and Derouin, F. Fungal contamination of food in hematology units. *J. Clin. Microbiol.*, 38, 4272–4273, 2000.
257. Leask, B. G. and Yarrow, D. *Pichia norvegensis* sp. nov. *Sabouraudia*, 61–63, 1976.
258. Sandven, P., Nilsen, K., Digranes, A., Tjade, T., and Lassen, J. *Candida norvegensis*: a fluconazole-resistant species. *Antimicrob. Agents Chemother.*, 41, 1375–1376, 1997.
259. Nho, S., Anderson, M. J., Moore, C. B., and Denning, D. W. Species differentiation by internally transcribed spacer

PCR and HhaI digestion of fluconazole-resistant *Candida krusei, Candida inconspicua,* and *Candida norvegensis* strains. *J. Clin. Microbiol.*, 35, 1036–1039, 1997.
260. Nolla-Salas, J., Torres-Rodriguez, J. M., Grau, S., et al. Successful treatment with liposomal amphotericin B of an intraabdominal abscess due to *Candida norvegensis* associated with a Gore-Tex mesh infection. *Scand. J. Infect. Dis.*, 32, 560–562, 2000.
261. Bille, J., Stockman, L., and Roberts, G. D. Detection of yeasts and filamentous fungi in blood cultures during a ten-year period (1972 to1981). *J. Clin. Microbiol.*, 16, 968, 1982.
262. Hopfer, R. L., Orengo, A., Chesnut, S., and Wenglar, M. Radiometric detection of yeasts in blood cultures of cancer patients. *J. Clin. Microbiol.*, 12, 329, 1980.
263. Horn, R., Wong, B., Kiehn, T. E., and Armstrong, D. Fungemia in a cancer hospital: changing frequency, earlier onset, and results of therapy. *Rev. Infect. Dis.*, 7, 646, 1985.
264. Prevost, E. and Bannister, E. Detection of yeast septicemia by byphasic and radiometric methods. *J. Clin. Microbiol.*, 13, 655, 1981.
265. Wherspann, P. and Fullbrandt, U. *Yarrowia lipolytica* (Wickerham et al) van der Walt and von Arx isolated from a blood culture. *Mykosen*, 28, 217, 1985.
266. Shin, J. H., Kook, H., Shin, D. H., et al. Nosocomial cluster of *Candida lipolytica* fungemia in pediatric patients. *Eur. J. Clin. Microbiol. Infect. Dis.*, 19, 344-349, 2000.
267. Sandhu, R. S., Randhawa, H. S., and Gupta, I. M. Pathogenicity of *Candida viswanathii* for laboratory animals: a preliminary study. *Sabouraudia*, 4, 37, 1965.
268. Viswanathan, R. and Randhawa, H. S. *Candida viswanathii* sp. nov., isolated from a case of meningitis. *Science & Culture*, 25, 86, 1959.
269. Sandhu, R. S. and Randhawa, H. S. On the re-isolation and taxonomic study of *Candida viswanathii*, Viswanathan et Randhawa. *Mycopath. Mycol. Applic.*, 18, 179, 1962.
270. Fell, J. W. and Meyer Sally, A. Systematics of yeast species in the *Candida parapsilosis* group. *Mycopath. Mycol. Applic.*, 32, 177, 1967.
271. van Uden, N. and Kolipinski, M. C. *Torulopsis haemulonii* nov. spec. a yeast from the Atlantic ocean. *Antonie van Leeuwenhoek*, 28, 78, 1962.
272. Lavarde, V., Daniel, F., Saez, H., Arnold, M., and Faguer, B. Peritonite mycosique a *Torulopsis haemulonii*. *Bul. Soc. Fr. Mycol. Méd.*, 13, 173, 1984.
273. Marjolet, M. *Torulopsis ernobii, Torulopsis haemulonii*: levures opportunistes chez l'immunodéprimé? *Bul. Soc. Fr. Mycol. Méd.*, 15, 143, 1986.
274. Kurtzman, C. P., Johnson, C. J., and Smiley, M. J. Determination of conspecificity of *Candida utilis* and *Hansenula jadinii* through DNA reassociation. *Mycologia*, 71, 844, 1979.
275. Kurtzman, C. P. Synonymy of the yeast genera *Hansenula* and *Pichia* demonstrated through comparisons of deoxyribonucleic acid and relatedness. *Antonie van Leeuwenhoek*, 50, 209, 1984.
276. Yamada, Y., Matsuda, M., and Mikata, K. The phylogenetic relationships of *Pichia jadinii*, formerly classified in the genus *Hansenula*, and related species based on the partial sequences of 18S and 26S ribosomal RNAs (*Saccharomycetaceae*). *Biosci. Biotechnol. Biochem.*, 59, 518, 1995.
277. Kogan, G., Sandula, J., and Simkovicova, V. Glucomannan from *Candida utilis*: structural investigation. *Folia Microbiol. (Praha)*, 38, 219, 1993.
278. Phaff, H. J. Biology of yeasts other than *Saccharomyces*, in *Biology of Industrial Microorganisms, Demain, A. L. and Solomon, N. A., Eds. Benjamin Cummings Publishing Co., Menlo Park, CA, 537, 1985.
279. Viviani, M. A., Tortorano, A. M., Piazza, T., Bassi, F., Grioni, A., and Langer, M. Candidosis surveillance in intensive care unit patients. *Bull. Soc. Fr. Mycol. Méd.*, 15, 121, 1986.
280. Holzcshu, D. L., Chandler, F. W., Ajello, L., and Ahearn, D. G. Evaluation of industrial yeasts for pathogenicity. *Sabouraudia*, 17, 71, 1979.
281. Hazen, K. C., Theisz, G. W., and Howell, S. A. Chronic urinary tract infection due to *Candida utilis*. *J. Clin. Microbiol.*, 37, 824–827, 1999.
282. Gunsilius, E., Lass-Florl, C., Kahler, C. M., Gastl, G., and Petzer, A. L. *Candida ciferrii*, a new fluconazole-resistant yeast causing systemic mycosis in immunocompromised patients. *Ann. Hematol.*, 80, 178–179, 2001.

22
Trichosporon beigelii

1. INTRODUCTION

The genus *Trichosporon* represents a group of imperfect filamentous yeast fungi of the family Cryptococcaceae, order Monilialis, which are normal flora of the respiratory and digestive tracts of humans and animals. As part of the normal flora of the human skin, *Trichosporon* spp. may cause benign cutaneous infections, known as white piedra, when the organisms penetrate the cells of the cuticle, forming whithish-yellow nodules on the hair folicles especially of the beard, axillary, and genital regions *(1)*. Other supeficial infections due to *T. beigelii* include onychomycosis *(2,3)*, and possibly otomycosis *(4)*. Torssander et al. *(5)* described anal colonization by *T. beigelii* in homosexual men, and white piedra of scrotal hair folicles. In the environment, *T. beigelii* has been implicated as the cause of hypersensitivity pneumonitis *(6,7)*.

T. beigelii (Kuchenmeister et Rabenhorst) Vuillemin is a common pathogen in humans and one of the causative agents of white piedra *(8,9)*, as well as potentially life-threatening localized visceral or disseminated trichosporonosis in immunocompromised hosts *(8,10–21)*.

In addition, *Trichosporon* spp. have been diagnosed in endocarditis *(22–27)*, endophthalmitis *(28)*, and endometritis *(29)* in immunocompetent hosts. Bottari et al. *(30)* presented a unusual case of esophageal stenosis complicated by gastrointestinal reflux due to *T. beigelii* in the absence of a pathologic predisposition or immunodeficiency. *T. beigelii* was also reported to cause disseminated infection in neonates with associated high mortality *(31,32)*.

There have been reports of trichosporonosis in HIV-positive individuals *(33–36)*. In two of these cases *(33,34)*, the patients had a bloodstream infection with *T. beigelii*. In a third case, the patient, who had chronic renal failure, developed peritonitis (with no evidence of disseminated disease) while on CAPD *(35)*.

Trichosporonosis is rapidly emerging as an opportunistic invasive fungal disease, with frequently fatal outcome (up to 64% *[8]*). Some non-neutropenic patients with trichosporoniasis have been reported to experience mortality rates as high as 78% *(14)*.

Immunocompromised patients, such as those with neoplastic disease (acute and chronic leukemia, multiple myeloma, solid tumors, aplastic anemia, and non-Hodgkin's lymphoma) have been at high risk for developing invasive trichosporonosis *(10–13,37–48)*. Other immunosuppressed conditions (solid organ *[19,49–51]* and bone-marrow *[18,20,52]* transplantation, prosthetic valve surgery, chronic active hepatitis, intravenous drug abuse, and cataract extractions) have also been reported to be predisposing factors for trichosporonosis. Studies by Wong et al. *(53)* demonstrated that trichosporonosis has been common among non-neutropenic patients with iron overload and hemochromatosis. Small clusters of infection has also been observed in low birth-weight neonates *(54,55)*.

The most likely portals of entry for *Trichosporon* spp. are the alimentary tract and the lungs *(14)*. Indwelling catheters (Hickman catheters, central venous catheters, and peripheral venous cannulae), and intravenous injections can be other potential portals of entry *(13,23,56,57)*.

From: Opportunistic Infections: Treatment and Prophylaxis
By: Vassil St. Georgiev © Humana Press Inc., Totowa, NJ

Trichosporonosis has been characterized by the presence of cutaneous lesions (discrete maculopapular erythematous skin rash) *(58)*, pulmonary and renal *(27,42,47,59–61)* involvement, peritonitis *(23,62–64)*, and chorioretinitis *(65)*. Disseminated trichosporonosis in granulocytopenic patients usually has a rapid onset of fever, fungemia, funguria, azotemia, pulmonary infiltrates, and cutaneous lesions with invasion of the kidney, lungs, skin, and other tissues *(66)*.

2. TREATMENT OF TRICHOSPORONOSIS

Even though amphotericin B has been widely used in the therapy of trichosporonosis *(10,13,62,67)*, its efficacy has not been clearly established because of the retrospective nature of most studies *(68)*. While successful amphotericin B therapy was achieved in most cases of patients recovering from myelosuppression, those patients with persistent and profound neutropenia have failed to recover *(14,69)*. In granulocytopenic patients, intravenous therapy with amphotericin B may be initiated at 0.5 mg/kg daily. In cases of refractory trichosporonosis, the daily dose regimen may be increased to 1.0 mg/kg or perhaps even higher *(8)*.

In addition to conventional amphotericin B, the therapeutic efficacies of liposomal amphotericin B and its deoxycholate have also been evaluated in experimental mouse trichosporonosis *(31,70)*. Liposome-encapsulated formulation may allow the administration of higher doses of amphotericin B with a reduced risk of nephrotoxicity.

Ujhelyi et al. *(62)* successfully treated *T. beigelii* peritonitis with intravenous amphotericin B and removal of the peritoneal dialysis catheter. The initial dose of the antibiotic, 15 mg daily, was escalated over 1-wk period to 35 mg daily; 2 wk later the dose was again escalated to 70 mg daily for a total dose of 1.0 g of amphotericin B. Flucytosine at a daily dose of 1.25 g (14 mg/kg), which was also added to the antifungal regimen, was seemingly not beneficial because of drug resistance and had to be discontinued *(62)*. Antifungal susceptibility testing of *T. beigelii* isolated from the patients showed MIC values against amphotericin B of 0.08, >100, 0.07/0.15, and 10.0 µg/mL *(62)*. Other antifungal agents successfully used to treat *Trichosporon*-induced CAPD peritonitis included oral fluconazole, oral ketoconazole, and intravenous miconazole given for periods of 18–40 d; in some cases, however, the dialysis catheter had to be removed *(23,63,64)*.

Alballaa et al. *(71)* described a fatal case of disseminated trichosporonosis due to *T. beigelii* in a patient with ALL despite therapy with amphotericin B. However, the fatal outcome may have been the result of lack of recovery of bone-marrow function rather than to drug tolerance *(66)*. Amphotericin B was started at 0.5 mg/kg daily, then increased to 1.0 mg/kg daily; 5-FC at a dose of 150 mg/kg daily was also added to the antifungal regimen. The susceptibility MIC values of a clinical isolate for amphotericin B, fluconazole, flucytosine, and miconazole were 0.78, >100, >100, and 1.56 µg/mL, respectively *(71)*.

Walsh et al. *(66)* also reported two cases of disseminated *T. beigelii* infection with persistent fungemia, that was refractory to amphotericin B; the MIC values of several clinical isolates for amphotericin B ranged from <0.14 to 1.16 µg/mL. It was postulated that inhibition alone, but not killing of resistant *T. beigelii* isolates, may be inadequate to cure trichosporonosis in granulocytopenic patients, in whom there are no granulocytes to facilitate host clearance and in whom fungicidal activity is needed *(66)*.

In several reports *(65,72)*, 5-FC has been shown to be effective in the treatment of trichosporonosis.

Anaissie et al. *(68)* studied the therapeutic efficacy of several azole antimycotics (fluconazole, miconazole, and SCH 39304) against trichosporonosis in patients with serious underlying disease (solid tumor and hematologic malignancies or immunosuppressive chemotherapy for liver transplantation), as well as in a murine model of disseminated disease. Fluconazole was found to be effective at the various dose regimens used (100–400 mg daily, or at 7.0 mg/kg, then 3.5 mg/kg). Miconazole was also found to be effective at daily doses of 1.2 g. SHC 39304 was given to a patient with ALL who, in addition to trichosporonosis, also had disseminated aspergillosis; at daily doses of 200 mg given for 5 wk, SCH 39304 eradicated trichosporonosis while evidence of aspergillosis was still present. In one case of acute prostetic valve endocarditis, however, fluconazole at daily doses of 400 mg failed to eradicate the fungus *(26)*.

A combination of intravenous miconazole (1.2 g) and oral norfloxacin (600 mg) even though effective had to be coupled with splenectomy in order to cure disseminated trichosporonosis in a patient with acute myelogenous leukemia (AML) *(17)*.

Canales et al. *(69)* reported a successful resolution of a case of *T. beigelii* pneumonia with itraconazole. Another azole, sulconazole has been recommended for the topical treatment of superficial infections of the skin *(73)*.

Although ketoconazole was reported to be effective in a patient with a history of intravenous drug abuse *(56)*, it failed to elicit response in a case of *T. beigelii*-related aortic valve endocarditis where the patient experienced a relapse 6 mo after treatment with 400 mg of ketoconazole daily *(24)*. In the latter case, amphotericin B (total of 250 mg) also failed to eradicate the pathogen.

Lowenthal et al. *(16)* described a case of disseminated *T. beigelii* infection in a bone-marrow transplant recipient who fully recovered following combination therapy comprising of amphotericin B, miconazole, and ketoconazole. Amphotericin B was administered intravenously for 6 d at a gradually increasing dose until it reached 20 mg. However, because of hepatic and renal toxicity, the patient was switched to intravenous miconazole (800 mg, t.i.d.) for 2 wk, followed by oral ketoconazole at 200 mg daily for an additional 4 wk on an outpatient basis.

Hajjeh and Blumberg *(74)* described a case of bloodstream infection due to *T. beigelii* in a burn patient. A combination of amphotericin B (0.5 mg/kg daily; total of 1.2 g) and flucytosine (100 mg/kg daily) successfully treated the mycosis. Recently, Cawley et al. *(21)* successfully treated a burn victim with a combination of amphotericin B and high dose of fluconazole. Patients with severe thermal injuries (over 40% of total body surface area) are known to have depressed humoral and cellular immune responses. In particular, burn victims are known to have a transient defect in neutrophil function that can be a major predisposing factor to opportunistic infections *(75–77)*. In addition, unwarranted changes also occur in other immune functions, including increased T-cell suppressor activity, decreased number and function of helper T cells, decreased IgG levels, and defects in the monocyte functions *(78)*.

3. *BLASTOSCHIZOMYCES CAPITATUS*

Trichosporon capitatum, long considered to be another pathogenic member of the genus *Trichosporon*, is now reclassified as *Blastoschizomyces capitatus (79)* (or *Geotrichum capitatum [80]*) based on photomicroscopic, cinematographic, and electron microscopic observations defining its "arthroconidia" as anneloconidia *(79)*. This new combination was established to accommodate two previous taxa, *Trichosporon capitatum* and *Blastoschizomyces pseudotrichosporon (81)* that were recognized to be con-specific *(79)*. In contrast to *T. capitatum*, *B. capitatus* consistently assimilates glucose but no other carbohydrates.

Because the deep infections caused by *T. beigelii* and *B. capitatus* appear similar both clinically and histopathologically, both are described in this chapter for consistency with previous reports *(8)*.

Disseminated infections caused by *B. capitatus* have been diagnosed and have involved immunocompromised patients *(82–93)*. By some accounts, within the past 10 years, nearly 50 cases *B. capitatus* infections have been diagnosed *(94)*. Most of the patients had acute leukemia or related disorders and had received chemotherapy treatment *(95,96)*. *B. capitatus* urinary infections in severely ill patients have also been reported *(97)*.

Recently, a case of *B. capitatus* onychomycosis in a healthy patient was described *(98)*. In another report *(99)*, a patient with no proven immunosuppression contracted *B. capitatus* infection through contamination of fluids for intravenous application.

3.1. Treatment of B. capitatus Infections

Due to *B. capitatus* resistance to currently used antifungal agents, this infection represents a therapeutic challenge and serious complication in the treatment of hematological malignancies *(94,100)*.

In a case of chronic meningeal trichosporonosis in an allogeneic bone-marrow recipient, oral fluconazole at 100–400 mg daily failed to eradicate *B. capitatus* after 11 mo of treatment *(92)*. The patient was immunosuppressed while receiving corticosteroid and cyclosporin A chemotherapy for chronic graft-vs-host disease. A similar clinical presentation was reported in an acute leukemia patient infected with *T. beigelii (101)*.

Because eradication of *B. capitatus* in severely immunosuppressed patients has been difficult to achieve *(102)*, continuous suppressive antifungal therapy may be necessary, especially in CNS infections, as has been previously established for *Cryptococcus neoformans* meningitis *(103–105)*.

Recently, Sanz et al. *(106)* reported three new cases of *B. capitatus* infection occuring in neutropenic patients with AML. All three patients were treated with amphotericin B, but only one survived after receiving a total of 1660 mg (1.3 mg/kg daily) over a 16-d period. In another case, a patient with clinical septicemia and multiorgan failure failed to respond to intravenous liposomal amphotericin B therapy *(100)*.

Despite aggressive antifungal therapy, the clinical response of hepatosplenic fungal infections due to neutropenia is often poor. To this end, DeMaio and Colman *(107)* described a case of hepatosplenic *B. capitatus* infection that responded to adjuvant interferon-γ (IFN-γ) therapy.

REFERENCES

1. Zaror, L. and Moreno, M. I. White piedra. Report of a case. *Rev. Med. Chil.*, 124, 593–596, 1996.
2. Fusaro, R. M. and Miller, N. G. Onychomycosis caused by *Trichosporon beigelii* in the United States. *J. Am. Acad. Dermatol.*, 11, 747, 1984.
3. Han, M. H., Choi, J. H., Sung, K. J., Moon, K. C., and Koh, J. K. Onychomycosis and *Trichosporon beigelii* in Korea. *Int. J. Dermatol.*, 39, 266–169, 2000.
4. Reiersol, S. *Trichosporon cutaneum* isolated from a case of otomycosis. *Acta Otol. Microbiol. Scand.*, 37, 459, 1955.
5. Torssander, J., Carlsson, B., and van Krogh, G. *Trichosporon beigelii*: an increased occurence in homosexual men. *Mykosen*, 28, 355, 1984.
6. Shimazu, K., Ando, M., Sakata, T., Yoshida, K., and Araki, S. Hypersensitivity pneumonitis induced by *Trichosporon cutaneum*. *Am. Rev. Respir. Dis.*, 130, 407, 1984.
7. Soda, K. Ando, M., Shimazu, K., Sakata, T., Yoshida, K., and Araki, S. Different classes of antibody activities to *Trichosporon cutaneum* antigen in summer-type hypersensitivity pneumonitis by enzyme-linked immunosorbent assay. *Am. Rev. Respir. Dis.*, 133, 83, 1986.
8. Walsh, T. J. Trichosporonosis. *Inf. Dis. Clin.*, 3, 43, 1989.
9. Kalter, D. C., Tschen, J. A., Cernoch, P. L., et al. Genital white piedra: epidemiology, microbiology, and therapy. *J. Am. Acad. Dermatol.*, 14, 982, 1986.
10. Gardella, S., Nomdedeu, B., Bombi, J. A., et al. Fatal fungemia with arthritic involvement caused by *Trichosporon beigelii* in a bone marrow transplant recipient. *J. Infect. Dis.*, 151, 566, 1985.
11. Gold, J. W. M., Poston, W., Mertelsmann, R., et al. Systemic infection with *Trichosporon cutaneum* in a patient with acute leukemia: report of a case. *Cancer*, 48, 2163, 1981.
12. Yung, C. W., Hanauer, S. B., Freitzin, D., Rippon, J. W., Shapiro, C., and Gonzalez, M. Disseminated *Trichosporon beigelii* (*cutaneum*). *Cancer*, 48, 2107, 1981.
13. Walsh, T. J., Newman, K. R., Moody, M., Wharton, R. C., and Wade, J. C. Trichosporonosis in patients with neoplastic disease. *Medicine (Baltimore)*, 65, 268, 1986.
14. Hoy, J., Hsu, K. C., Rolston, K., Hopfer, R. L., Luna, M., and Bodey, G.P. *Trichosporon beigelii* infection: a review. *Rev. Infect. Dis.*, 8, 959, 1986.
15. Anaissie, E., Bodey, G. P., Kantarjian, H., et al. New spectrum of fungal infections in patients with cancer. *Rev. Infect. Dis.*, 11, 369, 1989.
16. Lowenthal, R. M., Atkinson, K., Challis, D. R., Tucker, R. G., and Biggs, J. C., Invasive *Trichosporon cutaneum* infection: an increasing problem in immunosuppressed patients. *Bone Marrow Transplant.*, 2, 321, 1987.
17. Ogata, K., Tanabe, Y., Iwakuri, K., et al. Two cases of disseminated *Trichosporon beigelii* infection treated with combination antifungal therapy. *Cancer*, 65, 2793–2795, 1990.
18. Siegert, W., Henze, G., Wagner, J., et al. Invasive *Trichosporon cutaneum* (*beigelii*) infection in a patient with relapsed acute myeloid leukemia undergoing bone marrow transplantation. *Transplantation*, 46, 151, 1988.
19. Lussier, N., Laverdiere, M., Delorme, J., Weiss, K., and Dandavino, R. *Trichosporon beigelii* funguria in renal transplant recipients. *Clin. Infect. Dis.*, 31, 1299, 2000.

20. Grossi, P., Farina, C., Fiocchi, R., and Dalla Gasperina, D. Prevalence and outcome of invasive fungal infections in 1,963 thoracic organ transplant recipients: a multicenter retrospective study. Italian Study Group of fungal infections in thoracic organ transplant recipients. *Transplantation*, 70, 112, 2000.
21. Cawley, M. J., Braxton, G. R., Haith, L. R., Reilly, K. J., Guilday, R. E., and Patton, M. L. *Trichosporon beigelii* infection: experience in a regional burn victim. *Burns*, 26, 483-486, 2000.
22. Brahn, E. and Leonard, P. A. *Trichosporon cutaneum* endocarditis: a sequela of intravenous drug abuse. *Am. J. Clin. Pathol.*, 78, 792, 1982.
23. Reinhart, H. H., Urbanski, D. M., Harrington, S. D., and Sobel, J. D. Prosthetic valve endocarditis caused by *Trichosporon beigelii*. *Am. J. Med.*, 84, 355, 1988.
24. Thomas, D., Mogahed, A., Leclerc, J. P., and Grosgogeat, M. Prosthetic valve endocarditis caused by *Trichosporon cutaneum*. *Int. J. Cardiol.*, 5, 83, 1984.
25. Keay, S., Denning, D. W., and Stevens, D. A. Endocarditis due to *Trichosporon beigelii*: in vitro susceptibility of isolates and review. *Rev. Infect. Dis.*, 13, 383, 1991.
26. Martinez-Lacasa, J., Mana, J., Niubo, R., Rufi, G., Saez, A., and Fernandez-Nogues, F. Long-term survival of a patient with prosthetic valve endocarditis due to *Trichosporon beigelii*. *Eur. J. Clin. Microbiol.*, 10, 756, 1991.
27. Marier, R., Zakhireh, B., Downs, J., Wynne, B., Hammond, G. L., and Andriole, V. T. *Trichosporon cutaneum* endocarditis. *Scand. J. Infect. Dis.*, 10, 255, 1978.
28. Sheikh, H. A., Mahgub, S., and Badi, K. Postoperative endophthalmitis due to *Trichosporon cutaneum*. *Br. J. Ophthalmol.*, 58, 591, 1974.
29. Chan, R. M., Lee, P., and Wroblewski, J. Deep-seated trichonosporosis in an immunocompetent patient: a case report of uterine trichonosporonosis. *Clin. Infect. Dis.*, 31, 621, 2000.
30. Bottari, M., D'Amore, F., Buda, C. A., et al. Stenosing esophagitis caused by *Trichosporon beigelii*: presentation of a rare case. *G. Chir.*, 18, 344–347, 1997.
31. Sweet, D. and Reide, M. Disseminated neonatal *Trichosporon beigelii* infection: successful treatment with liposomal amphotericin B. *J. Infect.*, 36, 1998.
32. Yoss, B. S., Sauter, R. L., and Brenker, H. J. *Trichosporon beigelii*, a new neonatal pathogen. *Am. J. Perinatol.*, 14, 113–117, 1997.
33. Leaf, H. L. and Simberkoff, M. S. Invasive trichosporonosis in a patient with the acquired immunodeficiency syndrome. *J. Infect. Dis.*, 160, 356, 1989.
34. Nahass, G. T., Rosenberg, S. P., Leonardi, C. L., and Penneys, N. S. Disseminated infection with *Trichosporon beigelii*: report of a case and review of the cutaneous and histologic manifestations. *Arch. Dermatol.*, 129, 1020, 1993.
35. Parsonnet, J. *Trichosporon beigelii* peritonitis. *South. Med. J.*, 82, 1062, 1989.
36. Lascaux, A. S., Bouscarat, F., Descamps, V., et al. Cutaneous manifestations during disseminated trichosporonosis in an AIDS patient. *Ann. Dermatol. Venereol.*, 125, 111–113, 1998.
37. Nasu, K., Akizuki, S., Yoshiyama, K., Kikuchi, H., Higuchi, Y., and Yamamoto, S. Disseminated *Trichosporon* infection: a case report and immunohistochemical study. *Arch. Pathol. Lab. Med.*, 118, 191, 1994.
38. Alegre, A., Algora, M., Penalver, M. A., et al. Focal hepato-splenic mycosis caused by *Trichosporon beigelii* in a patient with acute leukemia. *Sangre*, 36, 311, 1991.
39. Yamauchi, K. and Sato, T. *Trichosporon beigelii* following busulfan-induced leucopenia. *Eur. Respir. J.*, 5, 594, 1992.
40. Fujishita, M., Kataoka, R., Kobayashi, M., and Miyoshi, I. Clinical features of 32 cases of fungal pneumonia. *Nippon Kyobu Shikkan Gakkai Zasshi*, 29, 420, 1991.
41. Hsu, K., Rolston, K., and Bodey, G. P. *Trichosporon* infection in cancer patients. *Proc. Annu. Meet. Am. Soc. Microbiol.*, American Society of Microbiology, Washington, DC, 370, 1985.
42. Kirmani, M., Tuazon, C. V., and Geelhoed, G. W. Disseminated *Trichosporon* infection: occurence in an immunosuppressed patient with chronic active hepatitis. *Arch. Intern. Med.*, 140, 277, 1980.
43. Libertin, C. R., Davies, N. J., Halper, J., Edson, R. S., and Roberto, G. D. Invasive disease caused by *Trichosporon beigelii*. *Mayo Clin. Proc.*, 58, 684, 1983.
44. Manzella, J. P., Berman, I. J., and Jukrilea, M. L. *Trichosporon beigelli* fungemia and cuttaneous dissemination, *Arch. Dermatol.*, 118, 343, 1982.
45. Saul, S. H., Khachatourian, T., Poorsattar, A., et al. Opportunistic *Trichosporon* pneumonia: association with invasive aspergillosis. *Arch. Pathol. Lab. Med.*, 105, 456, 1981.
46. Singer, C., Kaplan, M. H., and Armstrong, D. Bacteremia and fungemia complicating neoplastic disease: a study of 364 cases. *Am. J. Med.*, 62, 731, 1977.
47. Apaliski, S. J., Moore, M. D., Reiner, B. J., and Wald, E. R. Disseminated *Trichosporon beigelii* in an immunocompromised child. *Pediatr. Infect. Dis. J.*, 3, 451, 1984.
48. Ujiie, H., Teshima, H., Maeda, T., et al. Background and prognostic factors of fungemia in patients with hematological disease. *Kansenshogaku Zasshi*, 72, 912–917, 1998.
49. Murray-Leisure, K. A., Aber, R. C., Rowley, L. J., et al. Disseminated *Trichosporon beigelii* (*cutaneum*) infection in an artificial heart recipient. *J. Am. Med. Assoc.*, 256, 2995–2998, 1986.
50. Ness, M. J., Markin, R. S., Wood, R. P., Shaw, B. W., and Woods, G. L. Disseminated *Trichosporon beigelii* infection after orthotopic liver transplantation. *Am. J. Clin. Pathol.*, 92, 119, 1989.
51. Mirza, S. H. Disseminated *Trichosporon beigelii* infection causing skin lesions in a renal transplant patient. *J. Infect.*, 27, 67, 1993.
52. Erer, B., Galimberti, M., Lucarelli, G., et al. *Trichosporon beigelii*: a life-treatening pathogen in immunocompromised hosts. *Bone Marrow Transplant.*, 25, 745–749, 2000.

53. Wong, B., Bernard, E. M., Gold, J. W. M., and Armstrong, D. *Trichosporon* infection in three patients with leukemia: evidence for a permissive role for excess iron. *Proc. 22nd Intersci. Conf. Antimicrob. Agents Chemother.*, abstract # 7, 1982.
54. Fisher, D. J., Christy, C., Spafford, P., Maniscalco, W. M., Hardy, D. J., and Graman, P. S., Neonatal *Trichosporon beigelii* infection: report of a cluster of cases in a neonatal intensive care unit. *Pediatr. Infect. Dis. J.*, 12, 149, 1993.
55. Giacoia, G. P., *Trichosporon beigelii*: a potential cause of sepsis in premature infants. *South. Med. J.*, 85, 1247, 1992.
56. Moreno, S., Buzon, L., and Sanchez-Sousa, A. *Trichosporon capitatum* fungemia and intravenous drug abuse. *Rev. Infect. Dis.*, 9, 1202, 1987.
57. Finkelstein, R., Singer, P., and Leflcr, E. Catheter-related fungemia caused by *Trichosporon beigelii* in nonneutropenic patients. *Am. J. Med.*, 86, 133, 1989.
58. Pierard, G. E., Read, D., Pierard-Franchimont, C., Lother, Y., Rurangirwa, A., and Arrese Estrada, J. Cutaneous manifestations in systemic trichosporonosis. *Clin. Exp. Dermatol.*, 17, 79, 1992.
59. El-Ani, A. S. and Castillo, N. B. Disseminated infection with *Trichosporon beigelii*. *NY State Med. J.*, 84, 457, 1984.
60. Evans, H. L., Kletzel, M., Lawson, R. D., Frankel, L. S., and Hopfer, R.L. Systemic mycosis due to *Trichosporon cutaneum*: a report of two additional cases. *Cancer*, 45, 367, 1980.
61. Rose, H. D. and Kurup, V. P. Colonization of hospitalized patients with yeast-like organisms. *Sabouraudia*, 15, 251, 1977.
62. Ujhelyi, M. R., Raasch, R. H., van der Horst, C., and Mattern, W. D. Treatment of peritonitis due to *Curvularia* and *Trichosporon* with amphotericin B. *Rev. Infect. Dis.*, 12, 621, 1990.
63. Ahlmen, J., Edebo, L., Ericksson, C., Carlsson, L., and Torgersen, A. K. Fluconazole therapy for fungal peritonitis in continuous ambulatory peritoneal dialysis (CAPD): a case report. *Perit. Dial. Int.*, 9, 79, 1989.
64. Eisenberg, E. S., Leviton, I., and Soeiro, R. Fungal peritonitis in patients receiving peritoneal dialysis: experience with 11 patients and review of the literature. *Rev. Infect. Dis.*, 8, 309, 1986.
65. Walsh, T. J., Orth, D. H., Shapiro, C. M., Levine, R. A., and Keller, J. L. Metastatic fungal chorioretinitis developing during *Trichosporon* sepsis. *Ophthalmology*, 89, 152, 1982.
66. Walsh, T. J., Melcher, G. P., Rinaldi, M. G., et al. *Trichosporon beigelii*, an emerging pathogen resistant to amphotericin B. *J. Clin. Microbiol.*, 28, 1616, 1990.
67. Reyes, C. V., Stanley, M. M., and Rippon, J. W. *Trichosporon beigelii* endocarditis as a complication of peritoneovenous shunt. *Hum. Pathol.*, 16, 857, 1985.
68. Anaissie, E., Gokaslan, A., Hachem, R., et al. Azole therapy for trichosporonosis: clinical evaluation of eight patients, experimental therapy for murine infection, and review. *Clin. Infect. Dis.*, 15, 781, 1992.
69. Canales, M. A., Sevilla, J., Ojeda Gutierrez, E., and Hernandez Navarro, F. Successful treatment of *Trichosporon beigelii* pneumonia with itraconazole. *Clin. infect. Dis.*, 26, 999–1000, 1998.
70. Anaissie, E. J., Hachem, R., Karyotakis, N. C., et al. Comparative efficacies of amphotericin B, triazoles, and combination of both as experimental therapy for murine trichosporonosis. *Antimicrob. Agents Chemother.*, 38, 2541, 1994.
71. Alballaa, S., Bryce, E. A., Roberts, F. J., and Sekhon, A. Fatal trichosporonosis is not related to tolerance to amphotericin B. *Mycoses*, 34, 317, 1991.
72. Steer, P. L., Marks, M. I., Klite, P. D., and Eickhoff, T. C. 5-Fluorocytosine: an oral antifungal compound. A report on clinical and laboratory experience. *Am. J. Med.*, 76, 15, 1971.
73. Gugnani, H. C., Gugnani, A., and Malachy, O. Sulkonazole in the therapy of dermatomycoses in Nigeria. *Mycoses*, 40, 1,390,141, 1997.
74. Hajjeh, R. A. and Blumberg, H. M. Bloodstream infection due to *Trichosporon beigelii* in a burn patient: case report and review of therapy. *Clin. Infect. Dis.*, 20, 913, 1995.
75. McCabe, W. P., Rebuck, J. W., Kelly, A. P. Jr., and Ditmars, D. M. Jr. Leukocytic response as a monitor of immunodepression in burn patients. *Arch. Surg.*, 106, 155, 1973.
76. Alexander, J. W., Ogle, C. K., Stinnett, J. D., and Macmillan, B. G. A sequential, prospective analysis of immunologic abnormalities and infection following severe thermal injury. *Ann. Surg.*, 188, 808, 1978.
77. Yurt, R. W. and Shires, C. T. Burns, in *Principles and Practice of Infectious Diseases*, 3rd ed., Mandell, G. M., Douglas, R. G. Jr., and Bennett, J. E., Eds. Churchill Livingston, New York, 830, 1990.
78. Shelby, J. and Merrell, S. W. In vivo monitoring of postburn immune response. *J. Trauma*, 27, 213, 1987.
79. Salkin, I. F., Gordon, M. A., Samsonoff, W. A., and Rieder, C. L. *Blastoschizomyces capitatus*, a new combination. *Mycotaxon*, 22, 375, 1985.
80. Guého, E., de Hoog, G. S., Smith, M. T., and Meyer, S. A. DNA relatedness, taxonomy and medical significance of *Geotrichum capitatum*. *J. Clin. Microbiol.*, 25, 1191, 1987.
81. Salkin, I. F., Gordon, M. A., Samsonoff, W. A., and Rieder, C. L. *Blastoschizomyces pseudotrichosporon*, gen. et sp. nov. *Mycotaxon*, 14, 497,1982.
82. Martino, P., Venditti, M., Micozzi, A., et al. *Blastoschizomyces capitatus*: an emerging cause of invasive fungal disease in leukemic patients. *Rev. Infect. Dis.*, 12, 570, 1990.
83. Haupt, H. M., Merz, W. G., Beschorner, W. E., Vaughan, V. P., and Saral, R. Colonization and infection with *Trichosporon* species in the immunocompromised host. *J. Infect. Dis.*, 147, 199, 1983.
84. Oelz, O., Schaffner, A., Frick, P., and Schaer, G. *Trichosporon capitatum*: thrush-like oral infection, local invasion, fungemia, and metastatic abscess formation in a leukemic patient. *J. Infect.*, 6, 183, 1983.
85. Winston, D. J., Balsley, G. E., Rhodes, J., and Linné, S. R. Disseminated *Trichosporon capitatum* infection in an immunosuppressed host. *Arch. Intern. Med.*, 137, 1192, 1977.

86. Arnold, A. G., Gribbin, B., De Leval, M., Macartney, F., and Slack, M. *Trichosporon capitatum* causing recurrent fungal endocarditis. *Thorax*, 86, 478, 1981.
87. Ito, T., Ischikawa, Y., Fujii, R., et al. Disseminated *Trichosporon capitatum* infection in a patient with acute leukemia. *Cancer*, 61, 585, 1988.
88. Baird, D. R., Harris, M., Menon, R., and Stoddart, R. W. Systemic infection with *Trichosporon capitatum* in two patients with acute leukaemia. *Eur. J. Clin. Microbiol. Infect. Dis.*, 4, 62, 1985.
89. Deicke, P. and Gemeinhardt, H. Embolisch-metastatische pilzenzephalitis durch *Trichosporon capitatum* nach infusions-therapie. *Detsch. Gesundhitswesen*, 35, 673, 1980.
90. Wolff, M., Curran, Y., Bure, A., et al. Septicemie mortelle a *Trichosporon* sp. chez 3 malades immunodeprimes. *Presse Med.*, 25, 1201, 1986.
91. Baird, D. R., Harris, M., Menon, and Stoddart, R. W. Systemic infection *Trichosporon capitatum* in two patients with acute leukemia. *Eur. J. Clin. Microbiol.*, 4, 62, 1985.
92. Sicova-Mila, Z., Sufliarsky, J., and Krcméry, V. Jr. *Blastoschizomyces capitatus* fungemia in a compromised patient successfully treated with amphotericin. *J. Hosp. Infect.*, 40, 1131, 1992.
93. Ortiz, A. M., Sanz-Rodriguez, C., Culebras, J., et al. Multiple spondylodiscitis caused by *Blastoschizomyces capitatus* in an allogeneic bone marrow transplantation recipient. *J. Rheumatol.*, 25, 2276–2278, 1998.
94. Perez-Sanchez, I., Anguita, J., Martin-Rabadan, P., et al. *Blastoschizomyces capitatus* infection in acute leukemia patients. *Leuk. Lymphoma*, 39, 209–212, 2000.
95. Cheung, M. Y., Chiu, N. C., Chen, S. H., Liu, H. C., Ou, C. T., and Liang, D. C. Mandibular osteomyelitis caused by *Blastoschizomyces capitatus* in a child with acute myelogenous leukemia. *J. Formos. Med. Assoc.*, 98, 787–789, 1999.
96. Krcmery, V., Krupova, I., and Denning, D. W. Invasive yeast infections other than *Candida* ssp. in acute leukaemia. *J. Hosp. Infect.*, 41, 181–194, 1999.
97. Krcmery, S., Dubrava, M., and Krcmery, V., Jr. Fungal urinary tract infections in patients at risk. *Int. J. Antimicrob. Agents*, 11, 289–291, 1999.
98. D'Antonio, D., Romano, F., Iacone, A., et al. Onychomycosis caused by *Blastoschizomyces capitatus*. *J. Clin. Microbiol.*, 37, 2927–2930, 1999.
99. Mathews, M. S. and Sen, S. *Blastoschizomyces capitatus* infection after contaminantion for intravenous application. *Mycoses*, 41, 427–428, 1998.
100. Plum, G., Scheid, C., Franzen, C., Schutt-Gerowitt, H., Seifert, H., and Wickramanayake, P. D. Empirical liposomal amphotericin B therapy in a neutropenic patient: breakthrough of disseminated *Blastoschizomyces capitatus* infection. *Zentralbl. Bakteriol.*, 284, 361–366, 1996.
101. Surmont, I., Vergauwen, B., Marcelis, L., Verbist, L., Verhoef, G., and Boogaerts, M. First report of chronic meningitis caused by *Trichosporon beigelii*. *Eur. J. Clin. Microbiol. Infect. Dis.*, 9, 226, 1990.
102. Walling, D. M., McGraw, D. J., Merz, W. G., Karp, J. E., and Hutchins, G. M. Disseminated infection with *Trichosporon beigelii*. *Rev. Infect. Dis.*, 9, 1013, 1987.
103. Girmenia, C., Micozzi, A., Venditti, M., et al. Fluconazole treatment of *Blastoschizomyces capitatus* meningitis in an allogeneic bone marrow recipient. *Eur. J. Clin. Microbiol. Infect. Dis.*, 10, 752, 1991.
104. Venditti, M., Posteraro, B., Morace, G., and Martino, P. In vitro comparative activity of fluconazole and other antifungal agents against *Blastoschizomyces capitatus*. *J. Chemother.*, 3, 13, 1991.
105. Sugar, A. M. and Saunders, C. Oral fluconazole suppressive therapy of disseminated cryptococcosis in patients with acquired immunodeficiency syndrome. *Am. J. Med.*, 85, 481, 1988.
106. Sanz, M. A., Lopez, F., Martinez, M. L., et al. Disseminated *Blastoschizomyces capitatus* infection in acute myeloblastic leukaemia. *Support. Care Cancer*, 4, 291, 1996.
107. DeMaio, J. and Colman, L. The use of adjuvant-interferon-gamma therapy for hepatosplenic *Blastoschizomyces capitatus* infection in a patient with leukemia. *Clin. Infect. Dis.*, 31, 822–824, 2000.

23
Rhodotorula spp.

1. INTRODUCTION

Rhodotorula is a genus of imperfect pink-colored yeasts of the family Cryptococcaceae, subfamily Rhodotorulodae, which grow as globose budding fungi *(1)*.

Although *Rhodotorula* spp. have been rarely known to cause human disease *(2–5)*, a number of cases where the infection was clearly opportunistic have been reported, mainly in immunosuppressed patients *(6)* with cancer *(7–11)* and AIDS *(12–14)*, in patients undergoing continuous ambulatory peritoneal analysis (CAPD) *(15–19)*, and with indwelling catheters *(20)*. *Rhodotorula* infections can manifest as meningitis *(14,21)* endocarditis *(22)*, and ocular infections *(23–28)*. For systemic disease, mortality rates may reach 40–60% *(4,8,11,12,15,16,29–39)*.

2. TREATMENT OF *RHODOTORULA* INFECTIONS

In moderate cases, antifungal therapy and/or removal of infected catheters is generally effective *(10)*. Nevertheless, the fungus has been reported to provoke fatal endocarditis or meningitis and can probably cause septic shock.

Rhodotorula spp. were resistant to fluconazole *(8)*, miconazole *(8)*, and itraconazole *(8,40)* but susceptible to 5-fluorocytosine (5-FC) with minimum inhibitory concentrations (MICs) generally of less than 0.1 µg/mL. Thus, Kiehn et al. *(8)* assessed 9 clinical isolates of *Rhodotorula* for antifungal drug susceptibility and found MIC_{90} values of 1.6, 0.1, 0.8, 6.4, 3.2, >100, and <0.1 µg/mL for amphotericin B, amphotericin B-rifampin (10 µg/mL), ketoconazole, miconazole, itraconazole, fluconazole, and 5-FC, respectively.

5-FC is currently the recommended choice of treatment for such conditions *(32)*. Thus, Naveh et al. *(22)* have used 5-FC to successfully resolve a *Rhodotorula*-associated endocarditis.

Results from reported cases of *Rhodotorula* spp. fungemia have shown the efficacy of amphotericin B to be about 40% *(32)*. Lui et al. *(13)* used therapy with amphotericin B lipid complex to treat an AIDS patient with *R. rubra* fungemia.

Donald et al. *(41)* described a case of postoperative ventriculitis in an immunocompetent patient due to *R. rubra*. The patient fully responded to therapeutic regimen consisting of oral flucytosine (2.0 g, q.i.d., then reduced to 1.5 g, q.i.d. because of vomiting) and intravenous amphotericin B. The latter was given first as a test dose of 1.0 mg, followed by 13.7 mg (0.3 mg/kg) on the first day, then 33 mg (0.6 mg/kg) on the second day, and increasing over the next 7 d to a maximum of 50 mg daily total dose. After 5 wk, the intravenous therapy has been discontinued and oral flucloxacillin (2.0 g, q.i.d.) was given with rifampicin for five additional weeks. The flucytosine therapy lasted for 12 wk in total *(41)*.

The therapy of catheter-related *Rhodotorula* fungemia may or may not require the removal of the catheter in addition to antifungal chemotherapy. Because of the ability of host polymorphonuclear leukocytes to ingest and kill the pathogen *(4)*, in some patients, the removal of the catheter alone without antifungal chemotherapy has been sufficient to resolve the fungemia *(8)*. Kiehn et al. *(8)*

recommended that 0.7 mg/kg daily of amphotericin B be administered through all ports of the catheter for 2 wk if the catheter is not removed and for 1 wk if the catheter is removed.

Marinova et al. *(32)* have described a case of *Rhodototula* spp. fungemia in an immunocompromised pediatric patient secondary to neurosurgery. The infection was successfully treated with miconazole (600 mg daily) which was given for 6 d but then changed to intravenously administered 5-FC (2.0 g daily for 3 wk) because of unwarranted elevation of the liver enzyme levels.

Fluconazole failed to clear *R. rubra* fungemia in a profoundly neutropenic pediatric patient who died 2 d after the diagnosis of fungemia *(11)*.

A case of *R. minuta* central venous catheter infection with fungemia has been described in a patient with advanced AIDS, HIV nephropathy, end-stage renal disease requiring hemodialysis, and a permanent Quinton catheter in place for 6 mo *(36)*. At the time of the fungemia, the patient was taking oral fluconazole (100 mg daily) for a previous episode of *Candida* esophagitis. The catheter-associated *Rhodotorula* fungemia was successfully treated intravenously with 455 mg total dose of amphotericin B (0.6 mg/kg daily) given over a 25-d period without the removal of the catheter *(36)*. In another case *(42)*, *R. minuta* was isolated from the blood of a pediatric patient with AIDS, central nervous system (CNS) lymphoma, and systemic candidiasis; the patient died before antifungal therapy started.

R. minuta systemic infection with liver abscesses and bone-marrow involvement has been described in a leukemic patient who was successfully treated with 1.5 g total dose of amphotericin B and flucytosine *(43)*.

Guerra et al. *(26)* reported a case of deep keratomycosis due to *R. glutinis*. Although in this and other cases *(27)*, the infection was resolved by penetrating keratoplasty, these authors did not recommended it as a first procedure in the treatment of keratomycosis *(26)*. Rather, topical administration of pimaricin 5% or amphotericin B 0.15% would have been the more appropriate initial treatment and penetrating keratoplasty should be considered only after failure of the medical treatment *(44)*.

Fanci et al. *(45)* successfully treated with amphotericin B a case of *R. glutinis* fungemia in a patient with relapsed acute lymphatic leukemia (ALL) and persistent fever without any other clinical evidence.

REFERENCES

1. Phaff, H. J. and Ahern, D. G. *Rhodotorula* Harrison, in *The Yeasts*, 2nd ed., Lodder, J. Ed. North Holland, Amsterdam, 1187, 1970.
2. Kwon-Chung, K. J. and Bennett, J. E. Infections due to *Trichosporon* and other miscellaneous yeast-like fungi, in *Medical Mycology*, Kwon-Chung, K. J. and Bennett, J.E., Eds. Lea and Febiger, Philadelphia, 768, 1992.
3. Jennings, A. E. and Bennett, J. E. The isolation of red yeast-like fungi in a diagnostic laboratory. *J. Med. Microbiol.*, 5, 391, 1972.
4. Louria, D. B., Greenberg, S. M., and Molander, D. W. Fungemia caused by certain nonpathogenic strains of the family Cryptococcaceae. *N. Engl. J. Med.*, 263, 1281, 1960.
5. Cogate, A., Deodhar, L., and Cogate, S. Hydrosalpinx due to *Rhodotorula glutinis*: a case report. *J. Postgrad. Med.*, 33, 34, 1987.
6. Papadogeorgakis, H., Frangoulis, E., Papaeftathiou, C., and Katsambas, A. *Rhodotorula rubra* fungaemia in an immunosuppressed patient. *J. Eur. Acad. Dermatol. Venereol.*, 12, 169–170, 1999.
7. Kiehn, T. E., Edwards, F. F., and Armstrong, D. The prevalence of yeasts in clinical specimens from cancer patients. *Am. J. Clin. Pathol.*, 73, 518, 1980.
8. Kiehn, P., Gorey, E., Brown, A., Edwards, F., and Armstrong, D. Sepsis due to *Rhodotorula* related to use of indwelling central venous catheters. *Clin. Infect. Dis.*, 14, 841, 1992.
9. Paula, C. R., Sampaio, M. C. C., Birman, E. G., and Siqueira, A. M. Oral yeasts in patients with cancer of the mouth, before and during radiotherapy. *Mycopathologia*, 112, 119, 1990.
10. Alliot, C., Desablens, B., Garidi, R., and Tabuteau, S. Opportunistic infections with *Rhodotorula* in cancer patients treated by chemotherapy: two case reports. *Clin. Oncol. (R. Coll. Radiol.)*, 12, 115–117, 2000.
11. Manabe, A., Ebihara, Y., Saito, A., Takahashi, K., and Hosoya, R. Phagocytosis of fungi in the peripheral blood neutrophils of two children with cancer during treatment with fluconazole. *Rinsho Ketsueki*, 38, 669–673, 1997.
12. Walsh, T. J., Gonzalez, C., Roilides, E., et al. Fungemia in children infected with the human immunodeficiency virus: new epidemiologic patterns, emerging pathogens, and improved outcome with antifungal therapy. *Clin. Infect. Dis.*, 20, 900, 1995.

13. Lui, A. Y., Turett, G. S., Karter, D. L., Bellman, P. C., and Kislak, J. W. Amphotericin B lipid complex therapy in an AIDS patient with *Rhodotorula rubra* fungemia. *Clin. Infect. Dis.*, 27, 892–893, 1998.
14. Ahmed, A., Aggarwal, M., Chiu, R., Ramratnam, B., Rinaldi, M., and Flanigan, T. P. A fatal case of *Rhodotorula* meningitis in AIDS. *Med. Health R. I.*, 81, 22–23, 1998.
15. Benezra, D., Kiehn, T., Gold, J. W., Brown, A., Tubull, A, D, M., and Armstrong, D. Prospective study of infections in indwelling central venous catheters using quantitative blood cultures. *Am. J. Med.*, 85, 495, 1988.
16. Pennington, J. C. III, Hauer, K., and Miller, W. *Rhodotorula rubra* peritonitis in an HIV+ patient on CAPD. *Del. Med. J.*, 67, 184, 1995.
17. Eisenberg, E. S., Alpert, B. E., Weiss, R. A., Mittman, N., and Soeiro, R. *Rhodotorula rubra* peritonitis in patients undergoing continuous ambulatory peritoneal analysis. *Am. J. Med.*, 75, 349, 1983.
18. Johnson, R. I., Ramsey, P. G., Gallagher, P. G., and Ahmad, S. Fungal peritonitis in patients on peritoneal analysis: incidence, clinical features and prognosis. *Am. J. Nephrol.*, 5, 169, 1985.
19. Wong, V., Ross, L., Opas, L., and Lieberman, E. *Rhodotorula rubra* peritonitis in a child undergoing intermittent cycling peritoneal dialysis. *J. Infect. Dis.*, 157, 393, 1988.
20. Kiraz, N., Gulbas, Z., and Akgun, Y. Case report. *Rhodotorula rubra* fungaemia due to use of indwelling venous catheters. *Mycoses*, 43, 209–210, 2000.
21. Pore, R. S. and Chien, J. Meningitis caused by *Rhodotorula*. *Sabouraudia*, 14, 331, 1976.
22. Naveh, Y., Friedman, A., Merzbach, D., and Hashman, N. Endocarditis caused by *Rhodotorula* successfully treated with 5-fluorocytosine. *Br. Heart J.*, 37, 101, 1975.
23. Romano, A., Segal, E., and Ben-Tovim, T. Epithelial keratitis due to *Rhodotorula*. *Ophthalmologica*, 166, 353, 1973.
24. Francois, J. and Rijsselaere, M. Corneal infections by *Rhodotorula*. *Opthalmologica*. 178, 241–249, 1979.
25. Segal, E., Romano, A., Eylan, E., et al., *Rhodotorula rubra*, cause of eye infection. *Mykosen*, 18, 107, 1975.
26. Guerra, R., Cavallini, G. M., Longanesi, L., et al. *Rhodotorula glutinis* keratitis. *Int. Ophthalmol.*, 16, 187, 1992.
27. Casolari, C., Nanetti, A., Cavallini, G. M., et al., Keratomycosis with an unusual etiology (*Rhodotorula glutinis*): a case report. *Microbiologica*, 15, 83, 1992.
28. Panda, A., Pushker, N., Nainiwal, S., Satpathy, G., and Nayak, N. *Rhodotorula* sp. infection in corneal interface following lamellar keratoplasty: a case report. *Acta Ophthalmol. Scand.*, 77, 227, 1999.
29. Pinch, F. D. *Rhodotorula* septicemia. *Mayo Clin. Proc.*, 55, 258, 1980.
30. Shelburn, P. F. and Carey, J. *Rhodotorula* fungemia complicating staphylococcal endocarditis. *J. Am. Med. Assoc.*, 180, 38, 1962.
31. Lauria, D. B., Blevins, A., Armstrong, G. D., Burdich, R., and Lieberman, P. Fungemia caused by "nonpathogenic" yeasts. *Arch. Intern. Med.*, 119, 247, 1967.
32. Marinova, I., Szabadosova, V., Brandeburova, O., and Krcméry, V. Jr. *Rhodotorula* spp. fungemia in an immunocompromised boy after neurosurgery successfully treated with miconazole and 5-fluorocytosine: case report and review of the literature. *Chemotherapy*, 40, 287, 1994.
33. Kiehn, T. E. and Armstrong, D. Changes in the spectrum of organisms causing bacteremia and fungemia in immunocompromised patients due to venous access devices. *Eur. J. Clin. Microbiol. Infect. Dis.*, 9, 869, 1990.
34. Anaissie, E., Bodey, G. P., Kantarjian, H., et al. New spectrum of fungal infections in patients with cancer. *Rev. Infect. Dis.*, 11, 369, 1989.
35. Vartivarian, S. E., Anassie, E. J., and Bodey, G. P. Emerging fungal pathogens in immunocompromising patients: classification, diagnosis, and management. *Clin. Infect. Dis.*, 17(Suppl. 2), S487, 1993.
36. Goldani, L. Z., Craven, D. E., and Sugar, A. M. Central venous catheter infection with *Rhodotorula minuta* in a patient with AIDS taking suppressive doses of fluconazole. *J. Med. Vet. Mycol.*, 33, 267, 1995.
37. Sheu, M. J., Wang, C. C., Wang, C. C., Shi, W. J., and Chu, M. L. *Rhodotorula* septicemia: report of a case. *J. Formos. Med. Assoc.*, 93, 645, 1994.
38. Jiménez-Mejias, M. E., Ortiz Leyba, C., Jiménez Gonzalo, F. J., del Nozal, M., Campos, T., and Jiménez Jiménez, F. J. Fungemia caused by *Rhodotorula mucilaginosa* in relation to total parenteral nutrition. *Enferm. Infecc. Microbiol. Clin.*, 10, 543, 1992.
39. Samonis, G. and Bafaloukos, D. Fungal infections in cancer patients: an escalating problem. *In Vivo*, 6, 183, 1992.
40. Otcenasek, M. The in vitro susceptibility of some mycotic agents to a new orally active triazole, itraconazole. *J. Hyg. Epidemiol. Microbiol. Immunol.*, 34, 129, 1990.
41. Donald, F. E., Sharp, J. F., Firth, J. L., Crowley, J. L., and Ispahani, P. *Rhodotorula rubra* ventriculitis. *J. Infect.*, 16, 187, 1988.
42. Leibovitz, E., Rigaud, M., Chandwani, S., et al. Disseminated fungal infections in children infected with human immunodeficiency virus. *Pediatr. Infect. Dis. J.*, 10, 888, 1991.
43. Rusthoven, J. J., Feld, R., and Tuffnell, P. G. Systemic infection by *Rhodotorula* spp. in the immunocompromised host. *J. Infect.*, 8, 241, 1984.
44. Wood, T. O. and Williford, W. Treatment of keratomycosis with amphotericin B. *Am. J. Ophthalmol.*, 81, 847, 1976.
45. Fanci, R., Pecile, P., Martinez, R. L., Fabbri, A., and Nicoletti, P. Amphotericin B treatment of fungemia due to unusual pathogens in neutropenic patients: report of two cases. *J. Chemother.*, 9, 427–430, 1997.

24
Hansenula (Pichia) spp.

1. INTRODUCTION

The genus *Hansenula* (*Pichia*) belongs to the class Ascomycetes, order Endomycetales, family Saccharomycetaceae. To date, only two species of this genus have been implicated in human disease: *H. anomala* and *H. polymorpha* (1–4). *H. anomala* (also synonymous with *Pichia anomala* [5,6]), by far the most common human pathogen of the two, is an ascosporogenous yeast that represents the perfect (sexual) stage of *Candida* pelliculosa.

2. TREATMENT OF *HANSENULA* SPP. INFECTIONS

Of the *Hansenula* spp. infections described so far, the majority involved fungemia (2,7–9) and indwelling catheters (7,10–14). However, interstitial pneumonia (15), infectious endocarditis (3), urinary tract infection (16), and oral mucosal infection (17), have also been described.

H. anomala, which is rarely described as a pathogen in humans, may be the cause of morbidity and mortality among immunocompromised and other severely ill patients, and infants (1,2,7,10,18–24).

The predisposing factors for infections by *Hansenula* have been similar to those for *Candida* species (humoral and cell-mediated immune deficiencies, surgery, central venous catheters, broad-spectrum antibiotic and corticosteroid therapies) (7,18,25). The administration of hyperalimentation through an infected central intravascular catheter has been a particularly important risk factor because of the propensity of *Hansenula* spp. for a high-carbohydrate environment (7,24,26,27). Other risk factors playing role in *Hansenula* infections include previous use of steroids, chemotherapy, radiation therapy, and neutropenia (24).

In a study by Singh et al. (28) fungemia was detected in 22.8% of preterm neonates with predominance of *H. anomala* fungemia (62.5%); prematurity, male gender, broad spectrum antibiotic therapy, intubation, and higher colonizing rate were identified as significant risk factors for the development of fungemia.

Eradication of *Hansenula* spp. has generally been achieved by treatment with amphotericin B at daily doses of 0.1–1.0 mg/kg (8,9,12,14,21,22,25,29).

In a recent report, Kunova et al. (29) have described the successfull use of intravenous amphotericin B (1.0 mg/kg daily; total dose, 1.725 g) in the treatment of *H. anomala* fungemia in a patient with acute myelogenous leukemia (AML), after initial therapy with intravenous fluconazole (400 mg daily) failed to eradicate the yeast.

The aforementioned case corroborated the findings of two other studies (25,30). Thus, Alter and Farley (25) described a patient who developed *H. anomala* infection while receiving intravenous fluconazole therapy (6.0 mg/kg initially, followed by 4.0 mg/kg daily). Therapy with amphotericin B was initiated and maintained at a dose of 1.0 mg/kg daily (total cumulative dose, 15 mg/kg). The minimum inhibitory concentrations of a clinical isolate for amphotericin B, ketoconazole, 5-fluorocytosine, miconazole, and fluconazole were 0.8, 3.1, >100, 6.25, and 25 µg/mL, respectively, suggesting resistance of *H. anomala* to fluconazole *(25)*. In the other case *(30)*, the patient who was immunocompetent developed fungemia secondary to acute necrotizing pancreatitis. Daily treatment with 200 mg of fluconazole (amphotericin B was not given because of urinary excretion problems and elevated creatinine levels), failed to eradicate the yeast and the patient died.

It is thought that inhibition of the bacterial flora through the use of broad-spectrum antibiotics coupled with suppression of the more common fungal pathogens by use of fluconazole would permit natively resistant yeast species, such as *Hansenula* to emerge as pathogens (see also *Candida krusei* in Candidiasis). Thus, in an earlier report, Hirasaki et al. *(11)* reported the successful treatment of *H. anomala* fungemia in an adult cancer patient with intravenous fluconazole (200 mg daily; total dose, 3.0 g) given over 16 d, and removal of the central venous catheter. Yamada et al. *(13)* also reported that intravenous fluconazole (at 9.9–10 mg/kg daily) was efficacious in treating three cases of catheter-related *H. anomala* fungemia in children (coupled with removal of the catheter), even though in one of the cases the fungemia had developed while the patient was already receiving fluconazole. In a fourth case, however, fluconazole failed and was replaced with miconazole (10 mg/kg daily) and flucytosine (120 mg/kg daily) which led to clinical improvement.

Murphy et al. *(2)* described an outbreak of infection and colonization with *H. anomala* in a neonatal intensive care unit, where 10% of all admissions were colonized with the yeast; clinical infections included fungemia and ventriculitis. Treatment, which comprised of intravenous amphotericin B (initially at 100 µg/kg daily, later increased to 500 µg/kg daily) and flucytosine (initially given intravenously at 100 mg/kg daily and then enterally thereafter), lasted for 3 wk. In another case, *H. anomala* fungemia in an infant with gastric and cardiac complications was treated successfully with a combination of amphotericin B (0.1 mg/kg, q.i.d.; total dose, 20 mg/kg) and flucytosine (100 mg daily) *(9)*. However, Moses et al. *(18)* reported a case of an infant with invasive *H. anomala* disease who responded poorly to intravenous amphotericin B (1.0 mg/kg daily; total dose of 130 mg given over 31 d). The amphotericin B therapy was discontinued and oral ketoconazole was initiated at 5.0 mg/kg daily; the patient gradually defervesced and blood cultures became sterile after a 16-wk therapy *(18)*.

Goss et al. *(22)* reported the first case of *H. anomala* infection in a bone-marrow transplant recipient. The patient was treated with intravenous amphotericin B (1.0 mg/kg daily; cumulative dose, 680 mg) for 24 d, followed by prophylactic oral fluconazole (400 mg daily) for one additional week during treatment with corticosteroids. In a first report of urinary tract infection due to *H. anomala*, the patient (kidney-transplant recipient receiving treatment with immunosuppressive drugs) recovered spontaneously without antifungal therapy *(16)*.

In another case of transient *H. anomala* fungemaia that resolved without treatment, the infection was associated with intravenous drug abuse in a patient with AIDS *(30)*. Nevertheless, a clinical isolate was susceptible to amphotericin B, 5-fluorocytosine (5-FC), nystatin, ketoconazole, miconazole, and econazole with MIC values of 1.0, 0.062, 8.0, 2.0, 2.0, and 4.0 µg/mL, respectively *(31)*.

H. anomala was also isolated from the oral mucosa of a patient with acute stomatitis who was successfully treated with a 2-wk course of oral clotrimazole *(17)*.

The only clinical isolate of *H. polymorpha* tested in vitro for sensitivity to antifungal agents was susceptible to amphotericin B and miconazole (MIC values of 0.05 and 1.56 µg/mL, respectively), but resistant to 5-fluorocytosine (MIC >100 µg/mL) *(4)*.

REFERENCES

1. Wang, C. J. K. and Schwarz, J. The etiology of interstitial pneumonia: identification as *Hansenula anomala* of a yeast isolated from lungs of infants. *Mycopathol. Mycol. Applic.*, 9, 299, 1958.
2. Murphy, N., Damijanovic, V., Hart, C. A., Buchanan, C. R., Whitaker, R., and Cooke, R. W. Infection and colonization of neonates by *Hansenula anomala*. *Lancet*, 1, 291, 1986.
3. Nohinek, B., Zee-Cheng, C. S., Barnes, W., Dall, L., and Gibbs, H. R. Infective endocarditis of a bicuspid aortic valve caused by *Hansenula anomala*. *Am. J. Med.*, 82, 165, 1987.

4. McGinnis, M. R., Walker, D. H., and Folds, J. D. *Hansenula polymorpha* infection in a child with granulomatous disease. *Arch. Pathol. Lab. Med.*, 104, 290, 1980.
5. Polonelli, L., Conti, S., Campani, L., Gerloni, M., Morace, G., and Chezzi, C. Differential toxinogenesis in the genus *Pichia* detected by an anti-yeast killer toxin monoclonal antibody. *Antonie van Leeuwenhoek*, 59, 139, 1991.
6. Yamada, Y., Maeda, K., and Mikata, K. The phylogenetic relationship of the hat-shaped ascospore-forming, nitrate-assimilating *Pichia* species, formerly classified in the genus *Hansenula* Sydow et Sydow, based on the partial sequences of 18S and 26 S ribosomal RNSs (Saccharomycetaceae). *Biosci. Biotechnol. Biochem.*, 58, 1245, 1994.
7. Klein, A. S., Tortora, G. T., Malowitz, R., and Greene, W. H. *Hansenula anomala*: a new fungal pathogen: two cases and a review of the literature. *Arch. Intern. Med.*, 148, 121, 1988.
8. Milstoc, M. and Siddiqui, N. A. Fungemia due to *Hansenula anomala*. *NY State J. Med.*, 86, 541, 1986.
9. Sekhon, A. S., Kowalewska-Grochowska, K., Garg, A. K., and Vaudry, W. *Hansenula anomala* fungemia in an infant with gastric and cardiac complications with a review of the literature. *Eur. J. Epidemiol.*, 8, 305, 1992.
10. Haron, E., Anaissie, E., Dumpy, F., McCredie, K., and Fainstein, V. *Hansenula anomala* fungemia. *Rev. Infect. Dis.*, 10, 1182, 1988.
11. Hirasaki, S., Ijuchi, T., Fujita, N., Araki, S., Gotoh, H., and Nakagawa, M. Fungemia caused by *Hansenula anomala*: successful treatment with fluconazole. *Intern. Med.*, 31, 622, 1992.
12. Munoz, P., Garcia Leoni, M. E., Berenguer, J., Bernaldo de Quiros, J. C., and Bouza, E. Catheter-related fungemia by *Hansenula anomala*. *Arch. Intern. Med.*, 149, 709, 1989.
13. Yamada, S., Maruoka, T., Nagai, K., et al. Catheter-related infections by *Hansenula anomala* in children. *Scand. J. Infect. Dis.*, 27, 85, 1995.
14. Choy, B. Y., Wong, S. S., Chan, T. M., and Lai, K. N. *Pichia ohmeri* peritonitis in a patient on CAPD: response to treatment with amphotericin. *Perit. Dial. Int.*, 20, 91, 2000.
15. Csillag, A. and Brandstein, L. The role of *Blastomyces* in the aetiology of interstitial plasmocytic pneumonia of the premature infant. *Acta Microbiol. Hung.*, 2, 179, 1954.
16. Qadri, S. M. H., Al Dayel, F., Strampfer, M. J., and Cunha, B. A. Urinary tract infection caused by *Hansenula anomala*. *Mycopathologia*, 104, 99, 1988.
17. Kostiala, I., Kostiala, A. A. I., Elonen, E., Valtonen, V. V., and Vuopio, P. Comparison of clotrimazole and chlorhexidine in the topical treatment of acute fungal stomatitis in patients with hematological malignancies. *Curr. Ther. Res. Clin. Exp.*, 31, 752, 1982.
18. Moses, A., Maayan, S., Shvil, Y., et al. *Hansenula anomala* infections in children: from asymptomatic colonization to tissue invasion. *Pediatr. Infect. Dis. J.*, 10, 400, 1991.
19. Csillag, A., Brandstein, L., Faber, V., and Maczo, J., Adatok a koraszulottkori interstitialis pneumonia koroktanahoz, *Orv. Hetil.*, 94, 1303, 1953.
20. Dickensheets, D. L., *Hansenula anomala* infection, *Rev. Infect. Dis.*, 11, 507, 1989.
21. Lopez, F., Martin, M. L., and Paz y Sanz, M. A. Infeccion por *Hansenula anomala* en leucemia aguda. *Enferm. Infec. Microbiol. Clin.*, 8, 363, 1990.
22. Goss, G., Grigg, A., Rathbone, P., and Slavin, M. *Hansenula anomala* infection after bone marrow transplantation. *Bone Marrow Transplant.*, 14, 995, 1994.
23. Bergman, M. M., Gagnon, D., and Doern, G. V. *Pichia ohmeri* fungemia. *Diagn. Microbiol. Infect. Dis.*, 30, 229–231, 1998.
24. Thuler, L. C., Faivichenco, S., Velasco, E., Martins, C. A., Nascimento, C. R., and Castilho, I. A. Fungemia caused by *Hansenula anomala*: an outbreak in a cancer hospital. *Mycoses*, 40, 193–196, 1997.
25. Alter, S. J. and Farley, J. Development of *Hansenula anomala* infection in a child receiving fluconazole therapy. *Pediatr. Infect. Dis. J.*, 13, 158, 1994.
26. Cook, A. H., Ed. *The Chemistry and Biology of Yeasts*. Academic Press, Orlando, FL, 1958.
27. Sumitomo, M., Kawata, K., Kaminaga, Y., Ito, A., Makimura, K., and Yamaguchi, H. *Hansenula anomala* fungemia in a patient undergoing IVH-treatment with ascending colon carcinoma. *Kansenshogaku Zasshi*, 70, 198–205, 1996.
28. Singh, K., Chakrabarti, A., Narang, A., and Gopalan, S. Yeast colonization and fungemia in preterm neonates in a tertiary care center. *Indian J. Med. Res.*, 110, 169–173, 1999.
29. Kunova, A., Spanik, S., Kollar, T., Trupl, J., and Krcméry, V. Jr. Breakthrough fungemia due to *Hansenula anomala* in a leukemic patient successfully treated with amphotericin B. *Chemotherapy*, 42, 157–158, 1996.
30. Neumeister, B., Rockemann, M., and Marre, R. Fungaemia due to *Candida pelliculosa* in a case of acute pancreatitis. *Mycoses*, 35, 309, 1992.
31. Salesa, R., Burgos, A., Fernandez-Mazarrasa, C., Quindos, G., and Ponton, J. Transient fungaemia due to *Candida pelluculosa* in a patient with AIDS. *Mycoses*, 34, 327, 1991.

25
Dematiaceous Fungal Infections
Phaeohyphomycosis and Chromoblastomycosis

1. INTRODUCTION

The dematiaceous fungal infections are caused by the so-called "black" (darkly pigmented) or dematiaceous fungi *(1,2)*. The dematiaceous fungi are ubiquitous saprophytes in water, soil, and vegetation, and may be plant pathogens or airborne spores. They are characterized by the dark pigmentation of the mycelial structure, and most of them do not have a recognized mode of sexual reproduction *(3)*. However, upon histopathologic or direct examination of pathologic material, in many cases only a few hyphae have been visibly pigmented and sometimes a specific melanin stain was necessary to detect the presence of the pigment.

In addition to several human pathogens causing well-defined infections (sporotrichosis, onychomycosis, chromoblastomycosis, phaeohyphomycosis, fungal peritonitis), this group includes a significant number of ubiquitous environmental species, which may frequently contaminate the skin and occasionally become causative agents of opportunistic infections.

The dematiaceous fungi have become significant because of their broad spectrum of clinical features ranging in severity from superficial and mild to deep-seated, serious, and occasionally fatal outcome. In general, these infections are best characterized by a concept based on the combined clinical, pathologic, and mycologic relationships exhibited in these diseases. Another reason for their importance lies in the confusion surrounding the clinical nomenclature of diseases they represent, as well as the taxonomy of the various fungi classified as dematiaceous that show considerable pleomorphism both in vitro and in vivo *(4,5)*.

Currently, it is generally accepted that dematiaceous fungi produce three kinds of disease: phaeohyphomycosis, chromoblastomycosis, and mycetoma.

Over the years, terms such as chromomycosis, chromoblastomycosis, and phaeohyphomycosis have been applied to a variety of mycoses having distinctly different clinical, pathologic, and mycologic characteristics, thereby bringing misunderstanding, confusion, and lack of clarity and consistency in the terminology and conceptual basis for the entities known as chromoblastomycosis and phaeohyphomycosis *(6)*.

The term "chromoblastomycosis" was introduced by Terra et al. *(7)* in 1922 to discern a unique cutaneous fungal infection found in Brasil from the confusing clinical entity known as "dermatitis verrucosa." In 1935, Moore and de Almeida *(8)* proposed a new term "chromomycosis," as a replacement for the name "chromoblastomycosis," because they reasoned that the latter name has been misleading by implying that the etiologic agents grew as yeast in tissues. In the subsequent years, however, the term "chromomycosis" was inappropriately expanded from the original concept to include other mycoses caused by several different genera and species of dematiaceous fungi. To correct this problem and preserve the concept exemplified by the term "chromoblastomycosis" as originally conceived, Ajello et al. *(9)* coined a companion name "phaeohyphomycosis" to describe all mycotic infections caused by "black" fungi (containing melanin in their cell walls), which are clinically, pathologically, and mycologically distinct from classic chromoblastomycosis and black-grain mycetomata.

The fundamental difference between chromoblastomycosis and phaeohyphomycosis lies in the tissue form represented by their respective etiological agents. That is, in chromoblstomycosis, the fungi are characterized as large, muriform, thick-walled dematiaceous cells produced by fungus detained between a yeast-like and hyphal form *(5)*. In phaeohyphomycosis, the fungi exist as dark-walled ("black"), septate hyphal elements, pseudohyphae, or as solitary cells that divide either by budding, by septation in only one plane, or in various combinations of these *(10)*. Caligiorne et al. *(11)* compared genotypically various chromoblastomycosis and phaeohyphomycosis strains by using the random amplified polymorphic DNA (RAPD) technique. The data generated, which were subjected to a numerical taxonomy analysis, were used to create a phenogram enabling the investigators to cluster the strains according to their respective species.

According to current understanding, clinical chromoblastomycosis encompasses chronic, localized infections of the cutaneous and subcutaneous tissues that contain sclerotic bodies and histologically demonstrate hyperkeratotic pseudoepitheliomatous hyperplasia with keratolytic microabscess formation in the epidermis *(6)*. In contrast, phaeohyphomycosis is a broader term describing a heterogenous group of superficial, cutaneous and corneal, subcutaneous, and systemic mycoses that contain dematiaceous yeast-like cells; pseudohyphae-like elements, hyphae that may be short or elongated, regular, distorted to swollen in shape; or any combination of these form in tissue *(6)*. The term "chromomycosis" has been rejected for mycoses caused by dematiaceous fungi.

2. PHAEOHYPHOMYCOSIS

Phaeohyphomycosis is an umbrella term for all mycoses where the fungus is present in tissue with melanized filaments *(12–16)*. In its broadest definition, phaeohyphomycosis encompasses a wide group of opportunistic infections variously referred to by diferrent investigators as systemic chromoblastomycosis, subcutaneous chromoblastomycosis, cerebral chromoblastomycosis, hypodermomycosis, encephalomycosis, cystic chromomycosis, phaeomycotic cyst, keratochromomycosis. subcutaneous chromomycosis, cladosporiosis, cladosporoma, subcutaneous cystic granuloma, sporotrichosis (in part), phaeo-sporotrichose, cerebral dematiomycosis, cerebral chromycosis, and chromohyphomycosis—a confusing array of diseases *(17)* that underscores the important need for a consistent, unifying, and unambiguous terminology *(6)*.

During the past several decades, phaeohyphomycosis has been attributed to over 100 species and 60 genera of fungi in a variety of clinical syndromes, ranging from keratitis and solitary subcutaneous nodules to fulminant, rapidly fatal disseminated disease *(18,19)*.

Among the various agents of phaeohyphomycosis, fungi of the genera *Bipolaris* and *Exserohilum* have been closely associated as etiologic agents of human phaeohyphomycosis *(1,6,20)*. Other common etiologic agents of phaeohyphomycosis appear to be *Exophiala jeanselmei* and *Exophiala (Wangiella) dermatitidis (5,21–55)*. Both species have been recovered from plant materials, wood, and soil. Fungi known to cause cerebral phaeohyphomycosis include *Cladophialophora bantiana* (synonymous with *Xylohypha bantiana, Cladosporium bantianum*, and *C. trichoides*), *Phialophora pedrosoi*, and *Exophiala dermatitidis (56,57)*.

Phaeohyphomycosis concurrent with *Mycobacterium fortuitum* abscesses was described in a patient receiving corticosteroids for sarcoidosis *(58)*.

Both normal and immunocompromised hosts (renal *[59–61]* and kidney *[62]* transplant recipients, patients with malignancies, and diabetes *[63]*) can become infected (even premature infants *[64]*), and often the clinical disease that follows is characterized by invasive fungal growth. Date et al. *(65)* described a case of double infection of the same organ, echinococcosis associated with phaeohyphomycosis in the lungs.

Histological examination of subcutaneous phaeohyphomycosis revealed the presence of granulomatous lesions often surrounded by fibrious capsule and composed of multiple pyogranulomas *(10,13,66–68)*.

Disseminated phaeohyphomycosis, although still uncommon infection, has been on the increase in recent years with more dematiaceous species continually being added to the list of potential human pathogens *(18,69)*.

Surprisingly, there have been relatively very few cases of phaeohyphomycosis afflicting HIV-positive patients, mostly *Alternaria alternata* and *Exophiala jeanselmei*. Because HIV-induced immune deficiency affects primarily the T-cell population, the predominant mycoses in AIDS are those normally controlled by T lymphocytes. Primarily, granulocytes are involved in the control of fungi of hyalo- and phaeohyphomycosis and zigomycosis. Since those cell populations remain relatively intact, infections by these fungi have been rare and cannot be expected to rise significantly in variety and frequency in HIV-positive patients *(19)*.

In immunocompromised patients, the disease can disseminate through hematoghenous spread with extensive vascular invasion and necrosis *(20)*. Other reported cases of disseminated disease include dysmyelopoietic syndrome and neutropenia concurrent with multiple skin nodules (acute vasculitis) *(1,20,70)* and aortic insufficiency due to *E. rostratum* vegetation *(71)*. An immunocompetent child was diagnosed with *B. spicifera*-associated osteomyelitis of the femur and multiple brain abscesses *(72)*.

2.1. Treatment of Phaeohyphomycosis

The therapy of phaeohyphomycosis, which is usually carried out by surgery and antifungal chemotherapy, is difficult and often frustrating. The outcome of treatment of phaeohyphomycosis may often be influenced by the immunocompetence of the host, the site of infection, and the extent of involvement *(19,20,73–76)*. Patients with chronic sinusitis (allergic fungal sinusitis) may be at particular risk. The management of such patients can present formidable therapeutic problems, especially in immunocompromised hosts, because mortality rates are high regardless of the patient's immune status *(18,20,50,77)*.

In general, therapy with amphotericin B has been disappointing because of the high rates of failure and frequent relapses *(20,74,78)*. The therapeutic efficacy of ketoconazole and miconazole has been equally ineffective. However, the efficacy of itraconazole was more encouraging *(50,73,78–81)*. The recommended daily dosages of itraconazole may range from 50–600 mg; daily doses greater than 200 mg have been given twice daily *(50,82)*.

In addition, in several reports patients with cutaneous phaeohyphomycosis have also been successfully treated with terbinafine *(83)*. Newer azole agents, such as voriconazole, posaconazole, and raviconazole, have shown a broad spectrum of potent activity against dematiaceous fungi *(84–87)*.

2.1.1. Bipolaris spp. and Exserohilum spp. Phaeohyphomycosis

The last two decades have seen a dramatic increase in the frequency of phaeohyphomycosis caused by members of the genera *Bipolaris* Shoemaker and *Exserohilum* Leonard et Suggs *(1,20,72,88–100)*. In both immunocompetent and immunocompromised patients, infections associated with *B. australiensis (89)*, *B. hawaiiensis (91,93,96,98)*, *B. spicifera (20,72,88,100)*, *E. rostratum 90,101)*, *E. longirostratum (97)*, and *E. mcginnisii (99)* have been recognized as causing sinusitis, pansinusitis, endocarditis, cutaneous infections, and osteomyelitis. The first fatal human infection of meningoencephalitis related to *B. hawaiiensis* was reported by Fuste et al. *(93)* in 1973. In addition, *B. hawaiiansis* has been implicated as the cause of nasal obstruction and bone destruction *(96)*, pulmonary infection *(98)*, sinusitis *(1)*, and granulomatous encephalitis *(96)*.

Bipolaris species, particularly *B. spicifica* and *B. hawaiiensis* are associated most frequently with infections of the lower and upper respiratory tract, specifically the paranasal sinuses *(20,72,102,103)*. While *Bipolaris*-induced sinusitis in immunocompetent hosts may be an insidiously progressive infection that make take months or even years to evolve, in immunocompromised patients the disease may be more rapidly invasive. On the other hand, *Bipolaris* spp. seldom cause cutaneous ulcers in immunocompromised hosts *(104–106)*. These moulds have also been implicated as the cause of granulomatous encephalitis in immunocompetent hosts *(96)*. The fungi may also extend into the contiguous orbit with potential loss of vision *(73,102,107,108)*.

Therapy of *Bipolaris* infections depends upon the host and location of the infection *(19)*. In general, amphotericin B with or without 5-FC is used in treatment of severely immunocompromised patients with sinusitis, pneumonia, or fungemia. Koshi et al. *(92)* applied local excision of the crusted lesion followed by local application of 0.03% nystatin solution (q.i.d. in 2-mL aliquots) for 3 wk to cure nasal phaeohyphomycosis caused by *B. hawaiiensis* in an immunocompromised patient.

Itraconazole is being used increasingly for treatment of *Bipolaris* infections in immunocompetent hosts as well as in immunocompromised patients with refractory infections *(50)*. Where feasible, surgical resection of lesions should be performed *(1,109)*.

In cases of disseminated phaeohyphomycosis, complete surgical debridement appeared to be important in the treatment of locally invasive disease *(20)*. In addition, amphotericin B may prove useful in these patients as seen in a patient with disseminated *B. spicifera* skin lesions who responded promptly to the antibiotic given at 50 mg per dose, 3 times weekly, for a total of 750 g *(20)*. However, in another case of an immunosuppressed cardiac allograft recipient, *B. spicifica* involvement of the lung, pericardium, and the heart failed to respond to combination of amphotericin B and ketoconazole (800 mg, daily) *(20)*.

In the experience of Burges et al. *(110)* surgical debridement of an accessible focus of infection along with oral therapy with ketoconazole may provide adequate therapy of subcutaneous phaeohyphomycosis caused by *E. rostratum* in an immunocompetent patient.

In a case of localized *E. rostratum* (reported as *D. rostrata*) osteomyelitis, a patient responded after multiple relapses over a 5-yr period to surgical debridement and intravenous amphotericin B *(90)*. The ability of *Bipolaris* and *Exserohilum* spp. to penetrate the bone was demonstrated in other cases of bone invasion with disseminated disease *(72)* and sinusitis *(20,80,91)*.

In *Bipolaris*-induced meningoencephalitis, the onset of symptoms may be acute or subacute with polymorphonuclear or mononuclear pleocytosis of the cerebrospinal fluid (CSF) *(20,57)*. It is believed that central nervous system (CNS) involvement may result from fungal invasion through infected sinuses *(111)*. In one such case, a breast cancer patient with meningeal carcinomatosis and *Bipolaris* meningoencephalitis died after failing to respond to intravenous chloramphenicol following tentative diagnosis of bacterial meningitis *(20)*. In two other cases of *Bipolaris*-induced CNS infections *(93,112)*, one patient died without antifungal therapy and severe granulomatous and suppurative leptomeningitis with vasculitis *(93)*. In the second case *(112)*, the patient who showed granulomatous fungal encephalitis responded to combined therapy consisting of 5-FC and amphotericin B (a total of 2.0 g). Albeit cured, the patient was left with neurologic sequalae (residual seizure disorder and personality change) *(112)*. It should be noted, however, that in spite of its excellent CNS penetration, the therapeutic value of 5-FC is uncertain because of the observed in vitro resistance by *Bipolaris* species *(113)*.

Although pathologic evidence of bone invasion in *Bipolaris/Exserohilum* sinusitis may not always be present, there has been frequent radiographic data suggesting invasive disease *(20)*. Allergic rhinitis may be a risk factor for the development of *Bipolaris* sinusitis. Whether the use of corticosteroids increases the risk of infection is still not known. Treatment involved surgical debridement in addition to intravenous amphotericin B *(20)*. Surgical debridement alone was followed by a relapse *(72,91)*. Sinusitis has also been caused by dematiceous fungi other than *Bipolaris*, including *Curvalaria lunata (114)*, *Cladosporium (111)*, and *Alternaria (115,116)*. While complete surgical debridement seemed essential in the treatment of *Bipolaris/Exserohilum* sinusitis *(20,72)*, therapy with amphotericin B helped in preventing a relapse *(117)*.

Keratitis and corneal ulcers induced by *Bipolaris/Exserohilum* were related to *E. rostratum* (reported as *D. halodes*) *(94,101)*, *B. spicifera (94,118)*, and "*Helminthosporium*" (most likely to be

Bipolaris species) *(113,119,120)*. In all cases, patients presented with eye pain following trauma to the eye; corneal ulceration and inflammation with varying degree of visual deficit were also observed *(20)*. Topical amphotericin B *(113,118,119)*, pimaricin *(94,113)*, gentamicin *(94)*, 5-FC (flucytosine) *(20,113)*, nystatin/griseofulvin *(119)*, or tolnaftate *(113)* have been used to clear ulceration, occasionally after penetrating keratoplasty. In two cases, however, amphotericin B was apparently ineffective; in addition, intraocular amphotericin B caused severe local reaction and marginal efficacy against *Bipolaris*-associated keratitis *(20)*. On the other hand, pimaricin, a topical polyene antimycotic has shown promise in treating fungal keratitis. Visual acuity following treatment varied from normal to near blindness *(20,118,121)*.

Allergic bronchopulmonary disease related to *Bipolaris*/"Helminthosporium" invasion has been reported to present with a syndrome very similar to that caused by *Aspergillus*: productive cough, bronchospasm, bronchiectasis, localized pulmonary infiltrates, eosinophilia, and elevated IgE level *(2,20,95,121–124)*. Clinical improvement was seen with surgical resection *(95)* or with corticosteroid therapy *(2,20,122–124)*.

Pauzner et al. *(100)* described the first case of *B. spicifera* endocarditis in an immunocompetent patient with cryopreserved homograft aortic valve; the patient responded well to surgical and antifungal therapy.

2.1.2. Exophiala (Wangiella) dermatitidis *and* Exophiala *spp. Phaeohyphomycosis*

The preponderance of the cases of *Exophiala (Wangiella) dermatitidis*-related phaeohyphomycosis came from Japan *(5,22,24–26,38,46,125)* and recently, Korea *(126)*. This geographical localization may indicate the existence of virulence differences among strains, genetically based immunological susceptibility and propensity for environmental exposure *(19)*. Melanin is thought to contribute to the virulence of *E. dermatitidis* by preventing the pathogen to be killed in the phagolysosome of the neutrophils; however, the melanin did not influence the phagocytosis or the oxidative burst of the neutrophils involved *(127)*.

E. dermatitidis infections are usually chronic CNS or cutaneous disease. The manifestations of CNS infections are those of a local neurological deficit most often simulating a brain tumor or abscess *(19)*. The CSF was reported to show pleocytosis with a high eosinophil count but without peripheral blood eosinophilia *(126)*. Cutaneous lesions appear as chronic infections (usually without verrucoid hyperkeratosis) *(54,128)*, as well as subcutaneous cysts *(39,129,130)*.

Several cases describing pulmonary phaeohyphomycosis have also been reported *(131)*, including in patients with cystic fibrosis (CF) *(132,133)*. The symptoms consisted of chronic pneumonia, with cough, fever and pulmonary infiltrates, occasionally accompanied by hemoptysis. In addition, *E. dermatitidis* has been implicated in lesions of the digestive tract *(25)* and the lymph nodes *(22,25,32,38)*. Hiruma et al. *(46,125)* have described a case of systemic *E. dermatitidis* disease in which the infection first appeared as swelling of the cervical lymph nodes, followed by development of lesions in various organs, including the common bile duct and the brain. Surgical debridement, and repeated antifungal therapy with intravenous (drip infusion) miconazole (600 mg daily), oral flucytosine (12 g daily), and intralesional, intravenous (a total dose of 600 mg over a 3-mo period) and oral (4.8–7.2 g daily, with drug plasma level 1 yr after the start of oral therapy at 0.140 µg/mL) amphotericin B, did not prevent the systemic infection from recurring and the patient's death from respiratory failure *(125)*. While high oral doses of amphotericin B appeared to suppress fungal growth in the abdominal cavity, they were ineffective on the intracranial lesions.

Infections caused by *E. dermatitidis* have been notoriously resistant to antifungal therapy. Surgical excision is usually performed on small, localized cutaneous and subcutaneous lesions *(128)*. However, when the infection is widespread, or deep-seated, visceral and disseminated, chemotherapy with amphotericin B, flucytosin, or combination of both drugs has been recommended. Among newer antimycotics, ketoconazole, fluconazole, itraconazole, and terbinafine, have shown therapeutic promise *(52,128,134)*.

Pospisil et al. *(52)* described a case of corneal phaeohyphomycosis in a patient with von Recklinghausen's disease and immunodeficiency (lower T lymphocyte count). Despite treatment with amphotericin B, the patient was left blind in one eye.

Exophiala spp. and *E. jeanselmei* (conspecific with *Phialophora gougerotii*) *(135)*, in particular have been reported to cause both subcutaneous phaeohyphomycosis *(136–149)* and mycetomas with increasing frequency *(150–155)*, especially among patients with immune deficiencies *(156–158)* and transplant recipients *(61,159)*. Phaeohyphomycosis of the epididymis caused by *E. jeanselmei* has also been described *(160)*. The pathogen generally penetrates the skin by a traumatic inoculation with contaminated splinters or slivers of wood or other organic material *(145,161)*. Nosocomial *E. jeanselmei* pseudoinfection after sonography-guided aspiration of thoracic lesions has also been reported *(162)*.

In the majority of cases, *E. jeanselmei*-induced subcutaneous phaeohyphomycosis is characterized initially with solitary, discrete, asymptomatic, well-encapsulated subcutaneous nodules, and little involvement of the overlying epidermis *(6,145,163)*. Histological changes include the formation of extensive granulation tissue with abscesses that may enlarge into the sinuses. The fungus can be found as aggregates situated mostly in the center of the abscesses.

Despite its occurence in immunocompromised patients, *E. jeanselmei*-induced cutaneous and subcutaneous phaeohyphomycosis remain generally a localized disease that can be cured by surgical excision and antifungal therapy *(149,159)*.

Subcutaneous *E. jeanselmei* infection was reported to complicate cases of pulmonary tuberculosis *(164,165)*. In two cases involving renal *(61)* and kidney *(166)* transplant recipients, *E. jeanselmei* phaeohyphomycosis was concurrent with *Nocardia* infection.

Human cerebral infections with *Exophiala* spp. involving *E. jeanselmei* *(28,167)*, and one still-unclassified species *(168)* have also been reported. Although there are no apparent predisposing factors in cerebral phaeohyphomycosis, defective host immunity coupled with an environmental source of the organism may be important in establishing CNS *Exophiala* spp. infection in humans.

Hachisuka et al. *(59)* reported a case of *E. jeanselmei*-associated cutaneous phaeohyphomycosis in a renal transplant recipient. 5-Fluorocytosine at a total daily dose of 50 mg/kg (in two equally divided oral doses) successfully led to gradual decrease of the lesion in size, which completely disappeared 6 mo later. The serum concentration was 50.7 µg/mL 6 h after the administration of 2.0 g of the drug. Mauceri et al. *(138)* recommended higher dosage of flucytosine (150 mg/kg daily) conditional on patient's tolerance. In another case of postrenal transplantation of cutaneous phaeohyphomycosis caused by *E. jeanselmei*, Sindhuphak et al. *(169)* used surgical excision and oral ketoconazole (200–400 mg daily) for 2 yr to clear the lesions. South et al. *(140)* also recommended ketoconazole at 200 mg daily.

Recently, itraconazole has been increasingly used for the treatment of subcutaneous *E. jeanselmei* phaeohyphomycosis *(149,159,170–172)*. In vitro susceptibility testing has shown the drug to be effective against *Exophiala* spp. at concentrations of 0.0001–0.015 µg/mL (*E. jeanselmei*) *(171,173,174)*, 0.018–0.02 µg/mL (*E. spinifera*) *(50,136)*, and 0.018 µg/mL (*E. castellanii*) *(136)*. After initial surgical debridement, Whittle and Kominos *(171)* successfully applied a 4-mo course of oral itraconazole (200 mg, b.i.d.) to treat subcutaneous *E. jeanselmei* phaeohyphomycosis; the initial treatment with amphotericin B was discontinued because of renal insufficiency.

Chuan and Wu *(170)* used 200 mg daily of itraconazole for 2 mo, combined with incision and drainage to relieve the symptoms of subcutaneous phaeohyphomycosis in an elderly patient with systemic lupus erythematosus (SLE) who was being treated with prednisone. This case was one of several reports of subcutaneous phaeohyphomycosis developing in immunosuppressed patients as a result of prolonged steroid treatment; while most often lesions would remain solitary, in the immunosuppressed patient they may enlarge with frank tissue invasion or disseminate with fatal outcome *(170)*. However, in another case, Schwinn et al. *(172)* had to stop treatment of *E. jeanselmei* phaehyphomycotic cyst with a 200-mg daily regimen of itraconazole after 6 wk because of side effects (headache, gastrointestinal disorders, body weakness, and inreasing liver enzyme levels). In general, response to itraconazole treatment was found to be higher in patients with a shorter duration of illness and with no previous treatment *(79)*.

An elderly noninsulin dependent diabetic patient with *E. jeanselmei* pulmonary phaeohyphomycosis was treated successfully with oral ketoconazole (400 mg, daily) for 5 mo *(63)*.

E. jeanselmei var. *castellanii* was at one time considered to be a new species, *E. castellanii (175)*. However, currently it is considered to be a variant of *E. jeanselmei (176,177)*. Gold et al. *(136)* reported the first case of prosthetic valve endocarditis due to *E. castellanii* that was managed with surgical debridement and valve replacement, and chemotherapy consisting of amphotericin B (total of 1.6 g) and flucytosine (250 mg, q.i.d.). After recurrence (bilateral psoas abscesses), surgical drainage was applied, followed by a 6-mo course of amphotericin B (1.0 g total) and itraconazole (100 mg daily). Antifungal susceptibility testing showed that the organism was susceptible to amphotericin B (MIC = 0.58 µg/mL), flucytosine (MIC = 10.09 µg/mL or less), ketoconazole (MIC = 0.4 µg/mL), fluconazole (MIC = 2.5 µg/mL), and itraconazole (MIC = 0.018 µg/mL or less).

Intralesional amphotericin B (30–50 mg, weekly) was found to be helpful in the therapy of subcutaneous phaeohyphomycosis due to *E. moniliae (178)*.

E. spinifera can infect both animals *(179)* and humans *(136,180–185)*. The first case of human disease, reported by Rajam et al. *(185)*, involved a fatal infection in a child. In addition to cutaneous infection *(183)*, *E. spinifera* was identified as the etiologic agent of a systemic disease in a 9-yr-old child *(184)*. With regard to treatment of human *E. spinifera* pheohyphomycosis, one case proved fatal. In two cases, one of nasal granuloma and the other of pustular lesion on the forearm, the infections were diagnosed early and were successfully treated by surgical excision alone *(136)*. Reported antifungal therapy involved a combined treatment of ketoconazole and flucytosine which was effective, as well as itraconazole alone (after treatment with amphotericin B, ketoconazole, and flucytosine failed to elicit any clinical improvement). Rinaldi *(186)* reported a case of a renal-transplant recipient with recurrent subcutaneous nodules caused by *E. spinifera* who was successfully treated with repeated surgical excision of the lesions following a failed attempt with antifungal chemotherapy. In vitro susceptibility testing have shown the pathogen susceptible to amphotericin B (MIC = 0.14 µg/mL or less), flucytosine (MIC = 10.09 µg/mL or less), ketoconazole (MIC = 0.2 µg/mL), and itraconazole (MIC = 0.018 µg/mL or less) *(136)*.

2.1.3. Alternaria *spp. Phaeohyphomycosis*

Alternaria is a large genus with species usually found as soil saprophytes and plant pathogens, some of which can cause human infections. From all of the isolated *Alternaria* spp., *A. alternata* has been the most frequent cause of disease in humans *(187–195)*. According to one compilation of data *(196)*, *A. alternata* together with *Exophiala jeanselmei* were among the most common phaeoid fungi afflicting AIDS patients. Another species, *A. tenuissima*, has been identified in nearly one-third of the cases *(195,197–203)*. Other *Alternaria* spp. shown pathogenic to human include *A. dianthicola (204)*, *A. chartarum (205)*, *A. stemphyloides (206)*, *A. longipes (207)*, *A. infectoria (208,209)*, *A. alternata (195,210)*, and *A. chlamydospora (193,194)*.

Alternaria spp. have been identified as the causative agents of various clinical conditions including skin lesions *(14,189,197,207–209,211–217)*, hypersensitivity pneumonitis *(218)*, granulomatous lung disease *(219)*, allergic fungal sinusitis *(220,221)*, ocular infections *(222–225)*, peritonitis *(226)*, and osteomyelitis *(227,228)*. In general, *Alternaria* spp. infections are classified in four forms: superficial, cutaneous and corneal, subcutaneous, and systemic *(66,210)*.

Cutaneous alternariosis can no longer be considered a rare fungal infection *(189,197,211–216)*. Since 1933, when the first case was observed *(187)* this mycosis has been well-documented in numerous reports involving immunocompromised patients (those with Cushing's syndrome, kidney, liver and bone-marrow transplant recipients, with hematologic malignancies, chronic polyarthritis, discoid lupus erythematosus with leukopenia, primitive pulmonary hypertension, and nephrotic syndrome) *(187–190,192,200,209,211,217,229–241)*, although infections in immunocompetent individuals have also been recognized *(155,198,214,242)*. Cutaneous *Alternaria* infections have been distributed worldwide, including the Mediterranean region (Spain, France, Italy, Greece) and nearly all other European countries *(192,194,195,198,201,230,235,243)*, India *(193)*, Taiwan *(244)*, Japan, and the United States. Cutaneous alternariosis, which usually originate by a traumatic implantation of fungal spores, are relatively common in farmers *(207,235,245)*.

Phaeohyphomycosis caused by both *Alternaria* spp. and *Phaeosclera dematioides* has been reported by Slovak investigators *(68,245)*.

Clinical manifestations of cutaneous alternariosis include the presence of single or multiple, reddish brown, erythematous squamous, papulonodular or frankly nodular lesions with smooth or heaped-up surfaces *(229)*. Gerdsen et al. *(246)* described a cardiac-transplant patient who developed cutaneous alternariosis with a sporotrichoid distribution of the skin lesions.

Male and Pehamberger *(247)* classified cutaneous alternariosis into three types: endogenous, exogenous, and dermatopathic. In the endogenous form, the infection very likely is initially transmitted by inhalation, followed by hematogenous spread to the skin where the fungus causes typical verruciform or granulomatous lesions. In exogenous cutaneous alternariosis, the organisms are inoculated by trauma. The dermatopathic condition develops when *Alternaria* secondarily colonize preexisting lesions (e.g., steroid-treated facial eczema), in what appears to be nosoparasitism rather than genuine infection.

There have been numerous reports implicating corticosteroids as major pathogenic factor in cutaneous alternariosis. Higher levels of corticosteroids may be considered as a subjacent internal disease *(187,188,190,192,211,229,230,235)* such as the Cushing's syndrome *(215,237)*, or may be caused by other reasons *(187,191,201,234,236,244,248–250)*. In most instances, cutaneous alternariosis improved or healed after tapering of corticosteroid medication *(188,201,203,248,249,251)*, even without interruption of other chemotherapeutic regimens *(233)*. Richardson et al. *(252)* described one case of subcutaneous alternariosis of the foot in an immunocompromised patient on corticosteroid medication.

There have been several reports *(215,253,254)*, affiliating Cushing's syndrome with cutaneous alternariosis and other superficial mycoses *(255)*. The apparent cause for fungal infections in patients with Cushing's syndrome has been the immunosuppressive state of such patients due to the excessive endogenous glucocorticoid production associated with this syndrome, which serves as a predisposing factor *(215)*. Kasperlik-Zaluska and Bielunska *(191)* described a case of successful resolution of an unusual *A. alternata* cutaneous infection in a patient with the Cushing's syndrome related to mitotane medication. Because of the life-threatening signs of Cushing's syndrome, mitotane therapy (up to 6.0 g daily, for a total of 241 g over 5 wk) was implemented in order to reduce the endogenous high level of cortisol secretion. Because mitotane is not an antifungal drug and direct anti-*Alternaria* action would be highly unlikely, the resolution of alternariosis was attributed to the mitotane's inhibitory effect on steroidogenesis *(191)*. Guerin et al. *(215)* described the successful use of ketoconazole in the treatment of a patient suffering from both Cushing's syndrome and associated cutaneous alternariosis. To this end, Loli et al. *(256)* found that ketoconazole elicited rapid reduction of plasma and urinary cortisol levels and regression of clinical and biological abnormalities of the Cushing's syndrome. However, the place of ketoconazole in the therapy of Cushing's syndrome has not been well documented. Because ketoconazole does not remove the cause of increased corticotropin secretion, it cannot be considered to be the treatment of choice of the pituitary-dependent Cushing's disease. In addition, ketoconazole also failed when used for the treatment of Cushing's syndrome of peripheral origin *(257)*.

2.1.3.1. Therapy of Alternariosis

In general, ketoconazole, although being widely used to treat cutaneous alternariosis, has shown mixed success. It failed to resolve cutaneous lesions despite topical and systemic therapy in an immunocompromised patient with thrombocytopenic purpura *(235)* as well as in other cases *(200,232)*, but was reported to elicit positive responses in several different studies *(201,202,215,251)*. Bécherel et al. *(258)* used daily occlusive local ketoconazole therapy for 2 mo to heal cutaneous alternariosis in a renal-transplant recipient.

Amphotericin B (intralesional injections *[197,244]* and systemic *[190,192,200]*), miconazole *(259)*, oral ketoconazole *(260)*, and fluconazole *(248)* have also been reported to be effective sometimes. Thus, Benedict et al. *(212)* have described three cases of cutaneous alternariosis following solid organ transplantation that were successfully treated with intravenous amphotericin B or oral ketoconazole. Shearer and Chandrasekar *(261)* used intravenous amphotericin B (at 10 mg/kg for a total of 305 mg) to resolve skin lesions and cure lymphadenitis in a bone-marrow recipient; however, 10 d after discontinuation of therapy, the skin lesions reappeared and had to be surgically excised, followed by the additional administration of another 75 mg of amphotericin B *(261)*.

Viviani et al. *(229)* described cutaneous alternariosis caused by *A. tenuissima* in two patients with primitive myeloproliferative syndrome and lymphocytic lymphoma, respectively. Both cases were treated with a combination of surgical escision of lesions and therapy with ketoconazole at 200 mg, b.i.d. In the first case, because of low blood levels, the ketoconazole dosage had to be increased to 300 mg, b.i.d.; there was a disease relapse and dissemination leading to a fatal outcome. In the second case, drug levels in the blood were sufficiently high (1.6 µg/mL on the 9th day, at 2 h after the administration); there was no relapse despite continued corticosteroid therapy to control the underlying lymphocytic lymphoma.

Recently, several cases of cutaneous alternariosis have been successfully resolved with the use of daily oral doses of 100–200 mg of itraconazole *(188,190,194,199,207,210,211,214,230,248,262)*. Thus, Duffill and Coley *(188)* have recommended 100-mg daily oral itraconazole to treat *A. alternata* cutaneous phaeohyphomycosis in an elderly patient on prednisone medication (60 mg daily) for a nephrotic syndrome; while the prednisone dosage was tapered, the rash cleared following the itraconazole treatment. Oral itraconazole (400 mg, daily) was also used to treat multifocal cutaneous lesions due to *A. tenuissima (199)*.

Gené et al. *(207)* reported the first case of cutaneous phaeohyphomycosis due to *A. longipes* in a patient with underlying neoplastic disease. The patient was treated initially with oral ketoconazole (200 mg, b.i.d.) for 3 wk with no response, and then with oral itraconazole (100 mg, b.i.d.). After 2 mo of itraconazole therapy no new lesions developed. In vitro antifungal susceptibility testing of the same *A. longipes* isolate has shown susceptibility to amphotericin B, ketoconazole, miconazole, and itraconazole with MIC values of 0.29–0.58, 1.6, 2.5, and 0.24 µg/mL, respectively; the isolate was resistant to fluconazole (MIC = 40 µg/mL) and 5-FC (MIC >322.75 µg/mL) *(207)*.

Combined drug therapies, such as oral erythromycin with topical miconazole, have also been applied *(229)*.

Cutaneous infection by *Alternaria* spp. may also respond to surgical resection, especially when antifungal treatment is not effective.

Locally invasive sinonasal *Alternaria* infections in several immunocompetent patients have been described *(115,116,227,228,263)*. Morrison and Weisdorf *(264)* reported six cases of invasive sinonasal disease caused by *Alternaria* spp. that occured in bone-marrow transplant recipients. The infections, which were localized to the sinonasal region with no evidence of disseminated disease, were either asymptomatic (three of six patients) or the symptoms were mild and nonspecific (fever, headache, increased nasal secretions, nasal pain, and mild epistaxis). All patients received surgical debridement as well as therapy with amphotericin B for 5–61 d (median, 27). The total dose of the drug varied from 181 mg (in one patient who died 5 d after diagnosis) to 2.64 g; excluding the former patient, the mean total dose of amphotericin B was 1.952 mg. In addition, two patients received flucytosine and rifampin; granulocyte transfusions were administered to four patients, for periods of 1, 3, 3, and 16 d. The results of this combined therapy have shown the sinonasal alternariosis resolved in all surviving patients *(264)*. Invasive sinonasal alternariosis in patients with AIDS *(76)* and in neutropenic patients during therapy for hematologic malignancies have also been reported *(265,266)*.

A plant fungicide, imazalil, was used in the treatment of alternariosis involving the palate, nose and sinuses, which has been not responsive to conventional therapy *(267)*. The drug, which was used topically (instillation and irrigation) as well as orally (up to 1.2 g daily), arrested but did not cure the disease.

Recently, Halaby et al. *(208)* described a case of *A. infectoria* phaeohyphomycosis in a renal-transplant patient who developed pulmonary infiltrates and skin lesions. The treatment was successful and consisted of combination of surgical excision and a 28-d systemic antifungal therapy, first with itraconazole and subsequently with liposomal amphotericin B.

Ophthalmic infections associated with *Alternaria* spp. include blepharitis, conjunctivitis, keratomycosis, and endophthalmitis *(222,223,268–270)*. A case of chronic *A. alternata* endophthalmitis in a diabetic patient was completely resolved following treatment with systemic amphothericin B (up to 60 mg daily) and flucytosine (250 mg, q.i.d.) for 3 wk, combined with cycloplegic eyedrops 3 times daily *(222)*. In another case, a deep *Alternaria* keratomycosis with intraocular extension was successfully treated with topical 1% miconazole and oral fluconazole (200 mg, daily) *(223)*.

2.1.4. Phaeosclera dematioides Phaeohyphomycosis

In 1980, Sigler et al. *(271)* described *Phaeosclera dematioides* as a new dematiaceous fungus characterized by a bulblike masses of muriform cells, and by the conversion of short hyphal segments into sclerotic-like bodies. McGinnis et al. *(272)* were the first to describe *S. dematioides* as as the etiologic agent of phaeohyphomycosis in cattle causing nasal granulomas.

As an opportunistic pathogen in humans, *S. dematioides* was identified initially by Matsumoto et al. *(273)* in the pleural fluid of an AIDS patient, and shortly thereafter by Krempt-Lamprecht et al. *(274)* as subcutaneous lesion in a farmer.

In a third report, Slovak investigators presented a case of phaeohyphomycosis caused by strains of both *S. dematioides* and *Alternaria* spp *(68,245)*. Initially, the patient was treated with amphotericin B for 2 yr. After a 13-yr-long clinically asymptomatic remission, the patient relapsed; diabetes mellitus and asthma developed at this time. After pulse therapy with itraconazole (400 mg daily for 7 d, followed by a 21-d pause; therapeutic scheme repeated three times), the patient remained in stable clinical condition.

2.1.5. Curvularia spp. Phaeohyphomycosis

C. lunata (first described as *Acrothecium lunata [275]*) has been identified as pathogenic to humans, causing infections that include endocarditis, brain abscess *(276)*, skin and subcutaneous lesions *(277,278)*, onychomycosis, endophthalmitis *(279)*, keratitis *(279,280)*, pneumonia, disseminated disease, mycetoma, allergic bronchopulmonary disease, and sinusitis. The first two cases of human disease due to *C. lunata* were mycetomas in Africa *(281,282)*. Even though *C. pallescens* is commonly isolated from tropical regions of the world, infections by this species are very rare.

Although dissiminated *Curvularia* disease has been prevalent in immunocompromised patients, most cases of *C. lunata* sinusitis have been in immunocompetent hosts *(279,283–287)*.

Lampert et al. *(288)* were the first to describe a disseminated infection in an immunocompetent young adolescent patient; the lesions were initially detected in the lung but later metastasized to the brain. Inhalation of dirt was considered to be the most probable portal of entry, resulting in a primary pulmonary mycetoma with secondary cerebral metastasis. Treatment with amphotericin B and miconazole was described as moderately effective *(288)*. An invasive cutaneous infection caused by *C. pallescens* was cured by combination of surgical excision and oral ketoconazole for 7 mo *(289)*.

Allergic bronchopulmonary disease due to *C. senegalensis*, a rare saprophytic fungus, was desribed in an immunocompetent pediatric patient *(290)*. Prednisone therapy was initiated at a dose of 2.0 mg/kg (60 mg, daily). The dose regimen was decreased to 20 mg daily on alternate days after 3 mo, and subsequently tapered and discontinued after 6 mo of therapy. The patient remained asymptomatic 5 yr after completeion of therapy. According to deShazo and Swain *(291)*, isolation of *Curvularia* was second in frequency only to *Bipolaris* spp. as the organism recovered from patients with allergic fungal sinusitis.

Rinaldi et al. *(283)* described five cases of *C. lunata* paranasal sinusitis in immunocompetent patients with no underlying debilitating disease. All patients were treated with surgery (debridement and aeration) alone and fully recovered. The results of antifungal susceptibility varied depending on the medium used for testing, with the exception of 5-FC, to which all strains were resistant. The reported MIC values (at 24 h) were as follows: amphotericin B, 1.16 and 2.31 µg/mL; miconazole, 1.20 and 4.79 µg/mL; ketoconazole, 0.4 and >12.8 µg/mL; and 5-FC, >322.75 µg/mL *(283)*.

In another case of phaeohyphomycotic sinusitis due to *C. lunata*, the treatment involved an initial extensive surgical debridement by Caldwell-Luc operation, followed immediately by daily chemotherapy with intravenous amphotericin B (gradual daily increases to 50 mg). In addition, the sinuses were irrigated with 10 mg of amphotericin B daily by a catheter placed at the time of surgery. The antifungal medication was tolerated well by the patient who received a total of 1.0 g of the antibiotic intravenously, and another 200 mg administered into the sinuses in a 3-wk period. In this case, as well as with other *C. lunata* infections *(123,292,293)*, a peripheral eosinophilia was observed. In other reports involving *C. pallescens (288)*, *Drechslera hawaiiensis (123)*, and *Bipolaris spicifera* (a granulomatous encephalitis in which the CSF contained 30% eosinophils) *(112)*, the presence of eosinophilia has also been noticed. Whether or not the observed eosinophilia represented an inflammatory or hypersensitivity response to the fungus, or was indicative of an underlying allergic disorder, remained speculative *(284)*.

Ismail et al. *(293)* described an invasive *C. lunata*-associated pansinusitis presenting with extensive bone destruction and intracranial extension. The patient received numerous surgical procedures coupled with a 12-mo course of antifungal therapy consisting of 4.0 g of intravenous amphotericin B and a 8-mo course of 400 mg of oral ketoconazole daily.

A rare case of disseminated *C. lunata* disease involving infection of the lung and brain, as reported by de la Monte and Hutchins *(294)*, was successfully treated with intravenous amphotericin B (1.0 mg/kg daily, for a total of 3.4 g) for 6 wk. However, in two subsequent reports, Pierce et al. *(295,296)* elaborated on some additional therapeutic and clinical considerations involving the same case. Rather than 6 wk, as initially reported by de la Monte and Hutchins *(294)*, the patient had a long and complicated treatment course lasting 30 mo, during which a major clinical relapse occured and 12.2 g of amphotericin B (total dose over 30 mo) was given. In addition, immunologic studies have suggested that the infection was accompanied by an unexplained cell-mediated immune deficiency *(296)*. In three previously reported cases *(288,292,294)*, treatment of pulmonary and cerebral involvement of *Curvularia* was unsuccessful.

A pulmonary *Curvularia* infection in a profoundly immunosuppressed patient with megakaryocytic leukemia was successfully cured with amphotericin B *(297)*. The treatment consisted of initial surgical excision, followed by administration of 1.0 mg/kg of amphotericin B every other day for approx 1 mo; the therapy was then continued on an outpatient basis until a total dose of 2.5 g of amphotericin B was administered.

In a case involving an immunocompromised patient with granulocytic leukemia, *Curvularia* and *Alternaria* have been isolated from the nasal septum and tissue invasion was documented histologically *(265)*. The dual infection was managed without antifungal therapy (no evidence of distal organ involvement) following surgical excision of the nasal septum and spontaneous resolution of neutropenia.

Berlanga et al. *(298)* described a successful treatment of *Curvularia* infection with liposomal amphotericin B that developed in a patient with acute promyelocytic leukemia (AML type M3 on FAB classification). The latter condition showed resistance to primary chemotherapy but responded to treatment with all-*trans*-retinoic acid (a differentiation inducer of promyelocytic blast).

Bryan et al. *(299)* described a patient who developed *C. lunata*-induced endocarditis on a Carpentier-Edwards porcine heterograft with clinical involvement of the ring of the aortic valve and the aortic root. Because curative surgery was considered to be extremely high risk, the patient was treated with terbinafine (an allylamine antimycotic) after initial therapy with amphotericin B and ketoconazole failed to eradicate the fungus. Terbinafine at doses of 125 mg, b.i.d. was administered for nearly 7 yr without serious (hepatotoxicity) side effects. In vitro, a *C. lunata* isolate was susceptible to terbinafine with MIC value of 0.2 µg/mL *(300)*.

Curvularia keratitis typically presents as superficial feathery infiltration, rarely a visible pigmentation that gradually would become focally suppurative. By one account *(280)*, *Curvularia* was the third most prevalent filamentous fungus among corneal isolates and the most common dematiaceous mold. *C. sengalensis*, *C.lunata*, *C. pallescens*, and *C. prasadii* were the most frequent corneal isolates; all tested isolates were inhibited by 4.0 µg/mL or less of natamycin. While topical natamycin was used clinically for a median duration of 1 mo, delays in diagnosis beyond 1 wk doubled the average length of topical antifungal treatment ($p = 0.005$). Another recommended treatment of *Curvularia* keratitis consisted of topical miconazole every hour, daily subconjunctival injections of 5.0 mg of miconazole for 5 d, and oral ketoconazole (200 mg) once daily *(301)*. Topical and subconjunctival administration of miconazole produced good intraocular penetration both in humans *(302)* and a rabbit model *(303)*. Upon examination, the clinical differentiation between moniliaceous and dematiaceous keratomycoses can often be difficult; however, one helpful histologic distinction observed in dematiaceous (*C. lunata*) fungal keratitis has been the diffused brown pigmentation throughout the ulcer bed *(304)*.

Agrawal and Singh *(305)* reported the first case of cutaneous phaeohyphomycosis caused by *C. pallescens*. In vitro antifungal susceptibility testing showed that oxiconazole was the most active drug with an MIC value of 0.001 µg/mL, followed by amorolfine (MIC = 3.0 µg/mL), and ketoconazole (MIC = 30 µg/mL); itraconazole was ineffective *(305)*. One case of *Curvularia*-associated persistent subcutaneous infection was also reported by Subramanyam et al. *(306)*.

An invasive burn-wound *Curvularia* infection was successfully treated with a 10-d course of amphotericin B (1.0 mg/kg, daily) *(307)*. Yau et al. *(308)* described a case of a neonate with congenital heart disease in whom a sternal wound infection caused by *C. lunata* developed following cardiac surgery.

2.1.6. Ochroconis gallopava Phaeohyphomycosis

Ochroconis gallopava (synonymous with *Dactylaria constricta* var. *gallopavam*) is the etiologic agent of a seldom diagnosed but potentially lethal pulmonary and disseminated infection in immunocompromised patients *(176,309–311)*. *Ochroconis* is not known to cause systemic disease in immunocompetent hosts. In all reported cases, the patients had underlying immune deficiencies.

Most likely, the pathogen's portal of entry is the respiratory tract *(309)*. In addition, this phaeoid fungus is known to cause CNS infection in experimental murine models *(312)*. As compared to CNS phaeohyphomycosis due to *C. bantiana* and *E. dermatitidis*, the *O. gallopava*-associated CNS involvement has the tendency for causing ventriculitis *(313)*. This preference may also be observed in immunocompromised patients. In view of the absence of reliable distinguishing histologic features between *O. gallopava*, *C. bantiana*, *E. dermatitidis*, and *Phialophora pedrosoi* (*Fonsecaea pedrosoi*) *(313)*, a definitive identification of *O. gallopava* is important for timely therapy. Amphotericin B appears to be effective *(19)*.

Fukushiro et al. *(314)* reported the first human infection caused by *O. gallopava* in a patient with an acute myeloblastic leukemia (AML). A second disseminated fatal infection was described by Terreni et al. *(310)*. Although rare, human CNS involvement of *Ochroconis* has been reported *(315–318)*.

Using a *Dactylaria constricta*-infected mouse model, Dixon and Polak *(134)* found that invitro susceptibility testing had no predictive value for in vivo activity. Of the compounds tested, flucytosine was the most effective (at doses of 25–100 mg/kg), followed by amphotericin B (5–10 mg/kg), fluconazole (25–100 mg/kg), and ketoconazole (100 mg/kg). Nevertheless, amphotericin B remains the drug of choice.

Kralovic and Rhodes *(318)* described a case cerebral phaeohyphomycosis in a liver-transplant recipient in what appeared to be a nosocomially acquired infection. A 10-d treatment with amphotericin B (1.0 mg/kg) followed by itraconazole (400 mg daily) failed to resolve the infection and the patient died. In another fatal case of cerebral dactylariosis *(315)*, amphotericin B (0.5 mg/kg) and flucytosine (150 mg/kg) given for more than 2 wk, also failed to elicit a positive response. However, Vukmir et al. *(316)* treated successfully cerebral dactylariosis in a liver-transplant recipient using a combination of colloidal dispersion of amphotericin B (8.5 g total dose) and flucytosine for 4 wk, followed by itraconazole (200 mg, daily) for 1 yr.

Mancini and McGinnis *(309)* used amphotericin B alone at a dosage of 0.7 mg/kg (total of 811 mg) to cure *Dactylaria*-induced pulmonary phaeohyphomycosis.

Cerebral phaeohyphomycosis due to *O. gallopava* has also been reported *(310,313,319)*.

2.1.7. Phialophora spp. Phaeohyphomycosis

Phialophora spp. have a worldwide distribution and are considered the etiologic agent of a broad spectrum of clinical infections ranging from supeficial skin lesions to disseminated visceral involvement *(320–326)*. *Phialophora* appeared to have predilection causing infection in debilitated and immunocompromised patients, such as those with hematologic malignancies, SLE, solid organ transplantion, chronic renal failure, diabetes mellitus, and corticosteroid therapy *(137,223,327–332)*. However, even in severely immunosuppressed patients, *Phialophora* infections often tend to stay localized *(137,223,327,328,331)*. Using an experimental model of murine model of *P. verrucosa*, Gugnani et al. *(333)* observed that although cortisone-treated mice had more extensive lesions as compared to normal controls, the infection was rarely fatal.

Infection usually occurs through traumatic skin inoculation with contaminated matter, with the majority of lesions occuring on the feet and legs of outdoor workers *(334,335)*.

The course of *Phialophora* phaeohyphomycosis is subacute to chronic, with lesions developing over months to years *(336)*. Pruritis, although an uncommon manifestation, has also been observed *(322)*. Satellite lesions may also occur through lymphatic spread and, occasionally, hematologic dissemination to muscle, brain, or other visceral organs may also occur *(324)*.

In vitro susceptibility studies *(320–324,327,337,338)* have shown that while most *Phialophora* spp. were resistant to miconazole and flucytosine, several species were resistant to amphotericin B and ketoconazole *(338)*.

Corrado et al. *(339)* and Weitzman et al. *(340)* evaluated the susceptibilities of *Phialophora* spp. (*P. parasitica*, *P. richardsiae*, and *P. repens*) against amphotericin B, flucytosine, miconazole and ketoconazole. Their results showed that *P. parasitica* (see *Phaeoacremonium* spp. below) did not vary much in its response to each drug; while the MIC values against miconazole (2.5–10 µg/mL) were most uniform, *P. parasitica* proved notably resistant to ketoconazole (the MICs for the majority isolates were 40 µg/mL and over). The sensitivities of *P. richardsiae* (three clinical isolates) and *P. repens* (a single wood isolate) differed substantially from those of *P. parasitica*. These two species were very sensitive to amphotericin B, miconazole, and ketoconazole but resistant to flucytosine *(340)*.

For *P. richardsiae*, Ikai et al. *(327)* demonstrated MIC values of 3.13, 3.13, and 1.56 µg/mL for ketoconazole, miconazole, and amphotericin B, respectively. In animal model studies, however, Dixon and Polak *(134)* observed no correlation between in vitro susceptibility values and in vivo efficacy.

Treatment of both localized and systemic *Phialophora* infections has been difficult. Duggan et al. *(341)* described an extensive cutaneous *P. verrucosa*-induced infection in an AIDS patient. The disease failed to respond to ketoconazole (400 mg daily) but regression of lesions was achieved with itraconazole (200 mg daily). In another case of *P. verrucosa*-induced infection, an immunosuppressed patient presented with a subcutaneous phaeomycotic cyst involving the dorsum of the foot; the infection was treated with ketoconazole *(328)*. A case of subcutaneous *P. verrucosa* infection was completely resolved after initial treatment with fluconazole followed by oral itraconazole for 30 d, and local application of copper sulphate solution *(326)*.

In 1968, Schwartz and Emmons *(161)* described the first case of human phaeohyphomycosis (a subcutaneous abscess) caused by *P. richardsiae*. Since then, the organism has been isolated from lesions of subcutaneous tissues *(146,161,335,339)*, the lacrimal gland *(342)*, the olecranon bursa *(343)*, infected foot bone *(344)*, and from the prostate gland *(327)*. Ikai et al. *(327)* described a case of subcutaneous phaeohyphomycosis on the dorsum of the foot associated with *P. richardsiae*. The patient was treated with oral flucytosine and topical injection of amphotericin B, in combination with surgical excision of the subcutaneous abscess; however, the lesion immediately recurred.

Singh et al. *(337)* used topical clotrimazole cream twice daily for 15 d to cure a cutaneous lesions due to *P. richardsiae*; in vitro susceptibility testing showed a MIC value of 1.0 µg/mL (after 72 h) for clotrimazole against the same isolate. Amorolfine was the best drug against another clinical isolate of *P. richardsiae* with a MIC value of 0.1 µg/mL *(337)*.

A 3-mo course of itraconazole completely resolved *P. richardsiae*-induced cutaneous lesions in a pharmacologically immnunosuppressed patient *(345)*.

2.1.8. Phaeoacremonium *spp. Phaeohyphomycosis*

Phaeoacremonium spp. were previously classified as strains of *Phialophora parasitica*. In 1966, Crouss et al. *(346)* proposed the new hyphomycete genus *Phaeoacremonium* with *Phaeoacremonium parasiticum* (previously, *Phialophora parasitica*) as its type species. Two other hyphomyces pathogenic to humans, *Phaeoacremonium inflatipes* and *P. rubrigenum* were also classified under this genus. Morphologically, the genus *Phaeoacremonium* is intermediate between the genera *Acremonium* and *Phialophora*.

The majority of human infections caused by *Phaeoacremonium* spp. are acquired through traumatic inoculation, and involve subcutaneous abscesses, cysts, or chronic or acute arthritis in both immunocompromised and immunocompetent hosts *(9,331,340,347–352)*. Systemic infections, fungemia, or endocarditis have been rare *(353,354)*.

When subcutaneous lesions caused by *P. parasiticum* or *P. inflatipes* are localized and diagnosed early, total surgical excision is the most recommended treatment *(325,347,348)*. In this regard antifungal therapy so far has not been satisfactory because amphotericin B, 5-FC, ketoconazole, itraconazole, and terbinafine have been used in the past with variable success *(325,340,351,353)*.

Matsui et al. *(347)* described the first case of *P. rubrigenum* infection in an immunocompromised patient receiving corticosteroid therapy for malignant rheumatoid arthritis.

2.1.9. Hormonema dermatioides *Phaeohyphomycosis*

Coldiron et al. *(355)* described a rare cutaneous phaeohyphomycosis associated with *Hormonema dermatioides* in an immunocompetent patient. The lesions were cured with oral ketoconazole at 200 mg, b.i.d. given for 12 wk. Antifungal susceptibility measured at 24 h has demonstrated susceptibilities to amphotericin B (MIC = 0.29 µg/mL), ketoconazole (MIC = 0.8 µg/mL), itraconazole (MIC = 0.15 µg/mL), and fluconazole (MIC = 20 µg/mL) *(355)*.

2.1.10. Aureobasidium *spp. Phaeohyphomycosis*

A. pullulans is well-recognized as the etiologic agent of hypersensitivity pneumonitis *(356–361)*. In addition, the mold has also been diagnosed as the cause of cutaneous *(69,362–364)* and corneal *(365,366)* phaeohyphomycosis. The organism is most likely to enter through the respiratory tract or inoculation of the skin.

Jones and Christensen *(365)* described a corneal ulcer due to *A. pullulans* that was cured following a 3-wk course of topical 5% suspension of natamycin applied every hour; previous treatment with topical amphotericin B (2.5 mg/mL applied every 2 h for 5 d) failed to bring any improvement of the corneal thickness. Antifungal susceptibility testing of *A. pullulans* demonstrated sensitivity to amphotericin B, nystatin, natamycin, clotrimazole and miconazole at concentrations of 1.5, 12.5, 1.5, 6.0, and 0.75 µg/mL; the fungus was resistant to 5-FC (>50 µg/mL) *(365)*.

An unusual *A. pullulans* infection of the jaw was reported by Koppang et al. *(367)* in an immunocompetent patient. The fungus, which filled an intraosseous cavity, was successfully treated with daily oral doses of 10 mg of flucytosine given for 30 d; bone regeneration was evident 6 mo post-treatment.

Systemic infections with *Aureobasidium* spp. have also been reported *(69)* In one such case *(368)*, *A. pullulans* was repeatedly isolated from blood cultures of patient with AML. Treatment with amphotericin B (0.5 mg/kg daily; total 0.5 g) failed to eradicate the organism.

Salkin et al. *(369)* described an opportunistic vesceral infection of the spleen due to *A. pullulans* in a patient with disseminated lymphoma. Although the portal of entry and mode of dissemination were unclear, the patient's immunosuppression caused by the malignant lymphoproliferative disorder very likely allowed the secondary invasion of the fungus.

Krcméry et al. *(370)* reported *A. mansoni*-induced meningitis in a leukemic patient in what appeared to be the first case of *Aureobasidium* spp. CNS involvement. Intravenous amphotericin B was administered for 44 d for a total dose of 2.2 g. On d 6, the frequency of symptoms decreased, and on d 10 the patient was without meningitis-associated symptomatology.

2.1.11. Colletotrichum *spp. Phaeohyphomycosis*

The genus *Colletotrichum* is a typical plant pathogen characterized by the formation of acervular conidiomata when the fungus parasitizes in the plant tissue. The various species are differentiated from one another by the morphology of their conidia and setae. Of the currently known species, four *Colletotrichum* spp. (*C. dematium*, *C. gloeosporioides*, *C. coccodes*, and *C. graminicola*) have been identified as human pathogens *(18,371)*. Although rare, these infections are generally associated with some form of trauma. Clinical manifestations often include keratitis *(372–376)* or subcutaneous lesions, although a case of invasive infection has also been reported *(162)*.

Colletotrichum spp. may cause life-threatening phaeohyphomycosis in immunosuppressed patients *(374,377,378)*. Thus, O'Quinn et al. *(82)* described three cases of subcutaneous infections caused by *C. coccodes* (two patients) and *C. gloeosporidiosis* (one patient). Two of the cases were successfully resolved by intravenous amphotericin B (0.5 mg/kg, daily). The third patient (with *C. coccodes* infection) died after initial intravenous amphotericin B (1.0 mg/kg, daily), followed by oral flucytosine (1.5 g, daily), and oral itraconazole (200 mg, t.i.d.); all treatments failed, suggesting widely disseminated disease.

Castro et al. *(379)* reported the first case of a subcutaneous phaeohyphomycotic cyst caused by *C. crassipes*; the nodule was surgically excised.

2.1.12. Mycoleptodiscus indicus *Phaeohyphomycosis*

Mycoleptodiscus indicus (Sahni) Sutton is another tropical to subtropical dematiaceous hyphomycete, generally found to grow on leaves of different host plants *(380)*, that has been reported to cause a subcutaneous phaeohyphomycosis in an immunosuppressed patient *(381)*. The patient, who had Wegener's granulomatosis, had been treated over time with prednisone and methotrexate. The infection was successfully resolved over 18-d period with a total 1.5 g of amphotericin B. After the post-treatment culture remained fungus-negative, amphotericin B was substituted with itraconazole (200 mg, b.i.d.) for another 28 d *(381)*.

2.1.13. Phoma *spp. Phaeohyphomycosis*

The *Phoma* spp. represent dematiaceous Coelomyces that are usually soil-dwelling saprobes or plant pathogens. In a number of reports *(382–391)*, when grown on Sabouraud's agar, *Phoma* spp. produce dark brown broadly spreading colonies with globose-shaped pycnidia usually with a small papilla at its apex *(383)*.

The first case of human infection caused by *P. hibernica* (*P. herbarum* [392]) was described in 1970 by Bakerspigel *(385)*. Several other *Phoma* species (*P. eupyrena* [386], *P. minutispora* [387], *P. sorghina* [388], *P. minutella* [389], *P. oculo-hominis* [392], *P. cruris-hominis* [392], and *P. cava* [382]) were also isolated from human lesions. Immunocompromised patients are usually at risk *(382,393)*.

Hirsh et al. *(390)* successfully treated a case of *Phoma* subcutaneous phaeohyphomycosis with oral itraconazole at 200–400 mg daily for 3 mo. In another case, a *P. cava* nodular erythematous-violaceous skin hand lesions healed after therapy with amphotericin B followed by itraconazole *(382)*.

Zaitz et al. *(382)* reported a case of subcutaneous phaeohyphomycosis caused by *P. cava* in a patient presenting with pulmonary sarcoidosis and taking corticosteroids. After discontinuation of the latter, the patient healed following therapy with amphotericin B (cumulative dose of 610 mg) followed by itraconazole (400 mg, daily)

2.1.14. Pleurophomopsis *spp.* Phaeohyphomycosis

Pleurophomopsis spp. differ from members of the genus *Phoma* by the structure of the pycnidal wall, septate conidiophores, and the conidiogeneous phialide cells. The genus differs from the genus *Pyrenochaeta* by lacking setae. *Pleurophomopsis lignicoca* Petrak is a newly described human pathogen of the genus *Pleurophomopsis* that belongs to the dematiaceous Coelomycetes *(393,394)*.

Chabasse et al. *(393)* described a case of subcutaneous abscess due to *P. lignicola* in an asthma patient on prolonged corticosteroid therapy; the lesion was excised. In another case of an immunocompromised patient, *P. lignicola* multiple tissue abscesses covered the patient's entire left limb, in what appeared to be the first report of fatal soft-tissue infection *(394)*.

2.1.15. Pyrenochaeta *spp.* Phaeohyphomycosis

Pyrenochaeta spp. are widely distributed throughout the world; they grow on soil and vegetation. In humans they cause eumycetomas *(395–404)*. The species isolates from tissue lesions include *P. romeroi (395,396,398,399,401–404)*, *P. mackinnonii (396)*, and *P. ungui-homini (397)*.

Venugopal and Venugopal *(395)* successfully used oral ketoconazole at 400 mg daily for 8–24 mo to treat eumycetoma due to *P. romeroi*.

2.1.16. Geniculosporium *spp.* Phaeohyphomycosis

The genus *Geniculosporium* Chesters & Greenhalgh *(405)* is known as a conidial state (anamorph) of several genera in the Xylariaceae (e.g., *Anthostomella, Biscogniauxia, Euepixylon, Leprieuria, Phylacia,* and *Rosellina [406]*). Many of these saprophytic xylariaceous species, which caused wood decay but can also be found in soil, are widespread throughout the tropics, subtropics, and temperate zones, including Asia, Europe, and North America *(407,408)*.

Suzuki et al. *(409)* reported the first case of *Geniculosporium* spp. subcutaneous phaeohyphomycosis presenting as asymptomatic knee nodule, which, upon histological examination, revealed brownish hyphal elements in encapsulated puogranuloma. The lesion was excised, resulting in complete resolution of the infection.

2.1.17. Veronaea bothryosa *Phaeohyphomycosis*

The epidemiology and ecology of *Veronaea bothryosa* are unknown. It is thought that its distribution is worldwide likely as a saprophyte and/or plant pathogen. *V. bothryosa* is rarely isolated from human lesions. The first report of isolation was from a skin biopsy specimen from a Chinese specimen, but no clinical information was provided *(410)*. In the second report, the patient presented with cutaneous and oronasal ulceration *(411)*.

Foulet et al. *(412)* described a case of cutaneous *V. bothryosis* phaeohyphomycosis in a liver-transplant recipient that was successfully treated with 300 mg daily of oral itraconazole.

2.2. Cerebral Phaeohyphomycosis

Although it is not very common for dematiaceous fungi, they may exhibit neurotropism *(60,413)*. Two distinct conditions have been identified: 1) rhinocerebral phaeohyphomycosis, a typical secondary infection caused by airborne conidia that can germinate in the sinus and grow into the brain; and 2) cerebral phaeohyphomycosis, a primary infection by a fungus located exclusively in the brain parenchyma *(414)*. The main neurotropic isolates include *Cladophialophora bantiana* (Sacc) de Hoog et al. *(313,415–421)*, *Exophiala dermatitidis* (Kano) de Hoog *(24,55,125,313,419)*, *Ramichloridium obovoideum* (*R. mackenziei*) Campbell et Al-Hedaithy *(422)*, and *Ochroconis gallopava* (W. B. Cooke) de Hoog *(310,313,319,419,423)*, as well as the dematiaceous agents *Chaetomium attrobrunneum* Ames *(424,425)*, *Bipolaris spicifera* (Bainer) Subramanian *(418,419,426)*, *Bipolaris hawaiiensis* (M. B. Ellis) Uchida et Aragaki *(419,427,428)*, *Rhinocladiella atrovirens* Nannfeldt *(419,429)*, *Curvularia pallescens* Boedijn *(419,430,431)*, and *Fonsecaea pedrosoi* *(417,419,432,433)*. Morphologically, only *Rhinocladiela* and *Ramichloridium* form single-cell conidia with branched conidiophores. Conidiophores in *Ramichloridium* are unbranched.

In a recent report, another agent of phaeohyphomycosis, *Scopulariopsis* spp., was also identified as a causative agent of primary cerebral infections *(434)*.

2.2.1. Nodulisporium *spp. Phaeohyphomycosis*

The genus *Nodulisporium* is characterized by the presence of swollen conidiogenous areas and branching patterns of conidiogenous structures. It is an anamorph also associated in nature with many ascomycete species of the *Xylariaceae* family, especially *Xypoxylon*.

Indian researchers have diagnosed *Nodulisporium* spp. as the causative agent of a CNS infection in a male patient for the first time in humans *(371)*. The lesion and the involved fungus were located exclusively in the right medial temporo-parietal region. Surgical resection of the lesion combined with antifungal chemotherapy led to successful resolution.

2.2.2. Scopulariopsis *spp. Phaeohyphomycosis*

A fatal case of *Scopulariopsis obovoideum* in an immunocompetent patient has been described as a rapidly developed infection *(375)*. The disease presented as a single large lesion in the deep white matter of one temporal lobe. Four days after the surgical removal of the lesion, a large focus of cerebritis with massive invasion of fungi developed in each centrum semiovale around the ventriculostomy sites.

Phaeohyphomycosis due to *S. brumptii* in a liver-transplant recipient was described by Patel et al. *(435)*.

2.2.3. Ramichloridium *spp. Phaeohyphomycosis*

In 1937, Stahel *(436)* first reported the genus *Ramichloridium* as being responsible for leaf spots on bananas. In 1952, Binford et al. *(437)* described the first case of *Ramichloridium*-associated case of human cerebral phaeohyphomycosis.

R. obovoideum (*R. mackenziei*) is now recognized as a cause of cerebral abscesses in patients from the Middle East. In general, the prognosis is poor; the responses to antifungal therapy are temporary, with the medical and surgical treatment yet to be established *(438,439)*. To this end, Podnos et al. *(440)* reported a fatal case of cerebral *R. obovoideum* infection for which chemotherapy and surgical intervention both failed. Similarly, Sutton et al. *(438)* were unsuccessful in treating a fatal case of cerebral *R. obovoideum* with 200 mg itraconazole given twice daily.

2.2.4. Cladophialophora *spp. Phaeohyphomycosis*

Cladophialophora spp. are highly neurotropic species with *Cladophialophora bantiana* (also named *Xylohypha bantiana*, *Cladosporium bantianum*, *Cladosporium trichoides*, *Cladosporium trichoides* var. *chamidosporum*, and *Xylohypha emmonsii*) being the most commonly diagnosed pathogen *(416,441–443)*.

Naim-ur-Rahman et al. *(444)* reported a fatal case of multiple phaeohyphomycotic brain abscesses caused by *Cladosporium* spp. in an immunocompetent patient. The clinical course of the infection was characterized by spontaneous remissions and relapses despite continued chemotherapy with amphotericin B, flucytosine, and ketoconazole. Surgical intervention appeared to be the only treatment modality that seemed capable of prolonging the life or altering the course of the disease. An interesting transitory pulmonary phase of the phaeohyphomycosis resembling miliary tuberculosis was observed. The latter may help to explain the portal of entry and mode of fungal spread to the brain *(444)*.

In another case of fatal disseminated phaeohyphomycosis, *C. devriesii* was identified as the causative agent *(445)*.

Buiting et al. *(446)* treated successfully a *C. normodendrum*-associated foot mycetoma with curettage of fistulous ducts and administration of itraconazole.

A skin lesion caused by *C. cladosporiosis* was successfully cured with 600 mg daily of itraconazole oral solution for 6 mo. A 9-month treatment with terbinafine, although initially effective was followed by clinical and mycological relapse; there was no response to amphotericin B and flucytosine *(447)*. In another report, a case of subcutaneous phaeohyphomycosis caused by *C. cladosporiosis* was healed completely with oral fluconazole (150 mg, daily) *(448)*.

Cutaneous phaeohyphomycosis, caused by *C. oxysporum* and manifested as papulonodular lesions in the right leg, was reported in a patient with Cushing's syndrome *(449)*. The patient was initially treated with itraconazole, which led to clinical improvement, but mycological recovery was obtained after a course of ketoconazole, made necessary by the presence of pituitary adenoma.

2.2.4.1. CLADOPHIALOPHORA BANTIANA (XYLOHYPHA BANTIANA, CLADOSPORIUM BANTIANUM)

Cladophialophora bantiana is an infrequent but often fatal cause of infection of the CNS *(19,77,416,443,450)*. Clinical features of the infection include chronic headache, fever, and hemiparesis. Although pharmacological immunosuppression has not been considered to be an important predisposing factor, evidence from patients with previous history of systemic nocardiosis and facial phaeohyphomycosis caused by *Alternaria* spp. would suggest that some impairment of host immune responses may play a role as predisposing factors for *C. bantiana* infection.

Antifungal therapy did not significantly affected the outcome of infection, with survival rates reaching only 35% in all patients, and 45% for all neurosurgically treated patients *(19)*. Surgical resection still remains the single most important treatment of patients with *C. bantiana*-induced CNS phaeohyphomycosis, especially in those with solitary encapsulated masses that may be completely resected. Multifocal or nonencapsulated masses have poor prognosis despite antifungal chemotherapy. The clinical resistance to antimycotic agents has been consistent with data from experimental murine *C. bantiana* infection, where resistance to antifungal therapy was present *(416)*.

In 1952, Binford et al. *(451)* reported the first case of brain abscess caused by *C. bantiana*. Although the neurotropism of this phaeoid fungus has been well-documented *(451–459)*, its portal of entry has not been very apparent. The multiplicity of CNS lesions, however, support the concept of hematogenous spread *(452,460–462)*. The fungus showed remarkable affinity for glial tissue in both experimental animals and humans *(462)*. In several reports of CNS involvement, *Cladophialophora* spp. were isolated from systemic sites (skin, lung, ear, and paranasal sinus) *(455,460,463–467)*. Kim et al. *(468)* indicated that on occasion, the infections may be iatrogenic in nature. Buxi et al. *(469)* reported a case of unusual multiple, conglomerated brain abscesses due to *C. bantiana* with unique neuroimaging features.

Cases of paranasal sinus, ear, and pulmonary *C. bantiana* infections have also been reported *(470–472)*. The symptoms are largely nonspecific, with headache and papilledema being the most common manifestations *(451,461,473)*.

Although brain abscesses caused by *C. bantiana* have been observed predominantly in immunocompetent hosts (mostly males) *(455,474)*, one report of *C. bantiana* cerebral phaeohyphomycosis in a liver-transplant recipient, as well as in several other cases *(475–477)*, underscored the distinct possibility of immunocompromised patients being at higher risk of infection by this phaeoid mold *(470)*. Experimental models utilizing cortisone-treated mice seemed to support this concept *(478)*. Furthermore, cerebral *C. bantiana* infection has been associated with HIV infection, and listed as an indicator of the AIDS *(479)*.

Treatment of cerebral phaeohyphomycosis due to *C. bantiana* has been largely unsuccessful, with survival not expected to exceed 1 yr *(480)*, even though surgical excision has been performed in the majority of cases. Flucytosine has been used on several occasions *(417,473,477)*; amphotericin B in combination with flucytosine also proved unsuccessful *(415)*. After reviewing 26 cases of *C. bantiana*-associated CNS infections, Dixon et al. *(416)* came to the conclusion that neurosurgical resection of the lesion (with or without chemotherapy) remains the best option for cure and survival.

Dixon and Polak *(134)* conducted an in vivo study to assess drug activity against experimental infection of *C. bantiana* in mice. Overall, the best life-protecting activity was achieved with oral 5-FC, with ED_{50} values ranging from 50–100 mg/kg; the corresponding values for amphotericin B (subcutaneous administration), oral fluconazole, and oral ketoconazole were 25–100, 50–100, and 200 mg/kg, respectively. Previously, Block et al. *(481)*, using a similar murine model of cladosporiosis, found the survival values ranging from 40–100% depending on the fungal strain at 5 wk after infection in mice given 800 mg/kg of 5-FC. In addition to demonstrating differences in susceptibility to 5-FC by different strains of *C. bantiana*, the same investigators also showed that individual strains displayed dose-related responses in mortality rates over a dosage range of 100–800 mg/kg *(481)*.

Agressive antifungal chemotherapy with fluconazole (400 mg daily for 3 mo) in combination with surgery resulted in good clinical and radiologic outcome of multiple intracranial *C. bantiana*-induced mass lesions *(462)*.

Osiyemi et al. *(482)* described a cardiac-transplant recipient with pulmonary and cerebral *Cladophialophora* phaeohyphomycosis. Optimal management included both antifungal therapy and surgery. After initial treatment with amphotericin B lipid complex (10 mg/kg, daily for a total of 9.0 g) did not lead to clinical or radiographic improvement, surgical resection was performed, followed by amphotericin B lipid complex (5.0 mg/kg, daily) and liposomal amphotericin B (427 mg, q.i.d., i.v.) to improve CNS penetration. Two months after craniotomy, the liposomal amphotericin B was discontinued and itraconazole (200 mg, b.i.d., p.o.) was initiated. The patient died shortly thereafter.

Borges et al. *(475)* have described one of several known cases *(452,472,483)* of localized pulmonary involvement of *C. bantiana*. The patient had a history of steroid-treated inflammatory bowel disease. Surgical excision, which was curative, appeared to be the treatment of choice because antifungal chemotherapy had little effect on the course of infection. Brenner et al. *(472)* also described a rare case in which *C. bantiana* was repeatedly isolated from sputum of an AIDS patient having pulmonary infiltrates.

Patterson et al. *(484)* presented a case of cutaneous *C. bantiana* where the patient developed a nodule with pistule formation on the dorsum of the left hand; no trauma was reported. The lesion was successfully treated with itraconazole and surgical excision.

2.3. Fungal Peritonitis in Continuing Ambulatory Peritoneal Dialysis (CAPD)

Continuous ambulatory peritoneal dialysis (CAPD) has become a major therapeutic modality in the treatment of end-stage renal disease, complicated primarily by catheter malfunction and acute peritonitis *(485)*. It has been estimated that nearly 100% of patients will experience at least one episode of peritonitis during the first 3 yr of CAPD *(486)*. Among the opportunistic pathogens reported with increasing frequency as causes of peritonitis in CAPD patients, coagulative-negative staphylococcal bacteria have predominated. However to a lesser extent (less than 5%), fungi have also been implicated in CAPD peritonitis *(487)*, with *Candida albicans* being the most common (as high as 36.4%) *(488)*. *Curvularia* spp. were also diagnosed as causative agents of peritonitis in CAPD patients *(489–492)*, as well as *Alternaria* species *(493)*.

Several cases of CAPD peritonitis caused by *Bipolaris* species have also been reported *(20,226,494,495)*. Manifestations included abdominal pain, and in some instances fever and cloudy peritoneal fluid *(20,226)*. The most commonly applied therapy involved catheter removal and intraperitoneal amphotericin B alone, or in combination with flucytosine *(20)* or ketoconazole *(494)*; intraperitoneal, and then intravenous amphotericin B has also been used *(20,489,490)*.

In one such case described, the amphotericin B dose was escalated by 10 mg daily to reach 50 mg for a total of 1.0 g *(489)*. The results of antifungal susceptibility testing of *Curvularia* isolates from a patient with CAPD peritonitis have shown MIC values of 0.08, >100, 0.035/0.3, and 10/>80 µg/mL for amphotericin B, flucytosine, itraconazole, and fluconazole, respectively *(489)*. In another case, *Aureobasidium pullulans*-associated peritonitis in a CAPD patient was successfully treated with catheter removal and a prolonged course of intravenous amphotericin B, allowing for the resumption of CAPD *(496)*. Pritchard and Muir *(3)* also identified *Aureobasidium* spp. (*A. pullulans* and *A. melanogenum*) as causative agents of fungal peritonitis in CAPD patients.

In the absence of peritonitis, DeVault et al. *(485)* related a case of Tenckhoff catheter malfunction in a CAPD patient with a mechanical obstruction caused by colonization with *C. lunata*. Catheter removal alone was sufficient to eradicate the fungus because recurrence of colonization or peritonitis did not occur following the resumption of CAPD.

Several predisposing factors, such as antibiotic therapy *(487,497–500)*, immunosuppressive therapy, recent bacterial peritonitis, and the presence of bowel perforation *(497,499)*, may facilitate the development of fungal peritonitis. It has been estimated that between 55 and 100% of fungal peritoneal infections have been preceded by recent antibiotic use *(487,499,500)*.

Even though a number effective chemotherapeutic regimens have been described, high morbidity and mortality of fungal peritonitis remained a problem *(487,498)*. Among the antifungal agents used successfully to treat CAPD fungal peritonitis, amphotericin B, flucytosine, econazole, miconazole, and ketoconazole have been considered to be the most effective *(492,493,497,501–504)*. However, other factors, such as route of administration (systemic or intravenous), the dose, duration of therapy, and the use of combination antifungal therapy seem to be important for successful clinical resolution of fungal peritonitis *(267)*.

As part of the clinical management of fungal peritonitis in CAPD patients, the early removal of the dialysis catheter, in the opinion of many investigators, has been critical for consistant therapeutic success *(335,497,498,500–502)*. Although in a number of cases reported *(487,493,495,497,502–504)*, success has been achieved without removal of the catheter, and with the use of intraperitoneal antifungal therapy alone or in combination with systemic antifungal drugs, only about 50% of these patients returned to CAPD after the successful treatment of their peritonitis because of the development of multiple complications, such as relapse of infection, abscess formation, catheter obstruction, peritoneal adhesions, and fibrosis *(487,489,497,499)*.

3. CHROMOBLASTOMYCOSIS

Chromoblastomycosis is a subcutaneous mycotic disease also caused by dematiaceous fungi that normally occurs in patients living in tropical and subtropical regions, but is also being more frequently diagnosed in the US *(1,505,506)*. Its most characteristic feature is the presence of verrucous nodules on the distal extremities. The manifestations of chromoblastomycosis can often be confused with those of other diseases such as tertiary syphilis, phaeohyphomycosis, and cutaneous tuberculosis, among others.

In tissue, the chromoblastomycosis sclerotic bodies (also called "copper pennies") are chestnut-brown, cross-walled cells representing the tissue form of the fungus *(505)*. Initially, these sclerotic cells were thought to be budding yeasts, prompting the creating of the name "chromoblastomycosis." The terms phaeohyphomycosis and mycetoma (Madura foot) were created to delineate the other two mycoses caused by dematiaceous fungi but in which these pigmented sclerotic bodies were absent.

Chromoblastomycosis is not believed to be contagious, with no known human-to-human transmission. Because the fungal pathogen is a saprophyte growing in soil, decaying vegetation, and rotting wood (predominantly in tropical and subtropical regions), farm laborers make up the majority of those infected when trauma leads to inoculation of the pathogen *(1,505)*.

Padhye et al. *(507)* described a very rare case of chromoblasomycosis caused by *Exophiala spinifera (508)*. Histological examination of biopsied tissues showed thick-walled, internally septated, chestnut brown sclerotic bodies (muriform cells) within multinucleated giant cells present in the dermis that were characteristic for chromoblasomycosis. Initial treatment with itraconazole (200 mg, daily) and 5-FC (150 mg/kg, daily) followed by treatment with itraconazole (400 mg, daily) and heat resulted in marked improvement in the patient's lesions. These results have demonstrated that *E. spinifera*, an etiologic agent of phaeohyphomycosis, can cause more than one type of infection, and supports previous observations *(6)* that chromoblastomycosis and phaeohyphomycosis represent extremes of a continuum of infections. Other dematiaceous fungi (*Fonsecae pedrosoi*, *Phialophora verrucosa*, and *Exophiala jeanselmei*) have also been implicated as causative agents of both chromoblasomycosis and pheohyphomycosis *(6,509)*.

REFERENCES

1. McGinnis, M. R., Rinaldi, M. G., and Winn, R. E. Emerging agents of phaeohyphomycosis: pathogenic species of *Bipolaris* and *Exserohilum*. *J. Clin. Microbiol.*, 24, 250–259, 1986.
2. Halloran, T. J. Allergic bronchopulmonary helmintosporiosis. *Am. Rev. Respir. Dis.*, 128, 578, 1983.
3. Pritchard, R. C. and Muir, D. B. Black fungi: a survey of dematiaceous hyphomycetes from clinical specimens identified over a five year period in a reference laboratory. *Pathology*, 19, 281, 1987.
4. Matsumoto, T. and Ajello, L. Dematiaceous fungi potentially pathogenic to humans and lower animals, in *Handbook of Applied Mycology*, vol. 2, Arora, D. K., Ajello, L., and Mukerji, K. G., Eds. Marcel Dekker, New York, 117, 1991.
5. Matsumoto, T., Matsuda, T., McGinnis, M. R., and Ajello, L. Clinical and mycological spectra of *Wangiella dermatitidis* infections. *Mycoses*, 36, 145, 1993.
6. McGinnis, M. R. Chromoblastomycosis and phaeohyphomycosis: new concepts, diagnosis, and mycology. *J. Am. Acad. Dermatol.*, 8, 1-16, 1983.
7. Terra, F., Torres, M., da Fonseca, O., and Area Leao, A. E. Novo typo de dermatite verrucosa mycose por *Acrotheca* com associacao de leishmaniosa. *Brasil-Med.*, 2, 363, 1922.
8. Moore, M. and de Almeida, F. Etiologic agents of chromoblastomycosis (chromoblastomycosis of Terra, Torres, Fonseca and Leao, 1922), of North and South America. *Rev. Biol. Med.*, 6, 94, 1935.
9. Ajello, L., Georg, L. K., Steigbigel, R. T., and Wang, C. J. K. A case of phaeohyphomycosis caused by a new species of *Phialophora*. *Mycologia*, 66, 490–498, 1974.
10. Maekura, S., Sono, M., Teramura, K., et al. Subcutaneous phaeohyphomycosis of the right thumb. *Rinsho Byori*, 47, 976–979, 1999.
11. Caligiorne, R. B., Resende, M. A., Paiva, E., and Azavedo, V. Use of RAPD (random amplified polymorphic DNA) to analyze genetic diversity of dematiaceous fungal pathogens. *Can. J. Microbiol.*, 45, 408–412, 1999.
12. de Hoog, G. S. Significance of fungal evolution for the understanding of their pathogenicity, illustrated with agents of phaeohyphomycosis. *Mycoses*, 40(suppl. 2), 5-8, 1997.
13. Hurley, M. A. and Saffran, B. Subcutaneous phaeohyphomycosis: overview and case report. *J. Foot Ankle Surg.*, 36, 230–235, 1997.
14. Romano, C., Fimiani, M., Pellegrino, M., et al. Cutaneous phaeohyphomycosis due to *Alternaria tenuissima*. *Mycoses*, 39, 211-215, 1996.
15. Fotherhill, A. W. Identification of dematiaceous fungi and their role in human disease. *Clin. Infect. Dis.*, 22(Suppl. 2), S179–S184, 1996.
16. Rinaldi, M. G. Phaeohyphomycosis. *Dermatol. Clin.*, 14, 147–153, 1996.
17. Zaias, N. Chromomycosis. *J. Cutan. Pathol.*, 5, 155, 1978.
18. Revankar, S. G., Patterson, J. E., Sutton, D. A., Pullen, R., and Rinaldi, M. G. Disseminated phaeohyphomycosis: review of an emerging mycosis. *Clin. Infect. Dis.*, 34, 467–476, 2002.
19. Matsumoto, T., Ajello, L., Matsuda, T., Szaniszlo, P. J., and Walsh, T. J. Developments in hyalohyphomycosis and phaeohyphomycosis. *J. Med. Vet. Mycol.*, 32(Suppl. 1), 329–349, 1994.
20. Adam, R. D., Paquin, M. L., Petersen, E. A., et al. Phaeohyphomycosis caused by the fungal genera *Bipolaris* and *Exserohilum*: a report of 9 cases and review of the literature. *Medicine (Baltimore)*, 65, 203, 1986.
21. Kano, K. Uber die chromoblastomykose durch einen noch nicht als pathogen beschriebenen pilz: *Hormiscium dermatitidis* n. sp. *Aichi Igakkai Zasshi*, 41, 1657, 1934.
22. Mizogami, I., Yamashita, K., Kawakami, I., and Matsumoto, I. On a case of chromoblastomycosis (or chromomycosis) originating in oropharynx, with special reference of the etiologic agent. *Practica Otologica*, 52, 715, 1959.
23. Watanabe, S. Dematiaceous fungus infections. *Jpn. Med. J.*, 249, 31, 1961.
24. Shimazono, Y., Isaki, K., Torii, H., Otsuka, R., and Fukushiro, R. Brain abscess due to *Hormodendrum dermatitidis* (Kano) Conant, 1963: report of a case and review of the literature. *Folia Psych. Neurol. Japonica*, 17, 80–96, 1963.
25. Sugawara, M., Sobajima, Y., and Tamura, H. A case of generalized chromoblastomycosis. *Acta Pathol. Japonica*, 14, 239, 1964.
26. Takahashi, Y., Takahashi, S., Fukushi, G., Kobayashi, K. A case in which a pathogenic dematiaceous fungus forming a yeast-like colony was isolated from the liver. *Jpn. J. Med. Mycol.*, 7, 42, 1966.
27. Hori, S., Sakurane, T., Takagi, Y. A case of chromomycosis. *Jpn. J. Clin. Dermatol. Urol.*, 20, 1191, 1966.
28. Tsai, C. Y., Lu, Y. C., Wang, L. T., Hsu, T. L., and Sung, J. L. Systemic chromoblastomycosis due to *Hormodendrum dermatitidis* (Kano) Conant. *Am. J. Clin. Pathol.*, 46, 103, 1966.

29. Jen, T. M. Mycological study of *Hormodendrum dermatitidis* (*Fonsecaea dermatitidis*) isolated from the cervical lymph node of a Chinese in Taiwan (Formosa), China. *J. Formos. Med. Assoc.*, 65, 650, 1966.
30. Urabe, H., Yasumoto, K., and Nakashima, K. A case of chromoblastomycosis: probable involvement of central nervous system. *Jpn. J. Dermatol. Urol.*, 29, 1012, 1967.
31. Urabe, H. Nakama, T., and Nakahara, T. A case of chromoblastomycosis. *Jpn. J. Dermatol.*, 79, 775, 1969.
32. Hirayama, A., Takahashi, S., and Kasai, T. Chromomycosis of liver and brain. *Jpn. J. Med. Mycol.*, 12, 237, 1971.
33. Fujiwara, N., Mori, Y., Kamihata, S., Takami, T., Tsuru, K., and Mori, A. Six cases of chromomycosis. *Skin Research (Osaka)*, 14, 297, 1972.
34. Saruta, T. and Nakamizo, Y. A case of chromomycosis. *Nishinihon J. Dermatol.*, 35, 9, 1973.
35. Harada, S., Ueda, T., and Kusunoki, T. Systemic chromomycosis. *J. Dermatol. (Tokyo)*, 3, 13, 1976.
36. Watanabe, S., Takigawa, M., and Aoshima, T. A case of chromomycosis. *Jpn. J. Med. Mycol.*, 16, 231, 1976.
37. Matsuzaki, O., Furuya, H., and Saruta, T. Chromomycosis in siblings. *Jpn. J. Med. Mycol.*, 17, 239, 1977.
38. Honbo, S., Kiryu, H., Nishio, K., and Urabe, H. Chromomycosis exclusively involving lymph nodes. *Jpn. J. Med. Mycol.*, 19, 47, 1978.
39. Hohl, P. E., Holly, H. P. Jr., Prevost, E., Ajello, L., and Padhye, A. A. *Wangiella dermatitidis* infections in humans: first documented case from the United States with review of the literature. *Rev. Infect. Dis.*, 5, 854, 1983.
40. Levenson, J. E., Gardner, S. K., Duffin, R. M., and Pettit, T. H. Dematiaceous fungal keratitis following penetrating keratoplasty. *Ophthal. Surg.*, 15, 578, 1984.
41. Takase, T. Chromomycosis due to *Exophiala dermatitidis*: report of a case with asteroid tissue forms. *Jpn. J. Med. Mycol.*, 26, 81, 1985.
42. Vartian, C. V., Shlaes, D. M., Padhye, A. A., and Ajello, L. *Wangiella dermatitidis* endocarditis in an intravenous drug user. *Am. J. Med.*, 78, 703, 1985.
43. Scott, J. W., Luckie, J., Pfister, W. C., Standard, P. G., Bohan, C. A., and Breazeale, R. D. Phaeohyphomycotic cyst caused by *Wangiella dermatitidis*. *Mykosen*, 29, 243, 1986.
44. Cuce, L. C., Selebian, A., Porto, E., de Melo, N. T., and da Lacaz, C. Feo-hifomicose transplantada renal por *Exophiala dermatitidis* (Kano) de Hoog, 1977. *An. Bras. Dermatol.*, 61, 207, 1986.
45. Ventin, M., Ramirez, C., and Garau, J. *Exophiala dermatitidis* de Hoog from a valvular aortic prothesis. *Mycopathologia*, 99, 45, 1987.
46. Hiruma, M., Yamachi, K., Shimizu, T., Ohata, H., and Kukita, J. Systemic *Exophiala dermatitidis* infection. *Jpn. J. Med. Mycol.*, 29, 24, 1988.
47. Collee, G., Verhoef, L. M. H., van't Wout, J. W., Van Brummelen, P., Eulderink, F., and Dijkmans, B. A. C. Tenosynovitis caused by *Exophiala mansonii* in an immunocompromised host. *Arthritis Rheum.*, 31, 1213, 1988.
48. Crosby, J. H., O'Quinn, M. H., Steele, J. C. H., and Rao, R. N. Fine-needle aspiration of subcutaneous phaeohyphomycosis caused by *Wangiella dermatitidis*. *Diag. Cytopathol.*, 5, 293, 1989.
49. Barenfanger, J., Ramirez, F., Tewari, R. P., and Eagleton, L. Pulmonary phaeohyphomycosis in a patient with hemoptysis. *Chest*, 95, 1158, 1989.
50. Sharkey, P. K., Graybill, J. R., Rinaldi, M. G., et al. Itraconazole treatment of phaeohyphomycosis. *J. Am. Acad. Dermatol.*, 23, 577–586, 1990.
51. Margo, C. E. and Fitzgerald, C. R. Postoperative endophthalmitis caused by *Wangiella dermatitidis*. *Am. J. Ophthalmol.*, 110, 322, 1990.
52. Pospisil, L., Skorkovska, S., and Moster, M. Corneal phaeohyphomycosis caused by *Wangiella dermatitidis*. *Ophthalmologica*, 201, 128, 1990.
53. Matsumoto, T., Matsuda, T., and McGinnis, M. R. A previously undescribed synanomorph of *Wangiella dermatitidis*. *J. Med. Vet. Mycol.*, 28, 437, 1990.
54. Matsumoto, T., Matsuda, T., Padhye, A. A., Standard, P. G., and Ajello, L. Fungal melanonychia: unusual phaeohyphomycosis caused by *Wangiella dermatitidis*. *Clin. Exp. Dermatol.*, 17, 83, 1992.
55. Kenney, R. T., Kwon-Chung, K. J., Waytes, A. T., et al. Successful treatment of systemic *Exophiala dermatitidis* infection in a patient with chronic granulomatous disease. *Clin. Infect. Dis.*, 14, 235–242, 1992.
56. Bennett, J. E., Bonner, H., Jennings, A. E., and Lopez, R. I. Chronic meningitis caused by *Cladosporium trichoides*. *Am. J. Clin. Pathol.*, 59, 398–407, 1973.
57. Salaki, J. S., Louria, D. B., and Chmel, H. Fungal and yeast infections of the central nervous system: a clinical view. *Medicine (Baltimore)*, 63, 108–132, 1984.
58. Faulk, C. T. and Lesher, J. L. Jr. Phaeohyphomycosis and *Mycobacterium fortuitum* abscesses in a patient receiving corticosteroids for sarcoidosis. *J. Am. Acad. Dermatol.*, 33(2 Part 1), 309–311, 1995.
59. Hachisuka, H., Matsumoto, T., Kusihara, M., Nomura, H., Nakano, S., and Sasai, Y. Cutaneous phaeohyphomycosis caused by *Exophiala jeanselmei* after renal transplantation. *Int. J. Dermatol.*, 29, 198, 1990.
60. Arunkumar, M. J., Rajshekhar, V., Chandy, M. J., Thomas, P. P., and Jacob, C. K. Management and outcome of brain abscess in renal transplant recipients. *Postgrad. Med. J.*, 76, 207–211, 2000.
61. Sartorius, K. E., Baillie, G. M., Tiernan, R., and Rajagopalan, P. R. Phaeohyphomycosis from *Exophiala jeanselmei* with concomitant *Nocardia asteroids* infection in a renal transplant recipient: case report and review of the literature. *Pharmacotherapy*, 19, 995–1001, 1999.
62. Mesa, A., Henao, J., Gil, M., and Durango, G. Phaeohyphomycosis in kidney transplant patients. *Clin. Transplant.*, 13, 273–276, 1999.
63. Manian, F. A. and Brischetto, M. J., Pulmonary infection due to *Exophiala jeanselmei*: successful treatment with ketoconazole. *Clin. Infect. Dis.*, 16, 445, 1993.

64. Bryan, M. G., Elston, D. M., Hivnor, C., and Honl, B. A., Phaeohyphomycosis in a premature infant. *Cutis*, 65, 137–140, 2000.
65. Date, A., Mathews, M. S., Varma, S. K., and Korula, R. J., Echinococcosis with concurrent phaeohyphomycosis. *Mycoses*, 41, 429–430, 1998.
66. Clancy, C. J. and Nguen, M. H., Subcutaneous phaeohyphomycosis. *Clin. Infect. Dis.*, 25, 1065 & 1195, 1997.
67. Soomro, I. N. and Kennedy, A., Subcutaneous phaeohyphomycosis: infection with pigmented fungi. *J. Pak. Med. Assoc.*, 46, 156–158, 1996.
68. Pec, J., Palencarova, E., Plank, L., Straka, S., Pec, M., Jesenska, Z., and Filo, V., Phaeohyphomycosis due to *Alternaria* spp. and *Phaeosclera dematioides*: a histopathological study. *Mycoses*, 39, 217–221, 1996.
69. Fletcher, H., Williams, N. P., Nicholson, A., Rainford, L., Phillip, H., and East-Innis, A., Systemic phaeohyphomycosis in pregnancy and the puerperium. *West Indian Med. J.*, 49, 79–82, 2000.
70. Estes, S. A., Merz, W. G., and Maxwell, L. G., Primary cutaneous phaeohyphomycosis caused by *Drechslera spicifera*. *Arch. Dermatol.*, 113, 813, 1977.
71. Drouhet, E. and Dupont, B., Laboratory and clinical assessment of ketoconazole in deep-seated mycoses. *Am. J. Med.*, 74(Suppl. 1B), 30, 1983.
72. Sobol, S. M., Love, R. G., Stutman, H. R., and Pysher, T. J., Phaeohyphomycosis of the maxilloethmoid sinus caused by *Drechslera spicifera*: a new fungal pathogen. *Laryngoscope*, 94, 620, 1984.
73. Maskin, S. L., Fetchick, R. J., Leone, C. R., Sharkey, P. K., and Rinaldi, M. G., *Bipolaris hawaiiensis*-caused phaeomycotic orbitopathy. *Ophthalmology*, 96, 175, 1989.
74. Washburn, R. G., Kennedy, D. W., Begley, M. G., Henderson, D. K., and Bennett, J. E., Chronic fungal sinusitis in apparently normal hosts. *Medicine (Baltimore)*, 67, 231, 1988.
75. Noel, S. B., Greer, D. L., Abadie, S. M., Zachary, J. A., and Pankey, G. A., Primary cutaneous phaeohyphomycosis. *J. Am. Acad. Dermatol.*, 18, 1023, 1988.
76. Wiest, P. M., Wiese, K., Jacobs, M. R., et al. *Alternaria* infection in a patient with the acquired immunodeficiency syndrome: case report and review of invasive *Alternaria* infections. *Rev. Infect. Dis.*, 9, 799, 1987.
77. Gugnani, H. C., Ezeanolue, B. C., Khalil, M., Amoah, C. D., Ajuiu, E. U., and Oyewo, E., A. Fluconazole in the therapy of tropical deep mycoses. *Mycoses*, 38, 485–488, 1995.
78. Ganer, A., Arathoon, E., and Stevens, D. A. Initial experience in therapy for progressive mycoses with itraconazole, the first clinically studied triazole. *Rev. Infect. Dis.*, 9, 77, 1987.
79. Tucker, R. M., Williams, P. L., Arathoon, E. G., and Stevens, D. A. Treatment of mycoses with itraconazole. *Ann. NY Acad. Sci.*, 544, 451, 1988.
80. Frenkel, L., Kuhls, T. L., Nitta, K., et al. Recurrent *Bipolaris spicifera* following surgical and antifungal therapy. *Pediatr. Infect. Dis. J.*, 6, 1130, 1987.
81. Kotylo, P. K., Israel, K. S., Cohen, J. S., and Bartlett, M. S. Subcutaneous phaeohyphomycosis of the finger caused by *Exophiala spicifera*. *Am. J. Clin. Pathol.*, 91, 624, 1989.
82. O'Quinn, R. P., Hoffmann, J. L., and Boyd, A. S. *Colletotrichum* species as emerging opportunistic fungal pathogen: a report of 3 cases of phaeohyphomycosis and review. *J. Am. Acad. Dermatol.*, 45, 56-61, 2001.
83. Perez, A. Terbinafine: broad new spectrum of indications in several subcutaneous and systemic and parasitic diseases. *Mycoses*, 42(Suppl. 2), 111-114, 1999.
84. Cuenca-Estrela, M., Ruiz-Diez, B., Martinez-Suarez, J. V., et al. Comparative in vitro activity of voriconazole (UK-109,496) and six other antifungal agents against clinical isolates of *Scedosporium prolificans* and *Scedosporium apiospermum*. *J. Antimicrob. Microbiol.*, 43, 149–151, 1999.
85. Espinel-Ingroff, A. In vitro activity of the new triazole voriconazole (UK-109,496) against opportunistic filamentous and dimorphic fungi and common and emerging yeast pathogens. *J. Clin. Microbiol.*, 36, 198–202, 1998.
86. McGinnis, M. R., Pasarell, L., Sutton, D. A., et al. In vitro activity of voriconazole against selected fungi. *Med. Mycol.*, 36, 239–242, 1998.
87. McGinnis, M. R., Pasarell, L., Sutton, D. A., et al. In vitro evaluation of voriconazole against some clinically important fungi. *Antimicrob. Agents Chemother.*, 41, 1832–1834, 1997.
88. Rolston, K. V. I., Hopfer, R. L., and Larson, D. L. Infections caused by *Drechslera* species: case report and review of the literature. *Rev. Infect. Dis.*, 7, 525, 1985.
89. Lagerberg, T., Lundberg, G., and Melin, E. Biological and practical research in pine and spruce. *Svenska Skogsv. For Tidskr.*, 25, 145, 1927.
90. Ajello, L., Iger, M., Wybel, R., and Vigil, F. J. *Drechslera rostrata* as an agent of phaeohyphomycosis. *Mycologia*, 72, 1094, 1980.
91. Young, C. N., Swart, J. G., Ackermann, D., and Davidge-Pitts, K. Nasal obstruction and bone erosion caused by *Drechslera hawaiiensis*. *J. Laryngol. Otol.*, 92, 137, 1978.
92. Koshi, G., Anandi, V., Kurien, M., Kirubakaran, M. G., Padhye, A. A., and Ajello, L. Nasal phaeohyphomycosis caused by *Bipolaris hawaiiensis*. *J. Med. Vet. Mycol.*, 25, 397, 1987.
93. Fuste, F. J., Ajello, L., Threlkeld, R., and Henry, J. E. Jr. *Drechslera hawaiiensis*: causative agent of a fatal fungal meningo-encephalitis. *Sabouraudia*, 11, 59–63, 1973.
94. Forster, R. K., Rebell, G., and Wilson, L. A. Dematiaceous fungal keratitis. *Br. J. Ophthalmol.*, 59, 372, 1975.
95. Dolan, C. T., Weed, L. A., and Dines, D. E. Bronchopulmonary helminthosporiosis. *Am. J. Clin. Pathol.*, 53, 235, 1970.
96. Morton, S. J., Midthun, K., and Merz, W. G. Granulomatous encephalitis by *Bipolaris hawaiiensis*. *Arch. Pathol. Lab. Med.*, 110, 1183, 1986.

97. Drouhet, E., Guilmet, D., Kouvalchouk, J. F., et al. Premier cas humain de mycose a *Drechslera longirostrata*. *Nouv. Presse Med.*, 11, 3631, 1982.
98. Koenig, H., Warter, A., Bievre, C., De Waller, J., Weitzeblum, E., and Morand, G. Mycose pulmonaire a *Drechslera hawaiiensis*. *Bull. Soc. Fr. Mycol. Med.*, 13, 373, 1984.
99. Padhye, A. A., Ajello, L., Wieden, M. A., and Steinbronn, K. K. Phaeohyphomycosis of the nasal sinuses by a new species of *Exserohilum*. *J. Clin. Microbiol.*, 24, 245, 1986.
100. Pauzner, R., Goldschmied-Reouven, A., Hay, I., et al. Phaeohyphomycosis following cardiac surgery: case report and review of serious infection due to *Bipolaris* and *Exserohilum* species. *Clin. Infect. Dis.*, 25, 921-923, 1997.
101. Kanungo, R. and Srinivasan, R. Corneal phaeohyphomycosis due to *Excerohilum rostratum*. A case report and brief review. *Acta Ophthalmol. Scand.*, 74, 197-199, 1996.
102. Antoine, G. A. and Raternik, M. H. *Bipolaris*, a serious new fungal pathogen of the paranasal sinus. *Otolaryngol. Head Neck Surg.*, 100, 158, 1989.
103. Merz, W. G., Karp, J. E., Hoagland, M., Jettgoheen, M., Junkins, J. M., and Hood, A. F. Diagnosis and successful treatment of fusariosis in the compromised host. *J. Infect. Dis.*, 158, 1046, 1988.
104. Costa, A. R., Porto, E., Tabuti, A. H., and da Lacaz, C. Subcutaneous phaeohyphomycosis caused by *Bipolaris hawaiiensis*: a case report. *Rev. Inst. Med. Trop. Sao Paolo*, 33, 74, 1991.
105. Jacobson, M., Galetta, S. L., Atlas, S. W., Curtis, M. T., and Wulc, A. W. *Bipolaris*-induced orbital cellulitis. *J. Clin. Neuro-Ophthalmol.*, 12, 250, 1992.
106. Straka, B. F., Cooper, P. H., and Body, B. A. Cutaneous *Bipolaris spicifera* infection. *Arch. Dermatol.*, 125, 1383, 1989.
107. Jay, W. M., Bradsher, R. W., Lemay, B., Snyderman, N., and Angtuago, E. J. Ocular involvement in mycotic sinusitis caused by *Bipolaris*. *Am. J. Ophthalmol.*, 105, 366, 1988.
108. Kershaw, P., Freeman, R., Templeton, D., et al. *Pseudallescheria boydii* infection of the central nervous system. *Arch. Neurol.*, 47, 468, 1990.
109. McGinnis, M. R., Campbell, G., Gourley, W. K., and Lucia, H. L. Phaeohyphomycosis caused by *Bipolaris spicifera*: an informative case. *Eur. J. Epidemiol.*, 8, 383, 1992.
110. Burges, G. E., Walls, C. T., and Maize, J. C. Subcutaneous phaeohyphomycosis caused by *Exserohilum rostratum* in an immunocompetent host. *Arch. Dermatol.*, 123, 1346, 1987.
111. Brown, J. W. III, Nadell, J., Sanders, C. V., and Sardenga, L. Brain abscess caused by *Cladosporium trichoides* (Bantianum): a case with paranasal sinus involvement. *South. Med. J.*, 69, 1519, 1976.
112. Yoshimori, R. N., Moore, R. A., Itabashi, H. H., and Fujikawa, D. F. Phaeohyphomycosis of brain: granulomatous encephalitis caused by *Drechslera spicifera*. *Am. J. Clin. Pathol.*, 77, 363, 1982.
113. Krachmer, J. H., Anderson, R. L., Binder, P. S., Waring, G. O., Rousey, J. J., and Meeks, E. S. *Helminthosporium* corneal ulcers. *Am. J. Ophthalmol.*, 85, 666, 1978.
114. Berry, A. J., Kerkering, T. M., Giordano, A. M., and Chiacone, J. Phaeohyphomycotic sinusitis. *J. Pediatr. Infect. Dis.*, 3, 150, 1984.
115. Morgan, M. A., Wilson, W. R., Neel, H. B. III, and Roberts, G. D. Fungal sinusitis in healthy and immunocompromised individuals. *Am. J. Clin. Pathol.*, 82, 597, 1984.
116. Shugar, M. A., Montgomery, W. W., and Hyslop, N. E., Jr. *Alternaria* sinusitis. *Ann. Otol.*, 90, 251, 1981.
117. Shoemaker, R. A. Nomenclature of *Drechslera* and *Bipolaris*, grass parasites segregated from "*Helminthosporium*." *Can. J. Bot.*, 37, 879, 1959.
118. Zapater, R. C., Albesi, E. J., and Garcia, G. H. Mycotic keratitis by *Drechslera spicifera*. *Sabouraudia*, 13, 295, 1975.
119. Harris, R., Smith, R. E., Wood, T. R., and Biddle, M. *Helminthosporium* corneal ulcers. *Ann. Ophthalmol.*, 10, 729, 1978.
120. Chin, G. N. Corneal perforation due to *Helminthosporium* and *Mima polymorpha*. *Ann. Ophthalmol.*, 10, 607, 1978.
121. Matthiesson, A. M. Allergic bronchopulmonary disease caused by fungi other than *Aspegillus*. *Thorax*, 36, 719, 1981.
122. Glancy, J. J., Elder, J. L., and McAleer, R. Allergic bronchopulmonary fungal disease without clinical asthma. *Thorax*, 36, 345, 1981.
123. McAleer, R., Kroenert, D. B., Elder, J. L., and Froudist, J. H. Allergic bronchopulmonary disease caused by *Curvularia lunata* and *Drechslera hawaiiensis*. *Thorax*, 36, 338, 1981.
124. Hendrick, D. J., Ellithorpe, D. B., Lyon, F., Hattier, P., and Salvaggio, J. E. Allergic bronchopulmonary helminthosporiosis. *Am. Rev. Respir. Dis.*, 126, 935, 1982.
125. Hiruma, M., Kawada, A., Ohata, H., et al. Systemic phaeohyphomycosis caused by *Exophiala dermatitidis*. *Mycoses*, 36, 1–7, 1993.
126. Chang, C. L., Kim, D. S., Park, D. J., Kim, H. J., Lee, C. H., and Shin, J. H. Acute cerebral phaeohyphomycosis due to *Wangiella dermatitidis* accompanied by cerebrospinal fluid eosinophilia. *J. Clin. Microbiol.*, 38, 1965–1966, 2000.
127. Schnitzler, N., Peltroche-Llacsahuanga, H., Bestier, N., Zundorf, J., Lutticken, R., and Haase, G. Effect of melanin and carotenoids of *Exophiala* (*Wangiela*) *dermatitidis* on phagocytosis, oxidative burst, and killing by human neutrophils. *Infect. Immun.*, 67, 94–101, 1999.
128. Woollons, A., Darley, C. R., Pandian, S., Arnstein, P., Blackee, J., and Paul, J. Phaeohyphomycosis caused by *Exophiala dermatitidis* following intra-articular steroid injection. *Br. J. Dermatol.*, 135, 475–477, 1996.
129. Matsumoto, T., Padhye, A. A., Ajello, L., Standard, P. G., and McGinnis, M. R. Critical review of human isolates of *Wangiella dermatitidis*. *Mycologia*, 76, 232, 1984.
130. Scott, J. W., Luckie, J., Pfister, W. C., et al. Phaeohyphomycosis cyst caused by *Wangiella dermatitidis*. *Mykosen*, 29, 243, 1986.

131. Barenfanger, J., Ramirez, F., Tewari, R. P., and Eagleton, L. Pulmonary phaeohyphomycosis in a patient with hemoptysis. *Chest*, 95, 1158, 1989.
132. Haase, G., Skopnik, H., and Kusenbach, G., *Exophiala dermatitidis* infection in cystic fibrosis. *Lancet*, 336, 188, 1990.
133. Rath, P. M., Muller, K. D., Dermoumi, H., and Ansorg, R. A comparison of methods of phenotypic and genotypic fingerprinting of *Exophiala dermatitidis* isolated from sputum samples of patients with cystic fibrosis. *J. Med. Microbiol.*, 46, 757-762, 1997.
134. Dixon, D. M. and Polak, A. In vitro and in vivo drug studies with three agents of central nervous system phaeohyphomycosis. *Chemotherapy*, 33, 129, 1987.
135. McGinnis, M. R. and Padhye, A. A. *Exophiala jeanselmei*, a new combination for *Phialophora jeanselmei*. *Myxotaxon*, 1, 341, 1977.
136. Gold, W. L., Vellend, H., Salit, I. E., Campbell, I., Summerbell, R., Rinaldi, M., and Simor, E. Successful treatment of systemic and local infections to *Exophiala* species. *Clin. Infect. Dis.* 19, 339-341, 1994.
137. Di Salvo, A. F. and Chew, W. H. *Phialophora gougerotii*: an opportunistic fungus in a patient treated with steroids. *Sabouraudia*, 6, 241, 1968.
138. Mauceri, A. A., Cullen, S. L., Vandevelde, A. G., and Johnson, J. E. Flucytosine: an effective oral treatment for chromomycosis. *Arch. Dermatol.*, 109, 873, 1974.
139. Kotrajaras, R. and Chongsathien, S. Subcutaneous chromomycotic abscesses caused by *Phialophora gougerotii*. *Int. J. Dermatol.*, 18, 150, 1979.
140. South, D. A., Brass, C., and Stevens, D. A. Chromoblastomycosis: treatment with ketoconazole. *Arch. Dermatol.*, 117, 311, 1981.
141. Monroe, P. W. and Floyd, W. E. Chromohyphomycosis of the hand due to *Exophiala jeanselmei* - case report and review. *J. Hand Surg.*, 6, 370, 1981.
142. Hironaga, M., Mochizuki, T., and Watanabe, S. Cutaneous phaeohyphomycosis of the sole caused by *Exophiala jeanselmei* and its susceptibility to amphotericin B, 5-FC and ketoconazole. *Mycopathologia*, 79, 101, 1982.
143. Lisi, P. and Caraffini, S., Imported skin disease: a case of subcutaneous chromomycosis caused by *Phialophora gougerotii*. *Int. J. Dermatol.*, 22, 180, 1983.
144. Bambirra, E. A., Miranda, D., Nogueira, A. M., and Barbosa, C. S. P., Phaeohyphomycotic cyst: a clinicopathologic study of the first four cases described from Brasil. *Am. J. Trop. Med. Hyg.*, 32, 794, 1983.
145. Ziefer, A. and Connor, D. H. Phaeomycotic cyst: a clinico-pathologic study of twenty five patients. *Am. J. Trop. Med. Hyg.*, 29, 901, 1980.
146. Guèho, E., Bonnefoy, A., Luboinski, J., Petitt, J.-C, and de Hoog, G. S. Subcutaneous granuloma caused by *Phialophora richardsiae*: case report and review of the literature. *Mycoses*, 32, 219, 1989.
147. Sudduth, E. J., Crumbley, A. J. III, and Farrar, W. E. Phaeohyphomycosis due to *Exophiala* species: clinical spectrum of disease in humans. *Clin. Infect. Dis.*, 15, 639, 1992.
148. Sabbaga, E., Tedesco-Marchesi, L. M., Lacaz, C., et al. Subcutaneous phaeohyphomycosis due to *Exophiala jeanselmei*: report of 3 cases in patient with a kidney transplant. *Rev. Inst. Med. Trop. Sao Paolo*, 36, 175, 1994.
149. Xu, X., Low, D. W., Palevsky, H. I., and Elenitsas, R. Subcutaneous phaeohyphomycosis cysts caused by *Exophiala jeanselmei* in a lung transplant patient. *Dermatol. Surg.*, 27, 343-346, 2001.
150. Emmons, C. W. *Phialophora jeanselmei* comb. n. from mycetoma of the hand. *Arch. Pathol.*, 39, 364, 1945.
151. Nielsen, H. S., Conant, N. F., Weinberg, T., et al., Report of a mycetoma due to *Phialophora jeanselmei* and undescribed characteristics of the fungus. *Sabouraudia*, 6, 330, 1968.
152. Youngchaiyud, U., Thasnakorn, P., Chantarakul, N., et al., Maduromycosis of the hand due to *Phialophora jeanselmei*. *Southeast Asian J. Trop. Med. Public Health*, 3, 138, 1972.
153. Thammayya, A. and Sanyal, M. *Exophiala jeanselmei* causing mycetoma pedis in India. *Sabouraudia*, 18, 91, 1980.
154. Pupaibul, K., Sindhuphak, W., and Chindaporn, A. Mycetoma of the hand caused by *Phialophora jeanselmei*. *Mykosen*, 25, 321, 1981.
155. Lewis, G. M., Hopper, M. E., Sachs, W., Cormia, F. E., and Potelunas, C. B. Mycetoma-like chromoblastomycosis affecting the hand. *J. Invest. Dermatol.*, 10, 155, 1948.
156. Schnadig, V. J., Long, E. G., Washington, J. M., McNeely, M. C., and Troum, B. A. *Phialophora verrucosa*-induced subcutaneous phaehyphomycosis. *Arch. Cytol.*, 30, 425, 1986.
157. Zackheim, H. S., Halde, C., Goodman, R. S., Marchasin, S., and Buncke, H. J. Jr. Phaeohyphomycotic cyst of the skin caused by *Exophiala jeanselmei*. *J. Am. Acad. Dermatol.*, 12, 207, 1985.
158. Annessi, G., Cimitan, A., Zambruno, G., and DiSilverio, A. Cutaneous phaeohyphomycosis due to *Cladosporium cladosporioides*. *Mycoses*, 35, 243, 1992.
159. Clancy, C. J., Wingard, J. R., and Hong Nguyen, M. Subcutaneous phaeohyphomycosis in transplant recipients: review of the literature and demonstration of in vitro synergy between antifungal agents. *Med. Mycol.*, 38, 169-175, 2000.
160. Flynn, B. J., Bourbeau, P. P., Cera, P. J., Scicchitano, L. M., Jordan, R. L., and Yap, W. T. Phaeohyphomycosis of the epididymis caused by *Exophiala jeanselmei*. *J. Urol.*, 162, 492-493, 1999.
161. Schwartz, L. S. and Emmons, G. W. Subcutaneous cystic granuloma caused by a fungus of wood pulp (*Phialophora richardsiae*). *Am. J. Clin. Pathol.*, 49, 500, 1968.
162. Hsueh, P. R., Teng, L. J., Hsu, J. H., et al. Nosocomial *Exophiala jeanselmei* pseudoinfection after sonography-guided aspiration of thoracic lesions. *J. Formos. Med. Assoc.*, 100, 613-619, 2001.
163. Ravisse, P. and Vindas, A. J. R. Les kystes mycosiques: etude histopathologique. *Bull. Soc. Pathol. Exot.*, 74, 46, 1981.
164. Mita, Y., Dobashi, K., Nakazawa, T., and Mori, M. A case of pulmonary tuberculosis complicated with subcutaneous phaeohyphomycosis. *Kekkaku*, 75, 33-36, 2000.

165. Kim, H. U., Kang, S. H., and Matsumoto, T. Subcutaneous phaeohyphomycosis caused by *Exophiala jeanselmei* in a patient with advanced tuberculosis. *Br. J. Dermatol.*, 138, 351–353, 1998.
166. McCown, H. F. and Sahn, E. E. Subcutaneous phaeohyphomycosis and nocardiosis in a kidney transplant patient. *J. Am. Acad. Dermatol.*, 36 (5 Part 2), 863-866, 1997.
167. de Hoog, G. S. *Rhinocladiella* and allied genera in *Stud. Mycol.*, No. 15, Baarn: Centraalbureau voor Schimmelcultures, 1, 1977.
168. Tintelnot, K., de Hoog, G. S., Thomas, E., Steudel, W.-L., Huebner, K., and Seeliger, H. P. R. Cerebral phaeohyphomycosis caused by an *Exophiala* species. *Mycoses*, 34, 239, 1989.
169. Sindhuphak, W., MacDonald, E., Head, E., and Hudson, R. D. *Exophiala jeanselmei* infection in a postrenal transplant patient. *J. Am. Acad. Dermatol.*, 13, 877, 1985.
170. Chuan, M.-T. and Wu, M.-C. Subcutaneous phaeohyphomycosis caused by *Exophiala jeanselmei*: successful treatment with itraconazole. *Int. J. Dermatol.*, 34, 563, 1995.
171. Whittle, D. I. and Kominos, S. Use of itraconazole for treating subcutaneous phaeohyphomycosis caused by *Exophiala jeanselmei*. *Clin. Infect. Dis.*, 21, 1068, 1995.
172. Schwinn, A., Strohm, S., Helgenberger, M., Rank, C., and Bröcker, E.-B. Phaeohyphomycosis caused by *Exophiala jeanselmei* treated with itraconazole. *Mycoses*, 36, 445, 1993.
173. Van Cutsem, J., Van Gerven, F., and Janssen, P. A. J. Activity of orally, topically, and parenterally administered itraconazole in the treatment of superficial and deep mycoses: animal models. *Rev. Infect. Dis.*, 9(Suppl. 1), S15, 1987.
174. McGinnis, M. R. and Hilger, A. E., in *Laboratory Diagnosis of Infectious Diseases: Principle and Practice*, Balows, A., Hausler, W. J. Jr., and Lennette, E. H., Eds. Springer-Verlag, New York, 687, 1988.
175. Iwatsu, T., Nishimura, K., and Miyaji, M. *Exophiala castellanii* sp. nov. *Mycotaxon*, 20, 307–314, 1984.
176. Rossmann, S. N., Cernoch, P. L., and Davis, J. R. Dematiaceous fungi are an increasing cause of human disease. *Clin. Infect. Dis.*, 22, 73–80, 1996.
177. McGough, D. A. Clinical and laboratory aspects of the "black yeasts." *Clin. Microbiol. Newsl.*, 15, 145–151, 1993.
178. Matsumoto, T., Nishimoto, K., Kimura, K., Padhye, A. A., Ajello, L., and McGinnis, M. R. Phaeohyphomycosis caused by *Exophilia moniliae*. *Sabouraudia*, 22, 17, 1984.
179. Kettlewell, P., McGinnis, M. R., and Wilkinson, G. T. Phaeohyphomycosis caused by *Exophiala spinifera* in two cats. *J. Med. Vet. Mycol.*, 27, 257, 1989.
180. McGinnis, M. R., *Exophiala spinifera*, a new combination for *Phialophora spinifera*. *Mycotaxon*, 5, 337–340, 1977.
181. Padhye, A. A., Ajello, L., Chandler, F. W., Banos, J. E., Hernandex-Perez, E., Llerena, J., and Linares, L. M., Phaeohyphomycosis in El Salvador caused by *Exophiala* spinifera, *Am. J. Trop. Med. Hyg.*, 32, 799, 1983.
182. Padhye, A. A., Kaplan, W., Neuman, M. A., Case, P., and Radcliffe, G. N., Subcutaneous phaeohyphomycosis caused by *Exophiala spinifera*. *J. Med. Vet. Mycol.*, 22, 493, 1984.
183. Lacaz, C. da S., Porto, E., de Andrade, J. G., and de Tellhes Filo, F., Feohifomicose disseminada por *Exophiala spinifera*. *An. Bras. Dermatol.*, 59, 238, 1984.
184. Dai, W. L., Ren, Z. F., Wen, J. Z., et al. First case of systemic phaeohyphomycosis caused by *Exophiala spinifera* in China. *Chinese J. Dermatol.*, 20, 13,1987.
185. Rajam, R. V., Kandhari, K. C., and Thirumalacher, M. J. Chromoblastomycosis caused by a yeast-like dematiaceous fungus. *Mycopathol. Mycol. Appl.*, 9, 5, 1958.
186. Rinaldi, M. Recurrent *Exophiala spinifera* diagnosed in a patient with a renal allograft. *Mycology Observer*, 7, 1, 1987.
187. Chevrant-Breton, J., Boisseau-Lebreuil, M., Freour, E., Guiguen, G., Launois, B., and Guelfi, J. Les alternarioses cutanées humaines: a propos de 2 cas. Revie de la literature. *Ann. Dermatol. Venereol.*, 108, 653, 1981.
188. Duffill, M. B. and Coley, K. E. Cutaneous phaeohyphomycosis due to *Alternaria alternata* responding to itraconazole. *Clin. Exp. Dermatol.*, 18, 156, 1993.
189. Bang Pedersen, N., Mardh, P. A., Hallberg, T., and Jonsson, N. Cutaneous alternariosis. *Br. J. Dermatol.*, 94, 201, 1976.
190. Mirkin, L. D. *Alternaria alternata* infection of skin in a 6-year-old boy with aplastic anemia. *Pediatr. Pathol.*, 14, 757, 1994.
191. Kasperlik-Zaluska, A. A. and Bielunska, S. Effect of mitotane on *Alternaria alternata* infection in Cushing's syndrome. *Lancet*, 337, 53, 1991.
192. Rovira, M., Marin, P., Martin-Ortega, E., Montserrat, E., and Razman, L. *Alternaria* infection in a patient receiving chemotherapy for lymphoma. *Acta Haematol.*, 84, 98, 1990.
193. Singh, S. M., Naidu, J., and Pouranik, M. Ungual and cutaneous phaeohyphomycosis caused by *Alternaria alternata* and *Alternaria chlamydospora*. *J. Med. Vet. Mycol.*, 28, 275, 1990.
194. Romano, C., Paccagnini, E., and Difonzo, E. M. Onychomycosis caused by *Alternaria* spp. in Tuscany, Italy from 1985 to 1999. *Mycoses*, 44, 73–76, 2001.
195. Romano, C., Valenti, L., Miracco, C., et al. Two cases of cutaneous phaeohyphomycosis by *Alternaria alternata* and *Alternaria tenuissima*. *Mycopathologia*, 137, 65–74, 1997.
196. Ajello, L. Fungal infections in AIDS: a review. *L'Igiene Moderna*, 100, 288, 1993.
197. Iwatsu, T. Cutaneous alternariosis. *Arch. Dermatol.*, 124, 1822, 1988.
198. Di Silverio, A. and Sacchi, S. Cutaneous alternariosis: a rare chromoblastomycosis: report of a case. *Mycopathologia*, 95, 159, 1986.
199. Castanet, J., Lacour, J. P., Toussaint-Gary, M., Perrin, C., Rodot, S., and Ortonne, J. P. Infection cutanée pluri-focale a *Alternaria tenuissima*. *Ann. Dermatol. Venereol.* 122, 115–118, 1995.

200. Bouthenet, M. F., Guyenne, C., Bonnin, A., Camerlynck, P., and Lambert, D. Cas pour diagnostic. *Ann. Dermatol. Venereol.*, 120, 169, 1993.
201. Panagiotidou, D., Kapetis, E., Chrysomallis, F., et al. Deux cas d'altérnariose cutanée an Gréce. *J. Mycol. Med.*, 1, 1, 1991.
202. Camenen, I., De Closets, F., Vaillant, L., et al. Alternariose cutanée a *Alternaria tenuissima*. *Ann. Dermatol. Venereol.*, 115, 839, 1988.
203. Lulin, J., Lancien, G., Sandron, A., et al. Alternariose cutanée: a propos d'un nouveau cas. *Nouv. Dermatol.*, 9, 183, 1990.
204. Mitchell, A. J., Solomon, A. R., Beneke, E. S., and Anderson, T. F. Subcutaneous alternariosis. *J. Am. Acad. Dermatol.*, 8, 673–276, 1983.
205. Blanc, C., Lamey, B., and Lapalu, J. Alternariose cutanée chez, un transplante renal. *Bull. Soc. Fr. Mycol. Med.*, 13, 213, 1984.
206. Schillinger, F., Bressieux, J. M., Montagnac, R., and Hopfner, C. Les alternarioses humaines: analyse de la littérature a propos d'un cas personnel. *Semin. Hop. Paris*, 62, 1369, 1986.
207. Gené, J., Azon-Masoliver, A., Guarro, J., et al. Cutaneous phaeohyphomycosis caused by *Alternaria longipes* in an immunosuppressed patient. *J. Clin. Microbiol.*, 2774–2776, 1995.
208. Halaby, T., Boots, H., Vermeulen, A., et al. Phaeohyphomycosis caused by *Alternaria* infectoria in a renal transplant recipient. *J. Clin. Microbiol.*, 39, 1952–1955, 2001.
209. Laumaille, C., Le Gall, F., Degeilh, B., Guèho, E., and Huerre, M. Cutaneous *Alternaria infectoria* infection after liver transplantation. *Ann. Pathol.*, 18, 192–194, 1998.
210. Gianni, C., Cerri, A., and Crosti, C. Ungual phaeohyphomycosis caused by *Alternaria alternata*. *Mycoses*, 40, 219–221, 1997.
211. Repiso, T., Martin, N., Huguet, P., et al. Cutaneous alternariosis in a liver transplant recipient. *Clin. Infect. Dis.*, 16, 729, 1993.
212. Benedict, L. M., Kusne, S., Torre-Cisneros, J., and Hunt, S. J. Primary cutaneous fungal infection after solid organ transplantation: report of five cases and review. *Clin. Infect. Dis.*, 15, 17, 1992.
213. Wätzig, V. and Schmidt, U. Primäre kutane granulomatöse alternariose. *Hautarzt.*, 40, 718, 1989.
214. Lanigan, A. W. Cutaneous *Alternaria* infection treated with itraconazole. *Br. J. Dermatol.*, 127, 39, 1992.
215. Guerin, V., Barbaud, A., Duquenne, M., et al. Cushing's disease and cutaneous alternariosis. *Arch. Intern. Med.*, 151, 1863–1868, 1991.
216. Mardh, P. A. and Hallberg, T. *Alternaria alternata* as a cause of opportunistic fungal infection in man. *Scand. J. Infect. Dis. Suppl.*, 16, 36, 1978.
217. Badillet, G. Les alternarioses cutanées. Revue de la littérature. *J. Mycol. Med.*, 118, 59–71, 1991.
218. Schlueter, D. P., Fink, J. N., and Hensley, G. T. Wood-pulp workers' disease: a hypersensitivity pneumonia caused by *Alternaria*. *Ann. Intern. Med.*, 77, 907, 1972.
219. Lobritz, R. W., Roberts, T. H., Marrato, R. V., Carlton, P. K., and Thorp, D. J. Granulomatous pulmonary disease secondary to *Alternaria*. *J. Am. Med. Assoc.*, 241, 596, 1979.
220. Bartynski, J. M., McCaffrey, T. V., and Frigas, E. Allergic fungal sinusitis secondary to dematiaceous fungi - *Curvularia lunata* and *Alternaria*. *Otolaryngol. Head Neck Surg.*, 103, 32, 1990.
221. Manning, S. C., Schaefer, S. D., Close, L. G., and Vuich, F. Culture-positive allergic fungal sinusitis. *Arch. Otolaryngol. Head Neck Surg.*, 117, 174–178, 1991.
222. Rummelt, V., Ruprecht, K. W., Boltze, H. J., and Naumann, G. O. H. Chronic *Alternaria alternata* endophthalmitis following intraocular lens implantation. *Arch. Ophthalmol.*, 109, 178, 1991.
223. Chang, S.-W., Tsai, M.-W., and Hu, F.-R. Deep *Alternaria* keratomycosis with intraocular extension. *Am. J. Ophthalmol.*, 117, 544, 1994.
224. Simmons, R. B., Buffington, J. R., Ward, M., Wilson, L. A., and Ahearn, D. G. Morphology and ultrastructure of fungi in extended-wear soft contact lenses. *J. Clin. Microbiol.*, 24, 21, 1986.
225. Azar, P., Aquavella, J. V., and Smith, R. S. Keratomycosis due to an *Alternaria* species. *Am. J. Ophthalmol.*, 79, 881, 1975.
226. Moulsdale, M. T., Harper, J. M., and Thatcher, G. N. Fungal peritonitis: complication of continuous ambulatory peritoneal dialysis. *Med. J. Aust.*, 1, 88, 1981.
227. Garau, J., Diamond, R. D., Lagrotteria, L. V., and Kabins, S. A. *Alternaria* osteomyelitis. *Ann. Intern. Med.*, 86, 747, 1977.
228. Murtagh, J., Smith, J. W., and Mackowiak, P. A. Case report: *Alternaria* osteomyelitis: eight years of recurring disease requiring cyclic courses of amphotericin B for cure. *Am. J. Med. Sci.*, 293, 399, 1987.
229. Viviani, M. A., Tortorano, A. M., Laria, G., Giannetti, A., and Bignotti, G. Two cases of cutaneous alternariosis with a review of the literature. *Mycopathologia*, 96, 3, 1986.
230. Stenderup, J., Bruhn, M., Gadeberg, C., and Stenderup, A. Cutaneous alternariosis: case report. *Acta Pathol. Microbiol. Immunol. Scand.*, 95, 79, 1987.
231. Bourlond, A. and Alexandre, G. Dermal alternariosis in a kidney transplant recipient. *Dermatologica*, 168, 152, 1984.
232. Lévy-Klotz, B., Badillet, G., Cavelier-Balloy, B., Chemaly, P., Leverger, G., and Civatte, J. Alternariose cutanée au cours d'un SIDA. *Ann. Dermatol. Venereol.*, 112, 739, 1985.
233. Junkins, J. M., Beveridge, R. A., and Friedman, K. J. An unusual fungal infection in an immunocompromised oncology patient: cutaneous alternariosis. *Arch. Dermatol.*, 124, 1421 & 1424, 1988.

234. Sneeringer, R. M. and Haas, D. W. Cutaneous alternaria infection in a patient on chronic corticosteroids. *J. Tenn. Med. Assoc.*, 83, 15–17, 1990.
235. Chaidemenos, G. Ch., Mourellou, O., Karakatsanis, G., Koussidou, T., Panagiotidou, D., and Kapetis, E. Cutaneous alternariosis in an immunocompromised patient. *Cutis*, 56, 145, 1995.
236. Machet, L., Machet, M.-C., Maillot, F., Cotty, F., Vaillant, L., and Lorette, G. Cutaneous alternariosis occuring in a patient treated with local intrarectal corticosteroids. *Acta Derm. Venereol. (Stockholm)*, 75, 328, 1995.
237. Quieffin, J., Milleron, B., Billet, S., Roux, P., Blanchet, P., and Akoun, G. Alternariose cutanée chez un malade atteint de corticosurrenalome malin metastase. *Presse Med.*, 19, 1462, 1990.
238. Meyers, J. D. Infection in bone marrow transplant recipients. *Am. J. Med.*, 81(Suppl. 1A), 27, 1986.
239. Aloi, F. G., Cervetti, O., and Forte, M. *Alternaria* mycosis in a kidney transplant patient. *G. Ital. Dermatol. Venereol.*, 122, 35, 1987.
240. Morrison, V. A., Haake, R. J., and Weisdorf, D. J. The spectrum of non-*Candida* fungal infections following bone marrow transplantation. *Medicine (Baltimore)*, 72, 78, 1993.
241. Morrison, V. A., Haake, R. J., and Weisdorf, D. J. Non-*Candida* fungal infections after bone marrow transplantation: risk factors and outcome. *Am. J. Med.*, 96, 497, 1994.
242. Galgóczy, J., Simon, G., and Valyi-Nagy, T. Case report: human cutaneous alternariosis. *Mycopathologia*, 92, 77, 1985.
243. Simal, E., Navarro, M., Rubio, M. C., et al. Sobre ub caso de alternariasis cutanea. *Actas Dermosifilogr.*, 77, 252, 1986.
244. Chen, H. C., Kao, H. F., Hsu, M. L., and Lee, J. Y. Cutaneous alternariosis in association with scabies or iatrogenic Cushing's syndrome. *J. Formos. Med. Assoc.*, 91, 462, 1992.
245. Palencarova, E., Jesenska, Z., Plank, L., et al. Phaeohyphomycosis caused by *Alternaria* species and *Phaeosclera dematioides* Sigler, Tsuneda and Carmichael. *Clin. Exp. Dermatol.*, 20, 419–422, 1995.
246. Gerdsen, R., Uerlich, M., de Hoog, G. S., Bieber, T., and Horre, R. Sporotrichoid phaeohyphomycosis due to *Alternaria infectoria*. *Br. J. Dermatol.*, 145, 484–486, 2001.
247. Male, D. and Pehamberger, H. Secondary cutaneous mycoses caused by *Alternaria* species. *Hautarzl.*, 37, 94, 1983.
248. Machet, M. C., Stephanov, E., Estève, E., et al. Alternariose cutanée survenant au cours de l'évolution d'un pemphigus traité. *Ann. Pathol.*, 14, 186, 1994.
249. Miegeville, M., Bureau, B., Morin, O., Berthello, J. M., and Prost, A. Nouveau cas d'alternariose cutanée chez un malade sous corticotherapie. *Bull. Soc. Fr. Mycol. Med.*, 18, 329, 1989.
250. Miegeville, M., Dutartre, H., Bureau, B., Lajat, Y., and Avranche, P. Nouveau cas d'alternariose cutanée chez un malade sous corticotherapie. *J. Mycol. Med.*, 1, 160, 1991.
251. Aznar, R., Marigil, J., Puig de la Bellacasa, J., et al. Cutaneous alternariosis responding to ketoconazole. *Lancet*, 1, 667, 1989.
252. Richardson, A. A., Agger, W. A., Ringstrom, J. B., and Kemnitz, M. J. Subcutaneous alternariosis of the foot in a patient on corticosteroids. *J. Am. Podiatr. Med. Assoc.*, 83, 472, 1993.
253. del Palacio-Hernanz, A., Conde-Zurita, J. M., Reyes Pecharroman, S., and Rodriguez Noriega, A. A case of *Alternaria alternata* (Fr) Keissler infection of the knee. *Clin. Exp. Dermatol.*, 8, 641, 1983.
254. Male, O. and Pehamberger, H. Die kutane alternariose: fallberichte und literaturübersicht. *Mykosen*, 28, 278, 1985.
255. Findling, J. W., Tyrell, J. B., Aron, D. C., Fitzgerald, P. A., Young, C. W., and Sohne, P. G. Fungal infections in Cushing's syndrome. *Ann. Intern. Med.*, 95, 392, 1981.
256. Loli, P., Berselli, M. E., and Tagliaferri, M. Use of ketoconazole in the treatment of Cushing's syndrome. *J. Clin. Endocrinol. Metab.*, 63, 1365, 1986.
257. Diop, S. N., Warnet, A., Duet, M., Firmin, C., Mosse, A., and Lubetzki, J. Traitement prolongé de la maladie de Cushing par le kétoconazole: possibilité d'un échappement thérapeutique. *Presse Med.*, 18, 1325, 1989.
258. Bécherel, P.-A., Chosidow, O., and Francés, C. Cutaneous alternariosis after renal transplantation. *Ann. Intern. Med.*, 122, 71, 1995.
259. De Moragas, J. M., Prats, G., and Verger, G. Cutaneous alternariosis treated with miconazole. *Arch. Dermatol.*, 117, 292, 1981.
260. Singh, N., Chang, F. Y., Gayowski, T., and Marino, I. R. Infections due to dematiaceous fungi in organ transplant recipients: case report and review. *Clin. Infect. Dis.*, 24, 369, 1997.
261. Shearer, C. and Chandrasekar, P. H. Cutaneous alternariosis and regional lymphadenitis during allogeneic BMT. *Bone Marrow Transplant.*, 11, 497, 1993.
262. Benito, N., Moreno, A., Puig, J., and Rimola, A. Alternariosis after liver transplantation. *Transplantation*, 72, 1840–1843, 2001.
263. Diaz, M., Puente, R., and Trevino, M. A. Response of long-running *Alternaria alternata* infection to fluconazole. *Lancet*, 336, 513, 1990.
264. Morrison, V. A. and Weisdorf, D. J. *Alternaria*: a sinonasal pathogen of immunocompromised hosts. *Clin. Infect. Dis.*, 16, 265, 1993.
265. Loveless, M. O., Winn, R. E., Campbell, M., and Jones, S. R. Mixed invasive infection with *Alternaria* species and *Curvularia* species. *Am. J. Cin. Pathol.*, 76, 491, 1981.
266. Body, B. A., Sabio, H., Oneson, R. H., Johnson, C. E., Kahn, J., and Hanna, M. D. *Alternaria* infection in a patient with acute lymphocytic leukemia. *Pediatr. Infect. Dis. J.*, 6, 418, 1987.
267. Stiller, R. L. and Stevens, D. A. Studies with a plant fungicide, imazalil, with vapor-phase activity, in the therapy of human alternariosis. *Mycopathologia*, 93, 169, 1986.

268. Chin, G. N., Hyndiuk, R. A., Kwasny, G. P., and Schultz, R. O. Keratomycosis in Wisconsin. *Am. J. Ophthalmol.*, 79, 121, 1975.
269. Wenkel, H., Rummelt, V., Knorr, H., and Naumann, G. O. Chronic postoperative endophthalmitis following cataract extraction and intraocular lens implantation: report on nine patients. *Ger. J. Ophthalmol.*, 2, 419, 1993.
270. Ando, N. and Takatori, K. Keratomycosis due to *Alternaria alternata* corneal transplant infection. *Mycopathologia*, 100, 17, 1987.
271. Sigler, L., Tsuneda,A., and Carmichael, J. W. *Phaeotheca* and *Phaeosclera*, two genera of dematiaceous hyphomycetes and a redescription of *Sarcinomyces lindner*. *Mycotaxon*, 12, 449–467, 1981.
272. McGinnis, M. R., McKenzie, R. A., and Connole, M. D. *Phaeosclera dematioides*, a new etiologic agent of phaeohyphomycosis in cattle. *Sabouraudia*, 23, 133–135, 1985.
273. Matsumoto, T., Padhye, A. A., and Ajello, L. Medical significance of the so-called black yeast. *Eur. J. Epidemiol.*, 3, 87–95, 1987.
274. Krempl-Lamprecht, L., Luderschmidt, C., and Wehrmann, W. Chromomycosis caused by *Fonsecaea compacta* (Carrion 1940) followed by a secondary phaeohyphomycosis due to *Phaeosclera dematioides* (Sigler 1981). *Mykosen*, 30, 454–466, 1987.
275. Parmalee, J. A. The identification of the *Curvalaria* parasite of gladiolus. *Mycologia*, 48, 558, 1956.
276. Friedman, A. D., Campos, J. M., Rorke, L. B., Bruce, D. E., and Arbeter, A. M. Fatal recurrent curvularia brain abscess. *J. Pediatr.*, 99, 413, 1981.
277. Grieshop, T. J., Yarbrough, D. III, and Farrar, W. E. Case report: phaeohyphomycosis due to *Curvularia lunata* involving skin and subcutaneous tissue after an explosion at a chemical plant. *Am. J. Med. Sci.*, 305, 387, 1993.
278. Fernandez, M., Noyola, D. E., Rossmann, S. N., and Edwards, M. S. Cutaneous phaeohyphomycosis caused by *Curvularia lunata* and review of *Curvularia* infections in pediatrics. *Pediatr. Infect. Dis.*, 18, 727–731, 1999.
279. Kaushik, S., Ram, J., Chakrabarty, A., Dogra, M. R., Brar, G. S., and Gupta, A. *Curvularia lanata* endophthalmitis with secondary keratitis. *Am. J. Ophthalmol.*, 131, 140–142, 2001.
280. Wilhelmus, K. R. and Jones, D. B. *Curvularia* keratitis. *Trans. Am. Ophthalmol. Soc.*, 99, 111–130, 2001.
281. Baylet, J., Camain, R., and Segretain, G. Identification des agents des maduromycoses du Senegal et de la Mauritaine: description d'une espece nouvelle. *Bull. Soc. Path. Exot. Filiales*, 52, 448, 1959.
282. Mahgoub, E. S. Mycetomas caused by *Curvularia lunata*, *Madurella grisea*, *Aspergillus nidulans* and *Nocardia brasiliensis* in Sudan. *Sabouraudia*, 11, 179, 1973.
283. Rinaldi, M. G., Phillips, P., Schwartz, J. G., et al. Human *Curvularia* infections: report of five cases and review of the literature. *Diagn. Microbiol. Infect. Dis.*, 6, 27, 1987.
284. Berry, A. J., Kerkering, T. M., Giordano, A. M., and Chiancone, J. Phaeohyphomycotic sinusitis. *Pediatr. Infect. Dis. J.*, 3, 150, 1984.
285. Brummund, W., Kurup, V. P., Harris, G. J., Duncavage, J. A., and Arkins, J. A. Allergic sino-orbital mycosis: a clinical and immunologic study. *J. Am. Med. Assoc.*, 256, 3249, 1986.
286. McMillan, R. H. III, Cooper, P. H., Body, B. A., and Mills, A. S. Allergic fungal sinusitis due to *Curvularia lunata*. *Hum. Pathol.*, 18, 960, 1987.
287. Killingsworth, S. M. and Wetmore, S. J. *Curvularia/Drechslera* sinusitis. *Laryngoscope*, 100, 932, 1990.
288. Lampert, R. P., Hutto, J. H., Donnelly, W. H., and Shulman, S. T. Pulmonary and cerebral mycetoma caused by *Curvularia pallescens*. *J. Pediatr.*, 91, 603, 1977.
289. Berg, D., Garcia, J. A., Schell, W. A., Perfect, J. R., and Murray, J. C. Cutaneous infection caused by *Curvularia pallescens*: a case report and review of the spectrum of disease. *J. Am. Acad. Dermatol.*, 32(2 Part 2), 375, 1995.
290. Mroueh, S. and Spock, A. Allergic bronchopulmonary disease caused by *Curvularia* in a child. *Pediatr. Pulmonol.*, 12, 123, 1992.
291. deShazo, R. D. and Swain, R. E. Diagnostic criteria for allergic fungal sinusitis. *J. Allergy Clin. Immunol.*, 96, 24–35, 1995.
292. Rohwedder, J. J., Simmons, J. L., Colfer, H., and Gatmaitan, B. Disseminated *Culvularia lunata* infection in a football player. *Arch. Intern. Med.*, 139, 940, 1979.
293. Ismail, Y., Johnson, R. H., Wells, M. V., Pusavat, J., Douglas, K., and Arsura, E. L. Invasive sinusitis with intracranial extension caused by *Curvularia lunata*. *Arch. Intern. Med.*, 153, 1604, 1993.
294. de la Monte, S. M. and Hutchins, G. M. Disseminated curvularia infection. *Arch. Pathol. Lab. Med.*, 109, 872, 1985.
295. Pierce, N. F., Millan, J. C., and Bender, B. S. Disseminated *Curvularia* infection. *Arch. Pathol. Lab. Med.*, 110, 871, 1986.
296. Pierce, N. F., Millan, J. C., Bender, B. S., and Curtis, J. L. Disseminated *Curvularia* infection: additional therapeutic and clinical consideration with evidence of medical cure. *Arch. Pathol. Lab. Med.*, 110, 959, 1986.
297. Brubaker, L. H. Cure of *Curvularia* pneumonia by amphotericin B in a patient with megakaryotic leukemia. *Arch. Pathol. Lab. Med.*, 112, 1178, 1988.
298. Berlanga, J. J., Querol, S., Gallardo, D., Ferra, C., and Granena, A. Successful treatment of *Curvularia* sp. infection in a patient with primarily resistant acute promyelocytic leukemia. *Bone Marrow Transplant.*, 16, 617, 1995.
299. Bryan, C. S., Smith, C. W., Gerg, D. E., and Karp, R. B. *Curvularia lunata* endocarditis treated with terbinafine: case report. *Clin. Infect. Dis.*, 16, 30, 1993.
300. Corey, J. P. Allergic fungal sinusitis. *Otolaryngol. Clin. North Am.*, 25, 225, 1992.
301. Fitzsimons, R. and Peters, A. L. Miconazole and ketoconazole as a satisfactory first-line treatment for keratomycosis. *Am. J. Ophthalmol.*, 101, 605, 1986.

302. Foster, C. S. Miconazole therapy for keratomycosis. *Am. J. Ophthalmol.*, 91, 622, 1981.
303. Foster, C. S. and Stefanyszyn, M. Intraocular penetration of miconazole in rabbits. *Arch. Ophthalmol.*, 97, 1703, 1979.
304. Berger, S. T., Katsev, D. A., Mondino, B. J., and Pettit, T. H. Macroscopic pigmentation in a dematiaceous fungal keratitis. *Cornea*, 10, 272, 1991.
305. Agrawal, A. and Singh, S. M. Two cases of cutaneous phaeohyphomycosis caused by *Curvalaria pallescens*. *Mycoses*, 38, 301, 1995.
306. Subramanyam, V. R., Rath, C. C., Mishra, M., and Chhotrai, G. P. Subcutaneous infection due to *Curvalaria* species. *Mycoses*, 36, 449–450, 1993.
307. Still, J. M. Jr., Law, E. J., Pereira, G. I., and Singletary, E. Invasive burn wound infection due to *Curvularia* species. *Burns*, 19, 77, 1993.
308. Yau, Y. C., de Nanassy, J., Summerbell, R. C., Matlow, A. G., and Richardson, S. E. Fungal sternal wound infection due to *Curvularia lanata* in a neonate with congenital heart disease: case report and review. *Clin. Infect. Dis.*, 19, 735, 1994.
309. Mancini, M. C. and McGinnis, M. R. *Dactylaria* infection of a human being: pulmonary disease in a heart transplant recipient. *J. Heart Lung Transplant.*, 11, 827, 1992.
310. Terreni, A. A., Di Salvo, A. F., Baker, A. S., Crymes, W. B., Morris, P.R., and Dowd, A. H. Disseminated *Dactylaria gallopava* infection in a diabetic patient with chronic lymphocytic leukemia of the T-cell type. *Am. J. Clin. Pathol.*, 94, 104–107, 1990.
311. Kralovic, S. M. and Rhodes, J. C. Phaeohyphomycosis caused by *Dactylaria* (human dactylariosis): report of a case with review of the literature. *J. Infect.*, 31, 107–113, 1995.
312. Dixon, D. M., Walsh, T. J., Salkin, I. F., and Polak, A. *Dactylaria constricta*: another dematiaceous fungus with neurotropic potential in mammals. *J. Med. Vet. Mycol.*, 25, 55, 1987.
313. Walsh, T. J., Dixon, D. M., Polak, A., and Salkin, I. F. Comparative histopathology of *Dactylaria constricta*, *Fonsecaea pedrosoi*, *Wangiella dermatitidis*, and *Xylohypha bantiana* in experimental phaeohyphomycosis of the central nervous system. *Mykosen*, 30, 215–225, 1987.
314. Fukushiro, K. R., Udagawa, S., Kawashima, Y., and Kawamura, Y. Subcutaneous abscesses caused by *Ochroconis gallopavum*. *J. Med. Vet. Mycol.*, 24, 175, 1986.
315. Sides, E. H. III, Benson, J. D., and Padhye, A. A. Phaeohyphomycosis brain abscess due to *Ochroconis gallopavum* in a patient with malignant lymphoma of a large cell type. *J. Med. Vet. Mycol.*, 29, 317, 1991.
316. Vukmir, R. B., Kusne, S., Linden, P., et al. Successful treatment of cerebral phaeohyphomycosis due to *Dactylaria gallopava* in a liver transplant recipient. *Clin. Infect. Dis.*, 19, 714, 1994.
317. Prevost-Smith, E., Hutton, N., Padhye, A. A., Upshur, J. K., and Van Bakel, A. B. Fatal phaeohyphomycosis infection due to *Dactylaria gallopava* and *Scedosporium prolificans* in a cardiac transplant patient. *Proc. 93rd Annu. Meet. Am. Soc. Microbiol.*, abstract no. F-35, American Society for Microbiology, Washington, DC, 1993.
318. Kralovic, S. M. and Rhodes, J. C. Phaeohyphomycosis caused by *Dactylaria* (human dactylariosis): report of a case with review of the literature. *J. Infect.*, 31, 107, 1995.
319. Nieto-Rodriguez, J. A. and Kusne, S. Successful therapy for cerebral phaeohyphomycosis due to *Dactylaria gallopava*. *Clin. Infect. Dis.*, 23, 211, 1996 [see also: *Clin. Infect. Dis.*, 22, 73–80, 1996].
320. Gezuele, E., Mackinnon, J. E., and Conti-Diaz, I. A. The frequent isolation of *Phialophora verrucosa* and *Phialophora pedrosoi* from natural sources. *Sabouraudia*, 10, 266, 1972.
321. Dixon, D. M. and Polak-Wyss, A. The medically important dematiaceous fungi and their identification. *Mycoses*, 34, 1, 1991.
322. Matsumoto, T. and Matsuda, T. Chromoblastomycosis and phaeohyphomycosis. *Semin. Dermatol.*, 4, 240, 1985.
323. Pitrak, D. L., Koneman, E. W., Estupinan, R. C., and Jackson, J. *Phialophora richardsiae* infection in humans. *Rev. Infect. Dis.*, 10, 1195, 1988.
324. Wong, P. K., Ching, W. T. W., Kwon-Chung, K. J., and Meyer, R. D. Disseminated *Phialophora parasitica* infection in humans: case report and review. *Rev. Infect. Dis.*, 11, 770, 1989.
325. Pracharktam, R., Chongtrakool, P., Sriurairatana, S., and Sathapatayavongs, B. Mycetoma and phaeohyphomycosis caused by *Phialophora parasitica* in Thailand. *J. Med. Assoc. Thai.*, 83(Suppl. 1), S42–S45, 2000.
326. Tendolkar, U. M., Kerkar, P., Jerajani, H., Gogate, A., and Padhye, A. A. Phaeohyphomycotic ulcer caused by *Phialophora verrucosa*: successful treatment with itraconazole. *J. Infect.*, 36, 122–125, 1998.
327. Ikai, K., Tomono, H., and Watanabe, S. Phaeohyphomycosis caused by *Phialophora richardsiae*. *J. Am. Acad. Dermatol.*, 19, 478, 1988.
328. Schnadig, V. J., Long, E. G., Washington, J. M., McNeely, M. C., and Troum, B. A. *Phialophora verrucosa*-induced subcutaneous phaeohyphomycosis. *Acta Cytol.*, 30, 425, 1986.
329. Ahmad, S., Johnson, R. J., Hillier, S., Shelton, W. R., and Rinaldi, M. G. Fungal peritonitis caused by *Lecythophora mutabilis*. *J. Clin. Microbiol.*, 22, 182, 1985.
330. Iwatsu, T. and Miyaji, M. Subcutaneous cystic granuloma caused by *Phialophora verrucosa*. *Mycopathologia*, 64, 165, 1977.
331. Fincher, R. M. E., Fisher, J. F., Padhye, A. A., Ajello, L., and Steele, J. C. H. Subcutaneous phaeohyphomycotic abscess caused by *Phialophora parasitica* in a renal allograft recipient. *J. Med. Vet. Mycol.*, 26, 311–314, 1988.
332. Jha, V., Krishna, V. S., Chakrabarti, A., et al. Subcutaneous phaeohyphomycosis in a renal transplant recipient: a case report and review of the literature. *Am. J. Kidney Dis.*, 28, 137–139, 1996.

333. Gugnani, H. C., Obiefuna, M. N., and Ikerionwu, S. E. Studies on pathogenic dematiaceous fungi. II. Pathogenicity of *Fonsecaea pedrosoi* and *Phialophora verrucosa* for laboratory mice. *Mykosen*, 29, 505, 1986.
334. Rubin, H. A., Bruce, S., Rosen, T., and McBride, M. E. Evidence for percutaneous inoculation as the mode of transmission for chromoblastomycosis. *J. Am. Med. Dermatol.*, 25, 951, 1991.
335. Moskowitz, L. B., Cleary, T. J., McGinnis, M. R., and Thomson, C. B. *Phialophora richardsiae* in a lesion appearing as a giant cell tumor of the tendon sheath. *Arch. Pathol. Lab. Med.*, 107, 374, 1983.
336. Domsch, K. H., Grams, W., and Anderson, T. H. *Phialophora richardsiae*, in *Compendium of Soil Fungi*, vol. 1, Domsch, K. H., Grams, W., and Anderson, T. H., Eds. Academic Press, London, 628, 1980.
337. Singh, S. M., Agrawal, A., Naidu, J., de Hoog, G. S., and Figueras, M. J. Cutaneous phaeohyphomycosis caused by *Phialophora richardsiae* and the effect of topical clotrimazole in its treatment. *Antonie van Leeuwenhoek*, 61, 51, 1992.
338. Corrado, M. L., Kramer, M., Cummings, M., and Eng, R. H. Susceptibility of dematiaceous fungi to amphotericin B, miconazole, ketoconazole, flycytosine and rifampin alone or in combination. *Sabouraudia*, 20, 109, 1982.
339. Corrado, M. L., Weitzman, I., Stanek, A., Goetz, R., and Agyare, E. Subcutaneous infection with *Phialophora richardsiae* and its susceptibility to 5-fluorocytosine, amphotericin B and miconazole. *Sabouraudia*, 18, 97, 1980.
340. Weitzman, I., Gordon, M. A., Henderson, R. W., and Lapa, E. W. *Phialophora parasitica*, an emerging pathogen. *J. Med. Vet. Mycol.*, 22, 331–339, 1984.
341. Duggan, J. M., Wolf, M. D., and Kauffman, C. A. *Phialophora verrucosa* infection in an AIDS patient. *Mycoses*, 38, 215, 1995.
342. Listemann, H., Die kulturelle untersuchung eines tranensteines mit isolierung des pilzes *Phialophora richardsiae*. *Ernst Rodenwaldt Arch.*, 2, 45, 1975.
343. Torstrick, R. F., Harrison, K., Heckman, J. D., and Johnson, J. E. Chronic bursitis caused by *Phialophora richardsiae*. *J. Bone Joint Surg.*, 61, 772, 1979.
344. Yangco, B. G., TeStrake, D., and Okafor, J. *Phialophora richardsiae* isolated from infected human bone: morphological, physiological and antifungal susceptibility studies. *Mycopathologica*, 86, 103, 1981.
345. Tam, M. and Freeman, S. Phaeohyphomycosis due to *Phialophora richardsiae*. *Australas. J. Dermatol.*, 30, 37, 1989.
346. Crouss, P. W., Gams, W., Wingfield, M. J., and Van Wyk, P. S. *Phaeoacremonium* gen. nov. associated with wilt and decline diseases of woodly hosts and human infections. *Mycologia*, 88, 786–796, 1996.
347. Matsui, T., Nishimoto, K., Udagawa, S., Ishihara, H., and Ono, T. Subcutaneous phaeohyphomycosis caused by *Phaeoacremonium rubrigenum* in an immunosuppressed patient. *Nippon Ishinkin Gakkai Zasshi*, 40, 99–102, 1999.
348. Padhye, A. A., Davis, M. S., Baer, D., Reddick, A., Sinha, K. K., and Ott, J. Phaeohyphomycosis caused by *Phaeoacremonium inflatipes*. *J. Clin. Microbiol.*, 36, 2763–2765, 1998.
349. Kaell, A. T. and Weitzman, I. Acute monoarticular arthritis due to *Phialophora parasitica*. *Am. J. Med.*, 74, 19–22, 1983.
350. Lavarde, V., Bedrossian, J., De Bièvre, C., and Vacher, C. Un cas de phaeomycose a *Phialophora parasitica* chez un transplante. Deuxieme observation mondiale. *Bull. Soc. Fr. Mycol. Med.*, 11, 273–278, 1982.
351. Rowland, M. D. and Farrar, W. E. Case report: thorn-induced *Phialophora parasitica* arthritis treated successfully with synovectomy and ketoconazole. *Am. J. Med.*, 30, 393–395, 1987.
352. Ziza, J. M., Dupont, B., Boissonnas, A., et al. Osteo-arthrites a champignons noir (dematies). *Ann. Med. Interne*, 136, 393–397, 1985.
353. Heath, C. H., Lendrum, J. L., Wetherall, B. L., Wesselingh, S. L., and Gordon, D. L. *Phaeoacremonium parasiticum* infective endocarditis following liver transplantation. *Clin. Infect. Dis.*, 25, 1251–1252, 1997.
354. Wong, P. K., Wendell, T. W., Ching, W. T., Kwon-Chung, K. J., and Meyer, R. D. Disseminated *Phialophora parasitica* infection in humans: case report and review. *Rev. Infect. Dis.*, 11, 770–775, 1989.
355. Coldiron, B. M., Wiley, E. L., and Rinaldi, M. G. Cutaneous phaeohyphomycosis caused by a rare pathogen, *Hormonema dematioides*: successful treatment with ketoconazole. *J. Am. Acad. Dermatol.*, 23, 363, 1990.
356. Torok, M., De Weck, A. L., and Scherrer, M. Allergic alveolitis as a result of mould on a bedroom wall. *Schweiz. Med. Wochenschr.*, 3, 924, 1981.
357. Kersten, W. and Hoek, G. T. Mould allergy. *Wien Med. Wochenschr.*, 130, 275, 1980.
358. Storms, W. W. Occupational hypersensitivity lung diseases. *J. Occup. Med.*, 20, 823, 1978.
359. Blyth, W., Grant, I. W., and Blackadder, E. S. Fungal antigen as a cause of sensitization and respiratory disease in Scottish maltworkers. *Clin. Allergy*, 7, 549, 1977.
360. Velcovsky, H. G. and Graubner, M. Allergic alveolitis following inhalation of mould spores from pot plant earth. *Dtsch. Med. Wochenschr.*, 106, 115, 1981.
361. Metzger, W. J., Patterson, R., Fink, J., Semerdjian, R., and Roberts, M. Sauna-takers' disease: hypersensitivity pneumonitis due to contaminated water in a home sauna. *J. Am. Med. Assoc.*, 236, 2209, 1976.
362. Vermeil, C., Gordeef, A., Leroux, M. J., Morin, O., and Bouc, M. Blastomycose cheloidienne a *Aureobasidium pullulans* (de Bary) Arnoud en Bretagne. *Mycopathol. Mycol. Appl.*, 43, 35, 1981.
363. Gordeef, A. and Leroux, M.-J. Peut-on parler, en Bretagne, d'une blastomycose cutanée possible a *Aureobasidium pullulans*. I. Etude clinique et anatomopathologique. *Bull. Soc. Fr. Mycol. Med.*, 16, 19, 1969.
364. Cooke, W. B. An ecological life history of *Aureobasidium pullulans* (De Bary) Arnaud. *Mycopathol. Mycol. Appl.*, 12, 1, 1959.
365. Jones, F. R. and Christensen, G. R. *Pullaria* corneal ulcer. *Arch. Ophthalmol.*, 92, 529, 1974.
366. Ashikaga, Ueber eine besondere neve art von keratomykosis. *Klin. MBL Augenheilk.*, 66, 934, 1921.
367. Koppang, H. S., Olsen, I., Stuge, U., and Sandven, P. *Aureobasidium* infection of the jaw. *J. Oral Pathol. Med.*, 20, 191, 1991.

368. Kaczmarski, E. B., Liu Yin, J. A., Tooth, J. A., Love, E. M., and Delamore, I. W. Systemic infections with *Aureobasidium pullulans* in a leukemic patient. *J. Infect.*, 13, 289, 1986.
369. Salkin, I. F., Martinez, J. A., and Kemna, M. E. Opportunistic infection of the spleen caused by *Aureobasidium pullulans*. *J. Clin. Microbiol.*, 23, 828, 1986.
370. Krcméry, V. Jr., Spanik, S., Danisovicova, Z., and Blahova, M. *Aureobasidium mansoni* meningitis in a leukemia patient successfully treated with amphotericin B. *Chemotherapy*, 40, 70, 1994.
371. Umabala, P., Lakshmi, V., Murthy, A. R., Prasad, V. S., Sundaram, C., and Beguin, H. Isolation of a *Nodulisporium* species from a case of cerebral phaeohyphomycosis. *J. Clin. Microbiol.*, 39, 4213–4218, 2001.
372. Liesegang, T. J. and Forster, R. K. Spectrum of microbial keratitis in South Africa. *Am. J. Ophthalmol.*, 90, 38–47, 1980.
373. Liao, W. Q., Shao, J. Z., Li, S. Q., et al., *Colletotrichum dematium* caused keratitis. *Chin. Med. J. (Engl.)*, 96, 391–394, 1983.
374. Shukla, P. K., Khan, Z. A., Lal, B., Agrawal, P. K., and Srivastava, O. P. Clinical and experimental keratitis caused by *Colletotrichum* state of *Glomerella cingulata* and *Acrophialophora fusispora*. *Sabouraudia*, 21, 137–147, 1983.
375. Matsuzaki, O., Yasuda, M., and Ichinohe, M. Keratomycosis due to *Glomerella cingulata*. *Rev. Iber. Micol.*, 5(Suppl. 1), 30, 1988.
376. Ritterband, D. C., Shah, M., and Seedor, J. A. *Colletotrichum graminicola*: a new corneal pathogen. *Cornea*, 16, 362–364, 1997.
377. Midha, N. K. Y., Mirzanejad, Y., and Soni, M. *Colletotrichum* spp.: plant or human pathogen? *Antimicrob. Infect. Dis. Newsl.*, 15, 26–27, 1996.
378. Guarro, J., Svidzinski, T. E., Zaror, L., Forjaz, M. H., Gené, J., and Fischman, O. Subcutaneous hyalohyphomycosis caused by *Colletotrichum gloeosporioides*. *J. Clin. Microbiol.*, 36, 3060–3065, 1998.
379. Castro, L. G., da Silva Lacaz, C., Guarro, J., et al. Phaeohyphomycotic cyst caused by *Colletotrichum crassipes*. *J. Clin. Microbiol.*, 39, 2321–2324, 2001.
380. Sutton, B. C. *Pucciniopsis, Mycoleptodiscus* and *Amerodiscosiella*. *Trans. Br. Mycol. Soc.*, 60, 525–536, 1973.
381. Padhye, A. A., Davis, M. S., Reddick, A., Bell, M. F., Gearhart, E. D., and Von Moll, L. *Mycoleptodicus indicus*: a new etiologic agent of phaeohyphomycosis. *J. Clin. Microbiol.*, 33, 2796–2797, 1995.
382. Zaitz, C., Heins-Vaccari, E. M., de Freitas, R. S., et al. Subcutaneous phaeohyphomycosis caused by *Phoma cava*. Report of a case and review of the literature. *Rev. Inst. Med. Trop. Sao Paulo*, 39, 43–48, 1997.
383. Wilson, J. W. and Plunkett, O. A. *The Fungus Diseases of Man*, University of California Press, Los Angeles, 333, 1965.
384. Gordon, M. A., Salkin, I. F., and Stine, W. B. *Phoma (peyronellaea)* as zoopathogen. *Sabouraudia*, 13, 329–333, 1975.
385. Bakerspigel, A. The isolation of *Phoma hibernica* from a lesion on a leg. *Sabouraudia*, 7, 261–264, 1970.
386. Bakerspigel, A., Lowe, D., and Rostas, A. The isolation of *Phoma eupyrena* from a human lesion. *Arch. Dermatol.*, 117, 362–366, 1981.
387. Shulka, N. P., Rajak, R. K., Agarwal, G. P., et al. *Phoma minutispora* as a human lesion. *Mykosen*, 27, 255–258, 1984.
388. Rai, M. K. *Phoma sorghina* infection in a human being. *Mycopathologia*, 105, 167-170, 1989.
389. Baker, J. G., Salkin, I. F., Forgacs, P., et al. First report of subcutaneous phaeohyphomycosis of the foot caused by *Phoma minutella*. *J. Clin. Microbiol.*, 25, 2395–2397, 1987.
390. Hirsh, A. H. and Schiff, T. A. Subcutaneous phaeohyphomysis caused by an unusual pathogen: *Phoma species*. *J. Am. Acad. Dermatol.*, 34, 679–680, 1996.
391. Young, N. A., Kwon-Chung, K. J., and Freeman, J. Subcutaneous abscess caused by *Phoma* sp. resembling *Pyranochaeta romeroi*: unique fungal infection occurring in an immunosuppressed recipient of renal allograft. *Am. J. Clin. Pathol.*, 59, 810–816, 1973.
392. de Hoog, G. S., Guarro, J., Gené, J., and Figueras, M. J. *Atlas of Clinical Fungi*, 2nd ed. Centraalbureau voor Schimmelcultures, Utrecht, The Netherlands, 2000.
393. Chabasse, D., de Bièvre, C., Legrand, E., et al. Subcutaneous abscess caused by *Pleurophomopsis lignicola* Petr.: first case. *J. Med. Vet. Mycol.*, 33, 415–417, 1995.
394. Farina, C., Punithaligham, E., Ruggenenti, P., and Goglio, A. Phaeohyphomycotic soft tissue disease caused by *Plerophomopsis lignicola* in kidney transplant patient. *J. Med. Microbiol.*, 46, 699–703, 1997.
395. Venugopal, P. V. and Venugopal, T. V. Treatment of eumycetoma with ketoconazole. *Australas. J. Dermatol.*, 34, 27–29, 1993.
396. Romero, H. and Mackenzie, D. W. Studies on antigens from agents causing black grain eumycetoma. *J. Med. Vet. Mycol.*, 27, 303–311, 1989.
397. English, M. P. Infection of the fingernail by *Pyrenochaeta unguis-hominis*. *Br. J. Dermatol.*, 103, 91–93, 1980.
398. Thammayya, A., Sanyal, M., and Basu, N. *Pyrenochaeta romeroi* causing mycetoma pedis in India. *J. Indian Med. Assoc.*, 73, 66–67, 1979.
399. Destombes, P., Mariat, F., Rosati, L., and Segretain, G. Mycetoma in Somalia: results of a survey done from 1959 to 1964. *Acta Trop.*, 34, 355–373, 1977.
400. de Albornoz, M. B., Rodriguez-Garcilazo, Y. G., and Urdaneta-Gonzalez, D. Foot mycetoma of double etiology. *Sabouraudia*, 15, 187–193, 1977.
401. Segretain, G. and Destombes, P. Mycetomas caused by *Madurella grisei* and *Pyrenochaeta romeroi*. *Sabouraudia*, 7, 51–61, 1969.
402. Baylet, R., Camain, R., Chabal, J., and Izarn, R. Recent contribution to the study of mycetoma in Senegal. *Neotestudinarosatii. Pyrenochaeta romeroi. Aspergillus nidulans*. *Bull. Soc. Med. Afr. Noire Lang. Fr.*, 13, 311–313, 1968.

403. David-Chausse, J., Texier, L., Darrasse, H., and Moulinier, Autochthonous mycetoma of the foot to *Pyrenochaeta romeroi*. *Bull. Soc. Fr. Dermatol. Syphiligr.*, 75, 452–453, 1968.
404. Andre, M., Brumpt, V., Destombes, P., and Segretain, G. Fungal mycetoma with black grain due to *Pyrenochaeta romeroi* in Cambodia. *Bull. Soc. Pathol. Exot. Filiales*, 61, 108–112, 1968.
405. Chesters, C. G. C. and Greenhalgh, G. N. *Geniculosporium serpens* gen. et sp. nov., the imperfect state of *Hypoxilon serpens*. *Trans. Br. Mycol. Soc.*, 47, 393–401, 1964.
406. Laessøe, T. Index Ascomycetum 1. Xylariaceae. *Syst. Ascomycetum*, 13, 43–112, 1994.
407. Ellis, M. B. *Geniculosporium*, in *Dematiaceus Hyphomycetes*, Kew: Commonwealth Mycological Institute, 229–230, 1971.
408. Barron, G. L. *The Genera of Hyphomycetes From Soil*. Williams & Williams, Baltimore, 169–172, 1968.
409. Suzuki, Y., Udagawa, S., Wakita, H., et al. Subcutaneous phaeohyphomycosis caused by *Geniculosporium* species: a new fungal pathogen. *Br. J. Dermatol.*, 138, 346–350, 1998.
410. Nishimura, K., Miyaji, M., Taguchi, H., Wang, D. L., Li, R. Y., and Meng, Z. H. An ecological study on pathogenic dematiaceous fungi in China. *Proc. 4th Int. Symp. Research Center of Pathogenic Fungi*, 1st ed., Microbiology and Toxicology Laboratory, Tokyo, 17–20, 1989.
411. Ayadi, A., Huerre, M. R., and de Bièvre, C. Phaeohyphomycosis caused by *Veronaea bothryosa*. *Lancet*, 346, 1703–1704, 1995.
412. Foulet, F., Duvoux, C., de Bievre, C., Hezode, C., and Bretagne, S. Cutaneous phaeohyphomycosis caused by *Veronaea bothryosa* in a liver transplant recipient successfully treated with itraconazole. *Clin. Infect. Dis.*, 29, 689–690, 1999.
413. Moja, M., Muthuphei, M. N., van der Westhuizen, L. R., and Gladhill, R. F. Multiple infarcts in a patient with cerebral phaeohyphomycosis: CT and MRI. *Neuroradiology*, 42, 261–266, 2000.
414. Horré, R. and de Hoog, G. S. Primary cerebral infections by melanized fungi: a review. *Studies Mycol.*, 43, 176–193, 1999.
415. Sekhon, A. S., Galbraith, J., Mielke, B. W., Garg, A. K., and Sheehan, G. Cerebral phaeohyphomycosis caused by *Xylohypha bantiana*, with a review of the literature. *Eur. J. Epidemiol.*, 8, 387–390, 1992.
416. Dixon, D. M., Walsh, T. J., Merz, W. G., and McGinnes, M. R. Infections due to *Xylohypha bantiana* (*Cladosporium trichoides*). *Rev. Infect. Dis.*, 11, 515–525, 1989.
417. Middleton, F. G., Jurgenson, P. F., Utz, J. P., Shadomy, S., and Shadomy, H. J. Brain abscess caused by *C. trichoides*. *Arch. Intern. Med.*, 136, 444–448, 1976.
418. Biggs, P. J., Allen, R. L., Powers, M. M., and Holley, H. P. Phaeohyphomycosis complicating compound skull fracture. *Surg. Neurol.*, 25, 393–396, 1986.
419. Kwon-Chung, K. J. and Bennett, J. E., Eds. Medical Mycology, Lea & Fabiger, Philadelphia, 620–677, 1992.
420. Heney, C., Song, E., Kellen, A., Raal, F., Miller, S. D., and Davis, V. Cerebral phaeohyphomycosis caused by *Xylohypha bantiana*. *Eur. J. Clin. Microbiol. Infect. Dis.*, 8, 984–988, 1990.
421. Lacy, M. and Farr, W. *Cladiophialophora bantiana* brain abscess unresponsive to itraconazole and amphotericin B: case report, in *Focus in Fungal Infections 6*, Imedex USA, Inc., Alpharetta, GA, p. 41, abstract 41, 1996
422. Campbell, C. K. and Al-Hedaithy, S. S. A. Phaeohyphomycosis of the brain caused by *Ramichloridium mackenziei* sp. nov. in Middle Eastern countries. *J. Med. Vet. Mycol.*, 31, 325–332, 1993.
423. Vermeil, C., Morin, O., and Bouc, M., Peut-on parler, en Bretagne, d'une blastomycose cutanée possible a *Aureobasidium pullulans*. II. Etude mycologique. *Bull. Soc. Fr. Mycol. Med.*, 16, 20, 1969.
424. Abbott, S. P., Sigler, L., McAleer, R., McGough, D. A., Rinaldi, M. G., and Mizelli, G. Fatal cerebral mycoses caused by the ascomycete *Chaetomium strumarium*. *J. Clin. Microbiol.*, 33, 2692–2698, 1995.
425. Rinaldi, M. G., Inderlied, C. B., Mahnovski, V., et al. Fatal *Chaetomium atrobrunneum* Ames, 1949, systemic mycosis in a patient with acute lymphoblastic leukemia, *11th Congr. Intern. Soc. Human & Animal Mycology*, p. 107, abstract PS2.69, 1991.
426. Young, C. N., Swart, J. G., Ackerman, D., and Davidge-Pitts, K. Nasal obstruction and bone erosion caused by *Drechslera hawaiiensis*. *J. Laryngol. Otol.*, 92, 137–143, 1978.
427. Morton, S. J., Midthun, K., and Merz, W. G. Granulomatous encephalitis caused by *Bipolaris hawaiiensis*. *Arch. Pathol. Lab. Med.*, 110, 1183–1185, 1986.
428. Ruben, S. J., Scott, T. E., and Seltzer, H. M. Intracranial and paranasal sinus infection due to *Drechslera*. *South. Med. J.*, 80, 1057–1058, 1987.
429. del Palacio-Hernanz, A., Moore, M. K., Campbell, C. K., del Palacio-Medel, A., and Del Castillo, R. Infection of the central nervous system by *Rhinocladiella atrovirens* in a patient with acquired immunodeficiency syndrome. *J. Med. Vet. Mycol.*, 27, 127–130, 1989.
430. Lampert, R. P., Hutto, J. H., Donnelly, W. H., and Shulman, S. T. Pulmonary and cerebral mycetoma caused by *Curvularia pallescens*. *J. Pediatr.*, 91, 603–605, 1977.
431. Friedman, A. D., Campos, J. M., Rorke, L. B., Bruce, D. A., and Arbeter, A. M. Fatal recurrent *Curvularia* brain abscess. *J. Pediatr.*, 99, 413–415, 1981.
432. Al-Hedaithy, S. S. A., Jamjoom, Z. A. B., and Saeed, E. S. Cerebral phaeohyphomycosis caused by *Fonsecaea pedrosoi* in Saudi Arabia. *Acta Pathol. Microbiol. Scand.*, 96(Suppl. 3), 94–100, 1988.
433. Fukushiro, R. Chromomycosis in Japan. *J. Dermatol.*, 22, 221–229, 1983.
434. Hart, A. P., Sutton, D. A., McFeeley, P. J., and Kornfeld, M. Cerebral phaeohyphomycosis caused by a dematiaceous *Scopulariopsis* species. *Clin. Neuropathol.*, 20, 224–228, 2001.
435. Patel, R., Gustaferro, C. A., Krom, R. A., Wiesner, R. H., Roberts, G. D., and Paya, C. V. Phaeohyphomycosis due to *Scopulariopsis brumptii* in a liver transplant recipient. *Clin. Infect. Dis.*, 19, 198–200, 1994.
436. Stahel, G. The banana leaf spreckle in Surinam caused by *Chloridium musae* nov. spec. and other related banana diseases. *Trop. Agric.*, 14, 42–44, 1937.

437. Binford, C. H., Thompson, R. K., and Gorhan, M. E. Mycotic brain abscess due to *C. trichoides*, a new species. Report of a case. *Am. J. Clin. Pathol.*, 22, 535–542, 1952.
438. Sutton, D. A., Slifkin, M., Yakulis, R., and Rinaldi, M. G. U.S. case report of cerebral phaeohyphomycosis caused by *Ramichloridium obovoideum* (*R. mackenziei*): criteria for identification, therapy, and review of other known dematiaceus neurotoxic taxa. *J. Clin. Microbiol.*, 36, 708–715, 1998.
439. Jamjoom, A. B., Al-Hedaithy, S. A., Jamjoom, Z. A., et al. Intracranial mycotic infections in neurosurgical practice. *Acta Neurochir.*, 137, 78–84, 1995.
440. Podnos, Y. D., Anastasio, P., De La Maza, L., and Kim, R. B. Cerebral phaeohyphomycosis caused by *Ramichloridium obovoideum* (*Ramichloridium mackenziei*): case report. *Neurosurgery*, 45, 372–375, 1999.
441. Gugnani, H. C., Sidiqqui, N., and Magulike, M. O., Cerebral phaeohyphomycosis: report of a case from Nigeria. *Mycoses*, 41, 431–432, 1998.
442. Walz, R., Bianchin, M., Chaves, M. L., Cerski, M. R., Severo, L. C., and Londero, A. T., Cerebral phaeohyphomycosis caused by *Cladophialophora bantiana* in a Brazilian drug abuser. *J. Med. Vet. Mycol.*, 35, 427–431, 1997.
443. Mukherji, S. K. and Castillo, M., Cerebral phaeohyphomycosis caused by *Xylohypha bantiana*: MR findings. *AJR Am. J. Roentgenol.*, 164, 1304–1305, 1995.
444. Naim-Ur-Rahman, el Sheikh Mahgoub, Abu Aisha, H., Laajam, M., Yaqoub, B., and Chagla, A. H., Cerebral phaeohyphomycosis. *Bull. Soc. Pathol. Exot. Filiales*, 80, 320, 1987.
445. Mitchell, D. M., Fitz-Henley, M., and Horner-Bryce, J., A case of disseminated phaeohyphomycosis caused by *Cladosporium devriesii*. *West Indian Med. J.*, 39, 118, 1990.
446. Buiting, A. G., Visser, L. G., Barge, R. M., and van't Wout, J. W. Mycetoma of the foot: a disease from the tropics. *Ned. Tijdschr. Geneeskd.*, 137, 1513, 1993.
447. Vieira, M. R., Milheiro, A., and Pacheco, F. A., Phaeohyphomycosis due to *Cladosporium cladosporioides*. *Med. Mycol.*, 39, 135–137, 2001.
448. Gugnani, H. C., Sood, N., Singh, B., and Makkar, R., Case report. Subcutaneous phaeohyphomycosis due to *Cladosporium cladosporioides*. *Mycoses*, 43, 85–87, 2000.
449. Romano, C., Bilenchi, R., Allessandrini, C., and Miracco, C. Case report. Cutaneous phaeohyphomycosis caused by *Cladosporium oxysporum*. *Mycoses*, 42, 111–115, 1999.
450. Lirng, J. F., Tien, R. D., Osumi, A. K., Madden, J. F., McLendon, R. P., and Sexton, D. Cerebral phaeohyphomycosis complicated with brain abscess: a case report. *Zhonghua Yi Xue Za Zhi (Taipei)*, 55, 491–495, 1995.
451. Binford, C. H., Thompson, R. K., and Gorhan, M. E. Mycotic brain abscess due to *C. trichoides*, a new species: report of a case. *Am. J. Clin. Pathol.*, 22, 535, 1952.
452. Duque, O. Meningoencephalitis and brain abscess caused by *Cladosporium* and *Ponsecaea*: review of two cases and experimental studies. *Am. J. Clin. Pathol.*, 36, 505, 1961.
453. Felger, C. E. and Friedman, L. Experimental cerebral chromoblastomycosis. *J. Infect. Dis.*, 3, 1, 1962.
454. McGill, H. C. and Brueck, J. W. Brain abscess due to *Hormodendrum* species: report of third case. *Arch. Pathol.*, 62, 303, 1956.
455. Riley, O. and Mann, S. H. Brain abscess caused by *C. trichoides*: review of three cases and report of a fourth case. *Am. J. Clin. Pathol.*, 33, 525, 1960.
456. Segretain, G., Mariat, F., and Drouket, E. Sur *Cladosporium trichoides* isole d'une mycose cerebrale. *Ann. Inst. Pasteur*, 89, 465, 1955.
457. Desai, S. C., Bhatikar, M. L., and Mehta, R. S. Cerebral chromoblastomycosis due to *C. trichoides* (*bantianum*): part II. *Neurol. India*, 14, 6, 1966.
458. Dereymaeker, A. and De Somer, P. Arachnoidite fibro-purulente cerebello-cervical due a une moissiure (*Cladosporium*), *Acta Neurol. Psych. (Belgium)*, 55, 629, 1955.
459. Bobra, S. T. Mycotic abscess of the brain probably due to *Cladosporium trichoides*: report of the fifth case. *Can. Med. Assoc. J.*, 79, 657, 1958.
460. Horn, I. H., Wilanksy, D. L., Harland, A., and Blank, F. Neurogenic hypernatremia with mycotic brain granulomas due to *Cladosporium trichoides*. *Can. Med. Assoc. J.*, 83, 1314, 1960.
461. Sandhyamani, S., Bhatia, R., Mohopatra, L. N., and Roy, S. Cerebral cladosporiosis. *Surg. Neurol.*, 15, 431, 1981.
462. Türker, A., Altinörs, N., Aciduman, A., Demiralp, O., and Uluoglu, U. MPI findings and encouraging fluconazole treatment results of intracranial *Cladosporium trichoides* infection. *Infection*, 23, 60, 1995.
463. Barnola, J. and Ortega, A. A. *Cladosporium profunda*. *Mycopathol. Mycol. Appl.*, 15, 422, 1961.
464. Brown, J. W., Nadell, J., Sanders, C. V., and Sardenga, L. Brain abscess caused by *Cladosporium trichoides* (*bantianum*): a case with paranasal sinus involvement. *South. Med. J.*, 69, 1519, 1976.
465. Chrichlow, D. K., Enrile, F. T., and Memon, M. Y. Cerebelar abscess due to *Cladosporium trichoides* (*bantianum*): case report. *Am. J. Clin. Pathol.*, 60, 416, 1973.
466. King, A. B. and Collette, T. S. Brain abscess due to *Cladosporium trichoides*: report of the second case due to the organism. *Bull. Johns Hopkins Hosp.*, 91, 298, 1952.
467. Watson, K. C. Cerebral chromoblastomycosis. *J. Pathol. Bacteriol.*, 84, 233, 1962.
468. Kim, R. C., Hodge, C. D. Jr., Lamberson, H. V. Jr., and Weiner, L. B. Traumatic intracerebral implantation of *Cladosporium trichoides*. *Neurology*, 31, 1145, 1981.
469. Buxi, T. B., Prakash, K., Vohra, R., and Bhatia, D. Imaging in phaeohyphomycosis of the brain: case report. *Neuroradiology*, 38, 139, 1996.

470. Aldape, K. D., Fox, H. S., Roberts, J. P., Ascher, N. L., Lake, J. R., and Rowley, H. A. *Cladosporium trichoides* cerebral phaeohyphomycosis in a liver transplant recipient: report of a case. *Am. J. Clin. Pathol.*, 95, 499, 1991.
471. Wilson, E. Cerebral abscess caused by *Cladosporium bantiana*: case report. *Pathology*, 14, 91, 1982.
472. Brenner, S. A., Morgan, J., Rickert, P. D., and Rimland, D. *Cladophialophora bantiana* isolated from an AIDS patient with pulmonary infiltrates. *J. Med. Vet. Mycol.*, 34, 427–429, 1996.
473. Palaoglu, S., Sav, A., Basak, T., Yalcinlar, Y., and Scheithauer, B. W. Cerebral phaeohyphomycosis. *Neurosurgery*, 33, 894, 1993.
474. Goel, A., Satoskar, A., Desai, A. P., and Pandya, S. K. Brain abscess caused by *Cladosporium trichoides*. *Br. J. Neurosurg.*, 6, 591, 1992.
475. Borges, M. C., Warren,, S., White, W., and Pellettiere, E. V. Pulmonary phaeohyphomycosis due to *Xylohypha bantiana*. *Arch. Pathol. Lab. Med.*, 115, 627–629, 1991.
476. Musella, R. A. and Collins, G. H. Cerebral chromoblastomycosis: case report. *J. Neurosurg.*, 35, 219, 1971.
477. Seaworth, B. J., Kwon-Chung, K. J., Hamilton, J. D., and Perfect, J. R. Brain abscess caused by a variety of *Cladosporium trichoides*. *Am. J. Clin. Pathol.*, 79, 747, 1983.
478. Dixon, D. M., Merz, W. G., Elliott, H. L., and Macley, S. Experimental central nervous system phaeohyphomycosis following intranasal inoculation of *Xylohypha bantiana* in cortisone-treated mice. *Mycopathologia*, 100,145, 1987.
479. Ginzburg, H. M. and Macher, A. M. Clinical-pathological correlates of human immunodeficiency virus (HIV) infections: a conference summary. *Mod. Pathol.*, 1, 316, 1988.
480. Masini, T., Riviera, L., Capricci, E., and Arienta, C. Cerebral phaeohyphomycosis. *Clin. Neuropathol.*, 4, 246, 1985.
481. Block, E. R., Jennings, A. E., and Bennett, J. E. Experimental therapy of cladosporosis and sporotrichosis with 5-fluorocytosine. *Antimicrob. Agents Chemother.*, 3, 95, 1973.
482. Osiyemi, O. O., Dowdy, L. M., Mallon, S. M., and Cleary, T. Cerebral phaeohyphomycosis due to a novel species: report of a case and review of the literature. *Transplantation*, 71, 1343–1346, 2001.
483. Limsila, T., Stiltnimankarn, T., and Prayad, T. Pulmonary *Cladosporium*: report of a case. *J. Med. Assoc. Thai*, 53, 586, 1970.
484. Patterson, J. W., Warren, N. G., and Kelly, L. W. Cutaneous phaeohyphomycosis due to *Cladophialophora bantiana*. *J. Am. Acad. Dermatol.*, 40(2 Part 2), 364–366, 1999.
485. DeVault, G. A., Brown, S. T. III, King, J. W., Fowler, M., and Oberle, A. Tenckhoff catheter obstruction resulting from invasion by *Curvularia lunata* in the absence of peritonitis. *Am. J. Kidney Dis.*, 6, 124, 1985.
486. Peterson, P. K., Matzke, G., and Keane, W. F. Current concepts in the management of peritonitis in patients undergoing continuous ambulatory peritoneal dialysis. *Rev. Infect. Dis.*, 9, 604, 1987.
487. Johnson, R. J., Ramsey, P. G., Gallagher, N., and Ahmad, S. Fungal peritonitis in patients on peritoneal dialysis: incidence, clinical features and prognosis. *Am. J. Nephrol.*, 5, 169, 1985.
488. Ahlmen, J., Edebo, L., Ericksson, C., Carlsson, L., and Torgersen, A. K. Fluconazole therapy for fungal peritonitis in continuous ambulatory peritoneal dialysis (CAPD): a case report. *Perit. Dial. Int.*, 9, 79, 1989.
489. Ujhelyi, M. R., Raasch, R. H., van der Horst, C. M., and Mattera, W. D. Treatment of peritonitis due to *Curvularia* and *Trichosporon* with amphotericin B. *Rev. Infect. Dis.*, 12, 621, 1990.
490. Lopes, J. O., Alves, S. H., Benevenga, J. P., Brauner, F. B., Castro, M. S., and Melchiors, E. *Curvularia lunata* peritonitis complicating peritoneal dialysis. *Mycopathologia*, 127, 65, 1994.
491. Brackett, R. W., Shenouda, A. N., Hawkins, S. S., and Brock, W. B., *Curvularia* infection complicating peritoneal dialysis. *South. Med. J.*, 81, 943, 1988.
492. Guarner, J., Del Rio, C., Williams, P., and McGowan, J. E., Fungal peritonitis caused by *Curvularia lunata* in a patient undergoing peritoneal dialysis. *Am. J. Med. Sci.*, 298, 320, 1989.
493. Buchanan, W. E., Quinn, M. J., and Hasbargen, J. A., Peritoneal catheter colonization with *Alternaria*: successful treatment with catheter preservation. *Perit. Dial. Int.*, 14, 91, 1994.
494. Kerr, C. M., Perfect, J. R., Craven, P. C., et al. Fungal peritonitis in patients with continuous ambulatory peritoneal dialysis. *Ann. Intern. Med.*, 99, 334, 1983.
495. O'Sullivan, F. X., Stuewe, B. R., Lynch, J. M., et al. Peritonitis due to *Drechslera spicifera* complicating continuous ambulatory peritoneal dialysis. *Ann. Intern. Med.*, 94, 213, 1981.
496. Clark, E. C., Silver, S. M., Hollick, G. E., and Rinaldi, M. G. Continuous ambulatory peritoneal dialysis complicated by *Aureobasidium pullulans* peritonitis. *Am. J. Nephrol.*, 15, 353, 1995.
497. Eisenberg, E. S., Leviton, I., and Soeiro, R. Fungal peritonitis in patients receiving dialysis: experience with 11 patients and review of the literature. *Rev. Infect. Dis.*, 8, 309, 1986.
498. Tapson, J. S., Freeman M. R., and Wilkinson, R. The high morbidity of CAPD fungal peritonitis - description of 10 cases and review of treatment strategies. *Q. J. Med.*, 61, 1047, 1986.
499. Struijk, D. G., Krediet, R. T., Boeschoten, E. W., Rietra, P. J. G. M., and Arisz, L. Antifungal treatment of *Candida* peritonitis in continuous ambulatory peritoneal dialysis patients. *Am. J. Kidney Dis.*, 9, 66–70, 1987.
500. Kerr, C. M., Perfect, J. R., Craven, P. C., et al. Fungal peritonitis in patients on continuous ambulatory peritoneal dialysis. *Ann. Intern. Dis.*, 99, 334, 1983.
501. Ahmad, S., Johnson, R. J., Hillier, S., Shelton, W. R., and Rinaldi, M.G. Fungal peritonitis caused by *Lecythophora mutabilis*. *J. Clin. Microbiol.*, 22, 182, 1986.
502. Fabris, A., Biasioli, S., Chiaramonte, S., et al. An unusual form of *Fusarium verticillioides* peritonitis in a patient on chronic peritoneal dialysis. *Dialysis Transplant.*, 12, 644, 1983.

503. Cecchini, E., De Marchi, S., Panarello, G., et al. *Torulopsis glabrata* peritonitis complicating continuous peritoneal dialysis: successful management with oral 5-fluorocytosine. *Am. J. Kidney Dis.*, 4, 280, 1984.
504. Arfania, D., Everett, E. D., Nolph, K. D., and Rubin, J. Uncommon causes of peritonitis in patients undergoing peritoneal dialysis. *Arch. Intern. Dis.*, 141, 61, 1981.
505. Milam, C. P. and Fenske, N. A. Chromoblastomycosis. *Dermatol. Clin. North Am.*, 7, 219, 1989.
506. Burks, J. B., Wakabongo, M., and McGinnis, M. R. Chromoblastomycosis. A fungal infection primarily observed in the lower extremity. *J. Am. Podiatr. Med. Assoc.*, 85, 260–264, 1995.
507. Padhye, A. A., Hampton, A. A., Hampton, M. T., Hutton, N. W., Prevost-Smith, E., and Davis, M. S. Chromoblastomycosis caused by *Exophiala spinifera*. *Clin. Infect. Dis.*, 22, 331–335, 1996.
508. Barba-Gómez, J. F., Mayorga, J., McGinnis, M. R., González-Mendoza, A. Chromoblastomycosis caused by *Exophiala spinifera*. *J. Am. Acad. Dermatol.*, 26, 367–370, 1992.
509. Naka, W., Harada, T., Nishikawa, T., and Fukushiro, R. A case of chromoblastomycosis: with special reference to the mycology of the isolated *Exophiala jeanselmei*. *Mykosen*, 29, 445–452, 1986.

26
Hyalohyphomycosis

1. INTRODUCTION

The emerging filamentous fungal pathogens have been separated into two global disease entities: one with septate, hyaline hyphal tissue forms (hyalohyphomycosis), and the other with phaeoid, septate hyphal invasive forms (phaeohyphomycosis) *(1–4)*.

Caused by several molds (most frequently, *Pseudallescheria boydii, Fusarium moniliforme*, and *Scedosporium commune*), hyalohyphomycosis is increasingly becoming an opportunistic infection among neutropenic and immunocompromised patients (those with burns, leukemia, aplastic anemia, patients undergoing chemotherapy, and transplant recipients) *(5)*. Immunocompetent patients may also be affected *(6,7)*.

Cases of HIV-positive patients presenting with hyalohyphomycosis have also been reported *(8,9)*. Since the granulocytes, which are primarily involved in the control of the pathogens of hyalohyphomycosis, are relatively intact in HIV-infected patients, may be one reason for the fewer cases of hyalo- and phaeohyphomycosis in the HIV-infected population *(3)*.

Although definitive identification of hyalohyphomycosis-causing molds would require culture, they often can be identified provisionally in tissue sections by a combination of histologic features, including hyaline septate and and characteristic reproductive structures (phialides and phialoconidia). However, as pointed out by Liu et al. *(10)*, these morphologic features can be easily overlooked upon histologic examination and species like *Fusarium* and *Paecilomyces lilanicus* have been frequently misidentified in tissue sections as *Aspergillus* or *Candida* species. The use of adventitious sporulation *(11)* (the occurrence of mold reproductive in infected human tissue) may provide additional means for proper preliminary histopathologic identification of these molds as demonstrated for *Fusarium, Paecilomyces*, and *Acremonium* species *(10)*.

2. *PSEUDALLESCHERIA BOYDII* INFECTIONS

Pseudallescheria boydii is a homothallic fungus; its sexual reproduction occurs on a single thallus. However, many strains of *P. boydii*, when grown on routine isolation media, do not form an organ of sexual reproduction (cleistothecia). To produce cleistothecia, the organism has to be cultivated on either potato dextrose or cornmeal agar *(12)*.

P. boydii has been found to be the causative agent of white-grain mycetoma, pneumonia, or disseminated disease *(13–30)*. Other infections due to *P. boydii* include meningitis *(31–35)*; septicemia *(36)*; otomycosis *(37,38)*; prostatitis *(27)*; osteomyelitis and arthritis *(39–42)*; invasion of the conjunctiva, lacrimal glands, or the eyelids; corneal ulcers and endophthalmitis *(43)*; endocarditis *(26,44,45)*; and abscesses in the brain, kidney, thyroid *(46,47)*, prostate *(48)*, and the myocardium *(49)*. The infection has also been seen in patients with Cushing's disease *(39,50)*, renal failure *(51)*, and leukemia *(31,39,43,46,52–57)*. Over the years, there have been numerous reports of *P. boydii*-associated sinusitis in both immunocompetent and immunocompromised hosts *(52,53,58–62)*, ranging from chronic noninvasive form *(58,63)* and superficial invasion *(64)* to intracranial extension *(52)*.

Presently, *P. boydii* is recognized as an important cause of opportunistic infections in immunocompromised patients *(30,43)*. Central nervous system (CNS) involvement was reported on several occasions, presenting either as meningitis *(31–35)* or brain abscesses *(16,20,22,24,31,43,46, 52,54,56,57,65,66)*, including a unique case of fungoma (fungus ball) in the brain of patient with acute myelogenous leukemia (AML) *(67)*. In most cases, brain abscesses were the consequence of hematogenous dissemination of *P. boydii* from another site *(31,46,52,54,65,66)*, although in some instances *(20,43,56,57)* only brain involvement has been identified. Histopathologic studies have shown abscess formation in which necrotic brain tissue is being infiltrated by fungal hyphae. The observed extensive necrosis was in large part due to the propensity of *P. boydii* for blood-vessel invasion *(66)*, resulting in thrombosis and infarction.

In nearly all reported cases, the prognosis of *P. boydii* brain abscess has been extremely poor, and has resulted in the patient's death. Of the very few reported survivors, two were children treated with either amphotericin B or miconazole and complete surgical removal of the abscess *(56,67)*, and an adult immunocompetent patient who developed the disease as complication of infected central venous catheter *(22)*. In the latter case, a 2-mo course with the recommended intraventricular dose of miconazole (20 mg; 10 mg/mL) applied every 72 h and a surgical removal of the abscess led to the recovery; intrathecal or intraventricular therapy is considered necessary because of the poor penetration of the drug into the cerebrospinal fluid (CSF).

Fessler and Brown *(68)* described *P. boydii* infection of the superior sagital sinus in a patient with history of diabetes mellitus, chronic pancreatitis, and alcoholism, in what appeared to be the first reported case of hematogenous dissemination of this fungus that originated from the vascular structures into the CNS tissues. In addition to surgery, treatment with intravenous miconazole (500 mg, t.i.d.) for 55 d decreased the edema and the enhancement along the anterior aspect of the sagittal sinus.

Phillips et al. *(69)* reported the first case of chronic granulomatous disease complicated by disseminated pseudallescheriasis. Clinical response occured after prolonged therapy with intravenous miconazole (30 mg/kg divided into 3 daily doses) in association with recombinant interferon-γ (IFN-γ) (0.05 mg/m^2, 3 times weekly). The latter has been used as an immunoadjuvant in the management of patients with chronic granulomatous disease who have infections refractory to standard antimicrobial therapy *(70)*.

In a case of disseminated cutaneous *P. boydii* infection, a persistently neutropenic patient with AML failed to respond to liposomal amphotericin B at daily dose of 5.0 mg/kg; the patient died as a result of overwhelming fungal infection *(71)*. In contrast, a *P. boydii*-induced soft-tissue infection of the foot of an elderly patient with newly diagnosed acute myelomonocytic leukemia responded well to treatment with intravenous amphotericin B despite being resistant in vitro to the antibiotic *(72)*. Surgical debridement combined with itraconazole therapy was also reported to resolve successfully maduromycosis of the foot of an immunocompromised patient with acute myelocytic leukemia *(73)*.

Pulmonary infection is thought to originate with inhalation of *P. boydii* ascospores *(43)*. The disease course may vary from relatively benign noninvasive to destructive tissue invasion, with most patients presenting with allergic bronchopulmonary colonization, fungus ball (petriellidioma), or invasive pulmonary disease *(27–29,74)*. Pulmonary infections due to *P. boydii* are seldom diagnosed in immunocompetent hosts *(49,74)*. In one such case *(74)*, an immunocompetent patient with a history of chronic lung disease had developed invasive pulmonary pseudallescheriasis with extension to the adjacent bone, probably by acquiring *P. boydii* via pulmonary colonization. The treatment consisted of amphotericin B therapy at a dose of 0.5 mg/kg daily. The MIC values of amphotericin B, ketoconazole, and fluconazole for a clinical *P. boydii* isolate were 3.2, 6.4, and 100 μg/mL, respectively *(74)*.

In patients with chronic cystic or cavitary lung diseases (tuberculosis, sarcoidosis, bronchiectasis), the common course of pulmonary pseudallescheriasis has been that of a prolonged indolent disease. Fulminant, invasive lung infection usually occured in immunocompromised patients, such as those with malignancies (colon carcinoma, melanoma, leukemia), rheumatoid arthritis, sarcoidosis, or on corticosteroid and antibiotic therapies, thus confirming the opportunistic nature of the organism *(28)*.

In patients with localized pulmonary disease, surgical excision has been widely implemented. In addition, the pulmonary infection also appeared to respond to antifungal therapy with azole antimycotics. Seale and Hudson *(28)* reported one such case of invasive pulmonary infection, which was successfully treated with intravenous miconazole (300 mg, t.i.d.) for 30 d. Oral ketoconazole was also shown to be useful in the management of necrotizing pneumonia in a normal host *(49)*. However, Gumbart *(75)* reported a fatal *P. boydii* lung infection developed in a bone-marrow transplant recipient while on prophylactic ketoconazole therapy at 400 mg daily.

Goldberg et al. *(76)* described a rare case of simultaneous invasive pulmonary infection by *P. boydii* and *Aspergillus terrei* in a bone-marrow transplant recipient who was successfully treated with a combination of surgical debridement and oral itraconazole (200 mg, b.i.d.) given for 2 mo; initially, the patient was treated intravenously with a combination of amphotericin B (1.0 mg/kg daily) and miconazole (800 mg, t.i.d.); maintenance therapy with itraconazole (200 mg, b.i.d.) was also instituted. Antifungal susceptibility studies performed with a pulmonary *P. boydii* isolate showed MIC values of 0.39, 0.05, 5.0, and 0.018 µg/mL for ketoconazole, miconazole, fluconazole, and itraconazole, respectively *(76)*.

Because *P. boydii* has shown frequently resistance to amphotericin B and flucytosine *(77–79)*, the management of pulmonary infections in patients with leukemia may often be complicated and even fatal. To this end, oral ketoconazole (400 mg daily) given for 8 wk resolved *P. boydii* lung abscess in a leukemic patient despite a hematologic relapse and repeated episodes of granulocytopenia *(78)*. Although the susceptibility of *P. boydii* to miconazole *(54)* and ketoconazole *(80)* has been well-documented, strains resistant to both drugs have been reported *(16)*.

Whereas most invasive pseudallescheriasis infections have occurred in immunocompromised hosts, Hung et al. *(74)* described a case of an immunocompetent patient with invasive pulmonary pseudallescheriasis and subsequent contiguous extension to the ribs and spine.

Sphenoidal or maxillary sinusitis has been predominant *(62,64,65,81,82)* and management has been mainly through surgical intervention *(62,63)*. Two cases of *P. boydii* infections reported in AIDS patients have been reported *(83,84)*. In one of the them, the patient had a rapidly progressive native-valve endocarditis owing to the anamorph form *S. apiospermum (83)*, while the other case involved renal and pulmonary dissemination caused by *P. boydii (84)*.

Ophthalmic infections involving *P. boydii* involved endophthalmitis *(17,20,85–89)*, keratitis *(90–97)*, lacrimal gland, and orbital infections *(43)*. Several well-documented occurences of endophthalmitis secondary to *P. boydii*, all diagnosed in immunosuppressed patients, underscored the opportunistic nature of this fungus *(17,23,85–87,96)*. Glassman et al. *(85)*, described a patient with a long history of diabetes mellitus who suffered *P. boydii*-induced endophthalmitis following cataract extraction and postoperative corticosteroid therapy. The infection was successfully treated with amphotericin B eyedrops (4.0 mg/mL) given every hour *(85)*. The first instance of endogenous *P. boydii* endophthalmitis that occurred in a patient with lupus erythemathosus and on immunosuppressive medication was reported by Lutwick et al. *(54)*. Despite a partial vitrectomy coupled with intravitreal instillation of amphotericin B, followed by systemic therapy with intravenous miconazole, an enucleation of the globe was eventually required *(54)*.

In another case, a bilateral *P. boydii* endophthalmitis was diagnosed in a renal-transplant recipient also on immunosuppressive therapy *(17)*. Bilateral vitrectomy with initial intravitreal amphotericin B, followed by systemic therapy with miconazole, elicited only poor clinical response requiring enucleation of one eye, in spite of intravitreal miconazole therapy on the other eye; the patient died from brain abscess *(17)*. In two cases described by Pfeifer et al. *(23)*, intravitreal instillation of amphotericin B or miconazole was combined with systemic treatment with oral fluconazole (400 mg every 48 h). However, because therapeutic levels of fluconazole in the eye were difficult to achieve (the vitreous drug concentration reaching only 55% of the serum drug level), the fungus was not eradicated.

Postoperative *P. boydii* endophthalmitis was successfully managed with a combination of vitrectomy, corneoscleral resection, and a patch graft, in addition to intraocular, topical, and oral antifungal medication with ketoconazole (200 mg, t.i.d.) for 10 wk *(88)*.

Ruben *(98)* described what is believed to be the first case of *P. boydii* keratitis effectively treated with topical miconazole. In contrast, Bloom et al. *(95)* reported failure in a case of *P. boydii* keratitis after using a regimen consisting of 1% miconazole drops (every hour), oral itraconazole (200 mg daily), and a subconjunctival injection of miconazole (0.5 mL of 10 mg/mL solution). Following the lack of clinical improvement, the oral systemic therapy was changed to intravenous miconazole (600 mg, t.i.d.) to no avail; the eye eventually had to be eviscerated. Corticosteroids, either topical or systemic, have been recognized as aggravating fungal keratitis and should be avoided *(96)*.

Several occurrences of severe *P. boydii* corneoscleritis secondary to β-irradiation-induced scleral necrosis following pterygium excision *(90,91)* are discussed together with similar cases of *Scedosporium prolificans* corneoscleral infections (*see below*).

Mycetoma (also known as the Madura foot, from the city of Madurai, India where it was first described and for its predilection for the feet *[99]*), is a chronic suppurative fungal infection of the extremities that has been associated, along with other etiologic agents (Eumycetoma, Actinomycetoma, and Botryomycosis), with *P. boydii*. Mycetoma most often has been observed in tropical and hot temperate zones where it could be endemic (India, Central and South America, and parts of Africa). In United States, the highest incidence of mycetoma has been in the Southeast region, but it has also been reported as far north as New England and Canada *(99–101)*. Mycetoma is characterized by extensive tissue erosion, formation of draining fistulas and the presence of white grains *(24,102)*.

In several studies, oral ketoconazole has been used to treat *P. boydii* mycetoma *(80,100,101,103, 104)*. In one such case, an initial dose of 200 mg, b.i.d., was ineffective and had to be increased to 400 mg b.i.d., before a significant improvement was noticed *(100)*. Sheftel et al. *(101)* used *en bloc* resection and oral ketoconazole (600 mg daily for 8 d, then 400 mg daily for the remainder of a 4-mo course) to treat an unusual nontraumatic presentation of *P. boydii* soft-tissue abscess without draining sinus tracts. Aubock et al. *(104)* described a case of mycetoma of the lower leg with bone involvement, which, after an initial favorable response, could not be controlled with conventional therapy with ketoconazole (200 mg, b.i.d.) and ultimately necessitated amputation.

Pether et al. *(105)* described a case of acute pyogenic *P. boydii* foot infection treated sequentially with intravenous miconazole (600 mg, t.i.d.) and oral itraconazole (200 mg, daily).

P. boydii-associated arthritis and osteomyelitis have also been reported *(106–111)*. Ginter et al. *(42)* described a case of *P. boydii*-associated severe chronic arthritis, which, although without grains, had resulted in complete destruction of the cartilaginous surface. This case has been one of several similar reports describing post-traumatic arthritis of the knee joint caused by *P. boydii* in which the presence of fistulas was variable and grains remained absent *(40,112–114)*. The cases of *P. boydii*-produced arthritis have been remarkably similar to focal infections caused by *Scedosporium prolificans*, which has also the tendency to affect cartilage and joint areas and does not produce any fungal grains either *(115)*.

Because *P. boidii* has been almost invariably resistant to amphotericin B, therapy with azole antymicotics has been the most beneficial. Thus, in the aforementioned case by Ginter et al. *(42)*, the combination of miconazole and itraconazole was successful; miconazole was injected intravenously at 600 daily for the first 12 d, followed by 1.2 g of miconazole and 400 mg itraconazole (both given orally) for further 4 wk; then, itraconazole monotherapy at 200 mg was administered orally for the next 3 mo *(42)*. Treatment with itraconazole was also reported successful in two other cases of osteoarthritis *(113,114)*.

The in vitro susceptibility of *P. boydii* to miconazole has shown MIC values in the range of ≤0.8–1.0 mg/mL *(116)*. The recommended daily dose of miconazole, which depended on the severity and localization of the infection and the general condition of the patients, has been between 10 and 30 mg/kg *(42)*.

Ketoconazole at 200 mg, b.i.d. has been largely ineffective in treating *P. boydii* osteomyelitis *(40,106)*.

Hung and Norwood *(40)* described an interesting case of *P. boydii*-induced osteomyelitis in an immunocompetent patient who presented with no cutaneous or subcutaneous infection. Because osteomyelitis has been known to occur usually only after the soft tissue has been extensively involved *(117)*, this case (an insidious onset and an indolent course, basically symptom-free for the first 5 yr) should illustrate the possibility that after trauma and deep laceration, deep fungal infections can occur without cutaneous manifestations. A highly unusual *P. boydii*-related mycetoma of the scalp and osteomyelitis of the skull after craniotomy has been reported by Fernandez-Guerrero et al. *(41)*. The patient was cured by wide resection of the involved bone alone and without antifungal therapy. A post-craniotomy wound infection due to *P. boydii* was effectively treated with intravenous miconazole *(118)*.

One consequence of the Cushing's syndrome is the diminished capability of the host immune defense to resist a variety of infections [postoperative wound and pyogenic cutaneous infections, streptococcal sepsis, pneumonia, superficial cutaneous and mucosal fungal infections *(119)*, and *Pneumocystis carinii* pneumonia *(120)*]. To this end, Ansari et al. *(39)* also reported a case of *P. boydii*-induced arthritis and osteomyelitis associated with the Cushing's syndrome. The pathogen was successfully eradicated only after a combination therapy consisting of surgical debridement, long-term ketoconazole treatment (initially at 400 mg daily, then increased to 600 mg daily), and control of the endogenous hypercortisol production. The latter occurrence has been related to a marked increase in susceptibility to infections, especially those requiring cell-mediated immune defense *(119–121)*. There have been several studies aimed at elucidating the mechanism by which corticosteroids exert their immunomodulating effect. Fauci et al. *(122)* established that human peripheral blood lymphocytes are capable of expressing glucocorticoid receptors, and lymphopenia with selective affinity for T-cells is one well-known effect of corticosteroids. Furthermore, the corticosteroids can also reduce accumulation of inflammatory cells at sites of inflammation, and to inhibit cutaneous delayed hypersensitivity reactions by decreasing the recruitment of macrophages *(123)*, as well as to curtail the ability of lymphokines to recruit the cells necessary for expression of cellular immunity *(123)*. Most important, the latter has been essential for effective defense against fungal infections *(39)*.

3. *SCEDOSPORIUM* SPP. INFECTIONS

The genus *Scedosporium* comprises of two species of pathogenic hyphomycetes, *S. apiospermum* and *S. prolificans*.

S. apiospermum, the anamorph (asexual) state of *Pseudallescheria boydii* (teleomorph state), is an emerging cause of localized and disseminated mycotic infections *(12)*. To add more confusion to their taxonomic classification, over the past decades, both the anamorph and teleomorph states have undergone several name changes and have been referred to as *Petrellidium boydii*, *Allescheria boydii*, *Pseudallescheria sheari*, and *Monosporium apiospermum*. Because it is accepted that a fungal disease is named after the teleomorph stage (if known), the taxonomic designation *Scedosporium apiospermum* should be used only for those clinical isolates that are proven to lack a sexual state *(124)*. The organism is widespread and can be isolated from polluted water, sewage, soil, swamps, water-logged pastures, coastal tidelands, and poultry and cattle manure *(124)*.

The second species of the genus, *S. prolificans* (*S. inflatum*) is a recently recognized pathogen associated with osteomyelitis and arthritis, as well as localized and disseminated disease *(124–127)*.

Since the pathological features in tissue sections of both *Scedosporium* species can be easily confused with those of similar hyaline hyphomycetes (*Aspergillus* and *Fusarium* spp.), and because they have both shown resistance to a wide variety of antifungal agents, their precise identification becomes an important factor for successful clinical outcome *(12)*.

3.1. Scedosporium apiospermum

The risk factor for infection and the clinical course of *Scedosporium apiospermum*-associated hyalohyphomycosis are the same as those of the more frequently encountered *P. boydii* mycosis *(96,128–131)*. The portal of entry are the lungs and paranasal sinuses, or by traumatic inoculation.

S. apiospermum is almost always resistant to amphotericin B, and has shown variable resistance to flucytosine *(124,126,132)*.

In a report by Tadros et al. *(12)*, three different clinicopathologic cases of *S. apiospermum* have been described. The first case presented was a patient with underlying sickle-cell disease complicated with chronic *S. apiospermum* sinusitis. The second case involved an immunocompetent young adult with chronic osteomyelitis of the foot consistent with eumycotic white-grain mycetoma. The third case showed the propensity of *S. apiospermum* to act as an opportunistic pathogen in immunocompromised host; the patient, a bone-marrow transplant recipient, presented with fungal hyphae diffusely infiltrating the white matter and invading the blood vessels.

In another case, a patient with acute myeloblastic leukemia who, during consolidation chemotherapy developed lobar pneumonia due to *S. apiospermum*, had the lobar infiltrate cleared with high doses of itraconazole (600 mg, daily) after treatment with amphotericin B (1.0 mg/kg, daily) had failed *(133,134)*.

3.2. Scedosporium prolificans (S. inflatum)

Scedosporium prolificans (S. inflatum) is an emerging pathogen associated with localized soft-tissue and bone infections in immunocompetent hosts (most likely from traumatic inoculation), but frequently fatal disseminated infections in immunocompromised patients *(125,126,135–140)*.

The organism is an imperfect fungus, but, unlike *S. apiospermum*, its sexual state (teleomorph) is still unknown. In infected tissues, *S. prolificans* is indistinguishable by its morphological features from *S. apiospermum (P. boydii)*. However, when grown on standard nutrient agar, *S. prolificans* grows more rapidly, forming distinctive conidiogeneous cells and producing annelides with distinctly swollen bases; in addition, when compared to *S. apiospermum*, it is lacking the *Graphium* type of conidial state *(12)*.

S. prolificans was previously known as *Scedosporium inflatum*; the species was demonstrated to be conspecific with *Lomenospora prolificans* using DNA/DNA reassociation methods *(141)*. Having been isolated only from soil, the natural habitat of *S. prolificans* appears to be more limited as compared with *P. boydii (S. apiospermum) (125)*. In this context, Summerbell et al. *(142)* discussed the isolation of *S. prolificans* from hospital environment (potted plants) and its pathogenic potential as a nosocomial infection. It has also been reported to infect cats and horses *(125)*.

In 1984, Malloch and Salkin *(143)* described the first case of infection caused by *S. prolificans (S. inflatum)*. One likely portal of entry has been by penetrating trauma to the affected site *(115)* since most infections have been seen as localized infection of bone, joints, or soft tissues *(81,125,144,145)*.

Among immunocompromised patients, where dissemination is a distinct possibility *(146)*, the incidence of infections has been on the increase *(125,126,135–140,143,147–150)*. Diagnosis of disseminated disease due to *Scedosporium prolificans* is difficult to attain because its spectrum and symptoms strongly resemble those of pseudallescheriasis *(125,126)*. For example, cases of arthritis caused by *S. prolificans* and *P. boydii* have been nearly indistinguishable, even with mixed infection in the knee by both species being reported *(151)*. In view of the extreme drug tolerance by *S. prolificans*, early positive-culture identification of the pathogen should be essential. Furthermore, initial infections by *S. prolificans* may resemble pulmonary aspergillosis. Moreover, patients with disseminated disease may also present with fever, muscle tenderness, and papular cutaneous lesions, similar to those observed in acute hematogenous disseminated candidiasis *(3)*.

Despite antifungal therapy, the prognosis of disseminated *S. prolificans* infection is generally poor *(126,135–138,140,148–150)*.

Wise et al. *(135)* and Farag et al. *(136)* reported two fatal infections in immunocompromised patients, despite intravenous treatment in one of the cases *(135)* initially with amphotericin B (20 mg daily; increased to 30 mg daily), then with miconazole (600 mg, q.i.d.; increased to 800 mg, q.i.d.), and intravenous amphotericin B and flucytosine, in the second case *(136)*. Nielsen et al. *(149)* described another fatal outcome of disseminated *S. prolificans* infection in an immunocompromised patient where the clinical course was very similar to that of disseminated coccidioidomycosis, and the pathogen was resistant to amphotericin B (given intravenously initially at 1.0 mg/kg every 48 h; then increased to 1.4 mg/kg every 48 h, and flucytosine being added to the therapeutic regimen).

The major reason *S. prolificans* infections in immunocompromised patients have been very difficult to treat is that, contrary to *S. apiospermum*, this organism nearly always has been resistant to azole antimycotics (miconazole, itraconazole) and amphotericin B *(115,125,126,135,138,145)*. In vitro antifungal susceptibility studies have also shown *S. prolificans* to be repeatedly resistant to amphotericin B, miconazole, and ketoconazole *(115,125,135,152)*. In one of the studies *(147)*, the MIC values against amphotericin B, flucytosine, miconazole, ketoconazole, and itraconazole were ≥3.12, ≥3.12, 100, 100, and ≥100 µg/mL, respectively. These findings have been reflected in clinical settings where in the majority of serious cases of *S. prolificans* infections, treatment with amphotericin B has been unsuccessful *(115,125,138,140,145)*. Wilson et al. *(115)* suggested adjunctive topical or intra-articular administration of amphotericin B when the infections are localized.

There has been some anecdotal evidence that ketoconazole is effective in cases of chronic, recurrent osteomyelitis caused by *S. inflatum (115,145)*.

In view of the largely unseccessful antifungal chemotherapy, it appears that adequate debridement should be considered immediately *(115,145)*.

As an ocular pathogen, *S. prolificans* has been documented as the causative agent of metastatic endophthalmitis that required enucleation *(126)*. Furthermore, Sullivan et al. *(153)* and Moriarty et al. *(90,91)* have reported the development of *S. prolificans* sclerokeratitis in the setting of late scleral necrosis complicating pterygium surgery with adjunctive β-irradiation. Therapy with oral ketoconazole at 200 mg daily was unsuccessful and led to enucleation of the eye *(153)*. In view of the these and other reports, infective scleritis complicating scleral avascular necrosis following pterygium surgery *(154–157)* has become an increasingly recognized occurrence *(158)*.

4. *FUSARIUM* SPP. INFECTIONS

A systemic infection caused by ingestion of *Fusarium*-contaminated cereals was first reported in 1913 in Russia *(159)*, and again at the end of World War II, when as many as one million people may have been poisoned by infected grain *(160)*. The disease, known as the alimentary toxic aleukia in Russia *(159,160)*, and as akakabi-byo in Japan *(161)*, is characterized by initial gastrointestinal symptoms and weakness that culminate in aplastic anemia and death if ingestion of *Fusarium*-contaminated grain persists *(162,163)*. The disease results from the effects of fusarial mycotoxins and not from a systemic fungal infection *(159,164,165)*. Although in Russia, the alimentary toxic aleukia has been commonly owing to *F. sporotrichioides* and *F. poae (163)*, in Japan the causative agent has been *F. graminearum* and less often *F. nivale*, *F. poae*, and *F. oxysporum (161)*. Currently, *F. moniliforme* is the *Fusariium* species most often associated with basic human and animal dietary staples, such as corn *(166,167)*, and consequently most studied for the mycotoxins (moniliformins, fusarins, and fumonisins) it produces *(162)*. Another species causing human infections is *F. solani (168,169)*.

The increased use of immunosuppressive therapies, cytotoxic drugs in cancer patients, and the widespread use of antibiotics have resulted in increased incidence of newly recognized opportunistic pathogens, such as the *Fusarium* species *(4,170–176)*. In recent years, *Fusarium* spp. have emerged as important pathogens in community-acquired and nosocomial hyalohyphomycoses. Disseminated infections, when they have occurred, have been predominantly in immunocompromised patients *(177)*, such as those with hematologic malignancies *(168–171,173,174,176,178–194)*, organ-transplant recipients *(195,196)*, patients with chronic infectious mononucleosis syndrome *(197)*, and burn victims *(198–200)*.

Fusarium spp. have been reported to cause skin infections (necrotic, ecthyma gangrenosum-like or nodular lesions, or mycetomas) *(169,173,174,177,179,180,191,196,201–209)*, onychomycosis *(194)*, osteomyelitis *(210)*, septic arthritis *(211)*, extensive interdigital infection *(212)*, cystitis *(213)*, peritonitis *(214–216)*, brain abscess *(197,199)*, invasive sinusanal disease *(207,217–219)*, myocarditis

(220), endocarditis *(221)*, and ocular infections *(222–235)*. In diabetic patients, leg ulcers may allow this common soil saprophite to become imbedded in the subcutaneous tissue *(236)*. Fungemia has been variable, ranging from 11–50% in a small series of disseminated infections *(173,179)*; catheter-related fungemia has also been reported *(177)*. In some geographic regions of the world, especially the Western hemisphere, *Fusarium* (especially *F. solani*) has been the most common cause of keratomycosis *(226,237–247)*.

The portal of entry of *Fusarium* spp. is postulated to be the paranasal sinuses through inhalation of aerosolized conidia *(179)*, or through breaks of integummentary barriers, particularly in patients with *Fusarium*-associated onychomycosis *(4)*.

In the interaction of the immune system with *Fusarium* spp., the granulocytes and macrophages play essential roles in the defense against this pathogen. Thus, macrophages can inhibit the germination of conidia and the growth of hyphae, whereas granulocytes suppress the hyphal growth *(162)*.

Although invasive fusarial infections most frequently develop in patients with granulocytopenia, they seldom complicate HIV infections *(228,248)*. In neutropenic patients, the manifestations of *Fusarium* infections include fever, severe myalgia, maculonodular cutaneous lesions, fungemia, and occasionally pulmonary infiltrates *(170,192,249,250)*. Myoken et al. *(189)* have described an oral *F. moniliforme* infection in a granulocytopenic patient with acute myelogenous leukemia (AML) who developed necrotic ulceration of the gingiva, extending to the alveolar bone, but free of any active systemic lesions.

4.1. Treatment of Fusariosis

The therapy and outcome of *Fusarium* infections were dependent on the degree of invasion of the pathogen, and the status of the host. Superficial *Fusarium* infections usually respond to local treatment. However, there have often been cases refractory to antifungal therapy, as evidenced from experimental animal models *(251)* and humans, particulary in granulocytopenic patients *(170)*.

The prognosis in immunosuppressed patients with disseminated fusariosis is extremely poor. With very few exceptions *(172)*, the outcome was fatal for most patients, especially those with leukemia *(170,190,191,252)*. The treatment modalities recommended have included amphotericin B, flucytosine, rifampin, granulocyte transfusions, and local surgical debridement *(173,174,196,253)*. In general, the therapeutic efficacy of amphotericin B (1.2 mg/kg daily; 40 mg daily), fluconazole, and itraconazole in invasive fusarial infections in immunosuppressed hosts have been rather limited *(191,254)*. However, Cofrancesco et al. *(250)* and Viviani et al. *(255)* used liposomal amphotericin B (AmBisome®) at 3.0 mg/kg daily (total dose 3.85 g) to successfully eradicate *Fusarium* infection in a neutropenic patient with acute lymphoblastic leukemia; the initial treatment was with conventional amphotericin B (0.7–1.0 mg/kg daily; total dose 1.63 g). There was a complete regression of the pulmonary lesion.

Of the newer triazoles, SCH 39309 and D0870 have shown in vivo activity against *Fusarium* spp. *(171)*. However, because of unacceptable toxicity, SCH 39309 (also found active against invasive human fusariosis) is no longer being developed *(171,256)*.

The first disseminated *Fusarium* infection has been described in a child with acute lymphocytic leukemia by Cho et al. *(181)*. Dissemination to the eye occured hematogenously following initial colonization in the primary lesion. Treatment consisted of intravenous amphotericin B; the initial dose of 0.1 mg/kg was gradually increased within 1 wk to 1.0 mg/kg daily; the patient was maintained on this dose for a total of 8 wk. In addition, amphotericin B solution (1.0 mg/mL) was applied topically to the involved eye. In spite of the gradual improvement of skin and eye lesions, seizure activity and mental confusion remained unchanged and the patient died. The amphotericin B blood levels at 24 and 48 h were 0.59 and 0.24 µg/mL. In vitro amphotericin B sensitivity tests indicated a minimal inhibitory concentration (MIC) of 3.0 µg/mL *(181)*.

Venditti et al. *(180)* presented two cases of invasive *F. solani* infection in immunosuppressed patients with acute myelomonocytic and myelogenous leukemia, respectively; neither patient had an intravascular catheter in place. The first patient, despite continued treatment with systemic amphotericin B (total 4.5 g) and 5-fluorocytosine (5-FC) (180 mg/kg daily; total 720 g) and progressive improvement of skin lesions and myalgias, died in the setting of persistent granulocytopenia. The outcome was also fatal for the second patient, who despite systemic therapy with amphotericin B (total 2.66 g), continued to show profound and persistent granulocytopenia. Both patients experienced an insidious loss of vision that culminated in blindness in the first patient, apparently from hematogenous spread of *F. solani* to the eye *(183)* (also suggested by previous observations *[181,224]*).

Earlier studies established a relationship between the degree of leukopenia and the presence of infection in patients with acute leukemia *(257–260)* and various types of agranulocytosis *(261–263)*. Bodey et al. *(182)* studied the quantitative relationships between circulating leukocytes and infection in patients with acute leukemia *(264)*. The data showed that the incidence of infections in these patients decreased with increasing levels of circulating granulocytes and lymphocytes; a critical level was established for granulocytes (1,500 cells/mm^3) above which there was no further decrease in the incidence of infection. Because the risk of developing fungal infections is higher with increasing duration of granulocytopenia, recovery from granulocytopenia seems to be an important factor in survival after *Fusarium* infection in leukemic patients *(265–267)*.

Gutmann et al. *(183)* described a fatal case of systemic fusariosis in a patient with a myasthenic-like syndrome (Eaton-Lambert syndrome) and aplastic anemia. The Eaton-Lambert syndrome is characterized by proximal muscle weakness resulting from the blockade of the acetylcholine release from nerve terminals at the neuromuscular junction *(268)*. The systemic granulomatous infection caused by *F. oxysporum* was similar in many respects to alimentary toxic aleukia, although it was complicated by the therapeutic use of guanidine, a drug also known to cause bone-marrow suppression. The fact that other microbial derivatives produced a similar defect of acetylcholine release as seen in the Eaton-Lambert syndrome (e.g., neomycin, a *Streptomyces fradiae* metabolite) and bone-marrow suppression (e.g., chloramphenicol, derived from *S. venezuelae*), lent further support to the hypothesis that *Fusarium* mycotoxins may be one cause of the Eaton-Lambert syndrome, as well as aplastic anemia, as observed in this case *(183)*.

A disseminated *F. moniliforme* infection was described in a granulocytopenic patient with malignant lymphoma who was treated with cytotoxic drugs and corticosteroids *(178)*. The patient died following progressive renal and respiratory failure with diffuse alveolar infiltrates, massive gastrointestinal bleeding, and hypothermia. Steinberg et al. *(197)* described a patient with *F. oxysporum* brain abscess who developed meningitis. The outcome was fatal despite treatment with amphotericin B: an initial loading dose of 0.75 mg/kg, followed by 1.0 mg/kg daily; next, after the abscess was aspirated, an Ommaya reservoir has been placed to deliver intraventricular amphotericin B (0.1 mg every other day, then increased to 0.5 mg daily). In another case, a patient with B-type lymphoblastic lymphoma who underwent a bone-marrow transplantation and aggressive chemotherapy, developed a *Fusarium* onychomycosis *(269)* of the great toenail *(270)*. Septicemic fungal dissemination followed a lymphoma relapse, resulting in a fulminant and fatal disease despite the institution of amphotericin B therapy.

In a pancytopenic patient with disseminated fusariosis, Spielberger et al. *(271)* reported as safe and life-saving the combined use of amphotericin B, granulocyte transfusions, and granulocyte-macrophage colony-stimulating factor (GM-CSF). Also, a disseminated *F. proliferatum*-associated fusariosis in a patient with acute lymphocytic leukemia responded to an early, aggressive treatment consisting of granulocyte transfusion combined with chemotherapy comprising amphotericin B, ketoconazole, rifampin, and griseofulvin *(193)*. In yet another study, Hennequin et al. *(272)* used high doses of amphotericin B (1.5 mg/kg daily), flucytosine (200 mg/kg daily), and granulocyte colony-stimulating factor (G-CSF) as adjuvant therapy, to treat disseminated cutaneous fusariosis in a neutropenic child; the lesions progressively diminished and disappear after 15 d.

Even though a number of investigators have successfully used similar therapeutic regimens (high-dose amphotericin B, granulocyte transfusions, and intravenously administered GM-CSF) to treat other mycoses (*Candida albicans*-induced skin lesions, pulmonary aspergillosis) *(273–275)*, the benefit of granulocyte transfusions in the therapy of fungal infections still remains controversial *(276,277)*. Granulocyte transfusions, when given during amphotericin B treatment of invasive fungal infections in granulocytopenic patients, have raised concern about pulmonary complications from leukostasis *(6,278)*. The GM-CSF, which has been used to shorten the duration of granulocytopenia following chemotherapy-induced myelosuppression, also has the ability to activate neutrophils and to increase the cytotoxicity of macrophages *(279,280)*, as well as to impair neutrophil chemotaxis *(281,282)*.

Engelhard et al. *(283)* described a disseminated visceral fusariosis in a patient with T-type acute lymphoblastic leukemia who responded completely to amphotericin B-phospholipid complex (dimyristoyl phosphatidylcholine and dimyristoyl phosphatidylglycerol in a 7:3 ratio) administered at daily doses of 1.0–4.0 mg/kg (total dose 4.2 g). Wolff and Ramphal *(284)* also used a lipid complex of amphotericin B (0.5 mg/kg daily; total 11.89 g) to resolve disseminated cutaneous infection in a neutropenic patient with acute myelogenous leukemia. Of the various lipid complexes, amphotericin B desoxycholate has been the most widely used in neutropenic patients. However, the infusion of amphotericin B desoxycholate has often been poorly tolerated, and toxic effects were common. The toxicity has limited the maximum tolerable dose of amphotericin B desoxycholate to 0.7–1.5 mg/kg daily, which, in turn, may be suboptimal for clinical success in the treatment of some filamentous fungal infections *(284)*.

Krulder et al. *(187)* reported a patient with lymphoblastic non-Hodgkin's lymphoma who acquired a systemic *F. nygamai* infection during the granulocytopenic phase of cytostatic treatment. The patient survived after hematologic recovery and treatment with intravenous amphotericin B (total dose 543 mg).

The prognosis of *F. moniliforme* fungemia in children with neuroblastoma has been generally poor *(285)*. However, in one case *(5)*, treatment with amphotericin B at 1.0 mg/kg daily (total 132 mg; 11 mg/kg) administered over 2 wk resulted in rapid defervescence without any localization of the infection.

Fusarium infections are being increasingly reported in immunocompromised patients (acute leukemia or solid tumors) with indwelling central venous catheters *(188,192,286)*. A combined therapeutic modality consisting of removal of the catheter and amphotericin B therapy has usually produced an excellent response *(188)*. The first case of a Port-a-cath-related disseminated fusariosis in an HIV-infected patient was presented by Eljaschewitsch et al. *(248)*. Treatment with liposomal amphotericin B (AmBisome®) at a daily dose of 2.0 mg/kg for 2 wk was successful.

In another first occurence, Mohammedi et al. *(220)* described disseminated *F. oxysporum* infection presenting with fungal myocarditis. Despite antifungal therapy and hematologic recovery, the patient died of cardiogenic shock, with the myocardial involvement clearly contributing to the fatal outcome.

Fusarium spp. have been recognized as one of the most common pathogens associated with fungal keratitis *(226,230,232,235,237–247,287–289)*. Cases of keratitis in contact lens wearers have also been increasing in numbers *(7,162,242,290–292)*.

Although several *Fusarium* species (*F. epiphaeria, F. dimerum, F. moniliforme, F. nivale, F. oxysporum,* and *F. solani*) can induce keratomycosis, *F. solani* has been the most prevalent pathogen of eye infections. *Fusaria* corneal ulcers, when diagnosed early and when treatment is started immediately, have shown good prognosis for recovery *(226)*. Superficial fungal keratitis may be treated easily, but a scar will often remain: a leukoma of variable size that would diminish vision. In several reports *(282,293–296)*, *Fusarium* keratitis has been successfully treated with pimaricin (natamycin) as 5% suspension *(230)* or unguent *(297)* with 0.001% dexamethasone and 2% potassium iodide *(294,298)* applied topically every 2 h until infection sibsided. Donnenfeld et al. *(289)* reported a *Fusarium*-induced corneal perforation associated with corneal hydrops and contact lens wear in keratoconus.

Rowsey et al. *(225)* described a patient with *F. oxysporum* endophthalmitis, which responded to a combination treatment of vitrectomy, intravitreal and intravenous amphotericin B, and oral flucytosine. In order to prevent retinal necrosis, it was recommended that intravitreal amphotericin B (5.0 µg) be injected slowly into the midvitreous with a needle bevel toward the lens in a 0.1-mL volume *(225)*. With a vitreous volume of 4.0 mL, a central vitreous concentration of possibly 1.5 µg/mL of amphotericin B would be expected, which would be much higher than that available to the vitreous via the intravenous route alone *(299)*.

Patients with *Fusarium* keratitis have been known to develop endophthalmitis by direct extension from the corneal ulcer. However, Lieberman et al. *(224)* reported a case of an immunocompetent host in which *Fusarium* endophthalmitis developed without apparent primary corneal involvement, suggesting an endogenous origin (hematogenous spread following inhalation of fungal spores) of the infection. There have been a number of reports of endogenous endophthalmitis, which has been increasingly recognized in susceptible individuals *(228,229,231,233,300,301)*. For example, a bilateral endogenous *Fusarium* endophthalmitis was diagnosed in a patient with AIDS and cytomegalovirus (CMV) endophthalmitis; histopathologic examination showed a severe necrotizing acute and granulomatous reaction, with numerous fungal elements in the retina and uveal tract *(228)*. Despite intravitreous (two injections of 15 µg) and systemic (cumulative dose of 770 mg) treatment with amphotericin B and fluconazole therapy, the patient's endophthalmitis and mental status worsened and he died from disseminated fungal infection of the brain, lung, kidney, thyroid, and lymph nodes *(228)*. Disruption of the blood-retinal barriers from angiopathic findings related to AIDS or concurrent CMV retinitis may have contributed to the retinal involvement *(302)*.

In another case *(229)*, an intravenous drug abuser who had developed unilateral retinal infiltrates and retinal vasculopathy was successfully treated by a combination of pars plana vitrectomy and intravitreal and intravenous amphotericin B.

Fusarium-induced peritonitis associated with continuous ambulatory peritoneal dialysis (CAPD) has been reported on several occasions *(214–216,303)*. Successful treatment usually involved therapy with intravenous amphotericin B coupled with removal of the catheter *(214,216)*.

In another case of successful use of intravenous amphotericin B, an 8-wk course of the antibiotic (total dose of 1.76 g) was combined with repeated aspirations to resolve septic arthritis (finger joint infection) due to *F. solani* *(211)*.

Kurien et al. *(219)* described the first known cases of *F. solani* infections of the maxillary sinus with granuloma and oro-antral fistula in two immunocompetent hosts. Both patients responded to oral ketoconazole (200 mg daily) for 3 wk followed by a Caldwell-Luc operation. Ketoconazole was continued for 2 mo postoperatively. Successful use of oral ketoconazole has also been reported by Landau et al. *(304)* in a patient with leg ulcers due to *F. oxysporum*, by Baudraz-Rosselet et al. *(205)* in a patient with foot mycetoma, and by Ooi et al. *(206)* in the treatment of granuloma annulare-like skin lesion due to *F. roseum*.

A case of *Fusarium* eumycetoma that lasted for 18 yr improved significantly after 6 mo of oral itraconazole therapy (the initial dose of 100 mg daily was increased to 200 mg after 2 mo) *(305)*.

4.2. Fusarium napiforme

Melcher et al. *(176)* reported the first human hyalohyphomucosis caused by *Fusarium napiforme*, a species first isolated only from soil and grain in southern Africa and later in Australia. The distinguished clinical mycological characteristics of this opportunistic mold include unique turnip- or lemon-shaped microconidia. The case involved a patient previously diagnosed with acute myelogenous leukemia further complicated by pulmonary aspergillosis. The hyalohyphomycosis was disseminated and similar to other *Fusarium* infections.

5. *PHIALEMONIUM* SPP. INFECTIONS

Species of the genus *Phialemonium* spp. are pheoid fungi that cause lesions observed in both phaeo- and hyalohyphomycosis. Established in 1983 by Gams and McGinnis to accommodate selected hyphomycetes, *Phialemonium* represents an intermediate genus between *Acremonium* and *Phialophora (306)*. Initially, three species have been classified as belonging to the genus: *P. obovatum*, *P. curvatum*, and *P. dimorphosporum*.

In humans, *Phialemonium* are considered to be opportunistic pathogens that affect mainly the immunosuppressed population *(307–309)*. Recently, Heins-Vaccari et al. *(307)* described a *P. curvatum* lesions in a patient with multiple myeloma who had received an allogenic bone-marrow transplant. The infections underwent a 4-mo treatment with amphotericin B followed by ketoconazole, and surgical debridement; second prophylaxis with ketoconazole alone was maintained for an additional month, and no recurrence was observed. Previously, *P. curvatum* was isolated from the blood of two immunosuppressed patients, one of whom died; the second survived after successful treatment with itraconazole *(308)*.

P. obovatum was first reported to be an opportunistic fungus by McGinnis et al. *(310)*. The pathogen was isolated from cutaneous and subcutaneous tissues obtained from thermal burn wounds antemortem and from spleen tissue and three burn sites postmortem. Later, King et al. *(309)* described a *Phialemonium* spp. phaeohyphomycotic cyst in a renal-transplant recipient; surgical excision resolved the case without the need of antifungal therapy. In a second case from the same report, another renal-transplant recipient developed *P. obovatum* peritonitis; the patient was given intravenous amphotericin B for a total of 11 doses and oral ketoconazole for 4 d, which was later substituted with oral flucytosine until repeated peritoneal fluid cultures yielded no growth *(309)*.

6. *ACREMONIUM* SPP. INFECTIONS

Acremonium spp. are widespread fungi (soil, plant debris, rotting mushrooms) that have been increasingly associated with human infections *(311,312)*. Teleomorphs (perfect state) of *Acremonium* are found in several genera of ascomycetes such as *Emericellopsis*, *Hapsidospora*, *Nectria*, *Nectriella*, and *Pronectria*.

Although known for a long time, the *Acremonium* spp. often have not been reliably identified *(311,313,314)*. Thus, the name *Cephalosporium acremonium* of the genus *Cephalosporium*, has been applied to many different fungi; in most medical cases it was meant to imply *Acremonium kiliense*. Even today, the name *Cephalosporium acremonium* is still being used in the literature in reference to *Acremonium chrysogenum*, the source of the antibiotic cephalosporin. In another example of misidentification, *Cephalosporium serrae (315)* is currently considered to be a synonym for *Verticillium nigrescens (311)*.

Presently, all medically relevant fungi from this complex are identified as species of *Acremonium* or *Phialemonium (316)*. However, in view of the high degree of similarity between *Acremonium* and *Phialemonium (309)* as well as some other genera (*Fusarium*, *Cylindrocarpon*, and to a lesser degree *Lecythophora*), it is still possible that misidentification of some clinical isolates can occur.

Among the *Acremonium* spp., *A. kiliense* is the most frequent cause of human hyalohyphomycosis *(317–320)*. Other species associated with human disease include *A. strictum (321–324)*, *A. falciforme (325–334)*, *A. alabamense (335)*, *A. blochii*, *A. potronii (336,337)*, *A. atrogriseum (338)*, and *A. recifei (311,336,339–341)*.

The majority of reported infections produced by *Acremonium* spp. are mycetomas *(328,331–334,341,342)* and ocular infections *(317,318,326,327,336–338,340,343,344)*, and in recent years, localized (osteomyelitis, sinusitis, arthritis *[345]*, and peritonitis) or disseminated (pneumonia *[346,347]*, meningitis, endocarditis *[320,348]*, and cerebritis *[335]*) infections *(312)*. In a number of reports, cases of cutaneous *(319,349,350)*, subcutaneous *(330,339)*, and nail invasion *(351,352)* by *Acremonium* spp. have been described.

Immunosuppression is considered to be the main predisposing factor for *Acremonium* spp. infections *(329,353)* although immunocompetent persons could also be affected *(319,323,339)*. The majority of the disseminated infections have occurred in neutropenic *(321,324,350,354)* and immunosuppressed patients such as organ-transplant recipients *(325,330,333,355)*, those with myeloma or leukemia *(323,346)*, and patients receiving corticosteroid therapy; approximately half of the reported cases had a fatal outcome *(311,321)*.

Amphotericin B is the drug of choice for *Acremonium* hyalohyphomycosis. Other antifungal therapies included the use of flucytosin, fluconazole, miconazole, ketoconazole, itraconazole, and G-CSF most often in combination with surgical debridement *(323,340)*. However, in two cases of *Acremonium* keratitis, the infections were resolved with penetrating keratoplasty *(336–338)* after treatment with amphotericin B was unsuccessful *(336)*. Similarly, Weissgold et al. *(317)* also reported that in postoperative management of cataract surgery with delayed-onset *A. kiliense* endophthalmitis, the infection was recalcitrant to single-dose intravenous amphotericin B injections.

Combination therapy consisting of systemic itraconazole and terbinafine, topical terbinafine after nail-plate avulsion, and ciplopirox nail lacquer, was able to resolve *Acremonium* spp. onychomycosis in only 71.4% of patients *(351)* .

A 2-mo course of oral itraconazole (200 mg, daily) was successful in a case of subcutaneous *A. recifei* hyalohyphomycosis in an immunocompetent patient *(339)*. Oral itraconazole was also successful in resolving a case of *A. falciforme* mycetoma lesions *(328)*.

7. *SCOPULARIOPSIS* SPP. INFECTIONS

Scopulariopsis species were first described in 1907 *(356)*. Upon histological examination, these fungi, which are virtually identical to the *Aspergillus* spp. and very similar to *Penicillium* species, display as a primary feature broom-shaped conidiophores (seen only in culture) *(357)*.

Species indentified as human pathogens include *S. brevicaulis (358–362)*, *S. brumptii (358,362–366)*, *S. candida (358,362,363)*, *S. carbonaria (358,362,363)*, *S. fusca (358,362)*, and *S. coniingii (358,362,363)*, *S. brumptii* has been isolated from pulmonary nodules in an intravenous opium user with hypersensitivity pneumonitis *(366)*. A disseminated infection caused by *S. candida* has been diagnosed in a leukemic patient *(358)*.

Scopulariopsis spp. have been most frequently associated with onychomycosis, cutaneous, and subcutaneous infections *(358,362,367)*, and only in the last two decades or so with deep-tissue infections *(172,358,362,368–371)*, and ocular infections *(372–376)*.

Deep invasive infections with *Scopulariopsis* spp. such as invasive fungal sinusitis (which typically affects immunocompromised patients, those on intensive immunosuppressive chemotherapy and bone-marrow transplant recipients), are usually associated with a high mortality rate *(172,357,358,369,371)*.

7.1. Scopulariopsis brevicaulis

Scopulariopsis brevicaulis is a common nondermatophyte mold primarily known for causing onychomycosis *(351,359,362,377–381)*, cutaneous *(382–385)* and subcutaneous, and generalized infections, especially in immunocompromised patients *(357,360,385–388)*. Well-documented cases of invasive disease caused by *S. brevicaulis* include pneumonia and ear infections in leukemic patients *(358,370)*, a deeply necrotic lesion in the toe of a patient with aplastic anemia *(357)*, a subcutaneous infection involving an ankle *(389)*, and postulated skin lesions in both AIDS *(385)* and immunocompetent *(384)* patients.

Morphologic studies by Filipello Marchisio et al. *(361)* have shown that only 3 of 9 isolates of *S. brevicaulis* examined were keratinolytic by enzymatic digestion, demonstrating a rather low extent and rate of keratinolysis when compared with the efficiency of other keratinolytic fungi.

Although initially indicated for dermatophyte infections, terbinafine was found active against a broad spectrum of filamentous and dimorphic fungi, in most cases with a primary fungicidal action

(386). In addition, this allylamine antimycotic was also synergistic with azole antifungal agents against *S. brevicaulis* as well as *Candida* isolates and various non-*Candida* dematiaceous fungi *(390)*.

Itraconazole, when given either as continuous dosing (100 or 200 mg, daily) for 6–20 wk or as a 1-wk pulse dosing (200 mg b.i.d. for 1 wk per month) for 2–4 pulses, proved efficacious in the treatment of *S. brevicaulis* toenail onychomycosis *(377)*.

A granulomatous skin infection caused by *S. brevicaulis* was successfully treated with itraconazole and terbinafine for 19 mo; however, a relapse occurred 10 mo later *(391)*.

In a prospective, comparative, parallel-group, single-blind, randomized trial, the efficacy of itraconazole (pulse therapy given for 3 pulses, with each pulse consisting of 200 mg, b.i.d. for 1 wk with 3 wk off between successive pulses), terbinafine (250 mg, daily for 12 wk), fluconazole (150 mg, daily for 12 wk), griseofulvin (600 mg, b.i.d. for 1 yr), and ketoconazole (200 mg, daily for 4 mo) were evaluated in patients with *S. brevicaulis* toe onychomycosis. Overall, itraconazole and terbinafine have demonstrated efficacy in only some patients, whereas griseofulvine was found to be ineffective. With the availability of newer and more potent antifungal agents, ketoconazole and fluconazole are not recommended for toe onychomycosis given their potential to cause hepatic dysfunction and severe gastrointestinal events, respectively *(359)*.

In another disappointing report involving *S. brevicaulis* onychomycosis, three patients were treated with 4 pulses of itraconazole (400 mg, daily for 1 wk a month) and three patients received terbinafine at 250 mg, daily for 4 mo. Following mycological examination 8 mo after discontinuation of therapy, only one patient showed mycological cure, whereas the remaining five patients still carried *S. brevicaulis* in their nails *(378)*.

Treatment of *S. brevicaulis* plantar infection with itraconazole led to temporary improvement, but symptoms returned after treatment ceased; similar results were obtained with oral terbinafine *(383)*. However, according to Creus et al. *(392)* administration of itraconazole produced a dramatic and definitive cure of ulcerous granulomatous cheilitis with lymphatic invasion due to *S. brevicaulis*.

Local treatment of seven patients with toenail *S. brevicaulis* onychomycosis with 1% natamycin in 60% dimethylsulphoxide (DMSO) was largely successful in resolving the infection; the treatment of only one patient was ineffective *(381)*.

Miconazole, an imidazole antifungal agent, was used to treat a subcutaneous *Scopulariopsis* infection that progressed despite treatment with amphotericin B and itraconazole *(393)*. However, after intravenous miconazole was added to the regimen, the patient developed bradyarrhythmia, which progressed to ventricular fibrillation and death. The miconazole-induced cardiac arrhythmia was likely due to rapid intravenous administration, insufficient dilution, and the nature of the drug's vehicle, all important factors to consider in patients with underlying heart disease *(393)*.

Arrese et al. *(372)* described a case of unusual mold infection of human stratum corneum (unilateral scaly plantar lesions) by *S. brevicaulis (372)*. Another unusual case involved a posttraumatic fungal endophthalmitis resulting from *S. brevicaulis (373)*.

A case of fungal keratitis due to *S. brevicaulis* was successfully treated with topical amphotericin B and chloramphenicol without the need for surgical debridement *(374)*. Del Prete et al. *(375)* described fungal keratitis caused by *S. brevicaulis* in an eye previously suffering from herpetic keratitis; topical and oral administration of miconazole and scraping of the corneal infiltrate dispersed the infection *(375)*.

Migrino et al. *(387)* reported a fatal case of endocarditis caused by *S. brevicaulis*; the infection persisted despite two aortic valve replacements, debridement, and prolonged therapy with several antifungal agents. In another reported case of *S. brevicaulis* endocarditis, the infection was associated with Duran ring valvuloplasty *(394)*. To treat fungal prosthetic valve endocarditis, Muehrcke et al. *(395)* developed a strategy of treatment involving preoperative amphotericin B, radical debridement of infected tissue, reconstruction using biologic tissue whenever possible, and lifelong oral suppressive antifungal therapy.

7.2. Scopulariopsis acremonium

Scopulariopsis acremonium represents a saprophytic fungus only recently reported to cause invasive infection in humans. Ellison et al. *(368)* decribed a patient with acute myeloblastic leukemia who presented with invasive *S. acremonium* sinusitis shortly after completing a second course of chemotherapy. The case was resolved following definitive endoscopic sinus surgery including middle turbinate resection. The organism was found to be resistant in vitro to amphotericin B and fluconazole but sensitive to ketoconazole and itraconazole.

8. *MICROASCUS* SPP. INFECTIONS

The genus *Microascus* represents ascomycetous fungi whose identification is based primarily on the size and shape of the sexual fruiting structure (the perithecium) and its ascospores. Several *Microascus* species also display *Scopulariopsis* anamorphs (asexual forms), some of which are dematiaceous. Common *Microascus* spp. with dematiaceous *Scopulariopsis* anamorphs include *M. cinereus*, *M. cirrosus*, and *M. trigonosporus*. Conversely, the dematiaceous *Scopulariopsis* species *S. brumptii* did not appear to be associated with any known *Microascus* species *(396)*. Therefore, it is important, whenever a *Scopulariopsis* species is isolated, to consider the possibility of an associated *Microascus* teleomorph (the sexual stage) and to hold cultures for up to 6 wk for mature ascospore formation.

Other *Microascus* species that have been isolated from clinical specimens (mostly diseased skin, nail, and lung tissue) but with no evidence of pathogenicity, include *M. manginii*, and *M. lunasporus (397,398)*.

8.1. Microascus cinereus

Microascus cinereus is one of the most common 14 described species of *Microascus*. It has been recovered from soil *(399,400)* and stored grains (oats and corn) *(401)*.

M. cinereus is relatively uncommon in humans and animals, and has only recently been described by Marques et al. *(402)* as the sole pathogen of an invasive human infection causing chronic suppurative cutaneous granulomata in a patient with chronic granulomatous disease. The skin lesions appeared on the chest, back, and arm. After the patient was treated with 2.5 g of intravenous amphotericin B, the lesions resolved.

Baddley et al. *(396)* reported the first documented case of brain abscess caused by *M. cinereus* in a bone-marrow transplant recipient. The patient, who responded well to treatment with amphotericin B lipid complex (5.0 mg/kg, daily), itraconazole (400 mg, daily), and craniotomy, later died from secondary complications caused by graft-vs-host disease.

8.2. Microascus cirrosis

Microascus cirrosis Curzi represents the teleomorph (sexual, perfect form), whereas the dematiaceous *Scopulariopsis* sp. is its associated anamorph. This species, which is of interest because of its ability to cause invasive infection, is also dimatiaceous in both of its forms. Culturally, *M. cirrosis* is very close to *M. cinereus*, but differs in the darker color and less-stable habit.

Krisher et al. *(403)* isolated *M. corrosis* Curzi and its associated anamorphic state *Scopulariopsis* from the cutaneous lesion of a pediatric autologous bone-marrow transplant recipient in what appeared to be the first documented human infection by this species. The skin lesion resolved following treatment with liposomal amphotericin B (Amphocil) initiated at 6.0 mg/kg daily.

9. *PAECILOMYCES* SPP. INFECTIONS

The genus *Paecilomyces* represents asexual saprophytic molds related to *Penicillium* (Link) and *Aspergillus* and found worldwide in decaying vegetation and soil. It is thought by some investigators that *Paecilomyces* is the imperfect stage of the ascomycete *Byssochlamys (404–406)*.

P. lilacinus and *P. variotii*, the two most common *Paecilomyces* species causing human infections, are also emerging as serious opportunistic pathogens. *P. lilacinus* was found to be a contaminant in sterile solutions *(406–410)*. Two other species, *P. marquandii (411)* and *P. javanicus*, have also been associated with human disease.

Host vulnerability as a result of immunosuppression or therapies that involve surgical procedures *(412)* (organ *[413–416]* and bone-marrow *[417,418]* transplantations) and the use of prostethic materials *(419–422)* (or implants *[423]*) is generally considered to be an important predisposing factor for these opportunistic pathogens *(408,415,420,423,424)*. The association of *Paecilomyces* infections with prosthetic implants and surgery is remarkable and may be related to the resistance of the mature fungal conidia to most sterilization techniques. A Swiss epidemic in severely immunosuppressed patients (hematologic malignancies and transplant recipients) was traced to contaminated skin lotion *(425,426)*.

The most common site of *Paecilomyces* infection is the eye and the eye structures *(10,332,340,407,408,415,427–446)*. Skin and soft-tissue infections in immunocompromised hosts constitute the second largest group of human infections caused by *Paecilomyces* *(413,414,416,425,441,446–457)*.

Because *Paecilomyces* spp. have been implicated as the cause of allergic alveolitis in patients living in substandard urban dwellings in proximity to decaying wood, the possibility has been raised that inhalation of fungal spores into the lungs may be a likely route of parenchymal infection *(458)*. Cell-mediated granulomatous inflammation of the pulmonary parenchyma without pneumonia has resulted from chronic alveolitis *(459)*.

The *Paecilomyces* spp. are well-known for their resistance to sterilization methods leading to contamination of sterile solutions *(560–562)*. A major *P. lilacinus* endophthalmitis outbreak, which was registered in the United States *(407,408,442,445,463)*, was ultimately traced to a contaminated batch of neutralizing solution used to rinse the lenses during surgery *(408,445)*.

Increasingly, however, *Paecilomyces* spp. are being recognized as potential pathogens in immunocompromised hosts *(415,420,425,439,450,464,465)*, such as transplant recipients *(411,415,416,456)*, and patients with chronic granulomatous disease (CGD) *(466,466,467)*. CGD is a heterogenous group of disorders characterized by impaired ability of neutrophils to produce bactericidal and fungicidal oxygen metabolites (hydrogen peroxide, hypochlorous acid) necessary for killing catalase-positive organisms *(468–473)*.

Although rare, human *Paecilomyces* infections may also proceed with high morbidity and often with fatal outcome *(474)*. Thus, to date all reported cases of *Paecilomyces* endocarditis have had a fatal outcome *(422,456,475–479)*.

Specifically, *Paecilomyces* spp. have been associated with often lethal endocarditis after valve replacement *(422,475–479)*, mycotic infections of the skin *(416,439,457,480,481)*, keratitis *(432)*, onychomycosis *(482,483)*, pleural effusion, pneumonia *(464,484–487)* and lung abscesses *(488)*, sinusitis *(447,489–494)*, a lacrimal sac infection *(495)*, endophthalmitis *(407,408,429,442, 445,473,496)*, otitis media *(497)*, pyelonephritis *(498)*, a fatal case of ventriculoperitoneal shunt *(421)*, peritonitis in patients receiving CAPD *(419,499–501)*, and catheter-related fungemia *(418,420)*. In a unique case, Okhravi et al. *(430)* documented a progression to stromal keratitis from endogenous endophthalmitis secondary to *P. lilacinus*. This report highlights the difficulty of diagnosing endogenous fungal endophthalmitis presenting without risk factors and the difficulties of managing such cases using the antifungal agents presently available.

After analyzing data affecting 190 patients (aged 3–70 yr) with bronchial asthma in *Paecilomyces* infection, Akhunova *(502)* concluded that these fungi might play the role of a specific agent responsible for the development of bacterial asthma. It has been postulated that bronchial asthma may be provoked by a combination of hypersensitivity with participation of IgE defending the organism from the fungi persisting in the blood and pulmonary tissue, and biologically active substances produced by the fungal cells (exogenous phospholipase A2, in particular) *(502)*.

Hyalohyphomycosis

Suppression of cell-mediated immunity is one of the predisposing factors for infection *(464)*. In the case of patients with diabetes mellitus, the impaired activity and reduced concentration of the α-1 protease inhibitor (an endogenous lung antiprotease), may have a bearing on the ability of *Paecilomyces* spp., normally fungi with low pathogenicity, to infect the lung parenchyma *(503)*.

9.1. Treatment of Paecilomyces Infections

Results from in vitro susceptibility testing in animal models and humans *(408,409,440,445, 465,477)* have clearly indicated certain susceptibility trends. Thus, some *Paecilomyces* spp. (*P. lilacinus* and *P. marquandii*) have been found to be highly resistant to polyene antibiotics (amphotericin B) and flucytosine, while *P. variotii* was sensitive to both amphotericin B and flucytosine *(409,440,465)*. Because of such different sensitivities, species identification is important for the clinical outcome of the disease *(465)*. Although the in vitro susceptibilities of *Paecilomyces* spp. to various antifungal agents have been determined *(477,484)*, the lack of standartization and clinical correlation has markedly limited their usefulness *(504)*.

In clinical settings, amphotericin B has been widely used to treat *Paecilomyces* spp. infections. However, the clinical management of *Paecilomyces* hyalphyphomycosis may be complicated by reports that two species, *P. lilacinus* and *P. marquandii*, have shown high resistance to many antifungal drugs including amphotericin B and flucytosine *(415,426,452,456,476,489)*. Chan-Tack et al. *(417)* managed the successful clearance of *P. lilacinus* fungemia in a non-neutropenic bone-marrow transplant recipient, despite in vitro resistance to both amphotericin B and flucytosine. Similarly, a pediatric patient with CGD and abdominal-wall abscesses caused by *P. lilacinus* responded to treatment with amphotericin B *(466)*. On the other hand, *P. variotii* appeared to be universally susceptible to both amphotericin B and flucytosine *(415,456)*.

Itraconazole has been shown to converge in soft tissue collections of pus, making it particularly useful in the treatment of soft tissue infections *(505)*.

A case of *Paecilomyces* spp. keratitis was treated successfully with a combination of topical natamycin, intravenous miconazole (400 mg daily, for a total of 9.6 g over a 24-d period), a temporary conjunctival flap, and penetrating keratoplasty *(432)*.

9.1.1. Paecilomyces lilacinus

In a recent report, Domniz et al. *(427)* described successful treatment of *P. lilacinus* endophthalmitis by starting with an intravitreal injection of 50 µg/0.5 mL amphotericin B during the vitreal biopsy, then following with oral itraconazole (200 mg, b.i.d.), 5% topical natamycin every hour, 2.0 mg/mL of topical fluconazole every 2 h, three anterior chamber injections of 0.35 mL of 0.1%, and two amphotericin B injections to the interior chamber of 50 µg/mL each. Similarly, a case of *P. lilacinus* endophthalmitis was resolved with early vitrectomy, multiple intravitreal injections of ampho tericin B and miconazole, intravenous miconazole, and later oral itraconazole *(438)*.

Cutaneous *P. lilacinus* hyalohyphomycosis was successfully treated with a prolonged course of itraconazole (200 mg, daily for 3 mo) *(448)*.

Endoscopic sinus surgery combined with oral itraconazole for 6 mo effectively resolved a case of pansinusitis in an 8-yr-old child *(447)*.

P. lilacinus sinusitis in a patient with acute myeloid leukemia was resolved after surgical debridement and chemotherapy with amphotericin B and itraconazole (400 mg, daily) *(489)*.

In an earlier case, a child with CGD developed two unusual abdominal-wall abscesses due to *P. lilacinus*, an organism previously not known to cause infections in patients with CGD *(466)*. Contrary to the previously reported resistance of *P. lilacinus* to amphotericin B, the patient responded well to a 2-mo course of this antibiotic at initial daily doses of 0.5 mg/kg for 3 wk, followed by 1.0 mg/kg dose given 3 times weekly (total dose of 825 mg).

9.1.2. Paecilomyces variotii

Contrary to *P. lilanicus*-associated infections, the management of hyalohyphomycosis due to *P. variotii* is less problematic because of its susceptibility to antifungal chemotherapy with amphotericin B and itraconazole *(418)*, surgical intervention *(412)*, or the removal of prosthetic devices in combination with chemotherapy *(419,475)*.

A pediatric patient with chronic granulomatous disease was successfully treated with a 7-wk course of amphotericin B (0.8 mg/kg, daily for a total dose of 10 mg/kg), followed by 1 yr of therapy with itraconazole (100 mg, b.i.d.) *(456)*.

A case of *P. variotii* chronic suppurative otitis media responded to topical ketoconazole therapy *(497)*. In another report, *P. variotii* pyelonephritis complicating nephrolithiasis was resolved after therapy with cefamandole and tobramycin *(498)*.

Early removal of the dialysis catheter, intravenous amphotericin B or oral ketoconazole were used in the successful management of *P. variotii*-associated peritonitis in patients receiving CAPD *(419,501)*. *P. variotii* peritonitis in an infant on automated peritoneal dialysis was successfully treated with combined intraperitoneal and oral fluconazole, without removal of the peritoneal catheter *(500)*.

Byrd et al. *(464)* presented the first case of *P. variotii* pneumonia in a patient with diabetes mellitus as predisposing factor. The pneumonia responded poorly to oral ketoconazole (400 mg daily for 3 mo), and the chronic infiltrating process required administration of amphotericin B via a Hickman catheter to resolve.

9.1.3. Post-Transplantation Therapy of Paecilomyces Infections

The isolation of filamentous fungi with variable in vitro susceptibility to currently available antifungal drugs further complicates the therapeutic approach to post-transplantation antifungal treatment *(413,506)*.

Hilmarsdottir et al. *(414)* described cutaneous *P. lilacinus* hyalohyphomycosis in a renal-transplant recipient who responded to voriconazole treatment. *P. lilacinus*-associated hyalohy-phomycosis in a renal-transplant patient also responded well to oral griseofulvin (500 mg, daily) given for 45 d *(415)*. Oral griseofulvin has also been used successfully in an earlier case of skin infection by *P. lilacinus (457)*.

A heart-transplant recipient with *P. lilacinus* infection was successfully treated with terbinafine *(507)*. In another case of post-transplant infection, *P. variotii* was isolated from the airways of a pediatric patient with cystic fibrosis (CF) who underwent bilateral living-donor lobar lung transplantation *(508)*.

A case of *P. lilacinus* fungemia in a non-neutropenic adult, 120 d after bone-marrow transplant was cleared after treatment with amphotericin B and 5-FC despite in vitro resistance to these antifungal agents *(417)*.

Shing et al. *(418)* described a case of *P. variotii* catheter-related fungemia in an allogeneic bone-marrow transplant recipient receiving antifungal prophylaxis with fluconazole (50 mg daily). The successful treatment was achieved by removal of the central venous catheter and intravenous infusion of amphotericin B (initially at 0.5 mg/kg [11 mg, daily], followed by an increase to 1.0 mg/kg [23 mg/kg, daily] on d 14). Because of renal toxicity, amphotericin B was discontinued after 40 d of treatment and the therapy switched to oral itraconazole at 100 mg daily for 3 mo.

10. ACROPHIALOPHORA FUSISPORA INFECTIONS

Acrophialophora fusispora of the genus *Acrophialophora* was originally placed in the genus *Paecilomyces*. The genus *Acrophialophora* was first described by Edward in 1959 with the type species *A. nainiana* that was repeatedly recovered from Indian soil during the summer months *(509)*. The *Acrophialophora* species are considered similar to *Paecilomyces* in forming chains of ellipsoidal to fusiform conidia from basically swollen phialides that were borne either on conidiophores or directly from the vegetative hyphae, but differ in having colonies that become dark and in the development of phialides along the sides or at the tips of echinulate brown conidiophores *(510)*. Presently, *A. nainiana* and *A. levis* are considered as synonyms of *A. fusispora*.

A. fusispora is a thermotolerant, fast-growing fungus with a neurotropic potential and wide distribution in tropical and temperate regions growing well at 45°C or higher temperatures. It has been reported once from a human corneal infection *(511)* and implicated in disseminated infection involving the brain in two dogs *(512)*.

In 2000, al-Mohsen et al. *(428)* have described the first case of human cerebral brain abscess due to *A. fusispora* in a pediatric patient with acute lymphoblastic leukemia. The initial treatment included liposomal amphotericin B (6.0 mg/kg, daily, then increased to 10 mg/kg, daily), followed by the addition of itraconazole (7.5 mg/kg, daily); the patient also received G-CSF (5.0 µg/kg, daily) as adjunctive therapy. After clinical and radiological improvement (concomitant reduction in size of the brain abscess and resolution of the lung nodules) was achieved 8 mo later, amphotericin B was discontinued and itraconazole (15 mg/kg, daily) was given as suppressive therapy.

11. *ENGYODONTIUM ALBUM* INFECTIONS

Engyodontium album is a rather common inhabitant of waste and moist material, being relatively frequently isolated from paper, jute, linen, and painted walls. *E. album* may be considered as emerging opportunistic pathogen causing hyalohyphomycosis.

Over the past, its taxonomic status has undergone several changes. Initially it was included in the genus *Beauveria* (and known as *Beauveria alba*) but later transferred to the genus *Triticarchium*. Since 1978, a new genus, *Engyodontium* has been established with two species, *E. album* and *E. parvisporum (513)*. Later, Gams et al. *(514)* extended the genus *Engyodontium* to include six species. The *Engyodontium* species are characterized as having a denticulate rachis, conidiogenous cells in whorls, and colonies with no pigmentation. Using exoantigenic extracts, Sekhon et al. *(515)* established clear antigenic distinctness between *E. album* and the pathogenic *Beauveria bastiana* and other nonpathogenic species of the genus *Beauveria*. *E. album* is separated from *Triticarchium* species by its lack of pigmentation.

Augustinsky et al. *(516)* described the first case of native valve endocarditis due to *E. album*. Predisposing factors include the presence of a prosthetic valve or severe underlying valvular heart disease. Despite aggressive therapy with vancomycin and amphotericin B, the patient died.

Previously, infections reported to be caused by *E. album* included keratitis *(517)*, brain abscess *(518)*, and eczema vesiculosum *(519)*.

12. *BEAUVERIA BASSIANA* INFECTIONS

Fungi of the genus *Beauveria* are known as insect pathogens inhabiting the soil. This genus holds the distinction of being the first microorganism (back in 1835) shown to be pathogenic producing the muscardine dieases of silkworm *(520)*. Morphologically *Beauveria bassiana*, which is closely associated with the genus *Engyodontium* (*see above*), showed a characteristic zigzag configuration of the spore-bearing tip.

Beauveria bassiana has been very rarely reported to cause human infections. First, Freour et al. *(521)* described a case of pulmonary disease in young adult patient in whom *B. bassiana* was isolated from surgically excised lung tissue, and later, Drouhet et al. *(522)* reported a case of osteoarthritis caused by *Beauveria* sp. In 1985, Sachs et al. *(523)* isolated *B. bassiana* from the cornea of a patient that underwent progressive thinning following removal of a foreign body and after treatment with topical antibiotics and corticosteroids.

13. NON-*CANDIDA* MYCOSES AFTER SOLID ORGAN AND BONE-MARROW TRANSPLANTATIONS

In addition to *Candida* spp., *Aspergillus* and other non-*Candida* spp. have emerged as important causes of morbidity and mortality in patients with severe underlying diseases and compromised host immune defenses *(531,532)*, especially in solid organ and bone-marrow transplant recipients *(26,35,76,140,147,172,524–530)*.

The high incidence of mycoses has been related to multiple factors, such as prolonged granulocytopenia, broad-spectrum antimicrobial therapy known to permit fungal colonization and disrupt normal mucosal barriers, radiotherapy, and the use of central venous access devices. In addition, graft-vs-host disease (GVHD) and impaired cell-mediated immunity due to primary disease or its therapy have also contributed to the high frequency of fungal infections among these patients, especially after bone-marrow transplantation *(172,524)*. Thus, neutrophil dysfunction has been characterized after bone-marrow transplantation in patients with and without GVHD *(533)*. Treatment of GVHD, usually with prednisone and/or azathioprine, has been known to increase the degree of immunosuppression, thereby contributing to the neutrophil disorder. The latter, coupled with impairment of the lymphocyte functions after bone marrow transplantation *(534)* would create optimal host environment for the acquisition of fungal infections and their dissemination from sites that are only surface-colonized *(196)*.

Historically, *Candida* spp. have been the most frequently isolated fungi, followed by *Aspergillus* spp. *(535–539)*. However, in addition to an expending number of Zygomycetes, previously uncommon hyaline filamentous fungi (*Fusarium, Acremonium, Phialemonium, Pseudollescheria, Paecilomyces*, and *Scedosporium* spp.), dematiaceous filamentous fungi (*Cladophialophora bantiana, Dactylaria gallopava*, and *Bipolaris, Exophiala, Curvularia*, and *Alternaria* spp.) *(531,532)*, other non-*Candida* opportunistic fungi, including *Penicillium, Mucor, Histoplasma, Malassezia, Phialophora, Rhodotorula, Acremonium, Trichosporon, Moraxella*, and *Torulopsis* spp., have also emerged as invasive opportunistic agents in patients who underwent solid and bone-marrow organ transplantation *(13,26,76,140,147,195,172,174,196,265,524,525,527–529,540–546)*.

To determine the incidence, risk factors, and outcome of non-*Candida* fungal infections in the bone-marrow transplant population, Morrison et al. *(172,524)* studied a consecutive series of 1,186 patients from 1974–1989. The risk factors were analyzed with regard to clinical characteristics, such as age, sex, primary disease process, type of transplant, recipient cytomegalovirus (CMV) serostatus, time to engraftment, and the presence of graft-vs-host disease. The results of the study have shown that 10% of the patients (123 of 1,186) developed a non-*Candida* fungal infection within 180 d of transplant surgery. The majority of infections (85%) occured in allogeneic recipients, and 58% of patients were infected prior to white blood cell engraftment. Among the various non-*Candida* fungal pathogens, *Aspergillus* spp. were the most common isolates (70%), followed by *Fusarium* spp. (8%), and *Alternaria* spp. (5%). The percentages of single organ (or site) and dessiminated infections were similar (47 and 44%, respectively), whereas fungemia was observed in only 9% of patients. One of the discouraging statistics has been the mortality rate; only 17% of patients survived, with 68% of deaths related to the fungal infection. Furthermore, death was caused by a non-*Candida* fungus in 83% of those patients who died from fungal infections. Limited infections, such as fungemia, had the best clinical outcome, followed by infections of a single organ, whereas dessiminated infections were nearly all fatal. Among the different non-*Candida* species, *Aspergillus, Fusarium*, and *Scedosporium prolificans* have been the more virulent, more invasive, and therefore, highly likely to cause dessiminated and fatal infections *(140,172,524)*. Fungi that have the tendency to cause either localized infections (*Alternaria*) or isolated fungemia without disseminated disease (*Acremonium* spp., *Penicillium, Malassezia, Moraxella*) were associated with a better outcome *(172,524)*.

By invariate analysis, the allogeneic transplant, positive recipient CMV serostatus, delayed engraftment, and the recipient of greater than or equal to 18 yr, were identified as the major risk factors for non-*Candida* fungal infections *(172,524)*. The increased occurence of opportunistic mycoses in the allogeneic bone-marrow transplant population was likely related to the more intense preparative regimen and the more profound immunosuppressive effect of allografting. The increased risk among CMV-seropositive patients of developing deep mycoses stemmed from the CMV-induced suppression of both cell-mediated and humoral immune responses *(547,548)*. In addition, ongoing CMV infections may also disrupt normal integumentary barriers, such as the gastrointestinal and respiratory tracts, thus predisposing to invasive superinfections with colonizing fungi *(524)*.

Disseminated disease due to *Scedosporium prolificans* after bone-marrow transplantation has also been described *(75,549)*. Recently, *S. prolificans* have been implicated in the fatal outcome of two cases, one after a bone-marrow transplantation *(140)* and the other after a single-lung transplantation *(147)*. In the first case, the patient with acute myeloblastic leukemia underwent autologous bone-marrow transplantation. The fungal infection had developed during the severe neutropenia resulting from the conditioning preceding the marrow transplantation. The conditioning regimen included, in addition to busulfan and cyclophosphamide, also prophylaxis with oral fluconazole (100 mg daily). The *S. prolificans* isolate was resistant to amphotericin B, flucytosine, ketoconazole, and fluconazole with MIC values of 64, ≥128, 64, and 8.0 µg/mL, respectively *(140)*. In the second case, the patient received a single lung transplant *(147)*. Prophylactic anti-infective therapy with antibiotics (ticarcillin plus clavulanic acid and perfloxacin), acyclovir, and amphotericin B (0.3 mg/kg daily, i.v.) for 15 d, and postoperative treatment with intravenous amphotericin B (1.0 mg/kg daily) failed to thwart the fungal infection *(147)*. In a separate case of fatal *S. prolificans* disease, the patient who received a kidney transplant first developed a locally invasive infection that subsequently disseminated to the pleura *(144,145)*.

Opportunistic *Pseudallescheria boydii* infections have also been associated with several deaths after solid organ transplantions *(26,35,303)*. In one case of fatal orthotopic liver transplantion, the patient developed *P. boydii* endocarditis of the pulmonic valve *(26)*. To a large extent, pulmonic valve endocarditis has been identified with either congenital heart disease *(550)*, indwelling catheters (especially pulmonary artery catheters *[551]*), or in intravenous drug users (most often with a right-sided endocarditis of the tricuspid valve) *(550)*. What made this case highly unusual was that at autopsy the patient was found to have a vegetation on the pulmonic valve in addition to a septal abscess presented as endocardial mass along the left side of the septum, a rather unique association of pulmonic valve endocarditis with myocardial septal abscess *(26)*. Previously, *P. boydii* was reported as the cause of infection in one liver-transplant patient who acquired the infection nosocomially *(21)*.

Alsip and Cobbs *(35)* described a fatal *P. boydii* infection that disseminated to the central nervous system after cardiac transplant surgery; meningitis was the primary CNS manifestation, with no evidence of brain abscess. Amphotericin B, given both intravenously (20 mg daily) and intraventricularly (1.0 mg administered during ventriculostomy), and miconazole (600 mg, t.i.d.) failed to control the disseminated disease.

A mycotic aneurysm and visceral infection due to *Scedosporium apiospermum* in a kidney-transplant patient was described by Ben Hamida et al. *(525)*. Sequential therapy with intravenous fluconazole (400 mg daily) and intravenous miconazole (1.2 g daily) was unsuccessful and the patient died.

However, oral itraconazole was successful in the treatment of concurrent pulmonary *P. boydii* and *Aspergillus terreus* infections in a bone-marrow transplant recipient (see the preceding section) *(76)*.

Robertson et al. *(528)* described a patient who developed disseminated *Fusarium* infection with a secondary fungal endophthalmitis after an autologous bone-marrow transplant for acute myeloid leukemia. The fusariosis was successfully eradicated after neutrophil recovery by a prolonged systemic administration of amphotericin B combined with aggressive local therapy, including enucleation of the affected eye. In another case of disseminated *Fusarium* disease in a bone marrow transplant recipient, the infection caused by *F. proliferatum* was successfully treated with a combination of rifampin and amphotericin B, which acted in a synergistic manner to elicit a complete remission of infection although the neutrophil counts remained below 0.25×10^9 cells/L *(552)*.

Nucci et al. *(530)* studied the efficacy and safety of itraconazole in combination with amphotericin B to treat fungal infections (pulmonary aspergilloma, *Aspergillus fumigatus* sinusitis, fusariosis, and disseminated candidiasis) in neutropenic patients after bone-marrow transplant recovery.

In general, non-*Candida* fungal infections remain a substantial cause for morbidity and mortality among patients undergoing solid organ or bone-marrow transplantations *(196)*. In prevention of systemic aspergillosis, itraconazole at 200 mg daily has been effective only when adequate serum concentrations have been achieved *(542)*. None of the currently available oral antimycotics provides effective prophylaxis against *Fusarium*, *Pseudallescheria*, *Trichosporon*, and *Torulopsis (542)*. Therefore, early diagnosis, antifungal therapy, and transplant regimens incurring a shorter period of neutropenia may help to reduce the incidence and clinical impact of non-*Candida* infections.

14. PHARMACOKINETIC INTERACTIONS OF CYCLOSPORIN A WITH AZOLE ANTIMYCOTICS

Cyclosporin A, which is widely used in transplantaion surgeries to prevent organ rejections *(553)*, has frequently produced serious side effects as well as pharmacokinetic interactions with various antimicrobial agents, resulting in unwarranted changes of cyclosporin A blood concentrations that may often lead to either organ rejection or increase of toxicity *(554–560)*. Because the metabolic degradation of cyclosporin A is carried out primarily via the hepatic P-450 mixed function oxidase system *(561)*, cyclosporin A interactions with other drugs that involved modulation of the cytochrome P-450 system may significantly alter the clinical course after the transplantation surgery *(554)*. Thus, rifampin was found to accelerate the metabolism of cyclosporin A by inducing the P-450 system *(562)* leading to decrease in its blood levels *(557)* and eventually to organ rejection. Cimetidine *(563)* and ketoconazole *(554,558,559,564,565)*, on the other hand, were shown to inhibit the P-450 system, thereby increasing cyclosporin A concentrations and consequently enhancing its nephrotoxicity secondary to a reduced elimination.

In addition to inhibiting cytochrome P-450 enzymes, azole antimycotics such as clotrimazole, miconazole, and ketoconazole have also been found to induce certain hepatic cytochrome P-450 isoenzymes (P-450p, P-450b/e, P-450c/d, P-450j) *(566)* as evidenced by studies conducted both in animal models and humans *(549,566–573)*. The results have shown that different azole drugs interacted with various cytochrome P-450 isoenzymes in different ways. For example, whereas the glucocorticoid and aromatic hydrocarbon-responsive P-450p and P-450c/d isoenzymes, respectively, were induced by clotrimazole, miconazole, and ketoconazole, the phenobarbital-responsive P-450b/c isoenzyme was induced by clotrimazole and miconazole, but not ketoconazole. Also, the ethanol-responsive P-450j isoenzyme, although moderately induced by ketoconazole, was not affected by neither clotrimazole nor miconazole *(566)*.

When administered simultaneously to heart- and lung-transplant recipients, itraconazole interacted with cyclosporin A by raising its levels *(574)*; however, the results from in vitro *(549)* and in vivo *(575)* experiments were inconclusive and would not have predicted the results in humans.

Horton et al. *(554)* studied the interaction of cyclosporin A with the experimental triazole antimycotic agent SCH 39304 *(256)*. Although elevated cyclosporin A levels were noticed at the end of and after conclusion of the first course of SCH 39304 (d 119 through 122), they probably resulted from the increase in cyclosporin A dosage to 240 mg daily for d 112–118; it was unlikely that SCH 39304 have had a delayed inhibitory effect on the metabolism of cyclosporin A. In this context, the principle of competitive hepatic enzyme inhibition affirms that when a drug competitively inhibits the hepatic metabolism of another drug, an increase in the serum concentration of the inhibited drug should occur shortly after therapy is instituted, provided that the inhibitory agent reaches an effective inhibitory concentration *(576)*. However, there have been no previous increases in the cyclosporin A concentrations during the first course of treatment with SCH 39309 that could not be attributed to increases in the doses of cyclosporin A *(554)*.

Contrary to other azoles, the interaction of fluconazole with cyclosporin A produced conflicting results *(577–582)*. Thus, although data from some studies suggested increased cyclosporin A concentrations with or without nephrotoxicity *(580–582)*, others have indicated the absense of pharmacokinetic interaction between the two drugs *(554,577–579)*. In the studies indicating the presence of fluconazole-cyclosporin A interaction, fluconazole was used at higher doses. A fluconazole-cyclosporin A interaction, therefore, might have been a dose-dependent phenomenon *(554)*. In addition, fluconazole has a large distribution volume and long elimination half-life (22 h) *(552)*, which would allow its serum concentrations to accumulate over time. Another explanation for the contradictory results evaluating azole-cyclosporin A interactions may be the presence of interindividual variations in the hepatic metabolism of patients where some individuals may be more likely to either induce or inhibit certain cyctochrome P-450 isoenzymes by the azole antimycotics *(554)*.

REFERENCES

1. Mishra, S. K., Ajello, L., Ahearn, D. G., et al. Environmental mycology and its importance to public health. *J. Med. Vet. Mycol.*, 30(Suppl. 1), 287, 1992.
2. Ajello, L. Hyalohyphomycosis and phaeohyphomycosis: two global disease entities of public health importance. *Eur. J. Epidemiol.*, 2, 243, 1986.
3. Matsumoto, T., Ajello, L., Matsuda, T., Szaniszlo, P. J., and Walsh, T. J. Developments in hyalohyphomycosis and phaeohyphomycosis. *J. Med. Vet. Mycol.*, 32(Suppl. 1), 329, 1994.
4. Vartivarian, S. E., Anaissie, E. J., and Bodey, G. P. Emerging fungal pathogens in immunocompromised patients: classification, diagnosis, and management. *Clin. Infect. Dis.*, 17(Suppl. 2), S487, 1993.
5. Castagnola, E., Garaventa, A., Conte, M., Barretta, A., Faggi, E., and Viscoli, C. Survival after fungemia due to *Fusarium moniliforme* in a child with neuroblastoma. *Eur. J. Clin. Microbiol. Infect. Dis.*, 12, 308, 1993.
6. Dana, B. W., Durie, B. G. M., White, R. F., and Huestis, D. W. Concomitant administration of granulocyte transfusions and amphotericin B in neutropenic patients: absence of significant pulmonary toxicity. *Blood*, 57, 90, 1981.
7. Wilhelmus, K. R., Robinson, N. M., Font, R. A., Hamill, M. B., and Jones, D. B. Fungal keratitis in contact lens wearers. *Am. J. Ophthalmol.*, 106, 708, 1988.
8. Ajello, L. Fungal infections in AIDS: a review. *L'Igiene Moderna*, 100, 288, 1993.
9. Rosenthal, J., Katz, R., Du Bois, D. B., Morrissey, A., and Machicao, A. Chronic maxillary sinusitis associated with the mushroom *Schizophylum commune* in a patient with AIDS. *Clin. Infect. Dis.*, 14, 46, 1992.
10. Liu, K., Howell, D. N., Perfect, J. R., and Schell, W. A. Morphologic criteria for the preliminary identification of *Fusarium, Paecilomyces*, and *Acremonium* species by histopathology. *Am. J. Clin. Pathol.*, 109, 45–54, 1998 [see also: *Am. J. Clin. Pathol.*, 109, 1–2, 1998].
11. Schell, W. A. New aspects of emerging fungal pathogens: a multifaceted challenge. *Clin. Lab. Med.*, 15, 365–387, 1995.
12. Tadros, T. S., Workowski, K. A., Siegel, R. J., Hunter, S., and Schwartz, D. A. Pathology of hyalohyphomycosis caused by *Scedosporium apiospermum (Pseudallescheria boydii)*. *Hum. Pathol.*, 29, 1266–1272, 1998 [see also: *Hum. Pathol.*, 29, 1179–1180, 1998].
13. Anaissie, E., Bodey, G. P., Kantarjian, H., et al. New spectrum of fungal infections in patients with cancer. *Rev. Infect. Dis.*, 11, 369, 1989.
14. Berenguer, J., Diaz-Mediavilla, J., Urra, D., and Munoz, P. Central nervous system infection caused by *Pseudallescheria boydii*: case report and review. *Rev. Infect. Dis.*, 11, 890, 1989.
15. Cooper, C. R. and Salkin, I. F. Pseudallescheriasis, in *Fungal Infections and Immune Responses*, Murphy, J. W., Friedman, H., and Bendinelli, M., Eds. Plenum Press, New York, 335, 1993.
16. Fisher, J. F., Shadomy, S., Teabaut, J. R., et al. Near drowning complicated by brain abscess due to *Petriellidium boydii*. *Arch. Neurol.*, 39, 511, 1982.
17. Caya, J. G., Farmer, S. G., Williams, G. A., Franson, T. R., Komorowski, R. A., and Kies, J. C. Bilateral *Pseudallescheria boydii* endophthalmitis in an immunocompromised patient. *Wisconsin Med. J.*, 87, 11, 1988.
18. Hainer, J. W., Ostrow, J. H., and Mackenzie, D. W. R. Pulmonary monosporiosis: report of a case with precipitating antibody. *Chest*, 66, 601, 1974.
19. Kershaw, P., Freeman, R., Templeton, D., et al. *Pseudallescheria boydii* infection of the central nervous system. *Arch. Neurol.* 47, 468, 1990.
20. Yoo, D., Lee, W. H. S., and Kwon-Chung, K. J. Brain abscesses due to *Pseudallescheria boydii* association with primary non-Hodgkin's lymphoma of the central nervous system: a case report and literature review. *Rev. Infect. Dis.*, 7, 272, 1985.
21. Patterson, T. F., Andriole, V. T., Zervos, M. J., Therasse, D., and Kauffman, C. A. The epidemiology of pseudallescheriasis complicating transplantation: nosocomial and community-acquired infection. *Mycoses*, 33, 297, 1990.
22. Peréz, R. E., Smith, M., McClendon, J., Kim, J., and Eugenio, N. *Psedallescheria boydii* brain abscess: complication of an intravenous catheter. *Am. J. Med.*, 84, 359, 1988.
23. Pfeifer, J. D., Grand, M. G., Thomas, M. A., Berger, A. R., Lucarelli, M. J., and Smith, M. E. Endogenous *Pseudallescheria boydii* endophthalmitis: clinicopathologic findings in two cases. *Arch. Ophthalmol.*, 109, 1714, 1992.

24. Rippon, J. W. Pseudallescheriasis, in *Medical Mycology. The Pathogenic Fungi and the Pathogenic Actinomycetes*, 3rd ed., Rippon, J. W., Ed. W. B. Saunders, Philadelphia, 651, 1988.
25. Travis, L. B., Roberts, G. D., and Wilson, W. R. Clinical significance of *Pseudallescheria boydii*: a review of 10 years' experience. *Mayo Clinic Proc.*, 60, 531, 1985.
26. Welty, F. K., McLeod, G. X., Ezratty, C., Healy, R. W., and Karchmer, A. W. *Pseudallescheria boydii* endocarditis of the pulmonic valve in a liver transplant recipient. *Clin. Infect. Dis.*, 15, 858, 1992.
27. Arnett, J. C. and Hatch, H. B. Pulmonary allescheriasis. *Arch. Intern. Med.*, 135, 1250, 1975.
28. Seale, P. and Hudson, J. A. Successful medical treatment of pulmonary petriellidiosis, *South. Med. J.*, 78, 473, 1985.
29. McCarthy, D. S., Longbottom, J. L., Riddell, R. W., and Batten, J. C. Pulmonary mycetoma due to *Allescheria boydii*. *Am. Rev. Respir. Dis.*, 100, 213, 1969.
30. Guyotat, D., Piens, M. A., Bouvier, R., and Fiere. D., A case of disseminated *Scedosporium apiospermum* infection after bone marrow transplantation. *Mykosen*, 30, 151, 1987.
31. Forno, L. S. and Billingham, M. E. *Allescheria boydii* infection of the brain. *Pathology*, 106, 195, 1972.
32. Aronson, S. M., Benham, R., and Wolf, A. Maduromycosis of the central nervous system. *J. Neuropath. Exp. Neurol.*, 12, 158, 1953.
33. Benham, R. and Georg, L. K. *Allescheria boydii*, causative agent in a case of meningitis. *J. Invest. Derm.*, 10, 99, 1948.
34. Selby, R. Pachymeningitis secondary to *Allerschia boydii*. *J. Neurosurg.*, 36, 225, 1972.
35. Alsip, S. G. and Cobbs, C. G. *Pseudallescheria boydii* infection of the central nervous system in a cardiac transplant recipient. *South. Med. J.*, 79, 383, 1986.
36. Creitz, J. and Harris, H. W. Isolation of *Allescheria boydii* from spitum. *Am. Rev. Tuberc.*, 71, 126, 1955.
37. Travis, R. E., Ulrich, E. W., and Phillips, S. Pulmonary allescheriasis. *Ann. Intern. Med.*, 54, 151, 1961.
38. Blank, F. and Stuart, E. A. *Monosporium apiospermum sacc*. 1911 associated with otomycosis. *Can. Med. Assoc. J.*, 72, 601, 1955.
39. Ansari, R. A., Hindson, D. A., Stevens, D. A., and Kloss, J. G. *Pseudallescheria boydii* arthritis and osteomyelitis in a patient with Cushing's disease. *South. Med. J.*, 80, 90, 1987.
40. Hung, L. H. Y. and Norwood, L. A. Osteomyelitis due to *Pseudallescheria boydii*. *South. Med. J.*, 86, 231, 1993.
41. Fernandez-Guerrero, M. L., Barnés, P. R., and Alés, J. M. Postcraniotomy mycetoma of the scalp and osteomyelitis due to *Pseudallescheria boydii*. *J. Infect. Dis.*, 156, 855, 1987.
42. Ginter, G., de Hoog, G. S., Pschaid, A., et al. Arthritis without grains caused by *Pseudallescheria boydii*. *Mycoses*, 38, 369, 1995.
43. Winston, D. J., Jordan, M. C., and Rhodes, J. *Allescheria boydii*: infections in the immunosuppressed host. *Am. J. Med.*, 63, 830, 1977.
44. Davis, W. A., Isner, J. M., Bracey, A. W., Roberts, W. C., and Garagusi, V. F. Disseminated *Petriellidium boydii* and pacemaker endocarditis. *Am. J. Med.*, 69, 929, 1980.
45. Ogihara, A., Chino, M., Yoshino, H., et al. A case of prosthetic valve endocarditis due to *Scedosporium apiospermum*. *Nippon Naika Gakkai Zasshi*, 78, 432, 1989.
46. Rosen, F., Deck, J. H. N., and Rewcastle, N. B. *Allescheria boydii* unique systemic dissemination to thyroid and brain. *Can. Med. Assoc. J.*, 93, 1125, 1965.
47. de Ment, S. H., Smith, R. R., Karp, J. E., and Merz, W. G. Pulmonary, cardiac and thyroid involvement in disseminated *Pseudallescheria boydii*. *Arch. Pathol. Lab. Med.*, 108, 859, 1984.
48. Meyer, E. and Herrold, R. D. *Allescheria boydii* isolated from a patient with chronic prostatitis. *Am. J. Clin. Pathol.*, 35, 155, 1961.
49. Saadah, H. A. and Dixon, T. *Petriellidium boydii* (*Allescheria boydii*) necrotizing pneumonia in a normal host. *J. Am. Med. Assoc.*, 245, 605, 1981.
50. Collignon, P. J., Macleod, C., Packham, D. R. Miconazole therapy in *Pseudallescheria boydii* infection. *Australas. J. Dermatol.*, 26, 129, 1985.
51. Lichtman, D. M., Johnson, D. C., Mack, G. R., and Lack, E. E. Maduromycosis (*Allescheria boydii*) infection of the hand. *J. Bone Joint Surg. Am.*, 60, 546, 1978.
52. Bryan, C. S., DiSalvo, A. F., Kaufman, L., Kaplan, W., Brill, A. H., and Abbott, D. C. *Petriellidium boydii* infection of the sphenoid sinus. *Am. J. Clin. Pathol.*, 74, 846, 1980.
53. Schiess, R. J., Coscia, M. F., and McClellan, G. A. *Petriellidium boydii* pachymeningitis treated with miconazole and ketoconazole. *Neurosurgery*, 14, 220, 1984.
54. Lutwick, L. I., Galgiani, J. N., Johnson, R. H., and Stevens, D. A. Visceral fungal infections due to *Petriellidium boydii*. *Am. J. Med.*, 61, 632, 1976.
55. Shin, L. Y. and Lee, N. Disseminated petriellidiosis (allescheriasis) in a patient with refractory acute lymphoblastic leukemia. *J. Clin. Pathol.*, 37, 78, 1984.
56. Bell, W. E. and Myers, M. G. *Allescheria* (*Petriellidium*) *boydii* brain abscess in a child with leukemia. *Arch. Neurol.*, 35, 386, 1978.
57. Fry, V. G. and Young, C. N. A rare fungal brain abscess in an uncompromised host. *Surg. Neurol.*, 15, 446, 1981.
58. Agamanolis, D. P., Kalwinsky, D. K., Krill, C. E. Jr., Dasu, S., Halasa, B., and Galloway, P. G. *Fusarium* meningoencephalitis in a child with acute leukemia. *Neuropediatrics*, 22, 110, 1991.
59. Gluckman, S. J., Ries, K., and Abrutyn, E. *Allescheria* (*Petriellidium*) *boydii* sinusitis in a compromised host. *J. Clin. Microbiol.*, 5, 481, 1977.
60. Morgan, M. A., Wilson, W. R., Neel, H. B. III, and Roberts, G. D. Fungal sinusitis in healthy and immunocompromised individuals. *Am. J. Clin. Pathol.*, 82, 597, 1984.

61. Salitan, M. L., Lawson, W., Som, P. M., Bottone, E. J., and Biller, H. F. *Pseudallescheria* sinusitis with itracranial extension in a nonimmunocompromised host. *Otolaryngol. Head Neck Surg.*, 102, 745, 1990.
62. Winn, R. E., Ramsey, P. D., McDonald, J. C., and Dunlop, K. J. Maxillary sinusitis from *Pseudallescheria boydii*. *Arch. Otolaryngol.*, 109, 123, 1983.
63. Washburn, R. G., Kennedy, D. W., Begley, M. G., Henderson, D. K., and Bennett, J. E. Chronic fungal sinusitis in apparently normal hosts. *Medicine (Baltimore)*, 67, 231, 1988.
64. Mader, J. T., Ream, R. S., and Heath, P. W. *Petriellidium boydii* (*Allescheria boydii*) sphenoidal sinusitis. *J. Am. Med. Assoc.*, 239, 2368, 1978.
65. Dubeau, F., Roy, L. E., Allard, J., et al. Brain abscess due to *Petriellidium boydii*. *Can. J. Neurol. Sci.*, 11, 395, 1984.
66. Walker, D. H., Adamec, T., and Krigman, M. Disseminated petriellidiosis (allescheriosis). *Arch. Pathol. Lab. Med.*, 102, 158, 1978.
67. Anderson, R. L., Carroll, T. F., Harvey, R. T., and Myers, M. G. *Petriellidium* (*Allescheria*) *boydii* orbital and brain abscess treated with intravenous miconazole. *Am. J. Ophthalmol.*, 97, 771, 1984.
68. Fessler, R. G. and Brown, F. D. Superior sagittal sinus infection with *Petriellidium boydii*: case report. *Neurosurgery*, 24, 604, 1989.
69. Phillips, P., Forbes, J. C., and Speert, D. P. Disseminated infection with *Pseudallescheria boydii* in a patient with chronic granulomatous disease: response to gamma-interferon plus antifungal chemotherapy. *Pediatr. Infect. Dis. J.*, 10, 536, 1991.
70. The International Chronic Granulomatous Disease Cooperative Study Group. A controlled trial of interferon gamma to prevent infection in chronic granulomatous disease. *N. Engl. J. Med.*, 324, 509, 1991.
71. Bernstein, E. F., Schuster, M. G., Stieritz, D. D., Heuman, P. C., and Uitto, J. Disseminated cutaneous *Psedallescheria boydii*. *Br. J. Dermatol.*, 132, 456, 1995.
72. Cunningham, R. and Mitchell, D. C. Amphotericin B responsive *Scedosporium apiospermum* in a patient with acute myeloid leukaemia. *J. Clin. Pathol.*, 49, 93, 1996.
73. Ruxin, T. A., Steck, W. D., Helm, T. N., Bergfeld, W. F., and Bolwell, B. J. *Pseudallescheria boydii* in an immunocompromised host: successful treatment with debridement and itraconazole. *Arch. Dermatol.*, 132, 382,1996.
74. Hung, C. C., Chang, S. C., Yang, P. C., and Hsieh, W. C. Invasive pulmonary pseudallescheriasis with direct invasion of the thoracic spine in an immunocompetent patient. *Eur. J. Clin. Microbiol. Infect. Dis.*, 13, 749, 1994.
75. Gumbart, C. H. *Pseudallescheria boydii* infection after bone marrow transplantation. *Ann. Intern. Med.*, 99, 193, 1983.
76. Goldberg, S. L., Geha, D. J., Marshall, W. F., Inwards, D. J., and Hoagland, H. C. Successful treatment of simultaneous pulmonary *Pseudallescheria boydii* and *Aspergillus terreus* infection with oral itraconazole. *Clin. Infect. Dis.*, 16, 803, 1993.
77. Walsh, M., White, L., Atkinson, K., and Enno, A. Fungal *Pseudallescheria boydii* lung infiltrates unresponsive to amphotericin B in leukaemic patients. *Aust. N. Z. J. Med.*, 22, 265, 1992.
78. Mesnard, R., Lamy, T., Dauriac, C., and Le Prise, P.-Y. Lung abscess due to *Pseudallescheria boydii* in the course of acute leukaemia. *Acta Haematol.*, 87, 78, 1992.
79. Smith, A. G., Crain, S. M., Dejongh, C., Thomas, G. M., and Vigorito, R. D. Systemic pseudallescheriasis in a patient with acute myelocytic leukaemia. *Mycopathologia*, 90, 219, 1985.
80. Galgiani, J. N., Stevens, D. A., Graybill, J. R., Stevens, D. L., Tillinghast, A. J., and Levine, H. B. *Pseudallescheria boydii* infections treated with ketoconazole. *Chest*, 86, 219, 1984.
81. Guého, E. and de Hoog, G. S. Taxonomy of the medical species of *Pseudallescheria* and *Scedosporium*. *J. Mycol. Med.*, 118, 3, 1991.
82. Hecht, R. and Montgomerie, J. Z. Maxillary sinus infection with *Allescheria boydii* (*Petriellidium boydii*). *Johns Hopkins Med. J.*, 142, 107, 1978.
83. Raffanti, S. P., Fyfe, B., Carreiro, S., Sharp, S. E., Hyman, B. A., and Ratzan, K. R. Native valve endocarditis due to *Pseudallescheria boydii* in a patient with AIDS: case report and review. *Rev. Infect. Dis.*, 12, 993, 1990.
84. Scherr, G. R., Evans, S. G., Kiyabu, M. T., and Klatt, E. C. *Pseudallescheria boydii* infection in the acquired immunodeficiency syndrome. *Arch. Pathol. Lab. Med.*, 116, 535, 1992.
85. Glassman, M. I., Henkind, P., and Alture-Werber, E. *Monosporium apiospermum* endophthalmitis. *Am. J. Ophthalmol.*, 76, 821, 1973.
86. Stern, R. M., Zakov, Z, N., Meisler, D. M., Hall, G. S., and Martin, A. Endogenous *Pseudallescheria boydii* endophthalmitis: a clinicopathologic report. *Cleve. Clin. Q.*, 53, 197, 1986.
87. Meadow, W. L., Tripple, M. A., and Rippon, J. W. Endophthalmitis caused by *Pseudallescheria boydii*. *Am. J. Dis. Child.*, 135, 378, 1981.
88. Bouchard, C. S., Chaco, B., Cupples, H. P., Cavanagh, H. D., and Mathers, W. D. Surgical treatment for a case of postoperative *Pseudallescheria boydii* endophthalmitis. *Ophthal. Surg.*, 22, 98, 1991.
89. Stern, R. M., Zakov, Z. N., Meisler, D. M., Hall, G. S., and Martin, A. Endogenous *Pseudallescheria boydii* endophthalmitis: a clinicopathologic report. *Cleve. Clin. Q.*, 53, 197, 1986.
90. Moriarty, A. P., Crawford, G. J., McAllister, I. L., and Constable, I. J. Severe corneoscleral infection: a complication of beta irradiation scleral necrosis following pterygium excision. *Arch. Ophthalmol.*, 111, 947, 1993.
91. Moriarty, A. P., Crawford, G. J., McAllister, I. L., and Constable, I. J. Fungal corneoscleritis complicating beta-irradiation-induced scleral necrosis following pterygium excision. *Eye*, 7, 525, 1993.
92. Gordon, M. A., Valloton, W. W., and Groffead, G. S. Corneal sclerosis: a case of keratomycosis treated successfully with nystatin and amphotericin B. *Arch. Ophthalmol.*, 62, 758, 1959.
93. Matsuzaki, O. Ocular infection with a fungus from rice leaf. *Jpn. J. Med. Mycol.*, 10, 239, 1969.

94. Zapater, R. C. and Albesi, E. J. Corneal monosporiosis. *Ophthalmologica*, 178, 142, 1979.
95. Bloom, P. A., Laidlaw, D. A. H., Easty, D. L., and Warnock, D. W. Treatment failure in a case of fungal keratitis caused by *Pseudallescheria boydii*. *Br. J. Ophthalmol.*, 76, 367, 1992.
96. Ksiazek, S. M., Morris, D. A., Mandelbaum, S., and Rosenbaum, P. S. Fungal panophthalmitis secondary to *Scedosporium apiospermum* (*Pseudallescheria boydii*) keratitis. *Am. J. Ophthalmol.*, 118, 532-533, 1994.
97. Legeais, J. M., Blanc, V., Basset, D., et al. Severe keratomycosis: diagnosis and treatment. *J. Fr. Ophthalmol.*, 17, 568, 1994.
98. Ruben, S. *Pseudallescheria boydii* keratitis. *Acta Ophthalmol. (Copenh.)*, 69, 684, 1991.
99. Burns, E. L., Moss, E. S., and Brueck, J. W. Mycetoma pedis in the United States and Canada: with a report of three cases originating in Louisiana. *Am. J. Clin. Pathol.*, 15, 35, 1945.
100. Stierstorfer, M. B., Schartz, B. K., McGuire, J. B., and Miller, A. C. *Pseudallescheria boydii* mycetoma in Northern New England. *Int. J. Dermatol.*, 27, 383, 1988.
101. Sheftel, T. G., Mader, J. T., and Cierny, G. *Pseudallescheria boydii* soft tissue abscess. *Clin. Orthop.*, 215, 212, 1987.
102. Ajello, L. The isolation of *Allescheria boydii* Shear, an etiologic agent of mycetoma, from soil. *Am. J. Trop. Med. Hyg.*, 1, 227, 1952.
103. Drouhet, E. and Dupont, B. Chronic mucocutaneous candidiasis and other superficial and systemic mycoses successfully treated with ketoconazole. *Rev. Infect. Dis.*, 2, 606, 1980.
104. Aubock, J., Pichler, E., and Fritsch, P. Mycetoma caused by *Petriellidium boydii*: treatment with ketoconazole. *Hautarzt.*, 36, 453, 1985.
105. Pether, J. V. S., Jones, W., Greatorex, F. B., and Bunting, W. Acute pyogenic *Pseudallescheria boydii* foot infection sequentially treated with miconazole and itraconazole. *J. Infect.*, 25, 335, 1992.
106. Dellestable, F., Kures, L., Mainard, D., Pere, P., and Gaucher, A. Fungal arthritis due to *Pseudallescheria boydii* (*Scedosporium apiospermum*). *J. Rheumatol.*, 21, 766, 1994.
107. Hayden, G., Lapp, C., and Loda, F. Arthritis caused by *Monosporium apiospermum* treated with intra-articular amphotericin B. *Am. J. Dis. Child.*, 131, 927, 1977.
108. Kemp, H. B. S., Bedford, A. F., and Fincham, W. J. *Petriellidium boydii* infection of the knee: a case report. *Skeletal Radiol.*, 9, 114, 1982.
109. Dirschl, D. R. and Henderson, R. C. Patellar overgrowth after infection of the knee. *J. Bone Joint Surg.*, 73A, 940, 1991.
110. Halpern, A. A., Nagel, D. A., and Schurman, D. J. *Allescheria boydii* osteomyelitis following multiple steroid injections and surgery. *Clin. Orthop.*, 126, 232, 1977.
111. Gener, F. A., Kustimur, S., Sultan, N., and Sever, A. Fungus-induced arhtritis caused by *Scedosporium apiospermum* (*Pseudallescheria boydii*). *Z. Rheumatol.*, 50, 219, 1991.
112. Gener, F. A., Kustimur, S., Sultan, N., and Sever, A. Uber eine pilz-induzierte arthritis durch *Scedosporium apiospermum* (*Pseudallescheria boydii*). *Zeitschr. Rheumatol.*, 50, 219, 1991.
113. Piper, J. P., Golden, J., Brown, D., Broestler, J., and Grant, D. Successful treatment of *Scedosporium apiospermum* suppurative arthritis with itraconazole. *Pediatr. Infect. Dis. J.*, 9, 674, 1990.
114. Chatté, G., Boibieux, A., Bailly, M. P., et al., Osteoarthrite du genou a *Scedosporium apiospermum*: succès de l'itraconazole. *J. Mycol. Méd.*, 3, 111, 1993.
115. Wilson, C. M., O'Rourke, E. J., McGinnis, M. R., and Salkin, I. F. *Scedosporium inflatum*: clinical spectrum of a newly recognized pathogen. *J. Infect. Dis.*, 161, 102–107, 1990.
116. Van Cutsem, J. M. and Thienpont, D. Miconazole, a broad-spectrum antimycotic agent with antibacterial activity. *Chemotherapy*, 17, 391, 1972.
117. McCall, R. E. Maduromycosis *"Allescheria boydii"* septic arthritis of the knee: a case report. *Orthopedics*, 4, 1144, 1981.
118. Lazarus, H. S., Myers, J. P., and Brocker, R. J. Post-craniotomy wound infection caused by *Pseudallescheria boydii*: case report. *J. Neurosurg.*, 64, 153, 1986.
119. Findling, J. W., Tyrell, J. B., Aron, D. C., Fitzgerald, P. A., Young, C. W., and Sohnle, P. G. Fungal infections in Cushing's syndrome. *Ann. Intern. Med.*, 95, 392, 1981.
120. Anthony, L. B. and Greco, F. A. *Pneumocystis carinii* pneumonia: a complication of Cushing's syndrome. *Ann. Intern. Med.*, 94, 488, 1981.
121. Plotz, C. M., Knowlton, A. I., and Ragan, C. The natural history of Cushing's syndrome. *Am. J. Med.*, 13, 597, 1952.
122. Fauci, A. S., Dale, D. C., and Balow, J. E. Glucocorticosteroid therapy: mechanism of action and clinical consideration. *Ann. Intern. Med.*, 84, 304, 1976.
123. Balow, J. E. and Rosenthal, A. S. Glucocorticoid suppression of macrophage migration inhibitory factor. *J. Exp. Med.*, 137, 1031, 1973.
124. Kwon-Chung, K. J. and Bennett, J. E. Pseudallescheriasis and *Scedosporium* infection, in *Medical Mycology* Lea & Febiger, Philadelphia, 687–694, 1992.
125. Salkin, I. F., McGinnis, M. R., Dykstra, M. J., and Rinaldi, M. G. *Scedosporium inflatum*, an emerging pathogen. *J. Clin. Microbiol.*, 26, 498–503, 1988.
126. Wood, G. M., McCormack, J. G., Muir, D. B., et al. Clinical features of human infection with *Scedosporium inflatum*. *Clin. Infect. Dis.*, 14, 1027, 1992.
127. Schwartz, D. A. Pseudallescheriasis and scedosporiasis, in *Pathology of Infectious Diseases*, vol. 2, Connor, D. H., Chandler, F. W., Schwartz, D. A. et al., Eds. Appleton & Lange, Stamford, CT, 1073–1079, 1997.

128. Piper, J. P., Golden, J., Brown, D., et al. Successful treatment of *Scedosporium apiospermum* suppurative arthritis with itraconazole. *Pediatr. Infect. Dis.*, 9, 674–675, 1990.
129. Torok, L., Simon, G., Tapai, M., et al. *Scedosporium apiospermum* infection initiating lymphocutaneous sporotrichosis in a patient with myeloblastic-monocytic leukaemia. *Br. J. Dermatol.*, 133, 805–809, 1995.
130. Cunningham, R. and Mitchell, D. C. Amphotericin B responsive *Scedosporium apiospermum* infection in a patient with acute myeloid leukaemia. *J. Clin. Pathol.*, 49, 93–94, 1996.
131. Nomdedéu, J., Bruner, S., Martino, R., et al. Successful treatment of pneumonia due to *Scedosporium apiospermum* with itraconazole: case report. *Clin. Infect. Dis.*, 16, 731–733, 1993.
132. Vartivarian, S. E., Anaissie, E. J., and Bodey, G. P. Emerging fungal pathogens in immunocompromised patients: classification, diagnosis and management. *Clin. Infect. Dis.*, 17(Suppl. 2), S487–S491, 1993.
133. Nomdedéu, J., Brunet, S., Martino, R., Altés, A., Ausina, V., and Domingo-Albos, A. Successful treatment of pneumonia due to *Scedosporium apiospermum* with itraconazole: case report. *Clin. Infect. Dis.*, 16, 731, 1993.
134. Martino, R., Nomdedéu, J., Altés, A., et al. Successful bone marrow transplantation in patients with previous invasive fungal infections: report of four cases. *Bone Marrow Transplant.*, 13, 265, 1994.
135. Wise, K. A., Speed, B. R., Ellis, D. H., and Andrew, J. H. Two fatal infections in immunocompromised patients caused by *Scedosporium inflatum*. *Pathology*, 25, 187, 1993.
136. Farag, S. S., Firkin, F. C., Andrew, J. H., Lee, C. S., and Ellis, D. H. Fatal disseminated *Scedosporium inflatum* infection in a neutropenic immunocompromised patient. *J. Infect.*, 25, 201, 1992.
137. Guarro, J., Gaztelurrutia, L., Marin, J., and Barcena, J. *Scedosporium inflatum*, a new pathogenic fungus. *Enfermed. Infec. Microbiol. Clin.*, 9, 557, 1991.
138. Marin, J., Sanz, M. A., Sanz, G. F., et al. Disseminated *Scedosporium inflatum* infection in a patient with acute myeloblastic leukemia. *Eur. J. Clin. Microbiol. Infect. Dis.*, 10, 759, 1991.
139. Rosenthal, S. A., Weitzman, I., Salkin, I. F., and Kemna, M. Fungal sepsis caused by *Scedosporium inflatum*. *Mycol. Observer.*, 9, 1, 1989.
140. Salesa, R., Burgos, A., Ondiviela, R., Richard, C., Quindos, G., and Ponton, J. Fatal disseminated infection by *Scedosporium inflatum* after bone marrow transplantation. *Scand. J. Infect. Dis.*, 25, 389, 1993.
141. Guého, E. and de Hoog, G. S. Taxonomy of the medical species of *Pseudoallescheria* and *Scedosporium*. *J. Mycol. Med.*, 1, 3–9, 1991.
142. Summerbell, R. C., Krajden, S., and Kane, J. Potted plants in hospitals as reservoirs of pathogenic fungi. *Mycopathologia*, 106, 13, 1989.
143. Malloch, D. and Salkin, I. F. A new species of *Scedosporium* associated with osteomyelitis in humans. *Mycotaxon*, 21, 247, 1984.
144. Toy, E. C., Rinaldi, M. G., Savitch, C. B., and Leibovitch, E. R. Endocarditis and hip arthritis associated with *Scedosporium inflatum*. *South. Med. J.*, 83, 957, 1990.
145. Malekzadeh, M., Overturf, G. D., Auerbach, S. B., Wong, L., and Hirsch, M. Chronic, recurrent osteomyelitis caused by *Scedosporium inflatum*. *Pediatr. Infect. Dis. J.*, 9, 357, 1990.
146. Sparrow, S. A., Hallam, L. A., Wild, B. E., and Baker, D. L. *Scedosporium inflatum*: first case report of disseminated infection and review of the literature. *Pediatr. Hematol. Oncol.*, 9, 293, 1992.
147. Rabodonirina, M., Paulus, S., Thevenet, F., et al. Disseminated *Scedosporium prolificans* (*S. inflatum*) infection after single-lung transplantation. *Clin. Infect. Dis.*, 19, 138, 1994.
148. Tapia, M., Richard, C., Baro, J., et al. *Scedosporium inflatum* infection in immunocompromised haematological patients. *Br. J. Haematol.*, 87, 212, 1994.
149. Nielsen, K., Lang, H., Shum, A. C., Woodruff, K., and Cherry, J. D. Disseminated *Scedosporium prolificans* infection in an immunocompromised adolescent. *Pediatr. Infect. Dis. J.*, 12, 882, 1993.
150. Spielberger, R. T., Tegtmeier, B. R., O'Donnell, M. R., and Ito, J. I. Fatal *Scedosporium prolificans* (*S. inflatum*) fungemia following allogeneic bone marrow transplantation: report of a case in the United States. *Clin. Infect. Dis.*, 21, 1067, 1995.
151. Wild, B. E., Clemens, B. S., Holt, M. J. G., Gray, A., and Gatus, B. J. Successful treatment of *Scedosporium inflatum* and *Scedosporium apiospermum* osteomyelitis in 2 children. *Proc. XIIth ISHAM Congres*, Adelaide, abstract # D 38, 1994.
152. Gordon, M. A., Lapa, E. W., and Passero, P. G. Improved method for azole antifungal susceptibility testing. *J. Clin. Microbiol.*, 26, 1874, 1988.
153. Sullivan, L. J., Snibson, G., Joseph, C., and Taylor, H. R. *Scedosporium prolificans* sclerokeratitis. *Aust. N. Z. J. Ophthalmol.*, 22, 207, 1994.
154. Levine, D. J. Scleral complications following beta irradiation. *Arch. Ophthalmol.*, 112, 1016, 1994.
155. MacKenzie, F. D., Hirst, L. W., Kynarston, B., and Bain, C. Recurrence rate and complications after beta irradiation for pterygia. *Ophthalmology*, 98, 1776, 1991.
156. Alfonso, E. Surgical intervention in infectious keratoscleritis. *Arch. Ophthalmol.*, 112, 1017, 1994.
157. Levine, D. J. Beta irradiation of pterygium. *Ophthalmology*, 99, 841, 1992.
158. Farrell, P. L. R. and Smith, R. E. Bacterial corneoscleritis complicating pterygium excision. *Am. J. Ophthalmol.*, 107, 515, 1989.
159. Mayer, C. F. Endemic panmyelotoxicosis in the Russian grain belt: part one. The clinical aspects of alimentary toxic aleukia (ATA): a comprehensive review. *Military Surgeon*, Part 1, 173, 1953.
160. Marshall, E. The Soviet elephant grass theory. *Science*, 217, 2, 1982.

161. Saito, M. and Tatsuno, T. Toxins of *Fusarium nivale*, in *Microbial Toxins: Algal and Fungal Toxins*, vol. 7, Kadis, S., Ciegler, A., and Ajl, S., Eds. Academic Press, New York, 293, 1971.
162. Nelson, P. E., Dignani, M. C., and Anaissie, E. J. Taxonomy, biology, and clinical aspects of *Fusarium* species. *Clin. Microbiol. Rev.*, 7, 479–504, 1994.
163. Joffe, A. Z. Alimentary toxic aleukia, in *Microbial Toxins: Algal and Fungal Toxins*, vol. 7, Kadis, S., Ciegler, A., and Ajl, S., Eds. Academic Press, New York, 139, 1971.
164. Austwick, P. K. C. Mycotoxins. *Br. Med. Bull.*, 31, 222, 1975.
165. Wogan, G. N. Mycotoxins. *Ann. Rev. Pharmacol.*, 15, 437, 1975.
166. Marasas, W. F. O., Nelson, P. E., and Toussoun, T. A. *Toxigenic Fusarium Species: Identity and Mycotoxicology*. Pennsylvania State University Press, University Park, 1984.
167. Nelson, P. E. Taxonomy and biology of *Fusarium moniliforme*. *Mycopathologia*, 117, 29, 1992.
168. Costa, A. R., Valente, N. Y., Criado, P. R., Pires, M. C., and Vasconcellos, C. Invasive hyalohyphomycosis due to *Fusarium solani* in a patient with acute lymphocytic leukemia. *Int. J. Dermatol.*, 39, 717–718, 2000.
169. Repiso, T., Garcia-Patos, V., Martin, N., Creus, M., Bastida, P., and Castells, A. Disseminated fusariosis. *Pediatr. Dermatol.*, 118–121, 1996.
170. Anaissie, E., Kantarjian, H., Jones, P., et al. *Fusarium*: a newly recognized fungal pathogen in immunosuppressed patients. *Cancer*, 57, 2141, 1986.
171. Matsumoto, T., Ajello, L., Matsuda, T., Szaniszlo, P. J., and Walsh, T. J. Developments in the hyalohyphomycosis and phaeohyphomycosis. *J. Med. Vet. Mycol.*, 32(Suppl. 1), 329, 1994.
172. Morrison, V. A., Haake, R. J., and Weisdorf, D. J. The spectrum of non-*Candida* fungal infection following bone marrow transplantation. *Medicine (Baltimore)*, 72, 78–89, 1993.
173. Merz, W. G., Karp, J. E., Hoagland, M., Jettgoheen, M., Junkins, J. M., and Hood, A. F. Diagnosis and successful treatment of fusariosis in the compromised host. *J. Infect. Dis.*, 158, 1046, 1988.
174. Minor, R. L., Pfaller, M. A., Gingrich, R. D., and Burns, L. J. Disseminated *Fusarium* infections in patients following bone marrow transplantation. *Bone Marrow Transplant.*, 4, 653, 1989.
175. Guarro, J. and Gene, J. Opportunistic fusarial infections in humans. *Eur. J. Clin. Microbiol. Infect. Dis.*, 14, 741, 1995.
176. Melcher, G. P., McGough, D. A., Fothergill, A. W., Norris, C., and Rinaldi, M. G. Disseminated hyalohyphomycosis caused by a novel human pathogen, *Fusarium napiforme*. *J. Clin. Microbiol.*, 31, 1461–1467, 1993.
177. Richardson, S. E., Bannatyne, R. M., Summerbell, R. C., Milliken, J., Gold, R., and Weitzman, S. S. Disseminated fusarial infection in the immunocompromised host. *Rev. Infect. Dis.*, 10, 1171, 1988.
178. Young, N. A., Kwon-Chung, K. J., Kubota, T. T., Jennings, A. E., and Fisher, R. I. Disseminated infection by *Fusarium moniliforme* during treatment for malignant lymphoma. *Clin. Microbiol.*, 7, 589, 1978.
179. Anaissie, E., Kantarjian, H., Ro, J., et al. The emerging role of *Fusarium* infections in patients with cancer. *Medicine (Baltimore)*, 62, 77, 1988.
180. Venditti, M., Micozzi, A., Gentile, G., et al. Invasive *Fusarium solani* infections in patients with acute leukemia. *Rev. Infect. Dis.*, 10, 653, 1988.
181. Cho, C. T., Vats, T. S., Lowman, J. T., Brandsberg, J. W., and Tosh, F. E. *Fusarium solani* infection during treatment for acute leukemia. *J. Pediatr.*, 83, 1028, 1973.
182. Bodey, G. P., Buckley, M., Sathe, Y. S., and Freireich, E. J. Quantitative relationships between circulating leukocytes and infection in patients with acute leukemia. *Ann. Intern. Med.*, 64, 328, 1966.
183. Gutmann, L., Chou, S. M., and Pore, R. S. Fusariosis, myastenic syndrome, and aplastic anemia. *Neurology*, 25, 922, 1975.
184. Schneller, F. R., Gulati, S. C., Cunningham, I. B., O'Reilly, R. J., Schmitt, H. J., and Clarkson, B. D. *Fusarium* infections in patients with hematologic malignancies. *Leuk. Res.*, 14, 961, 1990.
185. Krcméry, V. Jr., Kunova, E., Jesenska, Z., et al., Invasive mold infections in cancer patients: 5 years' experience with *Aspergillus*, *Mucor*, *Fusarium* and *Acremonium* infections. *Support Care Cancer*, 4, 39, 1996.
186. Chevalet, P., Tiab, M., Miegeville, M., et al., Fusaria infection in patients with neutropenia: a propos of 3 cases. *Rev. Med. Interne*, 17, 474, 1996.
187. Krulder, J. W., Brimicombe, R. W., Wijermans, P. W., and Gams, W. Systemic *Fusarium nygamai* infection in a patient with lymphoblastic non-Hodgkin's lymphoma. *Mycoses*, 39, 121, 1996.
188. Velasco, E., Martins, C. A., and Nucci, M. Successful treatment of catheter-related fusarial infection in immunocompromised children. *Eur. J. Clin. Microbiol. Infect. Dis.*, 14, 697, 1995.
189. Myoken, Y., Sugata, T., Kyo, T., and Fujihara, M. Oral *Fusarium* infection in a granulocytopenic patient with acute myelogenous leukemia: a case report. *J. Oral Pathol. Med.*, 24, 237, 1995.
190. Rabodonirina, M., M., Piens, M. A., Monier, M. F., Guého, E., Fière, D., and Mojon, M. *Fusarium* infections in immunocompromised patients: case reports and literature review. *Eur. J. Clin. Microbiol. Infect. Dis.*, 13, 152, 1994.
191. Caux, F., Aractingi, S., Baurmann, H., et al. *Fusarium solani* cutaneous infection in a neutropenic patient. *Dermatology*, 186, 232, 1993.
192. Nucci, M., Spector, N., Lucena, S., et al. Three cases of infection with *Fusarium* species in neutropenic patients. *Eur. J. Clin. Microbiol. Infect. Dis.*, 11, 1160, 1992.
193. Helm, T. N., Longworth, D. L., Hall G. S., Bolwell, B. J., Fernandez, B., and Tonecki, K. Case report and review of resolved fusariosis. *J. Am. Acad. Dermatol.*, 23(2 Part 2), 393, 1990.
194. Arrese, J. E., Pierard-Franchimont, C., and Pierard, G. E. Fatal hyalohyphomycosis following *Fusarium* onychomycosis in an immunocompromised patient. *Am. J. Dermatopathol.*, 18, 196–198, 1996.
195. Mutton, K. J., Lucas, T. J., and Harkness, J. L. Disseminated *Fusarium* species. *Med. J. Aust.*, 2, 624, 1980.

196. Blazar, B. R., Hurd, D. D., Snover, D. C., Alexander, J. W., and McGlave, P. B. Invasive *Fusarium* infections in bone marrow transplant recipients. *Am. J. Med.*, 77, 645, 1984.
197. Steinberg, G. K., Britt, R. H., Enzmann, D. R., Finlay, J. L., and Arvin, A. M. *Fusarium* brain abscess: case report. *J. Neurosurg.*, 56, 598, 1983.
198. Wheeler, M. S., McGinnis, M. R., Schell, W. A., and Walker, D. H. *Fusarium* infection in burned patients. *Am. J. Clin. Pathol.*, 75, 304, 1981.
199. Abramowsky, C. R., Quinn, D., Bradford, W. D., and Conant, N. F. Systemic infection by *Fusarium* in a burned child. *J. Pediatr.*, 84, 561, 1974.
200. Becker, W. K., Cioffi, W. G. Jr., McManus, A. T., et al. Fungal burn wound infection: a 10-year experience. *Arch. Surg.*, 126, 44, 1991.
201. Benjamin, R. P., Callaway, J. L., Conant, N. F., and Durham, N. C. Facial granuloma associated with *Fusarium* infection. *Arch. Dermatol.*, 101, 598, 1970.
202. English, M. P. Invasion of the skin by non-dermatophyte filamentous fungi. *Br. J. Dermatol.*, 80, 282, 1968.
203. Destombes, P., Mariat, F., Rosati, L., and Segretain, G. Les mycétomes en Somalie - conclusions d'une enquéte menée de 1959 a 1964. *Acta Trop.*, 34, 355, 1977.
204. Peloux, Y. and Segretain, G. Mycetoma a *Fusarium*. *Bull. Fr. Mycol. Méd.*, 21, 31, 1966.
205. Baudraz-Rosselet, F., Monod, M., Borradori, L., et al. Mycetoma of the foot due to *Fusarium* sp. treated with oral ketoconazole. *Dermatology*, 184, 303, 1992.
206. Ooi, S. P., Chen, T. T., Huang, T. H., Chang, H. S., and Hsieh, H. Y. Granuloma annulare-like skin lesion due to *Fusarium roseum*: therapy with ketoconazole, *Arch. Dermatol.*, 123, 167, 1987.
207. Attapattu, M. C. and Anandakrishnan, C. Extensive subcutaneous hyphomycosis caused by *F. oxysporum*. *J. Med. Vet. Mycol.*, 24, 105, 1986.
208. Das, D. K., Khan, Z. U., Sheikh, Z. A., and Abdella, N. A. Subcutaneous hyalohyphomycosis due to *Fusarium oxysporum* diagnosed by cytology and culture of fine needle aspirates. *Acta Cytol.*, 45, 661–664, 2001.
209. Negroni, R., Martino, O., Robles, A. M., et al. A cutaneous ulcer induced by fungi of the genus *Fusarium*. *Rev. Soc. Bras. Med. Trop.*, 30, 323–328, 1997.
210. Bourguignon, R. L., Walsh, A. F., Flynn, J. C., Bare, C., and Spinos, E. *Fusarium* species osteomyelitis. *J. Bone Joint Surg.*, 58A, 722, 1976.
211. Jakle, C., Leek, J. C., Olson, D. A., and Robbins, D. L. Septic arthritis due to *Fusarium solani*. *J. Rheumatol.*, 10, 151, 1983.
212. Harris, J. J. and Downham, T. G. Unusual fungal infections associated with immunologic hyporeactivity. *Int. J. Dermatol.*, 17, 323, 1978.
213. Lazarus, J. A. and Schwartz, L. H. Infection of urinary bladder with an unusual fungus strain: *Fusarium*. *Urol. Cutan. Rev.*, 52, 185, 1948.
214. Kerr, C. M., Perfect, J. R., Craven, P. C., et al. Fungal peritonitis in patients on continuous ambulatory peritoneal dialysis. *Ann. Intern. Med.*, 99, 334, 1983.
215. Young, J. B., Ahmed-Jushuf, I. H., Brownjohn, A. M., Parsons, F. M., Foulkes, S. J., and Evans, E. G. Opportunistic peritonitis in continuous ambulatory peritoneal dialysis. *Clin. Nephrol.*, 22, 268, 1984.
216. Flynn, J. T., Meislich, D., Kaiser, B. A., Polinsky, M. S., and Baluarte, H. J. *Fusarium* peritonitis in a child on peritoneal dialysis: case report and review of the literature. *Perit. Dial. Int.*, 16, 52, 1996.
217. Valenstein, P. and Schell, W. A. Primary intranasal *Fusarium* infection: potential for confusion with rhinocerebral zygomycosis. *Arch. Pathol. Lab. Med.*, 110, 751, 1986.
218. Becelli, R., Sassano, P., Liberatore, G. M., Arcese, W., and Mengarelli, A. Surgical and local treatment in a case of fungal sinusitis in a patient with bone marrow aplasia. *Minerva Stomatol.*, 44, 171, 1995.
219. Kurien, M., Anandi, V., Raman, R., and Brahmadathan, K. N. Maxillary sinus fusariosis in immunocompetent hosts. *J. Laryngol. Otol.*, 106, 733, 1992.
220. Mohammedi, I., Gachot, B., Grossin, M., et al. Overwhelming myocarditis due to *Fusarium oxysporum* following bone marrow transplantation. *Scand. J. Infect. Dis.*, 27, 643, 1995.
221. Hsu, C. M., Lee, P. I., Chen, J. M., et al. Fatal *Fusarium* endocarditis complicated by hemolytic anemia and thrombocytopenia in an infant. *Pediatr. Infect. Dis. J.*, 13, 1146, 1994.
222. Forster, R. K., Zachary, I. G., Cottingham, A. J., and Norton, E. W. D. Further observations on the diagnosis, cause, and treatment of endophthalmitis. *Am. J. Ophthalmol.*, 81, 52, 1976.
223. Guss, R. B., Koenig, S., de la Pena, W., Marx, M., and Kaufman, H. E. Endophthalmitis after penetrating keratoplasty. *Am. J. Ophthalmol.*, 95, 651, 1983.
224. Lieberman, T. W., Ferry, A. P., and Bottone, E. J. *Fusarium solani* endophthalmitis without primary corneal involvement. *Am. J. Ophthalmol.*, 88, 764, 1979.
225. Rowsey, J. J., Acers, T. E., Smith, D. L., Mohr, J. A., Newson, D. L., and Rodriguez, J. *Fusarium oxysporum* endophthalmitis. *Arch. Ophthalmol.*, 97, 103, 1979.
226. Zapater, R. C. and Arrechea, A. Mycotic keratitis by *Fusarium*. *Ophthalmologica*, 170, 1, 1975.
227. Mohr, J. A., Nichols, N. B., Jones, J. H., Cherry, P., and Shaver, R. P. Fungal endophthalmitis. *South. Med. J.*, 66, 685, 1973.
228. Glasgow, B. J., Engstrom, R. E. Jr., Holland, G. N., Kreiger, A. E., and Wool, M. G. Bilateral endogenous *Fusarium* endophthalmitis associated with acquired immunodeficiency syndrome. *Arch. Ophthalmol.*, 114, 873, 1996.
229. Gabriele, P. and Hutchins, R. K. *Fusarium* endophthalmitis in an intravenous drug abuser. *Am. J. Ophthalmol.*, 122, 119, 1996.
230. Freidank, H. Hyalohyphomycoses due to *Fusarium* spp.: two case reports and review of the literature. *Mycoses*, 38, 69, 1995.

231. Louie, T., el Baba, F., Shulman, M., and Jimenez-Lucho, V. Endogenous endophthalmitis due to *Fusarium*: case report and review. *Clin. Infect. Dis.*, 18, 585, 1994.
232. Rosa, R. H. Jr., Miller, D., and Alfonso, E. C. The changing spectrum of fungal keratitis in South Florida. *Ophthalmology*, 101, 1005, 1994.
233. Comhaire-Poutchinian, Y., Berthe-Bonnet, S., Grek, V., and Cremer, V. Endophthalmitis due to *Fusarium*: an uncommon cause. *Bull. Soc. Belge Ophthalmol.*, 239, 75, 1990.
234. Vajpayee, R. B., Gupta, S. K., Bareja, U., and Kishore, K. Ocular atopy and mycotic keratitis. *Ann. Ophthalmol.*, 22, 369, 1990.
235. Duran, J. A., Malvar, A., Pereiro, M., and Pereiro, M. *Fusarium moniliforme* keratitis. *Acta Ophthalmol. (Copenhagen)*, 67, 710, 1989.
236. English, M. P. Observations on strains of *Fusarium solani*, *F. oxysporum*, *Candida parapsilosis* from ulcerated legs. *Sabouraudia*, 10, 35, 1972.
237. Foster, R. K. The diagnosis and management of keratomycosis: I. Cause and diagnosis. *Arch. Ophthalmol.*, 93, 975, 1975.
238. Garcia, N. P., Ascani, E., and Zapater, R. Queratomicosis por *Fusarium dimerum*. *Arch. Oftalmol. Buenos Aires*, 47, 332, 1972.
239. Gugnani, H. C., Talwar, R. S., Njoku-Obi, A. N. U., and Kodilinye, H. C. Mycotic keratitis in Nigeria: a study of 21 cases. *Br. J. Ophthalmol.*, 60, 607, 1976.
240. Jones, B. R. Principles in the management of oculomycosis. *Am. J. Ophthalmol.*, 79, 719, 1975.
241. Jones, D. B., Forster, R. K., and Rebell, G. *Fusarium solani* keratitis treated with natamycin (pimaricin): eighteen consecutive cases. *Arch. Ohthalmol.*, 88, 147, 1972.
242. Jones, D. B., Sexton, R., and Rebell, G. Mycotic keratitis in South Florida: a review of thirty-nine cases. *Trans. Ophthalmol. Soc. U. K.*, 89, 781, 1970.
243. Polack, F. M., Kaufman, E., and Newmark, E. Keratomycosis: medical and surgical management. *Arch. Ophthalmol.*, 85, 410, 1971.
244. Singh, G. and Malik, S. R. K. Therapeutic keratoplasty in fungal corneal ulcers. *Br. J. Ophthalmol.*, 56, 41, 1972.
245. Torres, M. A., Mohamed, J., Cavazos-Adame, H., and Martinez, L. A. Topical ketoconazole for fungal keratitis. *Am. J. Ophthalmol.*, 100, 293, 1985.
246. Zapater, R. C., de Arrachea, A., and Guevara, V. H. Queratomicosis por *Fusarium dimerum*. *Sabouraudia*, 10, 274, 1972.
247. Zapater, R. C., Brunzini, M. A., Albesi, E. J., and Silicarto, C. A. El genero *Fusarium* como agente etiologico de micosis ocularis: presentacion de 7 casos. *Arch. Oftalmol. Buenos Aires*, 51, 279, 1976.
248. Eljaschewitsch, J., Sandfort, J., Tintelnot, K., Horbach, I., and Ruf, B. Port-a-cath-related *Fusarium oxysporum* infection in an HIV-infected patient: treatment with liposomal amphotericin B. *Mycoses*, 39, 115, 1996.
249. Viscoli, C., Castagnola, E., Moroni, C., Garaventa, A., Manno, G., and Savioli, C. Infection with *Fusarium* species in two children with neuroblastoma. *Eur. J. Clin. Microbiol. Infect. Dis.*, 9, 773, 1990.
250. Cofrancesco, E., Boschetti, C., Viviani, M. A., et al. Efficacy of liposomal amphotericin B (AmBisome) in the eradication of *Fusarium* infection in a leukemic patient. *Haematologica*, 77, 280, 1992.
251. Legrand, C., Anaissie, E., Hashem, R., Nelson, P., Bodey, G. P., and Ro, J. Experimental fusarial hyalohyphomycosis in a murine model. *J. Infect. Dis.*, 164, 944, 1991.
252. Bushelman, S. J., Callen, J. P., Roth, D. N., and Cohen, L. M. Disseminated *Fusarium solani* infection. *J. Am. Acad. Dermatol.*, 32, 346, 1995.
253. Lupinetti, F. M., Giller, R. H., and Trigg, M. E. Operative treatment of *Fusarium* fungal infection of the lung. *Ann. Thor. Surg.*, 49, 991, 1990.
254. Anaissie, E. J., Kontoyiannis, D. P., Huls, C., et al. Safety, plasma concentrations, and efficacy of high-dose fluconazole in invasive mold infections. *J. Infect. Dis.*, 172, 599, 1995.
255. Viviani, M. A., Cofrancesco, E., Boschetti, C., Tortorano, A. M., and Cortellaro, M. Eradication of *Fusarium* infection in a leukopenic patient treated with liposomal amphotericin B. *Mycoses*, 34, 255, 1991.
256. Graybill, J. R. New antifungal agents. *Eur. J. Clin. Microbiol. Infect. Dis.*, 8, 402, 1989.
257. Miller, S. P. and Shanbrom, E. Infectious syndromes of leukemias and lymphomas. *Am. J. Med. Sci.*, 246, 420, 1963.
258. Silver, R. T., Beal, G. A., Schneiderman, M. A., and McCullough, N. B. The role of the mature neutrophil in bacterial infections in acute leukemia. *Blood*, 12, 814, 1957.
259. Baker, R. D. Leukopenia and therapy in leukemia as factors predisposing to fatal mycoses: mucormycosis, aspergillosis, and cryptococcosis. *Am. J. Clin. Pathol.*, 37, 358, 1962.
260. Francis, P. and Walsh, T. J. Approaches to management of fungal infections in cancer patients. *Oncology (Huntingt.)*, 6, 133, 144, 147, 1992.
261. Browne, E. A. and Marcus, A. J. Chronic idiopathic neutropenia. *N. Engl. J. Med.*, 262, 795, 1960.
262. Kostman, R. Infantile genetic agranulocytosis. *Acta Paediatr. (Stockholm)*, 45(Suppl. 105), 1, 1956.
263. Spaet, T. H. and Dameshek, W. Chronic hypoplastic neutropenia. *Am. J. Med.*, 13, 35, 1952.
264. Hersh, E. M., Bodey, G. P., Nies, B. A., and Freireich, E. J. The causes of death in acute leukemia: a study of 414 patients from 1954–1963. *J. Am. Med. Assoc.*, 193, 105, 1965.
265. Barrios, N. J., Kirkpatrick, D. V., Murciano, A., Stine, K., Van Dyke, R. B., and Humbert, J. R. Successful treatment of disseminated *Fusarium* infection in an immunocompromised child. *Am. J. Pediatr. Hematol. Oncol.*, 12, 319, 1990.

266. Merz, W. A., Karp, J. E., Hoagland, M., Jett-Goheen, M., Junkins, J. M., and Hood, A. F. Diagnosis and successful treatment of fusariosis in the compromised host. *J. Infect. Dis.*, 158, 1046, 1988.
267. Chaulk, C. P., Smith, P. W., Feagler, J. R., Verdirame, J., and Commers, J. R. Fungemia due to *Fusarium solani* in an immunocompromised child. *Pediatr. Infect. Dis. J*, 5, 363, 1986.
268. Lambert, E. H. and Elmqvist, D. Quantal components of end-plate potentials in the myasthenic syndrome. *Ann. NY Acad. Sci.*, 183, 183, 1971.
269. Dordain-Bigot, M. L., Baran, R., Baixench, M. T., and Bazex, J. *Fusarium* onychomycosis. *Ann. Dermatol. Venereol.*, 123, 191, 1996.
270. Arrese, J. E., Pierard-Franchimont, C., and Pierrard, G. E. Fatal hyalohyphomycosis following *Fusarium* onychomycosis in an immunocompromised patient. *Am. J. Dermatol.*, 18, 196, 1996.
271. Spielberger, R. T., Falleroni, M. J., Coene, A. J., and Larsen, R. A., Concomitant amphotericin B therapy, granulocyte transfusions, and GM-CSF administration for disseminated infection with *Fusarium* in a granulocytopenic patient. *Clin. Infect. Dis.*, 16, 528, 1993.
272. Hennequin, C., Benkerrou, M., Gaillard, J. L., Blanche, S., and Fraitag, S. Role of granulocyte colony-stimulating factor in the management of infection with *Fusarium oxysporum* in a neutropenic child. *Clin. Infect. Dis.*, 18, 490, 1994.
273. Montgomery, B., Bianco, J. A., Jacobsen, A., and Singer, J. W. Localization of transfused neutrophils to site of infection during treatment with recombinant human granulocyte-macrophage colony-stimulating factor and pentoxifylline. *Blood*, 78, 533, 1991.
274. Anaissie, E., Wong, E., Bodey, G. P., O'Brien, S., Gutterman, J., and Vadhan, S. Granulocyte-macrophage colony-stimulating factor plus amphotericin B for disseminated mycoses in neutropenic cancer patients. *Proc. 29th Intersci. Conf. Antimicrob. Agents Chemother.*, American Society for Microbiology, Washington, DC, abstract # 73, 1989.
275. Groll, A., Renz, S., Gerein, V., et al. Fatal haemoptysis associated with invasive pulmonary aspergillosis treated with high-dose amphotericin B and granulocyte-macrophage colony-stimulating factor (GM-CSF). *Mycoses*, 35, 67, 1992.
276. McCullough, J. Granulocyte transfusion, in *Neoplastic Diseases of the Blood*, Wiernik, P. H., Canellos, G. P., Kyle, R. A., and Schiffer, C. A., Eds. Churchill Livingstone, New York, 899, 1991.
277. Patoux-Pibouin, M., Couatarmanach, A., Le Gall, F., et al. Fusariose a *Fusarium solani* chez un adolescent leucémique. *Ann. Dermatol. Venereol.*, 119, 377, 1992.
278. Wright, D. G., Robichaud, K. J., Pizzo, P. A., and Deisseroth, A. B. Lethal pulmonary reactions associated with the combined use of amphotericin B and leukocyte transfusion. *N. Engl. J. Med.*, 304, 1185, 1981.
279. Kaplan, S. S., Zdziarski, U. E., Basford, R. E., Wing, E., and Shadduck, R. K. Effect of in vivo recombinant granulocyte-macrophage colony stimulating factor on peripheral blood granulocyte functions. *Clin. Res.*, 36, 566, 1988.
280. Wing, E. J., Magee, D. M., Kaplan, S. S., and Shadduck, R. K. Stimulation of human monocytes by recombinant human granulocyte-macrophage colony stimulating factor in patients with refractory metastatic carcinoma. *Clin. Res.*, 36, 422, 1988.
281. Peters, W. P., Stuart, A., Affronti, M. L., Kim, C. S., and Coleman, R. E. Neutrophil migration is defective during recombinant human granulocyte-macrophage colony stimulating factor infusion after autologous bone marrow transplantation in humans. *Blood*, 72, 1310, 1988.
282. Addison, I. E., Johnson, B., Devereux, S., Goldstone, A. H., and Linch, D. C. Granulocyte-macrophage colony-stimulating factor may inhibit neutrophil migration in vitro. *Clin. Exp. Immunol.*, 76, 149, 1989.
283. Engelhard, D., Eldor, A., Polacheck, I., et al. Disseminated visceral fusariosis treated with amphotericin B-phospholipid complex. *Leuk. Lymphoma*, 9, 385, 1993.
284. Wolff, M. A. and Ramphal, R. Use of amphotericin B lipid complex for treatment of disseminated cutaneous *Fusarium* infection in a neutropenic patient. *Clin. Infect. Dis.*, 20, 1568, 1995.
285. Viscoli, C., Castagnola, E., Moroni, C., Garaventa, A., Manno, G., and Savioli, C., Infection with *Fusarium* species in two children with neuroblastoma. *Eur. J. Clin. Microbiol. Infect. Dis.*, 9, 773, 1990.
286. Raad, I. and Hachem, R., Treatment of central venous catheter-related fungemia due to *Fusarium* oxysporum, *Clin. Infect. Dis.*, 20, 709, 1995.
287. Forster, R. K. and Rebell, G., Animal model of *Fusarium solani* keratitis. *Am. J. Ophthalmol.*, 79, 510, 1975.
288. Rihova, E., Havlikova, M., Boguszakova, J., and Pitrova, S. Keratomycoses. *Cesk. Slov. Oftalmol.*, 52, 164, 1996.
289. Donnenfeld, E. D., Schrier, A., Perry, H. D., et al. Infectious keratitis with corneal perforation associated with corneal hydrops and contact lens wear in keratoconus. *Br. J. Ophthalmol.*, 80, 409, 1996.
290. Donzis, P. B., Mondino, B. J., Weissman, B. A., and Bruckner, D. A. Microbial contamination of contact lens care systems. *Am. J. Ophthalmol.*, 104, 325, 1987.
291. Simmons, R. B., Buffington, J. R., Ward, M., Wilson, L. A., and Ahearn, D. G. Morphology and ultrastructure of fungi in extended-wear soft contact lenses. *J. Clin. Microbiol.*, 24, 21, 1986.
292. Strelow, S. A., Kent, H. D., Eagle, R. C. Jr., and Cohen, E. J. A case of soft contact lens related *Fusarium solani* keratitis. *Contact Lens Assoc. Ophthalmol. J.*, 18, 125, 1992.
293. Francois, J. and De Vos, E. Traitement des mycoses oculaires par la pimaricine. *Bull. Soc. Belge Ophthalmol.*, 195, 97, 1962.
294. Newmark, E., Ellison, A. C., and Kaufman, H. E. Pimaricin therapy of *Cephalosporium* and *Fusarium* keratitis. *Am. J. Ophthalmol.*, 69, 458, 1970.
295. Newmark, E., Ellison, A. C., and Kaufman, H. E. Combined pimaricin and dexamethasone therapy of keratomycosis. *Am. J. Ophthalmol.*, 71, 718, 1971.
296. Rippon, J. W. Mycotic infections of the eye: diagnosis and treatment. *Ophthalmol. Digest*, 34, 18, 1972.

297. Ellison, A. C., Newmark, E., and Kaufman, H. E. Chemotherapy of experimental keratomycosis. *Am. J. Ophthalmol.*, 68, 812, 1969.
298. Ellison, A. C. and Newmark, E. Potassium iodide in mycotic keratitis. *Am. J. Ophthalmol.*, 69, 126, 1970.
299. Green, W. R., Bennett, J. E., and Goos, R. D. Ocular penetration of amphotericin B: a report of laboratory studies and a case report of postsurgical *Cephalosporium* endophthalmitis. *Arch. Ophthalmol.*, 73, 769, 1965.
300. Patel, A. S., Hemady, R. K., Rodrigues, M., Rajagopalan, S., and Elman, M. J. Endogenous *Fusarium* endophthalmitis in a patient wuth acute lymphocytic leukemia. *Am. J. Ophthalmol.*, 117, 363, 1994.
301. Pflugfelder, S. C., Flynn, H. W. Jr., Zwickey, T. A., et al. Exogenous fungal endophthalmitis. *Ophthalmology*, 95, 19, 1988.
302. Glasgow, B. J. and Weisberger, A. K. A quantitative and cartographic study of retinal microvasculopathy in acquired immunodeficiency syndrome. *Am. J. Ophthalmol.*, 118, 46, 1994.
303. Chiaradia, V., Schinella, D., Pascoli, L., Tesio, F., and Santini, G. F. *Fusarium* peritonitis in peritoneal dialysis: report of two cases. *Microbiologica*, 13, 77, 1990.
304. Landau, M., Srebrnik, A., Wolf, R., Bashi, E., and Brenner, S. Systemic ketoconazole treatment for *Fusarium* leg ulcers. *Int. J. Dermatol.*, 31, 511, 1992.
305. Resnik, B. I. and Burdick, A. E. Improvement of eumycetoma with itraconazole. *J. Am. Acad. Dermatol.*, 33, 917, 1995.
306. Gams, W. and McGinnis, M. R. *Phialemonium*, a new anamorph genus intermediate between *Phialophora* and *Acremonium*. *Mycologia*, 75, 977-982, 1983.
307. Heins-Vaccari, E. M., Machado, C. M., Saboya, R. S., et al. *Phialemonium curvatum* infection after bone marrow transplantation. *Rev. Inst. Med. Trop. Sao Paulo*, 43, 163-166, 2001.
308. Guarro, J., Nucci, M., Akiti, T., et al. *Phialemonium* fungemia: two documented cases. *J. Clin. Microbiol.*, 37, 2493-2497, 1999.
309. King, D., Pasarell, L., Dixon, D. M., McGinnis, M. R., and Merz, W. G. A phaeohyphomycotic cyst and peritonitis by *Phialemonium* species and reevaluation of its taxonomy. *J. Clin. Microbiol.*, 31, 1804–1810, 1993.
310. McGinnis, M. R., Gams, W., and Goodwin, M. N. Jr. *Phialemonium obovatum* in a burned child. *J. Med. Vet. Mycol.*, 24, 51–55, 1986.
311. Guarro, J., Gams, W., Pujol, I., and Gené, J. *Acremonium* species: new emerging fungal opportunists - in vitro antifungal susceptibilities and review. *Clin. Infect. Dis.*, 25, 1222–1229, 1997.
312. Fincher, R. M., Fisher, J. F., Lovell, R. D., Newman, C. L., Espinel-Ingroff, A., and Shadomy, H. J. Infection due to the fungus *Acremonium (Cephalosporium)*. *Medicine (Baltimore)*, 70, 398–400, 1991.
313. Texier, L., Lahhourcade, Despinis, R., et al. Fungal granuloma due to a *Cephalosporium*. *Bull. Soc. Fr. Syphilgr.*, 79, 504–507, 1972.
314. Degeorges, M., Heintz, C., Valty, J., Drouhet, E., Acar, J. F., and Leduc, G. Infectious endocarditis due to *Listeria monocytogenes* and *Cephalosporium*. *Presse Med.*, 79, 1377–1380, 1971.
315. de Albornoz, M. B. *Cephalosporium serrae*, an etiologic agent of mycetoma. *Mycopathol. Mycol. Appl.*, 54, 485–498, 1974.
316. de Hoog, G. S. and Guarro, J. *Atlas of Clinical Fungi*. Baarn: Centralbureau voor Schimmelcultures, 720, 1995.
317. Weissgold, D. J., Maguire, A. M., and Brucker, A. J. Management of postoperative *Acremonium* endophthalmitis. *Ophthalmology*, 103, 749–756, 1996.
318. Fridkin, S. K., Kremer, F. B., Bland, L. A., Padhye, A., McNeil, M. M., and Jarvis, W. R. *Acremonium kiliense* endophthalmitis that occureed after cataract extraction in an ambulatory surgical center and was traced to an environmental reservoir. *Clin. Infect. Dis.*, 22, 222–227, 1996.
319. Lopes, J. O., Kolling, L. C., and Neumaier, W. Kerionlike lesion of the scalp due to *Acremonium kiliense* in a noncompromised boy. *Rev. Inst. Med. Trop. Sao Paulo*, 37, 365–368, 1995.
320. Lacaz Cda, S., Porto, E., Carneiro, J. J., Pazianni, I. O., and Pimenta, W. P. Endocarditis in dura mater prosthesis caused by *Acremonium kiliense*. *Rev. Inst. Med. Trop. Sao Paulo*, 23, 274–279, 1981.
321. Schell, W. A. and Perfect, J. R. Fatal, disseminated *Acremonium strictum* infection in a neutropenic host. *J. Clin. Microbiol.*, 34, 1333–1336, 1996.
322. Anadolu, R., Himioglu, S., Oskay, T., Boyvat, A., Peksari, Y., and Gurgey, E. Indolent *Acremonium Strictum* infection in an immunocompetent patient. *Int. J. Dermatol.*, 40, 451–453, 2001.
323. Warris, A., Wesenberg, F., Gaustad, P., Verweij, P. E., and Abrahamsen, T. G. *Acremonium strictum* fungemia in a paediatric patient with acute leukaemia. *Scand. J. Infect. Dis.*, 32, 442–444, 2000.
324. Krcméry, V., Jr., Fuchsberger, P., Trupl, J., et al. Fungal pathogens in etiology of septic shock in neutropenic patients with cancer (short communication). *Zentralbl. Bakteriol.*, 278, 562–565, 1993.
325. Yuen, K. Y., Woo, P. C., Liang, R. H., et al. Clinical significance of alimentary tract microbes in bone marrow transplant recipients. *Diagn. Microbiol. Infect. Dis.*, 30, 75–81, 1998.
326. Noble, R. C., Salgado, J., Newell, S. W., and Goodman, N. L. Endophthalmitis and lumbar diskitis due to *Acremonium falciforme* in a splenectomized patient. *Clin. Infect. Dis.*, 24, 277–278, 1997.
327. Cameron, J. A., Badawi, E. M., Hoffman, P. A., and Tabbara, K. F. Chronic endophthalmitis caused by *Acremonium falciforme*. *Can. J. Ophthalmol.*, 31, 367–368, 1996.
328. Lee, M. W., Kim, J. C., Choi, J. S., Kim, K. H., and Greer, D. L. Mycetoma caused by *Acremonium falciforme*: successful treatment with itraconazole. *J. Am. Acad. Dermatol.*, 32(5 Part 2), 897–900, 1995.
329. Lau, Y. L., Yuen, K. Y., Lee, C. W., and Chan, C. F. Invasive *Acremonium falciforme* infection in a patient with severe combined immunodeficiency. *Clin. Infect. Dis.*, 20, 197–198, 1995.

330. Miro, O., Ferrando, J., Lecha, V., and Campistol, J. M. Subcutaneous abscesses caused by *Acremonium falciforme* in a kidney transplant recipient. *Med. Clin. (Barc.)*, 102, 316, 1994.
331. Milburn, P. B., Papayanopulos, D. M., and Pomerantz, B. M. Mycetoma due to *Acremonium falciforme*. *Int. J. Dermatol.*, 27, 408–410, 1988.
332. McCormack, J. G., McIntyre, P. B., Tilse, M. H., and Ellis, D. H. Mycetoma associated with *Acremonium falciforme* infection. *Med. J. Aust.*, 147, 187–188, 1987.
333. Van Etta, L. L., Peterson, L. R., and Gerding, D. N. *Acremonium falciforme* (*Cephalosporium falciforme*) mycetoma in a renal transplant patient. *Arch. Dermatol.*, 119, 707–708, 1983.
334. Halde, C., Padhye, A. A., Haley, L. D., Rinaldi, M. G., Kay, D., and Leeper, R. *Acremonium falciforme* as a cause of mycetoma in California. *Sabouraudia*, 14, 319–326, 1976.
335. Wetli, C. V., Weiss, S. D., Clearly, T. J., and Gyori, E. Fungal cerebritis from intravenous drug abuse. *J. Forensic Sci.*, 29, 260–268, 1984.
336. Rodriguez-Ares, T., De Rojas Silva, V., Ferreiros, M. P., Becerra, E. P., Tome, C. C., and Sanchez-Salorio, M. *Acremonium* keratitis in a patient with herpetic neurotrophic corneal disease. *Acta Ophthalmol. Scand.*, 78, 107–109, 2000.
337. Forster, R. K., Rebell, G., and Stiles, W. Recurrent keratitis due to *Acremonium potronii*. *Am. J. Ophthalmol.*, 79, 126–128, 1975.
338. Read, R. W., Chuck, R. S., Rao, N. A., and Smith, R. E. Traumatic *Acremonium atrogriseum* keratitis following laser-assisted in situ keratomileusis. *Arch. Ophthalmol.*, 118, 418–421, 2000.
339. Zaitz, C., Porto, E., Heins-Vaccari, E. M., et al. Subcutaneous hyalohyphomycosis caused by *Acremonium recifei*: case report. *Rev. Inst. Med. Trop. Sao Paulo*, 37, 267–270, 1995.
340. Simonsz, H. J. Keratomycosis caused by *Acremonium recifei*, treated with keratoplasty, miconazole and ketoconazole. *Doc. Ophthalmol.*, 56, 131–135, 1983.
341. Koshi, G., Padhye, A. A., Ajello, L., and Chandler, F. W. *Acremonium recifei* as an agent of mycetoma in India. *Am. J. Trop. Med. Hyg.*, 28, 692–696, 1979.
342. Lacaz C. S., Porto, E., Cuce, L. C., and Salebian, A. Maduromycosis caused by *Cephalosporium acremonium*. Case report. *Rev. Inst. Med. Trop. Sao Paulo*, 21, 56–61, 1979.
343. Kennedy, S. M., Shankland, G. S., Lee, W. R., and Sekundo, W. Keratitis due to the fungus *Acremonium* (*Cephalosporium*). *Eye*, 8(Part 6), 692–694, 1994.
344. Pflugfelder, S. C., Flynn, H. W., Jr., Zwickey, T. A., et al. Exogenous fungal endophthalmitis. *Ophthalmology*, 95, 19–30, 1988.
345. Szombathy, S. P., Chez, M. G., and Laxer, R. M. Acute septic arthritis due to *Acremonium*. *J. Rheumatol.*, 15, 714–715, 1988.
346. Breton, P., Germaud, P., Morin, O., Audouin, A. F., Milpied, N., and Harousseau, J. L. Rare pulmonary mycoses in patients with hematologic disease. *Rev. Pneumol. Clin.*, 54, 253–257, 1998.
347. Miro, O., Campistol, J. M., Ribe, A., Nicolas, J. M., and Nadal, P. Pulmonary *Acremonium* abscesses and gastrointestinal tuberculosis manifested as massive upper gastrointestinal bleeding. *Nephrol. Dial. Transplant.*, 10, 1444–1446, 1995.
348. Heitmann, L., Cometta, A., Hurni, M., Aebischer, N., Tschan-Schild, I., and Billie, J. Right-sided pacemaker-related endocarditis due to *Acremonium* species. *Clin. Infect. Dis.*, 25, 158–160, 1997.
349. Grunwald, M. H., Cagnano, M., Mosovich, M., and Halevy, S. Cutaneous infection due to *Acremonium*. *J. Eur. Acad. Dermatol. Venereol.*, 10, 58–61, 1998.
350. Vasiloudes, P., Morelli, J. G., and Weston, W. L. Painful skin papules caused by concomitant *Acremonium* and *Fusarium* infection in a neutropenic child. *J. Am. Acad. Dermatol.*, 37, 1006–1008, 1997.
351. Tosti, A., Piraccini, B. M., and Lorenzi, S. Onychomycosis caused by nondermatophytic molds: clinical features and response to treatment of 59 cases. *J. Am. Acad. Dermatol.*, 42(2 Part 1), 217–224, 2000.
352. Gupta, A. K. and Summerbell, R. C. Combined distal and lateral sublingual and white superficial onychomycosis in the toenail. *J. Am. Acad. Dermatol.*, 41, 938–944, 1999 [see also: *J. Am. Acad. Dermatol.*, 44, 312, 2001].
353. Roilides, E., Bibashi, E., Acritidou, E., et al. *Acremonium* fungemia in two immunocompromised children. *Pediatr. Infect. Dis.*, 14, 548-550, 1995.
354. Brown, N. M., Blundell, E. L., Chown, S. R., Warnock, D. W., Hill, J. A., and Slade, R. R. *Acremonium* infection in a neutropenic patient. *J. Infect.*, 25, 73–76, 1992.
355. Uip, D. E., Amato Neto, V., Varejao Strabelli, T. M., et al. Fungal infections in 100 patients subjected to heart transplantation. *Arq. Bras. Cardiol.*, 66, 65–67, 1996.
356. Beneke, E. S. *Medical Mycology and Human Mycoses*. Star Publishing Co., Belmont, CA, 178-186, 1996.
357. Phillips, P., Wood, W. S., Phillips, G., and Rinaldi, M. G. Invasive hyalohyphomycosis caused by *Scopulariopsis brevicaulis* in a patient undergoing allogeneic bone marrow transplant. *Diagn. Microbiol. Infect. Dis.*, 12, 429–432, 1989.
358. Neglia, J. P., Hurd, D. D., Ferrieri, P., and Snover, D. C. Invasive *Scopulariopsis* in the immunocompromised host. *Am. J. Med.*, 83, 1163–1166, 1987.
359. Gupta, A. K. and Gregurek-Novak, T. Efficacy of itraconazole, terbinafine, fluconazole, griseofulvin and ketoconazole in the treatment of *Scopulariopsis brevicaulis* causing onychomycosis of the toes. *Dermatology*, 202, 235–238, 2001.
360. Martel, J., Faisant, M., Lebeau, B., Pinel, C., Feray, C., and Feuilhade, M. Subcutaneous mycosis due to *Scopulariopsis brevicaulis* in an immunocompromised patient. *Ann. Dermatol. Venereol.*, 128, 130–133, 2001.
361. Filipello Marchisio, V., Fusconi, A., and Querio, F. L. *Scopulariopsis brevicaulis*: a keratinophilic or a keratinolytic fungus? *Mycoses*, 43, 281–292, 2000.

362. Gupta, A. K., Gregurek-Novak, T., Konnikov, N., Lynde, C. W., Hofstader, S., and Summerbell, R. C. Itraconazole and terbinafine treatment of some nondermatophyte molds causing onychomycosis of the toes and a review of the literature. *J. Cutan. Med. Surg.*, 5, 2-6-210, 2001.
363. Filipello Marchisio, V. and Fusconi, A. Morphological evidence for keratinolytic activity of *Scopulariopsis* spp. isolates from nail lesions and the air. *Med. Mycol.*, 39, 287–294, 2001.
364. Patel, R., Gustaferro, C. A., Krom, R. A., Wiesner, R. H., Roberts, G. D., and Paya, C. V. Phaeohyphomycosis due to *Scopulariopsis brumptii* in a liver transplant recipient. *Clin. Infect. Dis.*, 19, 198–200, 1994.
365. Naidu, J., Singh, S. M., and Pouranik, M. Onychomycosis caused by *Scopulariopsis brumptii*. A case report and sensitivity studies. *Mycopathologia*, 113, 159–164, 1991.
366. Grieble, H. G., Rippon, J. W., Maliwan, N., and Daun, V. Scopulariopsosis and hypersensitivity pneumonitis in an addict. *Ann. Intern. Med.*, 83, 326–329, 1975.
367. Wang, D. L., Xu, C., and Wang, G. C. A case of mycetoma caused by *Scopulariopsis* maduromycosis. *Chin. Med. J. (Engl.)*, 99, 376–378, 1986.
368. Ellison, M. D., Hung, R. T., Harris, K., and Campbell, B. H. Report of the first case of invasive fungal sinusitis caused by *Scopulariopsis acremonium*: review of scopulariopsis infections. *Arch. Otolaryngol. Head Neck Surg.*, 124, 1014–1016, 1998.
369. Kriesel, J. D., Anderson, E. E., Gooch, W. M., and Pavia, A. T. Invasive sinonasal disease due to *Scopulariopsis candida*: case report and review of *Scopulariopsis*. *Clin. Infect. Dis.*, 19, 317–319, 1994.
370. Wheat, L. J., Bartlett, M., Ciccarelli, M., and Smith, J. W. Opportunistic *Scopulariopsis* pneumonia in an immunocompromised host. *South. Med. J.*, 77, 1608–1609, 1984.
371. Patel, R., Gustaferro, C. A., Krom, R. A., Weisner, R. H., Roberts, G. D., and Paya, C. V. Deep *Scopulariopsis* in the immunocompromised host. *31st Annu. Meet. Infect. Dis. Soc. America, (New Orleans)*, abstract 76, 1993.
372. Arrese, J. E., Pierard-Franchimont, C., and Pierard, G. E. Unusual mould infection of the human stratum corneum. *J. Med. Vet. Mycol.*, 35, 225–227, 1997.
373. Gariano, R. F. and Kalina, R. E., Posttraumatic fungal endophthalmitis resulting from *Scopulariopsis brevicaulis*. *Retina*, 17, 256–258, 1997.
374. Lotery, A. J., Kerr, J. R., and Page, B. A., Fungal keratitis caused by *Scopulariopsis brevicaulis*: successful treatment with topical amphotericin B and chloramphenicol without the need for surgical debridement. *Br. J. Dermatol.*, 78, 730, 1994.
375. Del Prete, A., Sepe, G., Ferrante, M., Loffredo, C., Masciello, M., and Sebastiani, A. Fungal keratitis due to *Scopulariopsis brevicaulis* in an eye previously suffering from herpetic keratitis. *Ophthalmologica*, 208, 333–335, 1994.
376. Ragge, N. K., Hart, J. C., Easty, D. L., and Tyers, A. G. A case of fungal keratitis caused by *Scopulariopsis brevicaulis*: treatment with antifungal agents and penetrating keratoplasty. *Br. J. Ophthalmol.*, 74, 561–562, 1990.
377. De Doncker, P. R., Scher, R. K., Baran, R. L., et al. Itraconazole therapy is effective for pedal onychomycosis caused by some nondermatophyte molds and in mixed infection with dermatophytes and molds: a multicenter study with 36 patients. *J. Am. Acad. Dermatol.*, 36(2 Part 1), 173–177, 1997.
378. Tosti, A., Piraccini, B. M., Stinchi, C., and Lorenzi, S. Onychomycosis due to *Scopulariopsis brevicaulis*: clinical features and response to systemic antifungals. *Br. J. Dermatol.*, 135, 799–802, 1996.
379. Frey, D. and Muir, D. B. Onychomycosis caused by *Scopulariopsis brevicaulis*. *Australs. J. Dermatol.*, 22, 123–126, 1986.
380. Onsberg, P. *Scopulariopsis brevicaulis* in nails. *Dermatologica*, 161, 259–264, 1980.
381. Onsberg, P. and Stahl, D. *Scopulariopsis* onychomycosis treated with natamycin. *Dermatologica*, 160, 57–61, 1980.
382. Gupta, A. K. and Elewski, B. E. Nondermatophyte causes of onychomycosis and superficial mycoses. *Curr. Top. Med. Mycol.*, 7, 87–97, 1996.
383. Ginarte, M., Pereiro, M. Jr., Fernandez-Redondo, V., and Toribio, J. Plantar infection by *Scopulariopsis brevicaulis*. *Dermatology*, 193, 149–151, 1996.
384. Cox, N. H. and Irving, B. Cutaneous "ringworm" lesions of *Scopulariopsis brevicaulis*. *Br. J. Dermatol.*, 129, 726–728, 1993.
385. Dhar, J. and Carey, P. B. *Scopulariopsis brevicaulis* skin lesions in an AIDS patient. *AIDS*, 7, 1283–1284, 1993.
386. Sellier, P., Monsuez, J. J., Lacroix, C., et al. Recurrent subcutaneous infection due to *Scopulariopsis brevicaulis* in a liver transplant recipient. *Clin. Infect. Dis.*, 30, 820–823, 2000.
387. Migrino, R. Q., Hall, G. S., and Longworth, D. L. Deep tissue infections caused by *Scopulariopsis brevicaulis*: report of a case of prosthetic valve endocarditis and review. *Clin. Infect. Dis.*, 21, 672–674, 1995.
388. Hagensee, M. E., Bauwens, J. E., Kjos, B., and Bowden, R. A. Brain abscess following marrow transplantation: experience at the Fred Hutchinson Cancer Research Center, 1984–1992. *Clin. Infect. Dis.*, 19, 402–408, 1994.
389. Sekhon, A. S., Williams, D. J., and Harvey, J. H. Deep *Scopulariopsis*: a case report and sensitivity studies. *J. Clin. Pathol.*, 27, 837–843, 1974.
390. Ryder, N. S. Activity of terbinafine against serious fungal pathogens. *Mycoses*, 42(Suppl. 2), 115–119, 1999.
391. Bruynzeel, I. and Starnik, T. M. Granulomatous skin infection caused by *Scopulariopsis brevicaulis*. *Am. J. Acad. Dermatol.*, 39(2 Part 2), 365–367, 1998.
392. Creus, L., Umbert, P., Torres-Rodriguez, J. M., and Lopez-Gil, F. Ulcerous granulomatous cheilitis with lymphatic invasion caused by *Scopulariopsis brevicaulis* infection. *J. Am. Acad. Dermatol.*, 31(5 Part 2), 881–883, 1994.
393. Coley, K. C. and Crain, J. L. Miconazole-induced fatal dysrhythmia. *Pharmacotherapy*, 17, 379–382, 1997.
394. Gentry, L. O., Nasser, M. M., and Kielhofner, M. *Scopulariopsis* endocarditis associated with Duran ring valvuloplasty. *Tex. Heart Inst. J.*, 22, 81–85, 1995.

395. Muehrcke, D. D., Lytle, B. W., and Cosgrove, D. M. 3rd Surgical and long-term antifungal therapy for fungal prosthetic valve endocarditis. *Ann. Thorac. Surg.*, 60, 538–543, 1995.
396. Baddley, J. W., Moser, S. A., Sutton, D. A., and Pappas, P. G. *Microascus cinereus* (*Anamorph scolulariopsis*) brain abscess in a bone marrow transplant recipient. *J. Clin. Microbiol.*, 38, 395–397, 2000.
397. Barron, G. L., Cain, R. F., and Gilman, J. C. The genus *Microascus*. *Can. J. Bot.*, 39, 1609–1631, 1961.
398. Schönborn, C. and Schmoranzer, H. Untersuchungen über schimmelpilzinfektionen der zehennägel. *Mykosen*, 13, 253–272, 1970.
399. Pandey, A., Agrawal, G. P., and Singh, S. M. Pathogenic fungi in soils of Jabalpur, India. *Mycoses*, 33, 116–125, 1990.
400. Youssef, Y., el-Din, A. A., and Hassanein, S. M. Occurrence of keratolytic fungi and related dermatophytes in soils in Cairo, Egypt. *Zentbl. Mikrobiol.*, 147, 80–85, 1992.
401. Lichtwardt, R. W., Barron, G. L., and Tiffany, L. H. Mold flora associated with deterioration of stored corn in Iowa. *Iowa State J. Sci.*, 13, 1–11, 1958.
402. Marques, A. R., Kwon-Chung, K. J., Holland, S. M., Turner, M. L., and Gallin, J. I. Suppurative cutaneous granulomata caused by *Microascus cinereus* in a patient with chronic granulomatous disease. *Clin. Infect. Dis.*, 20, 110–114, 1995.
403. Krisher, K. K., Holdridge, N. B., Mustafa, M. M., Rinaldi, M. G., and McGough, D. A. Disseminated *Microascus cirrosus* infection in pediatric bone marrow transplant recipient. *J. Clin. Microbiol.*, 33, 735–737, 1995.
404. Brown, A. H. S. and Smith, G. The genus *Paecilomyces* Bainier and its perfect stage *Byssochlamys* Westling. *Trans. Br. Mycological Soc.*, 40, 17–89, 1957.
405. Raper, K. B. and Thom, C., *A Manual of the Penicillia*. Williams & Williams, Baltimore, 284–288, 1949.
406. Samson, R. A. *Paecilomyces* and some allied hyphomycetes. *Studies in Mycology*, 6, 1–119, Centraalbureau voor Schimmelcultures, Baarn, The Netherlands, 1974.
407. Miller, G. R., Rebell, G., Magoon, R. C., Kulvin, S. M., and Forster, R. K. Intravitreal antimycotic therapy and the cure of mycotoc endophthalmitis caused by a *Paecilomyces lilacinus* contaminated pseudophakos. *Ophthalmic Surg.*, 9, 54–63, 1978.
408. O'Day, D. M. Fungal endophthalmitis caused by *Paecilomyces lilacinus* after intraocular lens implantation. *Am. J. Ophthalmol.*, 83, 130–131, 1977.
409. Gordon, M. A. *Paecilomyces lilacinus* (Thom) Samson, from systemic infection in an armadillo (*Dasypus novemcinctus*). *Sabouraudia*, 22, 109, 1984.
410. Barron, G. L. *The Genera of Hyphomycetes From Soil*. Williams & Wilkins, Baltimore, 54, 1978.
411. Naldi, L., Lovati, S., Farina, C., Gotti, E., and Cainelli, T. *Paecilomyces marquandii* cellulitis in a kidney transplant patient. *Br. J. Dermatol.*, 143, 647–649, 2000.
412. Athar, M. A., Sekhon, A. S., Mcgrath, J. V., and Malone, R. M. Hyalohyphomycosis caused by *Paecilomyces variotii* in an obstetrical patient. *Eur. J. Epidemiol.*, 12, 33–35, 1996.
413. Blackwell, V., Ahmed, K., O'Docherty, C., and Hay, R. J. Cutaneous hyalohyphomycosis caused by *Paecilomyces lilacinus* in a renal transplant patient. *Br. J. Dermatol.*, 143, 873–875, 2000.
414. Hilmarsdottir, I., Thorsteinsson, S. B., Asmundsson, P., Bodvarsson, M., and Arnadottir, M. Cutaneous infection caused by *Paecilomyces lilacinus* in a renal transplant patient: treatment with voriconazole. *Scand. J. Infect. Dis.*, 32, 331–332, 2000.
415. Castro, L. G., Salebian, A., and Sotto, M. N. Hyalohyphomycosis by *Paecilomyces lilacinus* in a renal transplant patient and a review of human *Paecilomyces* species infections. *J. Med. Vet. Mycol.*, 28, 15–26, 1990.
416. Harris, L. F., Dan, B. M., Lefkowitz, L. B. Jr., and Alford, R. H. *Paecilomyces* cellulites in a renal transplant patient: successful treatment with intravenous miconazole. *South Med. J.*, 72, 897–898, 1979.
417. Chan-Tack, K. M., Thio, C. L., Miller, N. S., Karp, C. L., Ho, C., and Merz, W. G. *Paecilomyces lilacinus* fungemia in an adult bone marrow transplant recipient. *Med. Mycol.*, 37, 57–60, 1999.
418. Shing, M. M., Ip, M., Li, C. K., Chik, K. W., and Yuen, P. M. *Paecilomyces variotii* fungemia in a bone marrow transplant patient. *Bone Marrow Transplant.*, 17, 281–283, 1996.
419. Marzec, A., Heron, L. G., Pritchard, R. C., et al. *Paecilomyces variotii* in peritoneal dialysate. *J. Clin. Microbiol.*, 31, 2392–2395, 1993.
420. Tan, T. Q., Ogden, A. K., Tillman, J., Demmler, G. J., and Rinaldi, M. G. *Paecilomyces lilacinus* catheter-related fungemia in an immunocompromised pediatric patient. *J. Clin. Microbiol.*, 30, 2479–2483, 1992.
421. Fagerburg, R., Suh, B., Buckley, H. R., Lorber, B., and Karian, J. Cerebrospinal fluid shunt colonization and obstruction by *Paecilomyces variotii*. Case report. *J. Neurosurg.*, 54, 257–260, 1981.
422. Haldane, E. V., MacDonald, J. L., Gittens, W. O., Yuce, K., and van Rooyen, C. E. Prosthetic valvular endocarditis due to the fungus *Paecilomyces*. *Can. Med. Assoc. J.*, 111, 963–965 & 968, 1974.
423. Young, V. L., Hertl, M. C., Murray, P. R., and Lambros, V. S. *Paecilomyces variotii* contamination in the lumen of a saline-filled breast implant. *Plast. Reconstr. Surg.*, 96, 1430–1434, 1995 [see also: *Plast. Reconstr. Surg.*, 98, 1323, 1996].
424. Murciano, A., Dommer, A., and Cohen, I., *Paecilomyces lilacinus* infection in an immunocompromised patient. *J. La State Med. Soc.*, 142, 35–37, 1990.
425. Itin, P. H., Frei, R., Lautenschlager, S., et al. Cutaneous manifestations of *Paecilomyces lilacinus* infection induced by a contaminated skin lotion in patients who are severely immunocompromised. *J. Am. Acad. Dermatol.*, 39, 401–409, 1998.
426. Orth, B., Frei, R., Itin, P. H., et al. Outbreak of invasive mycoses caused by *Paecilomyces lilacinus* from contaminated skin lotion. *Ann. Intern. Med.*, 125, 799–806, 1996.
427. Domniz, Y., Lawless, M., Sutton, G. L., Rogers, C. M., and Meagher, L. J. Successful treatment of *Paecilomyces lilacinus* endophthalmitis after foreign body trauma to the cornea. *Cornea*, 20, 109–111, 2001.

428. Al-Mohsen, I. Z., Sutton, D. A., Sigler, L., et al. *Acrophialophora fusispora* brain abscess in a child with acute lymphoblastic leukemia: review of cases and taxonomy. *J. Clin. Microbiol.*, 38, 4569–4576, 2000.
429. Lam, D. S., Koehler, A. P., Fan, D. S., Cheuk, W., Leung, A. T., and Ng, J. S. Endogenous fungal endophthalmitis caused by *Paecilomyces variotii*. *Eye*, 13(Part 1), 113–116, 1999.
430. Okhravi, N., Dart, J. K., Towler, H. M., and Lightman, S. *Paecilimyces lilacinus* endophthalmitis with secondary keratitis: a case report and literature review. *Arch. Ophthalmol.*, 115, 1320–1324, 1997.
431. Hirst, L. W. *Paecilomyces* keratitis. *Br. J. Ophthalmol.*, 79, 711, 1995 [see also: *Br. J. Dermatol.*, 78, 157–158, 1994].
432. Mizunoya, S. and Watanabe, Y., *Paecilomyces* keratitis with corneal perforation salvaged by a conjunctival flap and delayed keratoplasty. *Br. J. Ophthalmol.*, 78, 157–158, 1994 [see also: *Br. J. Ophthalmol.*, 79, 711, 1995].
433. Ohkubo, S., Torisaki, M., Higashide, T., Mochizuki, K., and Ishibashi, Y. Endophthalmitis caused by *Paecilomyces lilacinus* after cataract surgery: a case report. *Nippon Ganka Gakkai Zasshi*, 98, 103–110, 1994.
434. Legeais, J. M., Blanc, V., Basset, D., et al. Severe keratomycosis. Diagnosis and treatment. *J. Fr. Ophthalmol.*, 17, 568–573, 1994.
435. Hirst, L. W., Sebban, A., Whitby, R. M., Nimmo, G. R., and Stallard, K. Non-traumatic mycotic keratitis. *Eye*, 6(Part 4), 391–395, 1992.
436. D'Mellow, G., Hirst, L. W., Whitby, M., Nimmo, G., and Stallard, K. Intralenticular infections. *Ophthalmology*, 98, 1176–1378, 1991.
437. Minogue, M. J., Playfair, T. J., Gregory-Roberts, J. C., and Robinson, L. P. Cure of *Paecilomyces* endophthalmitis with multiple intravitreal injections of amphotericin B. Case report. *Arch. Ophthalmol.*, 107, 1281, 1989.
438. Levin, P. S., Beebe, W. E., and Abbott, R. L. Successful treatment of *Paecilomyces lilacinus* endophthalmitis following cataract extraction with intraocular lens implantation. *Opthalmic Surg.*, 18, 217–219, 1987.
439. Jade, K. B., Lyons, M. F., and Gnann, J. W. Jr. *Paecilomyces lilacinus* cellulites in an immunocompromised patient. *Arch. Dermatol.*, 122, 1169–1170, 1986.
440. Gordon, M. A. and Norton, S. W. Corneal transplant infection by *Paecilomyces lilacinus*. *Sabouraudia*, 23, 295–301, 1985.
441. Wolfson, J. S., Sober, A. J., and Rubin, R. H. Dermatologic manifestations of infections in immunocompromised patients. *Medicine (Baltimore)*, 64, 115–133, 1985.
442. Mosier, M. A., Lusk, B., Pettit, T. H., Howard, D. H., and Rhodes, J. Fungal endophthalmitis following intraocular lens implantation. *Am. J. Ophthalmol.*, 83, 1–8, 1977.
443. Rodrigues, M. M. and MacLeod, D. Exogenous fungal endophthalmitis caused by *Paecilomyces*. *Am. J. Ophthalmol.*, 79, 687–690, 1975.
444. Kozarsky, A. M., Stulting, D., Waring, G. O. III, Cornel, F. M., Wilson, L. A., and Cavanagh, L. A. Penetrating keratoplasty for exogenous *Paecilomyces* queratitis followed by postoperative endophthalmitis. *Am. J. Ophthalmol.*, 98, 552–557, 1984.
445. Pettit, T. H., Olson, R. J., Foos, R. Y., and Marin, W. J. Fungal endophthalmitis following intraocular lens implantation. *Arch. Ophthalmol.*, 98, 1025–1039, 1980.
446. Minogue, M. J., Francis, I. C., Quatermass, P., et al. Successful treatment of fungal keratitis caused by *Paecylomyces lilacinus*. *Am. J. Ophthalmol.*, 98, 626–627, 1984.
447. Nayak, D. R., Balakrishnan, R., Nainani, S., and Siddique, S. *Paecilomyces* fungus infection of the paranasal sinuses. *Int. J. Pediatr. Otorhinolaryngol.*, 52, 183–187, 2000.
448. Gutiérrez-Rodero, F., Morangon, M., Ortiz de la Tabla, V., Mayol, M. J., and Martin, C. Cutaneous hyalohyphomycosis caused by *Paecilomyces lilacinus* in an immunocompetent host successfully treated with itraconazole: case report and review. *Eur. J. Clin. Microbiol. Infect. Dis.*, 18, 814–818, 1999.
449. Castro, L. G. Cutaneous *Paecilomyces lilacinus* infection. *J. Am. Acad. Dermatol.*, 39, 516–517, 1998 [see also: *J. Am. Acad. Dermatol.*, 37(2 Part 1), 270–271, 1997].
450. Marchese, S. M. and Smoller, B. R. Cutaneous *Paecilomyces lilacinus* infection in a hospitalized patient taking corticosteroids. *Int. J. Dermatol.*, 37, 438–441, 1998.
451. Hecker, M. S., Weinberg, J. M., Bagheri, H., et al. Cutaneous *Paecilomyces lilacinus* infection: report of two novel cases. *J. Am. Acad. Dermatol.*, 37 (2 Part 1), 270–271, 1997 [see also: *J. Am. Acad. Dermatol.*, 39, 516–517, 1998.
452. Westenfeld, F., Alston, W. K., and Winn, W. C. Complicated soft tissue infection with prepatellar bursitis caused by *Paecilomyces lilacinus* in an immunocompetent host: case report and review. *J. Clin. Microbiol.*, 34, 1559–1562, 1996.
453. Castro, L. G. Sporotrichosis-like lesions caused by a *Paecilomyces* genus fungus. *Int. J. Dermatol.*, 34, 364, 1995 [see also: *Int. J. Dermatol.*, 33, 275–276, 1994].
454. Leigheb, G., Mossini, A., Boggio, P., Gattoni, M., Bornacina, G., and Griffanti, P. Sporotrichosis-like lesions caused by a *Paecilomyces* genus fungus. *Int. J. Dermatol.*, 33, 275–276, 1994.
455. Naidu, J. and Singh, S. M. Hyalohyphomycosis caused by *Paecilomyces variotii*: a case report, animal pathogenicity and "in vitro" sensitivity. *Antonie Van Leeuwenhoek*, 62, 225–230, 1992.
456. Williamson, P. R., Kwon-Chung, K. J., and Gallin, J. I. Successful treatment of *Paecilomyces variotii* infection in a patient with chronic granulomatous disease and a revie of *Paecilomyces* species infections. *Clin. Infect. Dis.*, 14, 1023–1026, 1992 [see also: *Clin. Infect. Dis.*, 15, 552–553, 1992].
457. Takayasu, S., Akagi, M., and Shimizu, Y. Cutaneous mycosis caused by *Paecilomyces lilacinus*. *Arch. Dermatol.*, 113, 1687–1690, 1977.
458. Bryant, D. H. and Rogers, P. Allergic alveolitis due to wood-rot fungi. *Allergy Proc.*, 12, 89, 1991.
459. Akhunova, A. M. and Shustova, V. I. *Paecilomyces* infection. *Probl. Tuberk.*, 8, 38, 1989.
460. Halde, C. and Okumoto, M. Ocular mycosis: a study of 82 cases. *Proc. 20th Int. Congr. Ophthalmol.*, Munich. Excerpta Medica International Congresses Series, 146, 705, 1966.

461. Rippon, J. W. *Medical Mycology: The Pathogenic Fungi and the Pathogenic Actinomycetes*, 3rd ed. W. B. Saunders, Philadelphia, 728, 1988.
462. Volna, F. and Maderova, E. *Paecilomyces lilacinus*-sensitivity to disinfectans. *Cesk. Epidemiol. Mikrobiol. Imunol.*, 39, 315, 1990.
463. Webster, R. G. Jr., Martin, W. J., Pettit, T. H., et al. Eye infection after plastic lens implantation. *Morbid. Mortal. Wkly Rep.*, 24, 437, 1975.
464. Byrd, R. P. J., Roy, T. M., Field, C. L., and Lynch, J. A. *Paecilomyces varioti*, pneumonia in a patient with diabetes mellitus. *J. Diab. Comp.*, 6, 150, 1992.
465. Weitzmann, I. Saprophytic molds as agents of cutaneous and subcutaneous infection in the immunocompromised host. *Arch. Dermatol.*, 122, 1161, 1986.
466. Silliman, C. C., Lawellin, D. W., Lohr, J. A., Rodgers, B. M., and Donowitz, L. G. *Paecilomyces lilacinus* infection in a child with chronic granulomatous disease. *J. Infect.*, 24, 191, 1992.
467. Sillevis Smitt, J. H., Leusen, J. H., Stas, H. G., Teeuw, A. H., and Weening, R. S. Chronic bullous disease of childhood and *Paecilomyces* lung infection in chronic granulomatous disease. *Arch. Dis. Child*, 77, 150–152, 1997.
468. Tauber, A. I., Borregaard, N., Simons, E., and Wright, J. Chronic granulomatous disease: a syndrome of phagocyte oxidase deficiencies. *Medicine (Baltimore)*, 62, 286, 1983.
469. Gallin, J. I. and Malech, H. L. Update on chronic granulomatous disease of childhood: immunotherapy and potential for gene therapy. *J. Am. Med. Assoc.*, 263, 1533, 1990.
470. Gallin, J. I., Malech, H. L., Weening, R. S., et al.. A controlled trial of interferon gamma to prevent infection in chronic granulomatous disease. *N. Engl. J. Med.*, 324, 509, 1991.
471. Hendrickson, D. H. and Krenz, M. M. Reagents and stains, in *Manual of Clinical Microbiology*, Balows, A., Ed. American Society for Microbiology, Washington, DC, 1290, 1991.
472. Mandell, G. L. and Hook, E. W. Leukocyte bactericidal activity in chronic granulomatous disease: correlation of bactericidal hydrogen peroxide production and susceptibility to intracellular killing. *J. Bacteriol.*, 100, 531, 1969.
473. Gallin, J. I., Buescher, E. S., Seligmann, B. E., Nath, J., Gaither, T., and Katz, P. Recent advances in chronic granulomatous disease. *Ann. Intern. Med.*, 99, 675, 1983.
474. Saberhagen, C., Klotz, S. A., Bartholomew, W., Drews, D., and Dixon, A. Infection due to *Paecilomyces lilacinus*: a challenging clinical identification. *Clin. Infect. Dis.*, 25, 1411–1413, 1997.
475. McClellan, J. R., Hamilton, J. D., Alexander, J. A., Wolfe, W. G., and Reed, J. B. *Paecilomyces variotii* endocarditis on a prosthetic aortic valve. *J. Thorac. Cardiovasc. Surg.*, 71, 472, 1976.
476. Silver, M. D., Tuffinel, P. G., and Bigelow, W. G. Endocarditis caused by *Paecilomyces variotii* affecting an aortic valve allograft. *J. Thorac. Cardiovasc. Surg.*, 61, 278, 1971.
477. Kalish, S. B., Goldschmidt, R., Li, C., et al. Infective endocarditis caused by *Paecilomyces varioti*. *Am. J. Clin. Pathol.*, 78, 249, 1982.
478. Allevato, P. A., Ohorodnik, J. M., Mezger, E., and Eisses, J. F. *Paecilomyces javanicus* endocarditis of native and prosthetic aortic valve. *Am. J. Clin. Pathol.*, 82, 247, 1984.
479. Uys, C. J., Don, P. A., Schrire, V., and Barnard, C. N. Endocarditis following cardiac surgery due to the fungus *Paecilomyces*. *S. Afr. Med. J.*, 37, 1276, 1963.
480. Harris, L. F., Dan, B. M., Lefhowitz, L. B. Jr., and Alford, R. H. *Paecilomyces* cellulitis in a renal transplant patient: successful treatment with intravenous miconazole. *South. Med. J.*, 72, 897, 1979.
481. Arai, H. and Endo, T. A case of deep mycosis *Fonseca pedrosoi* and *Paecilomyces lilacinus* following renal transplant. *Hifuka*, 31, 481, 1977.
482. Fletcher, C. L., Hay, R. J., Midgley, G., and Moore, M. Onychomycosis caused by infection with *Paecilomyces lilacinus*. *Br. J. Dermatol.*, 139, 1133–1135, 1998.
483. Fragner, P. and Krechlerova, M. *Paecilomyces* Bainier in onychomycosts. *Cesk. Dermatol.*, 47, 218–221, 1972.
484. Dharmasena, F. M. C., Davies, G. S. R., and Catovsky, D. *Paecilomyces varioti* pneumonia complicating hairy cell leukaemia. *Br. Med. J.*, 290, 967, 1985.
485. French, F. F. and Mallia, C. P. Pleural effusion caused by *Paecilomyces lilacinus*. *Br. J. Dis. Chest*, 66, 284, 1972.
486. Dekhkan-Khodzhaeva, N. A., Shamsiev, S. Sh., Shakirova, R. Yu., Macarova, G. I., and Mingbaeva, Sh. N. The role of *Paecilomyces* in the etiology of prolonged and recurrent bronchopulmonary diseases in children. *Pediatryia*, 9, 12, 1982.
487. Mormede, M., Texier, J., Gomez, F., Couprie, B., Fourche, J., and Martigne, C. Isolement d'un *Paecilomyces* (*P. lilacinus*) a partir d'un épanchement pleural. *Med. Malad. Infect.*, 14, 76, 1984.
488. Ono, N., Sato, K., Yokomise, H., and Tamura, K., Lung abscess by *Paecilomyces lilacinus*. *Respiration*, 66, 85–87, 1999.
489. Gucalp, R., Carlisle, P., Gialanella, P., Mitsudo, S., McKitrick, J., and Dutcher, J. *Paecilomyces sinusitis* in an immunocompromised adult patient: case report and review. *Clin. Infect. Dis.*, 23, 391–393, 1996.
490. Lawson, W. and Blitzer, A. Fungal infections of the nose and paranasal sinuses. Part II. *Otolaryngol. Clin. North Am.*, 26, 1037–1068, 1993.
491. Otcenasek, M., Jirousek, Z., Nozicka, Z., and Mencl, K. Paecilomycosis of the maxillary sinus. *Mykosen*, 27, 242, 1984.
492. Thompson, R. F., Bode, R. B., Rhodes, J. C., and Gluckman, J. L. *Paecilomyces varioti*: an unusual cause of isolated sphenoid sinusitis. *Arch. Otolaryngol. Head Neck Surg.*, 114, 567, 1988.
493. Rockhill, R. C. and Klein, M. D. *Paecilomyces lilacinus* as the cause of chronic maxillary sinusitis. *J. Clin. Microbiol.*, 11, 737, 1980.

494. Rowley, S. D. and Strom, C. G. *Paecilomyces* fungus infection of the maxillary sinus. *Laryngoscope*, 92, 332, 1982.
495. Henig, F. E., Lehrer, N., Gabbay, A., and Kurz, O. Paecilomycosis of the lacrimal sac. *Mykosen*, 16, 25, 1973.
496. Scott, I. U., Flynn, H. W. Jr., Miller, D., Speights, J. W., Snip, R. C., and Brod, R. D. Exogenous endophthalmitis caused by amphotericin B-resistant *Paecilomyces lilacinus*: treatment options and visual outcomes. *Arch. Ophthalmol.*, 119, 916–919, 2001.
497. Dhindsa, M. K., Naidu, J., Singh, S. M., and Jain, S. K. Chronic suppurative otitis media caused by *Paecilomyces variotii*. *J. Med. Vet. Mycol.*, 33, 59–61, 1995.
498. Sherwood, J. A. and Dansky, A. S. *Paecilomyces* pyelonephritis complicating nephrolithiasis and review of *Paecilomyces* infections. *J. Urol.*, 130, 526–528, 1983.
499. Crompton, C. H., Summerbell, R. C., and Silver, M. M. Peritonitis with *Paecilomyces* complicating peritoneal dialysis. *Pediatr. Infect. Dis. J.*, 10, 869, 1991.
500. Rinaldi, S., Fiscarelli, E., and Rizzoni, G. *Paecilomyces variotii* peritonitis in an infant on automated peritoneal dialysis. *Pediatr. Nephrol.*, 14, 365–366, 2000.
501. Kovac, D., Lindic, J., Lejko-Zupanc, T., et al. Treatment of severe *Paecilomyces varioti* peritonitis in a patient on continuous ambulatory peritoneal dialysis. *Nephtol. Dial. Transplant.*, 13, 2943, 1998.
502. Akhunova, A. M. Some pathogenetic mechanisms of bacterial bronchial asthma in paecilomycosis. *Klin. Med. (Mosk.)*, 78, 35–40, 2000.
503. Sandler, M., Gemperli, B. M., Hanekom, C., and Kuhn, S. H. Serum alpha 1-protease inhibitor in diabetes mellitus: reduced concentration and impaired activity. *Diabetes Res. Clin. Pract.*, 5, 249, 1988.
504. Galgiani, J. N. Progress in standardizing antifungal susceptibility tests. *Clin. Lab. Med.*, 9, 269, 1989.
505. Neijens, H. J., Frenkel, J., de Muinck Keizer-Schrama, S. M. P. F., Dzoljic-Danilovic, G., Meradji, M., and van Dongen, J. J. M. Invasive *Aspergillus* infection in chronic granulomatous disease: treatment with itraconazole. *J. Pediatr.*, 115, 1016, 1989.
506. Aguilar, C., Pujol, I., Sala, J., and Guarro, J. Antifungal susceptibilities of *Paecilomyces* species. *Antimicrob. Agents Chemother.*, 42, 1601–1604, 1998.
507. Clark, N. M. *Paecilomyces lilacinus* infection in a heart transplant recipient and successful treatment with terbinafine. *Clin. Infect. Dis.*, 28, 1169–1170, 1999.
508. Das, A., MacLaughlin E. F., Ross, L. A., et al. *Paecilomyces variotii* in a pediatric patient with lung transplantation. *Pediatr. Transplant*, 4, 328–332, 2000.
509. Edward, J. C. A new genus of the Moniliaceae. *Mycologia*, 51, 781–786, 1959.
510. Samson, R. A. and Mahmood, T. The genus *Acrophialophora* (fungi Moniliales). *Acta Bot. Neerl.*, 19, 804–808, 1970.
511. Shukla, P. K., Khan, Z. A., Lal, B., Agrawal, P. K., and Srivastava, O. P. Clinical and experimental keratitis caused by the *Collecorichum* state of *Glomerella cingulata* and *Acrophialophora fusispora*. *Sabouraudia*, 21, 137–147, 1983.
512. Welsh, R. D. and Ely, R. W. *Scopulariopsis chartarum* systemic mycosis in a dog. *J. Clin. Microbiol.*, 37, 2102–2103, 1999.
513. de Hoog, G. S. Notes on some fungicolous hyphomycetes and their relatives. *Persoonia*, 10(Part 1), 33–81, 1978.
514. Gams, W., de Hoog, G. S., and Samson, R. A. The hyphomycete genus *Engyodontium* - a link between *Verticillium* and *Aphanocladium*. *Persoonia*, 12(Part 2), 135–147, 1984.
515. Sekhon, A. S., Padhye, A. A., Kaufman, L., et al. Antigenic relationships among pathogenic *Beauveria bastiana* with *Engyodontium album* (=*B. alba*) and non-pathogenic species of the genus Beauveria. *Mycopathologia*, 138, 1–4, 1997.
516. Augustinsky J., Kammeyer, P., Husain, A., de Hoog, G. S., and Libertin, C. R. *Engyodontium album* endocarditis. *J. Clin. Microbiol.*, 28, 1479–1481, 1990.
517. McDonnell, P. J., Werblin, T. P., Sigler, L., and Green, W. R. Mycotic keratitis due to *Beauveria alba*. *Cornea*, 3, 213–216, 1984.
518. Seeliger, H. P. R. Infections of man by opportunistic molds - their identification and nomenclature of their diseases. *Mycosen*, 26, 587–598, 1983.
519. de Hoog, G. S. The genera *Beauveria*, *Isaria*, *Tritirachium* and *Acrodonium* gen. nov. *Stud. Mycol.*, 1, 1–41, 1972.
520. Bassi, A. Del male del segno calcinaccio o muscordino malattia che attigee: Bachi da set a Patel, Teorica Tip. Orcesi, Lodi, 1835, in *Medical Mycology- The pathogenic Fungi and the Pathogenic Actinomycetes*, Rippon, J. W., Ed. Saunders, Philadelphia, 467, 1974.
521. Freour, P., Lahourcade, M., and Chomy, P. Une mycose nouvelle: étude clinique et mycologique d'une localisation pulmonaire de *Beauvaria*. *Bull. Mem. Soc. Med. Hop. Paris*, 117, 197–206, 1966.
522. Drouhet, E., Dupont, B., Dompmartin, E., Heid, E., and Ravisse, P. Ketoconazole, a new imidazole active by the oral route in the superficial and systemic mycoses. *Bull. Soc. Fr. Mycoll. Med.*, 9, 53–57, 1980.
523. Sachs, S. W., Baum, J., and Mies, C. *Beauveria bassiana* keratitis. *Br. J. Ophthalmol.*, 69, 548–550, 1985.
524. Morrison, V. A., Haake, R. J., and Weisdorf, D. J. Non-*Candida* fungal infection: risk factors and outcome. *Am. J. Med.*, 96, 497, 1994.
525. Ben Hamida, M., Bedrossian, J., Pruna, A., Fouqueray, B., Metivier, F., and Idatte, J. M. Fungal mycotic aneurysms and visceral infection due to *Scedosporium apiospermum* in a kidney transplant patient. *Transplant. Proc.*, 25, 2290, 1993.
526. Lupinetti, F. M., Behrendt, D. M., Giller, R. H., Trigg, M. E., and de Alarcon, P. Pulmonary resection for fungal infection in children undergoing bone marrow transplantation. *J. Thorac. Cardiovasc. Surg.*, 104, 684, 1992.
527. Gamis, A. S., Gudnason, T., Giebink, G. S., and Ramsay, N. K. Disseminated infection with *Fusarium* in recipients of bone marrow transplants. *Rev. Infect. Dis.*, 13, 1077, 1991.
528. Robertson, M. J., Socinski, M. A., Soiffer, R. J., et al. Successful treatment of disseminated *Fusarium* infection after autologous bone marrow transplantation for acute myeloid leukemia. *Bone Marrow Transplant.*, 8, 143, 1991.

529. Mowbray, D. N., Paller, A. S., Nelson, P. E., and Kaplan, R. L. Disseminated *Fusarium solani* infection with cutaneous nodules in a bone marrow transplant patient. *Int. J. Dermatol.*, 27, 698, 1988.
530. Nucci, M., Pulcheri, W., Bacha, P. C., et al. Amphotericin B followed by itraconazole in the treatment of disseminated fungal infections in neutropenic patients. *Mycoses*, 37, 433, 1994.
531. Groll, A. H. and Walsh, T. J. Uncommon opportunistic fungi: new nosocomial threats. *Clin. Microbiol. Infect.*, 7(Suppl. 2), 8–24, 2001.
532. Walsh, T. J. and Groll, T. J. Emerging fungal pathogens: evolving challenges to immunocompromised patients for twenty-first century. *Transpl. Infect. Dis.*, 1, 247–261, 1999.
533. Clark, R. A., Johnson, F. L., Klebanoff, S. J., and Thomas, E. D. Defective neutrophil chemotaxis in bone marrow transplant patients. *J. Clin. Invest.*, 58, 22, 1976.
534. Witherspoon, R., Lum, L., Storb, R., and Thomas, E. D. Transplant-related immune deficiency in man, in *Recent Advances in Bone Marrow Transplantation*, Gale, R. P., Ed. A. R. Liss, New York, 473, 1983.
535. Meyers, J. D. Infection in recipients of bone marrow transplants, in *Current Clinical Topics in Infectious Diseases*, Remington, J. S. and Swartz, M. N., Eds. McGraw-Hill Co., New York, 262, 1985.
536. Tollemar, J., Ringdén, O., Boström, L., Nilsson, B., and Sundberg, B. Variables predicting deep fungal infections in bone marrow transplant recipients. *Bone Marrow Transplant.*, 4, 635, 1989.
537. Tollemar, J., Ringdén, O., Aschan, J., and Sundberg, B. Which bone marrow transplant recipients are at risk of acquiring life-threatening fungal infections? *Transplant. Proc.*, 22, 208, 1990.
538. Pirsch, J. D. and Maki, D. G. Infectious complications in adults with bone marrow transplantation and T-cell depletion of donor marrow. *Ann. Intern. Med.*, 104, 619, 1986.
539. Kusne, S., Dummer, J. S., Singh, N., et al. Infections after liver transplantation: an analysis of 101 consecutive cases. *Medicine (Baltimore)*, 67, 132, 1988.
540. Anaissie, E. J., Bodey, G. P., and Rinaldi, M. G. Emerging fungal pathogens. *Eur. J. Clin. Microbiol. Infect. Dis.*, 8, 323, 1989.
541. Anaissie, E. J. Opportunistic mycoses in the immunocompromised host: experience of a cancer center and review. *Clin. Infect. Dis.*, 14, 543, 1992.
542. Denning, D. W., Donnelly, J. P., Hellreigel, K. P., Ito, J., Martino, P., and van't Wout, J. W. Antifungal prophylaxis during neutropenia or allogeneic bone marrow transplantation: what is the state of the art? *Chemotherapy.*, 38(Suppl. 1), 43, 1992.
543. Ellis, M. E., Clink, H., Younge, D., and Hainau, B. Successful combined surgical and medical treatment of *Fusarium* infection after bone marrow transplantation. *Scand. J. Infect. Dis.*, 26, 225, 1994.
544. Drakos, P. E., Nagler, A., Or, R., et al. Invasive fungal sinusitis in patients undergoing bone marrow transplantation. *Bone Marrow Transplant.*, 12, 203, 1993.
545. Meyers, J. D. Fungal infections in bone marrow transplant patients. *Semin. Oncol.*, 17, 10, 1990.
546. June, C. H., Beatty, P. G., Shulman, H. M., and Rinaldi, M. G. Disseminated *Fusarium moniliforme* infection after allogeneic marrow transplantation. *South. Med. J.*, 79, 513, 1986.
547. Paulin, T., Ringdén, O., and Nilsson, B. Immunological recovery after bone marrow transplantation: role of age, graft-versus-host disease, prednisolone treatment and infections. *Bone Marrow Transplant.*, 1, 317, 1987.
548. Howard, R. J. and Najarian, J. S. Cytomegalovirus-induced immune suppression: I. Humoral immunity. *Clin. Exp. Immunol.*, 18, 109, 1974.
549. Lavrijsen, K., Van Houdt, J., Thijs, D., Meuldermans, W., and Heykants, J. Interaction of miconazole, ketoconazole and itraconazole with rat-liver microsomes. *Xenobiotica*, 17, 45, 1987.
550. Cassling, R. S., Rogler, W. C., and McManus, B. M. Isolated pulmonic valve infective endocarditis: a diagnostically elusive entity. *Am. Heart J.*, 109, 558, 1985.
551. Rowley, K. M., Clubb, K. S., Smith, G. J. W., and Cabin, H. S. Right-sided infective endocarditis as a consequence of flow-directed pulmonary-artery catheterization. *N. Engl. J. Med.*, 311, 1152, 1984.
552. Humphrey, M. J., Javons, S., and Trabit, M. H. Pharmacological evaluation of UK-49,858, a metabolically stable triazole antifungal drug, in animals and humans. *Antimicrob. Agents Chemother.*, 28, 648, 1985.
553. Keown, P. A., Stiller, C. R., Laupacis, A. L., et al. The effects and side effects of cyclosporine: relationship to drug pharmacokinetics. *Transplant. Proc.*, 24, 659, 1982.
554. Horton, C. M., Freeman, C. D., Nolan, P. E. Jr., and Copeland III, J. G. Cyclosporine interaction with miconazole and other azole-antimycotics: a case report and review of the literature. *J. Heart Lung Transplant.*, 11, 1127, 1992.
555. Yee, G. C. and McGuire, T. R. Pharmacokinetic drug interactions with cyclosporin (Part I). *Clin. Pharmacokinet.*, 19, 319, 1990.
556. Yee, G. C. and McGuire, T. R. Pharmacokinetic drug interactions with cyclosporin (Part II). *Clin. Pharmacokinet.*, 19, 400, 1990.
557. Cassidy, M. J., Van Zyl-Smit, R., Pascoe, M. D., Swanepoel, C. R., and Jacobson, J. E. Effect of rifampicin on cyclosporin A blood levels in a renal transplant recipient. *Nephron*, 41, 207, 1985.
558. Gumbleton, M., Brown, J. E., Hawksworth, G., and Whiting, P. H. The possible relationship between hepatic drug metabolism and ketoconazole enhancement of cyclosporine nephrotoxicity. *Transplantation*, 40, 454, 1985.
559. Shepard, J. H., Canafax, D. M., Simmons, R. L., and Najarian, J. S. Cyclosporine- ketoconazole: a potentially dangerous drud-drug interaction. *Clin. Pharm.*, 5, 468, 1986.
560. Sands, M. and Brown, R, B. Interactions of cyclosporine and antimicrobial agents. *Rev. Infect. Dis.*, 11, 691, 1989.
561. Maurer, G. Metabolism of cyclosporine. *Transplant. Proc.*, 27, 19, 1985.

562. Doble, N., Shaw, R., Rowland-Hill, C., Lush, M., Warnock, D. W., and Keal, E. E. Pharmacokinetic study of the interaction between rifampin and ketoconazole. *J. Antimicrob. Chemother.*, 21, 633, 1988.
563. Smith, S. R. and Kendall, M. J. Ranitidine versus cimetidine: a comparison of their potential to cause clinically important drug interactions. *Clin. Pharmacokinet.*, 15, 44, 1988.
564. Butman, S. M., Wild, J., Nolan, P., et al. Prospective study of the safety and financial benefit of ketoconazole as adjunctive therapy to cyclosporine after heart transplantation. *J. Heart Lung Transplant.*, 10, 351, 1991.
565. First, M. R., Weiskittel, P., Alexander, J. W., Schroeder, T. J., Myre, S. A., and Pesce, A. J. Concomittant administration of cyclosporin and ketoconazole in renal transplant recipients. *Lancet*, 2, 1198, 1989.
566. Hostetler, K. A., Wrighton, S. A., Molowa, D. T., Thomas, P. E., Levin, W., and Guzelian, P. S. Coinduction of multiple hepatic cytochrome P-450 proteins and their mRNAs in rats treated with imidazole antimycotic agents. *Mol. Pharmacol.*, 35, 279, 1989.
567. Sheets, J. J. and Mason, J. I. Ketoconazole: a potent inhibitor of cytochrome P-450- dependent drug metabolism in rat liver. *Drug Metab. Dispos.*, 12, 603, 1984.
568. Blyden, G. T., Abernethy, D. R., and Greenblatt, D. J. Ketoconazole does not impair antipyrine clearance in humans. *Int. J. Clin. Pharmacol. Ther. Toxicol.*, 24, 225, 1986.
569. Daneshmend, T. K., Warnock, D. W., Ene, M. D., et al. Multiple dose pharmacokinetics in man. *J. Antimicrob. Chemother.*, 12, 185, 1983.
570. Meredith, C. G., Maldonado, A. L., and Speeg, K. V. The effect of ketoconazole on hepatic oxidative drug metabolism in the rat in vivo and in vitro. *Drug Metab. Dispos.*, 13, 156, 1985.
571. La Delfa, I., Zhu, Q. M., Mo, Z., and Blaschke, T. F. Fluconazole is a potent inhibitor of antipyrine metabolism in vivo in mice. *Drug Metab. Dispos.*, 17, 49, 1989.
572. Pasanen, M., Taskinen, T., Iscan, M., Sotaniemi, E. A., Kairaluoma, M., and Peikonen, O. Inhibition of human hepatic and placental xenobiotic monooxygenases by imidazole antimycotics. *Biochem. Pharmacol.*, 37, 3861, 1988.
573. Hajek, K. K., Cook, N. I., and Novak, R. F. Mechanism of inhibition of microsomal drug metabolism by imidazole. *J. Pharmacol. Exp. Ther.*, 223, 97, 1982.
574. Kramer, M. R., Marshall, S. E., Denning, D. W., et al. Cyclosporine and itraconazole interaction in heart and lung transplant recipients. *Ann. Intern. Med.*, 113, 327, 1990.
575. Damanhouri, Z., Gumbleton, M., Nicholls, P. J., and Shaw, M. A. In-vivo effects of itraconazole on hepatic mixed-function oxidase. *J. Antimicrob. Chemother.*, 21, 187, 1988.
576. Powell, J. R. and Cate, E. W. Induction and inhibition of drug metabolism, in *Applied Pharmacokinetics: Principles of Therapeutic Drug Monitoring*, Evans, W. E., Schentag, J. J., and Jusko, W. J., Eds. Applied Therapeutics, Spokane, WA, 139, 1986.
577. Sugar, A. M., Saunders, C., Idelson, B. A., and Bernard, D. B. Interaction of fluconazole and cyclosporine. *Ann. Intern. Med.*, 110, 844, 1989.
578. Collignon, P., Hurley, B., and Mitchell, D. Interaction of fluconazole with cyclosporin. *Lancet*, 333, 1262, 1989.
579. Graves, N. M., Matas, A. J., Hiligoss, D. M., and Canafax, D. M. Fluconazole/cyclosporine interaction. *Clin. Pharmacol. Ther.*, 47, 208, 1990.
580. Ehninger, G., Jeschonek, K., Schuler, U., and Krüger, H. U. Interaction of fluconazole with cyclosporin. *Lancet*, 334, 104, 1989.
581. Conti, D. J., Tolkoff-Rubin, N. E., Baker, G. P. Jr., et al. Successful treatment of invasive fungal infection with fluconazole in organ transplant recipients. *Transplantation*, 48, 692, 1989.
582. Krüger, H. U., Schuler, U., Zimmerman, R., and Ehninger, G. Absence of significant interaction of fluconazole with cyclosporin. *J. Antimicrob. Chemother.*, 24, 781, 1989.

27
Histoplasma spp.

1. INTRODUCTION

The genus *Histoplasma* is a dimorphic fungus comprised of two pathogenic species, *H. falciminosum* (the causative agent of the equine disease) and *H. capsulatum*, which causes the disease in humans. *H. capsulatum*, in turn, is divided into two variants, *H. capsulatum* var. *capsulatum*, and *H. capsulatum* var. *duboisii* (1,2). *H. capsulatum* var. *capsulatum* is responsible for the classical or small form (in tissues, the yeast form reaches 2–4 µm in diameter) of histoplasmosis. It is endemic in various parts of the world (United States, the West Indies, Central and South America, Africa, India, and the Far East) with the exception of Europe, and presents with pulmonary and disseminated infection affecting largely the lungs, reticuloendothelial system, mucosal surfaces, and the skin (3). In the United States, the geographic distribution of *Histoplasma* covers large areas mainly along the Mississippi and Ohio River Valleys. Infection by *H. capsulatum* is carried out by airborn microconidia (spores), which are inhaled. After reaching the alveoli, the microconidia convert into the yeast phase at body temperature.

The second variant, *H. capsulatum* var. *duboisii* is the causative agent of the African or large form (in tissues, the yeast form is 12–20 µm in diameter) of histoplasmosis (4). The two variants differ in their antigenic compositions.

As a soil fungus, *H. capsulatum* with no known requirements for interacting with a mammalian host as part of an obligate lifecycle is well-adapted to be infectious and pathogenic to humans (5,6). The survival strategies of *H. capsulatum* in the human host include its ability to display various mechanisms for modulating its microenvironmental pH level, to resist host reactive oxygen and nitrogen intermediates and degradative enzymes, and to withstand nutrient starvation conditions, including acquisition of iron and calcium and biosynthesis of nucleic acid precursors.

2. EVOLUTION OF THERAPIES AND TREATMENT OF HISTOPLASMOSIS

In immunocompetent individuals, most cases of acute disease are asymptomatic and patients do not seek medical treatment. Even when symptomatic, the disease is expected to resolve quickly and without treatment. However, in immunocompromised patients, or when the infecting aerosol is large, the histoplasmosis could disseminate and become potentially lethal if not treated (7–9). Based on its severity, rate of progression, and histopathologic differences, progressive disseminated histoplasmosis may present as acute, subacute, or chronic (10–15). In the immunocompromised population, approx 66% suffered from chronic infection, whereas 22% and 12% present with the subacute and acute forms, respectively (16).

In immunocompetent hosts with acute disease and ventilatory failure, the preferred medication has been amphotericin B given in cumulative doses of 0.5–1.0 g. Such treatment is effective and patients usually respond within 1–2 wk (Table 1).

From: Opportunistic Infections: Treatment and Prophylaxis
By: Vassil St. Georgiev © Humana Press Inc., Totowa, NJ

Table 1
Treatment of Histoplasmosis in Immunocompetent Hosts[a]

Indication	Treatment
Acute infection	Observation
Acute infection with ventilatory failure	Amphotericin B: 0.5–1.0 g, i.v. (until improvement noted)
Cavitary infection	Itraconazole: 200–400 mg daily for 6 mo, p.o.; or ketoconazole: 400–800 mg daily for 6 mo, p.o.; or amphotericin B: 35 mg/kg, total dose, i.v.
Progressive disseminated	Amphotericin B: 0.5–1.0 g, i.v., until patient is stable, then itraconazole: 200–400 mg daily, p.o., for 6 mo; or amphotericin B: 40 mg/kg, i.v., total dose; or itraconazole: 200–400 mg, daily, p.o.; or ketoconazole: 200–400 mg, daily, p.o.; or fluconazole: 200–400 mg, daily, p.o.[b]

[a]Data taken from Sarosi and Davies (7), Dismukes et al. (18), and Wheat et al. (19). Some of the recommended dose regimens may reflect the personal preferences of the authors and therefore may remain controversial.
[b]Fluconazole should be used only if the patients cannot take itraconazole.

Since its introduction into clinic, itraconazole has become the drug of choice for most types of histoplasmosis with the exception of meningeal, endocarditis, and life-threatening pulmonary and disseminated infections (18,20,21). The recommended daily regimen is usually 200 mg, however, the dose may be increased to 400 mg (given twice daily) if patient failed to respond after several weeks of therapy at the lower dose.

So far, chronic cavitary pulmonary histoplasmosis has probably been the most difficult condition to treat because of the significant underlying chronic obstructive pulmonary disease found in patients with this condition (18,22). Other chronic forms of the disease such as fibrosing mediastinitis and broncholithiasis are unresponsive to pharmacologic treatment (23).

In immunocompromised host, histoplasmosis is potentially life-threatening, and amphotericin B remains the treatment of choice (7,9,23–25) (Table 2).

Hypercalcemia associated with disseminated histoplasmosis has been described in several reports (29–31). This condition has also been observed with other granulomatous diseases, such as sarcoidosis (32), tuberculosis (33–35), chronic berylliosis (36), and two disseminated mycoses: coccidioidomycosis (37), and candidiasis (38). Administration of vitamin D and calcium supplements should be avoided (30), because as described for other granulomatous diseases (33,34,38–40), hypercalcemia in disseminated histoplasmosis could be aggravated by these two treatments. It has been postulated that extrarenal conversion of vitamin D to its active $1\alpha,25$-dihydroxy metabolite may be the cause of the hypercalcemic condition (41–43). This increased conversion may take place within the granulomatous tissue itself (44) and the macrophages, in particular (45). Whereas the withdrawal of vitamin D and calcium supplements would lower the serum calcium levels (33,38,46), steroid therapy may also correct the hypercalcemia in granulomatous disease by decreasing the conversion of vitamin D to the pathogenic $1\alpha,25$-dihydroxy metabolite (39,47).

Fungal peritonitis is a well known risk in patients undergoing chronic ambulatory peritoneal dialysis (48). In the treatment of one such case involving histoplasma infection, the patient responded favorably to a combined therapy of fluconazole (200 mg loading dose; then, 100 mg daily), 5-fluorocytosine (5-FC) (50 mg/L were added to the dialysis fluid for 4 wk), and amphotericin B (30 mg for 10 d) (49).

In recent years, the use of methotrexate sodium to treat severe rheumatoid arthritis and psoriasis has been steadily increasing (50,51). In this context, with the escalating use of methotrexate medication, the incidence of opportunistic infections (varicella zoster [52,53], *Pneumocystis carinii* pneumonia [54–56], nocardiosis [57], cryptococcosis [58], and histoplasmosis [59,60]) in these patients

Table 2
Treatment of Histoplasmosis in Immunocompromised Hosts[a]

Indication	Treatment Without AIDS	Treatment With AIDS
Acute infection	Amphotericin B: 0.5–1.0 g, i.v., then itraconazole: 400 mg daily, p.o. for 6 mo	Amphotericin B: 0.5–1.0 g, i.v., then itraconazole: 400 mg daily for life
Acute infection with ventilatory failure	Amphotericin B: 1.0 g, i.v.; then, itraconazole: 400 mg daily, p.o., for 6 mo, or amphotericin B: 40 mg/kg cumulative dose, i.v.	Amphotericin B: 0.5–1.0 g, i.v.; then itraconazole: 400 mg daily, p.o., for life
Chronic cavitary infection	Itraconazole: 200–400 mg daily, p.o., for 6–24 mo 400 mg daily, p.o., for life Fluconazole: 200–400 mg, daily, p.o.; or ketoconazole: 200–800 mg, daily, p.o.[b]	Amphotericin B: 0.5–1.0 g, i.v.;then itraconazole:
Progressive disseminated	Amphotericin B: 1.0 g, i.v.; then, itraconazole: 400 mg daily, po, for 6 mo; or amphotericin B: 40 mg/kg cumulative dose, i.v. with itraconazole (400–600 mg, daily) (26)	Amphotericin B: 1.0 g, i.v.; then itraconazole: 400 mg daily, p.o., for life[c,d]; or liposomal amphotericin B, followed by maintenance therapy
CNS histoplasmosis	Amphotericin B: 0.7–1.0 mg/kg, daily (total: 35 mg/kg over 3–4 mo) [c,d]	Amphotericin B: 0.7–1.0 mg/kg, daily (total: 35 mg/kg over 3–4 mo) [c,d]
Granulomatous mediastinitis	Amphotericin B: 0.7–1.0 mg/kg, daily, then itraconazole (200 mg, once or twice daily)[e]	Amphotericin B: 0.7–1.0 mg/kg, daily, then itraconazole (200 mg, once or twice daily)[e]

[a]Data taken from Kauffman (8), Sarosi and Davies (7), Dismukes et al. (18), Wheat et al. (19), Graybill (27), and Drew (28). Some of the recommended dose regimens may reflect the personal preferences of the authors and therefore may remain controversial.

[b]Toxicity is more common in patients receiving the 800-mg dose and should be discouraged.

[c]Liposomal amphotericin B (AmBisome), 3.0–5.0 mg/kg, daily or every other day over a 3–4-mo period may be given to patients who have failed amphotericin B therapy, followed by fluconazole.

[d]Chronic fluconazole maintenance therapy (800 mg, daily) should be considered for patients who relapse. Itraconazole, although more active than fluconazole against *H. capsulatum* does not enter the CSF.

[e]Prednisone (40–80 mg, daily for 2 wk, may be considered for patients with major airway obstruction.

has also been on the rise. By inactivating the dihydrofolate reductase and ultimately blocking the DNA and amino acid biosynthesis (61) in rapidly proliferating cells, methotrexate therapy would lead to impairment of the cell-mediated immunity even when given at lower doses, thereby predisposing patients to opportunistic infections. Witty et al. (59) reported three cases of disseminated histoplasmosis in patients receiving low-dose methotrexate for psoriasis. All patients responded favorably to amphotericin B (total dose in the 2.0–3.0 g range), with one exception where the patient required long-term suppressive therapy because of persistent *Histoplasma* antigenuria.

Table 3
Prophylaxis Against Histoplasmosis in AIDS Patients[a]

Indication	Treatment	
	First choice	Alternative
Adults and adolescents		
Preventing first episode	Itraconazole capsule: 200 mg, p.o., daily	None
Preventing recurrence[b]	Itraconazole capsule: 200 mg p.o., b.i.d.	Amphotericin B: 1.0 mg/kg, i.v., weekly
Infants and children		
Preventing first episode	Itraconazole: 2.0–5.0 mg/kg, p.o., every 12–24 hrs[c]	None
Preventing recurrence[b]	Itraconazole: 2.0–5.0 mg/kg, p.o., every 12–48 h	Amphotericin B: 1.0 mg/kg, i.v., weekly

[a]Data taken from ref. *(62)*.
[b]Treatment should be initiated after therapy for acute disease.
[c]Not recommended for most children, but for use only in unusual circumstances.

2.1. Prophylaxis in Histoplasmosis

Prophylaxis against histoplasmosis should be considered for AIDS patients with CD4+ T-cell counts below 100 cells/µL and are at high risk due to occupational exposure or live in a community with a hyperendemic rate of histoplasmosis (>10 cases per 100 patient-years) (Table 3) *(62)*. Furthermore, patients who complete initial therapy for histoplasmosis should be considered for lifelong suppressive therapy.

Itraconazole prophylaxis (200 mg, daily) in HIV-infected patients showed promising results in a randomized, placebo-controlled, double-blind study *(63)*. While itraconazole significantly delayed time to onset of histoplasmosis ($p = 0.03$), a survival benefit was not demonstrated.

2.2. Histoplasmosis in AIDS Patients

Although not significantly different from the disease observed in non-HIV-infected individuals, disseminated histoplasmosis is a serious and potentially lethal infection in patients with AIDS *(64–66)*. Wheat et al. *(67)* and others *(10,68–74)* described a septicemia-like syndrome characterized by hypotension, renal and hepatic failure, respiratory insufficiency, and disseminated coagulopathy. Skin manifestations, which are seen in about 10% of cases, include pustular, folicular, maculopapular, and erythematous lesions with papulonecrotic centers *(10,73,75,76)* and pyoderma gangrenosum-like lesions *(24)*. Disseminated histoplasmosis may also present with pericarditis *(10)*, rhabdomyolysis *(67)*, pancreatitis *(67)*, chorioretinitis *(77)*, colonic masses *(10,69,78,79)*, mesenteric and omental nodules *(80)*, and thrombocytopenia *(81)*. Central nervous system (CNS) involvement in disseminated disease has also been reported (5–20% of patients) *(10,69)*, including encephalopathy, meningitis, and focal parenchymal lesions of the brain *(67,69)*. AIDS patients with CNS complications did not respond well to treatment as compared to those with other forms of disseminated disease (61–71% mortality rate) *(82,83)*.

Because in nearly half of the cases, AIDS patients will present with unexplained fever, accompanied by diffuse reticulonodular or interstitial pulmonary infiltrates *(10,67,84)*, misdiagnosis as miliary tuberculosis has been common in many such cases *(71,85)*. To this end, detection of *H. capsulatum* polysaccharide antigen (HPA) in the urine (90–96% of patients), blood (50–78%), and other body fluids showed promise as a rapid diagnostic tool for disseminated histoplasmosis *(86,87)*.

The HPA levels decreased with amphotericin B treatment but recurred in both the urine and blood at the time of relapse *(86,88)*. Graviss et al. *(89)* presented a clinical prediction model for differentiation of disseminated histoplasmosis and *Mycobacterium avium* complex (MAC) infection in febrile patients with AIDS. Positive predictors of *Histoplasma* infection by invariate analysis included the lactate dehydrogenase and alkaline phosphatase levels, and the white blood cell count.

Because of the severe clinical presentation as well as impaired cellular immune functions, AIDS patients may not always respond to treatment of histoplasmosis as well as other immunocompromised patients, and without life-long maintenance therapy the incidence of relapse has been an ever-present possibility. Because none of the currently available drugs for histoplasmosis is curative, the emphasis of treatment has been shifting from cure to disease suppression with the least toxic, best-tolerated, and most effective drug regimen *(28,90)*.

One therapy that is often recommended involves initial treatment with amphotericin B, followed by indefinite suppression with intermittent doses of amphotericin B or itraconazole *(70,82,91)*. Even though amphotericin B has been widely used, too often its toxicity and the discomfort due to the required intravenous or intrathecal administration were not well-tolerated. In these cases, alternative therapies with liposomal amphotericin B *(26)* or azole antifungals, especially itraconazole should be considered (Table 2) *(90)*. To this end, studies by Slain et al. *(92)* have shown that intravenously administered itraconazole offered a less toxic alternative for patients who are intolerant of or refractory to amphotericin B, or with pulmonary and extrapulmonary histoplasmosis, and patients unable to receive oral medication.

Treatment for AIDS patients who do not suffer from acute infection or meningeal involvement may include an initial daily regimen of 600 mg of itraconazole (200 mg three times daily) for 3 d, followed by 200-mg doses given twice daily. After 12 wk of treatment, a life-long maintenance therapy of 200 mg daily of itraconazole should be implemented *(8,9)*. In some cases, amphotericin B may become part of the entire treatment, or after being administered initially to most patients, therapy may be switched to itraconazole after a positive response is observed (cultures becoming negative for *H. capsulatum* concurrent with stable clinical condition) *(8)*.

Because anemia still remains one of the most common hematologic abnormalities associated with HIV infections *(93)*, one complication in AIDS patients receiving concomitant amphotericin B and zidovudine is that each of these drugs will also cause anemia, thus making multifactorial anemia a serious clinical condition in these patients. To this end, decreased endogenous erythropoietin levels have been observed in all of the aforementioned settings *(94,95)*. In a small study, Lancaster et al. *(96)* demonstrated that multifactorial anemia in AIDS patients with disseminated histoplasmosis receiving concomitant amphotericin B and zidovudine regimens can be corrected in some patients with the administration of recombinant human erythropoietin.

Itraconazole is also highly potent against histoplasmosis. It reaches high tissue concentrations, has prolonged drug clearance, and greater gastrointestinal tolerance than ketoconazole. However, its usefulness may be limited by acid-dependent absorption and limited cerebrospinal fluid (CSF) penetration *(97–102)*. When used in daily doses of 200–400 mg, itraconazole has shown clinical efficacy against pulmonary or disseminated infection in nearly 90% of patients without AIDS *(18,103,104)*. The British Society for Antimicrobial Chemotherapy Working Party has recommended the use of itraconazole at daily doses of 400 mg for 6 wk as an alternative therapy to amphotericin B for induction therapy for histoplasmosis, as well as the drug of choice for maintenance treatment *(105)*. With regard to its toxicity, however, at the 400-mg daily dose regimen, the adverse side effects of itraconazole have been more pronounced than those with a comparable dose of fluconazole, and included increased hepatic aminotransferase levels (in 5–10% of patients). At daily doses of 600 mg or more, other side effects may emerge, such as adrenal insufficiency and reversible idiosyncratic hepatitis.

Although it is well-tolerated, the potential exists for drug interactions involving itraconazole (mediated through the cytochrome P450 enzyme 3A4 system) that should be taken into consideration when itraconazole is used as part of a multidrug regimen *(21)*. Thus, in a report of two cases of patients receiving combination of itraconazole and rifampin, weight loss while taking the combination followed by weight gain after stopping rifampin, suggested the possibility of clinically significant drug interaction between these two drugs *(106)*.

Fluconazole, another of the newer triazole antimycotics, is water-soluble, easily absorbed, and showing high CSF penetrability *(102,107,108)*. However, in spite of some favorable clinical outcomes reported in treating histoplasmosis in immunocompetent hosts *(109)*, the role of fluconazole as primary therapy of histoplasmosis in AIDS patients has been very limited. In this regard, caution should be applied after in vivo experiments by Le Monte et al. *(110)* showed that when used in combination, fluconazole antagonized amphotericin B's reduction of fungal burden without reducing its effect on survival against histoplasmosis. Nevertheless, on several occasions fluconazole was used successfully for maintenance therapy in AIDS patients with disseminated histoplasmosis *(91,111,112)*; however, daily doses of less than 200 mg are considered inadequate *(27,113)*.

Because the *Histoplasma* antigen is reduced in the blood and urine during antifungal therapy, the antigen clearance was used to compare the activity of itraconazole and fluconazole *(114)*. In separate trials in AIDS patients where the clinical response to both drugs was similar (itraconazole, 85%; fluconazole, 74%), the more rapid clearance of fungemia suggested that itraconazole was the more effective agent. In sequential clinical trials in AIDS patients, the therapy with fluconazole failed in a higher proportion than did therapy with itraconazole most likely because of the development of resistance during therapy *(115)*.

The clearance of fungal burden following treatment of disseminated histoplasmosis with liposomal amphotericin B and itraconazole was compared in two separate trials of AIDS patients *(116)*. The more rapid clearance of fungemia supported the use of liposomal amphotericin B for initial treatment of moderately severe or severe histoplasmosis.

Ketoconazole has been inferior to both amphotericin B and the triazole antimycotics. It is generally ineffective, and should not be used as primary therapy for disseminated histoplasmosis in AIDS patients *(67,82,117,118)*. The ineffectiveness of ketoconazole may be the result of its poor absorption in AIDS patients caused by their high gastric pH *(119)*, as well as poor compliance associated with its gastrointestinal toxicity. However, there have been some positive results. Mello et al. *(120)* reported a single case of an HIV-positive patient with localized tonsilar infection and cervical adenopathy caused by *H. capsulatum*, who responded favorably to a 400-mg daily dose of ketoconazole administered over a 12-mo period. Given such positive clinical responses, oral ketoconazole treatment of HIV-positive patients with evidence of early, localized histoplasma infection may eventually be considered, but only if disseminated disease is not evident *(120)*.

Because there is consistently a high risk of relapse in AIDS patients with disseminated disease, life-long suppressive therapy is always warranted. After maintenance therapy was discontinued, the relapse rate among these patients was very high *(10,91,121)*. Even with chronic maintenance therapy with ketoconazole, the relapse rate was over 58%; by comparison, with amphotericin B the relapse rate was 19% *(70,82,122)*. In another study, maintenance therapy with amphotericin B, led to even better results: the relapse rate was only 5% (median follow-up, over 12 mo), with the amphotericin B doses ranging between 50 and 100 mg/kg administered weekly or every 2 wk *(91)*.

Wheat et al. *(123)* evaluated the efficacy of itraconazole in preventing relapse of histoplasmosis in 42 AIDS patients who had successfully completed induction therapy for disseminated histoplasmosis with amphotericin B (at least 15-mg/kg dose). The drug was found to be highly effective when given at 200-mg twice daily. Ninety-five percent remained relapse-free at follow-up evaluations for at least 52 wk. Only three patients failed to respond: one patient had discontuned medication because of toxicity (hypokalemia), and the other two relapsed. The antigen clearance from blood and urine correlated with the itraconazole clinical efficacy.

Fluconazole at 400 mg daily has also been recommended for maintenance therapy *(124)*. However, Pottage and Sha *(125)* reported a case of an HIV-positive patient with cryptococcosis who developed histoplasmosis while receiving suppressive fluconazole therapy for cryptococcal meningitis. The patient was treated successfully with amphotericin B, then switched to fluconazole (200 mg daily, orally) when he developed histoplasmosis. After being treated with amphotericin B for a second time, and again switched back to oral fluconazole (400 mg daily), the patient once more developed histoplasmosis.

2.3. Histoplasmosis in Transplant Recipients

Although not very frequently, progressive disseminated histoplasmosis has been diagnosed in patients from both endemic and nonendemic areas *(16)*. In 1983, Wheat et al. *(126)* described two large outbreaks of histoplasmosis in renal allograft recipients with incidence of infection reaching 2.1%. During a 4-yr period, Davies et al. *(127)* reported five cases of progressive disseminated disease in approx 1300 renal-transplant recipients. In general, the disease may follow-up a primary infection, or be a reactivation of previous infection owing to a great extent to the immunosuppressive effects of antirejection therapy *(127,128)*. Often, protracted fever and skin lesions are the most frequent symptoms of dessiminated disease. CNS involvement, although occasionally seen in AIDS patients, is relatively rare in transplant recipients *(16)*.

Before the introduction of the azole antimycotics, amphotericin B was used exclusively for treatment of disseminated histoplasmosis in transplant recipients. Sarosi et al. *(129)* suggested a regimen of 40 mg/kg for a cumulative dose of 2.0–2.5 g. However, because of its substantial toxicity, amphotericin B is not appropriate for renal allograft recipients and should be used with caution. Goetz and Jones *(130)* reported a case of disseminated histoplasmosis in a renal allograft recipient who was treated successfully with a short course of intravenous amphotericin B coupled with oral ketoconazole and rifampin, followed by a prolonged therapy with ketoconazole alone. The addition of rifampin was believed to increase the survival rate of nonimmunocompromised hosts against disseminated histoplasmosis when given in combination with amphotericin B, as demonstrated in murine histoplasmosis *(131)*. In nude mice, however, this combination not only did not offer any advantage over amphotericin B given alone, but was possibly deleterious *(132)*. In another combination, ketoconazole when given concomitantly with cyclosporin A (an immunosuppressive drug used in antirejection therapy) could adversely inhibit its metabolism resulting in unacceptable cyclosporin A-associated renal toxicity *(133)*.

2.4. Skin Manifestations of Histoplasmosis

Skin manifestations of histoplasmosis are part of the disseminated infection, and have been observed in 4–10% of the population *(10,11,134–136)* including HIV-infected patients *(24,137–141)*. In the latter cases, the preferred therapy has been with intravenous amphotericin B *(138)*.

Cutaneous lesions may appear on the head, trunk, or the extremities *(11,134,135,142–148)*, and will present as macules, papules, nodules, indurated plaques that ulcerate, purpura, abscesses, impetigo, eczematous or exfoliative dermatitis, cellulitis, or panniculitis *(135)*. In AIDS patients, some unusual skin manifestations, such as macular, blanching rashes, and papulonecrotic lesions, have also been observed *(149–151)*. In acute and subacute disseminated infections, the usual manifestations are indurated plaques that may develop as punched-out ulcers. Erythema nodosum and erythema multiforme have been observed as hypersensitivity reactions in acute pulmonary histoplasmosis *(142)*. Perianal ulcers, although rare, have also been described *(145,152)*. In one such case, the patient was treated with daily infusion of 0.4 mg/kg amphotericin B. After gradual clinical improvement, the ulcer healed completely after a total dose of 570 mg of amphotercin B *(152)*.

Navarro et al. *(151)* reported an unusual case of an immunosuppressed patient with systemic lupus erythematosus (SLE) and disseminated histoplasmosis presented with generalized cutaneous papulonodular lesions, which had evolved into vesicles with central necrosis that resembled molluscum contagiosum with an indurated erythematous halo. The patient was treated with intravenous amphotericin B (0.5 mg/kg daily) and oral 5-fluorocytosine (5-FC) (50 mg/kg daily). Because the clinical course was complicated by intractable hemolytic anemia (treated with prednisone, 20 mg daily), the 5-FC was discontinued and ketoconazole therapy (400 mg daily) was instituted for 14 mo; the dosage of amphotericin B was increased to 1.0 mg/kg daily for a total cumulative dose of 3.0 g.

In another case *(139)*, an HIV-infected patient with disseminated histoplasmosis who presented with ulcerated verrucous plaque localized above the upper lip was successfully treated with oral ketoconazole (400 mg daily) for 6 wk; the ketoconazole regimen was continued as a maintenance therapy. The possibility of human-to-human transmission of histoplasmosis has been postulated *(139)*.

Primary cutaneous histoplasmosis in an immunosuppressed patient with rheumatoid arthritis and receiving steroid therapy was successfully treated with 100-mg daily doses of fluconazole given for 2 mo *(136)*.

2.5. Gastrointestinal Histoplasmosis

Gastrointestinal involvement of histoplasmosis occurs in 70–90% of cases of disseminated disease, although it is infrequently encountered in patients with AIDS *(153–155)*. Its manifestations may be serious, such as perforation of the small intestines or the presence of large colonic polyps *(155–157)*. Gastrointestinal invasion is most likely due to hematogenous dissemination, but direct penetration of tissue may also occur. Because of its abundant lymphoid tissue, the ileocecal site has been most frequently involved.

Cimponeriu et al. *(158)* reported two cases of HIV-infected patients with gastrointestinal histoplasmosis, in which the radiographic and endoscopic mass lesions of the colon mimicked cancer; both patients were treated successfully with amphotericin B, followed by suppressive itraconazole therapy. In another report *(159)*, two HIV-infected patients with hemophilia A presented with hematochezia secondary to gastrointestinal infection with *H. capsulatum*. The patients responded to amphotericin B therapy, followed by itraconazole with no recurrence of bleeding.

Graham et al. *(160)* described two cases of AIDS patients with colonic structures secondary to histoplasmosis. Both patients were successfully treated with intravenous amphotericin B (each receiving a total dose of 2.0 g), followed by maintenance therapy with amphotericin B. Earlier, there were two reports *(78,161)* of AIDS patients diagnosed with the same condition, as well as another two reports *(162,163)* of histoplasmosis-induced colonic structures in non-AIDS patients.

Cappell and Manzione *(164)* described a patient with hyperglobulinemia E-recurrent infection (Job's syndrome) who developed colonic histoplasmosis and was successfully treated with 600-mg daily doses of ketoconazole for 2 mo. This report extends previous findings *(165–167)*, indicating that patients with Job's syndrome may be at higher risk of developing opportunistic fungal infections, including histoplasmosis.

2.6. Orofacial Manifestations of Histoplasmosis

Although cases of oral localized histoplasmosis have been observed in immunocompetent patients *(168)*, orofacial manifestations in histoplasmosis have been most frequently associated with disseminated disease *(11,169–172)*; some patients with pulmonary histoplasmosis may also present with oral lesions *(173,174)*. The most commonly affected sites in the upper aerodigestive tract are the tongue, palate, buccal mucosa or gingiva, and the larynx *(175,176)*. Generally, orofacial histoplasmosis appears as indurated ulcers or exophytic lesions and are often difficult to distinguish from carcinoma, sarcoidosis, tuberculosis, and other mycoses *(177)*. Rare cases have been reported with antral involvement *(178)* and invasion of the mandible *(179)*.

In disseminated disease, oral lesions have been seen especially in HIV-infected patients *(180–186)*, and in those with Hodgkin's lymphoma *(187)*.

Oropharyngeal ulcers have also been observed in 14–17% of patients with gastrointestinal histoplasmosis *(165,188)*. In two reported studies *(11,189)*, between 42 and 66% of patients with disseminated histoplasmosis presented with oropharyngeal disease, and 15–24% will have laryngeal lesions.

Although in most clinical settings laryngeal manifestations are associated with disseminated disease, there have been cases where the laryngeal lesions were believed to be primary *(190–198)*.

Hiltbrand and McGuirt *(173)* described a successful treatment of granulomatous lesions in the upper aerodigestive tract of a patient with chronic disseminated histoplasmosis with amphotericin B (2.0 g cumulative dose given over 4 mo), which remains the preferred choice of treatment *(176)*.

In two other reports *(199,200)*, histoplasmosis of the larynx was successfully cured with ketoconazole (200 mg three times daily, for 3 mo, and 400 mg daily for 11 wk, respectively).

Metronidazole and fluconazole have also been used to treat localized oral histoplasmosis in a patient with HIV infection *(183)*.

2.7. Ocular Histoplasmosis

Feman and Tilford *(201)* have estimated that nearly 100 patients are diagnosed each year with ocular histoplasmosis. In a retrospective study by Simmons and Mathews *(202)*, ocular histoplasmosis has been prevalent in 47% of cases of posterior uveitis reported in the Mississippi River Valley, an endemic area of the disease. However, intraocular tumors associated with disseminated histoplasmosis have been rare *(203–205)*.

Ocular histoplasmosis usually involves the appearance of discrete atrophic choroidal scars in the macula or midperiphery (known as histo spots), peripapillary atrophy, and choroidal neovascularization (multiple, peripheral, well-demarcated, atrophic-appearing lesions; peripapillary pigmentary lesions; and a macular diskiform lesion), which may lead to severe loss of central vision *(201,206–209)*. Ophthalmic lesions of this type are difficult to cure, although Feman et al. *(205)* reported one case where the lesion responded to intravenous amphotericin B (total dose of 1026 mg administered over a 32-d period) and topical drops of atropine and prednisolone acetate. The amphotericin B therapy was discontinued and treatment continued with oral ketoconazole for 9 additional months when the lesion appeared to be flat and atrophic-appearing.

In other treatments of ocular histoplasmosis, laser therapy itself has shown significant drawbacks by causing an absolute scotoma correlating with the site of the laser photocoagulation scar, as well as being not effective against subfoveal choroidal neovascularization. The latter condition was stabilized after photodynamic therapy *(208)*; submacular surgery for the removal of subfoveal choroidal neovascularization showed promising results *(206,209,210,211)*.

Martidis et al. *(212)* found corticosteroids (prednisone, triamcinolone) beneficial in managing subfoveal choroidal neovascularization secondary to presumed ocular histoplasmosis syndrome.

Gonzales et al. *(213)* reported the first case of clinically diagnosed endogenous endophthalmitis caused by *H. capsulatum* in an AIDS patient. Treatment consisted of intravenous and intravitreal amphotericin B, pars plana vitrectomy, and scleral buckling procedure.

Sen et al. *(214)* presented a case of an ulcerative eyelid histoplasmic lesion that responded to therapy.

2.8. Rheumatic Manifestations of Histoplasmosis

Rheumatic manifestations of histoplasmosis have been uncommon *(215)* and cases of arthritis and arthralgias have been diagnosed occasionally in the knee, ankle, wrist, and fingers *(216–227)*. Polyarticular joint infections were observed in several outbreaks of primary acute histoplasmosis *(216–220)* (6.3% of patients in one epidemic *[216]*). With a few exceptions, radiographic evaluation of involved joints did not show erosive lesions *(215)*. In spite of the high incidence of bone-marrow seeding in disseminated histoplasmosis, focal bone involvement, tenosynovitis, and arthritis have been rarely reported *(216,221–223)*.

Darouiche et al. *(215)* described a patient with solitary monoarticular histoplasmosis of the knee, which was successfully treated with oral fluconazole (200 mg daily for 9 mo) without requiring surgical intervention. In previously reported cases *(225–229)* of solitary articular histoplasmosis of the wrist, resolution of infection was achieved by a combination of surgical excision and intravenous amphotericin B (total doses ranging from 1.0–3.5 g).

Carpal tunnel syndrome due to *H. capsulatum* infection has been reported on several occasions *(222–227,230–232)*. This syndrome, commonly attributed to entrapment neuropathy of the median nerve at the wrist *(233)* and best known to be the result of work-related injuries *(234)*, may also be caused by various disorders, such as trauma, rheumatoid arthritis, gout, myxedema, acromegaly, pregnancy, amyloidosis, and infections *(235–238)*. Mascola and Rickman *(230)* described a case of recurrent carpal tunnel syndrome caused by histoplasma infection that was resolved successfully by surgical intervention and subsequent therapy with ketoconazole (400 mg daily) for 6 mo. In two of the previously reported cases *(225,232)*, in addition to surgery, treatment with amphotericin B (total doses of 3.5 and 1.0 g, respectively) was also applied.

2.9. Mediastinal Histoplasmosis

Sclerosing (fibrosing) mediastinitis is a condition of acute or chronic inflammation resulting in progressive fibrosis within the mediastinum *(239–244)*. It is a process of relentness proliferation of fibrous tissue that produces encroachment, entrapment, and eventual compression of mediastinal structures, such as the superior vena cava *(245)*, the azygos, innominate and pulmonary veins *(246)*, the pulmonary arteries *(247)*, and the esophagus and trachea *(248,249)*. Mediastinal fibrosis may be caused by a variety of pathogens, including *H. capsulatum (250–255)*. The recognition that mediastinal fibrosis may be associated with an underlying disease, such as fungal infection, has markedly improved the management of this difficult to treat condition, and reduced the necessity of surgical decompression of entrapped organs. Thus, Urchel et al. *(244)* successfully managed sclerosing mediastinitis in six patients with underlying disseminated histoplasmosis with 400-mg daily oral ketoconazole regimens.

Coss et al. *(256)* described a case of esophageal fistula complicating mediastinal histoplasmosis; the patient was successfully treated with amphotericin B (35 mg/kg administered over a 4-mo period). Esophageal involvement in patients with disseminated histoplasmosis is most likely due to hematogenous spread from a primary pulmonary infection *(257)*. In two previous occacions, Jenkins et al. *(258)*, and Sarosi and Davies *(259)* also used amphotericin B to treat patients with disphagia secondary to histoplasmosis.

A number of investigators *(260–263)* are still recommending surgical management of complications arising from mediastinal histoplasmosis because of lack of evidence to demonstrate active infection *(92)*. In addition, surgical intervention is favored over amphotericin B therapy because of several other factors, namely: (1) poor growth characteristics of *H. capsulatum* in the mediastinum; (2) the necessity for pathologic diagnosis of mediastinal masses; (3) the toxicity of amphotericin B; and (4) the potential prophylactic benefit of surgical excision of mediastinal granuloma to prevent fibrosis *(256)*. To this end, Cameron et al. *(264)* suggested the following criteria for nonoperative treatment of esophageal complications: (1) esophageal disruptions confined within the mediastinum, or between the mediastinum and the visceral lung pleura; (2) drainage of the cavity back into the esophagus; (3) minimal symptoms; and (4) minimal signs of clinical sepsis.

Heart involvement due to disseminated histoplasmosis may present with endocarditis or endarteritis *(11,265–280)*. Disseminated histoplasmosis is reported to be the third leading cause of fungal endocarditis *(281)*. Usually associated with severe patient morbidity and mortality, fungal endocarditis is difficult to diagnose because fungal pathogens are uncommonly isolated from routine blood cultures *(266)*. Histoplasmic endocarditis can affect not only normal cardiac valves but also grossly abnormal structures, such as diseased or prosthetic valves *(269,275,278,279)* and cardiac tumors *(265)*. In addition, infection of atheroma and aneurysms in great vessels and vascular drafts, has been reported *(265,282)*.

The recommended therapy for histoplasmic endocarditis is a combination of valve replacement and amphotericin B. Thus, Wilınshurst et al. *(283)* reported a case of histoplasmic endocarditis on a stenosed aortic valve presenting as dysphagia and weight loss. The patient was treated with intravenous amphotericin B (gradually increasing dose regimens to a maximum of 50 mg daily), beginning

4 d prior to aortic valve replacement; amphotericin B therapy was discontinued 50 d later because of excessive renal toxicity (total dose of 2.55 g), and oral itraconazole (400 mg daily) was instituted for the next 17 mo. In another report, however, Kanawaty et al. *(280)* described the first case of successful nonsurgical treatment of histoplasmic endocarditis involving a bioprosthetic valve using amphotericin B; a total dose of 4.0 g of the drug was infused via a Hickman catheter. Derby et al. *(284)* also treated a patient with endocarditis complicated with major arterial embolism with amphotericin B and without surgical intervention; the patient survived after receiving 4.8 g (total dose) of the drug. There have been several other reports *(11,268,270–272,277)* of histoplasmic endocarditis therapy consisting of amphotericin B alone and without surgical involvement.

2.10. Pulmonary Histoplasmosis and Pleural Effusions

Patients who inhale a large burden of organisms from the environment and those who are immunosuppressed may develop severe, life-threatening pneumonia *(285–287)*.

Chronic pulmonary histoplasmosis usually occurs in patients with preexisting severe chronic obstructive lung disease, such as emphysema and chronic bronchitis (285).

Complications of pulmonary histoplasmosis are mostly related to persistent mediastinal lymphodenopathy.

The occurence of pleural effusions associated with histoplasmosis is rarely seen (incidence rate of 0–6%) *(288–297)*. In pediatric patients (298–300), pleural effusion is sometimes diagnosed with concomitant pericarditis (301). Tutor et al. *(302)* reported a case of a child with pleural effusion presenting as chylothorax. The latter condition results from the escape of chyle from the lymphatic system into the thoracic cavity caused by an obstruction of lymph flow or a laceration of the thoracic duct.

After reviewing the cases of 32 children with acute pulmonary histoplasmosis, Kakos and Kilman *(296)* found no evidence of pleural effusion. It is not unusual for pleural fluid of patients with histoplasmosis to demonstrate eosinophilia (up to 17%) *(303–306)*, which in the majority of cases has been described as idiopathic *(307)*.

While, in general, pleural fluid cultures failed to grow the fungus, an exception was reported by Marshall et al. *(308)*, who were able to grow *H. capsulatum* from a pleural fluid of an AIDS patient. The failure to grow fungus from the pleural fluid of patients with histoplasmosis may support one of the proposed etiologies for the effusion, by being the result of antigen diffusing from the granulomatous foci located near the pleural space *(305)*.

For chronic pulmonary histoplasmosis, treatment with amphotericin B has been recommended for patients with progressive, disseminated disease, especially in immunocompromised hosts *(18)*. The management of pleural effusion would largely depend on the severity of the symptoms *(297)*. In symptomatic patients with a large pleural effusion, thoracentesis may be indicated to relieve symptoms and eliminate some of the other causes of pleural effusion *(298–301)*.

2.11. Histoplasmosis of the Central Nervous System

Although infrequent among patients with disseminated histoplasmosis, CNS involvement has been seen in 10–20%, and as high as 50% of immunocompromised hosts *(309–323)*. The condition can present as miliary or solitary granulomas of the brain, focal or diffuse cerebritis, or histoplasmic meningitis *(324)*. In the latter case, diagnosis may often be difficult since *H. capsulatum* is not readily grown from CSF samples and serology could be misleading *(317)*. In spite of the high incidence of meningeal histoplasmosis in both chronic and subacute disease, associated hydrocephalus has seldom been reported *(313,315,318)*.

Amphotericin B is widely used as therapy, but recurrence of infection is frequently observed *(69,324)*. In one report *(325)*, CNS histoplasmosis was cured in 61% of patients receiving at least 30 mg/kg of amphotericin B, as compared to 33% of those treated with lower doses. The higher dose regimens may be needed to overcome the poor penetration of the drug into CSF even in the presence of active meningitis *(326)*.

In AIDS patients, CNS histoplasmosis commonly presents as meningitis, single or multiple abscesses, or granulomas *(69)*. Tiraboschi et al. *(327)* treated one patient with chronic CNS histoplasmosis and hydrocephalus with oral fluconazole (200 mg daily for 6 wk; then 100 mg daily as maintenance therapy), after amphotericin B (20 mg/kg) failed to sterilize the CSF and reinfection resulted in recurrence of the hydrocephalus. Even though fluconazole easily penetrated the CSF and successfully sterilized it, transverse myelopathy still persisted, and shunting was needed to control the hydrocephalus *(327)*. High dose of intravenous fluconazole (800 mg, once daily) improved markedly the condition of an HIV-infected patient with multiple cerebral lesions caused by disseminated histoplasmosis *(328)*.

Kelly et al. *(329)* described a case of disseminated histoplasmosis presenting with multifocal cerebritis and intramedullary spinal histoplasmoma that was successfully treated with amphotericin B, resulting in nearly complete symptomatic recovery. In a previous report *(330)*, chronic administration of prednisone (as therapy for unrelated conditions) to a patient with spinal histoplasmosis was thought to have been the reason for the patient's relapse. Surgical intervention alone has also been used to treat spinal histoplasmosis successfully *(331,332)*.

In a report by Bamberger *(333)*, successful treatment of multiple cerebral histoplasmomas was achieved after treatment with itraconazole (200 mg, t.i.d. for 3 d, followed by 200 mg, b.i.d.) over 1-yr period.

A case of *H. capsulatum* involvement within the cutaneous nerves in patients with disseminated histoplasmosis and AIDS has also been described (334).

2.12. Adrenal Histoplasmosis

Several reports *(335–338)* have described adrenal histoplasmosis manifesting as bilateral adrenal masses; in one case, the patient after treatment with itraconazole made a complete recovery *(335)*. A unilateral adrenal histoplasmosis concurrent with hepatosplenomegaly and significant weigh loss was also reported *(339)*.

In a case of adrenal histoplasmosis manifested as Addison's disease, Rozenblit et al. *(340)* have found unusual CT features with magnetic resonance imaging correlation.

2.13. Musculoskeletal Histoplasmosis

Disseminated histoplasmosis has also been diagnosed as bone lesions *(341)*, although this is rare. de Fernandez et al. *(342)* presented a case of a patient with myelodysplasia and left tibial abscess caused by *H. capsulatum*. The patient, who showed no clinical evidence of pulmonary involvement, was successfully treated with itraconazole.

2.14. Histoplasmosis of the Thyroid

Infection of the thyroid by *H. capsulatum* has been reported, although rarely, as part of the disseminated disease. In one such case, Goldani et al. *(343)* presented a patient with a previous Hashimoto's disease and non-Hodgkin's lymphoma in which a diffuse enlarged thyroid gland with a large nodule was the only apparent locus of histoplasmosis; treatment with itraconazole (at 400 mg, daily) and chemotherapy for the lymphoma, followed by suppressive therapy with itraconazole (200 mg, daily) led to regression of the thyroid nodule and cervical adenopathy.

2.15. Genitourinary Histoplasmosis

Evidence of urogenital involvement of histoplasmosis, although rarely, has been reported *(6,344–355)*. The most involved organ was the kidney *(11,344,346,354)*. The ureter has been involved in only one reported case *(346)*, the bladder in two cases *(345,356)*, and the penis in six cases *(349–353,356)*. Disseminated histoplasmosis also occasionally may present as orchitis or epididymitis *(347,348,357)*. Ovarian histoplasmosis in a case of patient with SLE was reported by Isotalo et al. *(358)*.

In two cases described by Friskel et al. *(356)*, one of the patients presented with a ulcer of the bladder wall consistent with *Histoplasma* infection; the patient was given itraconazole (400 mg, daily), which led to total resolution. In the second case, a celibate patient with a history of severe rheumatoid arthritis and receiving methotrexate (13.5 mg once weekly) and prednisone (10 mg, daily) presented with a necrotic lesion of the penis; the patient was successfully treated with intravenous amphotericin B, then with lamellar amphotericin B, and finally with itraconazole for a total of 6 mo.

2.15.1. Prostatic Histoplasmosis

Disseminated histoplasmosis of the prostate gland, although uncommon, has been reported *(359–364)* including in HIV-positive patients *(365–367)*. Although in general most, if not all, of fungal prostatitis is the result of hematogenous dissemination, it is difficult to demonstrate conclusively whether prostatitis is caused directly by hematogenous seeding or is the result of epididymis or seminal vesicles by orthograde flow of seminal fluid *(368)*. Prostatic histoplasmosis, as with other mycotic prostatitis, may often resemble tuberculosis, neoplasms, benign prostatic hypertrophy, syphilis, or bacterial prostatitis *(364)*. Manifestations include dysuria, urinary outlet obstruction, perineal or suprapublic discomfort, hematuria, and hematospermia. Mawhorter et al. *(359)* described an unusual case of prostatic and CNS histoplasmosis in an immunocompetent patient.

Treatment strategies regarding prostatic histoplasmosis are limited *(359)*. To this end, surgical intervention may not be an option because of the the possibility of further dissemination *(359)*. The benefits of chemotherapy with amphotericin B, ketoconazole, itraconazole, or fluconazole are still unclear *(366)*, although fluconazole (in consolidation therapy for disseminated histoplasmosis with CNS involvement) and itraconazole have been shown to be effective in some cases *(369,370)*.

2.16. Childhood Histoplasmosis

A rare occurrence in immunocompetent infants and children, acute disseminated histoplasmosis is occasionally observed in immunosuppressed children *(11,345)* including those with AIDS *(287)*. Most cases of progressive disseminated histoplasmosis occur in immunosuppressed children usually complicating the management of hematologic malignancy (Hodgkin's disease, and acute and chronic lymphocytic leukemia) *(9,11,155,371)*.

Butler et al. *(372)* reviewed the clinical presentation and treatment of histoplasmosis among children hospitalized over a 21-yr period (1968–1988) in the Vanderbilt University Children's Hospital, serving an area in middle Tennessee with a high prevalence of endemic histoplasmosis. Of the 35 patients diagnosed with the disease, 83% ($n = 29$) had pulmonary/mediastinal infection, 14% ($n = 5$) had disseminated disease, and one patient (3%) had primary cutaneous histoplasmosis. While 80% ($n = 28$) of the patients did not received specific antifungal chemotherapy, five patients (14%) were treated with amphotericin B, one patient (3%) with ketoconazole, and one patient received an initial course of amphotericin B, followed by oral ketoconazole. Follow-up evaluations ranged from 1 mo to 15 yr (mean, 30.1 mo); persistency of symptoms existed in six patients, and two patients have been known to die of complications (disseminated pulmonary infection, and cardiopulmonary compromise due to mediastinal fibrosis, respectively) *(318)*. This survey, as well as other findings, have shown that mediastinal fibrosis although refractory to treatment, is relatively rare in children less than 10 yr old and will generally resolve spontaneously without residual damage *(373,374)*. Histoplasmic pericarditis has had more frequent manifestation in children than in adults *(301,372,375)*.

Another somewhat puzzling and still unexplained fact that came out of the Vanderbilt study *(372)* as well as from other groups *(11,376)*, was the apparently reduced incidence of pediatric disseminated histoplasmosis after 1970. Cases of primary cutaneous histoplasmosis among children are highly unusual and very rare *(372,377)*.

Rescorla et al. *(378)* described a case of otherwise normal child with acute obstruction of the common bile duct caused by histoplasmic lymphadenitis of the peripancreatic lymph nodes. The lymphadenitis was probably the result of duodenal ulcerations caused by histoplasmosis. The patient was treated with amphotericin B (1.0 mg/kg over 24 h) for 38 d; prednisone was started at a dose of 2.0 mg/kg/over 24 h for the first 7 d, 1.0 mg/kg/over 24 h for the ensuing 7 d, and tapered slowly thereafter. Two weeks after the regimen was initiated, the abdominal computerized tomographic (CT) scan showed complete resolution of mass. The rationale to employ a short course of steroids (prednisone) was to provide more rapid relief of the ductal obstruction and eventually to prevent later fibrotic changes to the duct *(378)*.

A case of acute disseminated histoplasmosis with multifocal choroiditis in an immunosuppressed child was successfully resolved with intravenous amphotericin B (1.0 mg/kg, daily) for 4 wk *(155)*.

Disseminated histoplasmosis in a 2-yr-old immunocompetent child was also treated successfully with amphotericin B *(379)*.

3. HOST IMMUNE DEFENSE AGAINST HISTOPLASMOSIS

Protective immunity against primary and secondary histoplasmosis is multifactorial and requiring cells of the innate and adaptive immune response. Effector mechanisms mediating the intracellular killing of the fungus involves cytokines (interferon-γ [IFN-γ], tumor necrosis factor-α [TNF-α]), and/or direct cytolytic activity by T- and natural killer (NK) cells *(380,381)*. In this regard, perforin-deficient knockout mice were found to have accelerated mortality and increased fungal burdan following a lethal or sublethal primary challenge, thereby establishing an essential role for perforin in the primary immunity systemic *Histoplasma* infection *(380)*.

Within 24 h of exposure, inhaled fungal microconidia would trigger an early nonimmune response by fungicidal neutrophils. It is, however, the cell-mediated immune response that is largely responsible for defense against histoplasmosis *(382)*. A vigorous cell-mediated immune response will usually begin to develop 10–21 d after the primary exposure. Development of specific cell-mediated immune response in immunocompetent hosts will frequently result in granuloma formation and containment of the pathogen. Therefore, without massive inhalational exposure, fungal virulence is generally low in immunocompetent patients *(28,67,84,383,384)*. However, reactivation of infection may occur, especially in immunocompromised patients. Macrophages will accumulate and attach to the pathogen through interaction with adherence-promoting proteins *(385)*. The mechanism(s) by which the histoplasmal yeasts manage to survive and proliferate inside the macrophages is still not well-understood. However, it is known that phagocytosis of the yeasts by human monocytes/macrophages would stimulate the respiratory burst *(385–387)* and the phagolysosomal fusion *(388)*. Even so, the ingested yeasts are still capable of multiplying within the phagolysosomes *(389–391)*.

In HIV-infected patients the immune responsiveness to *H. capsulatum* was depressed when the $CD4^+$ cell counts were between 200 and 500 cells/mm^3 but approached normal in those patients with $CD4^+$ cell counts of over 500 cells/mm^3 *(20)*.

Wu-Hsieh et al. *(392)* have examined the role of $CD8^+$ T-cell responses following viral infection in immunity to systemic histoplasmosis in mice. These and other results have shown that $CD8^+$ T cells can suppress immunity through different (perforin-dependent and -independent) mechanisms *(362,382)*.

Neutralization of endogenous granulocyte-macrophage colony-stimulating factor (GM-CSF) subverted the protective immune response to *H. capsulatum*, thereby proving to be essential for survival in primary but not secondary infection *(393)*.

Wheat et al. *(394)* reported several cases of systemic salmonellosis in patients with disseminated histoplasmosis. While generalized defects of the cellular immunity could have predisposed these patients to both histoplasmosis and salmonellosis, it has been postulated that histoplasma yeast parasitization of the macrophages ("macrophage blockade") would certainly impair their ability to resist other invasive intracellular pathogens, thus becoming, at least in part, a predisposing factor to systemic *Salmonella* infections *(394,395)*.

REFERENCES

1. Kwong-Chung, K. J. Sexual stage of *Histoplasma capsulatum*. *Science*, 177, 368, 1972.
2. Schwartz, J. Histoplasmosis, Praeger, New York, 1981.
3. Hay, R. J. Histoplasmosis. *Semin. Dermatol.*, 12, 310, 1993.
4. Williams, A. O., Lawson, E. A., and Lucas, A. O. African histoplasmosis due to *Histoplasma duboisii*. *Arch. Pathol.*, 92, 306,1971.
5. Woods, J. P., Heinecke, E. L., Luecke, J. W., et al. Pathogenesis of *Histoplasma capsulatum*. *Semin. Respir. Infect.*, 16, 91–101, 2001.
6. Retalack, D. M. and Woods, J. P. Molecular epidemiology, pathogenesis, and genetics of the dimorphic fungus *Histoplasma capsulatum*. *Microbes Infect.*, 1, 817–825, 1999.
7. Sarosi, G. A. and Davies, S. F. Concise review for primary-care physicians: therapy for fungal infections. *Mayo Clin. Proc.*, 69, 1111, 1994.
8. Kauffman, C. A. Newer developments in therapy for endemic mycoses. *Clin. Infect. Dis.*, 19(Suppl. 1), S28, 1994.
9. Wheat, L. J. Histoplasmosis: diagnosis and treatment. *Infect. Dis. Clin. Prac.*, 1, 277, 1992.
10. Johnson, P. C., Khardori, N., Najjar, A. F., Butt, F., Mansell, P. W., and Sarosi, G. A. Progressive disseminated histoplasmosis in patients with acquired immunodeficiency syndrome. *Am. J. Med.*, 85, 152, 1988.
11. Goodwin, R. A., Shapiro, J. L., Thurman, G. H., Thurman, S. S., and Des Prez, R. M. Disseminated histoplasmosis: clinical and pathological correlations. *Medicine (Baltimore)*, 59, 1, 1980.
12. Goodwin, R. A. Jr. and Des Prez, R. M. Histoplasmosis. *Am. Rev. Respir. Dis.*, 117, 929, 1987.
13. Davies, S. F., Khau, M., and Sarosi, G. A. Disseminated histoplasmosis in immunologically suppressed patients. *Am. J. Med.*, 65, 923, 1978.
14. Wheat, L. J., Slama, T. G., Norton, J. A., et al. Risk factors for disseminated and fatal histoplasmosis. *Ann. Intern. Dis.*, 96, 159, 1982.
15. Loyd, J. E., Des Prez, R. M., and Goodwin, R. A. *Histoplasma capsulatum*, in *Principle and Practice of Infectious Disease*, Mandell, G. L., Douglas, K. G., and Bennett, J. L., Eds. Churchill-Livingston, New York, 1989, 1985.
16. Zeluff, B. J. Fungal pneumonia in transplant recipients. *Semin. Respir. Infect.*, 5, 80, 1990.
17. Reddy, P., Gorelick, D. F., Brasher, C. A., and Larsh, H. Progressive disseminated histoplasmosis as seen in adults. *Am. J. Med.*, 48, 629, 1970.
18. Dismukes, W. E., Bradsher, R. W., Cloud, G. C., et al. Itraconazole therapy for blastomycosis and histoplasmosis. *Am. J. Med.*, 93, 489, 1992.
19. Wheat, J., Sarosi, G., McKinsey, D., et al. Practice guidelines for the management of patients with histoplasmosis. Infectious Diseases Society of America. *Clin. Infect. Dis.*, 30, 688-695, 2000.
20. Vail, G. M., Mocherla, S., Wheat, L. J., et al. Cellular immune response in HIV-infected patients with histoplasmosis. *J. Acqur. Immune Defic. Syndr.*, 29, 49–53, 2002.
21. Pierard, G. E., Arrese, J. E., and Pierard-Franchimont, C. Itraconazole. *Expert Opin. Pharmacother.*, 1, 287–304, 2000.
22. Goodwin, R. A., Owens, F. T., Snell, J. D., et al. Chronic pulmonary histoplasmosis. *Medicine (Baltimore)*, 55, 413, 1976.
23. Mocherla, S. and Wheat, L. J. Treatment of histoplasmosis. *Semin. Respir. Infect.*, 16, 141–148, 2001.
24. Laochumroonvorapong, P., DiCostanzo, D. P., Wu, H., Srinivasan, K., Abusamieh, M., and Levy, H. Disseminated histoplasmosis presenting as pyoderma gangrenosum-like lesions in a patient with acquired immunodeficiency syndrome. *Int. J. Dermatol.*, 40, 518–521, 2001.
25. Rao, R. D., Morice, W. G., and Phyliky, R. L. Hemophagocytosis in a patient with chronic lymphocytic leukemia and histoplasmosis. *Mayo Clin. Proc.*, 77, 287–290, 2002.
26. Rieg, G. K., Shah, P. M., Helm, E. B., and Just-Nubling, G. Case report. Successful therapy of disseminated histoplasmosis in AIDS with liposomal amphotericin B. *Mycoses*, 42, 117–120, 1999.
27. Graybill, J. R. Histoplasmosis and AIDS. *J. Infect. Dis.*, 158, 623, 1988.
28. Drew, R. H. Pharmacotherapy of disseminated histoplasmosis in patients with AIDS. *Ann. Pharmacother.*, 27, 1510, 1993.
29. Walker, J. V., Baran, D., Yakuk, N., and Freeman, R. B. Histoplasmosis with hypercalcemia, renal failure, and pulmonary necrosis. *J. Am. Med. Assos.*, 237, 1350, 1977.
30. Murray, J. J. and Heim, C. R. Hypercalcemia in disseminated histoplasmosis: aggravation by vitamin D. *Am. J. Med.*, 78, 881, 1985.
31. Liu, J. W., Huang, T. C., Lu, Y. C., et al. Acute disseminated histoplasmosis complicated with hypercalcaemia. *J. Infect.*, 39, 88–90, 1999.
32. Goldstein, R. A., Israel, H. L., Becker, K. L., and Moore, C. F. The infrequency of hypercalcemia in sarcoidosis. *Am. J. Med.*, 51, 21, 1970.
33. Shai, F., Baker, R. K., Addrizzo, J. R., and Wallach, S. Hypercalcemia in mycobacterial infection. *J. Clin. Endocrinol. Metab.*, 34, 251, 1972.
34. Abbasi, A. A., Chemplavi, J. K., Farah, S., Muller, B. F., and Arnstein, A. R. Hypercalcemia in active pulmonary tuberculosis. *Ann. Intern. Med.*, 90, 324, 1979.
35. Need, A. G., Phillips, P. J., Chiu, F. T. S., and Prisk, H. M. Hypercalcemia associated with tuberculosis. *Br. Med. J.*, 280, 831, 1980.
36. Stoekle, J. D., Hardy, H. L., and Weber, A. L. Chronic beryllium disease: long-term follow-up of sixty cases and selective review of the literature. *Am. J. Med.*, 46, 545, 1969.

37. Lee, J. C., Catanzaro, A., Parthemore, J. G., Roach, B., and Deftos, L. J. Hypercalcemia in disseminated coccidioidomycosis. *N. Engl. J. Med.*, 297, 431, 1977.
38. Kantarjian, H. M., Saad, M. F., Esteg, E. H., Sellin, R. V., and Samaan, N. A. Hypercalcemia in disseminated candidiasis. *Am. J. Med.*, 74, 721, 1983.
39. Bell, N. H., Stern, P. H., Pantzer, E., Sinha, T. K., and DeLuca, H. F. Evidence that increased circulating $1\alpha,25$-dihydroxyvitamin D is the probable cause for abnormal calcium metabolism in sarcoidosis. *J. Clin. Invest.*, 64, 218, 1979.
40. Stern, P. H., DeOlazzabal, J., and Bell, N. H. Evidence for abnormal regulation of circulating $1\alpha,25$-dihydroxyvitamin D in patients with sarcoidosis and normal calcium metabolism. *J. Clin. Invest.*, 66, 852, 1980.
41. Zimmerman, J., Holick, M. F., and Silver, J. Normocalcemia in a hypoparathyroid patient with sarcoidosis: evidence for parathyroid-hormone-independent synthesis of 1,25- dihydroxyvitamin D. *Ann. Intern. Med.*, 98, 338, 1983.
42. Barbour, G. L., Coburn, J. W., Slatopolsky, E., Norman, A. W., and Horst, R. L. Hypercalcemia in an anephric patient with sarcoidosis: evidence for extrarenal generation of 1,25-dihydroxyvitamin D. *N. Engl. J. Med.*, 305, 440, 1981.
43. Maeska, J. K., Batuman, V., Pablo, N. C., and Shakamuri, S. Elevated 1,25- dihydroxyvitamin D levels: occurence with sarcoidosis with end-stage renal disease. *Arch. Intern. Med.*, 142, 1206, 1982.
44. Mason, R. S., Frankel, T., Yuk-Luen, C., Lissner, D., and Posen, S. Vitamin D conversion by sarcoid lymph node homogenate. *Ann. Intern. Med.*, 100, 59, 1984.
45. Adams, J. S., Sharman, O. P., Gacad, M. A., and Singer, F. R. Metabolism of 25-hydroxyvitamin D3 by cultured pulmonary alveolar macrophages in sarcoidosis. *J. Clin. Invest.*, 72, 1856, 1983.
46. Anderson, J., Dent, C. E., Harper, C., and Philpot, G. R. Effect of cortisone on calcium metabolism in sarcoidosis with hypercalcemia. *Lancet*, 2, 720, 1954.
47. Zerwekh, J. E., Pak, C. Y. C., Kaplan, R. A., McGuire, J. L. Upchurch, K., Breslau, N., and Johnson, R. Jr., Pathogenic role of $1\alpha,25$-dihydroxyvitamin D in sarcoidosis and absorptive hypercalciuria: different response to prednisolone therapy. *J. Clin. Endocrinol. Metab.*, 51, 381, 1980.
48. Cheng, I. J. P., Fang, G. X., Chan, T. M., Chan, P. C. K., and Chan, M.K. Fungal peritonitis complicating peritoneal dialysis: report of 27 cases and review of treatment. *Q. J. Med.*, 265, 407, 1989.
49. Lim, W., Chau, S. P., Chan, P. C. K., and Cheng, I. K. P. *Histoplasma capsulatum* infection associated with continuous ambulatory peritoneal dialysis. *J. Infect.*, 22, 179, 1991.
50. Weinstein, G. D. Methotrexate. *Ann. Intern. Med.*, 86, 199, 1977.
51. Wilkens, R. F. and Watson, M. A. Methotrexate: a perspective of its use in the treatment of rheumatic disease. *J. Lab. Clin. Med.*, 100, 314, 1982.
52. Groff, G. D., Shenberger, K. N., Wilke, W. S., and Taylor, T. H. Low-dose oral methotrexate in rheumatoid arthritis: an uncontrolled trial and review of the literature. *Semin. Arthritis Rheum.*, 12, 333, 1983.
53. Weinstein, A., Marlowe, S., Korn, J., and Farouhar, F. Low-dose methotrexate treatment of rheumatoid arthritis. *Am. J. Med.*, 79, 331, 1985.
54. Perruquet, J. L., Harrington, T. M., and Davis, D. E. *Pneumocystis carinii* pneumonia following methotrexate therapy for rheumatoid arthritis. *Arthritis Rheum.*, 26, 1291, 1983.
55. Wallis, P. J. W., Ryatt, K. S., and Constable, T. J. *Pneumocystis carinii* pneumonia complicating low dose methotrexate treatment for psoriatic arthropathy. *Ann. Rheum. Dis.*, 48, 247, 1989.
56. Leff, R. L., Case, J. P., and McKenzie, R. Rheumatoid arthritis, methotrexate therapy, and pneumocystis pneumonia. *Ann. Intern. Med.*, 112, 716, 1990.
57. Keegan, J. M. and Byrd, J. W. Nocardiosis associated with low dose methotrexate for rheumatoid arthritis. *J. Rheumatol.*, 15, 1585, 1988.
58. Altx-Smith, M., Kendall, L. G. Jr., and Stamm, A. M. Cryptococcosis associated with low-dose methotrexate for arthritis. *Am. J. Med.*, 83, 179, 1987.
59. Witty, L. A., Steiner, F., Curfman, M., Webb, D., and Wheat, L. J. Disseminated histoplasmosis in patients receiving low-dose methotrexate therapy for psoriasis. *Arch. Dermatol.*, 128, 91, 1992.
60. Roy, V. and Hammerschmidt, D. E. Disseminated histoplasmosis following prolonged low- dose methotrexate therapy. *Am. J. Hematol.*, 63, 59-60, 2000.
61. Jolivet, J., Cowan, K., Curt, G., Clendeninn, N., and Chabner, B. The pharmacology and clinical use of methotrexate. *N. Engl. J. Med.*, 309, 1094, 1983.
62. U.S. Public Health Service (USPHS) and Infectious Diseases Society of America (IDSA). 1999 USPHS/IDSA guidelines for the prevention of opportunistic infections in persons infected with human immunodeficiency virus. *Infect. Dis. Obstet. Gynecol.*, 8, 5–74, 2000.
63. McKinsey, D. S., Wheat, L. J., Cloud, G. A., et al. Itraconazole prophylaxis for fungal infections in patients with advanced human immunodeficiency virus infection: randomized, placebo-controlled, double-blind study. National Institute of Allergy and Infectious Diseases Mycoses Study Group. *Clin. Infect. Dis.*, 28, 1049–1056, 1999.
64. Bilkenroth, U. and Holzhausen, H. J. Disseminated infection by *Histoplasma capsulatum* with AIDS. *Pathologe*, 22, 270–275, 2001.
66. Corti, M. E., Cendoya, C. A., Soto, I., et al. Disseminated histoplasmosis and AIDS: clinical aspects and diagnostic methods for early detection. *AIDS Patient Care*, 14, 149–154, 2000.
67. Wheat, L. J., Slama, T. G., and Zeckel, M. L. Histoplasmosis in the acquired immune deficiency syndrome. *Am. J. Med.*, 78, 203, 1985.
68. Salzman, S. H., Smith, R. L., and Aranda, C. P. Histoplasmosis in patients at risk for acquired immunodeficiency syndrome in a nonendemic setting. *Chest*, 93, 916, 1988.

69. Anaissie, E., Fainstein, V., Samo, T., Bodey, G. P., and Sarosi, G. A. Central nervous system histoplasmosis; an unappreciated complication of the acquired immunodeficiency syndrome. *Am. J. Med.*, 84, 215, 1988.
70. McKinsey, D. S., Gupta, M. R., Riddler, S. A., Driks, M. R., Smith, D. L., and Kurtin, P. J. Long-term amphotericin B therapy for disseminated histoplasmosis in patients with the acquired immunodeficiency syndrome (AIDS). *Ann. Intern. Med.*, 111, 655, 1989.
71. Huang, D. T., McGarry, T., Cooper, S., Saunders, R., and Andavolu, R. Disseminated histoplasmosis in the acquired immunodeficiency syndrome. *Arch. Intern. Med.*, 147, 1181, 1987.
72. Kaur, J. and Myers, A. M. Homosexuality, steroid therapy, and histoplasmosis. *Ann. Intern. Med.*, 99, 567, 1983.
73. Kalter, D. C., Tschen, J. A., and Klima, M. Maculopapular rash in a patient with acquired immunodeficiency syndrome. *Arch. Dermatol.*, 121, 1455, 1985.
74. Dietrich, P. Y., Pugin, P., Regamey, C., and Bille, J. Disseminated histoplasmsosis and AIDS in Switzerland. *Lancet*, 2, 752, 1986.
75. Johnson, P. C., Sarosi, G. A., Septimus, E. J., and Satterwhite, T. K. Progressive disseminated histoplasmosis in patients with the acquired immune deficiency syndrome: a report of 12 cases and a literature review. *Semin. Respir. Infect.*, 1, 1, 1986.
76. Hazelhurst, J. A. and Vismer, H. F. Histoplasmosis presenting with unusual skin lesions in acquired immunodeficiency syndrome (AIDS). *Br. J. Dermatol.*, 113, 345, 1985.
77. Macher, B. E., Rodriguez, M. M., Kaplan, W., et al. Disseminated bilateral chorioretinitis due to *Histoplasma capsulatum* in a patient with the acquired immunodeficiency syndrome. *Ophthalmology*, 92, 1159, 1985.
78. Haggerty, C. M., Britton, M. C., Dorman, J. M., and Marzoni, F. A. Jr. Gastrointestinal histoplasmosis in the acquired immunodeficiency syndrome. *West. J. Med.*, 143, 244, 1985.
79. Johnson, P. C. and Sarosi, G. A. AIDS and progressive disseminated histoplasmosis. *J. Am. Med. Assoc.*, 258, 202, 1987.
80. Alterman, D. D. and Cho, K. C. Histoplasmosis involving the omentum in an AIDS patient. *J. Compt. Assist. Tomogr.*, 12, 664, 1988.
81. Pasternak, J. and Bolivar, R. Bone marrow examination and culture in the diagnosis of acquired immunodeficiency syndrome (AIDS). *Arch. Intern. Med.*, 143, 1495, 1983.
82. Wheat, L. J., Connolly-Stringfield, P. A., Baker, R. L., et al. Disseminated histoplasmosis in the acquired immunodeficiency syndrome: clinical findings, diagnosis, and review of the literature. *Medicine (Baltimore)*, 69, 361, 1990.
83. Wheat, L. J. and Batteriger, B. E. Histoplasmosis. *Handbook Clin. Neurol.*, 8, 437, 1988.
84. Wheat, L. J. and Small, C. B. Disseminated histoplasmosis in AIDS. *Arch. Intern. Med.*, 144, 2147, 1984.
85. Greene, L., Peters, B., Lucas, S. B., and Pozniak, A. L. Extrapulmonary tuberculosis masking disseminated histoplasmosis in AIDS. *Sex Transm. Infect.*, 76, 54–56, 2000.
86. Wheat, L. J., Kohler, R. B., and Tewari, R. P. Diagnosis of disseminated histoplasmosis by detection of *Histoplasma capsulatum* antigen in serum and urine specimens. *N. Engl. J. Med.*, 314, 83, 1986.
87. Wheat, L. J., Connolly-Stringfield, P., Kohler, R. B., Frame, P. T., and Gupta, M. R. *Histoplasma capsulatum* polysaccharide antigen detection in diagnosis and management of disseminated histoplasmosis in patients with acquired immunodeficiency syndrome. *Am. J. Med.*, 87, 396, 1989.
88. Wheat, L. J., Connolly-Stringfield, P., Blair, R., et al. Effect of successful treatment with amphotericin B on *Histoplasma capsulatum* variety *capsulatum* polysaccharide antigen levels in patients with AIDS and histoplasmosis. *Am. J. Med.*, 92, 153, 1992.
89. Graviss, E. A., Vanden Heuvel, E. A., Lacke, C. E., Spindel, S. A., White, A. C. Jr., and Hamill, R. J. Clinical prediction model for differentiation of disseminated *Histoplasma capsulatum* and *Mycobacterium avium* complex infections in febrile patients with AIDS. *J. Acquir. Immune Defic. Syndr.*, 24, 30–36, 2000.
90. Sharkey-Mathis, P. K., Velez, J, Fetchick, R., and Graybill, J. R. Histoplasmosis in the acquired immunodeficiency syndeome (AIDS): treatment with itraconazole and fluconazole. *J. Acquir. Immune Defic. Syndr.*, 6, 809, 1993.
91. McKinsey, D. S., Gupta, M. R., Driks, M. R., Smith, D. L., and O'Connor, M. Histoplasmosis in patients with AIDS: efficacy of maintenance amphotericin B therapy. *Am. J. Med.*, 92, 225, 1992.
92. Slain, D., Rogers, P. D., Cleary, J. D., and Chapman, S. W. Intravenous itraconazole. *Ann. Pharmacother.*, 35, 720–729, 2001.
93. Zon, L. I., Arkin, C, and Groopman, J. E. Haematologic manifestations of the human immune deficiency virus (HIV). *Br. J. Haematol.*, 66, 251, 1987.
94. Spivak, J. L., Barnes, D. C., Fuchs, E., and Quinn, T. C. Serum immunoreactive erythropoietin in HIV-infected patients. *J. Am. Med. Assoc.*, 261, 3104, 1989.
95. Lin, A. C., Galdwasser, E., Bernard, E. M., and Chapman, S. W. Amphotericin B blunts erythropoietin response to anemia. *J. Infect. Dis.*, 161, 348, 1990.
96. Lancaster, D. J., Palte, S., and Ray, D. Recombinant human erythropoietin in the treatment of anemia in AIDS patients receiving concomitant amphotericin B and zidovudine. *J. Acquired Immune Defic. Syndr.*, 6, 533, 1993.
97. Negroni, R., Palmieri, O., Koren, F., Tiraboschi, I. N., and Galimberti, R. L. Oral treatment of paracoccidioidomycosis and histoplasmosis with itraconazole in humans. *Rev. Infect. Dis.*, 9(Suppl. 1), S47, 1987.
98. Cauteren, H., Heykants, J., Decoster, R., and Cauwenberg, G. Itraconazole: pharmacologic studies in animals and humans. *Rev. Infect. Dis.*, 9(Suppl. 1), S43, 1987.
99. Hay, R. J., Dupont, B, and Graybill, J. R. First international symposium on itraconazole: a summary. *Rev. Infect. Dis.*, 9(Suppl. 1), S1, 1987.
100. Van Cutsem, J., Van Gerven, F., and Janssen, P. A. J. Activity of orally, topically, and parenterally administered itraconazole in the treatment of superficial and deep mycosis: animal models. *Rev. Infect. Dis.*, 9(Suppl. 1), S15, 1987.

101. Ganer, A., Arathoon, E., and Stevens, D. A. Initial experience in therapy for progressive mycoses with itraconazole, the first clinically studied triazole. *Rev. Infect. Dis.*, 9(Suppl. 1), S77, 1987.
102. Saag, M. S. and Dismukes, W. E. Azole antifungal agents: emphasis on new triazoles. *Antimicrob. Agents Chemother.*, 32, 1, 1988.
103. Negroni, R., Robles, A. M., Arechavala, A., and Taborda, A. Itraconazole in human histoplasmosis. *Mycoses*, 32, 123, 1989.
104. Tucker, R. M., Williams, P. L., Arathoon, E. G., and Stevens, D. A. Treatment of mycoses with itraconazole. *Ann. NY Acad. Sci.*, 544, 51, 1988.
105. British Society for Antimicrobial Chemotherapy Working Party. Antifungal chemotherapy in patients with acquired immunodeficiency syndrome. *Lancet*, 340, 648, 1992.
106. Todd, J. R., Arigala, M. R., Penn, R. L., and King, J. W. Possible clinically significant interaction of itraconazole plus rifampin. *AIDS Patient Care*, 15, 505–510, 2001.
107. Baptist, S. J., Montana, J. B., Arden, S. B., Leon, L., and Dutel, M. Disseminated histoplasmosis in a man with AIDS. *NY State J. Med.*, 11, 664, 1985.
108. Humphrey, M. J., Jevon, S., and Tarbit, M. H. Pharmacokinetic evaluation of UK 49,858, a metabolically stable triazole antifungal drug, in animals and humans. *Antimicrob. Agents Chemother.*, 28, 648, 1985.
109. Diaz, M., Negroni, R., Montoro-Gei, F., et al. A Pan-American 5-year study of fluconazole therapy for deep mycoses in the immunocompetent host. *Clin. Infect. Dis.*, 14(Suppl. 1), S68, 1992.
110. Le Monte, A. M., Washum, K. E., Smedema, M. L., Schnizlein-Bick, C., Kohler, S. M., and Wheat, L. J. Amphotericin B combined with itraconazole or fluconazole for treatment of histoplasmosis. *J. Infect. Dis.*, 182, 545–550, 2000.
111. Smith, E., Franzmann, M., and Mathiesen, L. R. Disseminated histoplasmosis in Danish patients with AIDS. *Scand. J. Infect. Dis.*, 21, 573, 1989.
112. Graybill, J. R. Future directions of antifungal chemotherapy. *Clin. Infect. Dis.*, 14(Suppl. 1), S170, 1992.
113. Norris, S., McKinsey, D., Lancaster, D., and Wheat, J. Retrospective evaluation of fluconazole maintenance therapy for disseminated histoplasmosis in AIDS. *Proc. 32nd Intersci. Conf. Antimicrob. Agents Chemother.*, Anaheim, American Society for Microbiology, Washington, DC, abstract 1207, 1992.
114. Wheat, L. J., Connolly, P., Haddad, N., Le Monte, A., Brizendine, E., and Hafner, R. Antigen clearance during treatment of disseminated histoplasmosis with itraconazole versus fluconazole in patients with AIDS. *Antimicrob. Agents Chemother.*, 46, 248–250, 2002.
115. Wheat, L. J., Connolly, P., Smedema, M., Brezendine, E., Hafner, R., AIDS Clinical Trials Group and the Mycoses Study Group of the National Institute of Allergy and Infectious Diseases. Emergence of resistance to flucanazole as a cause of failure during treatment of histoplasmosis in patients with acquired immunodeficieny disease syndrome. *Clin. Infect. Dis.*, 33, 1910–1913, 2001.
116. Wheat, L. J., Cloud, G., Johnson, P. C., et al. Clearance of fungal burden during treatment of disseminated histoplasmosis with liposomal amphotericin B versus itraconazole. *Antimicrob. Agents Chemother.*, 45, 2354–2357, 2001.
117. Jones, P. G., Cohen, R. L., Batts, D. H., and Silva, J. Jr. Disseminated histoplasmosis, invasive pulmonary aspergillosis, and other opportunistic infections in a homosexual patient with acquired immune deficiency syndrome. *Sex Transm. Dis.*, 10, 202, 1983.
118. Salzman, S. H., Smith, R. L., and Aranda, C. P. Histoplasmosis in patients at risk for the acquired immunodeficiency syndrome in a nonendemic area. *Chest*, 93, 916, 1988.
119. Lake-Bakaar, G., Winston, T., Lake-Bakaar, D., et al. Gastropathy and ketoconazole malabsorption in the acquired immunodeficiency syndrome (AIDS). *Ann. Intern. Med.*, 109, 471, 1988.
120. Mello, K. A., Wheat, L. J., Lis, R., Donnelly, B., and Skolnik, P. R. Ketoconazole- responsive tonsilar infection due to *Histoplasma capsulatum* in an HIV-1-seropositive individual. *AIDS*, 5, 908, 1991.
121. Rawlinson, W. D., Packham, D. R., Gardner, F. J., and MacLeod, C. Histoplasmosis in the acquired immunodeficiency syndrome (AIDS). *Aust. N. Z. J. Med.*, 19, 707, 1989.
122. Nightingale, S. D., Parks, J. M., Pounders, S. M., Burns, D. K., Reynolds, J., and Hernandez, J. A. Disseminated histoplasmosis in patients with AIDS. *South. Med. J.*, 83, 624, 1990.
123. Wheat, J., Hafner, R., Wulfsohn, M., et al. Prevention of relapse of relapse of histoplasmosis with itraconazole in patients with the acquired immunodeficiency syndrome. *Ann. Intern. Med.*, 118, 610, 1993.
124. Stansell, J. J. D. Pulmonary fungal infections in HIV-infected persons. *Semin. Respir. Infect.*, 8, 116, 1993.
125. Pottage, J. C. Jr. and Sha, B. E. Development of histoplasmosis in a human immunodeficiency virus-infected patient receiving fluconazole. *J. Infect. Dis.*, 164, 622, 1991.
126. Wheat, L. J., Smith, E. J., Sathapatayavongs, B., et al. Histoplasmosis in renal allograft recipients: two large urban outbreaks. *Arch. Intern. Med.*, 143, 703, 1983.
127. Davies, S. F., Sarosi, G. A., Peterson, P. K., et al. Disseminated histoplasmosis in renal transplant recipients. *Am. J. Surg.*, 137, 686, 1979.
128. Jha, V., Sree Krishna, V., Varma, N., et al. Disseminated histoplasmosis 19 years after renal transplantation. *Clin. Nephrol.*, 51, 373–378, 1999.
129. Sarosi, G. A., Voth, D. W., Dahl, B. A., Doto, I. L., and Tosh, F. E. Disseminated histoplasmosis: results of long-term follow-up. *Ann. Intern. Med.*, 75, 511, 1971.
130. Goetz, M. B. and Jones, J. M. Combined ketoconazole and amphotericin B treatment of acute disseminated histoplasmosis in a renal allograft recipient. *South. Med. J.*, 78, 1368, 1985.
131. Kitahara, M., Kobayashi, G. S., and Medoff, G. Enhanced efficacy of amphotericin B and rifampicin combined treatment of murine histoplasmosis and blastomycosis. *J. Infect. Dis.*, 133, 663, 1976.

132. Williams, D. M., Graybill, J. R., and Drutz, D. J. Experimental chemotherapy of histoplasmosis in nude mice. *Am. Rev. Respir. Dis.*, 120, 837, 1979.
133. Ferguson, R. M., Sutherland, D. E. R., Simmons, R. L., and Najarian, J. S. Ketoconazole, cyclosporin metabolism, and renal transplantation. *Lancet*, 2, 882, 1982.
134. Studdard, J., Sneed, W. F., Taylor, J. R. Jr., and Campbell, G. D. Cutaneous histoplasmosis. *Am. Rev. Respir. Dis.*, 113, 689, 1976.
135. Dijkstra, J. W. E. Histoplasmosis. *Dermatol. Clin.*, 7, 251, 1989.
136. Romano, C., Castelli, A., Laurini, L., and Massai, L. Case report. Primary cutaneous histoplasmosis in an immunosuppressed patient. *Mycoses*, 43, 151–154, 2000.
137. Cohen, P. R., Bank, D. E., Silvers, D. N., and Grosmann, M. E. Cutaneous lesions of disseminated histoplasmosis in human immunodeficiency virus-infected patients. *J. Am. Acad. Dermatol.*, 23, 422, 1990.
138. Machado, A. A., Branco Coelho, I. C., Ferreira Roselino, A. M., et al. Histoplasmosis in individuals with acquired immunodeficiency syndrome (AIDS): report of six cases with cutaneous-mucosal involvement. *Mycopathologia*, 115, 13, 1991.
139. Cohen, P. R., Held, J. L., Grossman, M. E., Ross, M. J., and Silvers, D. N. Disseminated histoplasmosis as an ulcerated verrucous plaque in a human immunodeficiency virus-infected man: report of a case possibly involving human-to-human transmission of histoplasmosis. *Int. J. Dermatol.*, 30, 104, 1991.
140. Kucharski, L. D., Dal Pizzol, A. S., Fillus J. Neto, et al. Dissiminated cutaneous histoplasmosis and AIDS: case report. *Braz. J. Infect. Dis.*, 4, 255–261, 2000.
141. Bonifaz, A., Cansela, R., Novales, J., de Oca, G. M., Navarrete G., and Romo, J. Cutaneous histoplasmosis associated with acquired immunodeficiency syndrome (AIDS). *Int. J. Dermatol.*, 39, 35–38, 2000.
142. Madeiros, D. A., Marty, S. D., and Tosh, F. E. Erythema nodosum and erythema multiforme as clinical manifestations of histoplasmosis in a community outbreak. *N. Engl. J. Med.*, 274, 415, 1966.
143. Miller, H. E., Keddie, F. M., Johnstone, H. G., and Bostick, W. L. Histoplasmosis: cutaneous and membranous lesions, mycologic and pathologic observations. *Arch. Derm. Syphilol.*, 56, 715, 1947.
144. Farr, B., Beacham, B. E., and Stuk, N. O. Cutaneous histoplasmosis after renal transplantation. *South. Med. J.*, 74, 636, 1981.
145. Washburn, R. G. and Bennett, J. E. Reversal of adrenal glucocorticoid dysfunction in a patient with disseminated histoplasmosis. *Ann. Intern. Med.*, 110, 86, 1989.
146. Daman, L. A., Hashimoto, K., Kaplan, R. J., and Trent, M. G. Disseminated histoplasmosis in an immunosuppressed patient. *South. Med. J.*, 70, 355, 1977.
147. Abildgaard, W. H., Hargrove, R. H., and Kalivas, J. *Histoplasma* penicilitis. *Arch. Dermatol.*, 121, 914, 1985.
148. Johnson, C. A., Tang, C. K., and Tiji, R. M. Histoplasmosis of skin and lymph node and chronic lymphocytic leukemia. *Arch. Dermatol.*, 115, 336, 1979.
149. Strong, R. P. Study of some tropical ulcerations of skin with particular reference to their etiology. *Philippines J. Sci.*, 7, 91, 1986.
150. King, R. W., Kraikitpanich, S., and Lindeman, R. D., Subcutaneous nodules caused by *Histoplasma capsulatum*. *Ann. Intern. Med.*, 86, 586, 1977.
151. Navarro, E. E., Tupasi, T. E., Verallo, V. M., Romero, R. C., and Tuazon, C. U. Disseminated histoplasmosis with unusual cutaneous lesions in a patient from the Philippines. *Am. J. Trop. Med. Hyg.*, 46, 141, 1992.
152. Recondo, G., Sella, A., Ro, J. Y., Dexeus, F. H., Amato, R., and Kilbourn, R. Perianal ulcer in disseminated histoplasmosis. *South. Med. J.*, 84, 931, 1991.
153. Suh, K. N., Anekthananon, T., and Mariuz, P. R. Gastrointestinal histoplasmosis in patients with AIDS: case report and review. *Clin. Infect. Dis.*, 32, 483–491, 2001.
154. Flannery, M. T., Chapman, V., Cruz-Gonzales, I., Rivera, M., and Messina, J. L. Ileal perforation secondary to histoplasmosis in AIDS. *Am. J. Med. Sci.*, 320, 406–407, 2000.
155. Gumbs, M. A., Girishkumar, H., Yousuf, A., Levy, L., Patel, M., and Narasimha, V. Histoplasmosis of the small bowel in patients with AIDS. *Postgrad. Med. J.*, 76, 367–369, 2000.
156. Kane, S. and Brasitis, T. Histoplasmosis capsulatum as a new cause of lower gastrointestinal bleeding in common variable immunodeficiency. *Dig. Dis. Sci.*, 45, 2133–2135, 2000.
157. Lamps, L. W., Molina, C. P., West, A. B., Haggitt, R. C., and Scott, M. A. The pathologic spectrum of gastrointestinal and hepatic histoplasmosis. *Am. J. Clin. Pathol.*, 113, 64–72, 2000.
158. Cimponeriu, D., LoPresti, P., Lavelanet, M., et al. Gastrointestinal histoplasmosis in HIV infection: two cases of colonic pseudocancer and review of the literature. *Am. J. Gastroenterol.*, 89, 129, 1994.
159. Becherer, P. R., Sokol-Anderson, M., Joist, J. H., and Milligan, T. Gastrointestinal histoplasmosis presenting as hematochezia in human immunodeficiency virus-infected hemophilic patients. *Am. J. Hematol.*, 47, 229, 1994.
160. Graham, B. D., McKinsey, D. S., Driks, M. R., and Smith, D. L. Colonic histoplasmosis in acquired immunodeficiency syndrome. Report of two cases. *Dis. Colon Rectum*, 34, 185, 1991.
161. Keelan, C. and Imbert, M. Colonic histoplasmosis simulating Crohn's disease in a patient with AIDS. *Bol. Asoc. Med. P. R.*, 80, 248, 1988.
162. United States Public Health Service Cooperative Mycoses Study. Course and prognosis of untreated histoplasmosis. *J. Am. Med. Assoc.*, 177, 292, 1961.
163. Haws, C. C., Long, R. F., and Caplan, G. E. Histoplasmosis capsulatum as a cause of ileocolitis. *Am. J. Roentgenol.*, 128, 692, 1977.
164. Cappell, M. S. and Manzione, N. C. Recurrent colonic histoplasmosis after standard therapy with amphotericin B in a patient with Job's syndrome. *Am. J. Gastroenterol.*, 86, 119, 1991.

165. Cappell, M. S., Mandell, M., Grimes, M. M., and Neu, H. C. Gastrointestinal histoplasmosis. *Dig. Dis. Sci.*, 33, 353, 1988.
166. Hutto, J. O., Bryan, C. S., Greene, F. L., White, C. J., and Gallin, J. I. Cryptococcosis of the colon resembling Crohn's disease in a patient with the hyperimmunoglubulinemia E-recurrent infection (Job's syndrome). *Gastroenterology*, 94, 808, 1988.
167. Albert-Florr, J. J. and Granda, A. Ileocecal histoplasmosis mimicking Crohn's disease in a patient with Job's syndrome. *Digestion*, 33, 176, 1986.
168. Mignogna, M. D., Fedele, S., Lo Russo, L., Ruoppo, E., and Lo Muzio, L. A case of oral localized histoplasmosis in an immunocompetent patient. *Eur. J. Clin. Microbiol. Infect. Dis.*, 20, 753–755, 2001.
169. Miller, R. L., Gould, A. R., Skolnick, J. L., and Epstein, W. M. Localized oral histoplasmosis. *Oral Surg. Oral Med. Oral Pathol.*, 53, 367, 1982.
170. Hupp, J. R., Layne, J. M., and Glickman, R. S. Solitary palatal ulcer. *J. Oral Maxillofac. Surg.*, 43, 365, 1985.
171. Zain, R. B. and Ling, K. C. Oral and laryngeal histoplasmosis in a patient with Addison's disease. *Ann. Dent.*, 47, 31, 1988.
172. Clity, E., Aznar, C., Couppie, P., et al. Disseminated histoplasmosis detected by lingual and tonsillar erosions in an immunocompetent patient. *Ann. Dermatol. Venereol.*, 126, 709–711, 1999.
173. Hiltbrand, J. B. and McGuirt, W. F. Orophayngeal histoplasmosis. *South. Med. J.*, 83, 227, 1990.
174. Cobb, C. M., Schultz, R. E., Brewer, J. H., and Dunlap, C. L. Chronic pulmonary histoplasmosis with an oral lesion. *Oral Surg. Oral Med. Oral Pathol.*, 67, 73, 1989.
175. Donovan, J. O. and Wood, M. D. Histoplasmosis of the larynx. *Laryngoscope*, 94, 206, 1984.
176. Reibel, J. F., Jahrsdoerfer, R. A., Johns, M. M., and Cantrell, R. W. Histoplasmosis of the larynx. *Otolaryngol. Head Neck Surg.*, 90, 740–743, 1982.
177. Scully, C. and Paes de Almeida, O. Orofacial manifestations of the systemic mycoses. *J. Oral Pathol. Med.*, 21, 289, 1992.
178. Toth, B. B. and Frame, B. B. Oral histoplasmosis: diagnostic complications and treatment. *Oral Surg. Oral Med. Oral Pathol.*, 55, 597, 1983.
179. Dobleman, T. J., Scher, N., Goldman, M., and Doot, S. Invasive histoplasmosis of the mandible. *Head Neck Surg.*, 11, 81, 1989.
180. Fowler, C. B., Nelson, J. F., Henley, D. W., and Smith, B. R. Acquired immune deficiency syndrome presenting as a palatal perforation. *Oral Surg. Oral Med. Oral Pathol.*, 67, 313, 1989.
181. Huber, M. A., Hall, E. H., and Rathbun, W. A. The role of the dentist in diagnosing infection in the AIDS patient. *Milit. Med.*, 154, 315, 1989.
182. Oda, D., McDougal, L., Fritsche, T., and Worthington, P. Oral histoplasmosis as a presenting disease in acquired immunodeficiency syndrome. *Oral Surg. Oral Med. Oral Pathol.*, 70, 631, 1990.
183. Swindells, S., Durham, T., Jahansson, S. L., and Kaufman, L. Oral histoplasmosis in a patient infected with HIV. *Oral Surg. Oral Med. Oral Pathol.*, 77, 126, 1994.
184. Cohen, P. R. Oral histoplasmosis in HIV-infected patients. *Oral Surg. Oral Med. Oral Pathol.*, 78, 277, 1994.
185. Heinic, G. S., Greenspan, D. S., MacPhail, L. A., et al. Oral *Histoplasma capsulatum* infection in association with HIV infection: a case report. *J. Oral Pathol Med.*, 21, 85, 1992.
186. Gomes Ferreira, O., Vieira Fernandes, A., Sebastiao Borges, A., Simao Ferreira, M., and Mota Loyola, A. Orofacial manifestations of histoplasmosis in HIV-positive patients: a case report. *Med. Oral.*, 6, 101–105, 2001.
187. De Boom, G. W., Rhyne, R. R., and Correll, R. W. Multiple, painful oral ulcerations in a patient with Hodgkin's disease. *JADA*, 113, 807, 1986.
188. Miller, D. P. and Everett, E. D. Gastrointestinal histoplasmosis. *J. Clin. Gastroenterol.*, 1, 233, 1979.
189. Smith, J. W. and Utz, J. P. Progressive disseminated histoplasmosis: a prospective study of 26 patients. *Ann. Intern. Med.*, 75, 557, 1972.
190. Dean, L. W. Histoplasmosis of the larynx. *Arch. Otolaryngol. Head Neck Surg.*, 36, 390, 1942.
191. Van Pernis, P. A., Benson, M. E., and Holinger, P. H. Case reports: laryngeal and systemic histoplasmosis (Darling). *Ann. Intern. Med.*, 18, 384, 1943.
192. Parkes, M. and Burtoff, S. Histoplasmosis of the larynx: report of a case. *Med. Ann. D. C.*, 18, 641, 1949.
193. Roberts, S. E. and Forman, F. S. Histoplasmosis: a deficiency disease: report of two cases with laryngeal involvement. *Ann. Otol. Rhinol. Laryngol.*, 59, 809, 1950.
194. Hulse, W. F. Laryngeal histoplasmosis. *Arch. Otolaryngol. Head Neck Surg.*, 54, 65, 1951.
195. Hutchinson, H. E. Laryngeal histoplasmosis simulating carcinoma. *J. Path. Bact.*, 64, 309, 1952.
196. Burton, C. T. and Wallenborn, P. A. Histoplasmosis of the larynx. *Va. Med. Month.*, 80, 665, 1953.
197. Withers, B. T., Pappas, J. J., and Erickson, E. E. Histoplasmosis primary in the larynx. *Arch. Otolaryngol. Head Neck Surg.*, 77, 26, 1963.
198. Demaldent, J. E., Gentilini, M., Amat, C., and Manach, Y. A propos d'un cas d'histoplasmose laryngée. *Ann. Otolaryngol. Chir. Cervicofac.*, 95, 287, 1978.
199. Sataloff, R. T., Wilborn, A., Prestipino, A., Hawkshaw, M., Heuer, R. J., and Cohn, J. Histoplasmosis of the larynx. *Am. J. Otolaryngol.*, 14, 199, 1993.
200. Fletcher, S. M. and Prussin, A. J. Histoplasmosis of the larynx treated with ketoconazole: a case report. *Otolaryngol. Head Neck Surg.*, 103, 813, 1990.
201. Feman, S. S. and Tilford, R. H. Ocular findings in patients with histoplasmosis. *J. Am. Med. Assoc.*, 253, 2534, 1985.
202. Simmons, C. A. and Matthews, D. Prevalence of uveitis: a retrospective study. *J. Am. Optom. Assoc.*, 64, 386, 1993.
203. Maumenee, A. E. Clinical entities in uveitis. *Am. J. Ophthalmol.*, 69, 1, 1970.
204. Weingeist, T. A. and Watzke, R. C. Ocular involvement by *Histoplasma capsulatum*. *Int. Ophthalmol. Clin.*, 23, 33, 1983.

205. Feman, S. S., Pritchett, P., Johns, K., Weistrich, D. J., and Salmon, W. D. Intraocular tumor from disseminated histoplasmosis. *South. Med. J.*, 84, 780, 1991.
206. Ciulla, T. A., Piper, H. C., Xiao, M., and Wheat, L. J. Presumed ocular histoplasmosis syndrome: update on epidemiology, pathogenesis, and photodynamic, antiangiogenic, and surgical therapies. *Curr. Opin. Ophthalmol.*, 12, 442–449, 2001.
207. Ormerod, L. D., Qamar, T. U., Toller, K., Cooperstock, M. S., Caldwell, C. W., and Giangiacomo, J. Acute disseminated histoplasmosis with multifocal chroiditis in a child. *Pediatr. Infect. Dis.*, 19, 479–481, 2000.
208. Sickenberg, M., Schmidt-Erfurth, U., Miller, J. W., et al. A preliminary study of photodynamic therapy using verteporfin for choroidal neovascularization in pathologic myopia, ocular histoplasmosis syndrome, angioid streaks, and idiopathic causes. *Arch. Ophthalmol.*, 118, 327–336, 2000.
209. Uemura, A. and Thomas, M. A. Subretinal surgery for choroidal neovascularization in patients with high myopia. *Arch. Ophthalmol.*, 118, 344–350, 2000.
210. Cooper, B. A., Thomas, M. A., and Holekamp, N. M. Open retinotomy after submacular surgery. *Am. J. Ophthalmol.*, 130, 838–839, 2000.
211. Mann, E. S., Fogarty, S. J., and Kincaid, M. C. Choroidal neovascularization with granulomatous inflammation in ocular histoplasmosis syndrome. *Am. J. Ophthalmol.*, 130, 247–250, 2000.
212. Martidis, A., Miller, D. G., Ciulla, T. A., Danis, R. P., and Moorthy, R. S. Corticosteroids as an antiangiogenic agent for histoplasmosis-related subfoveal choroidal neovascularization. *J. Ocul. Pharmacol. Ther.*, 15, 425–428, 1999.
213. Gonzales, C. A., Scott, I. U., Chaudhry, N. A., et al. Endogenous endophthalmitis caused by *Histoplasma capsulatum* var. *capsulatum*: a case report and literature review. *Ophthalmology*, 107, 725–729, 2000.
214. Sen, S., Bajaj, M. S., and Vijayaraghavan, M. Histoplasmosis of the eyelids - a case report. *Indian J. Pathol. Microbiol.*, 42, 495–497, 1999.
215. Darouiche, R. O., Cadle, R. M., Zenon, G. J., Weinert, M. F., Hamill, R. J., and Lidsky, M. D. Articular histoplasmosis. *J. Rheumatol.*, 19, 1991, 1992.
216. Rosenthal, J., Brandt, K. D., Wheat, L. J., and Slama, T. G. Rheumatologic manifestations of histoplasmosis in the recent Indianapolis epidemic. *Arthritis Rheum.*, 26, 1065, 1983.
217. Friedman, S. J., Black, J. L., and Duffy, J. Histoplasmosis presenting as erythema multiforme and polyarthritis. *Cutis*, 34, 396, 1984.
218. Thornberry, D. K., Wheat, L. J., Brandt, K. D., and Rosenthal, J. Histoplasmosis presenting with joint pain and hilar adenopathy: pseudosarcoidosis. *Arthritis Rheum.*, 25, 1396, 1982.
219. Wheat, L. J., Slama, T. G., Eitzen, H. E., Kohler, R. B., French, M. L. V., and Biesecker, J. L. A large urban outbreak of histoplasmosis: clinical features. *Ann. Intern. Med.*, 94, 331, 1981.
220. Class, R. N. and Cascio, F. S. Histoplasmosis presenting as acute polyarthritis. *N. Engl. J. Med.*, 287, 1133, 1972.
221. Pfaller, M. A., Kyriakos, M., Week, P. M., and Kobayashi, G. S. Disseminated histoplasmosis presenting as an acute tenosynovitis. *Diagn. Microbiol. Infect. Dis.*, 3, 251, 1985.
222. Jones, P. G., Rolston, K., and Hopfer, R. L. Septic arthritis due to *Histoplasma capsulatum* in a leukaemic patient. *Ann. Rheum. Dis.*, 44, 128, 1985.
223. Van der Schee, A. C., Dinkla, B. A., and Festen, J. J. Gonarthritis as only manifestation of chronic disseminated histoplasmosis. *Clin. Rheumatol.*, 9, 92, 1990.
224. Key, J. A. and Large, A. M. Histoplasmosis of the knee. *J. Bone Joint Surg.*, 24, 281, 1942.
225. Omer, G. E. Jr., Lockwook, R. S., and Travis, L. O. Histoplasmosis involving the carpal joint: a case report. *J. Bone Joint Surg.*, 45A, 1699, 1963.
226. Perlman, R., Jubelirer, R. A., and Schwarz, J. Histoplasmosis of the common palmar tendon sheath. *J. Bone Joint Surg.*, 54A, 676, 1972.
227. Strayer, D. S., Gutwein, M. B., Herbold, D., and Bresilier, R. Histoplasmosis presenting as the carpal tunnel syndrome. *Am. J. Surg.*, 141, 286, 1981.
228. Schasfoort, R. A., Marck, K. W., and Houtman, P. M. Histoplasmosis in the wrist. *J. Hand Surg [Br]*, 24, 625–627, 1999.
229. Houtman, P. M., Marck, K. W., and Hol, C. Histoplasmosis of the wrist: a case report. *Reumatology (Oxford)*, 38, 906–907, 1999.
230. Mascola, J. R. and Rickman, L. S. Infectious causes of carpal tunnel syndrome: case report and review. *Rev. Infect. Dis.*, 13, 911, 1991.
231. Vanek, J. and Schwarz, J. The gamut of histoplasmosis. *Am. J. Med.*, 50, 89, 1971.
232. Randall, G., Smith, P. W., Korbitz, B., and Owen, D. R. Carpal tunnel syndrome caused by *Mycobacterium fortuitum* and *Histoplasma capsulatum*: report of two cases. *J. Neurosurg.*, 56, 299, 1982.
233. Phalen, G. S. The carpal-tunnel syndrome. Seventeen years' experience in diagnosis and treatment of six hundred fifty-four hands. *J. Bone Joint Surg.*, 48A, 211, 1966.
234. Baker, E. L. and Ehrenberg, R. L. Preventing the work-related carpal tunnel syndrome: physician reporting and diagnostic criteria. *Ann. Intern. Med.*, 112, 317, 1990.
235. Nakano, K. K. Entrapment neuropathies, in *Textbook of Rheumatoplogy*, 3rd ed., Kelley, W. N., Harris, E. D. Jr., Ruddy, S., and Sledge, C. B., Eds. W. B. Saunders, Philadelphia, 1845, 1989.
236. Biundo, J. J. Regional rheumatic pain syndromes, in *Primer on the Rheumatic Diseases*, Arthritis Foundation, Atlanta, GA, 263, 1988.
237. Klofkorn, R. W. and Steigerwald, J. C. Carpal tunnel syndrome as the initial manifestation of tuberculosis. *Am. J. Med.*, 60, 583, 1976.

238. Inglis, A. E., Straub, L. R., and Williams, C. S. Median nerve neuropathy at the wrist. *Clin. Orthop.*, 83, 48, 1972.
239. Dines, D. E., Bernatz, P. E., and Pairolero, P. C. Mediastinal granuloma and fibrosing mediastinitis. *Chest*, 75, 320, 1979.
240. Engleman, P., Liebow, A. A., Gmelich, J., and Friedman, P. J. Pulmonary hyalinizing granuloma. *Am. Rev. Respir. Dis.*, 115, 997, 1977.
241. Hewlett, T. H., Steer, A., and Thomas, D. E. Progressive fibrosing mediastinitis. *Ann. Thorac. Surg.*, 2, 345, 1966.
242. Light, A. M. Idiopathic fibrosis of mediastinum as discussion of three cases and a review of the literature. *Am. J. Clin. Pathol.*, 31, 78, 1978.
243. Schonengerdt, C. B., Suyemoto, R., and Main, F. B. Granulomatosis and fibrosing mediastinitis: a review and analysis of 180 cases. *J. Thorac. Cardiovasc. Surg.*, 57, 365, 1979.
244. Urchel, H. C. Jr., Razzuk, M. A., Netto, G. J., Disiere, J., and Chung, S. Y. Sclerosing mediastinitis: improved management with histoplasmosis titer and ketoconazole. *Ann. Thorac. Surg.*, 50, 215, 1990.
245. Doty, D. B. Bypass of superior vena cava. *J. Thorac. Cardiovasc. Surg.*, 83, 3326, 1982.
246. Arnett, E. N., Bacos, J. M., Marsh, H. B., Savage, D. D., Fulmer, J. D., and Roberts, W. C. Fibrosing mediastinitis causing pulmonary arterial hypertension without pulmonary venous hypertension. *Am. J. Med.*, 63, 634, 1977.
247. Trinkle, J. K. Fibrous mediastinitis presenting as mitral stenosis. *J. Thorac. Cardiovasc. Surg.*, 62, 161, 1970.
248. James, E. C., Harris, S. S., and Dillenburg, C. J. Tracheal stenosis: an unusual presenting complication of idiopathic fibrosing mediastinitis. *J. Thorac. Cardiovasc. Surg.*, 80, 410, 1980.
249. Zajtchuk, R., Strevey, T. E., Heydorn, W. H., and Treasure, R. L. Mediastinal histoplasmosis. *J. Thorac. Cardiovasc. Surg.*, 66, 300, 1973.
250. Ahmad, M., Weinstein, A. J., Hughes, J. A., and Cosgrove, D. E. Granulomatous mediastinitis due to aspergillus flavors in a nonimmunosuppressed patient. *Am. J. Med.*, 70, 887, 1981.
251. Drutz, D. J. and Catanzaro, A. Coccidioidomycosis. *Am. Rev. Respir. Dis.*, 117, 559, 1978.
252. Goodwin, R. A., Nickell, J. A., and Des Prez, R. Mediatinal fibrosis complicating healed primary histoplasmosis and tuberculosis. *Medicine (Baltimore)*, 51, 227, 1972.
253. Leong, A. S. Y. Granulomatous mediastinitis due to *Rhisopus* species. *Am. J. Clin. Pathol.*, 70, 103, 1978.
254. Stead, W. W. and Bates, J. H. Tuberculosis, *Harrison's Principles of Internal Medicine*, 10th ed., Petersdorf, R. G. et al., Eds. McGraw-Hill, New York, 1021, 1983.
255. Yacoub, M. H. and Thompson, V. C. Chronic idiopathic pulmonary hilar fibrosis. *Thorax*, 26, 365, 1971.
256. Coss, K. C., Wheat, L. J., Conces, D. J., Brashear, R. E., and Hull, M. T. Esophageal fistula complicating mediastinal histoplasmosis: response to amphotericin B. *Am. J. Med.*, 83, 343, 1987.
257. Lee, J. H., Newman, D. A., and Welsh, J. D. Disseminated histoplasmosis presenting with esophageal symptomatology. *Dig. Dis.*, 22, 831, 1977.
258. Jenkins, D. W., Fisk, D. E., and Byrd, R. B. Mediastinal histoplasmosis with esophageal abscess. *Gastroenterology*, 70, 109, 1976.
259. Sarosi, G. A. and Davies, S. F. Gastrointestinal involvement in histoplasmosis. *Pract. Gastroenterol.*, 8, 19, 1984.
260. Goodwin, R. A., Loyd, J. E., and Des Prez, R. M. Histoplasmosis in normal hosts. *Medicine (Baltimore)*, 60, 231, 1981.
261. Gilliland, M. D., Scott, L. D., and Walker, W. E. Esophageal obstruction caused by mediastinal histoplasmosis: beneficial results of operation. *Surgery*, 95, 59, 1984.
262. Schneider, R. P. and Edwards, W. Histoplasmosis presenting as an esophageal tumor. *Gastrointest. Endosc.*, 23, 158, 1977.
263. Dines, D. E., Payne, W. S., Bernatz, P. E., and Pairolero, P. C. Mediastinal granuloma and fibrosing mediastinitis. *Chest*, 75, 320, 1979.
264. Cameron, J. L., Kieffer, R. F., and Hendrix, T. R. Selective nonoperative management of contained intrathoracic disruptions. *Ann. Thorac. Surg.*, 27, 404, 1979.
265. Bradsher, R. W., Wickre, C. G., Savage, A, M., Harstone, W. E., and Alford, R. H. *Histoplasma capsulatum* endocarditis cured by amphotericin B combined with surgery. *Chest*, 78, 791, 1980.
266. Isotalo, P. A., Chan, K. L., Rubens, F., Beanlands, D. S., Auclair, F., and Veinot, J. P. Prosthetic valve fungal endocarditis due to histoplasmosis. *Can. J. Cardiol.*, 17, 297–303, 2001.
267. Gerber, H. J., Schoonmaker, F. W., and Vazquez, M. D. Chronic meningitis associated with *Histoplasma* endocarditis. *N. Engl. J. Med.*, 275, 74, 1966.
268. Hartley, R. A., Remsberg, J. R. S., and Sinaly, N. P. *Histoplasma* endocarditis. *Arch. Int. Med.*, 119, 527, 1967.
269. Weaver, D. K., Batsakis, J. G., Nishiyama, R. H., and Arbor, A. *Histoplasma* endocarditis. *Arch. Surg.*, 96, 19, 1968.
270. Segal, C., Wheeler, C. G., and Tompsett, R. *Histoplasma* endocarditis cured with amphotericin. *N. Engl. J. Med.*, 28, 206, 1969.
271. Matthay, R. A., Levin, D. C., Wicks, A. B., and Ellis, J. H. Jr. Disseminated histoplasmosis involving an aortofemoral prosthatic graft. *J. Am. Med. Assoc.*, 235, 1478, 1976.
272. Canlas, M. S. and Dillon, M. L. Jr. *Histoplasma capsulatum* endocarditis: report of a case following heart surgery. *Angiology*, 28, 454, 1977.
273. Olive, T., Lagier, A., Dumas, O., Bidart, J. M., and Bernard, P. M. Histoplasmose generalisée avec localosation laryngée et endocaroite. *Nouv. Presse Med.*, 7, 2262, 1978.
274. Rogers, E. W., Weyman, A. E., Noble, R. J., and Bruins, S. C. Left atrial myxoma infected with *Histoplasma capsulatum*. *Am. J. Med.*, 64, 683, 1978.
275. Alexander, W. J., Mowry, R. W., Cobbs, C. G., and Dismukes, W. E. Prosthetic valve endocarditis caused by *Histoplasma capsulatum*. *J. Am. Med. Assoc.*, 242, 1399, 1979.

276. Waterhouse, G., Burney, D. P., and Prager, R. L. *Histoplasma capsulatum*: endocarditis requiring aortic valve replacement for aortic insufficiency. *South. Med. J.*, 73, 683, 1980.
277. Blair, T. P., Waugh, R. A., Pollack, M., et al. *Histoplasma capsulatum* endocarditis. *Am. Heart J.*, 99, 783, 1980.
278. Gaynes, R. P., Gardner, P., and Causey, W. Prosthetic valve endocarditis caused by *Histoplasma capsulatum*. *Arch. Int. Med.*, 141, 1533, 1981.
279. Svirbely, J. R., Ayers, L. W., and Buesching, W. J. Filamentous *Histoplasma capsulatum* endocarditis involving mitral and aortic valve porcine bioprostheses. *Arch. Pathol. Lab. Med.*, 109, 273, 1985.
280. Kanawaty, D. S., Stalker, J. B., and Munt, P. W. Nonsurgical treatment of histoplasma endocarditis involving a bioprosthetic valve. *Chest*, 99, 253, 1991.
281. Weinstein, L., Pathogenesis of infectious endocarditis, in *Heart Disease: A Textbook of Cardiovascular Medicine*, 3rd ed., Braunwald, E., Ed. W. B. Saunders, Philadelphia, 1093, 1988.
282. Hawkins, S. S., Gregory, D. W., and Alford, R. H. Progressive disseminated histoplasmosis: favorable response to ketoconazole. *Ann. Intern. Med.*, 95, 446, 1981.
283. Wilmshurst, P. T., Venn, G. E., and Eykyn, S. J. *Histoplasma* endocarditis on a stenosed aortic valve presenting as dysphagia and weight loss. *Br. Heart J.*, 70, 565, 1993.
284. Derby, B. M., Coolidge, K., and Rogers, D. E. *Histoplasma capsulatum* endocarditis with major arterial embolism. *Arch. Intern. Med.*, 110, 101, 1962.
285. Kauffman, C. A. Pulmonary histoplasmosis. *Curr. Infect. Dis. Rep.*, 3, 279–285, 2001.
286. Martinez-Aparicio Hernandez, A., Sarduy Paneque, M., and Cepero Nogueira, M. Pulmonary histoplasmosis, complication in transplantation patients. *Arch. Bronconeumol.*, 36, 657–658, 2000.
287. Pecanha Martins, A. C., Costa Neves, M. L., Lopes, A. A., Querino Santos, N. N., Araujo, N. N., and Matos Pereira, K. Histoplasmosis presenting as acute respiratory distress syndrome after exposure to bat feces in a home basement. *Braz. J. Infect. Dis.*, 4, 103–106, 2000.
288. Curr, F. J. and Wier, J. A. Histoplasmosis, a review of one-hundred consecutively hospitalized patients. *Am. Rev. Respir. Dis.*, 77, 749, 1958.
289. Rubin, H., Furcolow, M. L., Yates, J. L., and Brasher, C. A. The course and prognosis of histoplasmosis. *Am. J. Med.*, 27, 278, 1959.
290. Baum, G. L. and Schwartz, J. Chronic pulmonary histoplasmosis. *Am. J. Med.*, 33, 873, 1962.
291. Palayew, M. J., Frank, H., and Sedlezsky, I. Histoplasmosis: our experience of seventy cases with follow-up study. *J. Can. Assoc. Radiol.*, 17, 142, 1966.
292. Brodsky, A. L., Gregg, M. B., Loewenstein, M. S., Kaufman, L., and Mallison, G. F. Outbreak of histoplasmosis associated with the 1970 Earth day activities. *Am. J. Med.*, 54, 333, 1973.
293. Ward, J. L., Weeks, M., Allen, D., et al. Acute histoplasmosis: clinical, epidemiologic and serologic findings of an outbreak associated with exposure to a fallen tree. *Am. J. Med.*, 66, 587, 1979.
294. Straus, S. E. and Jacobsen, E. S. The spectrum of histoplasmosis in a general hospital: a review of 55 cases diagnosed at Barnes Hospital between 1966 and 1977. *Am. J. Med. Sci.*, 279, 147, 1980.
295. Gustafson, T. L., Kaufman, L., Weeks, R., et al. Outbreak of acute pulmonary histoplasmosis in members of a wagon train. *Am. J. Med.*, 71, 759, 1981.
296. Kakos, G. S. and Kilman, J. W. Symptomatic histoplasmosis in children. *Ann. Thorac. Surg.*, 15, 622, 1973.
297. Quasney, M. W. and Leggiadro, R. J. Pleural effusion associated with histoplasmosis. *Pediatr. Infect. Dis. J.*, 12, 415–418, 1993.
298. Weissblith, M. Pleural effusion in histoplasmosis. *J. Pediatr.*, 88, 894, 1976.
299. Ericsson, C. D., Pickering, L. K., and Salmon, G. W. Pleural effusion in histoplasmosis. *J. Pediatr.*, 90, 327, 1977.
300. Brickman, H. F. Pleural effusion in histoplasmosis. *J. Pediatr.*, 90, 327, 1977.
301. Picardi, J. L., Kauffman, C. A., Schwarz, J., Holmes, J. C., Phair, J. P., and Fowler, N. O. Pericarditis caused by *Histoplasma capsulatum*. *Am. J. Cardiol.*, 37, 82, 1976.
302. Tutor, J. D., Schoumacher, R. A., and Chesney, P. J. Chylothorax associated with histoplasmosis in a child. *Pediatr. Infect. Dis. J.*, 19, 262–263, 2000.
303. Schub, H. M., Spivey, C. G., and Baird, G. D. Pleural involvement in histoplasmosis. *Am. Rev. Respir. Dis.*, 94, 225, 1966.
304. Brewer, P. L. and Himmelwright, J. P. Pleural effusion due to infection with *Histoplasma capsulatum*. *Chest*, 58, 76, 1970.
305. Swinburne, A. J., Fedullo, A. J., Wahl, G. W., and Fernand, B. Histoplasmoma, pleural fibrosis, and slowly enlarging pleural effusion in an asymptomatic patient. *Am. Rev. Respir. Dis.*, 135, 502, 1987.
306. Downey, E. F. Asymptomatic pleural effusion in histoplasmosis: case report. *Milit. Med.*, 147, 218, 1982.
307. Adelman, M., Albelda, S. M., Gottlieb, J., and Hoponik, E. F. Diagnostic utility of pleural fluid eosinophilia. *Am. J. Med.*, 77, 915, 1984.
308. Marshall, B. C., Cox, J. K., Carroll, K. C., and Morrison, R. E. Case report: histoplasmosis as a cause of pleural effusion in the acquired immunodeficiency syndrome. *Am. J. Med. Sci.*, 300, 98, 1990.
309. Schultz, D. M. Histoplasmosis of the central nervous system. *J. Am. Med. Assoc.*, 151, 549, 1953.
310. Shapiro, J. L., Lux, J. J., and Scrofkin, B. E. Histoplasmosis of the central nervous system. *Am. J. Pathol.*, 31, 319, 1955.
311. Cooper, R. A. and Goldstein, E. Histoplasmosis of the central nervous system: report of two cases and review of the literature. *Am. J. Med.*, 35, 45, 1963.
312. Ramseyer, J. C., Baker, R. N., and Tomiyasu, U. Ventriculovenous shunt in the treatment of obstructive hydrocephalus due to coccidioidomycotic meningitis. *Neurology*, 16, 701, 1966.

313. Fetter, B. F., Klintworth, G. K., and Hendry, W. S. *Mycoses of the Central Nervous System*. Williams & Wilkins, Baltimore, 1967.
314. Gelfand, J. A. and Bennett, J. E. Active histoplasma meningitis of 22 years duration. *J. Am. Med. Assoc.*, 233, 1294, 1975.
315. Enarson, D. A., Keys, T. F., and Onofrio, B. M. Central nervous system histoplasmosis with obstructive hydrocephalus. *Am. J. Med.*, 64, 895, 1978.
316. Laurence, R. M. and Goldstein, E. Histoplasmosis, in *Infections of the Nervous System. Part III. Handbook of Clinical Neurology*, vol. 35, Vinken, P. J. and Bruyn, G. W., Eds. North Holland, Amsterdam, 503, 1978.
317. Jacobson, E. S. and Straus, S. E. Reevaluation of diagnostic histoplasma serologies. *Am. J. Med. Sci.*, 281, 143, 1981.
318. Young, R. P., Gede, G., and Grinnell, V. Surgical treatment for fungal infections of the central nervous system. *J. Neurosurg.*, 63, 371, 1985.
319. Snyder, C. H. and White, R. S. Successful treatment of histoplasma meningitis with amphotercin B. *J. Pediatr.*, 58, 554, 1961.
320. Vos, M. J., Debets-Ossenkopp, Y. J., Claessen, F. A., Hazenberg, G. J., and Heimans, J. J. Cerebellar and medullar histoplasmosis. *Neurology*, 54, 1441, 2000.
321. Lanska, D. J. Cerebellar and medullar histoplasmosis. *Neurology*, 55, 1419, 2000.
322. Berard, H., Astoul, P., Frenay, C., Cuguilliere, A., Cho, K., and Boutin, C. Disseminated histoplasmosis caused by *Histoplasma capsulatum* with cerebral involvement occurring 13 years after the primary infection. *Rev. Mal. Respir.*, 16, 829-831, 1999.
323. Klein, C. J., Dinapoli, R. P., Temesgen, Z., and Meyer, F. B. Central nervous system histoplasmosis mimicking a brain tumor: difficulties in diagnosis and treatment. *Mayo Clin. Proc.*, 74, 803–807, 1999.
324. Kauffman, C. A., Israel, K. S., Smith, V. W., and White, A. C. Histoplasmosis in immunosuppressed patients. *Am. J. Med.*, 64, 923, 1978.
325. Wheat, L. J., Batteiger, B. E., and Sathapatayavongs, B. *Histoplasma capsulatum* infection of the central nervous system. *Medicine (Baltimore)*, 69, 244, 1990.
326. Louria, D. B. Some aspects of the absorption distribution and excretion of amphotericin B in man. *Antimicrob. Agents Chemother.*, 5, 295, 1958.
327. Tiraboschi, I., Casas Parera, I., Pikielny, R., Scattini, G., and Micheli, F. Chronic *Histoplasma capsulatum* infection of the central nervous system successfully treated with fluconazole. *Eur. Neurol.*, 32, 70, 1992.
328. Knapp, S., Turnherr, M., Dekan, G., Willinger, B., Stingl, G., and Rieger, A. A case of HIV-associated cerebral histoplasmosis successfully treated with fluconazole. *Eur. J. Clin. Microbiol. Infect. Dis.*, 18, 658–661, 1999.
329. Kelly, D. R., Smith, C. D., and McQuillen, M. P. Successful medical treatment of a spinal histoplasmoma. *J. Neuroimag.*, 4, 327, 1994.
330. Tan, V., Wilkins, P., Badve, S., Coppen, M., Lucas, S., Hay, R., and Schon, F. Histoplasmosis of the central nervous system. *J. Neurol. Neurosurg. Psychiatry*, 55, 619, 1992.
331. Voelker, J. L., Muller, J., and Worth, R. M. Intramedullary spinal *Histoplasma* granuloma: case report. *J. Neurosurg.*, 70, 959, 1989.
332. Bazan, C. and New, P. Z. Intramedullary spinal histoplasmosis: efficacy of gadolinium enhancement. *Neuroradiology*, 33, 190, 1991.
333. Bamberger, D. M. Successful treatment of multiple cerebral histoplasmomas with itraconazole. *Clin. Infect. Dis.*, 28, 915–916, 1999.
334. Rodriguez, G., Ordonez, N., and Motta, A. *Histoplasma capsulatum* var. *capsulatum* within cutaneous nerves in patients with disseminated histoplasmosis and AIDS. *Br. J. Dermatol.*, 144, 205–207, 2001.
335. Gohar, S., Sule, A., Gaitonde, S., et al. Adrenal histoplasmosis. *J. Assoc. Physicians India*, 49, 916–917, 2001.
336. Mahajan, R., Sharma, U., Trivedi, N., et al. *Histoplasma capsulatum* in adrenal gland aspirate - a case report. *Indian J. Pathol. Microbiol.*, 43, 165–168, 2000.
337. Lio, S., Cibin, M., Marcello, R., Viviani, M. A., and Ajello, L. Adrenal bilateral incidentaloma by reactivated histoplasmosis. *J. Endocrinol. Invest.*, 23, 476–479, 2000.
338. Giacaglia, L. R., Lin, C. J., Lucon, A. M., and Goldman, J. Disseminated histoplasmosis presenting as bilateral adrenal masses. *Rev. Hosp. Clin. Fac. Med. Sao Paulo*, 53, 254–256, 1998.
339. Singh, S. K., Bhadada, S. K., Singh, S. K., et al. Histoplasmosis: an unusual presentation. *J. Assos. Physicians India*, 48, 923–925, 2000.
340. Rozenblit, A. M., Kim, A., Tuvia, J., and Wenig, B. M. Adrenal histoplasmosis manifested as Addison's disease: unusual CT features with magnetic resonance imaging correlation. *Clin. Radiol.*, 56, 682–684, 2001.
341. Weinber, J. M., Ali, R., Badve, S., and Pelker, R. R. Musculoskeletal histoplasmosis. A case report and review of the literature. *J. Bone Joint Surg. Am.*, 83-A, 1718–1722, 2001.
342. de Fernandez, M. I., Negroni, R., and Arechavala, A. Tibial abscess caused by *Histoplasma capsulatum*. *Medicina (B. Aires)*, 61, 191–192, 2001.
343. Goldani, L. Z., Klock, C., Diehl, A., Monteiro, A. C., and Maia, A. L. Histoplasmosis of the thyroid. *J. Clin. Microbiol.*, 38, 3890–3891, 2000.
344. Salfelder, K., Brass, K., Doehnert, G., Doehnert, R., and Sauerteig, E. Fatal disseminated histoplasmosis: anatomic study of autopsy cases. *Virchows Arch. A Pathol. Anat.*, 350, 303–335, 1970.
345. Kauffman, C. A., Israel, K. S., Smith, J. W., White, A. C., Schwartz, J., and Brooks, G. F. Histoplasmosis in immunosuppressed patients. *Am. J. Med.*, 64, 923–932, 1978.

346. Kedar, S. S., Eldar, S., Abrahamson, J., and Boss, J. Histoplasmosis of kidney presenting as chronic recurrent renal disease. *Urology*, 31, 490–494, 1988.
347. Kauffman, C. A., Slama, T. G., and Wheat, L. J. *Histoplasma capsulatum* epididymitis. *J. Urol.*, 125, 434–435, 1981.
348. Monroe, M. Granulomatous orchitis due to *Histoplasma capsulatum* masquerading as sperm granuloma. *J. Clin. Pathol.*, 27, 929–930, 1974.
349. Sills, M., Schwartz, A., and Weg, J. G. Conjugal histoplasmosis: a consequence of progressive dissemination in the index case after steroid therapy. *Ann. Intern. Med.*, 79, 221–224, 1973.
350. Jayalakshmi, P., Goh, K. L., Soo-Hoo, T. S., and Daud, A. Disseminated histoplasmosis presenting as penile ulcer. *Aust. N. Z. J. Med.*, 20, 175–176, 1990.
351. Nayak, R. G., Ramnarayan, K., Rao, R. V., and Shenoy, M. G. A case of histoplasma posthitis. *Trop. Geogr. Med.*, 36, 309–311, 1984.
352. Mankodi, R. C., Kanvinde, M. S., and Mohapatra, L. N. Penile histoplasmosis: a case report. *Indian J. Med. Sci.*, 24, 354–356, 1970.
353. Preminger, B., Gerard, P. S., Lutwick, L., Frank, R., Minkowitz, S., and Plotkin, N. Histoplasmosis of the penis. *J. Urol.*, 149, 848–850, 1993.
354. Parsons, R. J. and Zarafonetis, C. J. D. Histoplasmosis in man: reports of seven cases and a review of 71 cases. *Arch. Intern. Med.*, 75, 1–23, 1945.
355. Wise, G. J., Talluri, G. S., and Marella, V. K. Fungal infections of the genitourinary system: manifestations, diagnosis, and treatment. *Urol. Clin. North Am.*, 26, 701–718, 1999.
356. Friskel, E., Klotz, S. A., Bartholomew, W., and Dixon, A. Two unusual presentations of urogenital histoplasmosis and a review of the literature. *Clin. Infect. Dis.*, 31, 189–191, 2000.
357. Schuster, T. G., Hollenbeck, B. K., Kauffman, C. A., Chensue, S. W., and Wei, J. T. Testicular histoplasmosis. *J. Urol.*, 164, 1652, 2000.
358. Isotalo, P. A., McCarthy, A. E., and Eidus, L. Ovarian histoplasmosis in systemic lupus erythematosus. *Pathology*, 32, 139–141, 2000.
359. Mawhorter, S. D., Curley, G. V., Kursh, E. D., and Farver, C. E. Prostatic and central nervous system histoplasmosis in an immunocompetent host: case report and review of the prostatic histoplasmosis literature. *Clin. Infect. Dis.*, 30, 595–598, 2000.
360. Bersack, S. R., Howe, J. S., and Rabson, A. S. Inflammatory pseudopolyposis of the small and large intestines with the Peutz-Jaghers syndrome in a case of diffuse histoplasmosis. *Urology*, 58, 73–78, 1958.
361. Rubin, H., Furcolow, M. L., and Yates, J. L. The course and prognosis of histoplasmosis. *Am. J. Med.*, 27, 278–288, 1959.
362. Miller, A. A., Ramsden, F., and Gaeke, M. R. Acute disseminated histoplasmosis of pulmonary origin probably contracted in Britain. *Thorax*, 16, 388–394, 1961.
363. Reddy, P. A., Sutaria, M., Brasher, C. A., and Christianson, C. S. Disseminated histoplasmosis: cutaneous (subcutaneous abscess), vesical and prostatic histoplasmosis. *South. Med. J.*, 63, 819–821, 1970.
364. Orr, W. A., Mulholland, S. G., and Walzak, M. P. Genitourinary tract involvement with systemic mycosis. *J. Urol.*, 107, 1047–1050, 1972.
365. Marans, H. Y., Mandell, W., Kislak, J. W., Starrett, B., and Moussouris, H. F. Prostatic abscess due to *Histoplasma capsulatum* in the acquired immunodeficiency syndrome. *J. Urol.*, 145, 1275–1276, 1991.
366. Zighelboim, J., Goldfarb, R. A., Mody, D., Williams, T. W., Bradshaw, M. W., and Harris, R. L. Prostatic abscess due to *Histoplasma capsulatum* in a patient with the acquired immunodeficiency syndrome. *J. Urol.*, 147, 166–168, 1992.
367. Shah, R. D., Nardi, P. M., and Han, C. C. *Histoplasma* prostatic abscess: rare cause in an immunocompromised patient. *AJR Am. J. Roentgenol.*, 166, 471, 1996.
368. Schwartz, J. Mycotic prostatitis. *Urology*, 19, 1–5, 1982.
369. Wheat, L. J., Batteiger, B. E., and Sathpatayavongs, B. *Histoplasma capsulatum* infections of the central nervous system: a clinical review. *Medicine (Baltimore)*, 69, 244–260, 1990.
370. Wheat, J. Histoplasmosis: experience during outbreaks in Indianapolis and review of the literature. *Medicine (Baltimore)*, 76, 339–354, 1997.
371. Odio, C. M., Navarrete, M., Carrillo, J. M., Mora, L., and Carranza, A. Disseminated histoplasmosis in infants. *Pediatr. Infect. Dis. J.*, 18, 1065–1068, 1999.
372. Butler, J. C., Heller, R., and Wright, P. F. Histoplasmosis during childhood. *South. Med. J.*, 87, 476, 1994.
373. Loyd, J. E., Tillman, B. F., Atkinson, J. B., and Des Prez, R. M. Mediastinal fibrosis complicating histoplasmosis. *Medicine (Baltimore)*, 67, 295, 1988.
374. Prager, R. L., Burney, D. P., Waterhouse, G., and Bender, H. W. Jr. Pulmonary, mediastinal, and cardiac presentations of histoplasmosis. *Ann.Thorac. Surg.*, 30, 385, 1980.
375. Wheat, L. J., Stein, L., Corya, B. C., et al. Pericarditis as a manifestation of histoplasmosis during two large urban outbreaks. *Medicine (Baltimore)*, 62, 110, 1983.
376. Leggiadro, R. J., Barrett, F. F., and Hughes, W. T. Disseminated histoplasmosis of infancy. *Pediatr. Infect. Dis. J.*, 7, 799, 1988.
377. Weinberg, G. A., Kleiman, M. B., Grosfeld, J. L., Weber, T. R., and Wheat, L. J. Unusual manifestations of histoplasmosis in childhood. *Pediatrics*, 72, 99, 1983.
378. Rescorla, F. J., Kleiman, M. B., and Grosfeld, J. L. Obstruction of the common bile duct in histoplasmosis. *Pediatr. Infect. Dis. J.*, 13, 1017, 1994.

379. Hasliza, M., Nur Atiqah, N. A., Lim, C. B., and Hussain, I. H. Disseminated histoplasmosis in a non-immunocompromised child. *Med. J. Malaysia*, 54, 120–124, 1999.
380. Zhou, P., Freidag, B. L., Caldwell, C. C., and Seder, R. A. Perforin is required for primary immunity to *Histoplasma capsulatum*. *J. Immunol.*, 166, 1968–1974, 2001.
381. Deepe, G. S. Jr. Immune response to early and late *Histoplasma capsulatum* infections. *Curr. Opin. Microbiol.*, 3, 359–362, 2000.
382. Newman, S. L. Cell-mediated immunity to *Histoplasma capsulatum*. *Semin. Respir. Infect.*, 16, 102–108, 2001.
383. Bonner, J. R., Alexander, W. J., Dismukes, W. E., et al. Disseminated histoplasmosis in patients with the acquired immune deficiency syndrome. *Arch. Intern. Med.*, 144, 2178, 1984
384. Spitzer, E. D., Keath, E. J., Travis, S. J., Painter, A. A., Kobayashi, G. B., and Medoff, G. Temperature-sensitive variants of *Histoplasma capsulatum* isolates from patients with acquired immunodeficiency syndrome. *J. Infect. Dis.*, 162, 258, 1990.
385. Bullock, W. E. and Wright, S. D. Role of the adherence-promoting receptors, CR3, LFA-1, and p150,95, in binding of *Histoplasma capsulatum* by human macrophages. *J. Exp. Med.*, 165, 195, 1987.
386. Newman, S. L., Bucher, C., Rhodes, J., and Bullock, W. E. Phagocytosis of *Histoplasma capsulatum* yeasts and microconidia by human cultured macrophages and alveolar macrophages: cellular cytoskeleton requirement for attachment and ingestion. *J. Clin. Invest.*, 85, 223, 1990.
387. Schnur, R. A. and Newman, S. L. The respiratory burst response to *Histoplasma capsulatum* by human neutrophils: evidence for intracellular trapping of superoxide anion. *J. Immunol.*, 144, 4765, 1990.
388. Newman, S. L., Gootee, L., Morris, R., and Bullock, W. E. Digestion of *Histoplasma capsulatum* yeasts by human macrophages. *J. Immunol.*, 149, 574, 1992.
389. Fleischmann, J., Wu-Hsieh, B., and Howard, D. H. The intracellular fate of *Histoplasma capsulatum* in human macrophages is unaffected by recombinant human interferon-γ. *J. Infect. Dis.*, 161, 143, 1990.
390. Newman, S. L., Gootee, L., Bucher, C., and Bullock, W. E. Inhibition of intracellular growth of *Histoplasma capsulatum* yeasts cells by cytokine-activated human monocytes and macrophages. *Infect. Immun.*, 59, 737, 1991.
391. Newman, S. L. and Gootee, L. Colony-stimulating factors activate human macrophages to inhibit the intracellular growth of *Histoplasma capsulatum* yeasts. *Infect. Immun.*, 60, 4593, 1992.
392. Wu-Hsieh, B. A., Whitmire, J. K., de Fries, R., Lin, J. S., Matloubian, M., and Ahmed, R. Distinct CD8 T cell functions mediate susceptibility to histoplasmosis during chronic viral infection. *J. Immunol.*, 167, 4566–4573, 2001.
393. Deepe, G. S. Jr., Gibbons, R., and Woodward, E. Neutralization of endogenous granulocyte- macrophage colony-stimulating factor subverts the protective immune response to *Histoplasma capsulatum*. *J. Immunol.*, 163, 4985–4993, 1999.
394. Wheat, L. J., Rubin, R. H., Harris, N., et al. Systemic salmonellosis in patients with disseminated histoplasmosis. *Arch. Intern. Med.*, 147, 561, 1987.
395. Kimberlin, C. L., Hariri, A. R., Hempel, H. O., and Goodman, N. L. Interactions between *Histoplasma capsulatum* and unusual circumstances.

28
African Histoplasmosis

1. INTRODUCTION

The dimorphic fungus *Histoplasma capsulatum* var. *duboisii* is the etiologic agent of African histoplasmosis. The disease has been limited largely to Central and Western Africa (especially Nigeria), and some other localized areas (the province of Natal in South Africa) *(1–5)*. Abrucio Neto et al. *(6)* described a case of African histoplasmosis diagnosed in Brasil. The patient, an immigrant from Angola, had cutaneous lesions. Earlier, Oddo et al. *(7)* reported the first case of *Histoplasma duboisii* in South America. Again, the patient lived in Africa before moving to Chile. Manfredi et al. *(8)* examined the epidemiologic and clinical features of African histoplasmosis in Europe and the role played by the emergence of the HIV pandemic and the progressively increasing rate of travel and immigration as risk factors for this infection in other part of the world *(9)*.

The yeast stage of *Histoplasma capsulatum* var. *duboisii* is relatively large and can reach size of 10–15 μm. Although occasional budding forms may be seen, hyphae are not present. While the natural reservoir of the fungus is unknown, it has been isolated from the soil and no animal source has been identified. Gugnani et al. *(10)* reported the isolation of the pathogen from soil admixed with bat guano and from the intestinal contents of a single bat in a sandstone cave in a rural area in Nigeria. To this end, Butler at al. *(11,12)* diagnosed *Histoplasma capsulatum* var. *duboisii* in baboons at a large primate colony in Texas. Infections are believed to occur secondary to traumatic inoculation into the skin *(2)*.

The African histoplasmosis has several manifestations that are seldom seen with *H. capsulatum* var. *capsulatum (13,14)*. Lungs do not usually contain clinically detectable lesions, although miliary infiltrates *(15)* and nodular lesions *(16)* have been described occasionally. The most common manifestations occur in bone and skin *(17–19)*.

Bone lesions, which tend to multiply, are particularly common in the rib, vertebra, femur, humeris, tibia, skull, and wrist *(18,20)*. A case of isolated osteomyelitis of the radius due to *H. capsulatum* var. *duboisii* has also been described *(21)*. Subcutaneous abscess from an underlying bone lesion has been one of the three cutaneous manifestations of this mycosis; the other two being subcutaneous granulomata and nodular lesions *(22)*.

Without other signs of the infection, African histoplasmosis (bone lesions *[21]* and colon *[23]*) often can be misdiagnosed as cancer.

2. MANAGEMENT OF AFRICAN HISTOPLAMOSIS AND EVOLUTION OF THERAPIES

The treatment of the disease is usually difficult and success is achieved only when therapy is initated early in the infection. The histologic appearance of the affected skin is characterized by epidermal atrophy with granulomatous infiltrate within the dermis, as well as acute and chronic infiltrates. A case of African histoplasmosis presented as an ulcer clinically mimicking squamous cell carcinoma, and eventually healed spontaneously *(24)*.

Dissemination could affect the subcutis, muscles, the reticuloendothelial system, mucous membranes, lungs, and the bone *(2)*. Cutaneous lesions may be manifested as either multiple painless or pruritic papules and nodules anywhere on the body surface. In the chronic form, the disease affects the mucous membranes and the gastrointestinal tract and is manifested by ulcerations of the nose, mouth, anus, and genitalia. Bone involvement is often seen, especially in the femur and vertebrae. In progressive disease, the reticuloendothelial system is also affected, resulting in enlargement of the liver and the lymph nodes. Dissemination occurs largely by the hematogenous route *(25)*. Contrary to infections caused by *Histoplasma capsulatum* var. *capsulatum*, pulmonary involvement of African histoplasmosis is not common and occurs only during disseminated disease *(2)*.

For years, intravenous amphotericin B has been considered the drug of choice in treating the disease *(26)* although it is not always curative and its toxicity may become very serious by causing irreversible renal damage in some patients.

Oral ketoconazole is less toxic and seems to be of therapeutic value *(27,28)*. Thus, Mabey and Hay *(29)* treated five patients (three children with disseminated disease, and two adults with localized cutaneous lesions) with ketoconazole at daily doses ranging from 5–15 mg/kg, depending on age and clinical conditions; in some cases amphotericin B was also used. Both patients with the cutaneous disease responded to treatment; of the three children with disseminated disease, one responded well, one responded initially but had a relapse, and one child did not respond to therapy *(4)*.

In a recent report of two cases of African histoplasmosis, the pathogen was located in the spine, causing dorsal spinal syndrome (spondylodiscitis) in both patients and a paraplegia in one case. Medical treatment, after surgical repair, consisted of ketoconazole with positive results after 12 mo *(30)*.

After its recent introduction into the clinic, itraconazole was used successfully in the treatment of several cases of African histoplasmosis *(31–33)*. Dupont and Drouhet *(34)* reported a case in which a patient, after falling repeatedly into relapses following treatments with amphotericin B and ketoconazole, was given oral itraconazole at daily doses of 100 mg for 6 mo. The patient remained well at 9 mo post-therapy. In another case *(35)*, the patient had no recurrence after itraconazole medication at a 2-yr follow-up examination. Bayles *(1)* reported on a case that presented with papular lesions resembling molluscum contagiosum, lymphadenopathy, and pulmonary and bone-marrow involvement. The initial therapy included 100 mg daily of itraconazole for 3 mo, increasing it afterwards to 200 mg daily for another 9 mo; the patient was free from skin lesions 3 yr later; however, the lung condition showed little change.

A case of African histoplasmosis where the patient had cutaneous lesions was successfully treated with itraconazole (100 mg daily) for 52 d; no recurrent skin lesions were observed during the 10-mo follow-up period *(6)*.

Eichmann and Schar *(36)* reported African histoplasmosis presenting as granulomatous and subsequently ulcerative nodules in the face of a HIV-2-positive patient with no signs of disseminated disease. The lesions were cleared by therapy with itraconazole (200 mg q. 24 h for 2 wk, subsequently 100 mg q. 24 h), as well as ketoconazole and Aqua Dalibour (A. zinco-cuprica) locally for 2 mo.

A case of African histoplasmosis manifesting as multiple osteomyelitis was successfully treated with oral fluconazole *(37)*.

Terbinafin was used to treat for 4 mo humeral, tibial, and cutaneous localizations of *H. capsulatum* var. *duboisii* in a child. The patient recovered without after-effects in the tibial localization, but did experience after-effects at the humeral localization *(20)*.

Localized orbital histoplasmosis due to *H. capsulatum* var. *duboisii* was successfully cured with 2 tablets daily of septrin (a combination of 80 mg trimethoprim and 400 mg sulfamethoxazole per tablet) and surgical drainage of the orbit *(38)*. Three previous reports *(39–41)* also indicated a complete or partial response of histoplasmosis to septrin alone or in combination with amphotericin B. Although the mechanism of action by which sulfamethoxazole and trimethoprim exerted their effects on histoplasma is not clearly understood, septrin could be an alternative to amphotericin B, especially in patients presenting with solitary or localized lesions *(38)*. However, in recent report, Salkind *(42)* have described the development of rash in response to trimethoprim-sulfamethoxazole administration in AIDS patients, as well as frank delirium in one patient. The latter resolved completely within 72 h of withdrawal of the drugs.

REFERENCES

1. Bayles, M. A. H. Tropical mycoses. *Chemotherapy*, 38(Suppl. 1), 27, 1992.
2. Gross, M. L. and Millikan, L. E. Deep fungal infections in the tropics. *Dermatol. Clin.*, 12, 695, 1994.
3. Vanbreuseghem, R. Reflexions sur l'histoplasmose africaine at l'histoplasmose americaine. *Mykosen*, 25, 171, 1982.
4. Williams, A. O., Lawson, E. A., and Lucas, A. O. African histoplasmosis due to *Histoplasma duboisii*. *Arch. Pathol.*, 92, 306, 1971.
5. Muotoe-Okafor, F. A., Gugnani, H. C., Gugnani, A., and Okafor, G. Antibodies to antigens of *Histoplasma, Blastomyces* and *Candida* in HIV patients and carriers in Nigeria. *Mycoses*, 43, 173–175, 2000.
6. Abrucio Neto, L., Takahashi, M. D. F., Salebian, A., and Cuce, L. C. African histoplasmosis: report of the first case in Brasil and treatment with itraconazole. *Rev. Inst. Med. Trop. Sao Paolo*, 35, 295, 1993.
7. Oddo, D., Etchart, M., and Thompson, L. *Histoplasma duboisii* (African histoplasmosis). An African case reported from Chile with ultrastructural study. *Pathol. Res. Pract.*, 186, 514, 1990.
8. Manfredi, R., Mazzoni, A., Nanetti, A., and Chido, F. Histoplasmosis capsulati and duboisii in Europe: the impact of the HIV pandemic, travel and immigration. *Eur. J. Epidemiol.*, 10, 675–681, 1994.
9. Nethercott, J. R., Schachter, R. K., Givan, K. F., and Ryder, D. E. Histoplasmosis due to *Histoplasma capsulatum* var. *duboisii* in a Canadian immigrant. *Arch. Dermatol.*, 114, 595–598, 1978.
10. Gugnani, H. C., Muotoe-Okafor, F. A., Kaufman, L., and Dupont, B. A natural focus of *Histoplasma capsulatum* var. *duboisii* is a bat cave. *Mycopathologia* 127, 151–157, 1994.
11. Butler, T. M. and Hubbard, G. B. An epizootic of histoplasmosis duboisii (African histoplasmosis) in an American baboon colony. *Lab. Anim. Sci.*, 41, 407–410, 1991.
12. Butler, T. M., Gleiser, C. A., Bernal, J. C., and Ajello, L. Case of disseminated African histoplasmosis in a baboon. *J. Med. Primatol.*, 17, 153–161, 1988.
13. Kwon-Chung, K. J. and Bennett, J. E. *Medical Mycology*. Lea & Febiger, Philadelphia, 487, 1992.
14. Aubry, P. and Lecamus, J. L. Les histoplasmoses. *Med. Trop. (Mars.)*, 46, 229–237, 1986.
15. Dupont, B., Drouhet, E., and Lapresle, C. Histoplasmosis généralisée a *Histoplasma duboisii*. *Nouv. Presse Med.*, 3, 1005, 1974.
16. Seeliger, H. P. R., Kracht, J., and Bikfalvi, A. Grosszellige (afrikanische) histoplasmamykose der lunge. *Dtsch. Med. Wochenschr.*, 105, 609, 1980.
17. Cockshott, W. P. and Lucas, A. O. *Histoplasma duboisii*. *Q. J. Med.*, 33, 223, 1964.
18. Williams, A. O., Lawson, E. A., and Lucas, A.O. African histoplasmosis due to *Histoplasma duboisii*. *Arch. Pathol.*, 92, 306, 1971.
19. Jones, R. C. and Goodwin, R. A. Jr. Histoplasmosis of bone. *Am. J. Med.*, 70, 864–866, 1981.
20. Bankole Sanni, R., Denoulet, C., Coulibaly, B., et al. A propos d'un cas ivoirien d'histoplasmose osseuse et cutanee a *Histoplasma capsulatum* var. *duboisii*. *Bull. Soc. Pathol. Exot.*, 91, 151–153, 1998.
21. Onwuasoigwe, O. and Gugnani, H. C. African histoplasmosis: osteomyelitis of the radius. *Mycoses*, 41, 105–107, 1998.
22. Lucas, A. O. Cutaneous manifestations of African histoplasmosis. *Br. J. Dermatol.*, 82, 435, 1970.
23. Khalil, M., Iwatt, A. R., and Gugnani, H. C. African histoplasmosis masquerading as carcinoma of the colon. Report of a case and review of literature. *Dis. Colon Rectum*, 32, 518–520, 1989.
24. Olasoji, H. O., Pindiga, U. H., and Adeosun, O. O. African histoplasmosis lip carcinoma: case report. *East Afr. Med. J.*, 76, 475–476, 1999.
25. Dietrich, P. Y., Billie, J., Fontolliet, C., and Regamey, C. Histoplasmose disseminee a *Histoplasma capsulatum* chez un patient presentantun syndrome d'immunodeficience acquise (SIDA). *Schweiz. Med. Wochenschr.*, 117, 1289–1296, 1987.
26. Lucas, A. O. Cutaneous manifestations of African histoplasmosis. *Br. J. Dermatol.*, 82, 435, 1970.
27. Drouhet, E. and Dupont, B. Laboratory and clinical assessment of ketoconazole in deep-seated mycoses. *Am. J. Med.*, 74(1B), 30–47, 1983.
28. Drouhet, E. and Dupont, B. Chronic mucocutaneous candidosis and other superficial and systemic mycoses successfully treated with ketoconazole. *Rev. Infect. Dis.*, 2, 606–619, 1980.
29. Mabey, D. C. W. and Hay, R. J. Further studies on the treatment of African histoplasmosis with ketoconazole. *Trans. R. Soc. Trop. Med. Hyg.*, 83, 560, 1989.
30. N'dri Oka, D., Varlet, G., Kakou, M., Zunon-Kipre, Y., Broalet, E., Ba Zeze, V. Spondylodiscitis due to *Histoplasma duboisii*. Report of two cases and review of the literature. *Neurochirurgie*, 47, 431–434, 2011.
31. De Rosso, J. Q. and Gupta, A. K. Oral itraconazole therapy for superficial, subcutaneous, and systemic infections. A panoramic view. *Postgrad. Med.*, Spec. No: 46–52, 1999.
32. Lortholary, O., Denning, D. W., Dupont, B. Endemic mycoses: a treatment update. *J. Antimicrob. Chemother.*, 43, 321–331, 1999.

33. Chandenier, J., Goma, D., Moyen, G., et al. Histoplasmose africaine a *Histoplasma capsulatum* var. *duboisii*: liens avec le SIDA a propos de cas congolais recents. *Sante*, 5, 227–234, 1995.
34. Dupont, B. and Drouhet, E. Early experience with itraconazole in vitro and in patients: pharmacokinetic studies and clinical results. *Rev. Infect. Dis.*, 9(Suppl. 1), S71–S76, 1987.
35. Drouhet, E. African histoplasmosis. *Baillieres Clin. Trop. Med. Commun. Dis.*, 4, 89, 1989.
36. Eichmann, A. and Schar, G. Afrikanische histoplasmose bei patient mit HIV-2 infektion. *Schweiz. Med. Wochenschr.*, 126, 765–769, 1996.
37. Onwuasoigwe, O. Fluconazole in the therapy of multiple osteomyelitis in African histoplasmosis. *Int. Orthop.*, 23, 82–84, 1999.
38. Ajayi, B. G. K., Osuntokun, B., Olurin, O., Kale, O. O., and Junaid, T. A. Orbital histoplasmosis due to *Histoplasma capsulatum* var. *duboisii*: successful treatment with septrin. *J. Trop. Med. Hyg.*, 89, 179–187, 1986.
39. MacLeod, W. M. Treatment of histoplasmosis. *Lancet*, 2, 363, 1970.
40. Brown, K. G. E., Molesworth, B. D., Boerrigter, F. G. G., and Tozer, R. A. Disseminated histoplasmosis duboisii in Malawi partial response to sulphonamide/trimethoprim combination. *East Afr. Med. J.*, 51, 584, 1974.
41. Egere, J. U., Gugnani, H. C., Okoro, A. N., and Suseelan, A. V. African histoplasmosis in Eastern Nigeria: report of two culturally proven cases treated with septrin and amphotericin B. *J. Trop. Med. Hyg.*, 81, 225, 1978.
42. Salkind, A. R. Acute delirium induced by intravenous trimethoprim-sulfamethoxazole therapy in a patient with the acquired immunodeficiency syndrome. *Hum. Exp. Toxicol.*, 19, 149–151, 2000.

29
Blastomyces dermatitidis

1. INTRODUCTION

Blastomycosis was originally believed to be endemic to North and Central America (U.S., Canada, Mexico, and Central America) until 1952, when a case was reported from Tunisia in which the pathogen was identified as *Scopulariopsis americana*, a synonym of *B. dermatitidis (1,2)*. Later, other cases of blastomycosis in Africa, South America, and Asia followed *(3–12)*.

In North America, blastomycosis is most frequently found in the regions of the Mississippi and Ohio River valleys, and the upper Midwestern states and Canadian provinces bordering the Great Lakes and the Saint Laurence River *(13–19)*. However, in a recent report, an HIV-related case of blastomycosis was diagnosed in Texas *(20)*. It appears that soil with a high organic content and low pH value may facilitate growth of the fungus. The proximity of water also appears to promote the growth of *B. dermatitidis (21–24)*. Although isolation of the fungus from natural soil was found to be difficult *(25,26)* Klein et al. *(15,23)* reported the isolation, on two separate occasions, of *B. dermatitidis* from soil in association with an epidemic of the infection.

Blastomycosis is generally considered to be a soil-borne infection. In humans, *B. dermatitidis* causes a mixed pyogenic and granulomatous disease *(27)*. The fungus has also been found in dogs *(28)*, cats, and other mammals *(29,30)*, where the prevalence and incidence of infection, especially in dogs and other mammals, has been similar to that in humans *(31,32)* and may be relevant to the correct diagnosis of human disease *(28,33)*.

Because the major route of human infection is most likely through the respiratory tract rather than the skin *(34–36)*, pulmonary blastomycosis is the most common condition of the disease *(18,19,37)*. Pulmonary manifestations include chronic cough and pleuritic pain, and radiographic appearance *(37,38)* of the infection may mimic bronchogenic lung carcinoma *(39)* or tuberculosis *(40)*. Laryngeal blastomycosis may occur in isolation from active pulmonary disease, and its signs, symptoms, clinical features, and pathological findings may mimic those of squamous cell carcinoma, thereby leading to misdiagnosis and inappropriate treatment with potential morbidity *(41)*.

When organs other than lungs are affected by the fungus, it has been nearly always by dissemination from a primary lesion in the lung *(42,43)*. Head and neck blastomycosis is often difficult to diagnose *(44)*. A case of chronic paronychia, osteomyelitis, and paravertebral abscess in a child with blastomycosis was recently reported *(43)*. Skin and soft-tissue involvement have also been involved *(45–47)*. Skin injuries caused by bites of infected dogs have been reported to result in cutaneous blastomycosis *(48)*. Cervical manifestation of blastomycosis presenting in a single abscessed cervical lymph node *(45)*, and blastomycosis of the petrous apex *(49)* have also been diagnosed. A case of recurrent CNS blastomycosis, although very rare, was described by Chowfin et al. *(50)*. In another case of CNS involvement, blastomycoma of the cerebellum was reported *(51)*.

Blastomycosis of the lumber spine, causing severe and crippling deformity, was treated early with aggressive chemotherapy and surgical reconstruction (abscess drainage, bone fusion, and posterior instrumentation) to prevent deformity *(52)*.

Li et al. *(53)* reported the clinical, cytologic, and histopathologic findings of a unique presentation of concomitant unilateral endophthalmitis and orbital cellulitis secondary to *B. dermatitidis* which, after initial response to treatment, deteriorated rapidly to no light perception in 3 mo; surgical enucleation and an orbital biopsy were performed.

Sexual transmission of blastomycosis has been described in at least two cases *(54,55)*. Person-to-person aerial transmission of the infection has never been reported.

Pulmonary blastomycosis in pregnant women has also been reported *(56–61)*. It is not unexpected that in such cases, the severity of infection may increase due to a depressed state of cell-mediated immunity likely to occur during pregnancy *(62)*. Intrauterine transmission to the fetus is very rarely observed *(61,63)*.

Recent progress in the genetic manipulations (gene-transfer techniques, selection markers, reported fusions, and targeting) has advanced the knowledge on the molecular basis of pathogenicity of *B. dermatitidis*, and in particular the importance of the mycelium-to-yeast transition and the crucial and complex role of the BAD1 and WI-1 adhesins *(64,65)*. Recent studies have pointed out the link between the phase-specific expression of WI-1 and the observation that transition to yeast cells is essential for the acquisition of pathogenicith by *B. dermatitidis (65)*.

In immunocompetent patients, blastomycosis will most likely produce clinical manifestations ranging from asymptomatic to mild influenza-like or atypical pneuminia syndrome *(21,66)*, or a rapidly progressive respiratory or systemic illness *(16)*. The long-term carriage of the organism also presents the potential for reactivation following the initial exposure *(67)*.

In immunocompromised hosts, however, the disseminated disease may be life-threatening and has been described in renal *(68–73)*, heart *(72)*, and bone-marrow *(72)* transplant recipients, patients receiving corticosteroids *(74,75)*, and patients with underlying hematologic malignancies or solid tumors *(75,76)*. In some earlier reports, the mortality rate from systemic blastomycosis was estimated to be between 70% and 80% *(77)*, and as high as 90% *(78)*.

Two cases of simultaneous infection with *B. dermatitidis* and *Cryptococcus neoformans* was reported *(79)*.

Presently, three clinical types of blastomycosis are most commonly described: pulmonary, disseminated, and cutaneous *(80,81)*.

2. AFRICAN BLASTOMYCOSIS

Results from several reports have shown the existence of both macro- and microscopic differences between *B. dermatitidis* strains isolated from North American and African patients *(820*. Initially described in the early 1950s *(1,2)*, cases of African blastomycosis have been described with increasing incidence *(83–85)*.

The capacity of *B. dermatitidis* to change its morphology from the mycelial form into yeast-like form has been clearly documented; on histopathologic examination, *B. dermatitidis* is almost always found only in the yeast-like form *(51)*. One of the major differences observed between the North American and African strains was that in the latter, the conversion of the mycelial (hyphal) into the yeast-like phase (M-Y conversion), achieved after 5–6 d of incubation at 37°C in Columbia ANC culture medium, was only partial. It was, rather, mycelial modification presented with marked swelling of the hyphae and a few budding yeast-like cells *(82,85,86)*. Vermeil et al. *(87)* demonstrated the lack of the sexual form in African *B. dermatitidis* strains and the loss of M-Y conversion in the older strains, confirming the suggestion of McGinnis *(88)* that total transformation is not necessary to classify a strain such as *B. dermatitidis*. However, with regard to clinical and immunologic characteristics, Vanbreuseghem et al. *(89)* proposed that there may be two different species involved. Because significant genetic diversity among clinical isolates of *B. dermatitidis* has been observed *(90)*, this may also underscore a similar environmental diversification.

Baily et al. *(91)* reviewed some of the clinical features, diagnosis, and treatment of blastomycosis in Africa. El Haouri et al. *(12)* reported what appeared the firsts case of chronic skin-localized granulomatosis caused by *B. dermatitidis* associated with malignant corticoadenoma; amphotericin B provided cure of the skin lesions.

3. ROLE OF HOST IMMUNE RESPONSE AGAINST *BLASTOMYCES DERMATITIDIS*

Inasmuch as antibodies to the fungus have been documented, they play little apparent role in the host defense against the pathogen *(92)*. Until now, the role of humoral response against human blastomycosis has not been fully evaluated because of the absence of a suitably active and specific antigen. Contrary to humoral immunity, however, cellular immunity is considered to be a major factor in preventing progressive disease caused by slow-growing, pathogenic fungi, such as *B. dermatitidis (35)*.

4. EVOLUTION OF THERAPIES AND TREATMENT OF BLASTOMYCOSIS

2-Hydroxystilbamidine (given intravenously) was the first therapeutic agent that was effective and reduced mortality from blastomycosis *(33,93)*. The total dose applied ranged between 12 and 16 g *(93)*. Although it still may be useful in a few cases, 2-hydroxystilbamidine is now seldom used and is of historical interest only. While it showed less toxicity than amphotericin B, 2-hydroxystilbamidine was also less effective; as compared to ketoconazole, it was less effective, but more toxic.

The toxicity of 2-hydroxystilbamidine is more likely to cause liver damage rather than the renal impairment associated with amphotericin B. Therefore, it is important that serum potassium levels are monitored closely. 2-Hydroxystilbamidine must be administered intravenously at recommended daily doses in adults of 225 mg and a total dose not exceeding 12–15 g *(93)*.

4.1. Amphotericin B

Since its introduction in 1956, amphotericin B has been the mainstay for treatment of various systemic mycoses. It is active against all types of blastomycosis, and dose regimens of 1.5–2.0 g should be adequate, especially in immunocompetent patients, and cases involving pulmonary blastomycosis with diffuse infiltrates and severe hypoxemia (a total cumulative dose of 500–1000 mg) (Table 1) *(81,94)*.

For treatment of meningeal blastomycosis, amphotericin B is the treatment of choice *(96–98,108–120)*. Also, amphotericin B should be used preferentially in patients with adult respiratory distress syndrome (ARDS) because of its quick onset of action *(59,60)*; up to 2.0 g total dose of the antibiotic has been recommended *(59,121)*. Clinical response towards the drug was between 66% and 93% depending on total dose and duration of treatment *(112,118,122,123)*.

The antibiotic is always administered intravenously with a total dose ranging from 25–35 mg/kg (as much as 2.5 g) *(121,124)*. Although intraventricular administration of amphotericin B has not been adequately evaluated, it may be useful in patients with obstructive hydrocephalus and rapid deterioration, or whenever the response to intravenous amphotericin B is unsatisfactory *(121)*. Lewis et al. *(125)* and Gottlieb et al. *(97)* cured disseminated choroidal blastomycosis after treatment with 2.0 of intravenous amphotericin B. Lopez et al. *(126)* used amphotericin B (0.5 mg/kg; total, 1260 mg) as primary systemic therapy combined with subconjunctival injections of miconazole (0.5 mg/ 0.5 mL) to treat intraocular blastomycosis.

Albert et al. *(127)* described a very unusual pediatric case of infection of the forearm synovium presenting as a soft-tissue mass without bone or skin involvement; the patient was treated successfully with surgical debridement of the mass combined with amphotericin B (0.7 mg/kg daily, i.v.) for 6 wk, followed by oral itraconazole (100 mg, b.i.d.) for another 12 wk.

Table 1
Recommended Therapies of Blastomycosis Infections (Single-Drug Regimens and Combinations) *(95)*

Drug or combination	Dose regimen (route of administration)	Clinical type	Duration of therapy
Amphotericin B	Total dose of 2.0 g (i.v.) *(95–97)*;	Chronic pulmonary[a]; extrapulmonary non-meningeal[a]; paranasal sinuses; choroidal	Until cure
	50 mg weekly (i.v.) *(98)* total dose of 2.0–3.0 g (i.v.) *(98)*; or 0.6–0.8 mg/kg, daily *(19)*	Meningeal[b,c]; acute[b]	Prolonged
Ketoconazole	400–800 mg daily (p.o.) *(99)*	Acute[a]; Chronic pulmonary[a]; extrapulmonary non-meningeal[a]	6 mo 6 mo 6 mo
Itraconazole	200–400 mg daily (p.o.) *(27,98,100–102)*	Acute[d]; Chronic pulmonary[a]; Meningeal[b]; Extrapulmonary non-meningeal[a]	6 mo 6 mo Prolonged 6 mo
	In children: 5–7 mg/kg (maximum: 200 mg daily) (p.o.)[e]	Pulmonary *(103)*	
Fluconazole	200–400 daily (p.o.) *(104)*	Nonmeningeal; non-life-threatening	6.7 mo (mean)
Amphotericin B Ketoconazole Itraconazole	500–1000 mg (i.v.)[f] 400–800 mg daily (p.o.) 400 mg daily (p.o.)	Acute with ventilatory failure *(95)*	Primary 6 mo 6 mo
Amphotericin B Itraconazole	500–1000 mg (i.v.)g 400 mg daily (p.o.)[b]	Acute *(98)*; Acute with ventilatory failure *(98)* Chronic pulmonary or extrapulmonary non-meningeal *(98)*	Primary 6 mo

[a] In immunocompetent patients.
[b] In immunocompromised patients.
[c] In cases of immunocompetent hosts, a total cumulative dose of 2.0–3.0 g is recommended *(98)*.
[d] In immunocompetent patients (however, with greater toxicity compared to itraconazole).
[e] In low birth-weight infants and children with fungal infections (disseminated candidiasis and aspergillosis), or chronic granulomatous disease, doses of 5.0–10 mg/kg of itraconazole have been used safely *(105–107)*.
[f] Amphotericin B is administered until patient's condition is stable, followed by either ketoconazole or itraconazole for a minimum of 6 additional months to complete therapy.
[g] In non-AIDS immunocompromised patients, the primary therapy is with amphotericin, then itraconazole for 6 mo; in AIDS patients, the follow-up treatment with itraconazole is for life.

Table 2
Toxic Side Effects of Drug Used to Treat Blastomycosis/Fungal Infections

Drug	Toxicity	Symptoms
Amphotericin B (132)	Dose-dependent	Nephrotoxicity (urinary abnormalities, hyposthenuria, azotemia, hypokalemia, nephrocalcinosis); normocytic, normochromic anemia (decreased erythropoietin levels and erythrocyte counts).
	Idiosyncratic	Flushing; rash; anaphylactic shock; acute liver failure; thrombocytopenia; vertigo; generalized pain; grand mal convulsion; ventricular fibrillation; cardial arrest; fever (in nearly all patients); chill (in nearly all patients).
Ketoconazole (133)		Nausea; vomiting; diarrhea; pruritis; rash; increased alkaline phosphatase; hyperlipidemia; inhibition of gonadal and adrenal steroid synthesis.
Itraconazole (133)		Asymptomatic liver function abnormalities; increased blood levels of urea nitrogen and serum levels of transaminase.
Fluconazole (134)		Nausea; headache; skin rash; vomiting; abdominal pain; diarrhea; hepatotoxicity; elevated serum transaminase levels; leukopenia; thrombocytopenia; reversible alopecia (135).
Miconazole (133)		Phlebitis; pruritis; nausea; fever; chill; rash; vomiting; anemia; decreased hematocrit (normoblastic hypoplasia); hyponatremia; anaphylaxis; ventricular tachycardia.

Relapse of blastomycosis following treatment with amphotericin B has been rare and appeared to be dose-dependent (118,128,129). In the majority of cases, relapse was observed shortly after completion of amphotericin B therapy (109), although in some patients, relapse occured as long as 9 yr after the treatment (1,100).

In spite of its clinical efficacy, the use of amphotericin B is limited because of serious side effects (130), such as azotemia (71%), anemia (53%), anorexia, nausea and vomiting (53%), fever and chills (49%), hypokalemia (37%), and thrombophlebitis (19%) (Table 2) (131). The toxicity of the antibiotic may become severe enough to require cessation of therapy. Some of the side effects of amphotericin B may be minimized by pretreatment of the patient with antihistamines, antipyretics, and antiemetics, but these drugs should never be mixed with the antibiotic (33).

In order to limit its unwarrented toxicity (132), amphotericin B has been either chemically modified (e.g., methyl ester formation) (136–139), or intercalated into lipid-based carriers (140), such as liposome encapsulation (141–152). Clemons and Stevens (153,154) compared the efficacies of amphotericin B lipid complex and a micellar amphotericin B-deoxycholate suspension (Fungizone®) against blastomycosis in a CD-1 mouse model. The lipid complex was a preparation of dimyristoyl phosphatidyl choline and dimyristoyl phosphatidyl glycerol (in a 7:3 molar ratio) containing 33 mol% of amphotericin B; the average particle size was 1.6–6.0 μm. The MIC (broth dilution) and minimum fungicidal concentration of fungizone against B. dermatitidis ATCC 26199 were 0.5 and 1.0 μg/mL; the corresponding values for the lipid complex were 0.25 and 1.0 μg/mL. All doses of each form prolonged survival ($p < 0.05$–0.001). Fungizone showed higher potency at doses of 0.8 mg/kg. However, the lipid complex of amphotericin B showed an overt toxicity at doses of 12.8 mg/kg and was superior ($p < 0.001$) to fungizone given at 2.0 mg/kg (a toxic dose) (153).

Recently, a novel heparin-coated hydrophilic preparation (AH) of amphotericin B hydrosomes was described (155). It represents a heparin-surfaced nonaparticles (mean diameter of 105 nm) designed to target the infected sites (lesions) by adhesion. Compared to fungizone, between 3 and 24 h post-injection AH accumulates threefold more in infected lungs of mice than in normal lungs, and showing sevenfold less toxicity. At doses of 4.8 mg/kg, AH cured 50–60% of B. dermatitidis-infected mice, whereas fungizone at a near lethal dose of 1.2 mg/kg cured none (155).

4.2. Azole Derivatives

4.2.1. Ketoconazole

While amphotericin B is used predominantly in patients who are acutely ill or imunocompromised, or when central nervous system (CNS) involvement has been diagnosed, since 1985 ketoconazole has been one of the primary therapeutic agents for all but the most severe cases of human blastomycosis (74,100,156–164). It was less effective in immunocompromised than immunocompetent patients (69,165).

The mechanism of action of ketoconazole involves interaction with cytochrome P-450 enzymes, which results in reduced levels of ergosterol, a major building block of the fungal cell membrane (166,167). Because ketoconazole competes with cyclosporin A for metabolism in the hepatic cytochrome P-450 system, there were some unpredictable elevated levels of cyclosporin A in some patients on immunosuppressive therapy (165).

Ketoconazole, which has the advantages of oral administration and lesser toxicity than most azole antimycotics, was shown to be effective against acute symptomatic blastomycosis. In clinical trials conducted by the NIAID Mycoses Study Group, of the 80 patients involved in the study, 89% were cured with a recommended dose regimen of 400 to 800 mg daily given for an average of 6 mo (Table 1) (158). Serum levels of the drug ranged from 3.32–6.2 μg/mL 2 h after an oral dose of 400 or 800 mg (158,159,168). At the lower dose of 400 mg daily, the relapse or primary failure rate was about 10% (74,158). Although it is difficult to predict which patients will develop a relapse, those with genitourinary involvement are more prone to do so, likely due to the lower concentration of ketoconazole in the urine and prostate (158). When the high-dose (800 mg daily) regimen is applied for at least 6 mo, the failure rate is negligible. However, adverse side effects such as anorexia, nausea or vomiting (29.1%), menstrual irregularities (16.2%), rash (9.7%), pruritis (9.7%), impotence or decreased libido (8.3%), gynecomastia (7.2%), and hepatic disfunction (2.9%) may also occur (Table 2) (74,158,167,133–135,169). The most severe toxicity of ketoconazole so far reported is hepatocellular damage; however, it has been very rarely observed (170).

There have been several studies (74,108,171) of patients who developed CNS blastomycosis while receiving ketoconazole. The patients who initially did not have CNS symptoms were treated for cutaneous and pulmonary blastomycosis that responded to ketoconazole. However, because of the poor ability of ketoconazole to penetrate the blood-brain barrier (BBB), it is possible that the therapeutic failure of the drug might have been caused by initially unrecognized CNS infection. Once diagnosed, CNS blastomycosis has been successfully treated with amphotericin B (108). Since the rate of asymptomatic CNS blastomycosis may be substantial (3–10% [110,111,116] and as high as 24% [36]), lumbar puncture or even cranial computed tomography (CT) have been recommended for all patients with disseminated blastomycosis before therapy with ketoconazole (171). Such initial evaluation may also be important because systemic asymptomatic blastomycosis was more frequent than previously thought *(172)*. Furthermore, blastomycomas, which are a common form of involvement when the CNS is infected by *B. dermatitidis*, may have a long asymptomatic phase *(173)*. Recently, Klein and Jones *(174)* described a radioimmunoassay for antibodies to the 120 kDa *B. dermatitidis* surface immunoprotein that may also prove useful in detecting early CNS involvement.

Hii et al. *(70)* described the successful use of high-dose ketoconazole in a renal-transplant recipient with pulmonary blastomycosis and evidence of systemic dissemination. The drug was given orally at 400 mg twice daily; random measuring produced ketoconazole levels of 3.22 and 4.56 µmol/L. Initiation of cyclosporin therapy was contraindicated because of its excessive nephrotoxicity *(175)*. Following the termination of ketoconazole medication, a relapse prompted the reinstitution of low-dose ketoconazole as chronic suppressive therapy *(70)*. Miliary blastomycosis in an HIV-positive patient with insulin-dependent diabetes mellitus was successfully treated with 800-mg daily doses of ketoconazole; follow-up at 3 mo showed complete clinical and radiologic resolution of the infection *(176)*.

A recent communication by Nouira et al. *(177)* described the successful use of ketoconazole in the treatment of one case of cutaneopulmonary blastomycosis, which is weakly endemic in Tunisia.

Despite its therapeutic activity, a number of reports *(69,74,75,164,178,179)* have indicated failures of ketoconazole to treat blastomycosis, including early (primary) failure as well as late (post-treatment) relapse, mainly due to poor patient compliance or early termination of therapy *(74,158,159,178)*, altered host immunity *(69)*, altered drug absorption *(180)*, and drug interactions *(181)*. Hebert et al. *(180)* described an unusual case in an otherwise healthy patient with pulmonary blastomycosis, in which therapy with oral ketoconazole resulted in failure with dissemination following a prolonged (5-mo) and apparently effective initial response to 400 mg daily of the drug.

4.2.2. Itraconazole

Itraconazole is a new triazole antifungal agent with a broad spectrum of activity against superficial and systemic mycosis. Like other azole antimycotics, its mechanism of action involves the impairment of ergosterol biosynthesis, resulting in damage of the permeability and other functions of the fungal cell wall *(182)*.

In preclinical studies, itraconazole, when given orally to mice at daily doses of 50–150 mg/kg, was protective against lethal infection of *B. dermatitidis*. Although the infection was not sterilized, itraconazole was found to be three times more potent than ketoconazole *(183)*.

Since its introduction to the clinic, itraconazole has become the treatment of choice for nonlife threatening *B. dermatitidis* infections occurring in immunocompetent individuals *(156)*.

At daily doses of 200 mg given to 42 patients (including 13 patients who had either progression of disease while earlier on ketoconazole medication, or a relapse following cure of blastomycosis with ketoconazole), all treated patients had a rapid initial response to the drug *(100)*. In the first documented case of blastomycosis in Namibia, a 42-yr-old man was successfully treated with itraconazole *(184)*.

A 3-wk course of oral itraconazole monotherapy (200 mg, once daily) elicited good clinical response (apyrexia and resolution of ascites) in a female patient with genital blastomycosis that presented as an ovarian tumor *(101)*.

In a multicenter, prospective, nonrandomized, open clinical trial involving 48 patients with blastomycosis, itraconazole was administered at daily doses ranging between 200 and 400 mg *(102)*. Patients receiving other systemic antifungal therapy were excluded. The observed success rate was 90% (43 of 48 patients); when patients were treated for more than 2 mo, the success rate was 95% (38 of 40). The median duration of a successful therapy was determined at 6.2 mo; the median duration of post-treatment evaluation for successfully treated patients was 11.9 mo.

So far, results have shown good absorption and effective oral activity of itraconazole in the treatment of nonmeningeal, non-life-treatening blastomycosis (Table 1) *(27,98,100–103,105–107,167,184–186)*. Ralph et al. *(187)* treated case of severe pulmonary blastomycosis with oral itraconazole.

The major advantage of itraconazole over ketoconazole was the lower rate of endocrinopathic toxicity (Table 2) *(167,184,188)*. Based on its efficacy and the absence of serious adverse side effects following prolonged treatment, itraconazole should replace amphotericin B as the drug of choice for therapy of acute non-life-threatening or chronic blastomycosis (Table 1) *(27,95,98,103,189)*.

4.2.3. Fluconazole

While an ongoing evaluation of fluconazole for treatment of nonacute blastomycosis is underway at daily doses of 200–400 mg, at least for now, it appears that the drug is not very effective in the management of blastomycosis *(167)*. For example, in a small number of patients, fluconazole at daily doses of 50 mg did not cure blastomycosis. It is possible, however, that this unsatisfactory result may be due to dose inadequacy rather than to deficiency of the drug *(35)*.

Nevertheless, Pearson et al. *(190)* described two cases of systemic blastomycosis that were successfully treated with fluconazole. One case involved infection of the respiratory tract and presumably the CNS, whereas the second case consisted only of pulmonary blastomycosis. Both patients received oral fluconazole given at 200 mg twice daily for 6 and 9 mo, respectively. The two patients had complete resolution of the disease and stayed asymptomatic for more than 6 mo after completion of therapy.

Taillan et al. *(191)* reported an unusual case of blastomycosis in the brain stem. The abscess was successfully treated with a combination of fluconazole and flucytosine *(192)*.

In a recently completed a multicenter, randomized, open-label pilot study *(104)*, two daily oral doses (200 and 400 mg) of fluconazole were found to be only moderately effective for the treatment of non-life threatening, nonmeningeal blastomycosis; the treatment was successful in 15 of 23 evaluable patients (65%), including 8 of 16 patients (63%) who received the 200-mg dose, and 7 of 10 (70%) patients treated with the 400-mg dose. The toxicity of the drug was minimal: rash, diarrhea, constipation, stomach cramps, mildly elevated liver function tests, and reversible alopecia *(135)* were each seen in one patient, and nausea was seen in four patients (Table 2) *(104)*. Overall, fluconazole appeared to be less effective than itraconazole for the treatment of blastomycosis.

4.2.4. Miconazole

Miconazole is an intravenously administered azole antimycotic with activity against *B. dermatitidis*. However, because of its adverse side effects, adequate trials have not been carried out *(100)*.

4.3. Treatment of Adult Respiratory Distress Syndrome (ARDS) Secondary to Blastomycosis

One unusual—and if left untreated, a potentially very dangerous or even fatal complication of blastomycosis is adult respiratory distress syndrome (ARDS) *(4,17,59,195–208)*. It is the pulmonary manifestation of a diffuse microcirculatory injury that results in exudation of a protein-rich fluid into the pulmonary interstitium and alveolary spaces *(209)*. Pulmonary fibroproliferation, is one of the leading causes of death in patients with late ARDS. However, its course may be reversed after therapy with high doses of corticosteroids (HDC). Results from large, prospective clinical investigations have indicated that short-course (48 h or less) of HDC therapy had no benefit when applied at the onset of ARDS *(210–214)*. However, HDC therapy has been reported effective if initiated in late-stage or chronic ARDS *(93,209,215–222)*. Thus, Meduri et al. *(209)* reported that prolonged treatment of nine patients with late ARDS with HDC, given intravenously, resulted in a marked and rapid improvement in the lung injury score ($p < 0.003$ at 5 d). An initial bolus dose of 2.0 mg/kg of methylprednisolone sodium succinate was followed by 2.0–3.0 mg/kg doses at 6-h intervals; the dose was tapered based on the patient's pulmonary physiologic response. Most complications of the HDC therapy were infections (*P. aeruginosa, P. maltophilia*); all patients had received gastrointestinal prophylaxis with intravenous ranitidine. Because of the immunosuppressive activity and impairment of wound healing of HDC, caution should be applied when considering such a therapy, especially in immunocompromised patients *(120)*.

Describing a case of overwhelming pulmonary blastomycosis associated with ARDS, Meyer et al. *(207)* recommended aggressive therapy in which the dose of amphotericin B should be increased as rapidly as possible—within 24 to 48 h—to a daily maintenance dose of 0.7–1.0 mg/kg (or a maximum of 70 mg). Because of the life-threatening potential of ARDS, amphotericin B should still remain as primary therapy for this condition.

REFERENCES

1. Broc, R. and Haddad, N. Tumeur bronchique a *Scopulariopsis americana*, determination precoce d'une maladie de Gilchrist. *Bul. Mem. Soc. Med. Des Hop. Paris*, 68, 679, 1952.
2. Vermeil, C., Gordeeff, A., and Haddad, N. Sur un cas Tunisien de mycose generalisee mortelle. *Ann. Inst. Pasteur*, 86, 636, 1954.
3. Bhagwandeen, S. B. North American blastomycosis in Zambia. *Am. J. Trop. Med.*, 23, 231, 1974.
4. Campos Magalhaes, M., Drouhet, E., and Destombes, P. Premier cas de blastomycose a *Blastomyces dermatitidis* observe au Mozambique. *Bul. Soc. Pathol. Exot. Fil.*, 61, 210, 1968.
5. Drouhet, E., Enjalbert, L., Planques, J., Bollinelli, R., Moreau, G., and Sabatier, A. A propos d'un cas de blastomycose a localisations multiples chez un Francais d'origine Tunisienne. *Bul. Soc. Pathol. Exot. Fil.*, 61, 202, 1968.
6. Emmons, C. W., Murray, I. G., Lurie, H. I., King, M. H., Tulloch, J. A., and Connor, D. H. North American blastomycosis: two autochthonous cases from Africa. *Sabouraudia*, 3, 306, 1964.
7. Fragoyannis, S., VanWyk, G., and Debeer, M. North American blastomycosis in South Africa. *S. Afr. Med. J.*, 51, 169, 1977.
8. Gatti, F., Renoirte, R., and Vandepitte, J. Premier cas de blastomycose nord-americaine observee au Congo (Leopoldville). *Ann. Soc. Belge Med. Trop.*, 44, 1057, 1964.
9. Rippon, J. W. *Medical Mycology*. W. B. Saunders, Philadelphia, 438, 1988.
10. Ibrahim, T. M. and Edinol, S. T. Pleural effusion from blastomycetes in an adult Nigerian: a case report. *Niger. Postgrad. Med. J.*, 8, 148–149, 2001.
11. Escovich, L. and Pilafis, M. Unusual clinical forms of south American blastomycosis. Report of two new cases. *Med. Oral.*, 4, 619–625, 1999.
12. El Haouri, M., Sedrati, O., Erragragui, Y., et al. Cutaneous blastomycosis revealing a corticoadenoma. *Ann. Dermatol. Venereol.*, 128, 253–256, 2001.
13. Kane, J., Righter, J., Krajden, S., and Lester, R. S. Blastomycosis: a new endemic region in Canada. *Can. Med. Assoc. J.*, 129, 728, 1983.
14. Kepron, N. W., Schoemperlen, C. B., Hershfield, E. S., Zylak, C.J., and Cherniack, R. M. North American blastomycosis in Central Canada: a review of 36 cases. *Can. Med. Assoc. J.*, 106, 243, 1972.
15. Klein, B. S., Vergeront, J. M., DiSalvo, A. F., Kaufman, L., and Davis, J. P. Two outbrakes of blastomycosis along rivers in Wisconsin: isolation of *Blastomyces dermatitidis* from riverbank soil and evidence of its transmission along waterways. *Am. Rev. Respir. Dis.*, 136, 1333, 1987.
16. Sarosi, G. A. and Davies, S. F. Blastomycosis. *Compr. Ther.*, 12, 31, 1986.
17. Lemos, L. B., Baliga, M., and Guo, M. Acute respiratory distress syndrome and blastomycosis: presentation of nine cases and review of the literature. *Ann. Diagn. Pathol.*, 5, 1–9, 2001.
18. Lemos, L. B., Guo, M., and Baliga, M. Blastomycosis: organ involvement and etiologic diagnosis. A review of 123 patients from Mississippi. *Ann. Diagn. Pathol.*, 4, 391–406, 2000.
19. Thompson, C. A., McEachern, R., and Norman, J. R. Blastomycosis as an etiology of acute lung injury. *South. Med. J.*, 91, 861–863, 1998.
20. Battle, S. E., Skillman, D. R., Maguire, J. H., and Bennett, K. S. Acquired immunodeficiency syndrome-related blastomycosis in an unusual geographic location. *Mil. Med.*, 166, 1026–1028, 2001.
21. Bradsher, R. W. Systemic fungal infections: diagnosis and treatment. I. Blastomycosis. *Infect. Dis. Clin. North Am.*, 2, 877, 1988.
22. Dismukes, W. E. Blastomycosis: leave it to beaver. *N. Engl. J. Med.*, 314, 575, 1986.
23. Klein, B. S., Vergeront, J. M., Weeks, R. J., et al. Isolation of *Blastomyces dermatitidis* in soil associated with a large outbreak of blastomycosis in Wisconsin. *N. Engl. J. Med.*, 314, 529, 1986.
24. McDonough, E. S., Wisniewski, T. R., Penn, L. A., Chan, D. M., and McNamara, W. J. Preliminary studies on conidial liberation of *Blastomyces dermatitidis* and *Histoplasma capsulatum*. *Sabouraudia*, 14, 199, 1976.
25. Denton, J. F., McDonough, E. S., Ajello, L., and Ausherman R. J. Isolation of *Blastomyces dermatitidis* from soil. *Science*, 133, 1126, 1961.
26. Tenenbaum, M. J., Greenspan, J., and Kerkering, T. M. Blastomycosis. *Crit. Rev. Microbiol.*, 9, 139, 1982.
27. Bradsher, R. W. Histoplasmosis and blastomycosis. *Clin. Infect. Dis.*, 22(Suppl. 2), S102, 1996.
28. Sarosi, G. A., Eckman, M. R., Davies, S. R., and Laskey, W. K. Canine blastomycosis as a harbinger of human disease. *Ann. Intern. Med.*, 91, 733, 1979.
29. McDonough, E. S. and Kuzma, J. F. Epidemiological studies on blastomycosis in the state of Wisconsin. *Sabouraudia*, 18, 173, 1980.
30. Sarosi, G. A. and Serstock, D. S. Isolation of *Blastomyces dermatitidis* from pigeon manure. *Am. Rev. Respir. Dis.*, 114, 1179, 1976.

31. Armstrong, C. W., Jenkins, S. R., Kaufman, L., Kerkering, T. M., Rouse, B. S., and Miller, G. B. Jr. Common-source outbreak of blastomycosis in hunters and their dogs. *J. Infect. Dis.*, 155, 568, 1987.
32. Furcolow, M. L., Chick, E. W., Busey, J. D., and Menges, R. W. Prevalence and incidence studies of human and canine blastomycosis. I. Cases in the United States, 1885–1968. *Am. Rev. Respir. Dis.*, 102, 60, 1970.
33. Steck, W. D. Blastomycosis. *Dermatol. Clin.*, 7, 241, 1989.
34. Emmons, C. W., Binford, C.H., and Utz, J. P. *Medical Mycology*. Lea & Febiger, Philadelphia, 309, 1970.
35. Bradsher, R. W. Blastomycosis. Fungal infections of the lung: update 1989. *Sem. Respir. Infect.*, 5, 105, 1989.
36. Schwartz, J. and Baum, G. L. Blastomycosis. *Am. J. Clin. Pathol.*, 21, 999, 1951.
37. Pondrom, J., Lee, P., and Stark, P. Diagnostic case study: radiographic findings in pulmonary blastomycosis. *Semin. Respir. Infect.*, 15, 336–338, 2000.
38. Patel, R. G., Patel, B., Petrini, M. F., Carter, R. R. 3rd, and Griffith, J. Clinical presentation, radiographic findings, and diagnostic methods of pulmonary blastomycosis: a review of 100 consecutive cases. *South. Med. J.*, 92, 289–295, 1999.
39. Wiesman, I. M., Podbielski, F. J., Hernan, M. J., Sekosan, M., and Vigneswaran, W. T. Thoracic blastomycosis and empyema. *JSLS*, 3, 75–78, 1999.
40. Koen, A. F. and Blumberg, L. H. North American blastomycosis in South Africa simulating tuberculosis. *Clin. Radiol.*, 54, 260–262, 1999.
41. Hanson, J. M., Spector, G., and El-Mofty, S. K. Laryngeal blastomycosis: a commonly missed diagnosis. Report of two cases and review of the literature. *Ann. Otol. Rhinol. Laryngol.*, 109, 281–286, 2000.
42. Schwartz, J. and Salfelder, K. Blastomycosis: a review of 152 cases. *Curr. Top. Pathol.*, 65, 165, 1977.
43. Muniz, A. E. and Evans, T. Chronic paronychia, osteomyelitis, and paravertebral abscess in a child with blastomycosis. *J. Emerg. Med.*, 19, 245–248, 2000.
44. Bergman, K. R., Sorensen, P., and Sinha, C. Disseminated blastomycosis presenting as neck mass. *Otolaryngol. Head Neck Surg.*, 122, 270–271, 2000.
45. Schweinfurth, J. M. and Powitzky, E. Cervical manifestation of blastomycosis. *Am. J. Otolaryngol.*, 22, 157–159, 2001.
46. Verma, K. K., Lakhanpal, S., Sirka, C. S., D'souza, P., Khaitan, B. B., and Banerjee, U. Disseminated mucocutaneous blastomycosis in a immunocompetent Indian patient. *J. Eur. Acad. Dermatol. Venereol.*, 14, 332–333, 2000 [see also: *J. Eur. Acad. Dermatol. Venereol.*, 14, 249–250, 2000].
47. Desai, A. P., Pandit, A. A., and Gupte, P. D. Cutaneous blastomycosis. Report of a case with diagnosis by fine needle aspiration cytology. *Acta Cytol.*, 41(Suppl.), 1217–1319, 1997.
48. Jaspers, R. H. Transmission of *Blastomyces* from animals to man. *J. Am. Vet. Med. Ass.*, 164, 8, 1974.
49. Blackledge, F. A. and Newlands, S. D. Blastomycosis of the petrous apex. *Otolaryngol. Head Neck Surg.*, 124, 347–349, 2001.
50. Chowfin, A., Tight, R., and Mitchell, S. Recurrent blastomycosis of the central nervous system: case report and review. *Clin. Infect. Dis.*, 30, 969–971, 2000.
51. Mirra, S. S., Trombley, I. K., and Miles, M. L. Blastomycoma of the cerebelum: an ultrastructural study. *Acta Neuropathol.*, 50, 109, 1990.
52. Hadjipavlou, A. G., Mader, J. T., Nauta, H. J., Necessary, J. T., Chaljub, G., and Adesokan, A. Blastomycosis of the lumbar spine: case report and review of the literature, with emphasis on diagnostic laboratory tools and management. *Eur. Spine J.*, 7, 416–421, 1998.
53. Li, S., Perlman, J. I., Edward, D. P., and Weiss, R. Unilateral *Blastomyces dermatitidis* endophthalmitis and orbital cellulites. A case report and literature review. *Ophthalmology*, 105, 1466–1470, 1998.
54. Craig, M. W., Davey, W. N., and Green, R. A. Conjugal blastomycosis. *Am. Rev. Respir. Dis.*, 102, 86, 1970.
55. Farber, E. R., Leahy, M. S., and Meadows, T. R. Endometrial blastomycosis acquired by sexual contact. *Obstet. Gynecol.*, 32, 195, 1968.
56. Daniel, L. and Salit, I. E. Blastomycosis during pregnancy. *Can. Med. Assoc. J.*, 131, 759, 1984.
57. Hager, H., Welt, S. I., Cardasis, J. P., and Alvarez, S. Disseminated blastomycosis in a pregnant woman successfully treated with amphotericin B: a case report. *J. Reprod. Med.*, 33, 485, 1988.
58. Ismail, M. A. and Lerner, S. A. Disseminated blastomycosis in a pregnant woman: a review of amphotericin B usage during pregnancy. *Am. Rev. Respir. Dis.*, 126, 350, 1982.
59. MacDonald, D. and Alguire, P. C. Adult respiratory distress syndrome due to blastomycosis during pregnancy. *Chest*, 98, 1527, 1990.
60. Neiberg, A. D., Mavromatis, F., Dyke, J., and Fayyad, A. *Blastomycosis dermatitidis* treated during pregnancy: a case report. *Am. J. Obstet. Gynecol.*, 128, 911, 1977.
61. Watts, E. A., Gard, P.D., and Tuthill, S. W. First reported case of intrauterine transmission of blastomycosis. *Pediatr. Infect. Dis. J.*, 2, 308, 1983.
62. Weinberg, E. D. Pregnancy-associated depression of cell-mediated immunity. *Rev. Infect. Dis.*, 6, 814, 1984.
63. Maxson, S., Miller, S. F., Tryka F., and Schutze, G. E. Perinatal blastomycosis: a review. *Pediatr. Infect. Dis. J.*, 11, 760, 1992.
64. Brandhorst, T. T., Rooney, P. J., Sullivan, T. D., and Klein, B. S. Using new genetic tools to study the pathogenesis of *Blastomyces dermatitidis*. *Trends Microbiol.*, 10, 25–30, 2002.
65. Klein, B. S. Molecular basis of pathogenicity in *Blastomyces dermatitidis*: the importance of adhesin. *Curr. Opin. Microbiol.*, 3, 339–349, 2000.
66. Sarosi, G. A., Hammerman, K. J., Tosh, F. E., and Kronenberg, R. S. Clinical features of acute pulmonary blastomycosis. *N. Engl. J. Med.*, 290, 540, 1974.
67. Ehni, W. Endogenous reactivation in blastomycosis. *Am. J. Med.*, 86, 831, 1989.

68. Butka, B. J., Bennett, S.R., and Johnson, A. C. Disseminated inoculation blastomycosis in a renal transplant recipient. *Am. Rev. Respir. Dis.*, 130, 1180, 1984.
69. Greene, N. B., Baughman, R. P., Kim, C. K., and Roselle, G. A. Failure of ketoconazole in an immunosuppressed patient with pulmonary blastomycosis. *Chest.*, 88, 640, 1985.
70. Hii, J. H., Legault, L., DeVeber, G., and Vas, S. I. Successful treatment of systemic blastomycosis with high-dose ketoconazole in a renal transplant recipient. *Am. J. Kidney Dis.*, 15, 595, 1990.
71. Pechan, W. B., Novick, A. C., Lalli, A., and Gephardt, G. Pulmonary nodules in a renal recipient. *J. Urol.*, 124, 111, 1980.
72. Serody, J. S., Mill, M. R., Detterbeck, F. C., Harris, D. T., and Cohen, M. S. Blastomycosis in transplant recipients: report of a case and review. *Clin. Infect. Dis.*, 16, 54, 1993.
73. Winkler, S., Stanek, G., Hübsch, P., et al. Pneumonia due to *Blastomyces dermatitidis*, in an European renal transplant recipient. *Nephrol. Dial. Transplant.*, 11, 1376, 1996.
74. Bradsher, R. W., Rice, D. C., and Abernathy, R. S. Ketoconazole therapy for endemic blastomycosis. *Ann. Intern. Med.*, 103, 872, 1985.
75. Recht, L. D., Davies, S. F., Eckman, M. R., and Sarosi, G. A. Blastomycosis in immunosuppressed patients. *Am. Rev. Respir. Dis.*, 125, 359, 1982.
76. Hasan, F. M., Jarrah, T., and Nassar, V. The association of adenocarcinoma in the lung and blastomycosis from an unusual geographic location. *Br. J. Dis. Chest*, 72, 242, 1978.
77. Bayer, A. S., Scott, V. J., and Guze, L. B. Fungal arthritis. IV. Blastomycotic arthritis. *Sem. Arthr. Rheum.*, 9, 145, 1979.
78. Logsdon, M. T. and Jones, H. E. North American blastomycosis: a review. *Cutis*, 24, 524, 1979.
79. Mounts, A. and Deepe, G. S. Simultaneous infection with *Blastomyces dermatitidis* and *Cryptococcus neoformans*. *Med. Mycol.*, 36, 47–50, 1998.
80. Georgiev, V. St. Treatment and experimental therapeutics of blastomycosis. *Int. J. Antimicrob. Agents*, 6, 1, 1995.
81. Mundey, K., Varkey, B., VanRuiswyk, J., Yang, F., and Schapira, R. M. Acute respiratory distress syndrome from blastomycosis. *WMJ*, 100, 40-42, 2001.
82. Mercantini, R., Marsella, R., Moretto, D., et al. Macroscopic and microscopic characteristics of an African *Blastomyces dermatitidis* strain. *Mycoses*, 38, 477, 1995.
83. Cohen, L. M., Golitz, L. E., and Wilson, M. L. Widespread papulae and nodules in an Ugandan man with acquired immunodeficiency syndrome: African blastomycosis. *Arch. Dermatol.*, 132, 821, 1996.
84. Raftopoulos, C., Flament-Duvant, J., Coremans-Pelseneer, J., and Noterman, J. Intracerebellar blastomycosis abscess in an African man. *Clin. Neurol. Neurosurg.*, 88, 209, 1986.
85. Frean, J. A., Carman, W. F., Crewe-Brown, H.-H., Culligan, G. A., and Young, C. N. *Blastomyces dermatitidis* infections in the RSA. *S. Afr. Med. J.*, 76, 13, 1989.
86. Lombardi, G., Padhye, A. A., and Ajello, L. *In vitro* conversion of African isolates of *Blastomyces dermatitidis* to their yeast form. *Mycoses*, 31, 447, 1988.
87. Vermeil, C., Morin, O., Miegeville, M., Marjolet, M., and Gordeeff, A. Maladie de Gilchrist et taxonomie fongique: un épineux problème. *Bull. Soc. Pathol. Exit.*, 74, 27, 1981.
88. McGinnis, M. R. *Laboratory Handbook of Medical Mycology*. Academic Press, New York, 479, 1980.
89. Vanbreuseghem, R., De Vroey, C., and Takashio, M. *Practical Guide to Medical and Veterinary Mycology*. Masson, Paris, 28, 1978.
90. Yates-Siilata, K. E., Sander, D. M., and Keath, E. J. Genetic diversity in clinical isolates of the dimorphic fungus *Blastomyces dermatitidis* detected by a PCR-based random amplified polymorphic DNA assay. *J. Clin. Microbiol.*, 33, 2171, 1995.
91. Baily, G. G., Robertson, V. J., Neill, P., Garrido, P., and Levy, L. F. Blastomycosis in Africa: clinical features, diagnosis, and treatment. *Rev. Infect. Dis.*, 13, 1005, 1991.
92. Zeluff, B. J. Fungal pneumonia in transplant recipients. *Sem. Respir. Infect.*, 5, 80, 1990.
93. Meduri, G. U., Chinn, A. J., Leeper, K. V., et al. Corticosteroid rescue treatment of progressive fibroproliferation in late ARDS: patterns of response and predictors of outcome. *Chest*, 105, 1516, 1994.
94. Ellis, D. Amphotericin B. *J. Antimicrob. Chemother.*, 49(Suppl. A), 7–10, 2002.
95. Sarosi, G. A. and Davies, S. F. Therapy for fungal infections. *Mayo Clin. Proc.*, 69, 1111, 1994.
96. Witzig, R. S., Quimosing, E. M., Campbell, W. L., Greer, D. L., and Clark, R. A. *Blastomyces dermatitidis* infection of the paranasal sinuses. *Clin. Infect. Dis.*, 18, 267, 1994.
97. Gottlieb, J. L., McAllister, I. L., Guttman, F. A., and Vine, A. K. Choroidal blastomycosis: a report of two cases. *Retina*, 15, 248, 1995.
98. Pappas, P. G., Threlkeld, M. G., Bedsole, G. D., Cleveland, K. O., Gelfand, M. S., and Desmukes, W. E. Blastomycosis in immunocompromised patients. *Medicine (Baltimore)*, 72, 311, 1993.
99. Saag, M. S. and Dismukes, W. E. Treatment of histoplasmosis and blastomycosis. *Chest*, 93, 848, 1988.
100. Bradsher, R. W. Blastomycosis. *Clin. Infect. Dis.*, 14(Suppl. 1), S82, 1992.
101. Mouzin, E. L. and Beilke, M. A. Female genital blastomycosis: case report and review. *Clin. Infect. Dis.*, 22, 718, 1996.
102. Dismukes, W. E., Bradsher, R. W., Cloud, G. C., et al. Itraconazole therapy for blastomycosis and histoplasmosis. *Am. J. Med.*, 93, 489, 1992.
103. Schutze, G. E., Hickerson, S. L., Fortin, E. M., et al. Blastomycosis in children. *Clin. Infect. Dis.*, 22, 496, 1996.
104. Pappas, P. G., Bradsher, R. W., Chapman, S. W., et al. Treatment of blastomycosis with fluconazole: a pilot study. *Clin. Infect. Dis.*, 20, 267, 1995.
105. Neijens, H. J., Frenkel, J., de Muinck Keiser-Schrama, S. M. P. F., Dzoljic-Danilovic, G., Meradji, M., and Dongen, J.

J. M. Invasive aspergillus infection in chronic gtanulomatous disease: treatment with itraconazole. *J. Pediatr.*, 115, 1016, 1989.
106. Bhandari, V. and Narang, A. Oral itraconazole therapy for disseminated candidiasis in low birth weight infants. *J. Pediatr.*, 120, 330, 1992.
107. Mony, R., Veber, F., Blanche, S., et al. Long-term itraconazole prophylaxis against aspergillus infections in thirty-two patients with chronic granulomatous disease. *J. Pediatr.*, 125, 998, 1994.
108. Pitrak, D. L. and Andersen, B. R. Cerebral blastomycoma after ketoconazole therapy for respiratory tract blastomycosis. *Am. J. Med.*, 86, 713, 1989.
109. Witorsch, P. and Utz, J. P. North American blastomycosis: a study of 40 patients. *Medicine (Baltimore)*, 47, 169, 1968.
110. Buchner, H. A. and Clawson, C. M. Blastomycosis of the central nervous system. II. A report of nine cases from the Veteran Administration Cooperative Study. *Am. Rev. Respir. Dis.*, 95, 820, 1967.
111. Gonyea, E. F. The spectrum of primary blastomycosis meningitis: a review of central nervous system blastomycosis. *Ann. Neurol.*, 3, 26, 1978.
112. Busey, J. F. Blastomycosis. III. A comparative study of 2-hydroxystilbamide and amphotericin B therapy. *Am. Rev. Respir. Dis.*, 105, 812, 1972.
113. Carmody, E. J. and Tappen, W. Blastomycosis meningitis: report of a case successfully treated with amphotericin B. *Ann. Intern. Med.*, 51, 139, 1959.
114. Kravitz, G. R., Davies, S. F., Eckman, M. R., and Sarosi, G. A. Chronic blastomycotic meningitis. *Am. J. Med.*, 71, 501, 1981.
115. Larkin, J. C., Young, J. M., and Sutliff, W. D. Clinicopathologic conference: systemic blastomycosis involving urinary tract and skin. *J. Tennesee Med. Ass.*, 66, 1141, 1973.
116. Lockwood, W. R., Allison, F., Batson, B. E., and Busey, J. F. The treatment of North American blastomycosis, ten years' experience. *Am. Rev. Respir. Dis.*, 100, 314, 1969.
117. Loudon, R. G. and Lawson, R. A. Systemic blastomycosis: recurrent neurological relapse in a case treated with amphotericin B. *Ann. Intern. Med.*, 55, 139, 1961.
118. Parker, J. D., Doto, I. L., and Tosh, F. E. A decade of experience with blastomycosis and its treatment with amphotericin B. *Am. Rev. Respir. Dis.*, 99, 895, 1969.
119. Rainey, R. L. and Harris, T. R. Disseminated blastomycosis with meningeal involvement. *Arch. Intern. Med.*, 117, 744, 1966.
120. Seaburg, J. H. and Dascomb, H. E. Results of the treatment of systemic mycosis. *J. Am. Med. Assoc.*, 188, 509, 1964.
121. Johnson, P. and Sarosi, G. Current therapy of major fungal diseases of the lung. *Infect. Dis. Clin. North Am.*, 5, 635, 1991.
122. Furcolow, M. C., Watson, K. A., Tisdall, O. F., Julian, W. A., Saliba, N. A., and Balows, A. Some factors affecting survival in systemic blastomycosis. *Dis. Chest*, 54, 285, 1968.
123. Phillips, J. R., Jones, S., Adamson, J. S., and Abernathy, R. S. Long-term follow-up of 101 patients with blastomycosis. *Am. Rev. Respir. Dis.*, 105, 1006, 1972.
124. Mikaelian, A. J., Varkey, B., and Grossman, T. W. Blastomycosis of the head and neck. *Otolaryngol. Head Neck Surg.*, 101, 489, 1989.
125. Lewis, H., Aaberg, T. M., Fary, D. R., and Stevens, T. S. Latent disseminated blastomycosis with choroidal involvement. *Arch. Ophthalmol.*, 106, 527, 1988.
126. Lopez, R., Mason, J. O., Parker, J. S., and Pappas, P. G. Intraocular blastomycosis: case report and review. *Clin. Infect. Dis.*, 18, 805, 1994.
127. Albert, M. C., Zachary, S. V., and Alter, S. Blastomycosis of the forearm synovium in a child. *Clin. Orthop.*, 317, 223, 1995.
128. Bradsher, R. W., Martin, M. R., Wilkes, T. D., Waltman, C., and Bolyard, K. Unusual presentations of blastomycosis: ten case summaries. *Infect. Med.*, 7, 10, 1990.
129. Sarosi, G. A. and Davies, S. F. Blastomycosis: state of the art. *Am. Rev. Respir. Dis.*, 120, 911, 1979.
130. Gallis, H. A., Drew, R. H., and Pickard, W. W. Amphotericin B: 30 years of clinical experience. *Rev. Infect. Dis.*, 12, 308, 1990.
131. Conant, N. F. and Howell, A. Similarity of the fungi causing South American blastomycosis (paracoccidial granuloma) and North American blastomycosis (Gilchrist's disease). *J. Invest. Dermatol.*, 5, 353, 1942.
132. Georgiev, V. St. Treatment and developmental therapeutics in aspergillosis. 1. Amphotericin B and its derivatives. *Respiration*, 59, 291, 1992.
133. Georgiev, V. St. Treatment and developmental therapeutics in aspergillosis. 2. Azoles and other antifungal drugs. *Respiration*, 59, 303, 1992.
134. Georgiev, V. St. Opportunistic/nosocomial infections: treatment and developmental therapeutics. II. Cryptococcosis. *Med. Res. Rev.*, 13, 507, 1993.
135. Pappas, P. G., Kauffman, C. A., Perfect, J., et al. Alopecia associated with fluconazole therapy. *Ann. Intern. Med.*, 123, 354, 1995; [see comment in *Ann. Intern. Med.*, 125, 153, 1996].
136. Ellis, W. G., Sobel, R. A., and Nielsen, S. L. Leukoencephalopathy in patients treated with amphotericin B methyl ester. *J. Infect. Dis.*, 146, 125, 1982.
137. Graybill, J. R. and Kaster, S. R. Experimental murine aspergillosis: comparison of amphotericin B and a new polyene antifungal drug, SCH 28191. *Am. Rev. Respir. Dis.*, 129, 292, 1984.
138. Hoeprich, P. D. Amphotericin B methyl ester and leukoencephalopathy: the other side of the coin. *J. Infect. Dis.*, 146, 173, 1982.

139. Lawrence, R. M. and Hoeprich, P. D. Comparison of amphotericin B and amphotericin B methyl ester: efficacy in murine coccidioidomycosis and toxicity. *J. Infect. Dis.*, 133, 168, 1976.
140. Cook, P. P. Amphotericin B lipid complex for the treatment of recurrent blastomycosis of the brain in a patient previously treated with itraconazole. *South. Med. J.*, 94, 548–549, 2001.
141. Graybill, J. R., Craven, P. C., Taylor, R. L., Williams, D. M., and Magee, W. E. Treatment of murine cryptococcosis with liposome-associated amphotericin B. *J. Infect. Dis.*, 145, 748, 1982.
142. Hopfer, R. L., Mills, K., Mehta, R., Lopez-Berestein, G., Fainstein, V., and Juliano, R. L. In vitro antifungal activities of amphotericin B and liposome-encapsulated amphotericin B. *Antimicrob. Agents Chemother.*, 25, 387, 1984.
143. Lopez-Berestein, G. Liposomes as carriers of antifungal drugs. *Ann. NY Acad. Sci.*, 544, 590, 1988.
144. Lopez-Berestein, G., Bodey, G. P., Fainstein, V., et al. Treatment of systemic fungal infections with liposomal amphotericin B. *Arch. Intern. Med.*, 149, 2533, 1989.
145. Patterson, T. F., Miniter, P., Dijkstra, J., Szoka, F., Ryan, J. L., and Andriole, V. T. Treatment of experimental invasive aspergillosis with novel amphotericin B/cholesterol-sulfate complexes. *J. Infect. Dis.*, 159, 717, 1989.
146. Shirhoda, A., Lopez-Berestein, G., Holbert, J. M., and Luna, M. A. Hepatosplenic fungal infection: CT and pathologic evaluation after treatment with liposomal amphotericin B. *Radiology*, 159, 349, 1986.
147. Szoka, F. C., Mulholland, D., and Barza, M. Effect of lipid composition and liposome size on toxicity and in vitro fungicidal activity of liposome-intercalated amphotericin B. *Antimicrob. Agents Chemother.*, 31, 421, 1987.
148. Taylor, R. L., Williams, D. M., Craven, P. C., Graybill, J. R., Drutz, D. J., and Magee, W. E. Amphotericin B in liposomes: a novel therapy for histoplasmosis. *Am. Rev. Respir. Dis.*, 125, 610, 1982.
149. Tremblay, C., Barza, M., Fiore, C., and Szoka, F. Efficacy of liposome-intercalated amphotericin B in the treatment of systemic candidiasis in mice. *Antimicrob. Agents Chemother.*, 26, 170, 1984.
150. Weber, R. S. and Lopez-Berestein, G. Treatment of invasive *Aspergillus* sinusitis with liposomal-amphotericin B. *Laryngoscope*, 97, 937, 1987.
151. Wiebe, V. J., and DeGregorio, M. W. Liposome-encapsulated amphotericin B: a promising new treatment for disseminated fungal infections. *Rev. Infect. Dis.*, 10, 1097, 1988.
152. Adler-Moore, J. and Proffitt, R. T. AmBisome: liposomal formulation, structure, mechanism of action and preclinical experience. *J. Antimicrob. Chemother.*, 49(Suppl. A), 21–30, 2002.
153. Clemons, K. V. and Stevens, D. A. Comparative efficacies of amphotericin B lipid complex and amphotericin B deoxycholate suspension against murine blastomycosis. *Antimicrob. Agents Chemother.*, 35, 2144, 1991.
154. Clemons, K. V. and Stevens, D. A. Therapeutic efficacy of a liposomal formulation of amphotericin B (AmBisome) against murine blastomycosis. *J. Antimicrob. Chemother.*, 32, 465, 1993.
155. Clemons, K. V., Ranney, D. F., and Stevens, D. A. A novel heparin-coated hydrophilic preparation of amphotericin B hydrosomes. *Curr. Opin. Investig. Drugs*, 2, 480–487, 2001.
156. Lortholary, O., Denning, D. W., and Dupont, B. Endemic mycoses: a treatment update. *J. Antimicrob. Chemother.*, 43, 321–331, 1999.
157. Witsell, D. L., Yarbrough, W. G., Garrett, C. G., and Weissler, M. C. Treatment of isolated laryngeal blastomycosis with ketoconazole. *N. C. Med. J.*, 55, 588, 1994.
158. Dismukes, W. E., Cloud, G., Bowles, C., et al. Treatment of blastomycosis and histoplasmosis with ketoconazole: result of a prospective, randomized clinical trial. *Ann. Intern. Med.*, 103, 861, 1985.
159. Dismukes, W. E., Stamm, A. M., Graybill, J. R., et al. Treatment of systemic mycoses with ketoconazole: emphasis on toxicity and clinical response in 52 patients. *Ann. Intern. Med.*, 98, 13, 1983.
160. Graybill, J. R. and Drutz, D. J. Ketoconazole: a major innovation for treatment of fungal disease. *Ann. Intern. Med.*, 93, 921, 1980.
161. Reynolds, R. J. and Burford, J. G. Blastomycosis, in *Conn's Current Therapy*, Rakel, R. E., Ed. W. B. Saunders, Philadelphia, 921, 1987.
162. Ahasan, H. A., Rahman, K. M., Chowdhury, M. A., Azhar, M. A., and Rafiqueuddin, A. K. Pulmonary blastomycosis. *Trop. Doct.*, 25, 83, 1995.
163. Hudson, C. P. and Callen, J. P. Systemic blastomycosis treated with ketoconazole. *Arch. Dermatol.*, 120, 536, 1984.
164. McManus, E. J. and Jones, J. M. The use of ketoconazole in the treatment of blastomycosis. *Am. Rev. Respir. Dis.*, 133, 141, 1986.
165. Ferguson, R. M., Sutherland, D. E. R., Simmons, R. L., and Najarian, J. S. Ketoconazole, cyclosporin metabolism, and renal transplantation. *Lancet*, 2, 882, 1982.
166. Abernathy, R. S. Amphotericin therapy of North American blastomycosis. *Antimicrob. Agents Chemother.*, 3, 208, 1967.
167. Saag, M. S. and Desmukes, W. E. Azole antifungal agents: emphasis on new triazoles. *Antimicrob. Agents Chemother.*, 32, 1, 1988.
168. Daneshmend, T. K., Warnock, D. W., Turner, A., and Roberts, C. J. C. Pharmacokinetics of ketoconazole in normal subjects. *J. Antimicrob. Chemother.*, 8, 299, 1981.
169. Pont, A., Graybill, J. R., Craven, P. C., et al. High-dose ketoconazole therapy and adrenal and testicular function in humans. *Arch. Intern. Med.*, 144, 2150, 1984.
170. Lewis, J. H., Zimmerman, H. J., Benson, G. D., and Ishak, K. G. Hepatic injury associated with ketoconazole therapy. *Gastroenterology*, 86, 503, 1984.
171. Yancey, R. W. Jr., Perlino, C. A., and Kaufman, L. Asymptomatic blastomycosis of the central nervous system with progression in patients given ketoconazole therapy: a report of two cases. *J. Infect. Dis.*, 164, 807, 1991.
172. Sugar, A. M., Alsip, S. G., Galgiani, J. N., et al. Pharmacology and toxicity of high dose ketoconazole. *Antimicrob. Agents Chemother.*, 31, 1874, 1987.

173. Turner, S., Kaufman, L., and Jalbert, M. Diagnostic assessment of an enzyme-linked immunosorbent assay for human and canine blastomycosis. *J. Clin. Microbiol.*, 23, 294, 1986.
174. Klein, B. S. and Jones, J. M. Isolation, purification, and radiolabeling of a novel 120-kD surface protein on *Blastomyces dermatitidis* yeasts to detect antibody in infected patients. *J. Clin. Invest.*, 85, 152–161, 1990.
175. Kahan, B. D. Cyclosporine nephrotoxicity: pathogenesis, prophylaxis, therapy and prognosis. *Am. J. Kidney Dis.*, 8, 323, 1986.
176. Herd, A. M., Greenfield, S. B., Thompson, W. S., and Brunham, R. C. Miliary blastomycosis and HIV infection. *Can. Med. Assoc. J.*, 143, 1329, 1990.
177. Nouira, R., Denguezli, M., Skhiri, S., et al. Cutaneopulmonary blastomycosis. *Ann. Dermatol. Venereol.*, 121, 180, 1994.
178. Thiele, J. S., Bueckner, H. A., and Cook, E. W. Failure of ketoconazole in two patients with blastomycosis. *Am. Rev. Respir. Dis.*, 128, 763, 1983.
179. Serneels, R. A., Marshall, G. S., Wampler, J., Miller, D., and Adams, G. Pulmonary sequestration with primary blastomycosis: failure of ketoconazole therapy after resection. *Chest*, 103, 1291, 1993.
180. Hebert, C. A., King, J. W., and George, J. B. Late dissemination of pulmonary blastomycosis during ketoconazole therapy. *Chest*, 95, 240, 1989.
181. Abadie-Kemmerly, S., Pankey, G. A., and Dalvisio, J. R. Failure of ketoconazole treatment of *Blastomyces dermatitidis* due to interaction of isoniazid and rifampin. *Ann. Intern. Med.*, 106, 844, 1988.
182. Zuckerman, J. M. and Tunkel, A. R. Itraconazole: a new triazole antifungal agent. *Infect. Control Hosp. Epidemiol.*, 15, 397, 1994.
183. Arathoon, E. G., Brummer, E., and Stevens, D. A. Efficacy of itraconazole in blastomycosis in a murine model and comparison with ketoconazole. *Mycoses*, 32(Suppl. 1), 109, 1989.
184. Brummer, E., Bhagavathula, P.R., Hanson, L. H., and Stevens, D. A. Synergy of itraconazole with macrophages in killing *Blastomyces dermatitidis*. *Antimicrob. Agents Chemother.*, 36, 2487, 1992.
185. Van Cauteren, H. J., Heykants, J., De Coster, R., and Cauwenbergh, G. Itraconazole: pharmacologic studies in animals and humans. *Rev. Infect. Dis.*, 9(Suppl.), 43, 1987.
186. Kauffman, C. A. Newer developments in therapy for endemic mycosis. *Clin. Infect. Dis.*, 19(Suppl. 1), S28, 1994.
187. Ralph, E. D., Plaxton, W. R., and Sharpe, M. D. Treatment of severe pulmonary blastomycosis with oral itraconazole: case report. *Clin. Infect. Dis.*, 29, 1336–1337, 1999.
188. Dismukes, W. E. Azole antifungal drugs: old and new. *Ann. Intern. Med.*, 109, 177, 1988.
189. Bayles, M. A. Tropical mycoses. *Chemotherapy*, 38(Suppl. 1), 27, 1992.
190. Pearson, G. J., Chin, T. W., and Fong, I. W. Case report: treatment of blastomycosis with fluconazole. *Am. J. Med. Sci.*, 303, 313, 1992.
191. Taillan, B., Ferrari, E., Cosnefroy, J. Y., et al. Blastomycosis localized in the brain stem. *Presse Med.*, 21, 207, 1992.
192. Taillan, B., Ferrari, E., Cosnefroy, J. Y., et al. Favourable outcome of blastomycosis of the brain stem with fluconazole and flucytosine treatment. *Ann. Med.*, 24, 71, 1992.
193. Skillrud, D. M. and Douglass, W. W. Survival in adult respiratory distress syndrome caused by blastomycosis infection. *Mayo Clin. Proc.*, 60, 266, 1985.
194. Thiele, J. S., Buechner, H. A., and Deshotels, S. J. Jr. Blastomycosis and the adult respiratory distress syndrome. *J. Louis. State Med. Soc.*,136, 38, 1984.
195. Unger, J. M., Peters, M. E., and Hinke, M. L. Chest case of the day. *Am. J. Roentgenol.*, 146, 1080, 1986.
196. Kubota, T. Acute respiratory distress syndrome. *Nippon Rinsho*, 60(Suppl. 1), 64-76, 2002.
197. Gerlach, H. Treatment of the acute respiratory distress syndrome (ARDS). *Dtsch. Med. Wochenschr.*, 126, 1173–1177, 2001.
198. Brower, R. G., Ware, L. B., Bethiaume, Y., and Mattay, M. A. Treatment of ARDS. *Chest*, 120, 1347–1367, 2001.
199. Craft, P. P. A case report of disseminated blastomycosis and adult respiratory distress syndrome. *J. Family Pract.*, 40, 597, 1995.
200. Recht. L. D., Davies, S. F., Eckman, M. R., and Sarosi, G. A. Blastomycosis in imunosuppressed patients. *Am. Rev. Respir. Dis.*, 125, 359, 1982.
201. Atkinson, J. B. and Curley, T. L. Pulmonary blastomycosis: filamentous forms in an immunocompromised patient with fulminating respiratory failure. *Hum. Pathol.*, 14, 186, 1983.
202. Griffith, J. E. and Campbell, G. D. Acute miliary blastomycosis presenting as fulminating respiratory failure. *Chest*, 75, 630, 1979.
203. Lockridge, R. S. and Glauser, F. L. Adult respiratory distress syndrome secondary to diffuse pulmonary blastomycosis. *South. Med. J.*, 72, 23, 1979.
204. Palmer, P. E. and McFadden, S. W. Blastomycosis. *N. Engl. J. Med.*, 279, 979, 1968.
205. Onal, E., Lopata, M., and Lourenco, R. V. Disseminated pulmonary blastomycosis in an immunosuppressed patient. *Am. Rev. Respir. Dis.*, 113, 83, 1976.
206. Arvanitakis, C., Sen, S. K., and Magnin, G. E. Fulminating fatal pneumonia due to blastomycosis. *Am. Rev. Respir. Dis.*, 105, 827, 1972.
207. Meyer, K. C., McManus, E. J., and Maki, D. G. Overwhelming pulmonary blastomycosis associated with the adult respiratory distress syndrome. *N. Engl. J. Med.*, 329, 1231, 1993.
208. Renston, J. P., Morgan, J., and Dimarco, A. F. Disseminated miliary blastomycosis leading to acute respiratory failure in an urban setting. *Chest*, 101, 1463, 1992.

209. Meduri, G. U., Belenchia, J. M., Estes, R. J., Wunderink, R. G., El Torky, M., and Leeper, K. V. Jr. Fibroproliferative phase of ARDS: clinical findings and effects of corticosteroids. *Chest*, 4, 943, 1991.
210. Bone, R. C., Fisher, C. J. Jr., Clemmer, T. P., Slotman, G. J., and Metz, C. A. Early methylprednisolone treatment for septic syndrome and the adult respiratory distress syndrome. *Chest*, 92, 1032, 1987.
211. Bernard, G. R., Luce, J. M., Sprung, C. L., et al. High- dose corticosteroids in patients with the adult respiratory distress syndrome. *N. Engl. J. Med.*, 317, 1565, 1987.
212. Weigelt, J. A., Norcross, J. F., Broman, K. R., and Snyder, W. H. Early steroid therapy for respiratory failure. *Arch. Surg.*, 120, 536, 1985.
213. Veterans Administration Systemic Sepsis Cooperative Study Group. Effect of high-dose glucocorticoid therapy on mortality in patients with clinical signs of systemic sepsis. *N. Engl. J. Med.*, 317, 659, 1987.
214. Luce, J. M., Montgomery, A. B., Marks, J. D., Turner, J., Metz, C. A., and Murray, J. F. Ineffectiveness of high-dose methylprednisolone in preventing parenchymal lung injury and improving mortality in patients with septic shock. *Am. Rev. Respir. Dis.*, 138, 62, 1988.
215. Mittermayer, C. H., Hassenstein, J., and Riede, U. N. Is shock-induced lung fibrosis reversible? A report on recovery from "Shock-lung." *Pathol. Res. Pract.*, 162, 73, 1978.
216. Passamonte, P. M., Martinez, A. J., and Singh, A. Pulmonary gallium concentration in the adult respiratory distress syndrome. *Chest*, 85, 828, 1984.
217. Ashbaugh, D. G. and Maier, R. V. Idiopathic pulmonary fibrosis in adult respiratory distress syndrome. *Arch. Surg.*, 120, 530, 1985.
218. Hooper, R. G. and Kearl, R. A. Established ARDS treated with a sustained course of adrenocortical steroids. *Chest*, 97, 138, 1990.
219. Hooper, R. G. and Kearl, R. A. Treatment of established ARDS: steroids, antibiotics, and antifungal therapy. *Chest*, 100, 137S, 1991.
220. Suter, P. M. ARDS treated with sustained adrenocortical steroids. *Chest*, 98, 1310, 1990.
221. Ho, S. L., Lewis, G. A., and Young, D. W. Recovery from adult respiratory distress syndrome after high dose corticosteroids. *Intensive Care Med.*, 17, 241, 1991.
222. Meduri, G. U. and Chinn, A. Fibroproliferation in late adult respiratory distress syndrome: pathophysiology, clinical and laboratory manifestations, and response to corticosteroid rescue treatment. *Chest*, 105(Suppl.), 127S, 1994.

30
Aspergillus spp.

1. INTRODUCTION

Aspergillosis may develop as a granulomatous, necrotizing, and cavitary disease that frequently affects the lungs *(1)*, but may also disseminate to other organs *(2)* The causative agents of the disease are fungi belonging to the genus *Aspergillus*. Several *Aspergillus* spp. have been implicated as human pathogens, namely, *A. fumigatus*, *A. niger*, *A. flavus*, *A. terreus*, *A. nidulans*, and *A. clavatus*. Recently, *A. ustus* has also emerged as an opportunistic pathogen in immunocompromised patients *(3)*.

In immunocompetent hosts the *Aspergillus* infection usually results in the development of allergic conditions such as asthma or allergic bronchopulmonary aspergillosis. In general, immunocompetent hosts will rarely develop invasive aspergillosis *(4–9)*. By comparison, the invasive disease is the primary manifestation in immunocompromised patients. Organs involved in disseminated disease include heart, kidney, CNS (sinocranial aspergilosis *[10]*), gastrointestinal tract, spleen, liver, thyroid gland, eye, and the pancreas. The genitourinary system can also be a source or target of disseminated aspergillosis *(11)*.

Major predisposing factors for invasive aspergillosis include hematologic malignancies *(12–20)* and prolonged neutropenia *(21,22)*, bone-marrow and solid organ transplantation *(18,23–48)* (lung recipients in particular *[49–55]*), prosthetic vascular graft *(56)*, chronic administration of adrenal corticosteroids *(57)*, diabetes *(58)*, the insertion of prosthetic devices, indwelling catheters *(59)*, and tissue damage due to prior infection or trauma. Invasive aspergillosis is also becoming an increasingly reported complication in AIDS patients *(60–67)*. There have also been reports of invasive aspergillosis in patients in intensive care units *(68–70)*, in particular those involving patients with chronic respiratory failure *(71)*.

The most common method of infection is through the respiratory tract, resulting in pneumonia followed by sinusitis. However, the pathogen may penetrate across all natural barriers, including cartilage, bone, and the blood vessels, where it may cause thrombosis and infarction *(72)*. *Aspergillus* spores may proliferate extensively in hospital ventilation systems *(72)*; airborne *Aspergillus* spp. related to air-filter change was assosiated with fatal invasive aspergillosis in two mechanically ventilated patients *(73)*.

Pulmonary aspergillosis may express itself into several forms, including: 1) invasive pulmonary aspergillosis (IPA); 2) allergic bronchopulmonary aspergillosis; 3) extrinsic alveolitis; and 4) saprophitic aspergillosis *(22,74,75)*. To this end, it has been reported that noninvasive pulmonary aspergillosis that passes through a period so active that it seems to resemble the invasive form for its entire clinical course *(76)*.

Although the lungs are the major portal of entry, invasion by *Aspergillus* may also occur through the paranasal sinuses, nose, palate, gastrointestinal tract, or skin *(77,78)*. Furthermore, the hematogenous spread shows no marked tissue tropism, and many different viscera (brain, kidneys, liver, thyroid, heart, intestines, esophagus, stomach, larynx) may have lesions *(79–81)*.

From: Opportunistic Infections: Treatment and Prophylaxis
By: Vassil St. Georgiev © Humana Press Inc., Totowa, NJ

In a cluster of cases of invasive aspergillosis in a transplant intensive care unit evidence was presented that debriding and dressing wounds infected with *Aspergillus* spp. may result in aerolization of spores and airborne person-to-person transmission *(70)*.

In immunocompromised patients, lesions containing hyphae within the blood vessels may produce infarction, edema, and hemorrhage *(77)*. Infection may also spread by contiguity. *Aspergillus*-associated osteomyelitis, although rare, have also been descibed *(82)* with the spine being most often affected *(83,84)*; it can been induced hematogenously, by contiguity, or by direct inoculation *(84)*.

Aspergillus infection following total joint arthroplasty may become an extremely serious complication *(85)*. In another severe complication, a fatal fungal abdominal aortic aneurysm developed as a sequel to concomitant prostatic and renal aspergillosis *(86)*.

A report of chronic necrotizing pulmonary aspergillosis *(72)* in patients with pneumoconiosis has emphasized the need to consider such possibility when chronic or progressive upper-lobe infiltrates and cavities are present *(87)*. *Aspergillus* tracheobronchitis is another uncommon clinical form of invasive aspergillosis, with the fungal infection limited exclusively or predominantly to the tracheobronchia tree *(88)*.

Recent data implied about an increase in the incidence of *Aspergillus* empyema thoracis, and the necessity for aggressive treatment of patient with this condition *(89)*.

Mazzoni et al. *(90)* described a case of apparently primary lymph node granulomatous aspergillosis. A survey of cases of primary aspergillosis has shown that granulomatous instead of exudative inflammation patterns have been observed in histologic sections only when neither major nor minor predisposing factors have been detected in the clinical history of the patients *(90)*.

Cases describing *A. fumigatus* pneumonia in patients with systemic lupus erythematosus (SLE) (an autoimmune disorder that has seldom been associated with *Aspergillus* infections *[91]*) have also been reported *(91–93)*. In one such case, Nenoff et al. *(92)* have described a patient with SLE who had been treated by antibiotics and high-dose corticosteroids (a primary risk factor), and developed a fatal peracute disseminated *A. fumigatus* disease involving the central nervous system (CNS). The typical clinical presentation has been fever and cough in patients with SLE and invasive aspergillosis previously treated with corticosteroids, immunosuppressive drugs, and broad-spectrum antibiotics *(91)*.

Pericardial and myocardial aspegillosis are rare manifestations of systemic aspergillosis and should be considered in any immunocompromised patient with long-lasting pulmonary infection, even in the absence of specific cardiac findings *(13)*. Another type of uncommon fungal involvement is pelvic aspergillosis with tubo-ovarian abscess in a renal-transplant recipient *(43)*.

Aspergillus peritonitis may also become complication of continuous ambulatory peritoneal dialysis (CAPD) *(94–96)*. In another case of infection involving indwelling device, Girmenia et al. *(97)* described intravenous catheter-related cutaneous aspergillosis and *A. fumigatus* fungemia in an HIV-positive patient with Burkitt-cell acute lymphocytic leukemia who developed pulmonary aspergillosis with a rapidly fatal outcome, despite recovery from neutropenia and improvement of the underlying malignancy. The unusual severity and rapid spread of the infection, despite normal neutrophil count and prompt antifungal therapy, underscored the risk of catheter-related cutaneous aspergillosis leading to severe deep-seated infection in immunocompromised patients *(97)*.

It is important to note that aspergillosis and mucormycosis *(98,99)*, two types of opportunistic fungal pneumonia, may often be clumped together because of their frequent occurrence in patients with leukemia and lymphoma and because they often invade vascular structures *(100,101)*. However, a number of characteristic radiographic abnormalities should facilitate an appropriate diagnosis and therapy *(100)*.

Tuberculosis is thought to be often associated with aspergillosis *(102,103)*. Furthermore, patients having chronic fibrosing pulmonary sarcoidosis would frequently develop cystic degeneration of the upper lobes as manifested by cysts and cavities *(104)*. Such preexisting parenchymal cavities are frequently the targets of *Aspergillus* colonization and proliferation, resulting in formation of pulmonary aspergilloma *(105,106)*. Fatal hemorrhage from such aspergillomas is considered to be the second most common cause of death in sarcoidosis *(104,107)*.

Aspergillus-related endophthalmitis has been reviewed *(108,109)*.

Cases involving *A. flavus*-related infections, which may often become fatal, include a rare anuria due to bilateral uretral obstruction by the fungus *(110)*, secondary cutaneous aspergillosis in a patient with acute myeloid leukemia following stem-cell transplantation *(12)*, renoureteric aspergilloma *(111)*, pericarditis *(112)*, endocarditis *(113,114)*, infection of the larynx in a patient with Felty's disease *(115)*, keratitis *(116)*, and infection of an aortic bypass *(117)*.

A. niger is one of several fungi implicated in otomycosis, a condition manifested by ear irritation, pruritis, and impairment of hearing *(2)*. The pathogen may invade the ear canal following another infection such as facial dermatophytosis *(2)*. In addition, a case of *A. niger*-associated renal abscess in a HIV-infected patient has also been reported *(65)*.

The first case of hepatitis due to *A. terreus* in an immunodeficient child occurred while the patient was receiving secondary prophylaxis with fluconazole after an episode of pulmonary candidiasis *(118)*. In other reports, *A. terreus* was the cause of fungal discitis in patient with leukemia *(18,19)*, and mycotic aneurysm of the thoracic aorta *(119)*. In an epidemiologic study involving frequently fatal cases of in-hospital *A. terreus* infections of patients with hematologic malignancies, the fungus was cultured from potted plants in the vicinity of the patients *(120)*.

It is not unusual for patients with *Aspergillus*-induced infections to remain asymptomatic with regard to lesion formation *(121)*. The most common symptom is hemoptysis, which has been observed in 50–85% of the patients *(122)*. Although the presence of precipitating antibodies to *Aspergillus* in the serum is found in virtually all immunocompetent patients *(123)*, in those with immune abnormalities, the presence of such antibodies may be an exception *(121)*. Therefore, chest roentgenograms should remain the single most important method of diagnosing pulmonary aspergillosis.

An unusual association of cutaneous *Aspergillus* and cytomegalovirus (CMV) infections in a liver-transplant recipient resulted in death of the patient in spite of treatment with ganciclovir, amphotericin B, and topical terbinafine cream *(124)*.

1.1. Aspergillus-*Related Spondylodiscitis*

Aspergillus spp.-related spondylodiscitis has been a well-defined condition *(17,19,57,125–128)*. Beckers et al. *(57)* described a patient with clinical signs of *Aspergillus* spondylodiscitis occurring 4 mo after the patient received daily inhalation corticosteroids for chronic obstructive pulmonary disease.

2. HOST IMMUNE RESPONSE TO ASPERGILLOSIS

Quantitative and qualitative defects in phagocytic activity render patients particularly susceptible to aspergillosis *(79,129–136)*. The major host defense against *Aspergillus* spp. are the pulmonary alveolar macrophages and peripheral blood polymorphonuclear and mononuclear phagocytes *(137)*. Macrophages have been shown to make up the first line of defense by ingesting and exterminating inhaled conidia of *Aspergillus*, thereby preventing their germination to hyphae *(138–140)*. If fungal hyphae are produced, then the second line of defense, the circulating phagocytes will damage and destroy hyphae by secreting microbicidal oxidative and nonoxidative metabolites *(138,140,141)*. The role of various cytokines on the phagocytic host defense against *Aspergillus* have only recently begun to be defined *(142–147)*.

Studies by Mehrad et al. *(148)* in immunocompetent and neutropenic mice have demonstrated that the macrophage protein-1-α (MIP-1-α) chemokine plays a critical role as mediator of host defense against *A. fumigatus* in the setting of neutropenia.

3. THERAPIES AND TREATMENT OF ASPERGILLOSIS

Among the treatment strategies for *Aspergillus* infections, amphotericin B remains the standard therapy for severe aspergillosis despite the fact that mortality in these patients remains high *(149,150)*. Alternative therapies include combination regimens and itraconazole *(149,150)*.

Pulmonary mycetoma is a characteristic clinical-radiological lesion due to colonization by *Aspergillus* and *Candida* species of preexisting pulmonary cavities following number of diseases *(106)*. Predisposing factors include sequelae of tuberculosis or lung abscess, bronchiectasis, bullous emphysema, leukemia/lymphoma, diabetes mellitus, corticosteroid and/or immunosuppressive therapy, and antiblastic chemotherapy. Treatment of aspergillomas should be dependent on the extension of the disease and clinical conditions of patients, but surgical resection combined with drug therapy, when possible, has been the treatment of choice. Since the first report by Gerstl et al. *(151)*, surgical resection of lesions has been one major option for therapy of aspergillomas *(152–156)*. However, drug therapy of *Aspergillus* infections *(157,158)* has been steadily increasing over the years, especially in those cases where other underlying pulmonary conditions (severe chronic obstructive lung diseases, emphysema, pulmonary fibrosis, and bilateral aspergilloma) may be severe enough to preclude surgical intervention.

The clinical aspects and treatment outcomes of 72 cases of *Aspergillus* sinusitis *(66,159,160)* were analyzed by Min et al. *(161)*, and over a 14-yr period revealed 60 cases of primary type and 12 cases of secondary type, with the maxillary and ethmoid sinuses most commonly affected in both types. Surgery was performed in most cases, and four of these patients after their surgery received chemotherapy with amphotericin B with or without flucytosine. In a single case report, Parker et al. *(162)* described aspergillosis of the sphenoid sinus and associated osteomyelitis of the skull base presenting as a pituitary mass. A postoperative *(67)* gallium (Ga) imaging showed intense uptake in the sphenoid sinus, which resolved after treatment with amphotericin B.

Sinusitis due to *Aspergillus* infection is also more frequently seen in HIV-positive patients *(163)*. In spite of aggressive surgical intervention and systemic antifungal therapy, the prognosis of this invasive infection in these patients is poor.

Allergic fungal rhinosinusitis associated with *Aspergillus* is manifested by a combination of nasal polyposis, crust formation, and sinus cultures yielding the fungus *(164,165)*.

When considering large-scale clinical trials relative to treatments of individual cases, it should be well-understood that multicenter clinical therapy involving a significant number of patients is by far the better choice for a study, because it will not only furnish the necessary information and clinical experience to put into focus the therapeutic efficacy of experimental anti-infectious drugs, but also provide viewpoint and directions necessary for future research. In this context, clinical reports describing treatments of limited number of patients or individual cases, when well-documented, may serve the useful purpose of shedding light on the antifungal activity of various agents, which may otherwise go unnoticed by those involved in drug research and development. In general, however, because of its limited scope, such information, even when valuable, should be viewed with caution in evaluating the therapeutic efficacy of a drug.

3.1. Amphotericin B

Although in the last 30 years or so amphotericin B has remained the drug of choice for treatment of aspergillosis (Table 1) *(157)*, toxicity problems have hindered considerably its use in immunocompromised patients, and its dosage regimens in neutropenic patients are thought to be not very well-defined *(46,166)*. On the positive side, a study by Moosa et al. *(167)* demonstrated that resistance to amphotericin B did not emerge during treatment for invasive aspergillosis.

In a recent study *(168)*, only 26% of cancer patients with aspergillosis when treated with amphotericin B survived their infections, and no patient with persistent neutropenia (<1000 neutrophils/mm^3) survived the infection. It should be emphasized that for the successful treatment of *Aspergillus*

Table 1
Treatment of *Aspergillus* Infections with Amphotericin B

Infection	Route of administration
Pulmonary aspergillosis	Intravenous
	Direct intracavitary instillation:
	transthoracic injection
	paste
	endobronchial instillation
	aerosol
Sinonasal aspergillosis	Intravenous: liposome-encapsulated
Aspergillus-induced endophthalmitis	Intravitreous; Intravenous
Aspergillus-induced peritonitis	Intraperitoneal
Aspergillus-induced empyema/bronchopleural fistula	Intrapleural

pneumonia in immunocompromised patients (even during profound neutropenia), early initiation of amphotericin B therapy is critical *(169,170)*; without prompt intervention, this condition has been frequently fatal, especially when an underlying malignancy did not remit or a bone-marrow recovery did not occur *(171,172)*.

A survey *(173)* of antifungal and surgical treatment of invasive aspergillosis involving 2,121 published cases has shown that the mortality from pulmonary aspergillosis in bone-marrow transplant recipients exceeded 94% regardless of the therapy applied; a similar mortality rate has been attributed to cerebral aspergillosis in all hosts. On average, the rate of response to amphotericin B has been 55%. The antibiotic when administered at daily a dose of 1.0 mg/kg in combination with 5-FC to neutropenic patients with pulmonary aspergillosis who did not received a bone-marrow transplant, lowered the mortality rate; however, relapses were common.

As therapy, the surgical resection of pulmonary tissue in cases of massive hemoptysis associated with pulmonary aspergilloma causes high morbidity and mortality in patients with inadequate pulmonary reserve *(107,121,174,175)*. An alternative therapy in such cases is provided by amphotericin B. For example, Shapiro et al. *(176)* reported the case of successful treatment of four patients with acute hemoptysis by a percutaneously placed catheter and intracavitary infusion of amphotericin B (total of 500 mg); *N*-acetylcysteine was also given in order to facilitate the dissolution of the fungus ball and to help clearing debris, and in one occasion, the instillation of aminocaproic acid was also utilized. Cochrane et al. *(177)* also used intracavitary amphotericin B to treat aspergilloma and recurrent hemoptysis. Intracavitary instillation of amphotericin B (delivered by a flexible fiberoptic bronchoscope) had a beneficial effect on a patient with chronic necrotizing pulmonary aspergillosis (an indolent locally invasive form of *Aspergillus* infection *(178)*.

A case of primary aspergilloma was treated with a total dose of 950 mg of amphotericin B over a period of 32 d; upon completion of therapy, the fungal mass has been reported to resolve *(179)*.

Fisher et al. *(180)* described a clinical study involving patients with invasive aspergillosis (with the majority of them having neutropenia and hematologic neoplasms as underlying disease) lasting for over 5 yr; the therapy comprised amphotericin B (181–1363 mg; mean 717.2 mg) and when necessary pneumonectomy or lobectomy. In another report *(170)*, two patients with *Aspergillus* pneumonia and hematologic neoplasia were successfully treated with amphotericin B (total of 1.8–2.0 g) for a period of 2 mo.

Invasive sinonasal aspergillosis can be severe and frequently, fatal infection in immunocompromised patients with hematologic malignancies *(101,181)*. It may result in bone erosion and extension into soft tissues of the cheek and orbit with facial pain and soft-tissue edema; intracranial extension, if it occurs, may be fatal *(182)*. Further complications include dissemination to noncontiguous structures (sinus, lung, viscera, and brain) leading to 50–80% mortality rate in immunocompromised patients *(180,183)*. Several cases of sinonasal aspergillosis have been reported that were managed by intravenous administration of amphotericin B in combination with surgery (Caldwell-Luc operation and antrostomy) in the invasive variety of the disease *(182)*. An immunocompromised patient with acute lymphoblastic leukemia who presented initially with aspergillosis of the nasopharynx responded rapidly to medication with amphotericin B *(184)*. Kusumoto et al. *(185)* discussed the use of intravenous amphotericin B combined with local lavage of amphotericin B in the treatment of aspergillosis of the maxillary sinus.

In a single case report, Ho et al. *(186)* described *Aspergillus*-induced endophthalmitis after a penetrating injury and primary repair of a scleral wound. Vitrectomy combined with intravitreous and intravenous amphotericin B (40–50 mg/kg daily) therapy for 34 d (total of 1560 mg) resulted in the preservation of useful vision in what appears to be the first successfully treated case of exogenous *Aspergillus* endophthalmitis. A case of localized aspergilloma of the eyelid responded to injections of amphotericin B directly into the lid granuloma *(187)*. Harris and Mill *(188)* used conservative debridement and local amphotericin B irrigation to treat orbital aspergillosis in a patient on a long-term immunosuppressive therapy. Endogenous *A. flavus*-induced endophthalmitis in association with severe periodontitis has been reported by Matsuo et al. *(189)*.

Stereotactic drainage of a bilateral *Aspergillus* brain abscess (craniotomy) combined with amphotericin B medication was applied to achieve a long-term survival in four of five patients *(190)*. A case of non-Hodgkin's lymphoma complicated with invasive CNS aspergillosis was treated with amphotericin B *(191)*.

Peritonitis is the most common observed complication of continuous ambulatory (or cycling) peritoneal dialysis *(192)*. Although the majority of infections are caused by Gram-positive bacteria, cases of peritonitis secondary to fungi have been on the increase; in one such report *(193)*, as many as 15% of all cases were fungus-related. All reported incidences were also fatal *(192)*. An individual case of successfully treated *Aspergillus*-related peritonitis in a child undergoing continuous cycling dialysis involved intraperitoneal administration of amphotericin B; the antibiotic was mixed in dialysate (1.0 mg/L of dialysate) in order to preserve the peritoneal dialysis therapy. In another case of *A. fumigatus*-associated peritonitis related to CAPD, the treatment consisted of removal of the catheter and intravenous administration of amphotericin B, followed by oral itraconazole *(94)*.

Scorodin et al. *(194)* presented a case of mixed empyema with bronchopleural fistula due to *Mycobacterium tuberculosis*, *A. fumigatus*, and *A. flavus*, which was resolved by administration of antituberculosis drugs and intrapleural amphotericin B (total of 575 mg) over a 4-wk period.

Conneally et al. *(195)* described the administration of nebulized amphotericin B (twice daily over a 12-mo period) as prophylaxis against invasive aspergillosis in granulocytopenic patients. The results, which were compared to historical controls (11.4% incidence of those at risks), suggested that after commencing prophylaxis, no cases of invasive aspergillosis had occurred *(195)*.

Aspergillus-associated laryngotracheobronchitis presenting as stridor in a patient with peripheral T-cell lymphoma responded to systemic treatment with amphotericin B *(196)*.

The toxicity of amphotericin B ranges from acute (idiosyncratic or dose-related) to chronic (Table 2) *(166,169)*. Usually, when the creatinine levels exceed 3.0–3.5 mg/dL, amphotericin B therapy should be ceased for several days and then reinstated at a lower dose. Premedication with acetaminophen and the addition of hydrocortisone sodium succinate (25–50 mg) to the infusion solution has been reported to reduce some of the toxicity of the antibiotic *(169)*.

3.1.1. Liposome-Encapsulated and Lipid-Based Formulations of Amphotericin B

The therapeutic effect of AmBisome® (a unilamellar liposomal formulation of amphotericin B) in systemic fungal infections was evaluated in several European studies *(197–199)*. In one clinical trial, the patients tested either had failed to respond to or tolerated alternatives, or who were in acute renal

Table 2
Toxicities of Amphotericin B

Dose-dependent
    Nephrotoxicity (urinary abnormalities, hyposthenuria,
        azotemia, hypokalemia, nephrocalcinosis)
    Normocytic, normochromic anemia (decreased
        erythropoietin levels and erythrocyte counts)
Idiosyncratic
    Flushing
    Rash
    Anaphylactic shock
    Acute liver failure
    Thrombocytopenia
    Vertigo
    Generalized pain
    Grand mal convulsion
    Ventricular fibrillation
    Cardiac arrest
    Fever (in nearly all patients)
    Chill (in nearly all patients)

failure. Although still preliminary, important findings emerging from these studies were that, in general, the liposomal amphotericin B did not display serious toxicity such as renal tubular damage, and that patients were able to tolerate doses of amphotericin B that significantly exceeded those used in conventional formulations. The reported cases of aspergillosis showed that 25% of the patients recovered clinically, another 25% were rated as clinically improved, and the remaining 50% were considered as clinical failures; the mycological efficacy of AmBisome resulted in 25% of patients being cured, 50% still having persistant cultures, and the remaining 25% not evaluated *(197)*. In a second trial, a low-dose therapy with AmBisome (1.0–2.2 mg/kg, i.v., daily) for 10 d led to fungal eradication in all patients *(198)*.

In another study, AmBisome was used to treat immunocompromised pediatric patients with invasive aspergillosis and candidiasis at a mean cumulative dose of 1.8 ± 1.3 g ($\pm$ SD) and for a median of 19 d; side effects were minimal and in those children treated for at least 1 wk, the overall cure rate was 86% *(200)*.

AmBisome was found to be most effective at doses up to 12.0 mg/kg with few side effects *(199)*. The safety, tolerance, and pharmacokinetics of high-dose AmBisome (7.5, 10.0, 12.5, and 15.0 mg/kg, daily) were evaluated in a Phase I–II clinical trial; daily doses as high as 15.0 mg/kg followed nonlinear saturation-like kinetics and were well-tolerated *(201)*.

Weber and Lopez-Berestein *(181)* also demonstrated that amphotericin B, when encapsulated in liposomes *(202)*, may become an effective and less toxic alternative to conventional amphotericin B therapy in patients with sinonasal aspergillosis who failed to respond to amphotericin B alone. In the reported trial, in six of seven patients, an underlying hematologic malignancy or aplastic anemia was also present. The initial dose of liposomal amphotericin B was 0.4 mg/kg (in sodium chloride suspension), administered intravenously over 10 min; depending on the patient's tolerance, the dose was gradually increased to 2 mg/kg daily for 3 wk (median dose 1.4 g; total of 280–4000 mg). The results showed that five of the patients were complete responders (four of them remained neutropenic throughout the therapy), with the response being rapid and leading to resolution of symptoms occurring within 4–5 d. Two of the patients did not respond. No severe renal or CNS toxicity was observed *(181)*. AmBisome was also used in the treatment of five pediatric patients with malignancies who developed invasive pulmonary aspergillosis during chemotherapy-induced neutropenia *(203)*. In addition to liposomal amphotericin B, the patients also received granulocyte colony-stimulating factor (G-CSF). Liposomal amphotericin B was well-tolerated in patients receiving high-doses of the antibiotic, such as those undergoing bone marrow or peripheral blood stem cell transplantation *(28)*. However, the use of liposomal amphotericin B to treat *A. fumigatus* infection in three lung-transplant recipients, although successful, was not free of undesired side effects and nephrotoxicity as suggested by previous results *(52)*.

A. flavus colonization of the renal pelvis and upper ureter of a patient with concomitant urinary schistosomiasis was successfully treated with liposomal amphotericin B *(204)*. In another *A. flavus* infection, an immunosuppressed pediatric patient with invasive pneumonia and endocarditis successfully responded to daily therapy with 10 mg/kg of liposomal amphotericin B *(114)*.

A patient with asthma, bronchopulmonary aspergillosis, pulmonary thromboembolic disease, and pulmonary hypertension who developed *A. fumigatus* empyema complicating pneumothorax and had failed to respond to intravenous and intrapleutal amphotericin B, improved promptly after changing treatment to nebulized liposomal amphotericin B and oral itraconazole *(205)*.

Hospenthal et al. *(206)* described the successful use of amphotericin B lipid complex in the treatment of invasive pulmonary aspergillosis complicating prolonged treatment-related neutropenia in acute myelogenous leukemia.

Mendicute et al. *(207)* treated three patients with *Aspergillus* keratomycosis with collagen shields impregnated with amphotericin B (0.50%) for 2 h at 25°C before application. The shields (replaced daily) were used in conjunction with amphotericin B (0.25%) eye drops, which were applied every 2 h. The collagen shields, as prepared, delivered adequate concentration of amphotericin B to the cornea and increased its tolerance. Xie et al. *(208)* considered penetrating keratoplasty as an effective treatment for fungal keratitis in cases that did not respond to antifungal therapy.

A case of massive intracerebral *A. flavus* invasive disease responded to combination of high-dose liposomal amphotericin B and cytokine therapy without surgery *(209)*.

The clinical response and safety (toxicity profile and maximum tolerated dose) of amphotericin B colloidal dispersion (Amphocil®) was evaluated in a Phase I dose-escalation trial in 75 bone-marrow transplant patients with invasive fungal infection primarily due to *Aspergillus* and *Candida (26)*. Escalating doses of 0.5–8.0 mg/kg in 0.5-mg/kg/patient increments were given up to 6 wk. There has been no infusion-related toxicities in 32% of patients; 52% had grade 2 and 5% had grade 3 toxicity. No appreciable renal toxicity was observed at any dose level. The estimated maximum tolerated dose was 7.5 mg/kg, defined by rigors and chills, and hypotension in three of five patients receiving 8.0 mg/kg of the drug *(26)*.

3.1.2. Routes of Administration

For treatment of pulmonary aspergillosis, amphotericin B may be applied by one of several routes (Table 1). Intravenous administration, although often used in earlier trials, is being viewed with reservation *(104)*. For example, Hammerman et al. *(210)*, when treating 71 patients with saprophitic pulmonary aspergillosis with intravenous amphotericin B, found that such treatment was no more advantageous than a pulmonary toilet regimen. This finding was corroborated by other researchers as well *(105,211)*, although in several reports *(212–214)* successful therapy involving intravenous administration of amphotericin B has been described.

Direct intracavitary instillation of amphotericin B is usually accomplished by repeated transthoracic injections into the cavity *(9)*. The drug is instilled in liquid form, but the use of a paste has also been recommended *(215)*. The drawbacks of intracavitary administration have included poor patient tolerance (development of fever), risk of pneumothorax, and relapse of infection in the cavity *(121)*. However, Hargis et al. *(216)* reported clinical improvement and stabilization in cases where a large dose of amphotericin B (500 mg) was instilled by intracavitary route in 50% dextrose in water. In general, however, endobronchial instillation of antifungal drugs had minimal success *(217,218)* and the possibility of relapse *(121)*.

Giron et al. *(219)* reported 30 cases of percutaneous treatment of symptomatic pulmonary aspergilloma by injection of amphotericin B paste in patients who were not considered to be operable because of severe respiratory failure. The preparation of the paste and the type of percutaneous injection were aimed at obtaining a complete filling of the cavity and creating anaerobic environment for the fungus. Shirai et al. *(220)* and Furuse et al. *(221)* also performed percutaneous instillation of amphotericin B to treat pulmonary aspergilloma.

In a rat model of pregressive pulmonary aspergillosis (characterized by hyphal bronchopneumonia), amphotericin B was administered as an aerosol (1.6 mg/kg given 2 d before infection) *(222)*. The application resulted in a markedly delayed mortality of the rats as compared to controls. When the same dose of aerosolized amphotricin B was administered as a treatment (1.6 mg/kg given 24 h after infection, and then daily of 6 d), it was found effective; 8 of 10 rats survived for 7 d, compared to only 1 of 10 controls. The colony counts in lung homogenates obtained 24 h after the infection showed an 80-fold reduction in the number of viable spores in rats, which received 6.4-mg/kg doses of aerosolized amphotericin B 2 d prior to infection *(222)*. Studies on the pharmacokinetics showed that 48 h after the administration of aerosolized amphotericin B at a single dose of 1.6 or 3.2 mg/kg, the mean lung concentrations of the antibiotic were 2.79 and 5.22 µg/mL, respectively. The beneficial action of aerosolized amphotericin B was likely due not only to its ability to kill inhaled spores but also to delay the progression of pulmonary aspergillosis by inhibiting mycelial proliferation *(222)*. In humans, pulmonary deposition of amphotericin B could also be achieved by using commercially available nebulizers; inhalations were well tolerated with little systemic absorption of the drug *(223)*.

Cahill et al. *(224)* reported a successful palliative treatment of *A. fumigatus* orbital mass in a patient with AIDS by direct injection of amphotericin B into the abscess cavity. This case of intraorbital administration was suggested as an alternative to surgical debridement.

A case of erythroleukemia associated with lung aspergilloma was successfully treated with continuous drip infusion of amphotericin B, which allowed for maintaining high lung-tissue drug levels *(225)*.

3.1.3. Combinations of Amphotericin B With Other Drugs

In addition to therapy with amphotericin B alone, a number of combinations with other drugs *(226)*, especially 5-FC *(58,227–231)* have also been used to treat *Aspergillus* infections (Table 3).

Although IPA occurs exclusively in severely immunocompromised patients, it is an increasingly recognized condition in apparently immunocompetent hosts. In the latter case, some potential risk factors (fibrotic lung disease, corticosteroid therapy, influenza, or psittacosis infection) may be present. If not treated early, the prognosis of IPA would remain poor for both immunocompromised and immunocompetent patients *(232)*. Rodenhuis et al. *(232)* reported a case of successful therapy of IPA in an immunocompetent patient by applying systemic treatment with amphotericin B and 5-FC together with inhalation of aerosolized amphotericin B. Apparently, the combination of the two drugs *(233)* acted locally, while the inhalation of amphotericin B helped to prevent continuing reinfection with 5-FC-resistant strains of *Aspergillus*. Spiteri et al. *(234)* also described a case of successful recovery of an immunocompetent patient with primary IPA (but no other detectable lung damage or underlying systemic disease) using combination of intravenous amphotericin B (initially 15 mg daily, increasing to 50 mg daily after 4 d) and oral 5-FC (200 mg/kg daily; total dose of 3 g daily, every 6 h); the therapy lasted for 8 wk.

Henze et al. *(235)* described a case of developed pulmonary and cerebral aspergillosis in an immunosuppressed patient who received antineoplastic treatment for CNS relapse of acute lymphoblastic leukemia. The combination therapy of intravenous amphotericin B (total dosage exceeded 500 mg) and oral flucytosine (100–150 mg/kg), which was supported by natamycin inhalations, resulted in complete regression of pulmonary infiltrates after treatment for 53 d. Some enlargement of the cerebral lesion was observed, but no viable organisms were present in the completely resected abscess after 4-wk treatment preceding neurosurgery *(235)*. Prolonged therapy with AmBisome and 5-fluorocytosine successfully eradicated brain abscess in a child with lymphoblastic anemia *(20)*.

Table 3
Combinations of Amphotericin B with Other Drugs

Combination	Indication
Amphothericin B (intravenous)/5-FC (oral)	Invasive pulmonary aspergillosis (IPA)
Amphotericin B (intravenous)/rifampin (oral)	Disseminated aspergillosis-chronic granulomatous disease
	Invasive pulmonary aspergillosis
Amphotericin B/Tetracyclines	In vitro assay
Amphotericn B/Nystatin (intrapleural instillation)	Pleural aspergillosis
Amphotericin B/Itraconazole	Invasive CNS aspergillosis

Combination therapy of intravenous amphotericin B (total of 1.3 g) and oral flucytosine (1.5-2.0 g, given 4 times daily) produced a rapid improvement and total eradication of *Aspergillus*-associated pneumonia *(236)*; the amphotericin B therapy was stopped after 2 mo, while 5-FC administration was continued alone at a dosage of 2.0 g (4 times daily) for another 3 mo.

Bogner et al. *(230)* described a successful treatment of *Aspergillus*-induced endocarditis with amphotericin B-flucytosine combination. The therapy commenced with daily intravenous injections of amphotericin B (increasing to 50 mg) combined with 1.5 g daily of oral 5-FC; a total of 1.1 g of amphotericin B and 41.5 g of 5-FC were given over a 5-wk period. A gradual decrease in symptoms and valve vegetation was observed.

In patients with acute leukemia, invasive *Aspergillus* rhinosinusitis may develop as a potentially lethal complication of chemotherapy-induced neutropenia. In the majority of cases, the causative agent is *A. flavus*. Talbot et al. *(231)* have recommended early treatment with aggressive surgery, high-dose amphotericin B and 5-FC; white blood cell transfusions may also be beneficial particularly in cases of bone-marrow recovery.

In view of the existing toxicity of both amphotericin B and flucytosine (especially the negative effect of the latter on the bone marrow), treatment of aspergillosis in terminally ill AIDS patients with combination amphotericin B-flucytosine should be applied with caution. Further, some of the gastrointestinal side effects of 5-FC may often superimpose on symptoms caused by HIV *(237,238)*.

In children with chronic granulomatous disease (CGD; an underlying immune disorder), therapy of disseminated aspergillosis with amphotericin B alone was only marginally effective and granulocyte transformations or a surgical excision was often required *(239–241)*. Corrado et al. *(242)* and Lizzarin and Capsoni *(239)* have recommended the combined use of rifampin and amphotericin B to manage disseminated aspergillosis in children with CGD. The therapy comprised intravenous amphotericin B (0.7 mg/kg daily) and oral rifampin (20 mg/kg daily) for 11 wk; hypokalemia was the only adverse side effect observed *(239)*.

A combination of rifampin and amphotericin B was successfully used in the therapy of one immunosuppressed patient (acute leukemia) with IPA; the patient received rifampin (600 mg daily for 3 wk) and a total dose of 1.8 g of amphotericin B *(243)*. Another case of pulmonary aspergillosis in a patient with acute leukemia that was managed by amphotericin B-rifampin has also been reported *(244)*.

Colp and Cook *(245)* reported a successful treatment of a patient with bronchopleural fistula and pleural aspergilloma by intrapleural instillation of amphotericin B (total of 750 mg over 1-mo period) and nystatin, followed by creation of an Eloesser flap for long-term drainage of the pleural space. In another example, a combination of amphotericin B and nystatin was applied topically for the treatment of aspergilloma *(215)*; the two antibiotics were used as a paste administered by intracavitary needling and instillation. It is thought that the paste covered the surface of the fungus ball and impaired the air supply coming to the pathogen *(215)*.

Combinations of amphotericin B and itraconazole have also been reported *(45,58,118,246)*. A patient with chronic necrotizing pulmonary aspergillosis complicated by a residual tuberculous cavity was treated successfully with oral itraconazole (200 mg daily) and inhaled amphotericin B (10 mg, q.i.d.). The serum concentration of amphotericin B was 0.09 µg/mL, which was equal to the level achieved after daily oral administration of 2.4 g of the antibiotic *(246)*. Similarly, amphotericin B at 1.0 mg/kg and itraconazole at 200 mg, daily, have also been used *(58)*.

A case of progressive disseminated aspergillosis in a bone-marrow transplant recipient—after failing to respond to liposomal amphotericin B (5.0 mg/kg, daily) given alone or in combination with itraconazole—responded well to high-dose amphotericin B (15 mg/kg, daily) and itraconazole *(45)*.

In another successful application, liposomal amphotericin B and oral itraconazole were combined with surgical excision of abscesses to cure invasive aspergillosis of the CNS in an immunosuppressed pediatric patient with acute lymphatic leukemia and multiple *Aspergillus* brain abscesses *(247)*.

Maesaki et al. *(248)* described a case of pulmonary aspergilloma that responded with complete dissapearance of the fungus ball on chest computerized tomography (CT) scan after treatment combination therapy of intravenous urinastatin (100,000 units) and intracavitary injection of amphotericin B.

3.2. Azole Derivatives

So far, published reports have indicated that the therapeutic efficacy of some azole antimycotics (clotrimazole, miconazole, and ketoconazole; Table 4) against various forms of aspergillosis is highly questionable. The observed lack of consistent antifungal effect coupled with the absence of large-scale clinical trials to show efficacy have virtually precluded their use in treatment of aspergillosis.

3.2.1. Clotrimazole

In one clinical case, Evans et al. *(250)* described the successful management of pulmonary aspergillosis in a child by using systemic therapy with clotrimazole at daily doses of 70 mg/kg for 45 d; previously, inhalation of nystatin (120,000 units daily) and cephalexin (750 mg daily), and irrigation of the pleural space with nystatin suspension (500,000 units) for 6 d failed to cure the disease. During therapy, clotrimazole was tolerated well *(250)*.

In a contradictory report, Milne *(249)* revealed the lack of mycologic and clinical improvement in four patients with bronchopulmonary aspergillosis treated with a daily dose of 100 mg/kg of clotrimazole for up to 3 mo. The observed maximum serum concentration of the drug was 0.17 µg/mL, whereas the MIC against *A. fumigatus* isolates was 1.0 µg/mL; this finding may be one reason for the lower therapeutic efficacy of clotrimazole.

Clinical experience from continuing oral administration of clotrimazole has shown an enhanced drug metabolism occuring after approx 2 wk of medication *(276)*. This inability to sustain adequate blood concentrations has proved to be a problem *(256)* for the systemic use of clotrimazole against various mycoses, including bronchopulmonary aspergillosis *(277)*.

Oral clotrimazole (60 mg/kg, daily for 127 d) had no beneficial effect on paranasal aspergilloma as reported by Mahgoub *(251)*; the drug also caused gastrointestinal side effects and disuria *(251)*.

Corneal infections caused by *A. fumigatus* are difficult to control, especially in cases when hypopyon is present. Jones et al. *(278)* described as successful the treatment of two such cases by using a combined therapy of topical (1% solution in arachis oil) and oral clotrimazole.

3.2.2. Miconazole

Although miconazole can be administered orally, it requires high doses (1.0 g) to achieve adequate blood concentrations of 1.16 mg/L at 2–4 h post-administration *(279)*. A more useful approach would be to inject the drug intravenously at 50 mg/kg every 8 h *(256)*.

Table 4
Azole Antimycotics in the Treatment of Aspergillosis

Azole/MIC (in µg/mL)	Indication (route of administration)	Side effects
Clotrimazole/1.0 (249)	Pulmonary aspergillosis (oral) (250)	Gastrointestinal, dysuria (251,252)
Miconazole/3.48 (253)	Pulmonary aspergillosis/hemoptysis (intracavitary instillation) (254)	Phlebitis, pruritis, nausea, fever, chill, rash, vomiting, anemia, decreased hematocrit (normoblastic hypoplasia), hyponatremia (255); anaphylaxis, ventricular tachycardia (256)
Ketoconazole/7.0 (257)	Chronic *Aspergillus* sinusitis (oral) (258), keratitis (topical) (252)	Nausea, vomiting, diarrhea, pruritis, rash, increased alkaline phosphatase, hyperlipidemia (259); inhibition of gonadal and adrenal steroid synthesis (260)
Itraconazole/ ≥0.07 (261)	Invasive aspergillosis (262–266), aspergilloma (267), allergic bronchopulmonary aspergillosis (267); chronic necrotizing pulmonary (247)	Superficial mycoses: nausea, headache, pyrosis, dysuria (268) Systemic mycosis: asymptomatic liver function abnormalities, increased blood levels of urea nitrogen and serum levels of transaminase (267)
BAY n 7133	Murine aspergillosis (oral) (269)	
Enilconazole/0.1–1.0 (270)	Avian aspergillosis (fumigation)(270)	Emesis, salivation, loss of body weight, decreased serum calcium, increased serum alkaline phosphatase (270)
Oxiconazole/10.0 (271)	*A. terreus*-induced keratitis (subconjunctival) (271)	
Saperconazole/0.1–1.0 (272)	Murine aspergillosis (oral, intravenous, intraperitoneal) (273)	No side effects observed (273)
SCH 39304	Murine pulmonary aspergillosis (oral) (274)	
SM-9164	Murine aspergillosis (oral, intravenous) (274)	
BAY R 3783	Murine pulmonary aspergillosis (275)	

Miconazole usually will not penetrate the urine, cerebrospinal fluid (CSF) or the joints in high concentrations. Its serum levels were determined by bioassay after intravenous injection of 200–600 mg to patients with deep-seated mycoses; peak concentrations of 1.0–1.6 µg/mL were reached at the end of the administration, followed by a rapid decrease of 25% (or less) after 7–8 h (280,281). When the serum levels were determined by high-pressure liquid chromatography (HPLC), the observed values tended to be higher than those determined by the bioassay, likely because the HPLC technique would measure not only the free but also the protein-bound miconazole (280).

Intrapleural administration of miconazole led only to partial improvement in a case of *Aspergillus*-induced empyema with bronchopleural fistula; for the complete treatment, lobectomy and decortication were also performed (282).

In another clinical application, parenteral miconazole was found to be very useful in the treatment of deep-seated aspergillosis of the respiratory tract (283). Hamamoto et al. (254) have tried intracavitary infusion of miconazole to cure a patient with pulmonary aspergillosis and recurrent hemoptysis (accompanied with tuberculosis and diabetes), who did not respond to surgical excision. Miconazole, which was infused through a catheter in eight treatments for a total of 50 mg, initiated lysis of the fungal ball.

A case of chronic necrotizing pulmonary aspergillosis effectively treated with miconazole inhalation was reported by Maeda *(284)*.

Clinical studies in Japan *(280)* on the therapeutic efficacy of miconazole showed a 84% cure rate for pulmonary aspergillosis and 83% for pulmonary aspergilloma.

3.2.3. Ketoconazole

Ketoconazole was the first azole antimycotic able to produce sustainable therapeutic concentrations after oral administration *(285)*. Even though ketoconazole did not penetrate the CSF and urine, it still managed to produce high recovery rates in various mycoses *(256)*.

Farquhar et al. *(258)* treated a case of chronic sinusitis attributed to *A. fumigatus* with oral ketoconazole (200 mg daily for 2 mo) with positive response.

Topical ketoconazole (2%) was used in the therapy of corneal infection induced by *A. flavus*; the drug, which was applied every 2 h for 17 d, healed the lesions completely *(286)*. Singh et al. *(287)* found oral ketoconazole effective in experimental corneal ulcer induced by injecting intralamellary spore suspension of *A. fumigatus* into the eye of previously immunosuppressed albino and black wild rabbits; a partial response, followed by relapse, was observed. O'Day et al. *(288)* described a case of deep corneal abscess caused by *Aspergillus* spp. that was successfully controlled by a combined corticosteroid-antifungal (amphotericin B, nystatin) medication, followed by penetrating keratoplasty.

Coriglione et al. *(289)* have described the first case of mycotic keratitis caused by *Neosartorya fischeri* var. *fischeri*, the teleomorph of *Aspergillus fischerianus*; ketoconazole failed to cure the infection.

3.2.4. Fluconazole

Oral fluconazole is a well-absorbed antimycotic, with over 70% of the administered dose detected in the serum *(290)*. The drug also penetrated the peritoneum and CSF in concentrations reaching those found in the serum. When administered to cancer patients in high-doses, neurologic toxicity by fluconazole was noticed only at daily doses of 2.0 g. The drug was well-tolerated at total daily doses of up to 1.6 g (average steady-state peak plasma concentration of 74.4 mg/L) *(291)*.

In general, with the exception of several anecdotal reports *(292–294)*, fluconazole has no activity against *Aspergillus* spp. *(295,296)*. Thus, patients at risk for that infection should be evaluated by chest radiograph, CT scanning, and cultures before initiating empiric fluconazole therapy.

3.2.5. Itraconazole

Itraconazole, a newly developed triazole-containing azole antimycotic, is a highly lipophilic substance that, similar to ketoconazole, is absorbed much better with food. It is poorly soluble in aqueous solutions and produces low serum concentrations (200–300 ng/mL after a single 100-mg dose) 2 h after administration. The drug avidly bound to plasma proteins *(297)*, and penetrated the urine and CSF at low concentrations. However, Niwa et al. *(298)* observed high concentrations of itraconazole in a case of pulmonary aspergillosis with aspergilloma; the drug, when given at 100 mg daily, produced plasma concentration of 249 ng/mL; concentrations in lung specimens and aspergilloma specimens obtained by thoractomy were 81 ng/g and 837 ng/g, respectively. These high concentrations may be explained with the increased itraconazole levels in purulent fluid, its ability to enter easily the aspergilloma through the root at the cavity wall, and the ability of itraconazole to dissolve in lipid derived from destroyed fungus *(298)*.

The activity of itraconazole is directed at the fungal cell periphery and cytoplasmic vacuoles in which lipid-like vesicles will assemble *(299)*. Drug-induced changes in the fungal cell are usually manifested by a marked increase in the cell volume, impaired cell division, and/or abortive hyphal outgrowth. Complete inhibition of the hyphal growth of *A. fumigatus* by itraconazole was achieved at concentration of ≥0.07 µg/mL (10^{-7} M) *(261)*. However, as with other azole antifungals, acquired itraconazole resistance in *Aspergillus* spp. has began to emerge *(300)*.

In a clinical trial conducted by Viviani et al. *(262)*, 9 of 35 patients with invasive aspergillosis when given oral itraconazole et doses of 100–400 mg were reported cured and another 12 patients showed marked improvement. The same investigators also found that a prolonged medication with itraconazole resulted in remission in 8 of 10 patients *(262)*. In general, positive response to treatment of invasive aspergillosis in immunocompromised patients (with leukemia, lymphoma, and heart-transplant recipients) were achieved by using relatively high doses of itraconazole (5 mg/kg or no less than 4 mg/kg) at least during the first 60 d of therapy *(262)*. This information makes it noteworthy to stress the difficulties encountered in evaluating a drug's antifungal efficacy because of the varying clinical characteristics of the infection and the changing immunological status of patients. During therapy, itraconazole was well-tolerated and serious side effects have not, so far, been encountered *(301)*. Kreisel *(302)* also recommended mean daily doses of 400 mg itraconazole for treatment of invasive aspergillosis.

The therapeutic efficacy of itraconazole was also evaluated in several studies involving a number of patients with pulmonary aspergillosis *(303–308)*. For example, itraconazole at daily oral doses of 100–200 mg was administered over a 5–20-mo period to four patients with pulmonary aspergillosis *(305)*. Improvement (as evidenced by CT, chest rentgenograms, as well as symptoms) was noticeable in two of the patients. Kramer et al. *(306)* have observed several cases of deep mucosal ulceration caused by invasive *Aspergillus*-induced tracheobronchitis in patients who received heart-lung and lung transplants; oral therapy with itraconazole was successful in five of six patients. A rare case of chronic pulmonary aspergillosis invading the thoracic wall responded well to itraconazole *(307)*.

Itraconazole, given orally once daily (200–400 mg), improves the outcome in patients with pulmonary aspergillosis, chronic necrotizing pulmonary aspergillosis, and invasive aspergillosis *(266,309)*. Overall, the drug showed more efficacy against the invasive and chronic necrotizing pulmonary aspergillosis; in aspergilloma it could be useful in unoperable cases *(309)*. A case of itraconazole (100 mg daily)-induced hypokalemia (serum potassium level at day 57, 2.33 mEq/L) with pulmonary aspergilloma has been reported; 31 d after discontinuation of therapy, the serum potassium level reached 3.57 mEq/L *(310)*.

Although surgical removal of endobronchial suture probably constitutes the key therapy for bronchial stump aspergillosis, Noppen et al. *(311)* found oral itraconazole beneficial in affecting clinical, histologic, and microbiologic improvement in three patients with BSA. Itraconazole, at 200 mg daily for 2–5 mo, cleared the infection or led to a marked improvement in immunocompetent patients with pulmonary aspergillosis *(264)*.

In another trial conducted by Denning et al. *(265)*, data were presented on the itraconazole therapy of 21 patients with invasive aspergillosis. Itraconazole was given orally, with 18 of the patients receiving 400 mg daily and the remaining three, 100–200 mg daily; 12 of 15 evaluable patients responded to the treatment. Furthermore, eight of the responders were immunocompromised (either with neutropenia or as renal-transplant recipients). The reported side effects of itraconazole were minimal *(265)*.

In a number of reports *(312–316)* itraconazole was found effective in the treatment of *Aspergillus* infections in patients with CGD. Treatment of one such infection with oral itraconazole at 16 mg/kg led to significant clinical improvement and nearly complete disappearance of intracerebral lesions *(312)*. The observed toxicity was confined to transient elevation of the alkaline phosphatase and γ-glutamyl transferase *(312)*. Itraconazole showed better efficacy than either amphotericin B given alone *(314)*, or combination of amphotericin B and flucytosine *(315)*. In the latter case, the failure was attributed to cytochrome B deficiency; using itraconazole instead led to considerable improvement in a short period of time *(315)*. A combination of itraconazole and interferon-γ (IFN-γ) *(316)* or IFN-γ alone *(317)* was used to successfully treat *Aspergillus* brain abscess in patients with CGD.

Witzig et al. *(318)* described a patient with diabetes and nephrotic syndrome with *A. flavus* mycetoma of the back, with the development of epidural abscess, diskitis, and vertebral osteomyelitis; decompressive laminectomy and a 14-mo course with itraconazole led to clinical cure.

There have been several other examples of clinical application of itraconazole involving individual cases. Thus, the drug was used to stabilize a case of sino-orbital aspergillosis after therapy with miconazole had failed *(319)*. In a similar report, oral itraconazole was used successfully to treat sino-orbital aspergillosis in an immunocompetent patient after two attempts with traditional therapeutic modalities (surgical debridement and intravenous amphotericin B) had failed *(320)*. Rowe-Jones and Freedman *(321)* successfully treated three cases of destructive sphenoid aspergillosis (two of which had intracranial extension) with surgery and adjuvant itraconazole therapy.

A patient with SLE who developed pneumonia caused by *A. fumigatus* rapidly responded to oral itraconazole at 200 mg given twice daily *(93)*.

Impens et al. *(322)* described medication with oral itraconazole as an alternative to surgical intervention for the treatment of aspergilloma in a case of necrotic small cell lung cancer (SCLC). Mori et al. *(323)* have used oral itraconazole (200 mg or more) to treat patients with aspergilloma; percutaneous intracavitary instillation of amphotericin B, performed in one patient, showed no efficacy.

Successful itraconazole therapy of aspergillosis in a cardiac-transplant patient has been reported *(324)*.

A deep traumatic keratomycosis with anterior chamber involvement due to *A. fumigatus* infection responded well to oral itraconazole and topical amphotericin B; apparently, itraconazole was able to penetrate both into the deeper layers of the cornea and the anterior chamber *(325)*. An *A. flavus*-induced onychomycosis was also successfully treated with oral itraconazole *(405)*.

Sanchez et al. *(327)* described a patient with chronic asthma who presented with cerebral abscesses due to *A. fumigatus* after being treated with corticosteroids; following therapy with high-dose itraconazole (800 mg daily for 5 mo, followed by 400 mg daily for an additional 4.5 mo) resulted in complete resolution of all lesions. The use of high-dose itraconazole may prove beneficial for high-risk patients with cerebral aspergillosis for whom conventional therapy had failed.

Other reports involved the clinical use of itraconazole in cases of *Aspergillus* spondylodiscitis *(125,126–128)*. It included a patient with *A. fumigatus*-induced spondylodiscitis who, after lumbar surgery, was treated successfully with itraconazole in combination with surgical debridement of the disc space *(126)*. Early recognition of this condition in immunocompromised hosts combined with itraconazole treatment alone (mean dose, 350 mg daily) *(125)* or in combination promises to be effective therapy. In another case, a patient with a long-standing ankylosing spondylitis who developed chronic necrotising pulmonary aspergillosis also responded to medication with itraconazole *(328)*.

According to Van Cutsem and Cauwenbergh *(329)*, data from the treatment of 251 evaluable patients with various manifestations of aspergillosis (allergic, aspergilloma, pulmonary, invasive pulmonary, disseminated) receiving a median daily oral dose of 200 mg itraconazole over a period of 91 d (median) have shown a global response between 46% (disseminated aspergillosis) and 74% (allergic aspergillosis), and negative mycology ranging between 25% (disseminated aspergillosis) and 76% (pulmonary aspergillosis). One reason that may explain the observed efficacy of itraconazole in treatment of aspergillosis is its good tissue penetration and its low minimum inhibitory concentration (MIC) value for *Aspergillus*.

The European experience with oral solution and intravenous itraconazole (Sporanox®) has demonstrated that in neutropenic patients with hematologic malignancies, the treatment with sporanox followed by oral itraconazole resulted in response or stable disease in two-third of patients with invasive pulmonary aspergillosis *(108)*. Furthermore, empiric treatment with sporanox followed by oral solution of itraconazole was at least as effective as, and significantly less toxic than, amphotericin B.

Several reports also point to failures of itraconazole to treat aspergillosis. Franco et al. *(31)* described a case of *Aspergillus* arthritis of the shoulder in a renal-transplant recipient who failed to respond to a single therapy with itraconazole; after initial clinical and roentgenologic improvements, the patient relapsed with a fatal neurologic involvement taking place. Gene et al. *(3)* reported a case of fatal cutaneous infection caused by *A. ustus* that also failed to respond to itraconazole. In another case, a presumably immunocompetent patient failed to respond to a 2-yr treatment by oral itraconazole (200 mg, daily) for a spinal epidural aspergillosis due to a lung aspergilloma. In spite of the long-term itraconazole treatment, the infection spread locally from lung aspergilloma to the epidural space *(8)*. In general, high morbidity and mortality is common in patients with *Aspergillus* spinal epidural abscess *(330)*.

Concomitant administration of itraconazole and digoxin resulted in interaction leading to a statistically significant increase in the half-life of digoxin which necessitated reduction of the digoxin dose by nearly 60%; monitoring digoxin, serum levels may have to be considered and nonspecific gastrointestinal symptoms should be carefully examined because such symptoms may indicate early digoxin toxicity *(331)*.

In a study by Wimberley et al. *(332)*, lung-transplant recipients on a combined itraconazole-cyclosporin A therapy when given the medications in a fed state with a carbonated beveridge (to increase the stomach acidity for enhanced absorption of itraconazole), needed a prolonged dosing interval for cyclosporin A as well as showing greater random blood concentrations of itraconazole.

3.3. Terbinafine

Schiraldi et al. *(333,334)* evaluated on a compassionate basis the clinical efficacy of terbinafine, a new allylamine antimycotic, in three immunocompetent patients affected by lower respiratory tract aspergillosis (one chronic empyema, and two chronic necrotizing aspergillosis) who were unresponsive to conventional antifungal therapies. The patients received terbinafine at daily doses ranging from 5.0–15 mg/kg according to their clinical status, for 3–5 mo depending on the clinical course of the disease and compliance *(333)*. At completion of therapy, one patient showed a negative anti-*A. fumigatus* precipitin together with eradication of the pathogen from the pleural cavity, which allowed a successful intrathoracic myo-omento-mammoplasty. In the other two patients, the fungus was also eradicated, the anti-*A. fumigatus* immunoprecipitins decreased, and clinical and radiologic findings significantly improved.

The use of terbinafine and itraconazole in the treatment of *Aspergillus* onychomycosis of the toes has been reviewed *(335)*.

Aspergillus versicolor infection of the external auditory canal was successfully treated with terbinafine *(336)*.

3.4. Caspofungin

Caspofungin acetate represents the first echinocandin antibiotic (a new class of glucan synthesis inhibitors) with broad range af fungicidal activity against a wide range of fungi, including *Aspergillus*, *Candida* and *Histoplasma* species *(337,338)*. Its mechanism of action involves the irreversible inhibition of 1,3-β-D-glucan synthase, preventing the formation of glucan polymers and disrupting the integrity of the fungal cell wall. Having an elimination of half-life of 9–10 h, caspofungin acetate is suitable for once-daily administration.

Caspofungin was found to be effective and well-tolerated in a multicenter noncomparative trial of patients with invasive aspergillosis *(338)*. The most common side effects included fever, nausea, vomiting, and complications associated with the vein into which caspofungin was infused.

In a study by Hoang *(337)*, 56 immunocompromised patients with refractory invasive aspergillosis were treated with one 70-mg dose of caspofungin acetate, then 50 mg once a day. In patients who received at least one dose of the drug, favorable response was observed in 41%. However, without adequate clinical trials to ascertain its efficacy and safety, it is still premature to add caspofungin acetate to the antifungal formulary.

3.5. Sodium (Potassium) Iodide Therapy of Aspergilloma

Oral administration of 24–30 g of potassium iodide to two patients with pulmonary aspergilloma was found to be therapeutically effective *(339)*. However, the presence of electrolytic imbalance (hypokalemia, elevation of serum carbon dioxide content, hyponatremia, hypocalcemia, and hypophosphatemia) resulting from the ingestion of large doses of iodide should preclude any casual approach to such treatment.

Ramirez *(340)* described as successful the therapy of two patients with symptomatic pulmonary aspergilloma by repeated endobronchial administration of amphotericin B and sodium iodide (total of 580 and 1200 mg, respectively) for periods of 29 d and 3 mo, respectively. In another case, 2% aqueous sodium iodide (total of 30 g for 29 d) was initiated 2 mo after a treatment with amphotericin B was completed *(340)*. The results suggested a more effective iodide therapy than amphotericin B in the management of pulmonary aspergilloma.

Adelson and Malcolm *(341)* also described as successful the treatment of mycetoma in one patient by applying percutaneous catheter for endocavitary instillation of sodium iodide; in this particular case, surgical excision was not recommended because the aspergilloma was superimposed on sarcoidosis.

3.6. Therapy of Allergic Bronchopulmonary Aspergillosis (ABPA)

Allergic bronchopulmonary aspergillosis (ABPA) is a pulmonary syndrome seen in patients with asthma and cystic fibrosis (CF), and is characterized by hypersensitivity to multiple antigens expressed by fungi, most commonly after chronic colonization of the bronchial mucos by *A. fumigatus* *(75,342–347)*. ABPA may present with diverse atypical syndromes, including paratracheal and hilar adenopathy, obstructive lung collapse, pneumothorax and bronchopleural fistula, allergic sinusitis, and pleural effusion.

Early diagnosis and treatment of ABPA is essential because inflammatory damage to the airways may be significantly reduced through the use of corticosteroids (initially with prednisone, starting at approx 0.5 mg/kg, daily *[348]*). The decision to taper steroids should be made on an individual basis, depending on the clinical course. If ABPA is left untreated, bronchiectasis causing permanent anatomic alteration of the airways may develop *(349)*. Successful therapy of ABPA is typically associated with a decline in total serum IgE *(348)*.

Chronic uncontrolled ABPA is well-known to cause extensive lung destruction as a result of type III immune response to *Aspergillus* antigen in the airways. Consequently, the reduction of antigen by antifungal therapy may lead to containment of lung damage, thereby limiting the progression of the disease. Shale et al. *(350)* conducted a 1-yr trial using ketoconazole in 10 patients with ABPA. The medication included 400 mg daily of the drug or placebo given orally in a double-blind fashion. In the treated group (six patients), concentrations of serum IgG specific for *A. fumigatus* were reduced significantly (mean change of 42%); by comparison, the remaining four patients who received placebo showed no meaningful change in their serum IgG concentrations (mean change of 10%).

In recent years, corticosteroid therapy of ABPA has emerged as the more successful approach for management of this condition. It is generally accepted that corticosteroids such as prednisolone and triamcinolone would act likely by suppressing the allergic inflammatory reactions and by decreasing the sputum production, thus making the bronchus less vulnerable to further fungal colonization *(351–353)*. For instance, when prednisolone was given at daily doses of >7.5 mg, it reduced the number of cases of recurrent consolidation *(353)*. The inhalation of corticosteroids is considered to be less efficient because of the presence of mucus plugging and obstruction, two common symptoms of ABPA *(354)*.

Corticosteroid drugs have been also applied to patients with symptoms of *Aspergillus* allergy (or classic ABPA) coexisting with aspergilloma *(355)*. A combination of ABPA with aspergilloma was treated with prednisolone with considerable improvement *(356)*. Davies and Somner *(357)* used prednisolone therapy to treat two cases of pulmonary aspergilloma following the failure of antibiotics and brilliant green to cure the disease. Because in both patients the reduction in purulent sputum was significant, it was postulated that prednisolone acted on a type III or an Arthus-type immune response involving antibody-antigen reaction in the cavity wall. Although Arthus reaction is commonly associated with ABPA, experimental evidence by Stevens et al. *(358)* lent support to the notion that in patients with aspergilloma, type III immune response may develop in the absence of clinical type I allergy.

Slavin et al. *(359)* treated two patients with ABPA with combination of oral corticosteroids and inhalation of amphotericin B. The therapy resulted in significant improvement as manifested by the clearing of pulmonary infiltrates, decrease in eosinophilia, weight gain, increase in vital capacity, negative sputum culture of *Aspergillus*, and the disappearance of precipitating antibody.

Recently, itraconazole was studied for its efficacy against ABPA *(303)*. Twice daily administration of 200 mg of the drug to patients for periods ranging from 1–6 mo (mean 3.9 mo) led, in general, to improvement of the pulmonary function with mean forced expiratory volume (FEV) increasing from 1.43 to 1.77 L/s, and mean forced vital capacity (FVC) increasing from 2.3 to 2.9 L in those treated for 2 mo or longer. The mean steady-state serum concentration of itraconazole was 5.1 µg/mL *(303)*.

Currently, for treatment of ABPA the inhalation of aerosolized amphotericin B *(360)*, nystatin *(361)*, natamycin *(362)*, or clotrimazole *(363)* has seen rather limited use because of frequent relapses that require repeated applications *(364)*. Radha and Viswanathan *(365)* described the treatment of seven patients with ABPA with hamycin, a polyene antibiotic isolated from *Streptomyces pimprina thirum*. The drug, which was administered at a dose of 25 mg, 4 times daily for 10 d, was reported efficacious and led to a marked alleviation of subjective symptoms and absence of fungus in the sputum.

In order to assess the steroid paring potential of natamycin, Currie et al. *(366)* conducted a controlled, double-blind trial of 20 patients with ABPA. The patients, already on a maintenance oral therapy with corticosteroids, were given 5.0 mg of natamycin or placebo by nebulizer twice daily for 1 yr; standardized reductions in the corticosteroid dosage were undertaken every 5 wk unless clinically contraindicated. The results showed no evidence of beneficial effect for natamycin.

Among other forms of treatment of ABPA *(268)*, immunotherapy through intradermal hyposensitization has had little success *(352)*. Similarly, medication with sodium chromoglycate, while ameliorating asthmatic symptoms, did not prevent recurrence in episodes of pulmonary infiltration of the fungal pathogen *(353)*.

A rarely reported case of concomitant allergic bronchopulmonary aspergillosis and allergic Aspergillus sinusitis has been reviewed *(367)*.

3.7. Therapy of Aspergillus-Induced Otomycosis

Of all *Aspergillus* spp., *A. niger* has been most commonly associated with *Aspergillus*-induced otitis externa. The latter condition is characterized with ear pain and hearing loss due to canal occlusion *(368,369)*. In addition, the external ear canal may also contain a black mass of moldy growth.

Local therapy of otomycosis may include the use of cresylate, alcohol, nystatin, amphotericin B, thymol, and gentian violet. Bezjak and Arya *(370)* treated five patients with topical nystatin ointment for 3–4 wk with clinical cure seen in three patients. In another case report *(371)*, dusting with nystatin powder (in combination with boric acid) was applied three times weekly for at least 3 wk.

Iodochlorhydroxyquine (as a powder) was found to be very effective when applied by insufflation into the infected auditory canal after removal of fungal growth; the treatment was followed by a regimen involving application three times daily of 3% iodochlorhydroxyquine lotion in the ear canal for 1 wk *(372)*. A combination of iodochlorhydroxyquine (1% in propylene glycol) with the corticosteroid flumethazone (0.02%) was also used to treat *Aspergillus*-induced otomycosis *(373)*.

According to Than et al. *(374)*, 10% 5-FC ointment was most effective in treating *Aspergillus* otitis externa. Previously, Schoneback and Zakrisson *(375)* and Youssef and Abdou *(376)* have described the topical application of 5-FC ointment as effective in treating otomycosis caused by *A. niger*, as many as 60% of all patients were reported cured.

Amphotericin B was found by Mc Gonigle and Jillson *(372)* to be a useful alternative in the therapy of *Aspergillus* otomycosis when applied topically as 3% solution (a three-drop dose). With other antibiotics such as oxytetracycline-polymyxin itic, complete cure of otomycosis was registered in 70% of the treated cases *(368)*.

The use of nitrofungin and clotrimazole in combination with 1% decamine ointment in the treatment of *A. niger*-induced otomycosis has been described *(377)*. Molina Utrilla et al. *(271)* compared the efficacy of iodine-povidone, chlotrimazole, and ciclopiroxolamine in the treatment of *Aspergillus*-induced otomycosis.

A. flavus, an unusual cause of malignant otitis, was identified in pure culture of tissue from two patients in which histologic examination revealed branching septate hyphae invading the temporal bone *(378)* Treatment with amphotericin B, followed by a more protracted course of itraconazole, resulted in an apparent cure.

A case of *A. terreus*-induced chronic bilateral suppurative otitis media presenting with otorrhoea, itching, mild deafness, heaviness in the ear and otalgia, has been reported by Tiwari et al. *(379)*; the infection responded well to topical ketoconazole therapy.

3.8. Therapy of Aspergillus-Induced Onychomycosis

In addition to dermatophytes and yeast fungi, *A. niger* and *A. fumigatus* were among several other pathogens (*Scopulariopsis brevicaulis*, *Hendersonula toruloidea*) implicated in human onychomycosis. Ulbricht and Worz *(272)* used topical 8% ciclopirox nail lacquer for maximum of 6 mo to achieve mycologic cure.

4. PROPHYLAXIS AGAINST ASPERGILLOSIS

Patients receiving allogeneic bone-marrow transplants are at high risk of developing aspergillosis. Post-transplant risk factors include severe graft-vs-host disease with concomitant high-dose corticosteroid therapy, and colonization with *Aspergillus* spp. To this end, using the experience of the Royal Melbourne Hospital, Grigg *(380)* recommended as prophylaxis of pre-transplant patients the use of granulocyte transfusions and AmBisome, and for post-transplant patients prophylaxis of oral itraconazole or, if it cannot be tolerated, AmBisome. Antifungal prophylaxis is usually discontinued upon resolution of neutropenia, when the prednisolone falls below 10 mg daily, or when *Aspergillus* colonization is no longer detected.

Prophylactic anti-*Aspergillus* therapy has also involved the use of azole antimycotics *(381)*. MacMillan et al. *(382)* conducted a clinical trial to determine the optimal dose and duration of fluconazole in antifungal prophylaxis in bone-marrow transplantation patients. Patients were randomly assigned to receive either high (400 mg, daily) or reduced (200 mg, daily) while being neutropenic. After neutrophil recovery, the patients were randomly assigned to receive maintenance therapy with either fluconazole (100 mg daily) or clotrimazole trochet (10 mg, q.t.d.) until 100 d after transplantation. The results have shown that both the high (400-mg) and low (200-mg) doses had similar efficacy in reducing the incidence of yeast colonization.

The role of itraconazole in antifungal prophylaxis has been limited by the low availability of the capsule formulation. However, the bioavailability of its oral solution is much improved as suggested by three multicenter trials using daily itraconazole solution at 5.0 mg/kg *(383)*. In an Italian study, when itraconazole solution was compared with placebo-proven, suspected, and superficial cases of aspergillosis were fewer in the itraconazole arm than with the placebo ($p = 0.035$). In a UK trial, where the itraconazole solution was compared with fluconazole suspension (100 mg, daily), no invasive aspergillosis occurred in the itraconazole group and there were more fungal deaths due to proven/

suspected infection in the fluconazole group than in the itraconazole group (0 vs 7, $p = 0.024$). In the third study, itraconazole was compared with amphotericin B capsules; however, there were no statistical differences between invasive fungal infections, *Aspergillus* infections, and mortality in the amphotericin B arm vs the itraconazole group *(383)*.

A historical comparison of prophylactic treatment of neutropenic patients with itraconazole and ketoconazole has been summarized by Tricot et al. *(263)* Of the 52 neutropenic patients receiving ketoconazole, 36.5% developed aspergillosis as compared with only 11.5% of the population (a total of 45 patients) receiving prophylactic itraconazole.

Results from the evaluation of nebulized amphotericin B as prophylaxis for *Aspergillus* infections in lung-transplant recipients and associated risk factors have shown the nebulized antibiotic to be efficient and safe in preventing infection, and that CMV disease increased the probality of *Aspergillus* infection *(384)*.

Prolonged secondary prophylaxis with liposomal amphotericin B showed no signs of toxicity after invasive aspergillosis following treatment for hematological malignancies *(385)*. Prophylaxis with amphotericin B lipid complex (1.0 mg/kg, daily) of patients requiring prolonged ICU treatment after orthotopic liver transplantation appears to be well-tolerated and may prevent invasive aspergillosis *(386)*.

Anti-*Aspergillus* prophylaxis in hematopoietic stem-cell transplant recipients has been reviewed by Marr *(387)*. Also, prevention of invasive aspergillosis in AIDS patients with sulfamethoxazole was reviewed by Afeltra et al. *(388)*.

5. ASPERGILLUS CHEVALIERI

Naidu and Singh *(389)* described the first three cases of cutaneous aspergillosis caused by *Aspergillus chevalieri*, a new opportunistic pathogen of human disease. The observed lesions were erythematous and hyperkeratotic with vesicopapular eruptions and scaling. Histopathologic examination revealed a granulomatous reaction showing polymorphonuclear leukocytes around the fungal hyphae, which were broad, septate, branched, and aggregated in the epidermal area.

In vitro, after 48 h of incubation, amphotericin B, 5-FC, ketoconazole, oxiconazole and the allylamine derivative, amorolfine showed MIC values against a clinical isolate of *A. chevalieri* of 0.1, 0.1, 1.0, 0.1, and 0.3 µg/mL, respectively *(389)*.

REFERENCES

1. Tomee, J. F. and van der Werf, T. S. Pulmonary aspergillosis. *Neth. J. Med.*, 59, 244–258, 2001.
2. Emmons, C. W., Binford, C. H., and Utz, J. P. *Medical Mycology*, 2nd ed. Lea & Febiger, Philadelphia, 256, 1970.
3. Gene, J., Azon-Masoliver, A., Guarro, J., et al. Cutaneous infection caused by *Aspergillus ustus*, an emerging opportunistic fungus in immunosuppressed patients. *J. Clin. Microbiol.*, 39, 1134–1136, 2001.
4. Sugimura, S., Yoshida, K., Oba, H., et al. Two cases of invasive pulmonary aspergillosis in non-immunocompromised hosts. *Nippon Kyobu Shikkan Gakkai Zasshi*, 32, 1032, 1994.
5. Muller, M., Fallen, H., and Zoller, L. Pulmonary aspergillosis in an immunocompetent female patient. *Dtsch. Med. Wochenschr.*, 119, 760, 1994 [see also: *Dtsch. Med. Wochenschr.*, 119, 1716 & 1717, 1994].
6. Valluri, S., Moorthy, R. S., Liggett, P. E., and Rao, N. A. Endogeneous *Aspergillus* endophthalmitis in an immunocompetent individual. *Int. Ophthalmol.*, 17, 131, 1993.
7. Ko, J. P., Kim, D. H., and Shepard, J. A. Pulmonary aspergillosis in an immunocompetent patient. *J. Thorac. Imaging*, 17, 70–73, 2002.
8. Jeanrot, C., Guigui, P., Groussard, O., and Deburge, A. Spinal epidural aspergillosis due to a lung aspergilloma despite long-term itraconazole treatment. *Rev. Chir. Orthop. Repatrice Appar. Mot.*, 87, 596–600, 2001.
9. Elgamal, E. A. and Murshid, W. R. Intracavitary administration of amphotericin B in the treatment of cerebral aspergillosis in a non-immunocompromised patient: case report and review of the literature. *Br. J. Neurosurg.*, 14, 137–141, 2000.
10. Murthy, J. M., Sundaram, C., Prasad, V. S., Purohit, A. K., Rammurti, S., and Laxmi, V. Aspergillosis of central nervous system: a study of 21 patients seen in a university hospital in South India. *J. Assos. Physicians India*, 48, 677–681, 2000.
11. Wise, G. J. Genitourinary fungal infections: a therapeutic conundrum. *Expert Opin. Pharmacother.*, 2, 121–126, 2001.
12. Nenoff, P., Kliem, C., Mittag, M., Horn, L. C., Niederwieser, D., and Haustein, U. F. Secondary cutaneous aspergillosis

due to *Aspergillus flavus* in an acute myeloid leukaemia patient following stem cell transplantation. *Eur. J. Dermatol.*, 12, 93–98, 2002.
13. Ozsahin, H., Wacker, P., Brundler, M. A., et al. Fatal myocardial aspergillosis in an immunosuppressed child. *J. Pediatr. Hematol. Oncol.*, 23, 456–459, 2001.
14. Nosari, A., Oreste, P., Cairoli, R., et al. Invasive aspergillosis in haematological malignancies: clinical findings and management for intensive chemotherapy completion. *Am. J. Hematol.*, 68, 231–236, 2001.
15. Buchheidt, D., Spiess, B., and Hehlmann, R. Systemic infections with *Aspergillus* species in patients with hematological malignancies: current serological and molecular diagnostic approaches. *Onkologie*, 24, 531–536, 2001.
16. Karthaus, M. and Bohme, A. Therapy of invasive organ mycoses in patients with systemic hematologic disease. *Wien Med. Wochenschr.*, 151, 80–88, 2001.
17. Takagi, K., Yoshida, A., Yamauchi, T., et al. Successful treatment of *Aspergillus* spondylodiscitis with high-dose itraconazole in a patient with acute myelogenous leukemia. *Leukemia*, 15, 1670–1671, 2001.
18. Park, K. U., Lee, H. S., Kim, C. J., and Kim, E. C. Fungal discitis due to *Aspergillus terreus* in a patient with acute lymphoblastic leukemia. *J. Korean Med. Sci.*, 15, 704–707, 2000.
19. Grandiere-Perez, L., Asfar, P., Foussard, C., Chennebault, J. M., Penn, P., and Degasne, I. Spondylodiscitis due to *Aspergillus terreus* during an efficient treatment against invasive pulmonary aspergillosis. *Intensive Care Med.*, 26, 1010–1011, 2000.
20. Ng, A., Gadong, N., Kelsey, A., Denning, D. W., Leggate, J., and Eden, O. B. Successful treatment of *Aspergillus* brain abscess in a child with acute lymphoblastic leukemia. *Pediatr. Hematol. Oncol.*, 17, 497–504, 2000.
21. Nucci, M., Pulcheri, W., Bacha, P. C., et al. Amphotericin B followed by itraconazole in the treatment of disseminated fungal infections in neutropenic patients. *Mycoses*, 37, 433, 1994.
22. Caillot, D., Mannone, L., Cuisenier, B., and Couaillier, J. F. Role of early diagnosis and aggressive surgery in the management of invasive pulmonary aspergillosis in neutropenic patients. *Clin. Microbiol. Infect.*, 7(Suppl. 2), 54–61, 2001.
23. Goldberg, S. L., Geha, D. J., Marshall, W. F., Inwards, D. J., and Hoagland, H. C. Successful treatment of simulataneous pulmonary *Pseudallescheria boydii* and *Aspergillus terreus* infection with oral itraconazole. *Clin. Infect. Dis.*, 16, 803, 1993.
24. Hadley, S. and Karchmer, A. W. Fungal infections in solid organ transplant recipients. *Infect. Dis. Clin. North Am.*, 9, 1045, 1995.
25. Marks, W. H., Florence, L., Lieberman, J., et al. Successfully treated invasive pulmonary aspergillosis associated with smoking marijuana in a renal transplant recipient. *Transplantation*, 61, 1771, 1996.
26. Bowden, R. A., Cays, M., Gooley, T., Mamelok, R. D., and van Burik, J. A. Phase I study of amphotericin B colloidal dispersion for the treatment of invasive fungal infections after marrow transplant. *J. Infect. Dis.*, 173, 1208, 1996.
27. Warnock, D. W. Fungal complications of transplantation: diagnosis, treatment and prevention. *J. Antimicrob. Chemother.*, 36(Suppl. B), 73, 1995.
28. Kruger, W., Stockschläder, M., Rüssmann, B., et al. Experience with liposomal amphotericin B in 60 patients undergoing high-dose therapy and bone marrow or peripheral blood stem cell transplantation. *Br. J. Haematol.*, 91, 684, 1995.
29. Choi, S. S., Milmoe, G. J., Dinndorf, P. A., and Quinones, R. R. Invasive *Aspergillus* sinusitis in pediatric bone marrow transplant patient: evaluation and management. *Arch. Otolaryngol. Head Neck Surg.*, 121, 1188, 1995.
30. Cassuto-Viguier, E., Mondain, J. R., Van Elslande, L., et al. Fatal outcome of *Aspergillus* fumigatus arthritis in a renal transplant recipient. *Transplant. Proc.*, 27, 2461, 1995.
31. Franco, M., Van Elslande, L., Robino, C., et al. *Aspergillus* arthritis of the shoulder in a renal transplant recipient: failure of itraconazole therapy. *Rev. Rhum. Engl. Ed.*, 62, 215, 1995.
32. Hagensee, M. E., Bauwens, J. E., Kjos, B., and Bowden, R. A. Brain abscess following marrow transplantation: experince at the Fred Hutchinson Cancer Research Center, 1984–1992. *Clin. Infect. Dis.*, 19, 402, 1994.
33. Collins, L. A., Samore, M. H., Roberts, M. S., et al. Risk factors for invasive fungal infections complicating orthotopic liver transplantation. *J. Infect. Dis.*, 170, 644, 1994.
34. Wang, S. S., Chu, S. H., Lee, Y. C., Chang, S. C., and Yang, P. C. Successful treatment of invasive pulmonary aspergillosis. *Transplant. Proc.*, 26, 2329, 1994.
35. Saah, D., Drakos, P. E., Elidan, J., Braverman, I., Or, R., and Nagler, A. Rhinocerebral aspergillosis in patients undergoing bone marrow transplantation. *Ann. Otol. Rhinol. Laryngol.*, 103, 306, 1994.
36. O'Donnell, M. R., Schmidt, G. M., Tegmeier, B. R., et al. Prediction of systemic fungal infection in allogeneic marrow recipients: impact of amphotericin prophylaxis in high-risk patients. *J. Clin. Oncol.*, 12, 827, 1994.
37. McWhinney, P. H., Kibbler, C. C., Hamon, M. D., et al. Progress in the diagnosis and management of aspergillosis in bone marrow transplantation: 13 years' experience. *Clin. Infect. Dis.*, 17, 397, 1993.
38. Holt, R. I., Kwan, J. T., Sefton, A. M., and Cunningham, J. Successful treatment of concomitant pulmonary nocardiosis and aspergillosis in an immunocompromised renal patient. *Eur. J. Clin. Microbiol. Infect. Dis.*, 12, 110, 1993.
39. Paya, C. V. Fungal infections in solid-organ transplantations. *Clin. Infect. Dis.*, 16, 677, 1993.
40. Monteforte, J. S. and Wood, C. A. Pneumonia caused by *Nocardia nova* and *Aspergillus fumigatus* after cardiac transplantation. *Eur. J. Clin. Microbiol. Infect. Dis.*, 12, 112, 1993.
41. Grow, W. B., Moreb, J. S., Roque, D., et al. Late onset of invasive aspergillus infection in bone marrow transplant patients at a university hospital. *Bone Marrow Transplant.*, 29, 15–19, 2002.
42. Watanabe, C., Yajima, S., Taguchi, T., et al. Successful unrelated bone marrow transplantation for a patient with chronic granulomatous disease and associated resistant pneumonitis and *Aspergillus* osteomyelitis. *Bone Marrow Transplant.*, 28, 83–87, 2001.

43. Kim, S. W., Nah, M. Y., Yeum, C. H., et al. Pelvic aspergillosis with tubo-ovarien abscess in a renal transplant recipient. *J. Infect.*, 42, 215–217, 2001.
44. Barnes, C., Berkovitz, R., Curtis, N., and Waters, K. *Aspergillus* laryngotracheobronchial infection in a 6-year-old girl following bone marrow transplantation. *Int. J. Pediatr. Otorhinolaryngol.*, 59, 59–62, 2001.
45. Kontoyiannis, D. P., Andersson, B. S., Lewis, R. E., and Raad, I. I. Progressive disseminated aspergillosis in a bone marrow transplant recipient: response with a high-dose lipid formulation of amphotericin B. *Clin. Infect. Dis.*, 32, E94–E96, 2001.
46. Jantunen, E., Ruutu, P., Piilonen, A., Volin, L., Parkkali, T., and Ruutu, T. Treatment and outcome of invasive *Aspergillus* infections in allogeneic BMT recipients. *Bone Marrow Transplant.*, 26, 759–762, 2000.
47. Jantinen, E., Piilonen, A., Volin, L., et al. Diagnostic aspects of invasive *Aspergillus* infections in allogenic BMT recipients. *Bone Marrow Transplant.*, 25, 867–871, 2000.
48. Ho, P. L. and Yuen, K. Y. Aspergillosis in bone marrow transplant recipients. *Crit. Rev. Oncol. Hematol.*, 34, 55–69, 2000.
49. Yeldandi, V., Laghi, F., McCabe, M. A., et al. *Aspergillus* and lung transplantation. *J. Heart Lung Transplant.*, 14, 883, 1995.
50. Tomee, J. F., Mannes, G. P., van der Bij, W., et al. Serodiagnosis and monitoring of *Aspergillus* infections after lung transplantation. *Ann. Intern. Med.*, 125, 197, 1996.
51. Heurlin, N., Bergstrom, S. E., Winiarski, J., et al. Fungal pneumonia: the predominant lung infection causing death in children undergoing bone marrow transplantation. *Acta Paediatr.*, 85, 168, 1996.
52. Mannes, G. P., van der Bij, W., and de Boer, W. J. Liposomal amphotericin B in three lung transplant recipients. *J. Heart Lung Transplant.*, 14, 781, 1995.
53. Flume, P. A., Egan, T. M., Paradowski, L. J., Detterbeck, F. C., Thompson, J. T., and Yankaskas, J. R. Infectious complications of lung transplantation: impact of cystic fibrosis. *Am. J. Respir. Crit. Care Med.*, 149, 1601, 1994.
54. Mehrad, B., Paciocco, G., Martinez, F. J., Ojo, T. C., Iannettoni, M. D., and Lynch, J. P. 3rd. Spectrum of *Aspergillus* infection in lung transplant recipients: case series and review of the literature. *Chest*, 19, 169–175, 2001.
55. Gilbey, J. G., Chalermskulrat, W., and Aris, R. M. *Aspergillus* endocarditis in a lung transplant recipient. A case report and review of the transplant literature. *Ann. Transplant.*, 5, 48–53, 2000.
56. Collazos, J., Mayo, J., Martinez, E., and Ibarra, S. Prosthetic vascular graft infection due to *Aspergillus* species: case report and literature review. *Eur. J. Clin. Microbiol. Infect. Dis.*, 20, 414–417, 2001.
57. Beckers, E. A. and Strack van Schijndel, R. J. *Aspergillus* spondylodiskitis in a patient with chronic obstructive pulmonary disease. *Eur. J. Intern. Med.*, 13, 139–142, 2002.
58. Nenoff, P., Kellermann, S., Horn, L. C., et al. Case report. Mycotic arteritis due to *Aspergillus fumigatus* in a diabetic with retrobulbar aspergillosis and mycotic meningitis. *Mycoses*, 44, 407–414, 2001.
59. Berner, R., Sauter, S., Michalski, Y., and Niemeyer, C. M., Central venous catheter infection by *Aspergillus fumigatus* in a patient with B-type non-Hodgkin lymphoma, *Med. Pediatr. Oncol.*, 27, 202, 1996.
60. Meyohas, M. C., Roux, P., Poirot, J. L., Meynard, J. L., and Frottier, J. Aspergillosis in acquired immunodeficiency syndrome. *Pathol. Biol. (Paris)*, 42, 647, 1994.
61. Keating, J. J., Rogers, T., Petrou, M., et al. Management of pulmonary aspergillosis in AIDS: an emerging clinical problem. *J. Clin. Pathol.*, 47, 805, 1994.
62. Libanore, M., Pastore, A., Frasconi, P. C., et al. Invasive multiple sinusitis by *Aspergillus fumigatus* in a patient with AIDS. *Int. J. STD AIDS*, 5, 293, 1994.
63. Tumbarello, M., Ventura, G., Caldarola, G., Morace, G., Cauda, R., and Ortona, L. An emerging opportunistic infection in HIV patients: a retrospective analysis of 11 cases of pulmonary aspergillosis. *Eur. J. Epidemiol.*, 9, 638, 1993.
64. Lortholary, O., Meyohas, M. C., Dupont, B., et al. Invasive aspergillosis in patients with acquired immunodeficiency syndrome: report of 33 cases. *Am. J. Med.*, 95, 177, 1993.
65. Blanco Espinosa, A., Moreno Izarra, J., Regueiro Lopez, J. C., Anglada Curado, F. J., and Requena Tapia, M. J. Renal abscess in patients with HIV infection in the era of highly active antiretroviral therapy. *Actas Urol. Esp.*, 25, 396–399, 2001.
66. Keller, M. J. and Sax, P. E. *Aspergillus* sinusitis in two HIV-infected men. *AIDS Clin. Care*, 9, 94, 100, 1997.
67. Stanford, D., Boyle, M., and Gillespie, R. Human immunodeficiency virus-related primary cutaneous aspergillosis. *Australas. J. Dermatol.*, 41, 112–116, 2000.
68. Le Conte, P., Blanloeil, Y., Germaud, P., Morin, O., and Moreau, P. Invasive aspergillosis in intensive care. *Ann. Fr. Anesth. Reanim.*, 14, 198, 1995 [see also: *Ann. Fr. Anesth. Reanim.*, 14, 454, 1995].
69. Blanloeil, Y., Francois, T., Germaud, P., et al. Invasive aspergillosis in surgical intensive care patients. *Ann. Fr. Anesth. Reanim.*, 12, 379, 1993.
70. Pegues, D. A., Lasker, B. A., McNeil, M. M., Hamm, P. M., Lundal, J. L., and Kubak, B. M. Cluster of cases of invasive aspergillus in a transplant intensive care unit: evidence of person- to-person airborne transmission. *Clin. Infect. Dis.*, 34, 412–416, 2002.
71. Pouchelon, E., Murris-Espin, M., Didier, A., et al. Invasive pulmonary aspergillosis in 4 patients with acute decompensation of chronic respiratory insufficiency. *Rev. Mal. Respir*, 10, 325, 1993.
72. Bodey, G. P. and Vartivarian, S. Aspergillosis. *Eur. J. Clin. Microbiol. Infect.*, 8, 413, 1989.
73. Pittet, D., Huguenin, T., Dharan, S., et al. Unusual cause of lethal pulmonary aspergillosis in patients with chronic obstructive pulmonary disease. *Am. J. Respir. Crit. Care Med.*, 154, 541, 1996.
74. Logan, P. M. and Muller, N. L. High-resolution computed tomography and pathologic findings in pulmonary aspergillosis: a pictorial essay. *Can. Assoc. Radiol. J.*, 47, 444, 1996.

75. Denning, D. W. Chronic forms of pulmonary aspergillosis. *Clin. Microbiol. Infect.,* 7(Suppl. 2), 25-31, 2001.
76. Ikeue, T., Nishiyama, H., Yokomise, H., et al. A case of non-invasive pulmonary aspergillosis that rapidly deteriorated. *Nihon Kokyuki Gakkai Zasshi,* 39, 582–586, 2001.
77. Kwon-Chung, K. J. and Bennett, J. E. *Medical Mycology.* Lea & Febiger, Philadelphia, 217, 1992.
78. de Aquino, M. Z., Brasciner, A., Cristofani, L. M., et al. Aspergillosis in immunocompromised children with acute myeloid leukemia and bone marrow aplasia: report of two cases. *Rev. Inst. Med. Trop. Sao Paolo,* 36, 465, 1994.
79. Young, R. C., Bennett, J. E., Vogel, C. L., Carbone, P. P., and DeVita, V. T. *Aspergillus* - the spectrum of the disease in 98 patients. *Medicine (Baltimore),* 49, 107, 1970.
80. Nong, H., Li, J., and Huang, G. Aspergillosis of the larynx. *Chung Hua Erh Pi Yen Hou Ko Tsa Chih,* 30, 111, 1995.
81. Viale, P., Di Matteo, A., Sisti, M., Voltolini, F., Paties, C., and Alberici, F. Isolated kidney localization of invasive aspergillosis in a patient with AIDS. *Scand. J. Infect. Dis.,* 26, 767, 1994.
82. Hovi, L., Saarinen, U. M., Donner, U., and Lindqvist, C. Opportunistic osteomyelitis in the jaws of children on immunosuppressive chemotherapy. *J. Pediatr. Hematol. Oncol.,* 18, 90, 1996.
83. Liu, Z., Hou, T., Shen, Q., Liao, W., and Xu, H. Osteomyelitis of sacral spine caused by *Aspergillus* versicolor with neurologic defects. *Chin. Med. J.,* 108, 472, 1995.
84. D'Hoore, K. and Hoogmartens, M. Vertebral aspergillosis: a case report and review of the literature. *Acta Orthop. Belg.,* 59, 306, 1993.
85. Baumann, P. A., Cunningham, B., Patel, N. S., and Finn, H. A. *Aspergillus fumigatus* infection in a mega prosthetic total knee arthroplasty: salvage by staged reimplantation with 5-year follow-up. *J. Arthroplasty,* 16, 498–503, 2001.
86. Ansari, M. S. Nabi, G., Singh, I., Hemal, A. K., and Bhan, A. Mycotic abdominal aortic aneurysm: a fatal sequel to concomitant prostatic and renal aspergillosis. Case report and review of the literature. *Urol. Int.,* 66, 36–37, 2001.
87. Kato, T., Usami, I., Morita, H., et al. Chronic necrotizing pulmonary aspergillosis in pneumoconiosis: clinical and radiologic findings in 10 patients. *Chest,* 121, 118–127, 2002.
88. Routsi, C., Platsouka, E., Prekates, A., Rontogianni, D., Paniara, O., and Roussos, C. *Aspergillus* bronchitis causing atelectasis and acute respiratory failure in an immunocompromised patient. *Infection,* 29, 243–244, 2001.
89. Ko, S. C., Chen, K. Y., Hsueh, P. R., Luh, K. T., and Yang, P. C. Fungal empyema thoracis: an emerging clinical entity. *Chest,* 117, 1672–1678, 2000.
90. Mazzoni, A., Ferrarese, M., Manfredi, R., Facchini, A., Sturani, C., and Nanetti, A. Primary lymph node invasive aspergillosis. *Infection,* 24, 37, 1996.
91. Gonzalez-Crespo, M. R. and Gomez-Reino, J. J. Invasive aspergillosis in systemic lupus erythematosus. *Semin. Arthritis Rheum.,* 24, 304, 1995.
92. Nenoff, P., Horn, L.-C., Mierzwa, M., et al. Peracute disseminated fatal *Aspergillus fumigatus* sepsis as a complication of corticoid-treated systemic lupus erythematosus. *Mycoses,* 38, 467, 1995.
93. Collazos, J., Martinez, E., Flores, M., and Mayo, J. *Aspergillus* pneumonia successfully treated with itraconazole in a patient with systemic lupus erythematosus. *Clin. Invest.,* 72, 920, 1994.
94. Tanis, B. C., Verburgh, C. A., van't Wout, J. W., and van der Pijl, J. W. *Aspergillus* peritonitis in peritoneal dialysis: case report and a review of the literature. *Nephrol. Dial. Transplant.,* 10, 1240, 1995 [see also: *Nephrol. Dial. Transplant.,* 10, 1124, 1995].
95. Miles, A. M. and Barth, R. H. *Aspergillus* peritonitis: therapy, survival, and return to peritoneal dialysis. *Am. J. Kidney Dis.,* 26, 80, 1995.
96. Nguyen, M. H. and Muder, R. R. *Aspergillus* peritonitis in a continuous ambulatory peritoneal dialysis patient: case report and review of the literature. *Diagn. Microbiol. Infect. Dis.,* 20, 99, 1994.
97. Girmenia, C., Gastaldi, R., and Martino, P. Catheter-related cutaneous aspergillosis complicated by fungemia and fatal pulmonary infection in an HIV-positive patient with acute lymphocytic leukemia. *Eur. J. Clin. Microbiol. Infect. Dis.,* 14, 524, 1995.
98. Baker, R. D. Pulmonary mucormycosis. *Am. J. Pathol.,* 32, 287, 1956
99. Jurgens Mestre, A., Martinez Vecina, V., Peiro Cabrera, G., et al. Mucormycosis of paranasal sinuses: benign type. Report of one case. *Acta Otorrinolaringol. Esp.,* 45, 117–120, 1994.
100. Libshitz, H. I. and Pagani, J. J. Aspergillosis and mucormycosis: two types of opportunistic fungal pneumonia. *Radiology,* 140, 301, 1981.
101. Borges, V. Neto, Medeiros, S., Ziomkowski, S., and Machado, A. Successful treatment of mucormycosis and *Aspergillus* sp. rhinosinusitis in an immunocompromised patient. *Braz. J. Infect. Dis.,* 2, 209–211, 1998.
102. British Thoracic and Tuberculosis Association. Aspergilloma and residual cavities: the result of a resurvey. *Tubercle,* 51, 227, 1970.
103. Kueh, Y. K., Chionh, S. B., Ti, T. Y., Tan, W. C., and Lee, Y. S. Tuberculosis and invasive pulmonary aspergillosis in a young woman with a myelodysplastic syndrome. *Singapore Med. J.,* 36, 107, 1995.
104. Freundlich, I. M., Libshitz, H. I., Glassman, L. M., and Israel, H. L. Sarcoidosis: typical and atypical thoracic manifestations and complications. *Clin. Radiol.,* 21, 376, 1970.
105. Israel, H. L. and Ostrow, A. Sarcoidosis and aspergillosis. *Am. J. Med.,* 47, 243, 1969.
106. Mariotta, S., Giuffreda, E., Tramontano, F., Treggiari, S., Ricci, A., and Schmid, G. Therapeutic approach in pulmonary mycetoma. Analysis of 27 patients. *Panminerva Med.,* 43, 161–165, 2001.
107. Israel, H. L., Lenchner, G. S., and Atkinson, G. W. Sarcoidosis and aspergilloma: the role of surgery. *Chest,* 82, 430, 1982.

108. Potter, M. European experience with oral solution and intravenous itraconazole. *Oncology (Huntingt.)*, 15(11 Suppl. 9), 27–32, 2001.
109. Bagnoud, M., Baglivo, E., Hengstler, J., Safran, A. B., Pournaras, C. J., and Leuenberger, P. Endogenous fungal endophthalmitis: results of antifungal treatment with and without vitrectomy. *Klin. Monatsbl. Augenheilkd.*, 218, 398–400, 2001.
110. Kueter, J. C., MacDiarmid, S. A., and Redman, J. F. Anuria due to bilateral ureteral obstuction by *Aspergillus flavus* in an adult male. *Urology*, 59, 601, 2002.
111. Perez-Arellano, J. L., Angel-Moreno, A., Belon, E., Frances, A., Santana, O. E., and Martin- Sanchez, A. M. Isolated renouretic aspergilloma due to *Aspergillus flavus*: case report and review of the literature. *J. Infect.*, 42, 163–165, 2001.
112. Gokahmetoglu, S., Koc, A. N., and Patiroglu, T. Case report. Fatal *Aspergillus flavus* pericarditis in a patient with acute myeloblastic leukaemia. *Mycoses*, 43, 65–66, 2000.
113. Demaria, R. G., Durrleman, N., Rispail, P., et al. *Aspergillus flavus* mitral valve endocarditis after lung abscess. *J. Heart Valve Dis.*, 9, 786–790, 2000.
114. Rao, K. and Saha, V. Medical management of *Aspergillus flavus* endocarditis. *Pediatr. Hematol. Oncol.*, 17, 425–427, 2000.
115. Morelli, S., Sgreccia, A., Bernardo, M. L., Della Rocca, C., Gallo, A., and Valesini, G. Primary aspergillosis of the larynx in a patient with Felty's disease. *Clin. Exp. Rheumatol.*, 18, 523–524, 2000.
116. Sridhar, M. S., Garg, P., Bansal, A. K., and Gopinathan, U. *Aspergillus flavus* keratitis after laser in situ keratomileusis. *Am. J. Ophthalmol.*, 129, 802–804, 2000.
117. Marroni, M., Cao, P., Repetto, A., Prattichizzo, L., Parlani, G., and Fiorio, M. *Aspergillus flavus* infection of an aortic bypass. *Eur. J. Clin. Microbiol. Infect. Dis.*, 20, 439–441, 2001.
118. Trachana, M., Roilides, E., Gompakis, N., Kanellopoulou, K., Mpantouraki, M., and Kanakoudi-Tsakalidou, F. Case report. Hepatic abscesses due to *Aspergillus terreus* in an immunodeficient mice. *Mycoses*, 44, 415–418, 2001.
119. Silva, M. E., Malogolowkin, M. H., Hall, T. R., Sadeghi, A. M., and Krogstad, P. Mycotic aneurysm of the thoracic aorta due to *Aspergillus terreus*: case report and review. *Clin. Infect. Dis.*, 31, 1144–1148, 2000.
120. Lass-Florl, C., Rath, P., Niederwieser, D., et al. *Aspergillus terreus* infections in haematological malignancies: molecular epidemiology suggests association with in-house plants. *J. Hosp. Infect.*, 46, 31–35, 2000.
121. Glimp, R. A. and Bayer, A. S. Pulmonary aspergilloma: diagnostic and therapeutic consideration. *Arch. Intern. Med.*, 143, 303, 1983.
122. Flye, M. W. and Sealy, W. C. Pulmonary aspergilloma: a report of its occurrence in two patients with cyanotic heart disease. *Ann. Thorac. Surg.*, 20, 196, 1975.
123. Longbottom, J. L., Pepys, J., and Clive, F. T. Diagnostic precipitin test in *Aspergillus* pulmonary mycetoma. *Lancet*, 1, 588, 1964.
124. Wong, J., McCracken, G., Ronan, S., and Aronson, I. Coexistent cutaneous *Aspergillus* and cytomegalovirus infection in a liver transplant recipient. *J. Am. Acad. Dermatol.*, 44(2 Suppl.), 370–372, 2001.
125. Cortet, B., Richard, R., Deprez, X., et al. Aspergillus spondylodiscitis: successful conservative treatment in 9 cases. *J. Rheumatol.*, 21, 1287, 1994.
126. Peters-Christodoulou, M. N., de Beer, F. C., Bots, G. T., Ottenhoff, T. M., Thomson, J., and van't Hout, J. W. Treatment of postoperative *Aspergillus fumigatus* spondylodiscitis with itraconazole. *Scand. J. Infect. Dis.*, 23, 373, 1991.
127. Richard, R., Lucet, L., Mejjad, O., et al. Aspergillus spondylodiscitis: apropos of 3 cases. *Rev. Rhum. Ed. Fr.*, 60, 45, 1993.
128. Cortet, B., Deprez, X., Triki, R., et al. Aspergillus spondylodiscitis: apropos of 5 cases. *Rev. Rhum. Ed. Fr.*, 60, 37, 1993.
129. Roilides, E., Dimitriadou, A., Kadiltsoglou, I., et al. IL-10 exerts suppressive and enhancing effects on antifungal activity of mononuclear phagocytes against *Aspergillus fumigatus*. *J. Immunol.*, 158, 322, 1997.
130. Walsh, T. J. Invasive aspergillosis in patients with neoplastic diseases. *Semin. Respir. Infect.*, 5, 111, 1990.
131. Cohen, M. S., Isturiz, R. E., Malech, H. L., et al. Fungal infection in chronic granulomatous disease: the importance of the phagocyte in defense against fungi. *Am. J. Med.*, 71, 59, 1981.
132. Denning, D. W., Follansbee, S. E., Scolaro, M., Norris, S., Edelstein, H., and Stevens, D. A. Pulmonary aspergillosis in the acquired immunodeficiency syndrome. *N. Engl. J. Med.*, 324, 654, 1991.
133. Rowen, J. L., Correa, A. G., Sokol, D. M., Hawkins, H. K., Levy, M. L., and Edwards, M. S. Invasive aspergillosis in neonates: report of five cases and literature review. *Pediatr. Infect. Dis. J.*, 11, 576, 1992.
134. Weinberger, M., Elattar, I., Marshall, D., et al. Patterns of infection in patients with aplastic anemia and the emergence of *Aspergillus* as a major cause of death. *Medicine (Baltimore)*, 71, 24, 1992.
135. Brooks, R. G., Hofflin, J. M., Jamieson, S. W., Stinson, E. B., and Remington, J. S. Infectious complications in heart-lung transplant recipients. *Am. J. Med.*, 79, 412, 1985.
136. Morrison, V. A., Haake, R. J., and Weisdorf, D. J. The spectrum of non-*Candida* fungal infections following bone marrow transplantation. *Medicine (Baltimore)*, 72, 78, 1993.
137. Waldorf, A. R. and Diamond, R. D. Aspergillosis and mucormycosis, in *Immunology of the Fungal Disease*, Cox, R. A. Ed. CRC Press, Boca Raton, 29, 1989.
138. Schaffner, A., Douglas, H., and Braude, A. Selective protection against conidia by mononuclear and mycelia by polymononuclear phagocytes in resistance to *Aspergillus*: observations on these two lines of defense in vivo and in vitro with human and mouse phagocytes. *J. Clin. Invest.*, 69, 617, 1982.
139. Waldorf, A. R., Levitz, S., and Diamond, R. D. In vivo bronchoalveolar macrophage defense against *Rhizopus oryzae* and *Aspergillus fumigatus*. *J. Infect. Dis.*, 150, 752, 1984.

140. Levitz, S., Selsted, M. E., Ganz, T., Lehrer, R. I., and Diamond, R. D. In vitro killing of spores and hyphae of *Aspergillus oryzae* by rabbit neutrophil cationic peptides and bronchoalveolar macrophages. *J. Infect. Dis.*, 154, 483, 1986.
141. Diamond, R. D., Krzesicki, R., Epstein, B., and Jao, W. Damage to hyphal forms of fungi by human leukocytes in vitro: a possible host defense mechanism in aspergillosis and mucormycosis. *Am. J. Pathol.*, 91, 313, 1978.
142. Polak-Wyss, A. Protective effect of human granulocyte colony-stimulating factor on *Cryptococcus* and *Aspergillus* infections in normal and immunosuppressed mice. *Mycoses*, 34, 205, 1991.
143. Rex, J. H., Bennett, J. E., Gallin, J. I., Malech, H. L., Decarlo, E. S., and Melnick, D. A. In vivo interferon-γ therapy augments the in vitro ability of chronic granulomatous disease neutrophils to damage *Aspergillus* hyphae. *J. Infect. Dis.*, 163, 849, 1991.
144. Roilides, E., Holmes, A., Blake, C., Venzon, D., Pizzo, P. A., and Walsh, T. J. Antifungal activity of elutriated human monocytes against *Aspergillus fumigatus* hyphae: enhancement by granulocyte-macrophage colony-stimulating factor and interferon-γ. *J. Infect. Dis.*, 170, 894, 1994.
145. Roilides, E., Sein, T., Holmes, A., Blake, C., Pizzo, P. A., and Walsh, T. J. Effects of macrophage colony-stimulating factor on antifungal activity of mononuclear phagocytes against *Aspergillus fumigatus*. *J. Infect. Dis.*, 172, 1028, 1995.
146. Roilides, E., Uhlig, K., Venzon, D., Pizzo, P. A., and Walsh, T. J. Granulocyte colony-stimulating factor and interferon-γ enhance the oxidative responses and the damage caused by human neutrophils to *Aspergillus fumigatus* hyphae in vitro. *Infect. Immun.*, 61, 1185, 1993.
147. Walsh, T., Gonzalez, C., Lyman, C., et al. Human recombinant macrophage colony-stimulating factor augments pulmonary host defense against *Aspergillus fumigatus*. *Proc. Annu. Mtg. Am. Soc. Microbiol.*, American Society for Microbiology, Washington, D.C., abstract # F-27 (p. 593), 1994.
148. Mehrad, B., Moore, T. A., and Standiford, T. J. Macrophage inflammatory protein-1 alpha is a critical mediator of host defense against invasive pulmonary aspergillosis in neutropenic hosts. *J. Immunol.*, 165, 962–968, 2000.
149. Patterson, T. F., Kirkpatrick, W. R., White, M., et al. Invasive aspergillosis. Disease spectrum, treatment practices, and outcomes. I3 Aspergillus Study Group. *Medicine (Baltimore)*, 79, 250–260, 2000 [see also: *Medicine (Baltimore)*, 79, 281–282, 2000].
150. Stevens, D. A., Kan, V. L., Judson, M. A., et al. Practice guidelines for diseases caused by *Aspergillus*. Infectious Diseases Society of America. *Clin. Infect. Dis.*, 30, 696–709, 2000 [see also: *Clin. Infect. Dis.*, 32, 321, 2001].
151. Gerstl, B., Weidmen, W. H., and Newmann, A. V. Pulmonary aspergillosis: report of two cases. *Ann. Intern. Med.*, 28, 662, 1948.
152. Klossek, J. M., Peloquin, L., Fourcroy, P. J., Ferrie, J. C., and Fontanel, J. P. Aspergillomas of the sphenoid sinus: a series of 10 cases treated by endoscopic sinus surgery. *Rhinology*, 34, 179, 1996.
153. Klossek, J. M., Serrano, E., Peloquin, L., Percodani, J., Fontanel, J.-P., and Pessey, J.-J. Functional endoscopic sinus surgery and 109 mycetomas of paranasal sinuses. *Laryngoscope*, 107, 112, 1997.
154. Klinjongol, C., Chanyasawath, S., Pakdirat, B., and Pakdirat, P. One-stage surgical treatment of pulmonary aspergilloma with cavernostomy and muscle transposition flap: a case report. *J. Med. Assoc. Thai.*, 78, 692, 1995.
155. Robinson, L. A., Reed, B. C., Galbraith, T. A., Alonso, A., Moulton, A. L., and Fleming, W. H. Pulmonary resection for invasive *Aspergillus* infections in immunocompromised patients. *J. Thorac. Cardiovasc. Surg.*, 109, 1182, 1196, 1995.
156. Pidhorecky, I., Urschel, J., and Anderson, T. Resection of invasive pulmonary aspergillosis in immunocompromised patients. *Ann. Surg. Oncol.*, 7, 312–217, 2000.
157. Georgiev, V. St. Opportunistic/nosocomial infections: treatment and developmental therapeutics. I. Aspergillosis. *Respiration*, 59, 291, 1992.
158. Georgiev, V. St. Opportunistic/nosocomial infections: treatment and developmental therapeutics. II. Azoles and other antifungal drugs. *Respiration*, 59, 303, 1992.
159. Karci, B., Burhanoglu, D., Erdem, T., Hilmioglu, S., Inci, R., and Veral, A. Fungal infections of the paranasal sinuses. *Rev. Laryngol. Otol. Rhinol. (Bord.)*, 122, 31–35, 2001.
160. Rizk, S. S., Kraus, D. H., Gerresheim, G., and Mudan, S. Aggressive combination treatment for invasive fungal sinusitis in immunocompromised patients. *Ear Nose Throat J.*, 79, 278–280, 2000.
161. Min, Y. G., Kim, H. S., Kang, M. K., and Han, M. H. Aspergillus sinusitis: clinical aspects and treatment outcomes. *Otolaryngol. Head Neck Surg.*, 115, 49, 1996.
162. Parker, K. M., Nicholson, J. K., Cezayirli, R. C., and Biggs, P. J. Aspergillosis of the sphenoid sinus: presentation as a pituitary mass and postoperative gallium-67 imaging. *Surg. Neurol.*, 45, 354, 1996.
163. Teh, W., Matti, B. S., Marisiddaiah, H., and Minamoto, G. Y. Aspergillus sinusitis in patients with AIDS: report of three cases and review. *Clin. Infect. Dis.*, 21, 529, 1995.
164. Marple, B. F. Allergic fungal rhinosinusitis: current theories and management strategies. *Laryngoscope*, 111, 1006–1119, 2001.
165. Jaing, T. H., Yang, C. P., Hung, I. J., Chiu, C. H., and Hsueh, C. Successful treatment of invasive *Aspergillus* rhinosinusitis in a child with acute myeloid leukemia. *J. Otolaryngol.*, 29, 257–259, 2000.
166. Bodey, G. P. Fungal infections in cancer patients. *Ann. NY Acad. Sci.*, 544, 431, 1988.
167. Moosa, M. Y., Alangaden, G. J., Manavathu, E., and Chandrasekar, P. H. Resistance to amphotericin B does not emerge during treatment for invasive aspergillosis. *J. Antimicrob. Chemother.*, 49, 209–213, 2002.
168. Maksymiuk, A. W., Thongprasert, S., Hopfer, R., Luna, M., Fainstein, V., and Bodey, G. P. Systemic candidiasis in cancer patients. *Am. J. Med.*, 77(4D), 20, 1984.
169. Aisner, J., Schimpff, S. C., and Wiernik, P. H. Treatment of invasive aspergillosis: relation of early diagnosis and treatment to response. *Ann. Intern. Med.*, 86, 539, 1977.

170. Pennington, J. E. Successful treatment of *Aspergillus* pneumonia in hematologic neoplasia. *N. Engl. J. Med.*, 295, 426, 1976.
171. Pizzo, P. A. Infectious complications in the child with cancer. I. Pathophysiology of the compromised host and the initial evaluation and management of the febrile cancer patient. *J. Pediatr.*, 98, 341, 1981.
172. Pizzo, P. A. Infectious complications in the child with cancer. II. Management of specific infectious organisms. *J. Pediatr.*, 98, 513, 1981.
173. Denning, D. W. and Stevens, D. A. Antifungal and surgical treatment of invasive aspergillosis: review of 2,121 published cases. *Rev. Infect. Dis.*, 12, 1147, 1990.
174. Jewkes, J., Kay, P. H., Paneth, M., and Citron, K. M. Pulmonary aspergilloma: analysis of prognosis in relation to haemoptysis and survey of treatment. *Thorax*, 38, 572, 1983.
175. Pagano, L., Ricci, P., Nosari, A., et al. Fatal haemoptysis in pulmonary filamentous mycosis: an underdevaluated cause of death in patients with acute leukaemia in haematological complete remission: a retrospective study and review of the literature. *Br. J. Haematol.*, 89, 500, 1995.
176. Shapiro, M. J., Albelda, S. M., Mayock, R. L., and McLean, G. K. Severe hemoptysis associated with pulmonary aspergilloma: percutaneous intracavitary treatment. *Chest*, 94, 1255, 1988.
177. Cochrane, L. J., Morano, J. U., Norman, J. R., and Mansel, J. K. Use of intracavitary amphotericin B in a patient with aspergilloma and recurrent hemoptysis. *Am. J. Med.*, 90, 654, 1991.
178. Bennett, M. R., Weinbaum, D. L., and Fiehler, P. C. Chronic necrotizing pulmonary aspergillosis treated by endobronchial amphotericin B. *South. Med. J.*, 83, 829, 1990.
179. Rodriguez, V., Bardwil, J. M., and Bodey, G. P. Primary aspergilloma cured with amphotericin B. *South. Med. J.*, 64, 396, 1971.
180. Fisher, B. D., Armstrong, D., Yu, B., and Gold, J. W. M. Invasive aspergillosis: progress in early diagnosis and treatment. *Am. J. Med.*, 71, 571, 1981.
181. Weber, R. S. and Lopez-Berestein, G. Treatment of invasive aspergillosis sinusitis with liposomal-amphotericin B. *Laryngoscope*, 97, 937, 1987.
182. Bahadur, S., Kacker, S. K., D'Souza, B., and Chopra, P. Paranasal sinus aspergillosis. *J. Laryngol. Otol.*, 97, 836, 1983.
183. Schwartz, R. S., Macintosh, F. R., Schrier, S. L., and Greenberg, P. L. Multivariate analysis of factors associated with invasive fungal disease during remission induction therapy for acute myelogenous leukemia. *Cancer*, 53, 411, 1984.
184. Lashley, P. M., Callender, D. P., Graham, A. C., Gopwani, H., and Garriques, S. Aspergillosis in a patient with acute lymphoblastic leukaemia. *West Indian Med. J.*, 40, 37, 1991.
185. Kusumoto, S., Matsuda, A., Fukuda, M., et al. Aspergillosis of the maxillary sinus in a patient with Ph1 positive acute lymphoblastic leukemia: a case report. *Rinsho Ketsueki*, 31, 1512, 1990.
186. Ho, P. C., Tolentino, F. I., and Baker, A. S. Successful treatment of exogenous aspergillus endophthalmitis: a case report. *Br. J. Ophthalmol.*, 68, 412, 1984.
187. Harrell, E. R., Wolter, J. R., and Gutow, R. F. Localized aspergilloma of the eyelid: treatment with local amphotericin B. *Arch. Ophthalmol.*, 76, 322, 1966.
188. Harris, G. L. and Mill, B. R. Orbital aspergillosis: conservative debridement and local amphotericin irrigation. *Ophthal. Plast. Reconstr. Surg.*, 5, 207, 1989.
189. Matsuo, T., Nakagawa, H., and Matsuo, N. Endogenous *Aspergillus* endophthalmitis associated with periodontitis. *Ophthalmologica*, 209, 109, 1995.
190. Goodman, M. L. and Coffey, R. J. Stereotactic drainage of *Aspergillus* brain abscess with long-term survival: case report and review. *Neurosurgery*, 24, 96, 1989.
191. Shuper, A., Levitsky, H. I., and Cornblath, D. R. Early invasive CNS aspergillosis: an easily missed diagnosis. *Neuroradiology*, 33, 183, 1991.
192. Kravitz, S. P. and Berry, P. L. Successful treatment of *Aspergillus* peritonitis in a child undergoing continuous cycling peritoneal dialysis. *Arch. Intern. Med.*, 146, 2061, 1986.
193. Kerr, C., Perfect, J., Craven, P., et al. Fungal peritonitis in patients of continuous ambulatory peritoneal dialysis. *Ann. Intern. Med.*, 99, 334, 1983.
194. Skorodin, M. S., Gergans, G. A., Zvetina, J. R., and Siever, J. R. Xenon-133 evidence of bronchopleural fistula healing during treatment of mixed aspergillosis and tuberculosis empyema. *J. Nucl. Med.*, 23, 688, 1982.
195. Conneally, E., Cafferkey, M. T., Daly, P. A., Keana, C. T., and McCann, S. R. Nebulized amphotericin B as prophylaxis against invasive aspergillosis in granulocytopenic patients. *Bone Marrow Transplant.*, 5, 403, 1990.
196. Kuo, P. H., Lee, L. N., Yang, P. C., Chen, Y. C., and Luh, K. T. Aspergillus laryngotracheobronchitis presenting as stridor in a patient with peripheral T cell lymphoma. *Thorax*, 51, 869, 1996.
197. Hay, R. J. Use of ambisome, liposomal amphotericin B, in systemic fungal infections: preliminary findings of a European multicenter study, *in Recent Progress in Antifungal Chemotherapy*, Yamaguchi, H., Kobayashi, G. S., and Takahashi, H., Eds. Marcel Dekker, New York, 323, 1992.
198. Lequaglie, C. Liposomal amphotericin B (AmBisome): efficacy and safety of low-dose therapy in pulmonary fungal infections. *J. Antimicrob. Chemother.*, 49(Suppl. A), 49–50, 2002.
199. Chopra, R. AmBisome in the treatment of fungal infections: the UK experience. *J. Antimicrob. Chemother.*, 49(Suppl. A), 43–47, 2002.
200. Ringdèn, O. and Tollemar, J. Liposomal amphotericin B (AmBisome) treatment of invasive fungal infections in immunocompromised children. *Mycoses*, 36, 187, 1993.
201. Walsh, T. J., Goodman, J. L., Pappas, P., et al. Safety, tolerance, and pharmacokinetics of high-dose liposomal ampho-

tericin B (AmBisome) in patients infected with *Aspergillus* species and other filamentous fungi: maximum tolerated dose study. *Antimicrob. Agents Chemother.*, 45, 3487–3496, 2001.
202. Mehta, R., Lopez-Berestein, G., Hopfer, R., Mills, K., and Juliano, R. L. Liposomal amphotericin B is toxic to fungal cells but not to mammalian cells. *Biochem. Biophys. Acta*, 770, 230, 1984.
203. Dornbusch, H. J., Urban, C. E., Pinter, H., et al. Treatment of invasive pulmonary aspergillosis in severely neutropenic children with malignant disorders using liposomal amphotericin B (AmBisome), granulocyte colony-stimulating factor, and surgery: report of five cases. *Pediatr. Hematol. Oncol.*, 12, 577, 1995.
204. Khan, Z. U., Gopalakrishnan, G., al-Awadi, K., et al. Renal aspergilloma due to *Aspergillus flavus*. *Clin. Infect. Dis.*, 21, 210, 1995.
205. Purcell, I. F. and Corris, P. A. Use of nebulised liposomal amphotericin B in the treatment of *Aspergillus fumigatus* empyema. *Thorax*, 50, 1321, 1995.
206. Hospenthal, D. R., Byrd, J. C., and Weiss, R. B. Successful treatment of invasive aspergillosis complicating prolonged treatment-related neutropenia in acute myelogenous leukemia with amphotericin B lipid complex. *Med. Pediatr. Oncol.*, 25, 119, 1995.
207. Mendicute, J., Ondarra, A., Eder, F., et al., The use of collagen shields impregnated with amphotericin B to treat *Aspergillosis* keratomycosis. *CLAO J.*, 21, 252, 1995.
208. Xie, L., Dong, X., and Shi, W. Treatment of fungal keratitis by penetrating keratoplasty. *Br. J. Ophthalmol.*, 85, 1070–1074, 2001.
209. Ellis, M., Watson, R., McNabb, A., Lukic, M. L., and Nork, M. Massive intracerebral aspergillosis responding to combination high dose liposomal amphotericin B and cytokine therapy without surgery. *J. Med. Microbiol.*, 51, 70–75, 2002.
210. Hammerman, K. J., Sarosi, G. A., and Tosh, F. E. Amphotericin B in the treatment of saprophytic forms of pulmonary aspergillosis. *Am. Rev. Respir. Dis.*, 109, 57, 1974.
211. Kilman, J. W., Ahn, C., Andrews, N. C., and Klassen, K. Surgery for pulmonary aspergillosis. *J. Thorac. Cardiovasc. Surg.*, 57, 642, 1969.
212. Reddy, P. A., Christianson, C. S., Brasher, C. A., Larsh, H., and Sutaria, M. Comparison of treated and untreated pulmonary aspergilloma: an analysis of 16 cases. *Am. Rev. Respir. Dis.*, 101, 928, 1970.
213. Peer, E. T. Case of aspergillosis treated with amphotericin B. *Dis. Chest*, 38, 222, 1960.
214. Tabeta, H. and Moriya, T. A case of chronic necrotizing pulmonary aspergillosis in which intravenous infusion of amphotericin B was effective. *Nippon Kyobu Shikkan Gakkai Zasshi*, 33, 342, 1995.
215. Krakowka, P., Traczyk, K., Walczak, J., Halweg, H., Elsner, Z., and Pawlicka, L. Local treatment of aspergilloma of the lung with a paste containing nystatin and amphotericin B. *Tubercle*, 51, 184, 1970.
216. Hargis, J. L., Bone, R. C., Stewart, J., Rector, N., and Hiller, F. C. Intracavitary amphotericin B in the treatment of symptomatic pulmonary aspergillosis. *Am. J. Med.*, 68, 389, 1980.
217. Henderson, A. H. and Pearson, J. E. G. Treatment of bronchopulmonary aspergillosis with observation on the use of natamycin. *Thorax*, 23, 519, 1968.
218. Ramirez, R. J. Pulmonary aspergillosis. *N. Engl. J. Med.*, 271, 1281, 1964.
219. Giron, J., Poey, C., Fajadet, P., et al., Palliative percutaneous treatment under x-ray computed tomographic control of inoperable pulmonary aspergilloma: apropos of 30 cases. *Rev. Mal. Respir.*, 12, 593, 1995.
220. Shirai, T., Taniguchi, M., Imokawa, S., Sugiura, W., Sato, A., and Genma, H. Usefulness of percutaneous instillation of antifungal agents for pulmonary aspergilloma. *Kekkaku*, 70, 9, 1995.
221. Furuse, F., Nakanishi, Y., Kotoh, H., et al., Percutaneous intracavitary treatment of pulmonary aspergilloma - clinical efficacy and prognosis. *Nippon Kyobu Shikkan Gakkai Zasshi*, 32, 538, 1994.
222. Schmitt, H. J., Bernard, E. M., Haeuser, M., and Armstrong, D. Aerosol amphotericin B is effective for prophylaxis and therapy in a rat model of pulmonary aspergillosis. *Antimicrob. Agents Chemother.*, 32, 1676, 1988.
223. Beyer, J., Schwartz, S., Barzen, G., et al. Use of amphotericin B aerosols for the prevention of pulmonary aspergillosis. *Infection*, 22, 143, 1994.
224. Cahill, K. V., Hogan, C. D., Koletar, S. L., and Gersman, M. Intraorbital injection of amphotericin B for palliative treatment of *Aspergillus* orbital abscess. *Ophthal. Plast. Reconstr. Surg.*, 10, 276, 1994.
225. Inai, K., Ueda, T., Kagawa, D., Iwasaki, H., and Nakamura, T. A case of erythroleukemia associated with lung aspergilloma successfully treated with continuous drip infusion of amphotericin B. *Kansenshogaku Zasshi*, 69, 602, 1995.
226. Maesaki, S., Kawamura, S., Miyazaki, Y., Tomono, K., Tashiro, T., and Kohno, S. Effect of sequential combination of amphotericin B and azole antifungal agents against *Aspergillus fumigatus*. *J. Infect. Chemother.*, 5, 125–129, 1999.
227. Gevender, S., Rajoo, R., Goga, I. E., and Charles, R. W. *Aspergillus* osteomyelitis of the spine. *Spine*, 16, 746, 1991.
228. Yokoyama, S., Taniguchi, H., Kondo, Y., Matsumoto, K., and Okada, A. A case of bronchopulmonary aspergillosis recurring in a residual tuberculosis cavity. *Kekkaku*, 64, 579, 1989.
229. Saral, R. *Candida* and *Aspergillus* infections in immunocompromised patients: an overview. *Rev. Infect. Dis.*, 13, 487, 1991.
230. Bogner, J. R., Luftl, S., Middeke, M., and Spengel, F. Successful drug therapy in *Aspergillus* endocarditis. *Dtsch. Med. Wochenschr.*, 115, 1833, 1990.
231. Talbot, G. H., Huang, A., and Provencher, M. Invasive aspergillus rhinosinusitis in patients with acute leukemia. *Rev. Infect. Dis.*, 13, 219, 1991.
232. Rodenhuis, S., Beaumont, F., Kauffman, H. F., and Sluiter, H. J. Invasive pulmonary aspergillosis in a nonimmunosuppressed patient: successful management with systemic amphotericin and flucytosine and inhaled amphotericin. *Thorax*, 39, 78, 1984.

233. Shadomy, S., Wagner, G., Espinel-Ingroff, A., and Davis, B. A. In vitro studies with combinations of 5-fluorocytosine and amphotericin B. *Antimicrob. Agents Chemother.*, 8, 117, 1975.
234. Spiteri, M. A., McCall, J., and Clarke, S. W. Successful management of primary invasive pulmonary aspergillosis. *Br. J. Dis. Chest*, 80, 297, 1986.
235. Henze, G., Aldenhoff, P., Stephani, U., Grosse, G., Kazner, E., and Staib, F. Successful treatment of pulmonary and cerebral aspergillosis in an immunosuppressed child. *Eur. J. Pediatr.*, 138, 263, 1982.
236. Codish, S. D., Tobias, J. S., and Hannigan, M. Combined amphotericin B-flucytosine therapy in *Aspergillus* pneumonia. *J. Am. Med. Assoc.*, 241, 2418, 1979.
237. Donahue, R. E., Johnson, M. M., Zon, L. I., Clark, S. C., and Groopman, J. E. Suppression of in vitro haematopoiesis following human immunodeficiency virus infection. *Nature*, 326, 200, 1987.
238. Kotler, D. P., Gaetz, H. P., Lange, M., Klein, E. B., and Holt, P. R. Enteropathy associated with acquired immunodeficiency syndrome. *Ann. Intern. Med.*, 101, 421, 1984.
239. Lazzarin, A. and Capsoni, F. Disseminated aspergillosis. *Am. J. Dis. Child.*, 136, 136, 1982.
240. Raubitschek, A. A., Levin, A. S., Stites, D. P., Phillips, J. C., and Ahonkhai, V. I. Normal granulocyte infusion therapy for aspergillosis in chronic granulomatous disease. *Pediatrics*, 51, 230, 1973.
241. Elgefors, B., Haugstvedt, S., Brorsson, J. E., and Esbjorner, E. Disseminated aspergillosis treated with amphotericin B and surgery in a boy with chronic granulomatous disease. *Infection*, 8, 174, 1980.
242. Corrado, M. L., Cleri, D., Fikrig, S. M., Shaw, E. B., and Fudenberg, H.H. Aspergillosis in chronic granulomatous disease: therapeutic consideration. *Am. J. Dis. Child.*, 134, 1092, 1980.
243. Beyt, B. E. Jr., Cannon III, R. O., and Tuteur, P. G. Successful treatment of invasive pulmonary aspergillosis in the immunocompromised host. *South. Med. J.*, 71, 1164, 1978.
244. Ribner, B., Keusch, G. T., Hanna, B. A., and Perloff, M. Combination amphotericin B- rifampin therapy for pulmonary aspergillosis in a leukemic patient. *Chest*, 70, 681, 1976.
245. Colp, C. R. and Cook, W. A. Successful treatment of pleural aspergillosis and bronchopleural fistula. *Chest*, 68, 96, 1975.
246. Sato, A., Nakatani, K., Matsushita, Y., et al., Chronic necrotizing pulmonary aspergillosis treated with itraconazole and inhaled amphotericin B. *Nippon Kyobu Shikkan Gakkai Zasshi*, 33, 1141, 1995.
247. Coleman, J. M., Hogg, G. G., Rosenfeld, J. V., and Waters, K. D. Invasive central nervous system aspergillosis: cure with liposomal amphotericin B, itraconazole, and radical surgery - case report and review of the literature. *Neurosurgery*, 36, 858, 1995.
248. Maesaki, S., Kohno, S., Tanaka, K., et al. A case of pulmonary aspergilloma successfully treated with combination therapy of intracavitary injection of amphotericin B and intravenous administration of urinastatin. *Nippon Kyobu Shikkan Gakkai Zasshi*, 31, 1327, 1993.
249. Milne, L. J. R. Mycological studies in the use of clotrimazole in bronchopulmonary aspergillosis and neonatal and vaginal candidiasis. *Postgrad. Med. J.*, 50(Suppl. 1), 20, 1974.
250. Evans, E. G. V., Watson, D. A., and Mattews, N. R. Pulmonary aspergilloma in a child treated with clotrimazole. *Br. Med. J.*, 4, 599, 1971.
251. Mahgoub, E. S. Laboratory and clinical experience with clotrimazole (BAY b 5097). *Sabouraudia*, 10, 212, 1972.
252. Tettenborn, D. Akute toxizitat und lokale vertraglichkeit von clotrimazole. *Arzneimit.-Forsch.*, 22, 1272, 1972.
253. Dixon, D., Wagner, G. E., Shadomy, S., and Shadomy, H. J. In vitro comparison of the antifungal activities of R 34,000, miconazole and amphotericin B. *Chemotherapy*, 24, 364, 1978.
254. Hamamoto, T., Watanabe, K., and Ikemoto, H. Endobronchial miconazole for pulmonary aspergilloma. *Ann. Intern. Med.*, 98, 1030, 1983.
255. Heel, R. C., Brogden, R. N., Pakes, G. E., Speight, T. M., and Avery, G. S. Miconazole: a preliminary review of its therapeutic efficacy in systemic fungal infections. *Drugs*, 19, 7, 1980.
256. Hay, R. J. Historical perspectives and projected needs for systemic azole antifungals, in *Recent Progress in Antifungal Chemotherapy*, Yamaguchi, H., Kobayashi, G. S., and Takahashi, H., Eds. Marcel Dekker, New York, 173, 1992.
257. Maryniak, D. M., Mullen, G. B., Allen, S. D., Mitchell, J. T. Kinsolving, C. R., and Georgiev, V. St., Studies on antifungal agents, In vitro activity of novel *cis*-5-alkoxy (or acyloxy)alkyl-3-phenyl-3-(1H-imidazol-1-ylmethyl)-2-methylisoxazolidine derivatives. *Arzneimit.-Forsch.*, 40, 95, 1990.
258. Farquhar, D. L., Munro, J. F., Milne, J. R., and Piris, J. Ketoconazole and fungal sinusitis. *Scott. Med. J.*, 29, 192, 1984.
259. Heel, R.C., Brogden, R. N., Carmine, A., Morley, P. A., Speight, T. M., and Avery, G. S. Ketoconazole: a review of its therapeutic efficacy in superficial and systemic fungal infections. *Drugs*, 23, 1, 1982.
260. Sonino, N. The use of ketoconazole as an inhibitor of steroid production. *N. Engl. J. Med.*, 317, 812, 1987.
261. Van Cutsem, J., Van Gerven, F., Van de Ven, M. A., Borgers, M., and Janssen, P. A. J. Itraconazole, a new triazole that is orally active against aspergillosis. *Antimicrob. Agents Chemother.*, 26, 527, 1984.
262. Viviani, M. A., Tortorano, A. M., Langer, M., et al. Experience with itraconazole in cryptococcosis and aspergillosis. *J. Infect.*, 18, 151, 1989.
263. Tricot, G., Joosten, E., Boogaerts, M. A., Vande Pitte, J., and Cauwenbergh, G. Ketoconazole versus itraconazole for antifungal prophylaxis in patients with severe granulocytopenia: preliminary results of two nonrandomized studies. *Rev. Infect. Dis.*, 9(Suppl. 1), S94, 1987.
264. Dupont, B. and Drouhet, E. Early experience with itraconazole in vitro and in patients: pharmacokinetic studies and clinical results. *Rev. Infect. Dis.*, 9(Suppl. 1), S71, 1987.
265. Denning, D. W., Tucker, R. M., Hanson, L. H., and Stevens, D. A. Treatment of invasive aspergillosis with itraconazole. *Am. J. Med.*, 86, 791, 1989.

266. Utili, R., Zampino, R., De Vivo, F., et al. Improved outcome of pulmonary aspergillosis in heart transplant recipients with early diagnosis and itraconazole treatment. *Clin. Transplant.*, 14(4 Part 1), 282–286, 2000.
267. Lebeau, B., Pelloux, H., Pinel, C., Michallet, M., Gout, J. P., Pison, C., Delormas, P., Bru, J., P., Brion, J. P., Ambroise-Thomas, P., and Grillo, R. Itraconazole in the treatment of aspergillosis: a study of 16 cases. *Mycoses*, 37, 171, 1994.
268. Cauwenbergh, G., De Doncker, P., Stoops, K., De Dier, A. M., Goyvaaerts, H., and Schuermans, V. Itraconazole in the treatment of human mycoses: review of three years of clinical experience. *Rev. Infect. Dis.*, 9(Suppl. 1), S146, 1987.
269. Graybill, J. R., Kaster, S. R., and Drutz, D. J. Treatment of experimental murine aspergillosis with BAY n 7133. *J. Infect. Dis.*, 148, 898, 1983.
270. Thienpont, D., Van Cutsem, J., Van Cauteren, H., and Marsboom, R. The biological and toxicological properties of imazalil. *Arzneimit.-Forsch.*, 31, 309, 1981
271. Molina Utrilla, R., Lao Luque, J., Perello Scherdel, E., Companyo Hermo, C., and Casamitjana Claramunt, F. Otomycosis: case reports of 18 months in the General University Hospital of the Valle de Hebron in Barcelona. *An. Otorrinolaringol. Ibero Am.*, 21, 255, 1994.
272. Ulbricht, H. and Worz, K. Therapy with ciclopirox lacquer of onychomycoses caused by molds. *Mycoses*, 37(Suppl. 1), 97, 1994.
273. Van Cutsem, J., Van Gerven, F., and Janssen, P. A. Oral and parenteral therapy with saperconazole (R 66905) of invasive aspergillosis in normal and immunocompromised animals. *Antimicrob. Agents Chemother.*, 33, 2063, 1989.
274. Tanio, T., Ohashi, N., Saji, I., and Fukusawa, M. SM-9164, an active enantiomer of SM- 8668 (SCH 39304): oral and parenteral activity in systemic fungal infection models, in *Recent Progress in Antifungal Chemotherapy*, Yamaguchi, H., Kobayashi, G. S., and Takahashi, H., Eds. Marcel Dekker, New York, 473, 1992.
275. Hector, R. F. and Yee, E. Evaluation of BAY R 3783 in rodent models of superficial and systemic candidiasis, meningeal cryptococcosis, and pulmonary aspergillosis. *Antimicrob. Agents Chemother.*, 34, 448, 1990.
276. Holt, R. J. and Newman, R. L. Mycological studies in the use of clotrimazole in bronchopulmonary aspergillosis and neonatal and vaginal candidiasis. *Postgrad. Med. J.*, 50(Suppl. 1), 20, 1974.
277. Crompton, G. K. and Milne, L. J. Treatment of bronchopulmonary aspergillosis with clotromazole. *Br. J. Dis. Chest*, 67, 301, 1973.
278. Jones, B. R., Richards, A. B., and Clayton, Y. M. Clotrimazole in the treatment of ocular infection by *Aspergillus fumigatus*. *Postgrad. Med. J.*, 50(Suppl. 1), 39, 1974.
279. Bolaert, J., Daneels, R., Van Landuyt, H., and Symoens, J. Miconazole plasma levels in healthy subjects and in patients with impaired renal function. *Chemotherapy*, 6, 165, 1976.
280. Ito, A. Therapeutic results with miconazole in Japan, in *Recent Progress in Antifungal Chemotherapy*, Yamaguchi, H., Kobayashi, G. S., and Takahashi, H., Eds. Marcel Dekker, New York, 183, 1992.
281. Uchida, K. and Yamaguchi, H. Bioassay for miconazole and its levels in human body fluids. *Chemotherapy*, 32, 541, 1984.
282. Mukae, H., Iwamoto, M., Tagawa, H., et al. A case of *Aspergillus* empyema with bronchopleural fistula. *Nippon Kyobu Shikkan Gakkai Zasshi*, 28, 1482, 1990.
283. Watanabe, A., Ohizumi, K., Motomiya, M., et al., Therapeutic efficacy of miconazole on deep- seated fungal infections in the respiratory tract system. *Jpn. J. Antibiot.*, 43, 1392, 1990.
284. Maeda, T. A case of chronic necrotizing pulmonary aspergillosis effectively treated with miconazole inhalation. *Nippon Kyobu Shikkan Gakkai Zasshi*, 32, 168, 1994.
285. Huang, Y. C., Colaizzi, J. L., Bierman, R. H., Woestenborghs, R., and Heykants, J. Pharmacokinetics and dose proportionality of ketoconazole in normal volunteers. *Antimicrob. Agents Chemother.*, 30, 206, 1986.
286. Torres, M. A., Mohamed, E., Cavazos-Adame, H., and Martinez, L. A. Topical ketoconazole for fungal keratitis. *Am. J. Ophthalmol.*, 100, 293, 1985.
287. Singh, S. M., Khan, R., Sharma, S., and Chatterjee, P. K. Clinical and experimental mycotic corneal ulcer caused by *Aspergillus fumigatus* and the effect of oral ketoconazole in the treatment. *Mycopathologia*, 106, 133, 1989.
288. O'Day, D. M., Moore, T. E. Jr., and Aronson, S. B. Deep fungal corneal abscess: combined corticosteroid therapy. *Arch. Ophthalmol.*, 86, 414, 1971.
289. Coriglione, G., Stella, G., Gafa, L., et al. *Neosartorya fischeri* var. *fischeri* (Wehmer) Malloch and Cain 1972 (anamorph: *Aspergillus fischerianus* Samson and Gams 1985) as a cause of mycotic keratitis. *Eur. J. Epidemiol.*, 6, 382, 1990.
290. Humphrey, M. J., Jevons, S., and Tarbit, M. H. Pharmacokinetic evaluation of UK 49,858, a metabolically stable triazole antifungal in animals and humans. *Antimicrob. Agents Chemother.*, 28, 648, 1985.
291. Anaissie, E. J., Kontoyiannis, D. P., Hule, C., et al. Safety, plasma concentrations, and efficacy of high-dose fluconazole in invasive mold infections. *J. Infect. Dis.*, 172, 599, 1995.
292. Onist, P. and Tauris, P. Short-term curative treatment of *Aspergillus fumigatus* pneumonia with fluconazole. *Scand. J. Infect. Dis.*, 22, 749, 1990.
293. Yoneda, R. A clinical study of fluconazole in pulmonary aspergillosis. *Jpn. J. Antibiot.*, 42, 40, 1989.
294. Takamoto, M., Ishibashi, T., Shinoda, A., et al., A clinical study on fluconazole against pulmonary mycosis associated with respiratory diseases. *Jpn. J. Antibiot.*, 47, 1145, 1994 [correction in *Jpn. J. Antibiot.*, 48, 162, 1995].
295. Nakashima, M. The clinical study of fluconazole against pulmonary mycosis: effects of fluconazole on pulmonary cryptococcosis and aspergillosis, and its pharmacokinetics in patients. *Jpn. J. Antibiot.*, 42, 127, 1989.
296. Winston, D. J., Hathorn, J. W., Schuster, M. G., Schiller, G. J., and Territo, M. C. A multicenter, randomized trial of fluconazole versus amphotericin B for empiric antifungal therapy of febrile neutropenic patients with cancer. *Am. J. Med.*, 108, 282–289, 2000 [see also: *Am. J. Med.*, 108, 343–345, 2000].

297. Heykants, J., Van Peer, A., Van de Velde, V., et al. The clinical pharmacokinetics of itraconazole: an overview. *Mycoses*, 32(Suppl. 1), 67, 1989.
298. Niwa, H., Yamakawa, Y., Kondo, K., et al., A high concentration of itraconazole in an aspergilloma. *Nippon Kyobu Shikkan Gakkai Zasshi*, 34, 67, 1996.
299. Borgers, M. and Van de Ven, M. A. Degenerative changes in fungi after itraconazole treatment. *Rev. Infect. Dis.*, 9(Suppl. 1), S33, 1987.
300. Dannaoui, E., Borel, E., Monier, M. F., Piens, M. A., Picot, S., and Persat, F. Acquired itraconazole resistance in *Aspergillus fumigatus*. *J. Antimicrob. Chemother.*, 47, 333–340, 2001.
301. Warnock, D. W. Itraconazole and fluconazole: new drugs for deep fungal infection. *J. Antimicrob. Chemother.*, 24, 275, 1989.
302. Kreisel, W. Therapy of invasive aspergillosis with itraconazole: our own experiences and review of the literature. *Mycoses*, 37(Suppl. 2), 42, 1994.
303. Denning, D. W., Van Wye, J. E., Lewiston, N. J., and Stevens, D. A. Adjunctive therapy of allergic bronchopulmonary aspergillosis with itraconazole. *Chest*, 100, 813, 1991.
304. Niimi, T., Kajita, M., and Saito, H. Necrotizing bronchial aspergillosis in a patient receiving neoadjuvant chemotherapy for non-small cell lung carcinoma. *Chest*, 100, 277, 1991.
305. Kamei, K., Kohno, N., Tabeta, H., et al. The treatment of pulmonary aspergilloma with itraconazole. *Kansenshogaku Zasshi*, 65, 808, 1991.
306. Kramer, M. R., Denning, D. W., Marshall, S. E., et al. Ulcerative tracheobronchitis after lung transplantation: a new form of invasive aspergillosis. *Am. Rev. Respir. Dis.*, 144, 552, 1991.
307. Milleron, B., Roger, V., Roux, P., et al. Semi-invasive aspergillosis with involvement of the thoracic wall cured by itraconazole. *Rev. Pneumol. Clin.*, 46, 175, 1990.
308. Watanabe, T., Kuriyama, K., and Kamei, K. Case of pulmonary aspergillosis successfully treated with itraconazole. *Jpn. J. Antibiot.*, 53, 103–106, 2000.
309. Dupont, B. Itraconazole therapy in aspergillosis: study in 49 patients. *J. Am. Acad. Dermatol.*, 23, 607, 1990.
310. Yamamoto, T., Suzuki, K., Yamakoshi, M., Tamamoto, T., and Ariga, K. A case of itraconazole-induced hypokalemia with pulmonary aspergilloma. *Kansenshogaku Zasshi*, 69, 1413, 1995.
311. Noppen, M., Claes, I., Maillet, B., Meysman, M., Monsieur, I., and Vincken, W. Three cases of bronchial stump aspergillosis: unusual clinical presentations and beneficial effect of oral itraconazole. *Eur. Respir. J.*, 8, 477, 1995.
312. Kloss, S., Schuster, A., Schroten, H., Lamprecht, J., and Wahn, V. Control of proven pulmonary and suspected CNS aspergillus infection with itraconazole in a patient with chronic granulomatous disease. *Eur. J. Pediatr.*, 150, 483, 1991.
313. Neijens, H. J., Frenkel, J., de Muinck Keiser-Schrama, S. M., Dzoljic-Danilovic, G., Meradji, M., and van Dongen, J. J. Invasive *Aspergillus* infection in chronic granulomatous disease: treatment with itraconazole. *J. Pediatr.*, 115, 1016, 1989.
314. van't Wout, J. W., Raven, E. J., and van der Meer, J. M. Treatment of invasive aspergillosis with itraconazole in a patient with chronic granulomatous disease. *J. Infect.*, 20, 147, 1990.
315. Lamprecht, J., Kuhn, A. G., and Sauer, S. *Aspergillus* mastoiditis in infected granulomatosis: a case report. *Laryngorhinootologia*, 69, 341, 1990.
316. Saulsbury, F. T. Successful treatment of *Aspergillus* brain abscess with itraconazole and interferon-gamma in a patient with chronic granulomatous disease. *Clin. Infect. Dis.*, 32, E137–E139, 2001.
317. Touza Rey, F., Martinez Vazquez, C., Alonso Alonso, J., Mendez Pineiro, M. J., Rubianes Gonzalez, M., and Crespo Casal, M. The clinical response to interferon-gamma in a patient with chronic granulomatous disease and brain abscesses due to *Aspergillus fumigatus*. *An. Med. Interna*, 17, 86–87, 2000.
318. Witzig, R. S., Greer, D. L., and Hyslop, N. E. Jr. *Aspergillus flavus* mycetoma and epidural abscess successfully treated with itraconazole. *J. Med. Vet. Mycol.*, 34, 133, 1996.
319. Gresenguet, G., Belec, L., Testat, J., Lesbordes, J. L., Dupont, B., and Georges, A. J. Pseudotumoral naso-sinusal aspergillosis stabilized by itraconazole. *Med. Trop. (Mars.)*, 49, 73, 1989.
320. Massry, G. G., Hornblass, A., and Harrison, W. Itraconazole in the treatment of orbital aspergillosis. *Ophthalmology*, 103, 1467, 1996.
321. Rowe-Jones, J. M. and Freedman, A. R. Adjuvant itraconazole in the treatment of destructive sphenoid aspergillosis. *Rhinology*, 32, 203, 1994.
322. Impens, N., De Greve, J., De Beule, K., Meysman, M., De Beuckelaere, S., and Schandevyl, W. Oral treatment with itraconazole of aspergilloma in cavitary lung cancer. *Eur. Respir. Dis.*, 3, 837, 1990.
323. Mori, T., Ebe, T., Isonuma, H., et al. Aspergilloma: comparison of treatment methods and prognoses. *J. Infect. Chemother.*, 6, 233–239, 2000.
324. De Laurenzi, A. Aspergillosis in a cardiac transplant patient successfully treated with itraconazole. *Clin. Transpl.*, 321, 1989.
325. Villard, C., Lacroix, C., Rabot, M. H., Rovira, J. C., and Jacquemin, J. L. Severe *Aspergillus* keratomycosis treated with itraconazole per os. *J. Fr. Ophthalmol.*, 12, 323, 1989.
326. Scher, R. K. and Barnett, J. M. Successful treatment of *Aspergillus flavus* onychomycosis with oral itraconazole. *J. Am. Acad. Dermatol.*, 23, 749, 1990.
327. Sanchez, C., Mauri, E., Dalmau, D., Quintana, S., Aparicio, A., and Garau, J. Treatment of cerebral aspergillosis with itraconazole: do high doses improve the prognosis? *Clin. Infect. Dis.*, 21, 1485, 1995.
328. Elliott, J. A., Milne, L. J., and Cumming, D. Chronic necrotizing pulmonary aspergillosis treated with itraconazole. *Thorax*, 44, 820, 1989.
329. Van Cutsem, J. and Cauwenbergh, G. Results of itraconazole treatment in systemic mycoses in animals and man, in

Recent Progress in Antifungal Chemotherapy, Yamaguchi, H., Kobayashi, G. S., and Takahashi, H., Eds. Marcel Dekker, New York, 203, 1992.
330. Gupta, P. K., Mahapatra, A. K., Gaind, R., Bhandari, S., Musa, M. M., and Lad, S. D. *Aspergillus* spinal epidural abscess. *Pediatr. Neurosurg.*, 35, 18–23, 2001.
331. Sachs, M. K., Blanchard, L. M., and Green, P. J. Interaction of itraconazole and digoxin. *Clin. Infect. Dis.*, 16, 400, 1993 [see also: *Clin. Infect. Dis.*, 18, 259, 1994].
332. Wimberley, S. L., Haug, M. T. 3rd, Shermock, K. M., et al. Enhanced cyclosporine-itraconazole interaction with cola in lung transplant recipients. *Clin. Transplant.*, 15, 116–122, 2001.
333. Schiraldi, G. F., Lo Cicero, S. L., Colombo, M. D., Rossato, D., Ferrarese, M., and Soresi, E. Refractory pulmonary aspergillosis: compassionate trial with terbinafine. *Br. J. Dermatol.*, 134(Suppl. 46), 25, 39, 1996.
334. Schiraldi, G. F., Colombo, M. D., Harari, S., et al. Terbinafine in the treatment of non-immunocompromised compassionate cases of bronchopulmonary aspergillosis. *Mycoses*, 39, 5, 1996.
335. Gupta, A. K., Gregurek-Novak, T., Konnikov, N., Lynde, C. W., Hofstader, S., and Summerbell, R. C. Itraconazole and terbinafine treatment of some nondermatophyte molds causing onychomycosis of the toes and a review of the literature. *J. Cutan. Med. Surg.*, 5, 206–210, 2001.
336. Rotoli, M., Sascaro, G., and Cavalieri, S. *Aspergillus* versicolor infection of the external auditory canal successfully treated with terbinafine. *Dermatology*, 202, 143, 2001.
337. Hoang, A. Caspofungin acetate: an antifungal agent. *Am. J. Health Syst. Pharm.*, 58, 1206–1217, 2001.
338. Keating, G. M. and Jarvis, B. Caspofungin. *Drugs*, 61, 1121–1131, 2001.
339. Utz, J. P., German, J. L., Louria, D. B., Emmons, C. W., and Bartter, F. C. Pulmonary aspergillosis with cavitation: iodide therapy associated with unusual electrolyte imbalance. *N. Engl. J. Med.*, 260, 264, 1959.
340. Ramirez, R. J. Pulmonary aspergilloma. *N. Engl. J. Med.*, 271, 1281, 1964.
341. Adelson, H. T. and Malcolm, J. A. Endocavitary treatment of pulmonary mycetomas. *Am. Rev. Respir. Dis.*, 98, 87, 1968.
342. O'Connor, T. M., O'Donnell, A., Hurley, M., and Bredin, C. P. Allergic bronchopulmonary aspergillosis: a rare cause of pleural effusion. *Respirology*, 6, 361–363, 2001.
343. Vlahakis, N. E. and Aksamit, T. R. Diagnosis and treatment of allergic bronchopulmonary aspergillosis. *Mayo Clin. Proc.*, 76, 930–938, 2001.
344. Wark, P. A. and Gibson, P. G. Allergic bronchopulmonary aspergillosis: new concepts of pathogenesis and treatment. *Respirology*, 6, 1–7, 2001.
345. Elphick, H. and Southern, K. Antifungal therapies for allergic bronchopulmonary aspergillosis in people with cystic fibrosis. *Cochrane Database Syst. Rev.*, (4), CD002204, 2000.
346. Vilar, M. E., Najib, N. M., Chowdhry, I., et al. Allergic bronchopulmonary aspergillosis as presenting sign of cystic fibrosis in an elderly man. *Ann. Allergy Asthma Immunol.*, 85, 70–73, 2000.
347. D'Urzo, A. D. and McIvor, A. R. Case report: allergic bronchopulmonary aspergillosis in asthma. *Can. Fam. Physician*, 46, 882–884, 2000.
348. Judson, M. A. and Stevens, D. A. Current pharmacotherapy of allergic bronchopulmonary aspergillosis. *Expert Opin. Pharmacother.*, 2, 1065–1071, 2001.
349. Greenberger, P. A. Diagnosis and management of allergic bronchopulmonary aspergillosis. *Allergy Proc.*, 15, 335, 1994.
350. Shale, D. J., Faux, J. A., and Lane, D. J. Trial of ketoconazole in non-invasive pulmonary aspergillosis. *Thorax*, 42, 26, 1987.
351. Rosenberg, M., Patterson, R., and Mintzer, R. Clinical and immunologic criteria for the diagnosis of allergic bronchopulmonary aspergillosis. *Ann. Intern. Med.*, 86, 405, 1977.
352. McCarthy, D. S. and Pepys, J. Allergic bronchopulmonary aspergillosis: clinical immunology. 1. Clinical features. *Clin. Allergy*, 1, 261, 1971.
353. Safirstein, B. H., D'Souza, M., Simon, G., Tai, E. H.-C., and Pepys, J. Five-year follow-up of allergic bronchopulmonary aspergillosis. *Am. Rev. Respir. Dis.*, 108, 450, 1973.
354. Pingleton, W. W., Hiller, F. C., Bone, R. C., Kerby, G. R., and Ruth, W. E. Treatment of allergic aspergillosis with triamcinolone acetonide aerosol. *Chest*, 71, 782, 1977.
355. Glimp, R. A. and Bayer, A. S. Pulmonary aspergulloma: diagnosis and therapeutic consideration. *Arch. Intern. Med.*, 143, 303, 1983.
356. Shah, A., Khan, Z. U., Chaturvedi, S., Ramchandran, S., Randhawa, H. S., and Jaggi, O. P. Allergic bronchopulmonary aspergillosis with coexistent aspergilloma: a long-term follow up. *J. Asthma*, 26, 109, 1989.
357. Davies, D. and Somner, A. R. Pulmonary aspergilloma treated with corticosteroids. *Thorax*, 27, 156, 1972.
358. Stevens, E. A. M., Hilvering, C., and Orrie, N. G. M. Inhalation experiments with extracts of *Aspergillus fumigatus* on patients with allergic aspergillosis and aspergilloma. *Thorax*, 25, 11, 1970.
359. Slavin, R. G., Million, L., and Cherry, J. Allergic bronchopulmonary aspergillosis: characterization of antibodies and results of treatment. *J. Allergy*, 46, 150, 1970.
360. Slavin, R. G., Stanczyk, D. J., Lonigro, A. J., and Broun, G. O. Allergic bronchopulmonary aspergillosis: a North American rarity. *Am. J. Med.*, 47, 306, 1969.
361. Stark, J. E. Allergic pulmonary aspergillosis successfully treated with inhalation of nystatin. *Dis. Chest*, 51, 96, 1967.
362. Henderson, A. H. and Pearson, J. E. G. Treatment of bronchopulmonary aspergillosis with observation on the use of natamycin. *Thorax*, 23, 519, 1968.
363. Crompton, G. K. and Milne, L. J. R. Treatment of bronchopulmonary aspergillosis with clotrimazole. *Br. J. Dis. Chest*, 67, 301, 1973.

364. Patterson, T. F., Kirkpatrick, W. R., White, M., et al. *Proc. 36th Inresci. Conf. Antimicrob. Agents Chemother.*, American Society for Microbiology, Washington, DC, abstract # LM38, 1996.
365. Radha, T. G. and Viswanathan, R. Allergic bronchopulmonary aspergillosis. *Respiration*, 36, 104, 1978.
366. Currie, D. C., Lueck, C., Milburn, H. J., et al. Controlled trial of natamycin in the treatment of allergic bronchopulmonary aspergillosis. *Thorax*, 45, 447, 1990.
367. Shah, A., Panchal, N., and Agarwal, A. K. Concomitant allergic bronchopulmonary aspergillosis and allergic *Aspergillus* sinusitis: a review of an uncommon association*. *Clin. Exp. Allergy*, 31, 1896–1905, 2001.
368. Lopez, L. and Evans, R. P. Drug therapy of aspergillosis otitis externa. *Otolaryngol. Head Neck Surg.*, 88, 649, 1980.
369. Lohoue Petmy, J., Bengono Toure, G., and Founda Onana, A. A study of otomycoses in Yaounde. *Rev. Laryngol. Otol. Rhinol. (Bord.)*, 117, 119, 1996.
370. Bezjak, V. and Arya, O. P. Otomycosis due to *Aspergillus niger*. *East. Afr. Med. J.*, 47, 247, 1970.
371. Gregson, A. E. W. and LeTouche, C. J. The significance of mytotic infection in the etiology of otitis externa. *J. Laryngol. Otol.*, 75, 167, 1961.
372. Mc Gonigle, J. J. and Jillson, O. F. Otomycosis: an entity. *Arch. Dermatol.*, 95, 45, 1967.
373. Bear, V. D. Otitis externa: immediate and long-term results with flumethasone pivalate/iodochlorhydroxyquine ear drugs. *Med. J. Aust.*, 1, 273, 1969.
374. Than, K. M., Naing, K. S., and Min, M. Otomycosis in Burma, and its treatment. *Am. J. Trop. Med. Hyg.*, 29, 620, 1980.
375. Schoneback, J. and Zakrisson, J. E. Topical 5-fluorocytosine therapy in otomycosis. *J. Laryngol. Otol.*, 88, 227, 1974.
376. Youssef, Y. A. and Abdou, M. H. Studies on fungus infection of the external ear. II. On the chemotherapy of otomycosis. *J. Laryngol. Otol.*, 81, 1005, 1967.
377. Pavlenko, S. A. Otomycosis in the Kuznetsk region and organization of medical services for this group of population. *Vestn. Otorinolaringol.*, 70, 1990.
378. Gordon, G. and Giddings, N. A. Invasive otitis externa due to *Aspergillus* species: case report and review. *Clin. Infect. Dis.*, 19, 866, 1994.
379. Tiwari, S., Singh, S. M., and Jain, S. Chronic bilateral suppurative otitis media caused by *Aspergillus terreus*. *Mycoses*, 38, 297, 1995.
380. Grigg, A. Prophylaxis and treatment of patients with aspergillosis: an overview, including the Royal Melbourne Hospital experience. *J. Antimicrob. Chemother.*, 49(Suppl. A), 75–80, 2002.
381. Hamacher, J., Spiliopoulos, A., Kurt, A. M., and Nicod, L. P. Pre-emptive therapy with azoles in lung transplant patients. Geneva Lung Transplantation Group. *Eur. Respir. J.*, 13, 180–186, 1999.
382. MacMillan, M. L., Goodman, J. L., DeFor, T. E., and Weisdorf, D. J. Fluconazole to prevent yeast infections in bone marrow transplantation patients: a randomized trial of high versus reduced dose, and determination of the value of maintenance. *Am. J. Med.*, 112, 369–379, 2002.
383. Kibbler, C. C. Antifungal prophylaxis with itraconazole oral solution in neutropenic patients. *Mycoses*, 42(Suppl. 2), 121–124, 1999.
384. Monforte, V., Roman, A., Gavalda, J., et al. Nebulized amphotericin B prophylaxis for *Aspergillus* infection in lung transplantation: study of risk factors. *J. Heart Lung Transplant.*, 20, 1274–1281, 2001.
385. Mele, L., Pagano, L., Equitani, F., and Leone, G. Case report. Secondary prophylaxis with liposomal amphotericin B after invasive aspergillosis following treatment for haematological malignancy. *Mycoses*, 44, 201–203, 2001.
386. Singhal, S., Ellis, R. W., Jones, S. G., et al. Targeted prophylaxis with amphotericin B lipid complex in liver transplantation. *Liver Transplant.*, 6, 588–595, 2000.
387. Marr, K. A. Antifungal prophylaxis in hematopoietic stem cell transplant recipients. *Oncology (Huntingt.)*, 15(11 Suppl. 9), 1519, 2001.
388. Afeltra, J., Meis, J. F., Mouton, J. W., and Verweij, P. E. Prevention of invasive aspergillosis in AIDS by sulfamethoxazole. *AIDS*, 15, 1067–1068, 2001.
389. Naidu, J. and Singh, S. M. *Aspergillus chevalieri* (Mangin) Thom and Church: a new opportunistic pathogen of human cutaneous aspergillosis. *Mycoses*, 37, 271, 1994.

31
Coccidioides immitis

1. INTRODUCTION

Coccidioidomycosis is a systemic fungal infection generally considered to be endemic for localized areas of the Western Hemisphere, in the so-called "Lower Sonoran Life Zone" (the semiarid section of southwestern United States and Mexico), and Central and South America (1–9). As recent reports have suggested, however, because of increased exposure to the pathogen, mainly because of expanded travel and tourism to endemic areas, incidence of coccidioidomycosis have been diagnosed in various other parts of the United States and the world (10–19).

While *Coccidioides immitis* is a dimorphic fungus, it actually infiltrates the host with a multifarious range of fungal morphotypes (20). Thus, although the diagnostic pathologic finding in tissue is expected be a mature endosporulating spherule, hyphal structures can also be found in pathologic specimens (21,22). Further, Nosanchuk et al. (23) presented a case of pulmonary coccidioidomycosis in which there were no intact spherules, but the characteristic barrel-shaped arthrospores predominantly present in tissue and cultures positively identified the organism as *C. immitis*.

Infections due to *C. immitis* usually begin in the lungs usually initiated by the airborne arthroconidia, a desiccated, diasarticulated mycelial fragment measuring between 2 and 4 µ. Despite the initial pulmonary portal of entry, endotracheal- and endobronchial-acquired coccidioidomycosis have also been described (24).

Although in the immunocompetent host, the majority of infections are asymptomatic, in a number of cases, miliary manifestations (25) as well as a subacute influenza-like transient illness characterized by fatigue, cough, chest pain, sore throat and headache (26), have been observed and usually resolve spontaneously.

In immunocompromised patients, however, coccidioidomycosis can lead to serious complications because of dissemination (27,28). If not treated, disseminated coccidioidomycosis is often life-threatening. Among the risk factors that predispose to dissemination, race is important. As compared with Caucasians, Asians (particularly Filipinos) and African Americans have shown an increased risk of dissemination.

With the increase of cancer chemotherapy, organ and bone-marrow transplantations, the use of corticosteroids, and the advent of the AIDS pandemic, the incidence of coccidioidomycosis resulting from reactivation of dormant infections has been on the rise. Other predisposition factors for dissemination of the disease include pregnancy, especially during the third trimester and the peripartum period (2,29), Hodgkin's disease (30), some genetic factors, such as race and ethnic background (Filipino, African-American, Hispanic, Native American, and oriental extraction) (31–36), and specific blood groups and histocompatability types (37,38). Thus, data by Louie et al. (39) supported the hypothesis that host genes, in particular HLA class II and the ABO blood group, influenced the susceptibility to severe coccidioidomycosis.

Even though neonatal coccidioidomycosis has been reported *(40,41)*, infants of infected mothers are usually uninfected *(2)*. With the exception of pregnant women *(42)*, disseminated coccidioidomycosis in males seems to be more prevalent than in women *(1,43)*. Age is probably a risk factor only in infants, young children, and adults over 50 yr of age *(35,44–48)*. Diabetics may also be at high risk. Although there is no strong evidence to demonstrate a higher rate of dissemination in diabetics than in nondiabetics, the rate of pulmonary complications among diabetic patients is definetely higher *(49,50)*.

Pulmonary complications resulting from coccidioidomycosis may include pleural involvement *(18,51)*, interstitial dermatitis *(52)*, as well as adult respiratory distress syndrome (ARDS), formation of cavities and nodules, empyema *(53)*, and peritonitis *(54)*. Extrapulmonary dissemination of infection include skin lesions *(55)*, abscesses, arthritis, osteomyelitis, and meningitis *(2)*; the latter is one of the most serious complication of coccidioidomycosis. In addition, coccidioidal infection can be observed in the thyroid *(56)*, eye *(57,58)*, sella turcica *(59)*, larinx *(60–62)*, external ear *(63,64)*, liver *(65–67)*, intestinal tract *(68)*, peritoneum *(69,70)*, prosthetic grafts of the femoral artery *(71)*, placenta during pregnancy *(72)* and the female genital tract *(73–75)*, as well as various urogenital disorders *(76–79)*. Hypercalcemia associated with *C. immitis* dissemination was also described *(80,81)*. Treatment with pamidronate was reported to easily resolve this condition *(81)*.

Constrictive pericarditis in the setting of disseminated coccidioidomycosis can be fatal despite antifungal therapy and pericardectomy *(82)*.

A case describing coccidioidomycosis associated with Sweet syndrome (likely related to Th-1 lymphocyte proliferation) has been reported *(83)*.

An unusual case of a female patient manifesting genital coccidioidomycosis, Addison's disease and sigmoid loop abscess due to *C. immitis*, was described by Chowfin and Tight *(75)*.

2. IMMUNE RESPONSES TO HUMAN COCCIDIOIDOMYCOSIS

In regard to innate resistance, arthroconidia (the infectious propagale of *C. immitis*) and newly released endospores would elicit an intense cellular infiltrate comprised predominantly of polymorphonuclear cells. Ingestion of cells is followed by a respiratory burst, and although arthroconidia are susceptible to the products of oxidative burst and cationic peptides, less than 20% of the phagocytized cells are killed *(84)*.

The high immunogenicity of *C. immitis* would trigger acquired immunity consisting of both humoral responses and cell-mediated immunity. Patients with progressive disease usually display a polyclonal B-cell activation with increased levels of IgG and IgE antibodies as well as circulating C1q-binding immune complexes consisting of *C. immitis* antigen and anti-*Coccidioides* IgG *(85–88)*. The IgE antibodies were shown to be directed against *C. immitis* antigens and to directly correlate with the disease involvement *(84)*.

Using T27K, a coccidioidal antigen preparation protective in mice but not previously studied in humans, Ampel et al. *(89)* carried out whole blood flow cytometry experiments with donors showing various clinical forms of coccidioidomycosis. The obtained data indicated that there was a specific human cellular immune response to T27K as a coccidioidal antigen. Further, a membranous outer wall component (SOWgp), another major cell surface-expressed antigen of *C. immitis*, was found to elicit both humoral and cellular immune responses in patients with coccidioidal infection *(90)*.

A *C. immitis* proline-rich antigen described by Peng et al. *(91)* has been found among genetically and geographically diverse *C. immitis* isolates *(80)*.

3. EVOLUTION OF THERAPIES AND TREATMENT OF COCCIDIOIDOMYCOSIS

The way therapeutic strategies and treatment of coccidioidomycosis have been determined depended to a large extent on the seriousness of infection after complete evaluation, and the immune status of the patient *(92)*. In the majority of cases, patients with uncomplicated acute pulmonary

Table 1
Treatment of Coccidioidomycosis in the Immunocompetent Host[a]

Indication	Clinical Stage	Treatment
Acute infection		
Low-risk for dissemination		None
High-risk for dissemination	Rapid progression	Amphotericin B: 1.5–2.0 g total dose, i.v.
	Slow progression	Fluconazole: 400–800 mg daily for 6–12 mo, p.o.
Thin-walled cavity	Symptomatic, enlarging	Fluconazole: 400 mg daily for 6 mo, p.o.; or resection
	High-risk	Fluconazole: 400 mg daily for 6 mo, p.o.; or resection
Ruptured cavity with empyema and pneumothorax		Amphotericin B: 1.5–2.5 g total dose, i.v.
Rapidly progressive miliary		Amphotericin B: 2.0–3.0 g total dose, i.v.
Meningeal infection	Patient awake	Fluconazole: 400–600 mg daily for 1 yr or longer, p.o.
	Patient confused	Amphotericin B: 2.0–3.0 g (systemically + intracisternally 3× weekly until cultures negative, then decreased frequency); with improvement: fluconazole (400–800 mg daily, p.o., for 1 year or longer)

[a]Data taken from Sarosi and Davies *(93)*, Einstein and Johnson *(36)*, and Johnson and Sarosi *(95)*. Some of the recommended dose regimens may reflect the personal preferences of the authors, and therefore, may remain controversial.

coccidioidomycosis or asymptomatic coccidioidal lung nodules may recover without treatment. However, immediate therapy is required in immunocompromised patients (especially those with AIDS) to prevent morbidity (e.g., destroyed joints) and mortality due to hypoxemia, dissemination, or meningitis *(2,43,93)*. Patients with severe primary pulmonary infections having a prolonged fever or prostration, persistent adenopathy, or extensive or progressive coccidioidomycotic pneumonia should also be treated, as well as the very young or the very old, patients with diabetis, and those with underlying malignancies or concurrent lung diseases *(2)*. Persistent thin-walled cavities are commonly observed in acute pulmonary infections. Treatment of such cavities is strongly advised when they begin to enlarge or when symptoms, such as productive cough and/or hemoptysis begin to develop *(93,94)*.

For years, intravenous amphotericin B has been the most efficacious drug for treating coccidioidomycosis in patients with extensive and rapidly progressive primary disease and at risk of developing dissemination, or in those already having disseminated disease (Table 1) *(36,93,95)*.

Because of the potential seriousness of its side effects, amphotericin B should always be applied with caution, especially in severely ill patients. In general, a total dose of 1.0–2.0 g of the antibiotic may be used in an attempt to prevent dissemination; the drug is given in 50-mg increments as either once-daily or three times weekly infusions administered over 1–2 h. In cases of meningeal infection, amphotericin B should be administered by direct lumbar or protracted intracisternal injection, or by using ventricular or the cisternal Ommaya reservoir *(96)*; the average tolerated dose is 0.5 mg *(36)*.

Koehler et al. *(97)* used amphotericin B lipid complex to successfully treat a case of disseminated coccidioidomycosis after intolerance and toxicity precluded therapy with other antifungal agents.

After their introduction into the clinic, the oral azole antimycotics (ketoconazole, fluconazole, and most recently itraconazole) have been used extensively to treat less severe cases of the disease. Currently, treatment with fluconazole (400–800 mg, daily) is recommended to prevent disease progression in high-risk patients with acute coccidioidomycosis, and in cases of meningeal infection *(36,93,98)*. Ketoconazole has been used orally in mild to moderate but stable infections at doses of 400 mg daily from 3 mo to several years *(36)*. The recommended dose regimens for itraconazole in patients with nonmeningeal coccidioidomycosis are 100 mg daily given for periods of up to 39 mo *(99)*.

A randomized, double-blind, clinical trial was conducted to compare the efficacies of oral fluconazole and itraconazole in the therapy of progressive, nonmeningeal coccidioidomycosis *(100)*. At the doses studied (fluconazole, 400 mg, daily; itraconazole, 200 mg, b.i.d.), neither of the drugs showed statistically superior efficacy although there was a trend toward slightly greater efficacy with itraconazole at the doses studied.

Data by Jiang et al. *(101)* indicated that co-administration of interleukin-12 (IL-12) expression vector with antigen 2 cDNA enhanced the induction of protective immunity against *C. immitis*.

Surgical intervention of coccidioidomycosis has also been considered as an alternative management of the disease *(102)*.

3.1. Coccidioidomycosis in Immunocompromised Hosts and AIDS Patients

Among the various opportunistic mycoses, infections caused by *C. immitis* have become a distinct possibility in patients who live in or have travelled to endemic areas of the disease *(103)*. The most important factor associated with the risk for developing clinically active coccidioidomycosis is a CD4+ peripheral blood lymphocyte count of less than 250 cells/μL *(104)*. If the infection is not treated immediately, the underlying immunodeficiencies associated with AIDS account for its high morbidity and mortality rate in those patients. Because of the sustained immune depression characteristic of AIDS, a complete eradication of the disease, even after a prolonged treatment, is virtually imposible with the currently available chemotherapeutics. Difffuse pulmonary infections and coccidioidal meningitis remain the most common and most dangerous manifestations of disseminated coccidioidomycosis in AIDS. Thus, in cases of diffuse pulmonary coccidioidomycosis, the mortality rate in HIV-infected patients within 1 mo of diagnosis may reach as high as 70%, and at this point, it is not clear whether treatment will alter disease outcome *(105)*. It is highly recommended that a lifelong therapy for such patients is initiated as soon as the CD4+ lymphocyte count become less than 200 cells/μL. One major management strategy would be to control the initial infection as effectively as possible, followed by indefinite suppressive chemotherapy aimed to prevent relapse (Table 2) *(106)*. The initial therapy, especially in diffuse pulmonary disease and coccidioidal meningitis, should include treatment with amphotericin B. The recommended daily regimens vary between 0.5 and 1.0 mg/kg (usually between 40 and 60 mg daily for adults) *(106)*.

Although a decline in frequency is possible, few data are available regarding the incidence of coccidioidomycosis since the initiation of the highly active antiretroviral therapy (HAART) *(104)*.

For meningeal coccidioidal infections, amphotericin B is administered repeatedly into the cerebrospinal space and the treatment may last for months or even years. In this regard, the less toxic oral fluconazole has emerged as an attractive alternative to intrathecal therapy with amphotericin B. Also, oral therapy (400 mg daily) with fluconazole and itraconazole should be considered for other forms of disseminated disease when the patient is clinically stable *(105)*. Both fluconazole and itraconazole are recommended for long-term suppressive chemotherapy usually at daily doses of 400 mg. Zar and Fernandez *(107)* reported failure of 400-mg daily maintenance dose of oral ketoconazole to prevent recurrence of infection in an AIDS patient. For patients who do not respond to or cannot tolerate azole therapy, treatment with amphotericin B should be considered *(105)*.

Table 2
Treatment of Coccidioidomycosis in Immunocompromised Hosts[a]

Indication	Clinical stage	Treatment Without AIDS	Treatment With AIDS
Acute infection	Rapid progression	Amphotericin B:1.5–2.0 g total dose, i.v.	Amphotericin B: 1.0–2.0 g; then, 400–800 mg for life, p.o.
	Slow progression	Fluconazole: 400 mg daily for 6–12 mo, p.o.	Fluconazole: 800 mg daily for life, p.o.
Thin-walled cavity		Fluconazole: 400–800 mg daily for 6–12 mo, p.o.	Fluconazole: 400–800 mg daily for life, p.o.
Ruptured cavity with empyema and pneumothorax		Amphotericin B: 1.5–2.0 g total dose, i.v.; then, fluconazole (400–800 mg daily for 1 year), p.o.	Amphotericin B: 2.0–3.0 g total dose, i.v.; then, fluconazole for life, p.o.
Rapidly progressive miliary		Amphotericin B: 2.0–3.0g total dose, i.v.	Amphotericin B: 2.0–3.0 g total dose, i.v.; then, fluconazole for life, p.o.
Meningeal infection	Patient awake	Fluconazole: 400–800 mg daily, p.o., likely for life	Fluconazole: 400–800 mg, p.o. for life; or amphotericin B 2.0–3.0 g (systemically + intracisternally 3× weekly); once awake and cultures negative: fluconazole (400–800 mg p.o., for life)
	Patient confused	Amphotericin B:2.0–3.0 g total dose (systemically + intracisternally 3× weekly until cultures negative; then, fluconazole (400–800 mg, for life)	

[a]Data taken from Sarosi, G. A. and Davies, S. F. (93) and Johnson P. and Sarosi, G. (95) Some of the recommended dose regimens may reflect the personal preferences of the authors, and therefore, may remain controversial.

In one of many complications with AIDS patients, it is not uncommon to have concurrent pulmonary infections with *C. immitis* and *Pneumocystis carinii (108,109)*. In such cases, the diagnosis of *C. immitis* could be delayed or missed. In cases of *P. carinii* pneumonia (PCP), AIDS patients are often treated in the early stage of the infection with combination of anti-PCP agents (trimethoprim-sulfamethoxazole [TMP-SMX]) and adjuvant corticosteroids *(110–113)*. However, the use of corticosteroids in patients with PCP concurrent with coccidioidal pneumonia may be to risky in this setting because corticosteroids have been previously associated with severe, disseminated progression of coccidioidomycosis in patients without HIV disease *(114)*. To this end, Mahaffey et al. *(115)* reported two cases of concurrent pulmonary coccidioidomycosis and PCP in which the coccidioidal infection was not immediately recognized and the patients received TMP-SMX medication combined with oral prednisone (40 mg daily); in both patients, the therapy led to clinical worsening associated with the development of a reticulonodular pulmonary infiltrate. Such distinct nodular pattern is visible on chest roentgenograms; because it is uncommon for PCP, the nodular pattern should be used as a diagnostic tool for coccidioidomycosis *(115)*.

3.2. Cutaneous Manifestations

Cutaneous manifestations have been observed in nearly half of all symptomatic infections involving *C. immitis* *(1,94,116–118)*. In addition, virtually all cases of dissemination involved the development of morphologically highly variable skin lesions *(119)*. There are three distinct cutaneous pattern of coccidioidal skin manifestations: toxic erythema, erythema nodosum, and erythema multiforme.

Primary cutaneous coccidioidomycosis, a skin infection acquired percutaneously, has been very rarely observed (1–2% of total cases) *(1)*. Its entry route is similar to other subcutaneous mycoses and results in a primary complex resembling that of tuberculosis (lymphangitis and adenitis). In patients who are predisposed or are immunodeficient, a granulomatous lesion is established that is similar in appearance to verrucous tuberculosis, or the infection may follow the route of the regional lymph nodes as in lymphangitine sporotrichosis *(120–122)*.

Facial lesions are commonly observed and may carry the risk of a greater CNS involvement *(123)*. In an earlier report, Newland and Komisar *(124)* presented a case in which a slowly enlarging supraclavicar mass with cutaneous extension was the only evidence of disseminated coccidioidal infection; therapy with parenteral amphotericin B proved to be effective. Lavalle et al. *(125)* described mycological and clinical cure of a large coccidioidal forehead lesion 2 mo after amphotericin B therapy was instituted.

One strategy that could be pursued in treatment of disseminated coccidioidomycosis involving the skin is to achieve clinical stabilization with either amphotericin B or some of the newer azole antimycotics, followed by a longer term of suppressive therapy if needed to reduce the likelihood of relapse *(1,126)*. To this end, Bonifaz et al. *(122)* reported a successful treatment of a patient with primary cutaneous coccidioidomycosis with itraconazole, given at a daily dose of 200 mg (b.i.d.) for 5 mo.

Reevaluating the potential seriousness of primary cutaneous coccidioidomycosis if left untreated, Winn *(55)* indicated the need for early recognition of this condition, and the prompt use of suppressive intravenous amphotericin B therapy until local tissue resistance and systemic immunity have contained the infection within the initial cutaneous site, leading to complete healing of the primary lesion and its associated lymphodenopathy.

3.3. Coccidioidomycosis in Pregancy and Early Infancy

Pregnant women are at high risk for coccidioidal infections *(127,128)*. The dissemination rate is 40–100 times that of the general population and reaches its peak during the second and third trimesters. After the first cases of disseminated coccidioidomycosis in pregnant women were reported back in the 1940s *(129–131)*, it has become a major cause of mortality ranging between 20% and 60% *(30,132)*. The increased risk of dissemination is likely consequence of the relative immunosuppression observed in women during pregnancy, as well as the agonistic effect of 17-β-estradiol and progesterone in the serum of pregnant women on coccidial growth *(133,134)*. Reactivation or exacerbation of a chronic low-grade infection during pregnancy has been reported in patients previously treated for disseminated disease; in both reported cases, the patients have been insulin-dependent diabetics *(135,136)*.

In 1998, Arsura et al. *(137)* made the observation (later supported by others *[138]*) that pregnant women who developed erythema nodosum were less likely to have disseminated coccidioidomycosis. Erythema nodosum, which represents a delayed hypersensitivity reaction (cell-mediated immunity) in the subcutaneous fat in response to various bacterial, viral, fungal, and chemical antigens *(139)*, would typically appear in association with a positive intradermal skin reaction to a purified protein derivative (e.g., coccidioidin) in patients infected by their respective etiological agents *(138,139)*.

Disseminated coccidioidomycosis in early infancy has been relatively rare *(140–150)*, with aspiration of infectious vaginal secretions during birth being the major mode of transmission *(149,151)*. So far, in cases of neonatal coccidioidomycosis there has been no evidence presented of transplacen-

Coccidioides immitis

tal infection because extensive coccidioidal placentitis was found without transmission of infection to the fetus; the placenta is thought to be impermeable to the coccidioidal spherule because of its large size (40–70 µm) *(140,152,153)*. However, intrauterine transmission of coccidioidomycosis has been reported *(154)*. In another case, the acquisition of infection was also thought to have occurred by maternal-fetal transmission *(155)*.

Golden et al. *(156)* described a case of *C. immitis* disseminated chorioretinis in a 7-wk-old infant. Therapy involved gradually increasing dosages of intravenous amphotericin B until a daily maintenance dose of 1.0 mg/kg was reached. An additional 50-mg/kg course of amphotericin B was administered over 3.5-mo period; follow-up examinations at 4.5 and 6.5 mo revealed no further change in the retinal lesion *(156)*.

In over 100 cases of coccidioidomycosis in pregnant women reported so far *(127)*, over half of them have been cases of disseminated infections, which were treated with intravenous amphotericin B with favorable maternal and neonatal outcomes *(135,157–162)*. Recommended dose regimens begin with a test dose of 1.0 mg, followed by sequential dose increases of 5–10 mg every other day to reach a total dose of 50 mg every other day (maximum dose of 0.5–1.5 mg/kg every other day) *(127)*. In case of emergency, following the 1.0-mg test dose, a 25-mg dose can be administered with subsequent rapid increases to the desired dosage *(127)*. During chemotherapy, the effects of amphotericin B should be monitored by weekly tests on electrolytes, hematocrit, and renal function (blood urea nitrogen and creatinine). Decreased creatinine levels indicate an early nephrotoxicity *(163)*.

3.4. Coccidioidomycosis in Transplant Recipients

Although primary coccidioidal infections are acquired in endemic areas, in immunocompromised hosts reactivation of the disease can develop months or even years later *(156,164)*. Among organ-transplant recipients, disseminated disease is common and has substantial morbidity *(165)*. In cases when organ transplantations are needed, the question has been raised whether they should be even considered in endemic areas for coccidioidomycosis *(166,167)*. Because endogenous reactivation is a distinct possibility, caution should be used with patients with a history of symptomatic coccidioidomycosis before transplant surgery is deliberated, especially in cases where extrapulmonary infections have been involved *(168)*. To this end, Hall et al. *(169)* proposed that before any transplantation surgery is performed, certain markers relevant to this problem should be examined. First will be the measurement of coccidioidal serum antibodies in patients with any endemic exposure. Patients having had previous history of coccidioidal pulmonary infections or with reactive coccidioidal serologies may benefit from receiving antifungal chemotherapy following the surgery. In addition, serologic surveillance and antifungal therapy should be considered during periods of increased immunosuppression, which may occur during the treatment of rejection episodes *(169)*.

Amphotericin B and antifungal azoles remained the mainstay of therapy.

3.4.1. Cardiac Transplant Recipients

In cardiac-transplant recipients, coccidioidal infections, although seldom, have been reported *(166,169–172)*. Similarly, coccidioidomycosis of the myocardium has been very rarely observed *(173)*. However, in patients on immunosuppressive therapy (either a two-drug regimen of prednisone-azathioprine or prednisone-cyclosporin A, or the triple-drug regimen of cyclosporin A-prednisone-azathioprine), the likelihood of primary or recurrent mycoses with higher rate of dissemination and mortality should not be underestimated. Therefore, screening for exposure to *C. immitis* before cardiac transplantation is performed is important.

Hall et al. *(174)* conducted a retrospective analysis of 199 patients who underwent transplantation in Arizona during a 6-yr period. The data showed that although in endemic area, the incidents of coccidioidomycosis among heart-transplant recipients accounted for only 4.5% of the population. In cases of either past medical history or positive serology, 200 mg of oral ketoconazole was applied twice daily beginning immediately after transplantation and maintained indefinitely. Vartivarian et al. *(171)* described a case of reactivated disseminated coccidioidomycosis in a orthotopic cardiac-transplant recipient, presented with invasion of the cardiac graft. The patient, who received immunosuppressive medication but not antifungal therapy, died. At the time of transplanation, it was not known that coccidioidomycosis was apparently acquired during a brief visit to an endemic area several years prior to the surgery.

In all earlier reports (before the introduction of the newer triazole antimycotics), the postoperative antifungal chemotherapy in the presence of prior clinical history of primary coccidioidal pneumonia or detectable coccidioidal serum antibodies at the time of surgery, consisted mainly of ketoconazole (200 mg daily), or amphotericin B (100 mg given to a child over a 4-mo period); no relapses have been observed at follow-up monitoring *(169)*. Even so, the more effective fluconazole and itraconazole should be considered first for controlling recurrence of infection.

3.4.2. Renal Transplant Recipients

Although systemic fungal infections have been frequently diagnosed in renal allograft recipients subjected to immunosuppressive therapy *(175,176)*, cases of disseminated coccidioidomycosis, because of the endemic nature of the disease, have been rare *(177–182)*. However, if not treated, as in other transplant recipients, such infections usually have high mortality rate. According to Cohen et al. *(177)*, predisposing factors for disseminated coccidioidomycosis in renal-transplant recipients living in Arizona, included gender (males have been found to be at higher risk than females), and blood group (either B or AB, or a combination of both). Dissemination was manifested with pneumonia (59%), arthritis (24%), meningitis (12%), and pyelonephritis (6%). However, these conclusions should be viewed with caution since the study involved a limited number of patients and was conducted in only one localized endemic area. Amphotericin B (total dose of 1.5–2.7 g) was used to treat the pulmonary dissemination; the results were disappointing because relapse occured in all patients treated. Ketoconazole was also used as an alternative *(177)*.

Chandler et al. *(183)* described a case of disseminated coccidioidomycosis with choroiditis in which an apparent healed focus of pulmonary infection was reactivated after treatment with corticosteroids and immunosupressive therapy after renal transplantation. The following treatment with systemic polymyxin, methicillin, amphotericin B, and gentamicin sulfate proved unsuccessful and the patient died.

3.4.3. Liver Transplant Recipients

Disseminated fungal infections in recipients of liver allografts have a particularly poor prognosis *(184–189)*. Disseminated *C. immitis* infection was first diagnosed in a liver transplant recipient in 1990 *(190)*. The reported case was unusual because the infection was not clinically suspected until the spherules of the pathogen were fortuitously detected in a percutaneous liver biopsy. Therapy with amphotericin B proved unsuccessful and the patient died.

3.4.4. Bone-Marrow Transplant Recipients

Riley et al. *(191)* reported three cases of coccidioidomycosis (one pulmonary and two disseminated) in allogeneic bone-marrow transplant recipients. All three patients had been in an area endemic for *C. immitis* prior to the bone-marrow transplantation. The treatment consisted mainly of intravenous amphotericin B. Both patients with disseminated infection died; the patient with localized pulmonary disease survived. One major impediment in managing coccidioidomycosis in bone marrow transplant recipients is the difficulty in diagnosing the infection. In treating such cases, one recommendation made was to reduce immunosuppressive medication as much as possible in order to allow for increased doses of amphotericin B *(191)*. The question of whether itraconazole, high doses of fluconazole, or liposomal amphotericin B would be most efficacious in these patients is still not resolved *(191)*.

3.5. Ocular Coccidioidomycosis

Although relatively rare, ocular coccidioidomycosis has been diagnosed not only in patients with progressive disseminated illness, but also in patients with very little or no systemic involvement *(192)*. Usually it is confined to the anterior segment and adnexa *(193)*. In general, the ocular dissemination of coccidioidomycosis is presented as either: (1) extraorbital disease, involving the optic nerve and cranial nerve lesions; (2) extraocular disease, manifested as nonspecific phlyctenular conjunctivitis, episcleritis, scleritis, and fungal granulomata of the lids and orbit; or (3) intraocular disease, manifested as anterior uveitis (iris and ciliary body) or posterior uveitis (choroid), or both, as well as occasional retinal and vitreous manifestations *(192,194)*.

It has been reported *(195–198)* that initial therapy with topical and systemic corticosteroids led to improvement in the ocular lesions. However, further evidence has suggested that continuation of such therapy may, in fact, exacerbate the ocular inflammation or as the corticosteroids were being tapered to cause progressive destruction of the eye *(183,196–198)*.

Since its introduction into the clinic in 1955 and in subsequent years, amphotericin B has been used extensively in the therapy of ocular coccidioidomycosis *(192,199)*. The antibiotic can be used topically to treat external ocular infection as aqueous suspension at concentrations of 1–5 mg/mL, instilled one drop every 30 min; however, severe local irritations may frequently occur with its topical use *(200)*. When injected intravenously, amphotericin B has shown poor intraocular penetration unless used in large doses, which, in turn, would increase its hepato- and nephrotoxicity. In the therapy of corneal ulcers and endophthalmitis, the antibiotic may be used by conjunctival and subconjunctival routes in doses ranging from 0.75–5.0 mg in a 1.0-mL aqueous suspension *(200,201)*. In the latter route, the injection is painful and may cause yellowing of the conjunctiva with a nodular formation *(202)*.

In treating a case of macular coccidioidomycosis, Lamer et al. *(203)* used amphotericin B in daily doses ranging from 20–50 mg given for 1 mo; by the end of the period, the lesion was cicatricial. It is important to mention that macular dissemination in coccidioidomycosis differs from that in histoplamosis both funduscopically and angiographically *(203,204)*.

Miconazole has also been utilized to treat ocular coccidioidomycosis. Blumenkranz and Stevens *(199)* found that at doses of 400–1000 mg, given three times daily for a period of 1 mo, miconazole was ineffective in preventing the development of new lesions. In fact, new retinal lesions had developed, which were later reversed with the institution of amphotericin B therapy. Overall, in the reported study, miconazole was inferior to amphotericin B in the treatment of intraocular fungal infection *(199)*.

3.6. Acute Respiratory Failure

Acute respiratory failure in coccidioidomycosis is a rather serious complication occuring usually in the setting of a disseminated illness *(181,205–221)*. In the majority of cases, there was one or more predisposing factors for disseminated illness.

In 1972, Knapp et al. *(222)* described a patient with primary pulmonary coccidioidomycosis who developed acute respiratory failure. Recently, two more such cases caused by primary pulmonary coccidioidomycosis have been described *(223)*. The acute failure is believed to be the consequence of an intense exposure to arthrospore-laden dust and massive inoculation with the pathogen. The proliferating fungus and the associated immune-mediated response would have caused the resulting lung injury *(224,225)*. Both patients survived after treatment with intravenous amphotericin B (total doses, 2.8 and 2.0 g, respectively); oral ketoconazole was also administered to one of the patients *(223)*.

3.7. Coccidioidal Peritonitis and Gastrointestinal Dissemination

Peritonitis is a rare complication of disseminated pulmonary coccidioidomycosis *(213,226–228)*, which is likely to occur by hematogenous dissemination at the time of the primary pulmonary infection *(228)*. Jamidar et al. *(70)* described an HIV-positive patient with a very rare AIDS-defining peritoneal coccidioidomycosis. The patient, who presented with ascites, low serum-ascites albumin gradient, and laparoscopy showing peritoneal implants that grew *C. immitis*, was discharged after 2 wk of amphotericin B therapy with greatly reduced amount of ascites; 6 mo later, the patient remained afibrile with no clinically detectable ascites.

So far, excluding autopsy series, only 15 cases of coccidioidal peritonitis have been reported *(68,226,228–230)*, and only one of these occured in an AIDS patient who had a history of alcohol-induced cirrhosis, portal hypertension, and secondary hypersplenism *(70)*.

Amphotericin B was used widely for treatment of coccidioidal peritonitis even when there was no evidence for additional sites of dissemination. On the negative side, a lack of peritoneal clearance in a patient with fungal peritonitis given systemically amphotericin B has been reported *(231)*. However, the dose regimen of amphotericin B still remains largely empiric and is dependent on the overall clinical response, sequential serologies, and the immunological status of patients *(68,232)*.

C. immitis is commonly believed not to spread into the gastrointestinal tract with the possible exception of some widely disseminated terminal stages of the disease. However, Weisman et al. *(68)* reported a unique case of gastrointestinal dissemination where histologic and culture evidence were presented to demonstrate invasion of the pathogen into chylous ascites, the mesentery, as well as into the entire length of the small bowel. As with the case of coccidioidal peritonitis, the gastrointestinal infiltration was likely the result of an initial hematogenous dissemination. The initial treatment of the patient consisted of intravenous amphotericin B (total dose, 4.25 g); in spite of the observed progressive clinical improvement, there has been recurrence of the disease. Following persistent renal toxicity, the amphotericin B medication was ceased and oral ketoconazole was instituted for 1 mo at 400 mg daily, folowed by increased dosage for an additional month. Both drugs failed, and stools continued to be positive for *C. immitis*. Next, itraconazole therapy was initiated. Repeated endoscopy 3 mo after initiation of itraconazole showed nearly total resolution of the intraluminal duodenal disease, and stablization in the patient's clinical condition with minimal persistent ascites *(68)*.

3.8. Coccidioidal Infections of Bones and Joints

Coccidioidomycosis involving the bones and joints is a very common occurence during dissemination *(233)*. As sometimes referred to as "desert rheumatism," it is reportedly present in 10–50% of cases involving extrathoracic infection *(234–237)*. The most affected sites of bone involvement included the ends of the long bones and bony prominences, as well as the spine and pelvis. However, diagnosis and treatment may pose difficult problems. Data from a retrospective study involving 24 patients with 44 separate skeletal lesions caused by *C. immitis* showed that a successful outcome was more likely in those patients treated by a combination of chemotherapy and surgical intervention, rather than chemotherapy alone *(238–244)*. Patients with a complement fixation serum antibody titer ratio of 1:128 or less were more likely to fail chemotherapy alone ($p < 0.01$) *(244)*. There were earlier studies done before the availability of the newer generation of triazole antimycotics, with treatment regimens consisting of intravenous amphotericin B (total dose, 3.0–4.9 g *[245]*) or oral ketoconazole (400–800 mg daily for a minimum of several months) *(246)*. Both drugs have been shown to produce detectable levels in the joints *(246,247)*. Synovial infection were more likely to improve as a result of ketoconazole medication than osteomyelitis *(246)*.

Buckley and Burkus *(248)* presented a case of coccidioidal osteomyelitis of a tarsal bone that was successfully treated with local surgical debridement followed by a long-term treatment with ketoconazole.

Magnetic resonnance imaging (MRI) studies of 15 patients with diagnosed vertebral column coccidioidomycosis were retrospectively reviewed to determine the MR features of coccidioidal spondylitis *(249)*.

A case of musculoskeletal coccidioidomycosis involving the wrist has also been described *(250)*. In a rare finding, disseminated coccidioidomycosis of the medial cuneiform was also reported *(27)*. as well as coccidioidomycosis in the hand mimicking a metacarpal enchondroma *(251)*.

3.9. Genitourinary Coccidioidomycosis

Genitourinary involvement is commonly observed in disseminated coccidioidomycosis. Autopsy results have shown renal involvement in as many as 60% of patients suffering from disseminated infection *(213,227)*. Although less frequent, other sites of coccidioidal involvement include the kidney, adrenal, prostate, scrotal content, psoas, and the retroperitoneum *(213,217)*.

3.9.1. Coccidioidomycosis of the Prostate

A number of clinically diagnosed cases of coccidioidal dissemination in the prostate have been described *(227,252–261)*. Earlier treatment included intravenous amphotericin B or ketoconazole *(252,254,257,258)*. Surgical procedures (transuretral resection *[254,257,258]*) have also been part of the therapy. The clinical outcome was dependent on the presence or absence of other sites of dissemination. When dissemination confined within the prostate gland had good prognosis for recovery, in general, the presence of extragenital dissemination was associated with high mortality rate *(259)*.

3.9.2. Infection of Intrascrotal Contents With or Without Prostatic Involvement

Coccidioidal infection of the scrotal contents have been reported on a numerous occasions *(253,255,262–271)*. The most common manifestations have been the development of a scrotal mass representing either granuloma or an abscess in the epididymus, and the presence of a sinus tract. In the mostly early reports, treatment was usually surgical, with only one patient treated with a combination of surgery and intravenous amphotericin B *(270)*.

3.9.3. Bladder Involvement

Bladder involvement is a very rare manifestation of systemic coccidioidomycosis *(79)*. In one such case, Weinberg at al. *(272)* found the mycelial phase of the fungus in the bladder. The patient was treated with ketoconazole and showed no clinical symptoms one year after the therapy. In another case report, Kuntze et al. *(79)* treated one patient with 2.0 g of amphotericin B followed by 200 mg of oral ketoconazole every morning for 1 yr; at the 4-yr follow-up examination, the patient was still asymptomatic.

3.9.4. Other Coccidioidal Genitourinary Involvement

Infection of the female reproductive organ is also a rare manifestation of systemic coccidioidomycosis *(79,273)*. It may be presented as pelvic inflammatory disease, pelvic mass, infertility, abdominal pain, hypermenorrhea, or vaginal discharge. The disease is usually associated with coccidioidal peritonitis. In earlier reported cases, the recommended therapy has been combination of surgical excision and systemic therapy *(274,275)*.

3.10. Coccidioidal Infection of Arterial Prosthesis

Schwartz et al. *(276)* reported a case of disseminated coccidioidomycosis involving bilateral infection of femoral artherial prosthetic grafts and miliary pulmonary disease. Although the occurence of vasculitis complicating coccidioidal meningitis has been previously reported *(277)*, what made this case highly unusual is that for the first time arterial involvement (whether native or prostetic) of *C. immitis* was described in sites remote from the CNS. In the ensuing systemic chemotherapy (coupled with repeated percutaneous aspiration of the perivascular fluid collections), the patient failed to respond to ketoconazole and was intolerant to amphotericin B. However, treatment with oral fluconazole (200–400 mg daily for 9 mo) led to clinical resolution; a life-long maintenance therapy with fluconazole (400-mg daily dose) was also instituted *(276)*.

3.11. Coccidioidal Infections of CNS

Coccidiodal meningitis is a severe infection that even with antifungal treatment can result in death *(278,279)*. It can cause severe mechanical complications including hydrocephalus *(280)* and increased intracranial pressure *(281)*.

Although the hyphal (soil) form of *C. immitis* has been found rarely in humans, several reports have described cases in which hyphae were discovered in brain tissue and the spinal cord *(21,22)*. It appeared that the presence of CNS plastic devices might be associated with morphological reversion of *C. immitis* to its saprophytic form.

A rare case of coccidioidal meningitis complicated with massive dural and cerebral venous thrombosis and tissue arthroconidia has been reported *(282)*.

As compared to amphotericin B, the advent of antifungal azoles did not bring improvement in therapy, leaving amphotericin B as the treatment of choice. Thus, ketoconazole either alone or in combination with intrathecal miconazole has been used in children with coccidioidal meningitis and was effective only in some cases *(283,284)*. Itraconazole's poor bioavailability with oral administration (the need of an acidic stomach for adequate absorption) and its limited penetration into CNS *(285)* coupled with the lack of intravenous formulation have significantly curtailed its usefulness in coccidioidal meningitis, especially in severely ill patients.

In order to achieve success, intra-cerebrospinal fluid (CSF) therapy with amphotericin B because of toxicity problems requires much more careful clinical management. As an alternative, the intrathecal administration of amphotericin B has been recommended *(286)*. However, relapses of meningitis after cessation of intrathecal amphotericin B have been reported, even after years of quiescence.

Oral fluconazole has also been used for therapy of coccidioidal meningitis. In adults, the recommended dose is 400–600 mg, daily *(287)*; in children, the usual dosage of fluconazole is 3–12 mg/kg, daily *(281)*. In general, fluconazole has been less potent than itrathecal amphotericin B in eradicating coccidioidal meningitis, in that meningitis recurred in most cases when fluconazole treatment was ceased *(288–290)*.

Cases of vasculitis complicating coccidioidal meningitis have increasingly being described *(291,292)*. Histologically, two types of vascular inflammation have so far been recognized. The first type represents a transmural inflammatory process of the intracranial blood vessels that is observed in the early course of the disease. Encroachment of the vessel lumen may result in thrombosis. Two cases of disseminated coccidioidomycosis complicated by fatal subarachnoid hemorrhage were reported by Erly et al. *(292)*. The second type of vascular inflammation occurs within a chronic disease and is associated with intimal thickening and luminal occlusion but with little inflammation *(291)*.

Currently, there are no established therapies for coccidioidal vasculitis *(291)*. The use of corticosteroids is still controversial, whereas agents that block the pathologic process (omega-3 oils and pentoxyfylline) may be of interest.

4. PROPHYLAXIS OF COCCIDIOIDOMYCOSIS

Patients who have completed initial treatment for an acute episode of coccidioidomycosis should receive lifelong suppressive therapy (secondary prophylaxis or chronic maintenance therapy) consisting of either 400 mg daily of oral fluconazole or 200 mg of oral itraconazole twice daily *(293)*. Alternative therapy with amphotericin B (1.0 mg/kg, i.v., once weekly) has also been recommended.

The recommended prophylaxis in HIV-positive infants and children to prevent recurrence of coccidioidomycosis consists of daily oral fluconazole at 6.0 mg/kg. As alternative therapy, either amphotericin B (1.0 mg/kg, i.v., once weekly) or itraconazole (2.0–5.0 mg, p.o., every 12–48 h) have been recommended *(293)*.

5. VACCINE STUDIES IN HUMANS

Although vaccine studies thus far have largely yielded disappointing results, supportive evidence exist to demonstrate the feasibility and need of developing a vaccine for coccidioidomycosis *(84)*. Most persons who had recovered from benign or asymptomatic infection developed a solid state of immunity to exogenous re-infection. Another factor is the presence of a well-defined target population of persons who are genetically predisposed to developing disseminated disease as well as persons who have a high probability of exposure based on their occupation. Also, because the saprobic phase of *C. immitis* is geographically limited, delineating the areas of potential infection would be possible.

Early experiments in animal models have established that killed spherules induced protection against death (but not infection) following pulmonary challenge with *C. immitis* arthroconidia *(294–297)*. However, the following studies in healthy, skin-test-negative volunteers to evaluate the efficacy of this approach in humans while showing vaccine toleration rendered unacceptable levels of toxicity with doses of 10 mg or more; recipients of doses of 2.7 mg of the vaccine (given intramuscularly in one to three injections) showed localized tenderness or induration at the site of injection *(298–301)*. A larger randomized, double-blind, multicenter study conducted between 1980 and 1985 and involving 2867 healthy, skin-test-negative volunteers who received three intramuscular injections of 1.75 mg of killed spherules or sterile saline, respectively, showed no clinical benefits in the vaccinated group *(84,302)*.

REFERENCES

1. Hobbs, E. R. Coccidioidomycosis. *Dermatol. Clin.*, 7, 227, 1989.
2. Galgiani, J. N. Coccidioidomycosis. *West. J. Med.*, 159, 153, 1993.
3. Centers for Disease Control and Prevention. Coccidioidomycosis among persons attending the world championship of model airplane flying: Kern County, California, October 2001. *J. Am. Med. Assoc.*, 287, 312, 2002.
4. Coccidioidomycosis among persons attending the world championship of model airplane flying: Kern County, California, October 2001. *MMWR Morb. Mortal. Wkly Rep.*, 50, 1106–1107, 2001.
5. Centers for Disease Control and Prevention. Coccidioidomycosis in workers at an archeologic site: Dinosaur National Monument, Utah, June–July, 2001. *J. Am. Med. Assoc.*, 286, 3072–3073, 2001.
6. Coccidioidomycosis in workers at an archeologic site: Dinosaur National Monument, Utah, June–July. *MMWR Morbid. Mortal. Wkly Rep.*, 50, 1005–1008, 2001.
7. Rosenstein, N. E., Emery, K. W., Werner, S. B., et al. Risk factors for severe pulmonary and disseminated coccidioidomycosis: Kern County, California, 1995–1996. *Clin. Infect. Dis.*, 32, 708–715, 2001.
8. Leake, J. A., Mosley, D. G., England, B., et al. Risk factors for acute symptomatic coccidioidomycosis among elderly persons in Arizona, 1996-1997. *J. Infect. Dis.*, 181, 1435–1440, 2000.
9. Vaz, A., Pineda-Roman, M., Thomas, A. R., and Carlson, R. W. Coccidioidomycosis: an update. *Hosp. Pract. (Off Ed.)*, 33, 105–108, 113–115, 119–120, 1998.
10. Hughes, C. V. and Kvale, P. A. Pleural effusion in Michigan caused by *Coccidioides immitis* after travel to an endemic area. *Henry Ford Hosp. Med. J.*, 37, 47, 1989.
11. Babycos, P. B. and Hoda, S. A. A fatal case of disseminated coccidioidomycosis in Louisiana. *J. La State Med. Soc.*, 142, 24, 1990.
12. Taylor, G. D., Boettger, D. W., Miedzinski, L. J., and Tyrrell, D. L. J. Coccidioidal meningitis acquired during holidays in Arizona. *Can. Med. Assoc. J.*, 142, 1388, 1990.
13. Sekhon, A. S., Isaac-Renton, J., Dixon, J. M., Stein, L., and Sims, H. V. Review of human and animal cases of coccidioidomycosis diagnosed in Canada. *Mycopathologia*, 113, 1, 1991.
14. Ito, H., Itaoka, T., Onuki, T., Yokoyama, N., and Nitta, S. A case of pulmonary coccidioidomycosis. *Nippon Kyobu Geka Gakkai Zasshi*, 39, 1222, 1991.
15. Cayce, W. R. Cases from the aerospace medicine residents' teaching file; case #47: primary pulmonary coccidioidomycosis. *Aviat. Space Environ. Med.*, 62, 1200, 1991.
16. Lefler, E., Weiler-Ravell, D., Merzbach, D., Ben-Izhak, O., and Best, L. A. Traveler's coccidioidomycosis: case report of pulmonary infection diagnosed in Israel. *J. Clin. Microbiol.*, 30, 1304, 1992.
17. Futsuki, Y., Nagashima, S., Yamamoto, Y., et al. An imported case of primary pulmonary coccidioidomycosis. *Kansenshogaku Zasshi*, 74, 580–584, 2000.
18. Fohlman, J., Sjolin, J., Bennich, H., Chryssanthou, E., Von Rosen, M., and Petrini, B. Coccidioidomycosis as imported atypical pneumonia in Sweden. *Scand. J. Infect. Dis.*, 32, 440–441, 2000.
19. Radkar, G. and Hospenthal, D. Unusual presentation of pulmonary coccidioidomycosis in a traveler. *Hawaii Med. J.*, 59, 238–239, 2000.
20. Cole, G. T. and Sun, S. H. Arthroconidium-spherule-endospore transformation in *Coccidioides immitis*, arthroconidium-spherule-endospore transformation in *Coccidioides immitis* parasitic cycle in vivo. *J. Med. Vet. Mycol.*, 24, 183–192, 1985.
21. Hagman, H. M., Madnick, E. G., D'Agostino, A. N., et al. Hyphal form in the central nervous system of patients with coccidioidomycosis. *Clin. Infect. Dis.*, 30, 349–353, 2000.
22. Zepeda, M. R., Kobayashi, G. K., Appleman, M. D., and Navarro, A. *Coccidioides immitis* presenting as a hyphal form in cerebrospinal fluid. *J. Natl. Med. Assoc.*, 90, 435–436, 1998.
23. Nosanchuk, J. D., Snedeker, J., and Nosanchuk, J. S. Arthroconidia in coccidioidoma: case report and literature review. *Int. J. Infect. Dis.*, 3, 32–35, 1998.

24. Polesky, A., Kirsch, C. M., Snyder, L. S., et al. Airway coccidioidomycosis - report of cases and review. *Clin. Infect. Dis.*, 28, 1273–1280, 1999.
25. Arsura, E. L. and Kilgore, W. B. Miliary coccidioidomycosis in the immunocompetent. *Chest*, 117, 404–409, 2000.
26. Yozwiak, M. L., Lundergan, L. L., Kerrick, S. S., and Galgiani, J. N. Symptoms and routine laboratory abnormalities associated with coccidioidomycosis. *West. J. Med.*, 149, 419, 1988.
27. Fishco, W. D. and Blocher, K. S. Disseminated coccidioidomycosis masquerading as tendonitis. *J. Am. Podiatr. Med. Assoc.*, 90, 508–511, 2000.
28. Robertson, S., Kovitz, K. L., and Moroz, K. Disseminated coccidioidomycosis. The role of cytology in multidisciplinary clinical approach and diagnosis. *J. La State Med. Sci.*, 151, 409–413, 1999.
29. Peterson, C. M., Schuppert, K., Kelly, P. C., and Pappagianis, D. Coccidioidomycosis and pregnancy. *Obstet. Gynecol. Surv.*, 48, 149, 1993.
30. Deresinski, S. C. and Stevens, D. A. Coccidioidomycosis in compromised hosts: experience at Stanford University Hospital. *Medicine (Baltimore)*, 54, 377, 1974.
31. Gifford, M. A., Buss, W. C., Douds, R. J., Miller, H. E., and Tupper, R. B. Data on coccidioides fungus infection: Kern County, Bakersfield, Calif. *Kern County Dept. Public Health Annual Report.*, 39, 1936.
32. Huppert, M. Racism in coccidioidomycosis? *Am. Rev. Respir. Dis.*, 118, 797, 1978.
33. Pappagianis, D., Lindsay, S. Beall, S., and Williams, P. Ethnic background and the clinical course of coccidioidomycosis. *Am. Rev. Respir. Dis.*, 120, 959, 1979.
34. Williams, P. L., Sable, D. L., Mendez, P., and Smyth, L. T. Symptomatic coccidioidomycosis following a severe natural dust storm. *Chest*, 76, 566, 1979.
35. Johnson, W. M. Racial factors in coccidioidomycosis: mortality experience in Arizona: a review of the literature. *Ariz. Medicine*, 39, 18, 1982.
36. Einstein, H. E. and Johnson, R. H. Coccidioidomycosis: new aspects of epidemiology and therapy. *Clin. Infect. Dis.*, 16, 349, 1993.
37. Deresinski, S. C., Pappagianis, D., and Stevens, D. A. Association of ABO blood group and outcome of coccidioidal infection. *Sabouraudia*, 17, 261, 1979.
38. Cohen, I. M., Galgiani, J. N., Potter, D., and Ogden, D. A. Coccidioidomycosis in renal replacement therapy. *Arch. Intern. Med.*, 142, 489, 1982.
39. Louie, L., Ng, S., Hajjeh, R., et al. Influence of host genetics on the severity of coccidioidomycosis. *Emerg. Infect. Dis.*, 5, 672–680, 1999.
40. Shafai, T. Neonatal coccidioidomycosis in premature twins. *Am. J. Dis. Child.*, 132, 634, 1978.
41. Bernstein, D. I., Tipton, J. R., Schott, S. F., and Cherry, J. D. Coccidioidomycosis in a neonate: maternal-infant transmission. *J. Pediatr.*, 99, 752, 1981.
42. Caldwell, J. W., Arsura, E. L., Kilgore, W. B., Garcia, A. L., Reddy, V., and Johnson, R. H. Coccidioidomycosis in pregnancy during an epidemic in California. *Obstet. Gynecol.*, 95, 236–239, 2000.
43. Bronnimann, D. A. and Galgiani, J. N. Coccidioidomycosis. *Eur. J. Clin. Microbiol. Infect. Dis.*, 8, 466, 1989.
44. Willet, F. M. and Weiss, A. Coccidioidomycosis in southern California: report of a new endemic area with a review of 100 cases. *Ann. Intern. Med.*, 23, 349, 1945.
45. Lonky, S. A., Catanzaro, A., Moser, K. M., and Einstein, H. Acute coccidioidal pleural effusion. *Am. Rev. Respir. Dis.*, 114, 681, 1976.
46. Bronnimann, D. A., Adam, R. D., Galgiani, J. N., et al. Coccidioidomycosis in the acquired immunodeficiency syndrome. *Ann. Intern. Med.*, 106, 372, 1987.
47. Bouza, E., Dreyer, J. S., Hewitt, W. L., and Meyer, R. D. Coccidioidal meningitis. *Medicine (Baltimore)*, 60, 139, 1981.
48. Bloom, J. W., Camilli, A. E., and Barbee, R. A. Disseminated coccidioidomycosis: a ten-year experience, in *Coccidioidomycosis*, Einstein, H. E. and Catanzaro, A., Eds. The National Foundation of Infectious Diseases, Washington, DC, 369, 1985.
49. Einstein, H. E., Chia, J. K. S., and Meyer, R. D. Pulmonary infiltrate and pleural effusion in a diabetic man. *Clin. Infect. Dis.*, 14, 955, 1992.
50. Salkin, D. and Said, A. Reinfection with coccidioidomycosis. *Clin. Infect. Dis.*, 17, 1066, 1993.
51. Takamura, M. and Stark, P. Diagnostic case study. Coccidioidomycosis: pleural involvement. *Semin. Respir. Infect.*, 16, 280–285, 2001.
52. DiCaudo, D. J. and Connolly, S. M. Interstitial granulomatous dermatitis associated with pulmonary coccidioidomycosis. *J. Am. Acad. Dermatol.*, 45, 840–845, 2001.
53. Feldman, B. S. and Snyder, L. S. Primary pulmonary coccidioidomycosis. *Semin. Respir. Infect.*, 16, 231–237, 2001.
54. Phillips, P. and Ford, B. Peritoneal coccidioidomycosis: case report and review. *Clin. Infect. Dis.*, 30, 971–976, 2000.
55. Winn, W. A. Primary cutaneous coccidioidomycosis. Reevaluation of its potentiality based on study of three new cases. *Arch. Dermatol.*, 92, 221–228, 1965.
56. Loeb, J. M., Livermore, B. M., and Wofsy, D. Coccidioidomycosis of the thyroid. *Ann. Intern. Med.*, 91, 409, 1979.
57. Rodenbiker, H. T. and Ganley, J. P. Ocular coccidioidomycosis. *Surv. Ophthalmol.*, 24, 263, 1980.
58. Moorthy, R. S., Rao, N. A., Sidikaro, Y., and Foos, R. Y. Coccidioidomycosis iridocyclitis. *Ophthalmology*, 101, 1923, 1994.
59. Scanarini, M., Rotillo, A., Rigobello, L., Pomes, A., Parenti, A., and Alessio, L. Primary intracellar coccidioidomycosis simulating a pituitary adenoma. *Neurosurgery*, 28, 748, 1991.
60. Ward, P. H., Berci, G., Morledge, D., and Schwartz H. Coccidioidomycosis of the larinx in infants and adults. *Ann. Otol. Rhinol. Laryngol.*, 86, 655, 1977.

61. Hajare, S., Rakusan, T. A., Kalia, A., and Strunk, C. L. Laryngeal coccidioidomycosis causing airway obstruction. *Pediatr. Infect. Dis. J.*, 8, 54, 1989.
62. Boyle, J. O., Coulthard, S. W., and Mandel, R. M. Laryngeal involvement in dissiminated coccidioidomycosis. *Arch. Otolaryngol. Head Neck Surg.*, 117, 433, 1991.
63. Harvey, R. P., Pappagianis, D., Cochran, J., and Stevens, D. A. Otomycosis due to coccidioidomycosis. *Arch. Intern. Med.*, 138, 1434, 1978.
64. Busch, R. F. Coccidioidomycosis of the external ear. *Otolaryngol. Head Neck Surgery*, 107, 491, 1992.
65. Craig, J. R., Hillberg, R. H., and Balchum, O. J. Disseminated coccidioidomycosis - diagnosis by biopsy of liver. *West. J. Med.*, 122, 171, 1975.
66. Howard, P. F. and Smith, J. W. Diagnosis of disseminated coccidioidomycosis by liver biopsy. *Arch. Intern. Med.*, 143, 1335, 1983.
67. Zangerl, B., Edel, G., von Manitius, J., Schmidt-Wilcke, H. A. Coccidioidomycosis as the cause of granulomatous hepatitis. *Med. Klin.*, 93, 170–173, 1998.
68. Weisman, I. M., Moreno, A. J., Parker, A. L., Sippo, W. C., and Liles, W. J. Gastrointestinal dissemination of coccidioidomycosis. *Am. J. Gastroenterol.*, 81, 589, 1986.
69. Ampel, N. M., White, J. D., Varanasi, U. R., et al. Coccidioidal peritonitis associated with ambulatory peritoneal dialysis. *Am. J. Kidney Dis.*, 11, 512, 1988.
70. Jamidar, P. A., Campbell, D. R., Fishback, J. L., and Klotz S. A. Peritoneal coccidioidomycosis associated with human immunodeficiency virus infection. *Gastroenterology*, 102, 1054, 1992.
71. Schwartz, D. N., Fihn, S. D., and Miller, R. A. Infection of an arterial prosthesis as the presenting manifestation of disseminated coccidioidomycosis: control of disease with fluconazole. *Clin. Infect. Dis.*, 16, 486, 1993.
72. McCaffree, M. A., Altshuler, G., and Benirschke, K. Placental coccidioidomycosis without fetal disease. *Arch. Pathol. Lab. Med.*, 102, 512, 1078.
73. Bylund, D. J., Nanfro, J. J., and Marsh, W. L. Jr. Coccidioidomycosis of the female genital tract. *Arch. Pathol. Lab. Med.*, 110, 232, 1986.
74. Saw, E. C., Smale, L. E., Einstein, H., and Huntington, R. W. Jr. Female genital coccidioidomycosis. *Obstet. Gynecol.*, 45, 199, 1975.
75. Chowfin, A. and Tight, R. Female genital coccidioidomycosis (FGC), Addison's disease and sigmoid loop abscess due to *Coccidioides immitis*: case report and review of the literature on FGC. *Mycopathologia*, 145, 121–123, 1999.
76. Conner, W. T., Drach, G. W., and Bucher, W. C. Jr. Genitourinary aspects of disseminated coccidioidomycosis. *J. Urol.*, 113, 82, 1975.
77. Frangos, D. N. and Nyberg, L. M. Jr. Genitourinary fungal infections. *West. Med. J.*, 79, 455, 1986.
78. Dunne, W. M. Jr., Ziebert, A. P., Donahoe, L. W., and Standard, P. Unexpected laboratory diagnosis of latent urogenital coccidioidomycosis in a nonendemic area. *Arch. Pathol. Lab. Med.*, 110, 236, 1986.
79. Kuntze, J. R., Herman, M. H., and Evans, S. G. Genitourinary coccidioidomycosis. *J. Urol.*, 140, 370, 1988.
80. Ali, M. Y., Gopal, K. V., Llarena, L. A., and Taylor, H. C. Hypercalcemia associated with infection by *Cryptococcus neoformans* and *Coccidioides immitis*. *Am. J. Ed. Sci.*, 318, 419–423, 1999.
81. Westphal, S. A. Disseminated coccidioidomycosis associated with hypercalcemia. *Mayo Clin. Proc.*, 73, 893–894, 1998.
82. Faul, J. L., Hoang, K., Schmoker, J., Vagelos, R. H., and Berry, G. J. Constrictive pericarditis due to coccidioidomycosis. *Ann. Thorac. Surg.*, 68, 1407–1409, 1999.
83. Holemans, X., Levecque, P., Despontin, K., and Maton, J. P. First report of coccidioidomycosis associated with Sweet syndrome. *Presse Med.*, 29, 1282–1284, 2000.
84. Cox, R. A. and Magee, D. M. Protective immunity in coccidioidomycosis. *Res. Immunol.*, 149, 417–428, 506–507, 1998.
85. Cox, R. A. and Arnold, D. A. Immunoglobulin E in coccidioidomycosis. *J. Immunol.*, 123, 194–200, 1979.
86. Cox, R. A., Baker, B. S., and Stevens, D. A. Specificity of immunoglobulin E in coccidioidomycosis and correlation with disease involvement. *Infect. Immun.*, 37, 609–616, 1982.
87. Yoshinoya, S., Cox, R. A., and Pope, R. M.,' Immune complexes in coccidioidomycosis. Detection and characterization. *J. Clin. Invest.*, 66, 655–663, 1980.
88. Cox, R. A., Pope, R. M., and Stevens, D. A. Immune complexes in coccidioidomycosis. Correlation with disease involvement. *Am. Rev. Respir. Dis.*, 126, 439–443, 1982.
89. Ampel, N. M., Kramer, L. A., Kerekes, K. M., Johnson, S. M., and Pappagianis, D. Assessment of the human cellular immune response to T27K, a coccidioidal antigen preparation, by flow cytometry of whole blood. *Med. Mycol.*, 39, 315–320, 2001.
90. Hung, C. Y., Ampel, N. M., Christian, L., Seshan, K. R., and Cole, G. T. A major cell surface antigen of *Coccidioides immitis* which elicits both humoral and cellular immune responses. *Infect. Immun.*, 68, 584–593, 2000.
91. Peng, T., Orsborn, K. I., Orbach, M. J., and Galgiani, J. N. Proline-rich vaccine candidate antigen of *Coccidioides immitis*: conservation among isolates and differential expression with spherule maturation. *J. Infect. Dis.*, 179, 518–521, 1999.
92. Galgiani, J. N. Coccidioidomycosis: a regional disease of national importance. Rethinking approaches for control. *Ann. Intern. Med.*, 130(4 Part 1), 293–300, 1999.
93. Sarosi, G. A. and Davies, S. F. Concise review for primary-care physicians. Therapy for fungal infections. *Mayo Clin. Proc.*, 69, 1111, 1994.
94. Werner, S. B., Pappagianis, D., Heindl, I., and Mickel, A. An epidemic of coccidioidomycosis among archeology students in Northern California. *N. Engl. J. Med.*, 286, 507, 1972.
95. Johnson, P. and Sarosi, G. Current therapy of major fungal diseases of the lung. *Infect. Dis. Clin. North Am.*, 5, 635, 1991.

96. LaPage, E. Using a ventricular reservoir to instill amphotericin B. *J. Neurosci. Nurs.*, 25, 212, 1993.
97. Koehler, A. P., Cheng, A. F., Chu, K. C., Chan, C. H., Ho, A. S., and Lyon, D. J. Successful treatment of disseminated coccidioidomycosis with amphotericin B lipid complex. *J. Infect.*, 36, 113–115, 1998.
98. American Thoracic Society. Treatment of fungal infection. *Am. Rev. Respir. Dis.*, 120, 1393, 1979.
99. Graybill, J. R., Stevens, D. A., Galgiani, J. N., Dismukes, W. E., Cloud, G. A, and the NIAID Mycoses Study Group. Itraconazole treatment of coccidioidomycosis. *Am. J. Med.*, 89, 282, 1990.
100. Galgiani, J. N., Catanzaro, A., Cloud, G. A., et al. Comparison of oral fluconazole and itraconazole for progressive, nonmeningeal coccidioidomycosis. A randomized, double-blind trial. *Mycoses Study Group, Ann. Intern. Med.*, 133, 676–686, 2000.
101. Jiang, C., Magee, D. M., and Cox, R. A. Coadministration of interleukin 12 expression vector with antigen 2 cDNA enhances induction of protective immunity against *Coccidioides immitis*. *Infect. Immun.*, 67, 5848–5853, 1999.
102. Connelly, M. B. and Zerella, J. T. Surgical management of coccidioidomycosis in children. *J. Pediatr. Surg.*, 35, 1633–1634, 2000.
103. Kappe, R., Levitz, S., Harrison, T. S., Ruhnke, M., Ampel, N. M., and Just-Nubling, G. Recent advances in cryptococcosis, candidiasis, and coccidioidomycosis complicating HIV infection. *Med. Mycol.*, 36(Suppl. 1), 207–215, 1998.
104. Ampel, N. M. Coccidioidomycosis among persons with human immunodeficiency virus infection in the era of highly active antiretroviral therapy (HAART). *Semin. Respir. Infect.*, 16, 257–262, 2001.
105. McNeil, M. M. and Ampel, N. M. Opportunistic coccidioidomycosis in patients infected with human immunodeficiency virus: prevention issues and priorities. *Clin. Infect. Dis.*, 21(Suppl. 1), S111, 1995.
106. British Society For Antimicrobial Chemotherapy Working Party. Antifungal chemotherapy in patients with acquired immunodeficiency syndrome. *Lancet*, 340, 648, 1992.
107. Zar, F. A. and Fernandez, M. Failure of ketoconazole maintenance therapy for disseminated coccidioidomycosis in AIDS. *J. Infect. Dis.*, 164, 824, 1991.
108. Bronnimann, D. A., Adam, R. D., Galgiani, J. N., et al. Coccidioidomycosis in the immunodeficiency syndrome. *Ann. Intern. Med.*, 106, 372, 1987.
109. Fish, D. G., Ampel, N. M., Galgiani, J. N., et al. Coccidioidomycosis during human immunodeficiency virus infection: a review of 77 patients. *Medicine (Baltimore)*, 69, 384, 1990.
110. Bozzette, S. A., Sattler, F. R., Chiu, J., et al. A controlled trial of early adjunctive treatment with corticosteroids for *Pneumocystis carinii* pneumonia in the acquired immunodeficiency syndrome. *N. Engl. J. Med.*, 323, 1451, 1990.
111. Gagnon, S., Boota, A. M., Fischl, M. A., Baier, H., Kirksey, O. W., and La Voie, L. Corticosteroids as adjunctive therapy for severe *Pneumocystis carinii* in the acquired immunodeficiency syndrome: a double-blind, placebo-controlled trial. *N. Engl. J. Med.*, 323, 1444, 1990.
112. MacFadden, D. K., Edelson, J. D., Hyland, R. H., Rodriguez, C. H., Innouye, T., and Rebuck, A. S. Corticosteroids as adjunctive therapy in treatment of *Pneumocystis carinii* pneumonia in patients with acquired immunodeficiency syndrome. *Lancet*, 1, 1477, 1987.
113. Montaner, J. S., Lawson, L. M., Levitt, N., Belzberg, H., Schechter, M. T., and Ruedy, J. Corticosteroids prevent early deterioration in patients with moderately severe *Pneumocystis carinii* pneumonia and the acquired immunodeficiency syndrome (AIDS). *Ann. Intern. Med.*, 113, 14, 1990.
114. Ampel, N. M., Ryan, K. J., Carry, P. J., Wieden, M. A., and Schifman, R.B. Fungemia due to *Coccidioides immitis*: an analysis of 16 episodes in 15 patients and a review of the literature. *Medicine (Baltimore)*, 65, 312, 1986.
115. Mahaffey, K. W., Hippenmeyer, C. L., Mandel, R., and Ampel, N. M. Unrecognized coccidioidomycosis complicating *Pneumocystis carinii* pneumonia in patients infected with the human immunodeficiency virus and treated with corticosteroids. *Arch. Intern. Med.*, 153, 1496, 1993.
116. Harvey, W. C. and Greendyke, W. H. Skin lesions in acute coccidioidomycosis. *Am. Fam. Physician*, 2: 81, 1970.
117. Lundergan, L. L., Kerrick, S. S., and Galgiani, J. N. Coccidioidomycosis at a university outpatient clinic: a clinical description, in *Coccidioidomycosis: Proceedings of the 4th International Conference on Coccidioidomycosis*, San Diego, 1984, National Federation of Infectious Diseases, Washington DC, 47, 1985.
118. Ohashi, D. K., Ruppe, J. P., Courrege, M. L., and Kletter, G. G. Coccidioidomycosis in a patient with atopic dermatitis. *N. C. Med. J.*, 59, 76–78, 1998.
119. Huntington, R. W. Jr. Coccidioidomycosis - a great imitator disease. *Arch. Pathol. Lab. Med.*, 110, 182, 1986.
120. Bonifaz, A. Coccidioidomycosis, in *Micologia Medica Basica*, Mendez, C., Ed. Mexico, DF, 215, 1991.
121. Rippon, J. W. Coccidioidomycosis, in *Medical Mycology*, 3rd ed. W. B. Saunders, Philadelphia, 433, 1988.
122. Bonifaz, A., Saul, A., Galindo, J., and Andrade, R. Primary cutaneous coccidioidomycosis treated with itraconazole. *Int. J. Dermatol.*, 33, 720, 1994.
123. Meyer, R. D. Cutaneous and mucosal manifestations of the deep mycotic infections. *Acta Derm. Venereol. (Stockholm)*, 121(Suppl.), 52, 1986.
124. Newland, Y. and Komisar, A. Coccidioidomycosis of the head and neck. *Ear Nose Throat J.*, 65, 55, 60.
125. Lavalle, P., Suchil, P., De Ovando, F., and Reynoso, S. Itraconazole for deep mycosis: preliminary experience in Mexico. *Rev. Infect. Dis.*, 9(Suppl. 1), S64, 1987.
126. Drutz, D. J. Amphotericin B in the treatment of coccidioidomycosis. *Drugs*, 26, 337, 1983.
127. Peterson, C. M., Schuppert, K., Kelly, P.C., and Pappagianis, D. Coccidioidomycosis and pregnancy. *Obstet. Gynecol.*, 48, 149, 1993.
128. Ie, S., Rubio, E. R., Alper, B., and Szerlip, H. M. Respiratory complications of pregnancy. *Obstet. Gynecol. Surv.*, 57, 39–46, 2002.
129. Farness, O. J. Coccidioidomycosis. *J. Am. Med. Assoc.*, 116, 1749, 1941.

130. Mendenhall, J. C., Black, W. C., and Pottz, G. E. Progressive (disseminated) coccidioidomycosis during pregnancy. *Rocky Mountain Med. J.*, 45, 472, 1948.
131. Smale, L. E. and Birsner, J. W. Maternal deaths from coccidioidomycosis. *J. Am. Med. Assoc.*, 140, 1152, 1949 [correction, *J. Am. Med. Assoc.*, 141, 212, 1949].
132. Pappagianis, S. Epidemiology of coccidioidomycosis, in *Coccidioidomycosis: A Text*, Stevens, D. A., Ed. Plenum Medical Book Co., New York, 80, 1980.
133. Drutz, D. J., Huppert, M., Sun, S. H., and McGuire, W. L. Human sex hormones stimulate the growth and maturation of *Coccidioides immitis*. *Infect. Immunol.*, 32, 897, 1981.
134. Powell, B. L., Drutz, D. J., Huppert, M., and Sun, S. H. Relationship of progesterone and estradiol-binding proteins in *Coccidioides immitis* to coccidioidal dissemination in pregnancy. *Infect. Immunol.*, 40, 478, 1983.
135. Walker, M. P. R., Brody, C. Z., and Resnick, R. Reactivation of coccidioidomycosis in pregnancy. *Obstet. Gynecol.*, 79, 815, 1992.
136. Mongan, E. S. Acute disseminated coccidioidomycosis. *Am. J. Med.*, 24, 820, 1958.
137. Arsura, E. L., Kilgore, W. B., and Ratnayake, S. N. Erythema nodosum in pregnant patients with coccidioidomycosis. *Clin. Infect. Dis.*, 27, 1201–1203, 1998.
138. Braverman, I. M. Protective effects of erythema nodosum in coccidioidomycosis. *Lancet*, 353, 168, 1999.
139. Braverman, I. M. *Skin Signs of Systemic Disease*, 3rd ed. W. B. Saunders, Philadelphia, 349-353, 1998.
140. Spark, R. P. Does transplacental spread of coccidioidomycosis occur? Report of a neonatal fatality and review of the literature. *Arch. Pathol. Lab. Med.*, 105, 347–350, 1981.
141. Townsend, T. E. and McKey, R. W. Coccidioidomycosis in children. *Am. J. Dis. Child.*, 86, 51-53, 1953.
142. Hyatt, H. W. Coccidioidomycosis in a 3-week-old infant. *Am. J. Dis. Child.*, 105, 93–98, 1963.
143. Bernstein, O. I., Tipton, J. R., Schott, S. F., and Cherry, J. D. Coccidioidomycosis in a neonate: maternal-fetal transmission. *J. Pediatr.*, 99, 752, 1981.
144. Cohen, R. Coccidioidomycosis: case studies in children. *Arch. Pediatr.*, 66, 241, 1949.
145. Christian, J., Sarre, S., Peers, J., Salazar, E., and Rosario, J. Pulmonary coccidioidomycosis in a twenty-one day old infant. *Am. J. Dis. Child*, 92, 66–74, 1956.
146. Larwood, T. Maternal-fetal transmission of coccidioidomycosis, *Trans. 7th Annu. Meet. Veterans Administration-Armed Forces Coccidioidomycosis Study Group*, Wayne, L., Ed. Veterans Adminsistration, 28–29, 1962.
147. Smale, L. and Waechter, K. Dissemination of coccidioidomycosis in pregnancy. *Am. J. Obstet. Gynecol.*, 107, 356–361, 1970.
148. Shafai, T. Neonatal coccidioidomycosis in premature twins. *Am. J. Dis. Child*, 132, 634, 1978.
149. Bernstein, D., Tipton, J., Schott, S., and Cherry, J. Coccidioidomycosis in a neonate: maternal-infant transmission. *J. Pediatr.*, 99, 752–754, 1981.
150. Child, D., Newell, J., Bjelland, J., and Spark, R. Radiographic findings of pulmonary coccidioidomycosis in neonates and infants. *Am. J. Roentgenol.*, 145, 261–263, 1985.
151. Saw, E., Smale, L., Einstein, F., and Huntington, R. Female genital coccidioidomycosis. *Obstet. Gynecol.*, 45, 199–202, 1975.
152. Cohen, R. Placental *Coccidioides*: proof that congenital *Coccidioides* is nonexistent. *Arch. Pediatr.*, 68, 59–66, 1951.
153. McCaffree, M., Altshuler, G., and Benirschke, K. Placental coccidioidomycosis without fetal disease. *Arch. Pathol. Lab. Med.*, 102, 512–514, 1978.
154. Charlton, V., Ramsdell, K., and Sehring, S. Intrauterine transmission of coccidioidomycosis. *Pediatr. Infect. Dis.*, 18, 561–563, 1999.
155. Linsangan, L. C. and Ross, L. A. *Coccidioides immitis* infection of the neonate: two routes of infection. *Pediatr. Infect. Dis. J.*, 18, 171–173, 1999.
156. Golden, S. E., Morgan, C. M., Bartley, D. L., and Campo, R. V. Disseminated coccidioidomycosis with chorioretinitis in early infancy. *Pediatr. Infect. Dis. J.*, 5, 272, 1986.
157. Sanford, W. G., Rasch, J. R., and Stonehill, R. B. A therapeutic dillema: the treatment of disseminated coccidioidomycosis with amphotericin B. *Ann. Intern. Med.*, 56, 533, 1962.
158. Hadsall, F. J., and Acquarelli, M. J. Disseminated coccidioidomycosis presenting as facial granulomas in pregnancy: a report of two cases and a review of the literature. *Laryngoscope*, 83, 51, 1973.
159. McCoy, M. J., Ellenberg, J. F., and Killam, A. P. Coccidioidomycosis complicating pregnancy. *Am. J. Obstet. Gynecol.*, 140, 739, 1980.
160. Peterson, C. M., Johnson, S. L., Kelly, J. V., and Kelly, P. C. Coccidioidal meningitis and pregnancy: a case report. *Obstet. Gynecol.*, 73, 835, 1989.
161. Catanzaro, A. Pulmonary mycosis in pregnant women. *Chest*, 86, 155, 1984.
162. Wack, E. E., Ampel, N. M., and Galgiani, J. N. Coccidioidomycosis during pregnancy. *Chest*, 94, 376, 1988.
163. Stevens, D. A. Chemotherapy of coccidioidomycosis, in *Coccidioidomycosis: A Text*, Stevens, D. A., Ed. Plenum Medical Book Co., New York, 253, 1980.
164. Logan, J. L., Blair, J. E., and Galgiani, J. N. Coccidioidomycosis complicating solid organ transplantation. *Semin. Respir. Infect.*, 16, 251–256, 2001.
165. Blair, J. E. and Logan, J. L. Coccidioidomycosis in solid organ transplantation. *Clin. Infect. Dis.*, 33, 1536-1544, 2001.
166. Zeluff, B. J. Fungal pneumonia in transplant recipients. *Semin. Respir. Infect.*, 5, 80, 1990.
167. Peterson, P. K. Pulmonary mycosis in organ transplant recipients, in *Fungal Diseases of the Lung*, Sarosi, G. A. and Davies, S. F., Eds. Grune & Stratton, Orlando, 283, 1986.

168. Tripathy, U., Yung, G. L., Kriett, J. M., Thistlethwaite, P. A., Kapelanski, D. P., and Jamieson, S. W. Donor transfer of pulmonary coccidioidomycosis in lung. *Ann. Thor. Surg.*, 73, 306–308, 2002.
169. Hall, K. A., Copeland, J. G., Zukoski, C. F., Sethi, G. K., and Galgiani, J. N. Markers of coccidioidomycosis before cardiac or renal transplantation and the risk of recurrent infection. *Transplantation*, 55, 1422, 1993.
170. Britt, R. H., Enzmann, D. R., and Remington, J. S. Intracranial infection in cardiac transplant recipients. *Ann. Neurol.*, 9, 107, 1981.
171. Vartivarian, S. E., Coudron, P. E., and Markowitz, S. M. Disseminated coccidioidomycosis: unusual manifestations in a cardiac transplantation patient. *Am. J. Med.*, 83, 949, 1987.
172. Calhoun, D. D. L., Galgiani, J. N., Zukoski, C., and Copeland, J. G. Coccidioidomycosis in recent renal or cardiac transplant recipients, in *Coccidioidomycosis: Proceedings of the 4th Int. Conf. Coccidioidomycosis.* National Foundation for Infectious Diseases, Washington, DC, 312, 1985.
173. Stevens, D. A., *Coccidioides immitis*, in *Principles and Practice of Infectious Diseases*, Mandell, G. L., Douglas, R. G., and Bennett, J. E., Eds. John Wiley & Sons, New York, 1485, 1985.
174. Hall, K. A., Sethi, G. K., Rosado, L. J., Martinez, J. D, Huston, C. L., and Copeland, J. G. Coccidioidomycosis and heart transplantation. *J. Heart Lung Transplant.*, 12, 525, 1993.
175. Rifkind, D., Marchioro, T. L., Schneck, S. A., and Hill, R. B. Jr. Systemic fungal infections complicating renal transplantation and immunosuppressive therapy. *Am. J. Med.*, 43, 28, 1967.
176. Tolkoff-Rubin, N. E. and Rubin, R. H. Opportunistic fungal and bacterial infection in the renal transplant recipient. *J. Am. Soc. Nephrol.*, 2(Suppl. 3), S264, 1992.
177. Cohen, I. M., Galgiani, J. N., Potter, D., and Ogden, D. A. Coccidioidomycosis in renal therapy. *Arch. Intern. Med.*, 142, 489, 1982.
178. Seltzer, J., Broaddus, V. C., Jacobs, R., and Golden, J. A. Reactivation of coccidioides infection. *West. J. Med.*, 145, 96, 1986.
179. Hart, P. D., Russell, E., and Remington, J. S. The compromised host and infection. II. Deep fungal infection. *J. Infect. Dis.*, 120, 169, 1969.
180. Schroter, G. P. J, Bakshanden, K., Husberg, B. S., and Weil, R. Coccidioidomycosis and renal transplantation. *Transplanation*, 23, 485, 1977.
181. Deresinski, S. C. and Stevens, D. A. Coccidioidomycosis in compromised hosts. *Medicine (Baltimore)*, 54, 377, 1974.
182. Murphy, M., Drash, A. L., and Donnelly, W. H. Disseminated coccidioidomycosis associated with immunosuppressive therapy following renal transplantation. *Pediatrics*, 48, 144, 1971.
183. Chandler, J. W., Kalina, R. E., and Milan, D. F. Coccidioidal choroiditis following renal transplantation. *Am. J. Ophthalmol.*, 74, 1080, 1972.
184. Colonna, J. O., Winston, D. J., Brill, J. E., et al. Infectious complications in liver transplant recipients. *Arch. Surg.*, 123, 360, 1988.
185. Dummer, S. J., Hardy, A., Poorsattar, A., and Ho, M. Early infections in kidney, heart and liver transplant recipients on cyclosporine. *Transplantation*, 36, 259, 1983.
186. Ho, M., Wajszczuk, C. P., Hardy, A., et al. Infections in kidney, heart, and liver transplant recipients on cyclosporine. *Transplant. Proc.*, 15(Suppl. 1), 2768, 1983.
187. Kusne, S., Dummer, J. S., Singh, N., et al. Infections after liver transplantation: an analysis of 101 consecutive cases. *Medicine (Baltimore)*, 67, 132, 1988.
188. Schroter, G. P. J., Hoelscher, M., Putnam, C. W., Porter, K. A., and Starzl, T. E. Fungus infections after liver transplantation. *Ann. Surg.*, 186, 115, 1977.
189. Wajszczuk, C. P., Dummer, J. S., Ho, M., et al. Fungal infections in liver transplant recipients. *Transplantation*, 40, 347, 1985.
190. Dodd, L. G. and Nelson, S. D. Disseminated coccidioidomycosis detected by percutaneous liver biopsy in a liver transplant recipient. *Am. J. Clin. Pathol.*, 93, 141, 1990.
191. Riley, D. K., Galgiani, J. N., O'Donnell, M. R., Ito, J. I., Beatty, P. G., and Evans, T. G. Coccidioidomycosis in bone marrow transplant recipients. *Transplantation*, 56, 1531, 1993.
192. Rodenbiker, H. T. and Ganley, J. P. Ocular coccidioidomycosis. *Surv. Ophthalmol.*, 24, 263, 1980.
193. Blumenkranz, M. S. and Stevens, D. A. Endogenous coccidioidal endophthalmitis. *J. Ophthalmol.*, 87, 974, 1980.
194. Cunningham, E. T. Jr., Seiff, S. R., Berger, T. G., Lizotte, P. E., Howes, E. L. Jr., and Horton, J. C. Intraocular coccidioidomycosis diagnosed by skin biopsy. *Arch. Ophthalmol.*, 116, 674–677, 1998.
195. Brown, W. C., Kellenberger, R. E., and Hudson, K. E. Granulomatous uveitis associated with disseminated coccidioidomycosis. *Am. J. Ophthalmol.*, 45, 102, 1958.
196. Cutler, J. E., Binder, P. S., Paul, T. O., and Beamis, J. F. Metastatic coccidioidal endophthalmitis. *Arch. Ophthalmol.*, 96, 689, 1978.
197. Hagele, A. J., Evans, D. J., and Larwood, T. R. Primary endophthalmic coccidioidomycosis: report of a case of exogenous primary coccidioidomycosis of the eye diagnosed prior to enucleation, in *Coccidioidomycosis* Ajello, L., Ed. University of Arizona Press, Tucson, AZ, 37, 1967.
198. Petitt, T. H., Learn, R. N., and Foos, R. Y. Intraocular coccidioidomycosis. *Arch. Ophthalmol.*, 77, 655, 1967.
199. Blumenkranz, M. S. and Stevens, D. A. Therapy of endogenous fungal endophthalmitis: miconazole or amphotericin B for coccidioidal and candidal infection. *Arch. Ophthalmol.*, 98, 1216, 1980.
200. American Medical Association Department of Drugs. *American Medical Association Drug Evaluations*, PSG Publishing Co., Littleton, MA, 824, 968, 1977.

201. Allen, H. F. Amphotericin B and exogenous mycotic endophthalmitis after cataract extraction. *Arch. Ophthalmol.*, 88, 640, 1972.
202. Bell, R. W. and Ritchey, M. C. Subconjunctival nodules after amphotericin B injection. *Arch. Ophthalmol.*, 90, 402, 1973.
203. Lamer, L., Paquin, F., Lorange, G., Bayardelle, P., and Ojeimi, G. Macular coccidioidomycosis. *Can. J. Ophthalmol.*, 17, 121, 1982.
204. Alexander, P. B. and Coodley, E. L. Disseminated coccidioidomycosis with intraocular involvement. *Am. J. Ophthalmol.*, 64, 283, 1967.
205. Bayer, A.S., Yoshikawa, T. T., Galpin, J. E., and Guze, L. R. Unusual syndromes of coccidioidomycosis: diagnostic and therapeutic considerations. *Medicine (Baltimore)*, 55, 131, 1976.
206. Harris, R. E. Coccidioidomycosis complicating pregnancy. Report of 3 cases and review of the literature. *Obstet. Gynecol.*, 28, 400, 1966.
207. Andersen, F. C. and Cuckian, J. C. Systemic lupus erythematosus associated with fatal pulmonary coccidioidomycosis. *Tex. Rep. Biol. Med.*, 26, 94, 1968.
208. Berry, C. Z., Goldberg, L. C., and Shepard, W. L. Systemic lupus erythematosus complicated by coccidioidomycosis. *J. Am. Med. Assoc.*, 206, 1083, 1968.
209. Conger, J., Farrell, T., and Douglas, S. Lupus nephritis complicated by fatal disseminated coccidioidomycosis. *Calif. Med.*, 118, 60, 1973.
210. Hileman, W. T. Disseminated coccidioidomycosis occurence in a patient receiving steroid therapy for rheumatoid arthritis: a case report. *Ariz. Med.*, 20, 268, 1963.
211. Farness, O. J. Some unusual aspects of coccidioidomycosis, in *Coccidioidomycosis*, Ajello, L., Ed. University of Arizona Press, Tucson, AZ, 23, 1967.
212. Winn, W. R., Finegold, S. M., and Huntington, R. W. Coccidioidomycosis with fungemia, in *Coccidioidomycosis*, Ajello, L., Ed. University of Arizona Press, Tucson, AZ, 93, 1967.
213. Huntington, R. W., Waldmann, W. J., Sargent, J. A., O'Connell, H., Wybel, R., and Croll, D. Pathological and clinical observations on 142 cases of fatal coccidioidomycosis with necropsy, in *Coccidioidomycosis*, Ajello, L., Ed. University of Arizona Press, Tucson, AZ, 143, 1967.
214. Castellot, J. J., Creveling, R. L., and Pitts, F. W. Fatal miliary coccidioidomycosis complicating prolonged prednisone therapy in a patient with myelofibrosis. *Ann. Intern. Med.*, 52, 254, 1960.
215. Johnson, W. M. Coccidioidomycosis mortality in Arizona, in *Coccidioidomycosis. Current Clinical and Diagnostic Status*, Ajello, L., Ed. Symposia Specialists, Miami, 33, 1977.
216. Rowland, V. S., Westfall, R. E., and Hinchcliffe, W. A. Fatal coccidioidomycosis: analysis of host factors, in *Coccidioidomycosis. Current Clinical and Diagnostic Status*, Ajello, L., Ed. Symposia Specialists, Miami, 91, 1977.
217. Huntington, R. W. Acute fatal coccidioidal pneumonia, in *Coccidioidomycosis. Current Clinical and Diagnostic Status*, Ajello, L., Ed. Symposia Specialists, Miami, 127, 1977.
218. Rowland, V. S., Westfall, R. E., Hinchcliffe, W. A., and Jarrett, P. B. Acute respiratory failure in miliary coccidioidomycosis, in *Coccidioidomycosis. Current Clinical and Diagnostic Status*, Ajello, L., Ed. Symposia Specialists, Miami, 139, 1977.
219. Allen, W. G., Olsen, G. N., and Yergin, B. M. Disseminated coccidioidomycosis respiratory failure presenting in Florida. *J. Fla. Med. Assoc.*, 68, 356, 1981.
220. Johnson, W. M., and Gall, E. P. Fatal coccidioidomycosis in collagen vascular disease. *J. Rheumatol.*, 10, 79, 1983.
221. Land, C. A., Dorn, G. L., and Hill, J. M. The isolation of disseminated *Coccidioides immitis* by an improved blood culture technique, in *Coccidioidomycosis. Current Clinical and Diagnostic Status*, Ajello, L., Ed. Symposia Specialists, Miami, 19, 1977.
222. Knapp, W. A., Seeley, T. T., and Reuben, E. H. Fatal coccidioidomycosis: report of two cases. *Calif. Med.*, 116, 86, 1972.
223. Larsen, R. A., Jacobson, J. A., Morris, A. H., and Benowitz, B. A. Acute respiratory failure caused by primary pulmonary coccidioidomycosis: two case reports and a review of the literature. *Am. Rev. Respir. Dis.*, 131, 797, 1985.
224. Drutz, D. J. and Huppert, M. Coccidioidomycosis: factors affecting the host parasite interaction. *J. Infect. Dis.*, 147, 372, 1983.
225. Huppert, M, Sun, S. H., Gleason-Jordan, I., and Vukovich, K. R. Lung weights parallels disease severity in experimental coccidioidomycosis. *Infect. Immun.*, 14, 1356, 1976.
226. Ruddock, J. C. and Hope, R. B. Coccidioidal peritoneoscopy. *J. Am. Med. Assoc.*, 113, 2054, 1939.
227. Forbus, W. and Bestebreurtje, A. M. Coccidioidomycosis study of 95 cases of disseminated type with special reference to the pathogenesis of disease. *Milit. Surg.*, 99, 653, 1946.
228. Saw, E. C., Shields, S. J., Comer, T. P., and Huntington, R. W. Jr. Granulomatous peritonitis due to *Coccidioides immitis*. *Arch. Surg.*, 108, 369, 1974.
229. Crum, R. B. Peritoneal coccidioidomycosis. *Arch. Surg.*, 78, 91, 1959.
230. Chen, K. T. K. Coccidioidal peritonitis. *Am. J. Clin. Pathol.*, 80, 514, 1983.
231. Muther, R. S. and Bennett, W. M. Peritoneal clearance of amphotericin B and 5- fluorocytosine. *West. J. Med.*, 133, 157, 1980.
232. Einstein, H. Coccidioidomycosis. *Basic Respir. Dis.*, 9, 1, 1980.
233. Acree, T., Abreo, F., and Bagby, J. Coccidioidomycosis of the knee diagnosed by fine-needle aspiration: a case report. *Diagn. Cytopathol.*, 19, 110–112, 1998.
234. Drutz, D. J. and Catanzaro, A. Coccidioidomycosis: Part I. *Am. Rev. Respir. Dis.*, 117, 559, 1978.
235. Drutz, D. J. and Catanzaro, A. Coccidioidomycosis: Part II. *Am. Rev. Respir. Dis.*, 117, 727, 1978.

236. Resnick, D. and Niwayama, G. *Diagnosis of Bone and Joint Disorders*, W. B. Saunders, Philadelphia, 1988.
237. Bernreuter, W. K. Coccidioidomycosis of bone: a sequela of desert rheumatism. *Arthr. Rheum.*, 32, 1608, 1989.
238. Bisla, R. S. and Taber, T. H. Coccidioidomycosis of bone and joints. *Clin. Orthop.*, 121, 196, 1976.
239. Rettig, A. C., Evanski, P. M., Waugh, T. R., and Prietto, C. A. Coccidioidal synovitis of the knee, a report of four cases and review of the literature. *Clin. Orthop.*, 132, 187, 1978.
240. Stein, S. R., Leukens, C. A. Jr., and Bagg, R. J. Treatment of coccidioidomycosis infection of bone with local amphotericin B suction - irrigation, report of a case. *Clin. Orthop.*, 108, 161, 1975.
241. Winter, W. G. Jr., Larson, R. K., Honeggar, M. M., Jacobsen, D. T., Pappagianis, D. T., and Huntington, R. W. Jr. Coccidioidal arthritis and its treatment - 1975. *J. Bone Joint Surg.*, 57A, 1152, 1975.
242. Winter, W. G. Jr., Larson, R. K., Zettas, J. P., and Libke, R. Coccidioidal spondylitis. *J. Bone Joint Surg.*, 60A, 240, 1978.
243. Thorpe, C. D. and Spout, H. J. Coccidioidal osteomyelitis in a child's finger. *J. Bone Joint Surg.*, 67A, 330, 1985.
244. Bried, J. M. and Galgiani, J. N. *Coccidioides immitis* infections in bones and joints. *Clin. Orthop. Relat. Res.*, 311, 235, 1986.
245. Mitlar, R. P. and Bates, J. H. Amphotericin B toxicity. A follow-up report of 53 patients. *Ann. Intern. Med.*, 71, 1089, 1969.
246. Galgiani, J. N. Ketoconazole in the treatment of coccidioidomycosis. *Drugs*, 26, 355,1983.
247. Noyes, F. R., McCabe, J. D., and Fekety, F. R. Jr. Acute candida arthritis. Report of a case and use of amphotericin B. *J. Bone Joint Surg.*, 55A, 169, 1973.
248. Buckley, S. L. and Burkus, J. K. Coccidioidomycosis of the first cuneiform: successful treatment utilizing local debridement and long-term ketoconazole therapy. *Foot & Ankle*, 6, 300, 1986.
249. Olson, E. M., Duberg, A. C., Herron, L. D., Kissel, P., and Smilovitz, D. Coccidiodal spondylitis: MR finding in 15 patients. *AJR Am. J. Roentgenol.*, 171, 785-789, 1998.
250. Akin, J. R. Diagnostic dillema. Musculoskeletal coccidioidomycosis involving the left wrist. *Am. J. Med.*, 111, 236 & 239, 2001.
251. Huang, J. I., Seeger, L. L., and Jones, N. F. Coccidioidomycosis fungal infection in the hand mimicking a metacarpal enchondroma. *J. Hand Surg.*, 25, 475–477, 2000.
252. Gritti, E. J., Cook, F. E. Jr., and Spencer, H. B. Coccidioidomycosis granuloma of the prostate: a rare manifestation of the disseminated disease. *J. Urol.*, 89, 249, 1963.
253. Weitzner, S. Coccidioidomycosis of prostate and epididymis. *Southwest. Med. J.*, 49, 67, 1968.
254. Bellin, H. J. and Bhagavan, S. Coccidioidomycosis of the prostate gland. *Arch. Pathol.*, 96, 114, 1973.
255. Gottesman, J. E. Coccidioidomycosis of prostate and epididymis with urethrocutaneous fistula. *Urology*, 4, 311, 1974.
256. Petersen, E. A., Friedman, B. A., Growder, E. D., and Rifkind, D. Coccidioidouria: clinical significance. *Ann. Intern. Med.*, 85, 34, 1976.
257. Sung, J. P., Sun, S. S. Y., and Crutchlow, P. F. Coccidioidomycosis of the prostate gland and its therapy. *J. Urol.*, 121, 127, 1979.
258. Price, M. J., Lewis, E. L., and Carmalt, J. E. Coccidioidomycosis of prostate gland. *Urology*, 19, 653, 1982.
259. Chen, K. T. K. and Schiff, J. J. Coccidioidomycosis of the prostate. *Urology*, 25, 82, 1985.
260. Lawrence, M. A., Ginsberg, D., Stein, J. P., Kanel, G., and Skinner, D. G. Coccidioidomycosis prostatitis associated with prostate cancer. *BJU Int.*, 84, 372-373, 1999.
261. Niku, S. D., Dalgleish, G., and Devendra, G. Coccidioidomycosis of the prostate gland. *Urology*, 52, 127, 1998.
262. Weyrauch, H. M., Normand, F. W., and Bassett, J. B. Coccidioidomycosis of the genital tract. *Calif. Med.*, 72, 465, 1950.
263. Rohn, J. G., Davilla, J. C., and Gibson, T. E. Urogenital aspects of coccidioidomycosis: review of the literature and report of two cases. *J. Urol.*, 65, 660, 1951.
264. Amromin, G. and Blumenfeld, C. M. Coccidioidomycosis of the epididymis: a report of two cases. *Calif. Med.*, 78, 136, 1953.
265. Pace, J. M. Coccidioidomycosis of the epididymis. *South. Med. J.*, 48, 259, 1955.
266. Bodner, H., Howard, A. H., and Kaplan, J. H. Coccidioidomycosis of the spermatic cord; roentgen therapy: report of a case. *J. Int. Coll. Surg.*, 36, 530, 1959.
267. Stewart, B. G. Epidymitis and prostatitis due to coccidioidomycosis: a case report with 5- year follow up. *J. Urol.*, 91, 280, 1964.
268. Cheng, S. F. Bilateral coccidioidal epididymitis. *Urology*, 3, 362, 1974.
269. Conner, W. T., Drach, G. W., and Bucher, W. C. Jr. Genitourinary aspects of disseminated coccidioidomycosis. *J. Urol.*, 113, 82, 1975.
270. Chen, K. T. K. Coccidioidomycosis of the epididymis. *J. Urol.*, 130, 978, 1983.
271. Liao, J. C. and Reiter, R. E. Coccidioidomycosis presenting as testicular mass. *J. Urol.*, 166, 1396, 2001.
272. Weinberg, M. G., Galgiani, J. N., Switzer, R. W., and Vega, E. Coccidioidomycosis of the urinary bladder, in *Coccidioidomycosis*, Einstein, H. E. and Catanzaro, A., Eds. The National Foundation for Infectious Diseases, Washington DC, 355, 1985.
273. Salgia, K., Bhatia, L., Rajashekaraiah, K. R., Zangan, M., Hariharan, S., and Kallick, C. A. Coccidioidomycosis of the uterus. *South. Med. J.*, 75, 614, 1982.
274. Saw, E. C., Smale, L. E., Einstein, H., and Huntington, R. W. Jr. Female genital coccidioidomycosis. *Obstet. Gynecol.*, 45, 199, 1975.
275. Parker, P. and Adcock, L. L. Pelvic coccidioidomycosis. *Obstet. Gynecol. Surv.*, 36, 225, 1981.

276. Schwartz, D. N., Fihn, S. D., and Miller, R. A. Infection of an arterial prosthesis as the presenting manifestation of disseminated coccidioidomycosis: control of disease with fluconazole. *Clin. Infect. Dis.*, 16, 486, 1993.
277. Williams, P. L., Johnson, R., Pappagianis, D., et al. Vasculitic and encephalitic complications associated with *Coccidioides immitis* infection of the central nervous system in humans: report of 10 cases and review. *Clin. Infect. Dis.*, 14, 673, 1992.
278. Nino Oberto, S., Ponce de Leon, A., and Sierra Madero, J. *Coccidioides immitis*: primary infection of the central nervous system. Case report and literature review. *Rev. Invest. Clin.*, 51, 43–48, 1999.
279. Arsura, E. L., Kilgore, W. B., Caldwell, J. W., Freeman, J. C., Einstein, H. E., and Johnson, R. H. Association between facial cutaneous coccidioidomycosis and meningitis. *West. J. Med.*, 169, 13–16, 1998.
280. Romeo, J. H., Rice, L. B., and McQuarrie, I. G. Hydrocephalus in coccidioidal meningitis: case report and review of the literature. *Neurosurgery*, 47, 773-777, 2000.
281. Saitoh, A., Homans, J., and Kovacs, A. Fluconazole treatment of coccidioidal meningitis in children: two case reports and review of the literature. *Pediatr. Infect. Dis.*, 19, 1204–1208, 2000.
282. Kleinschmidt-Demasters, B. K., Mazowiecki, M., Bonds, L. A., Cohn, D. L., and Wilson, M. L. Coccidioidomycosis meningitis with massive dural and cerebral venous thrombosis and tissue arthroconidia. *Arch. Pathol. Lab. Med.*, 124, 310–314, 2000.
283. Shehab, Z. M., Britton, H., and Dunn, J. H. Imidazole therapy of coccidioidal meningitis in children. *Pediatr. Infect. Dis. J.*, 7, 40-44, 1988.
284. Harrison, H. R., Galgiani, J. N., Reynolds, A. F. Jr., Sprunger, L. W., and Friedman, A. D. Amphotericin B and imidazole therapy for coccidioidal meningitis in children. *Pediatr. Infect. Dis. J.*, 2, 216–221, 1983.
285. Craven, P. C., Graybill, J. R., Jorgensen, J. H., Dismukes, W. E., and Levine, B. E. High-dose ketoconazole for treatment of fungal infections of the central nervous system. *Ann. Intern. Med.*, 98, 160–167, 1983.
286. Stevens, D. A. and Shatsky, S. A. Intrathecal amphotericin in the management of coccidioidal meningitis. *Semin. Respir. Infect.*, 16, 263–269, 2001.
287. Galgiani, J. N., Catanzaro, A., Cloud, G. A., et al., Fluconazole therapy for coccidioidal meningitis. The NIAID Mycoses Study Group. *Ann. Intern. Med.*, 119, 28–35, 1993.
288. Dewsnup, D. H., Galgiani, J. N., Graybill, J. R., et al. Is it safe to stop azole therapy for *Coccidioides immitis* meningitis? *Ann. Intern. Med.*, 124, 305–310, 1996.
289. Oldfield, E. C. III, Bone, W. D., Martin, C. R., Gray, G. C., Olson, P., and Schillaci, R. F. Prediction of relapse after treatment of coccidioidomycosis. *Clin. Infect. Dis.*, 25, 1205–1210, 1997.
290. Stevens, D. A. Adequacy of therapy for coccidioidomycosis. *Clin. Infect. Dis.*, 25, 1211–1212, 1997.
291. Williams, P. L. Vasculitic complications associated with coccidioidal meningitis. *Semin. Respir. Infect.*, 16, 270–279, 2001.
292. Erly, W. K., Labadie, E., Williams, P. L., Lee, D. M., Carmody, R. F., and Seeger, J. F. Disseminated coccidioidomycosis complicated by vasculitis: a cause of fatal subarachnoid hemorrhage in two cases. *AJNR Am. J. Neuroradiol.*, 20, 1605–1608, 1999.
293. U.S. Public Health Service (USPHS) and Infectious Diseases Society of America (IDSA), 1999 USPHS/IDSA guidelines for the prevention of opportunistic infections in persons infected with human immunodeficiency virus. *Infect. Dis. Obstet, Gynecol.*, 8, 5–74, 2000.
294. Kong, Y. M. and Levine, H. B. Experimentally induced immunity in the mycoses. *Bacteriol. Rev.*, 31, 35–53, 1967.
295. Levine, H. B., Cobb, J. M., and Smith, C. E. Immunogenicity of spherule-endospores vaccines of *Coccidioides immitis* for mice. *J. Immunol.*, 87, 218–227, 1961.
296. Levine, H. B., Miller, R. L., and Smith, C. E. Influence of vaccination on respiratory coccidioidal disease in Cynomolgous monkeys. *J. Immunol.*, 89, 241–251, 1962.
297. Levine, H. B., Kong, Y. M., and Smith, C. E. Immunization of mice to *Coccidioides immitis*: doses, regimen and spherulation stage of killed spherule vaccines. *J. Immunol.*, 94, 132–142, 1965.
298. Levine, H. B. and Smith, C. E. The reactions of eight volunteers injected with *Coccidioides immitis* spherule vaccine: first human trials, in *Coccidioidomycosis*, Ajello, L., Ed. University of Arizone Press, Tucson, AZ, 197-200, 1967.
299. Pappagianis, D., Levine, H. B., and Smith, C. E. Further studies on vaccination of human volunteers with killed *Coccidioides immitis*, in *Proc. 2nd Coccidioidomycosis Symposium*, Ajello, L., Ed. Symposium Specialists, Miami, FL, 201-210, 1967.
300. Pappagianis, D. and Levine, H. B. The present status of vaccination against coccidioidomycosis in man. *Am. J. Epidemiol.*, 102, 30–41, 1975.
301. Williams, P. L., Sable, D. L., Sorgen, S. P., et al. Immunological responsiveness and safety associated with the *C. immitis* spherule vaccine in volunteers of white, black, and Filipino ancestry. *Am. J. Epidemiol.*, 119, 591–602, 1984.
302. Pappagianis, D. and the Valley Fever Vaccine Study Group. Evaluation of the protective efficacy of the killed *Coccidioides immitis* spherule vaccine in humans. *Am. Rev. Respir. Dis.*, 148,656–600, 1993.

32
Paracoccidioides brasiliensis

1. INTRODUCTION

Paracoccidioidomycosis is a systemic mycosis characterized by primary pulmonary lesions with dissemination to many visceral organs. Secondary lesions appear frequently as ulcerative granulomas of the buccal and nasal mucosa with extension to the skin, lymph nodes, adrenals, and by generalized lymphangitis *(1)*. The disease may often become severe and even fatal, especially in immunocompromised patients, such as those with AIDS *(2–5)*. In addition, subclinical infections have been documented in healthy individuals living in regions where the disease is endemic, namely the countries of Central and South America (most often in Brasil, Venezuela, and Colombia, as well as in Ecuador, Uruguay, and Argentina but not in the Guyanas, Surinam, and Chile) *(5–8)*. Only one case (in Trinidad *[9]*) has been reported in the Caribbean islands.

A new monotypic genus, *Lacazia*, with *L. loboi* as the type species, was recently proposed by Taborda et al. *(10)* to accommodate the obligate etiologic agent of lobomycosis in mammals and humans *(11)*. The continued placement of *L. loboi* in the genus *Paracoccidioides* as *Paracoccidioides loboi* O.M. Fonseca et Lacaz was found to be taxonomically inappropriate *(11)*. The older name *Loboa loboi* Ciferri at al. was considered to be a synonym of *Paracoccidioides brasiliensis (10)*. In a similar vein, mycologic and immunochemical data have clearly demonstrated that *Paracoccidioides cerebriformis*, a species first described in 1935, also does not belong to the genus *Paracoccidioides (12)*.

Paracoccidioidomycosis affects most often adults between 30 and 60 yr of age, and is rarely observed in children (3%) and young adults (10%). It occurs more frequently in males than in females, with an overall ratio in endemic regions of 13:1 *(5)*; this ratio is even larger (150:1) in Colombia, Ecuador, and Argentina *(13)*. A strong argument supporting the importance of female hormonal influences in paracoccidioidomycosis was the finding that there was no sex prevalence in children with overt disease *(14–17)*.

Two distinct clinical forms of paracoccidioidomycosis are currently defined: the acute (subacute) juvenile form (3–5% of all cases), and the chronic adult form (over 90% of patients). The chronic form is predominantly manifestated with mucocutaneous lesions. Furthermore, depending on the evolution and localization of lesions, the chronic form may also be manifested with uni- or multifocal developments *(18)*. The juvenile form is usually more severe, with rapid progression, and involvement of the reticuloendothelial system (spleen, liver, lymph nodes, and bone marrow) *(5,19–22)*. In children, it is characterized with high morbidity and mortality, which is probably related to an antigen-specific immunodeficiency *(23)*. Although the basis for virulence in *P. brasiliensis* is not completely understood, some evidence suggested the presence of morphological difference found after animal passage of fungal isolates obtained from patients with acute and chronic disease *(24)*.

Although oropharyngeal paracoccidioidomycosis may be fairly common as first presentation of the disease (even with relatively small number of reports *[25–29]* in support), cases of oral lesions caused by *P. brasiliensis* have been extremely rare and, so far, associated only with patients who

From: Opportunistic Infections: Treatment and Prophylaxis
By: Vassil St. Georgiev © Humana Press Inc., Totowa, NJ

have lived in or visited Brazil, Paraguay, or Venezuela *(30–33)*. One case of submandibular lymph node paracoccidioidomycosis has been diagnosed in an HIV-infected patient *(34)*.

The most common affected sites of oral disease have been the alveolar and gingival mucosa, and the palate *(30–33,35)*. The infection, which often remains subclinical or localized, may occasionally disseminate *(36)*.

Miranda Aires et al. *(37)* described a case of paracoccidioidomycosis in a HIV-positive patient with a rather unusual clinical presentation that included primarily massive bone lesion but did not include the lymphatic and disseminated disease described in this population.

Two cases of palpebral (eyelid) paracoccidioidomycosis have been reported and viewed as what could be the first manifestation of the disease *(38)*. Other uncommon localizations of paracoccidioidomycosia include the scrotum (verrucous lesions) *(39)*, and the knee (osteoarthritis) *(40)* where the patients showed no signs of systemic disease.

Remission of paracoccidioidomycosis is frequently related to extensive pulmonary fibrosis *(25,41,42)*. The fibrotic sequelae may still persist even after successful therapy *(25,43)*.

2. HOST IMMUNE RESPONSE TO PARACOCCIDIOIDOMYCOSIS

In both clinical forms of paracoccidioidomycosis, the cell-mediated immune responses are abnormal, and the lack of specific therapy is often associated with high mortality rate *(16,44–46)*.

In general, there is a strong correlation between inhibition of cell-mediated immune responses and the acute progressive form of paracoccidioidomycosis *(47–50)*, especially in the disseminated form of the disease *(49)*. It is thought that the fungal infection is primarily responsible for the impairment of cell-mediated immunity, which, in turn, will contribute to disease progression *(5)*. The observed reversal in cell-mediated immunity functions after successful antifungal therapy lent credence to this hypothesis *(50,51)*. Factors associated with impairment of cell-mediated immunity that have been studied include unidentified host-produced inhibitory factors in human plasma *(50,52)*, circulating immune complexes *(53–57)*, and imbalance in T-cell subsets *(58,59)*.

Silva and Figueiredo *(60)* observed significantly increased levels of tumor necrosis factor-α (TNF-α) in patients with paracoccidioidomycosis, suggesting that it may play a role in the host defense mechanism, especially in regulating the production of interferon-γ (IFN-γ) or some other cytokines critical for the host defense against *P. brasiliensis*.

The production of IFN-γ, which is impaired in patients with paracoccidioidomycosis during active disease, is restored after clinical remission, underscoring the cellular immune deficiency seen in these patients *(61)*.

As compared to controls, significantly lower cytotoxic activity of circulating natural killer (NK) cells recovered from *P. brasiliensis*-infected patients (both treated and untreated), has also been observed *(62)*. Jimenez and Murphy *(63)* found that murine NK cells were able to inhibit in vitro the growth of *P. brasiliensis*; thus, disturbance in the immune effector functions of these cells may be an important factor in the host resistance against *P. brasiliensis*.

Hyporeactive proliferative responses of patient's peripheral blood lymphocytes (PBLs) to *P. brasiliensis* antigens or mitogens has been another immunologic reaction reported in several studies *(49,50,52,64,65)*.

Rezkallah-Iwasso et al. *(66)* reported that patients with active paracoccidioidomycosis had a decreased number of T cells expressing interleuken-2 (IL-2) receptors.

Earlier studies of patients with paracoccidioidomycosis have revealed no hindrance of antibody production but rather a hyperactive humoral immunity as evidenced by the increased serum levels of IgG, IgE, and IgA, which is indicative of a polyclonal activation of the system *(67)*. This increment in antibody production may be due at least in part to the pathogenicity of the fungal strain. As demonstrated by Singer-Vermes et al. *(68)*, in B10.A mice, intermediate and slightly virulent *P. brasiliensis* strains induced weak IgG antibody production, whereas the most virulent isolates induced strong specific humoral response.

Studies on human histocompatibility complexes (HLA antigens) in paracoccidioidomycosis have produced different correlations *(7)*. The HLA-A9, HLA-B13, and HLA-B40 histocompatibility antigens have been commonly described in infected patients. The A9 antigen was especially prevalent in the unifocal pulmonary form, whereas the B40 antigen was associated with both the uni- and multifocal form, suggesting a genetic influence on the susceptibility and the development of the various clinical forms of paracoccidioidomycosis. Dias et al. *(69)* found no evidence of association between a specific HLA antigen and paracoccidioidomycosis. To this end, de Restrepo et al. *(70)* demonstrated the association of HLA-A9 and HLA-B13 in Colombian patients with the disease, whereas a preferential correlation with HLA-B13 was described in Venezuelan patients *(71)*. Furthermore, Lacerda et al. *(72)* discovered the presence of HLA-B40 at significantly higher level than in controls in 83 Brazilian patients with paracoccidioidomycosis. Results by de Messias et al. *(73)* demonstrated that MHC class III products, especially the nonexpressed C4B allele (C4B:Q0), were also markedly elevated in comparison with controls, and associated with both the chronic uni- and multifocal forms, and thereby in a position to influence the course of disease. Taken together, all these findings underscored the involvement of the HLA system in the genetic susceptibility to paracoccidioidomycosis as well as the importance of ethnic variability in this association *(7)*.

Munk et al. *(74)* showed that during reactivation of paracoccidioidomycosis, the classical complement system was activated, as evidenced by the presence of circulating C4d component.

3. PARACOCCIDIOIDOMYCOSIS IN THE IMMUNOCOMPROMISED HOST

In various reported cases of patients with compromised immune functions (organ transplant recipients *(75)*, cancer chemotherapy *(76)*, AIDS *[77–80]*), infection with *P. brasiliensis* or reactivation of latent paracoccidioidomycosis remained a threat, especially in areas of disease endemicity *(8,75,76,81–84)*.

After the spread of the AIDS epidemic, the greatest incidence in HIV-positive and AIDS cases has occured in regions endemic for *P. brasiliensis*. However, in Brasil, the reported number of AIDS patients with paracoccidioidomycosis has been surprisingly small *(34,77–79,85,86)*. The majority of these patients were adult males, and all presented with the acute and subacute juvenile form of the disease (not regularly observed in patients older than 25 yr). The patients had multifocal involvement, with the reticuloendothelial system being implicated in the majority of cases. An unusual presenation of paracoccidioidomycosis in AIDS patients has been a case of a solitary pulmonary nodular lesion, illustrating that restricted lung lesions also can be found and diagnosed in immunodeficient patients *(80)*.

One possible explanation for the low incidence of paracoccidioidomycosis among AIDS patients is lack of exposure; AIDS has been a predominantly urban disease, whereas paracoccidioidomycosis occurs mainly in rural areas *(87)*. Although the reported findings did not make clear whether AIDS should be considered a predisposing factor for reactivation of latent paracoccidioidomycosis or acquisition of primary disease, in non-AIDS patients the juvenile form of paracoccidioidomycosis has been associated with a marked decrease in cell-mediated immunity *(18)*.

Shikanai-Yasuda et al. *(88)* described four patients who have developed immunodeficiency secondary to juvenile paracoccidioidomycosis, probably due to enteric protein loss and/or malabsorption and malnutrition *(89–91)*. Several concurrent infections (*Campilobacter foetus* sepsis, and *Shigella flexneri* and *Staphylococcus* infections) have been diagnosed, thus underscoring the possibility of associated infections to occur even after clinical and serological remission of paracoccidioidomycosis.

4. TREATMENT OF PARACOCCIDIOIDOMYCOSIS

4.1. Sulfonamides

Until 1940, the year sulfamidopyridine was introduced *(92)*, paracoccidioidomycosis was considered to be an incurable disease. Subsequently, other sulfonamide drugs were used, and sulfadiazine, which was shown to be effective in over 60% of patients *(93)*, is occasionally still being used *(94)*. The sulfonamides are administered orally (usually sulfadiazine every 6 h, and sulfamethoxypyridazine every 12 h) at daily doses of 3.0–5.0 g for rapidly eliminated drugs and 1.0 g for slowly eliminated drugs *(95)*. Blood levels of 50 mg/L should be maintained *(83,96)*.

Benard et al. *(78)* treated successfully an AIDS patient initially with sulfadiazine (6.0 g daily for 4 mo) followed by ketoconazole (400 mg daily for another 4 mo); a maintenance dose of sulfadoxine (1.0 g daily) was instituted afterwards. A significant improvement of abnormalities was observed at the end of 3 mo, with the pulmonary infiltrate, respiratory symptoms, cutaneous rash, and the hepatomegaly all dissolved.

In spite of their low cost and relatively low toxicity (occasional crystaluria with hematuria) *(93,95)*, the sulfonamides have two significant drawbacks: long periods of treatment required (up to 5 yr), and the significant rate of relapse *(91,97)*. In addition, there is also the possibility of fungal resistance to sulfonamides *(98)*, especially after early discontinuation of therapy *(83)*.

The use of trimethoprim-sulfonamide combinations has been recommended as alternative to sulfonamides in patients with sulfadiazine-resistant isolates *(99,100)*. Cotrimazine (trimethoprim-sulfadiazine) was reported useful in the treatment of cerebral paracoccidioidomycosis because both drugs could penetrate the cerebrospinal blood barrier well *(100)*. Barraviera et al. *(101)* evaluated the acetylator phenotype (genetic factors linked to liver metabolism), renal function, and serum sulfadiazine levels in patients with paracoccidioidomycosis treated with cotrimazine; approx 95% of patients had adequate sulfadiazine levels (over 40 µg/mL) with the highest levels measured in those qualified as slow acetylators.

Another combination, trimethoprim-sulfamethoxazole (co-trimoxazole) has also been used in the treatment of paracoccidioidomycosis *(102–104)*. The therapeutic efficacy of co-trimoxazole appeared to be similar to that of other sulfonamides; it may be used in patients with sulfonamide-resistant paracoccidioidomycosis. The usual dose of co-trimoxazole is one tablet, twice daily, for 12 mo *(102)*.

4.2. Amphotericin B

Amphotericin B was introduced in the therapy of paracoccidioidomycosis in 1958 and immediately proved to be more effective than the sulfonamides *(44,95,105,106)*. Following amphotericin B treatment, remission has been observed in 50–60% of patients. Amphotericin B is administered intravenously at an initial daily dose of 0.2 mg/kg; the dosage is increased to up to 0.8 mg/kg daily until a total dose of 1.5–2.0 g is reached. The relapse rate following amphotericin B therapy has also been relatively high: as many as 18% of patients *(44,97,107)*. In addition, the unwarranted toxicity of the antibiotic and difficulties with its administration would require physician supervision, which is not always available in areas of endemicity *(5)*. It is usually recommended that after amphotericin B treatment, a prolonged oral sulfonamide therapy be implemented to maintain remission under control *(44,94,97,108)*. Bakos et al. *(77)* used successfully a 3-wk course of amphotericin B (total, 3.0 g) to treat disseminated paracoccidioidomycosis with skin lesions in a patient with AIDS.

Shikanai-Yasuda et al. *(109)* reported a rare case of severe juvenile paracoccidioidomycosis manifested as cholestatic jaundice, lymph node enlargement, and an unusual form of polyserositis associated with portal hypertension secondary to schistosomiasis, as well as bacteremias caused by *Escherichia coli* and *Staphylococcus aureus* and post-transfusional hepatitis C. The patient was treated with amphotericin B (reaching a total dose of 2.0 g), followed by maintenance therapy with itraconazole for 1 yr; the hepatosplenic schistosomiasis was treated with oxamniquine *(109)*.

While amphotericin B desoxycholate is considered one of the most effective treatments for disseminated paracoccidioidomycosis, the use of amphotericin B colloidal dispersion as the initial induction of therapy failed to cure the infection *(110)*. Thus, four adult patients with the juvenile form of paracoccidioidomycosis when given 3 mg/kg daily of the antibiotic colloidal dispersion for at least 28 d relapsed within 6 mo. Possible reasons for the observed failure may include dose, duration, or reduced efficacy of this lipid formulation of amphotericin B *(110)*.

4.3. Azole Derivatives

The introduction of the orally administered azole antimycotics, especially ketoconazole *(43,111)* and itraconazole, has not only improved the prognosis of, but also facilitated the therapy of, paracoccidioidomycosis *(5,95)*.

Miconazole was the first azole antifungal drug used in the treatment of paracoccidioidomycosis *(112,113)*. In clinical trials involving 40 patients, the drug was administered intravenously at daily doses of 600 mg, or orally at daily doses of 3.0 g. Remission was observed in 25 patients, improvement in 11 patients, and no changes in 2 patients. Side effects (which prompted discontinuation of therapy in two patients) included mainly diarrhea and venous thrombosis, and less frequently anemia, purpura, pruritis, and tachycardia.

Intravenous econazole was also used successfully in four cases of paracoccidioidomycosis at daily doses of 600 mg; oral administration was also applied at daily doses of 1.0 g. The duration of therapy was 6–12 mo *(112)*.

Treatment with ketoconazole at daily doses of 200–400 mg for 1 yr or less resulted in disease remission in more than 90% of cases *(5,102,114)*. Most external lesions resolved within 3–6 mo concurrent with gradual clearing of lung lesions *(43,111)*; however, fibrosis was unaffected by therapy *(42,115)*. The relapse rate 3 yr after therapy was ceased, remained relatively low (11%) as compared to earlier therapies *(95,116)*. One requirement for proper ketoconazole treatment is the maintenance of acidic gastric pH in order for the drug to be properly absorbed.

The side effects of ketoconazole included gastrointestinal and endocrine (gynecomastia, decreased libido) disorders *(43,111)*. In addition, patients on ketoconazole therapy had decreased activity of antioxidant enzymes (glucose 6-phosphate dehydrogenase, glutathione reductase) *(117)*, necessitating close monitoring of patients with erythrocyte enzyme abnormalities during treatment with ketoconazole. In patients with concurrent tuberculosis receiving rifampin *(95)*, the ketoconazole levels became markedly reduced and their monitoring has been recommended *(5)*.

Currently, the drug of choice for the treatment of paracoccidioidomycosis is itraconazole *(5,102,114,118–120)*. Its higher activity allows for both shorter duration of therapy (6 mo) and lower daily doses (100 mg) but as the case with ketoconazole *(43)*, itraconazole did not arrest the progression of paracoccidioidic fibrotic sequalae *(25)*. Because itraconazole showed low toxicity (it did not interfere with the endocrine metabolism *[25,121]*) and relapses occured at a lower level (3–5%) than with ketoconazole *(121,122)*, it has been recommended in the treatment of cases of the severe juvenile form of paracoccidioidomycosis *(22)*. As with ketoconazole, itraconazole requires an acid pH for its proper absorption. Consequently, antacids and β-blockers have been contraindicated during therapy *(121)*. In a recent report, Borgia et al. *(119)* described a long-term therapy of a patient with paracoccidioidomycosis starting with an initial dose of 400 mg daily for 2 mo, then reducing it to 200 mg daily; after 2 yr of therapy there was complete regression of the pulmonary lesions and of the osteolytic area of the left knee of the patient.

Among the other triazole antifungals, fluconazole and sapeconazole have been studied extensively for their efficacy against paracoccidioidomycosis. Diaz et al. *(123)* reported fluconazole to be highly active because its water solubility allowed for rapid penetration into the fluid compartments of the patient, as well as for the opportunity of its parenteral administration. In another study *(113)*, fluconazole was used in 37 patients at a daily dose of 200–400 mg for at least 6 mo. Significant clinical improve-

Table 1
Currently Used Therapies for Paracoccidioidomycosis

Drug	Daily dose	Duration of therapy	Relapse rate (in %)
Sulfonamides[a]			
Sulfadiazine	3.0–5.0 g (adults)	3–5 yr	35
	0.2 g/kg (children)		
Sulfamethoxypyridazine	500 mg		
Amphotericin B[b]	0.5–0.75 mg (total dose: 1.5–2.0 g)	3–4 mo	38
Ketoconazole[a]	200 mg	6–12 mo	11
Itraconazole[a]	100 mg	3–6 mo	3.5

[a]Oral administration.
[b]Intravenous dose per treatment. Sulfonamide therapy is recommended to follow amphotericin B treatment.

ment was observed in 34 patients; however, one sudden death also occurred. Co-trimoxazole therapy has been recommended as a means to prevent relapses following fluconazole treatment *(113)*.

When used orally at 100 mg daily, saperconazole elicited prompt responses, resolution of symptoms, and healing of mucocutaneous lesions in less than 2 mo; X-ray alterations also improved early (3–6 mo) *(124)*.

The currently used therapies of paracoccidioidomycosis are summarized in Table 1 *(5,102)*.

4.3.1. Adrenocortical Dysfunction in Paracoccidioidomycosis and Azole Therapy

The adrenal glands are important target organs for *P. brasiliensis (125–133)*, with the development of adrenal lesions contributing to the severity of symptoms. Autopsy results have demonstrated adrenal involvement in 80–95% of patients *(125–128)*. In nonfatal cases, adrenal involvement has been diagnosed in as many as 48% of patients *(134–138)*.

The spectrum of manifestations evolved from overt Addison's syndrome to diminished functional reserve *(134–137,139)*; Del Negro et al. *(135)* found significant hypoadrenalism in as many as 44% of such cases. In another study *(130)*, a high percentage of patients with paracoccidioidomycosis presented with increased plasma renin activity, reduced aldosterone response to adrenocorticotropic hormone (ACTH) or to postural stimulation, as well as with low or subnormal plasma dehydroepiandrosterone sulfate (DHEA-S) levels.

Patients treated with ketoconazole seemed to manage less well in terms of adrenal function compared to controls; in one such study *(129)*, 44% had a decreased adrenal reserve. It is well-known that ketoconazole can adversely affect the adrenal steroid biosynthesis by lowering serum cortisol levels and blunting the response of corticotropin infusion *(139,140)*. In addition, ketoconazole suppressed the testosterone biosynthesis and lowered its concentrations *(140–142)*, largely as the result of selective inhibition of the mitochondrial P-450-mediated enzyme synthesis *(143–145)*. Although ketoconazole also displaced dihydrotestosterone and estradiol from sex hormone-binding globulins, it did not affect the cortisol binding to serum proteins *(145)*. It should also be noted that the ketoconazole effects on the steroid biosynthesis are dose-dependent and reversible 8–16 h after discontinuation of therapy.

Francesconi do Valle et al. *(131)* questioned the concept of irreversibility of the adrenal function damage in paracoccidioidomycosis and the necessity of initiating replacement corticoid therapy for the rest of the patient's life. These investigators reported that following specific ketoconazole or sulfonamide therapy (1–2 yr), patients with adrenal insufficiency experienced complete recovery of adrenal function.

4.4. Immunostimulansts in the Treatment of Paracoccidioidomycosis

In a comparative study involving moderately-to-seriously ill patients with paracoccidioidomycosis, Meira et al. *(146)* used antifungal therapy together with intravenous glucan (β-1,3-polygucose) as an immunostimulant (once weekly for 1 mo, followed by monthly doses of 10 mg for 11 more mo). The results have indicated that patients who received glucan, in spite of being more seriously ill, had a stronger and more favorable response to antifungal therapy.

REFERENCES

1. Emmons, C. W., Binford, C. H., and Utz, J. P. *Medical Mycology*, 2nd ed. Lea & Febiger, Philadelphia, 330, 1970.
2. Goldani, L. Z. and Sugar, A. M. Paracoccidioidomycosis and AIDS: an overview. *Clin. Infect. Dis.*, 21, 1275, 1995.
3. Marques, S. A., Conterno, L. O., Sgarbi, L. P., et al. Paracoccidioidomycosis associated with acquired immunodeficiency syndrome: report of seven cases. *Rev. Inst. Med. Trop. Sao Paolo*, 37, 261, 1995.
4. de Lima, M. A., Silva-Vergara, M. L., Demachki, S., and dos Santos, J. A. Paracoccidioidomycosis in a patient with human immunodeficiency virus: a necropsy case. *Rev. Soc. Bras. Med. Trop.*, 28, 279, 1995.
5. Brummer, E., Castaneda, E., and Restrepo, A. Paracoccidioidomycosis: an update. *Clin. Microbiol. Rev.*, 6, 89, 1993.
6. Restrepo, A. *Paracoccidioides brasiliensis*, in *Principles and Practice of Infectious Diseases*, Mandell, G. L. D., Douglas, G. R., and Bennett, J. E., Eds. Churchill Livingstone, London, 2021, 1990.
7. San-Blas, G. Paracoccidioidomycosis and its etiologic agent *Paracoccidioides brasiliensis. J. Med. Vet. Mycol.*, 31, 99, 1993.
8. Blotta, M. H., Mamoni, R. L., Oliveira, S. J., et al. Endemic regions of paracoccidioidomycosis in Brazil: a clinical and epidemiologic study of 584 cases in the southeast region. *Am. J. Trop. Med. Hyg.*, 61, 390–394, 1999.
9. Janky, N., Raju, G. C., and Barrow, S. Paracoccidioidomycosis in Trinidad. *Trop. Geogr. Med.*, 39, 83, 1987.
10. Taborda, P. R., Taborda, V. A., and McGinnis, M. R., *Lacazia loboi gen.* nov., comb. Nov., the etiologic agent of lobomycosis [published erratum appears in *J. Clin. Microbiol.*, 38, 2026, 2000]. *J. Clin. Microbiol.*, 37, 2031–2033, 1999.
11. Burns, R. A., Roy, J. S., Woods, C., Padhye, A. A., and Warnock, D. W. Report of the first human case of lobomycosis in the United States. *J. Clin. Microbiol.*, 38, 1283–1285, 2000.
12. Lacaz C. da S., Vidal, M. S., Pereira, C. N., et al. *Paracoccidioides cerebriformis* Moore, 1935. Mycologic and immunochemical study. *Rev. Inst. Med. Trop. Sao Paulo*, 39, 141–144, 1997.
13. Borelli, D., Prevalence of systemic mycoses in Latin America, *Proc. Int. Mycoses,* publ. # 205 (p. 28), Pan American Health Organization, Washington, DC.
14. Greer, D. L. and Restrepo, A., La epidemiologia de la paracoccidioidomicosis. *Bol. Of. Sanit. Panam.*, 83, 428, 1977.
15. Londero, A. T. and Melo, I. S., Paracoccidioidomycosis in childhood: a critical review. *Mycopathologia*, 82, 49, 1983.
16. Londero, A. T. and Ramos, C. D. Paracoccidioidomicose: estudo clinico-micologico de 260 casos observados no interior do Estado do Rio Grande do Sul. *J. Pneumol. (Brasil)*, 16, 129, 1990.
17. Marques, S. A., Franco, M., Mendes, R. P., et al. Aspectos epidemiologicos da paracoccidioidomicose na area endemica de Botucatu (Sao Paolo-Brasil). *Rev. Inst. Med. Trop. Sao Paolo*, 25, 87, 1983.
18. Franco, M. Host-parasite relationships in paracoccidioidomycosis. *J. Med. Vet. Mycol.*, 25, 5, 1987.
19. Franco, M. F., Montenegro, R. G., Mendes, R. P., Marcos, S. A., Dillon, N. L., and Mota, N. G. S. Paracoccidioidomycosis: a recently proposed classification of its clinical forms. *Rev. Soc. Bras. Med. Trop.*, 20, 129, 1987.
20. Giraldo, R., Restrepo, A., Gutierrez, F., et al. Pathogenesis of paracoccidioidomycosis: a model based on the study of 46 patients. *Mycopathologia*, 58, 63, 1976.
21. Montenegro, M. R. G. Formas clinicas de paracoccidioidomicose. *Rev. Inst. Med. Trop. Sao Paolo*, 28, 203, 1986.
22. Ochoa, M. T., Franco, L., and Restrepo, A. Caracteristicas de la paracoccidioidomicosis infantil: informe de cuatro casos. *Medicina U.P.B. (Madelin)*, 10, 97, 1991.
23. Benard, G., Orii, N. M., Marques, H. H. S., et al. Severe acute paracoccidioidomycosis in children. *Pediatr. Infect. Dis. J.*, 13, 510, 1994.
24. Svidzinski, T. I., Miranda Neto, M. H., Santana, R. G., Fischman, O., and Colombo, A. L. *Paracoccidioides brasiliensis* isolates obtained from patients with acute and chronic disease exhibit morphological differences after animal passage. *Rev. Inst. Med. Trop. Sao Paulo*, 41, 279–283, 1999.
25. Naranjo, M. S., Trujillo, M., Munera, M. I., Restrepo, P., Gomez, I., and Restrepo, A. Treatment of paracoccidioidomycosis with itraconazole. *J. Med. Vet. Mycol.*, 28, 67, 1990.
26. Londero, A. T., Ramos, C. D., and Lopes, J. O. S. Progressive pulmonary paracoccidioidomycosis: a study of 34 cases observed in Rio Grande do Sul (Brazil). *Mycopathologia*, 63, 53, 1978.
27. de Almeida, O. P., Jorge, J., Scully, C., and Bozzo, L. Oral manifestations of paracoccidioidomycosis (South American blastomycosis). *Oral Surg. Oral Med. Oral Pathol.*, 72, 430, 1991.
28. Lazow, S. K., Seldin, R. D., and Solomon, M. P. South American blastomycosis of the maxilla: report of a case. *J. Oral Maxillofac. Surg.*, 48, 68, 1990.
29. Kwon-Chung, K. J. and Bennett, J. E. Paracoccidioidomycosis, in *Medical Mycology*. Lea & Febiger, Philadelphia, 594, 1992.

30. Sposto, M. R., Mendes-Giannini, M. J., Moraes, R. A., Branco, F. C., and Scully, C. Paracoccidioidomycosis manifesting as oral lesions: clinical, cytological and serological investigation. *J. Oral Pathol. Med.*, 23, 85, 1994.
31. Lazow, S. K., Seldin, R. D., and Solomon, M. P. South American blastomycosis of the maxilla: report of a case. *J. Oral Maxillofac. Surg.*, 48, 68, 1990.
32. Almeida, O. D. P., Jorge, J., Scully, C., and Bozzo, L. Oral manifestations of paracoccidioidomycosis (South American blastomycosis). *Oral Surg. Oral Med. Oral Pathol.*, 72, 430, 1991.
33. Sposto, M. R., Scully, C., de Almeida, O. P., Jorge, J., Graner, E., and Bozzo, L. Oral paracoccidioidomycosis: a study of 36 South American patients. *Oral Surg. Oral Med. Oral Pathol.*, 75, 461, 1993.
34. Goldani, L. Z., Coelho, I. C., Machado, A. A., and Martinez, R. Paracoccidioidomycosis and AIDS. *Scand. J. Infect. Dis.*, 23, 393, 1991.
35. Joseph, E. A., Mare, A., and Irving, W. R. Oral South American blastomycosis in the USA. *Oral Surg. Oral. Med. Oral Med. Pathol.*, 21, 732, 1966.
36. Restrepo, A., Robledo, M., Gutierrez, F., San Clemente, M., Castaneda, E., and Calle, G. Paracoccidioidomycosis (South American blastomycosis): a study of 39 cases observed in Medellin, Colombia. *Am. J. Trop. Med. Hyg.*, 19, 68, 1970.
37. Miranda Aires, E., Costa Alves C. A., Ferreira, A. V., et al. Bone paracoccidioidomycosis in an HIV-positive patient. *Braz. J. Infect. Dis.*, 1, 260–265, 1997.
38. Burnier, S. V. and Sant'Anna, A. E. Palpebral paracoccidioidomycosis. *Mycopathologia*, 140, 29–33, 1997.
39. Tomimori-Yamashita, J., Tagliolatto, S., Porro, A. M., Ogawa, M. M., Michalany, N. S., and Camargo, Z. P. Paracoccidioidomycosis: an uncommon localization in the scrotum. *Mycoses*, 40, 415–418, 1997.
40. Silvestre, M. T., Ferreira, M. S., Borges, A. S., Rocha, A., de Souza, G. M., and Nishioka, S. A. Monoartrite de joelho como manifestacao isolada de paracoccidioidomicose. *Rev. Soc. Bras. Med. Trop.*, 30, 393–395, 1997.
41. Campos, E. P., Padovani, C. R., and Cataneo, A. M. J. Paracoccidioidomicose: estudo radiologico e pulmonar de 58 casos. *Rev. Inst. Med. Trop. Sao Paolo*, 33, 267, 1991.
42. Guitierez, F., Silva, M., Pelaez, F., Gomez, I., and Restrepo, A. The radiological appearances of pulmonary paracoccidioidomycosis and the effect of ketoconazole therapy. *J. Pneumol. (Brasil)*, 11, 1, 1985.
43. Restrepo, A., Gomez, I., Cano, E., et al. Treatment of paracoccidioidomycosis with ketoconazole: a 3-year experience. *Am. J. Med.*, 78, 48, 1985.
44. Dillon, N. L., Sampaio, S. A. P., Habermann, M. C., et al. Delayed results of treatment of paracoccidioidomycosis with amphotericin B plus sulfonamides versus amphotericin B alone. *Rev. Inst. Med. Trop. Sao Paolo*, 28, 265, 1986.
45. Lacaz, C. S., Porto, E., and Martins, J. E. C. Paracoccidioidomicose, in *Micologia Médica*, 8th ed. Servier Editora, Sao Paolo, Brasil, 248, 1991.
46. Terra, G. M. F., Rios-Goncalvez, A. J., Londero, A. T., et al. Paracoccidioidomicose em criancas ABP. *Arq. Bras. Med.*, 65, 8, 1991.
47. Mendes, E. and Raphael, A. Impaired delayed hypersensitivity in patients with South American blastomycosis. *J. Allergy*, 47, 17, 1971.
48. Mendes, N. F., Musatti, C. C., Leao, R. C., Mendes, E., and Naspitz, C. K. Lymphocyte cultures and skin allograft survival in patients with South American blastomycosis. *J. Allergy Clin. Immunol.*, 48, 17, 1971.
49. Mota, N. G. S., Rezkallah-Iwasso, M. T., Peracoli, M. T. S., et al. Correlation between cell-mediated immunity and clinical forms of paracoccidioidomycosis. *Trans. R. Soc. Trop. Med. Hyg.*, 79, 765, 1985.
50. Restrepo, A., Restrepo, M., Restrepo, F., Aristizabal, L. H., Monkada, L. H., and Vélez, H. Immune responses in paracoccidioidomycosis: a controlled study of 16 patients before and after treatment. *Sabouraudia*, 16, 151, 1978.
51. Mok, P. W. Y. and Greer, D. L. Cell-mediated immune responses in patients with paracoccidioidomycosis. *Clin. Exp. Immunol.*, 28, 89, 1977.
52. Musatti, C. C., Rezkallah-Iwasso, M. T., Mendes, E., and Mendes, N. F. In vivo and in vitro evaluation of cell-mediated immunity in patients with paracoccidioidomycosis. *Cell. Immunol.*, 24, 365, 1976.
53. Arango, M., Oropeza, F., Anderson, O., Contreras, C., Bianco, M., and Yarzabal, L. Circulating immune complexes and in vitro reactivity in paracoccidioidomycosis. *Mycopathologia*, 79, 153, 1982.
54. Chequeur-Bou-Habib, D., Daniel-Ribeiro, C., Banic, D. M., Francescone do Valle, A. C., and Galvao-Castro, B. Polyclonal B cell activation in paracoccidioidomycosis. *Mycopathologia*, 108, 89, 1989.
55. Chequer-Bou-Habib, D., Ferreira-da-Cruz, M. F., Oliveira-Neto, M. P., and Galvao-Castro, B. The possible role of circulating immune complexes in paracoccidioidomycosis. *Braz. J. Med. Biol. Res. Braz. Biol.*, 22, 205, 1989.
56. Silva, M. R., Campos, D. S., Taboada, D. C., et al. Imunologia da paracoccidioidomicose. *An. Bras. Dermatol.*, 56, 227, 1981.
57. Chequer-Bou-Habib, D., Ferreira-da-Cruz, M., and Galvao-Castro, B. Immunosuppressive effect of paracoccidioidomycosis sera on the proliferative response of normal mononuclear cells: identification of a *Paracoccidioides brasiliensis* 34-kDa polypeptide in circulating immune complexes. *Mycopathologia*, 119, 65, 1992.
58. Moscardi-Bacchi, M., Soares, A., Mendes, R., Marques, S., and Franco, M. In situ localization of T lymphocyte subsets in human paracoccidioidomycosis. *J. Med. Vet. Mycol.*, 27, 149, 1989.
59. Mota, N. G. S., Peracoli, M. T. S., Mendes, R., et al. Mononuclear cell subsets in patients with different clinical forms of paracoccidioidomycosis. *J. Med. Vet. Mycol.*, 26, 105, 1988.
60. Silva, C. L. and Figueiredo, F. Tumor necrosis factor in paracoccidioidomycosis patients. *J. Infect. Dis.*, 164, 1033, 1991.
61. Karhawi, A. S., Colombo, A. L., and Salomao, R. Production of IFN-gamma is impaired in patients with paracoccidioidomycosis during active disease and is restored after clinical remission. *Med. Mycol.*, 38, 225–229, 2000.

62. Peracoli, M. T. S., Soares, A. M. V. C., Mendes, R. P., Marques, S. A., Pereira, P. C. M., and Rezkallah-Iwasso, M. T. Studies of natural killer cells in patients with paracoccidioidomycosis. *J. Med. Vet. Mycol.*, 29, 373, 1991.
63. Jimenez, B. E. and Murphy, J. W. In vitro effects of natural killer cells against *Paracoccidioides brasiliensis* yeast phase. *Infect. Immun.*, 46, 552, 1984.
64. Da Costa, J. C., Pagnano, P. M. G., Bechelli, L. M., Fiorillo, A. M., and Liina Filho, E. C. Lymphocyte transformation test in patients with paracoccidioidomycosis. *Mycopathologia*, 84, 55, 1983.
65. Bava, A. J., Mistchenko, A. S., Palacios, M. F., et al. Lymphocyte subpopulations and cytokine production in paracoccidioidomycosis patients. *Microbiol. Immunol.*, 35, 167, 1991.
66. Rezkallah-Iwasso, M. T., Peracoli, M. T. S., Mendes, R. P., et al. Defective expression of interleukin-2 (IL-2) receptors in patients with paracoccidioidomycosis. *Resumenes IV Encuentro Internacional Sobre Paracoccidioidomicosis*, Caracas, Venezuela, abstract I-21, 1989.
67. Arango, M. and Yarzabal, L. T-cell dysfunction and hyperimmunoglobulinemia E in paracoccidioidomycosis. *Mycopathologia*, 79, 115, 1982.
68. Singer-Vermes, L. M., Burger, E., Franco, M. F., Di Bacchi, M. M., Mendes-Giannini, M. J., and Calich, V. L. Evaluation of the pathogenicity and immunogenicity of seven *Paracoccidioides brasiliensis* isolates in susceptible inbred mice. *J. Med. Vet. Mycol.*, 27, 71, 1989.
69. Dias, M. F., Pereira, A, C. Jr., Pereira, A. Jr., and Alves, M. S. The role of HLA antigen in the development of paracoccidioidomycosis. *J. Eur. Acad. Dermatol. Venereol.*, 14, 166–171, 2000.
70. de Restrepo, F. M., Restrepo, M., and Restrepo, A. Blood groups and HLA antigens in paracoccidioidomycosis. *Sabouraudia*, 21, 35, 1983.
71. Gonzalez, N. M., Albornoz, M., Rios, R., and Prado, L. Paracoccidioidomycosis y sui relacion con el sistema HLA. II Encontro sobre paracoccidioidomicose, Brasil, Resumos adicionais, 1983.
72. Lacerda, G. B., Arce-Gomez, B., and Telles, F. Q. Increased frequency of HLA-B40 in patients with paracoccidioidomycosis. *J. Med. Vet. Mycol.*, 26, 253, 1988.
73. de Messias, I. J. T., Reis, A., Brenden, M., Queiroz-Telles, F., and Mauff, G. Association of major histocompatibility complex class III complement components C2, BF, and C4 with Brazilian paracoccidioidomycosis. *Compl. Inflamm.*, 8, 288, 1991.
74. Munk, M. E., Kajdacsy-Balla, A., Del Negro, G., Cuce, L. C., and Dias da Silva, W. Activaton of human complement system in paracoccidioidomycosis. *J. Med. Vet. Mycol.*, 30, 317, 1992.
75. Sugar, A. M., Restrepo, A., and Stevens, D. A. Paracoccidioidomycosis in the immunocompromised host: report of a case and review of the literature. *Am. Rev. Respir. Dis.*, 129, 340, 1984.
76. Severo, L. C., Londero, A. T., Geyer, G. R., and Porto, N. S. Acute pulmonary paracoccidioidomycosis in an immunosuppressed patient. *Mycopathologia*, 68, 171, 1979.
77. Bakos, L., Kronfeld, M., Hampe, S., Castro, I., and Zampese, M. Disseminated paracoccidioidomycosis with skin lesions in a patient with acquired immunodeficiency syndrome. *J. Am. Acad. Dermatol.*, 20, 854, 1989.
78. Benard, G., Bueno, J. P., Yamashiro-Kanashiro, E. H., et al. Paracoccidioidomycosis in a patient with HIV infection: immunological studies. *Trans. R. Soc. Trop. Med. Hyg.*, 84, 151, 1990.
79. Goldani, L. Z., Martinez, R., Landell, G. A. M., Machado, A. A., and Coutinho, V. Paracoccidioidomycosis in a patient with acquired immunodeficiency syndrome. *Mycopathologia*, 105, 71, 1989.
80. dos Santos, J. W., Costa, J. M., Cechella, M., Michel, G. T., de Figueiredo, C. W., and Londero, A. T. An unusual presentation of paracoccidioidomycosis in an AIDS patient: a case report. *Mycopathlogia*, 142, 139–142, 1998.
81. Bodey, G. P. Infections in cancer patients. *Cancer Treat. Rev.*, 2, 89, 1975.
82. Rutala, P. G. and Smith, J. W. Coccidioidomycosis in potentially compromised hosts: the effect of immunosuppressive therapy in dissemination. *Am. J. Med. Sci.*, 275, 283, 1978.
83. Machado Filho, R. and Miranda, J. L. Consideracoes relativas a blastomicose sul-americana: evolucao, resultados consecutivos. *Hospital (Rio de Janeiro)*, 61, 375, 1961.
84. Rappoport, A., Santos, I. C., Andrade-Sobrinho, J., Faccio, C. H., and Menucelli, R. Importancia da blastomicose sul-americana no diagnostico con as neoplasias malignas de cabeca e pescoso. *Rev. Bras. Cab. Pesc.*, 1, 13, 1974.
85. Hadad, D. J., Pires, M. F. C., Petry, T. C., et al. *Paracoccidioides brasiliensis* isolated from blood in an AIDS patients. *Proc. XIth Congr. Int. Soc. Human Animal Mycol. (ISHAM)*, Montreal, Canada, abstract # PS2.104 (p. 116), 1991.
86. Pedro, R., Aoki, F. H., Boccato, R. S., et al. Paracoccidioidomicose e infeccao pelo virus da imunodeficiencia humana. *Rev. Inst. Med. Trop. Sao Paolo*, 31, 119, 1989.
87. Lacaz, C. S., Ueda, M., Del Negro, G., et al. Pesquisa de anticorpos HIV-1 em pacientes com paracoccidioidomicose ativa. *An. Bras. Dermatol.*, 65, 105, 1990.
88. Shikanai-Yasuda, M. A., Cotrim Segurado, A. A., Pereira Pinto, W., et al. Immunodeficiency secondary to juvenile paracoccidioidomycosis: associated infections. *Mycopathologia*, 120, 23, 1992.
89. Andrade, D. R., Hutzler, R. U., Carvalho, S. A., Rosenthal, C., Carvalho, M. A. B., and Ferreira, J. M. Hipoproteinemia em pacientes com paracoccidioidomicose do tubo digestivo e sistema linfatico abdominal. *Rev. Hosp. Clin. Fac. Med. Sao Paolo*, 31, 174, 1976.
90. Laudanna, A. A., Betarello, A., Van Bellen, B., and Kieffer, J. South American blastomycosis as a cause of malabsorption and protein-losing enteropathy. *Arq. Gastroent. Sao Paolo*, 12, 195, 1975.
91. Troncon, L. E. A., Martinez, R., Meneghelli, U. G., Oliveira, R. B., and Iazzigi, N. Perda intestinal de proteinas na paracoccidioidomocose. *Rev. Hosp. Clin. Fac. Med. Sao Paolo*, 36, 172, 1982.
92. Ribeiro, O. D. Nova terapeutica para blastomicose. *Publ. Med.*, 12, 36, 1940.

93. Borelli, D. Terapia de la paracoccidioidomicosis, valor actual de los antiguas tratamientos. *Rev. Argent. Micol. Suppl.*, 13, 1987.
94. Del Negro, G. Tratamiento de paracoccidioidomicose. *Rev. Assoc. Med. Bras.*, 20, 231, 1974.
95. Restrepo, A. Paracoccidioidomycosis (South American blastomycosis), in *Antifungal Drug Therapy: a Complete Guide to the Practitioner*, Jacobs, P. H. and Nall, L., Eds. Marcel Dekker, New York, 181, 1990.
96. Machado Filho, J. and Miranda, J. L. Consideracoes relativas a 238 casos consecutivos de blastomicose sulamericana: contribuicao para o seu estudo epidemiologico. *Hospital (Rio de Janeiro)*, 55, 721, 1959.
97. Borelli, D. Terapia de la paracoccidioidomicosis: valor actual de los tratamientos. *Rev. Argent. Micol. Suppl.*, 13, 1987.
98. Restrepo, A. and Arango, M. D. In vitro susceptibility testing of *Paracoccidioides brasiliensis* to sulfonamides. *J. Clin. Microbiol.*, 18, 190, 1980.
99. Lopez, C. F. and Armond, S. Ensaio terapeutico en casos sulforesistentes de blastomicose sul-americana. *Hospital (Rio de Janeiro)*, 73, 253, 1967.
100. Barraviera, B., Mendes, R. P., Machado, J. M., Pereira, P. C. M., Souza, M. J., and Meira, D. A. Evaluation of treatment of paracoccidioidomycosis with cotrimazine (combination of sulfadiazine and trimethoprim): preliminary report. *Rev. Inst. Med. Trop. Sao Paolo*, 31, 53, 1989.
101. Barraviera, B., Pereira, P. C. M., Mendes, R. P., Machado, J. M., Lima, C. R. G., and Meira, D. A. Evaluation of acetylator phenotype, renal function and serum sulfadiazine levels in patients with paracoccidioidomycosis treated with cotrimazine (a combination of sulfadiazine and trimethoprim). *Mycopathologia*, 108, 107, 1989.
102. Negroni, R. Paracoccidioidomycosis (South American blastomycosis, Lutz's mycosis). *Int. J. Dermatol.*, 32, 847, 1993.
103. Mercano, C. and Negroni, R. Paracoccidioidomycosis: aspectos terapeuticos. *Interciencia (Venezuela)*, 15, 227, 1990.
104. Silva, C. E., Cordeiro, A. F., Gollner, A. M., Cupolilo, S. M., Quesado-Filgueiras, M., and Curzio, M. F. Patacoccidioidomicose do sistema nervoso central: relato de caso. *Arq. Neuropsiquiatr.*, 58, 741–747, 2000.
105. Lacaz, C. S. and Sampaio, S. A. P. Tratamento de blastomicose sulamericana com anfotericina B: resultados preliminares. *Rev. Paulista Med.*, 52, 443, 1958.
106. Campos, E. V., Sartori, J. C., Hetch, M. L., and Franco, M. F. Clinical and serologic features of 47 patients with paracoccidioidomycosis treated by amphotericin B. *Rev. Inst. Med. Trop. Sao Paolo*, 26, 179, 1984.
107. Dillon, N. L. and Marques, S. A. Vantagens e desvantagens da amfotericina B no tratamento da paracoccidioidomicose. *An. Bras. Dermatol.*, 65, 226, 1990.
108. Benard, G., Neves, C. P., Gryschek, R. C. B., and Duarte, A. J. S. Severe juvenile type paracoccidioidomycosis in an adult. *J. Med. Vet. Mycol.*, 33, 67, 1994.
109. Shikanai-Yasuda, M. A., Benard, G., Duarte, M. I. S., Leite, O. H. M., Eira, M., and Mendes-Giannini, M. J. S. Polyserositis in a patient with acute paracoccidioidomycosis and hepatosplenic schistosomiasis. *Mycopathologia*, 130, 75, 1995.
110. Dietze, R., Fowler, V. G., Jr., Steiner, T. S., Pecanha, P. M., and Corey, G. R. Failure of amphotericin B colloidal dispersion in the treatment of paracoccidioidomycosis. *Am. J. Trop. Med. Hyg.*, 60, 837–839, 1999.
111. del Negro, G. Tratamento, controle de cura, profilaxia, in *Paracoccidioidomicose: Blastomicose Sul-Americana*, Del Negro, G., Lacaz, C. de S., and Fiorillo, A. M., Eds. Sarvier, Sao Paolo, 271, 1982.
112. Negroni, R. Azole derivatives in the treatment of paracoccidioidomycosis. *Ann. NY Acad. Sci.*, 544, 497, 1988.
113. Negroni, R. Azoles in the treatment of paracoccidioidomycosis, in *Fungal Dimorphism*, Janssen Research Foundation, University of Cambridge, UK, 105, 1992.
114. Negroni, R. Estado actual del empleo del ketoconazol en paracoccidioidomicosis (ketoconazol: 6 anos despues). *Rev. Argent. Micol.*, 1(Suppl.), 21, 1987.
115. Restrepo, A., Gomez, I., Cano, L. E., Arango, M. D., and Robledo, M. A. Post-therapy status of paracoccidioidomycosis patients treated with ketoconazole. *Am. J. Med.*, 78, 53, 1985.
116. Robledo, M. A., Gomez, I., Gutierrez, F., Cano, L. E., and Restrepo, A. Evaluacion a largo plazo de pacientes con paracoccidioidomycosis tratados con ketoconazol. *Acta Med. Colomb.*, 10, 155, 1985.
117. Barraviera, B., Mendes, R., Pereira, P. C. M., Machado, J. M., Curi, P. R., and Meira, D. A. Measurement of glucose 6-phosphate dehydrogenase and glutathione reductase activity in patients with paracoccidioidomycosis treated with ketoconazole. *Mycopathologia*, 104, 87, 1988.
118. Restrepo, A., Gomez, I., Robledo, J., Patino, M. M., and Cano, L. E. Itraconazole in the treatment of paracoccidioidomycosis: a preliminary report. *Rev. Infect. Dis.*, 9, 851, 1987.
119. Borgia, G., Reynaud, L., Cerini, R., et al. A case of paracoccidioidomycosis: experience with long-term therapy. *Infection*, 28, 119-120, 2000.
120. Martins, R., Marques, S., Alves, M., Fecchio, D., and de Franco, M. F. Serological follow-up of patients with paracoccidioidomycosis treated with itraconazole using Dot-blot, ELISA and western-blot. *Rev. Inst. Med. Trop. Sao Paulo*, 39, 261–269, 1997.
121. Negroni, R., Robles, A. M., Arechavala, A., and Tiraboschi, I. N. Resultados del tratamiento con itraconazol por via oral en la paracoccidioidomicosis. *Rev. Argent. Micol. Suppl.*, 27, 1987.
122. Munera, M. I., Naranjo, M. S., Gomez, I., and Restrepo, A. Seguimiento post-terapia de pacientes con paracoccidioidomycosis tratados con itraconazol. *Medicina U.P.B. (Medellin)*, 8, 33, 1989.
123. Diaz, M., Negroni, R., Montero-Gei, F., et al. A Pan American 5-year study of fluconazole therapy for deep mycoses in the immunocompetent host. *Clin. Infect. Dis.*, 14(Suppl.), S68, 1992.
124. Franco, L., Gomez, I., and Restrepo, A. Treatment of subcutaneous and systemic mycoses with a new orally-administered triazole, saperconazole R-66905. *Int. J. Dermatol.*, 31, 725, 1992.

125. Angelo-Ortega, A. and Polak, L. Paracoccidioidomycosis, in *The Patological Anatomy of the Mycosis*, Baker, R. D., Ed. Springer-Verlag, Berlin, 507, 1970.
126. Brass, K. Observaciones sobre la anatomia patologica, patogenesis y evolucion de la paracoccidioidomicosis. *Mycopathologia*, 37, 119, 1969.
127. Salfelder, K., Doehnert, G., and Doehnert, H. D. Paracoccidioidomycosis: anatomic study with complete autopsies. *Virchows Arch. Pathol. Anat.*, 348, 51, 1969.
128. Pena, C. E. Deep mycotic infections in Colombia: a clinico-pathologic study of 102 patients. *Am. J. Clin. Pathol.*, 47, 505, 1967.
129. Abad, A., Gomez, P., Velez, P., and Restrepo, A. Adrenal function in paracoccidioidomycosis: a prospective study in patients before and after ketoconazole therapy. *Infection*, 14, 22, 1986.
130. Moreira, A. C., Martinez, R., Castro, M., and Elias, L. L. K. Adrenocortical dysfunction in paracoccidioidomycosis: comparison between plasma β-lipotrophin/adrenocorticotrophin levels and adrenocortical tests. *Clin. Endocrinol.*, 36, 545, 1992.
131. Francesconi do Valle, A. C., Cotrim, M. R., Cuba, G. J., Wanke, B., and Tendrich, M. Recovery of adrenal function after treatment of paracoccidioidomycosis. *Am. J. Trop. Med. Hyg.*, 48, 626, 1993.
132. Tendrich, M., Wanke, B., Vaisman, M., et al. Funcao da cortex adrenal em pacientes com paracoccidioidomicose: estudo atraves da dosagem radioimunologica do ACTH plasmatico. *Arq. Bras. Med.*, 61, 223, 1987.
133. Colombo, A. L. Estudo prospectivo da avaliacao funcional do cortex adrenal em pacientes com paracoccidioidomicose. *MA Thesis Sao Paolo*, Escola Paulista de Medicina, 1, 1989.
134. Del Negro, G., Wajchenberg, B. L., Pereira, V. G., et al. Addison's disease associated with South American blastomycosis. *Ann. Intern. Med.*, 58, 189, 1961.
135. Del Negro, G., Melo, E. H. L., Rodbard, P., Melo, M. R., Layton, J., Washslicht-Rodbard, H. Limited adrenal reserve in paracoccidioidomycosis: cortisol and aldosterone responses to 1-24 ACTH. *Clin. Endocrinol.*, 13, 553–559, 1980.
136. Costa, V. R., Mendes, T. I. A., and Scherman, J. Sindrome de Addison asociado a blastomicose sulamericana: a presentaceo de tres casos. *Rev. Bras. Med.*, 29, 224, 1978.
137. Marsiglia, I. and Pinto, J. Adrenal cortisol insufficiency associated with paracoccidioidomycosis (South American blastomycosis): report of four cases. *J. Clin. Endocrinol. Metabol.*, 26, 1109, 1966.
138. Torres, C. M., Duarte, E., Guimaraes, J. P., and Moreira, L. F. Destructive lesions of the adrenal gland in South American blastomycosis (Lutz disease). *Am. J. Pathol.*, 28, 145, 1952.
139. Osa, S. R., Peterson, R. E., and Roberts, R. E. Recovery of adrenal reserve following treatment of disseminated South American blastomycosis. *Am. J. Med.*, 71, 298, 1981.
140. Pont, A., Graybill, J. R., Craven, P. C., et al. High dose ketoconazole therapy and adrenal and testicular function in humans. *Arch. Intern. Med.*, 144, 2150, 1984.
141. Schurmeyerth, T. H. and Nieschlag, E. Effect of ketoconazole and other imidazole fungicides on testosterone biosynthesis. *Acta Endocrinol.*, 105, 275, 1982.
142. Pont, A., Williams, P. L., Azhar, S., et al. Ketoconazole blocks testosterone synthesis. *Arch. Intern. Med.*, 142, 2137, 1982.
143. Kowal, L. The effect of ketoconazole on steroidogenesis in cultured mouse adrenal cortex tumor cells. *Endocrinology*, 112, 1541, 1983.
144. Loose, D. S., Kan, P. B., Hirst, M. A., Marcus, R. A., and Feldman, D. Ketoconazole blocks adrenal steroidogenesis by inhibiting cytochrome P 450-dependent enzymes. *J. Clin. Invest.*, 71, 1495, 1983.
145. Santen, R. J., vanden Bossche, H., Symoens, J., Brugmans, J., and De Coster, R. Site of action of low dose ketoconazole on androgen biosynthesis in men. *J. Clin. Endocrinol. Metabol.*, 57, 732, 1983.
146. Meira, D. A., Pereira, P. C., Marcondes-Machado, J., et al. The use of glucan as immunostimulant in the Treatment of paracoccidioidomycosis. *Am. J. Trop. Med. Hyg.*, 55, 496–503, 1996.

33
Penicillium marneffei

1. INTRODUCTION

Although fungi of the genus *Penicillium* are widely distributed in nature and at present several hundred species have been identified *(1,2)*, infections in humans caused by these fungi have seldom been described *(3)*. Among the species pathogenic to humans, *Penicillium citrinum*, *P. commune*, *P. crustaceum*, *P. expansum*, *P. glaucum*, and *P. spinulosum* were reported to cause infections in the urinary tract *(4)*, lung *(5)*, brain *(5)*, ear and sinus *(6)*, cornea *(7)*, and the heart *(8–10)*. *P. notatum* was reported as the causative agent of a chronic infection of the paranasal sinuses *(11)*.

However, *P. marneffei* is by far the most pathogenic of all *Penicillium* spp. *(12–21)*. The infection with *P. marneffei* (also known as penicilliosis marneffei [22,23]) has been reported to affect both immunocompetent *(12,15,21,22,24–26)* and immunocompromised *(12,13,27–29)* hosts. With the advance of the AIDS pandemic, penicilliosis marneffei has emerged as an AIDS-defining opportunistic infection in HIV-infected persons *(30,31)*, especially in Southeast Asia *(16–19,21,32–44)*. Although environmental and epidemiological studies have yet to determine the cause for the hightened virulence of *P. marneffei*, one characteristic distinguishes this fungus from other *Penicillium* species, in that while the latter grow as monomorphic molds bearing typical asexual propagules (conidia), *P. marneffei* is thermally dimorphic (mold and arthroconidial phases) *(45)*. Although its reservoir in nature is still unknown, it seems likely that inhalation may be the route of entry leading to infection *(46)*. Recurrence of the disease is common; even after successful primary treatment, the relapse rate for this potentially fatal systemic opportunistic disease is about 50% *(47)*.

In addition to HIV infection, patients at increased risk include those with lymphoproliferative disorders *(14)*, bronchiectasis and tuberculosis *(23)*, autoimmune disorders, receiving corticosteroid therapy *(22)*, and malignancies (especially Hodgkin's lymphoma). In two reports *(48,49)*, *Penicillium* species have been identified as the etiologic agents of peritonitis in patients receiving continuous ambulatory peritoneal dialysis (CAPD). Fungal colonies were observed on the inner surface of the CAPD catheter. Cases of *Penicillium* spp. causing endophthalmitis were also reported *(50,51)*.

Most often, penicilliosis affects the reticuloendothelial system, causing deep-seated infections that are either focal or disseminated *(21)*. Localized superficial human infection has also been described *(52)*.

Penicilliosis marneffei is usually disseminated and progressive and frequently starts suddenly with chills, persistent fever, painful cough, and pleurisy *(12,35,44)*. In HIV-positive patients, the disease is often manifested with fever, weight loss and anemia, lymphadenopathy and hepatomegaly, and pulmonary symptoms; oropharyngeal and genital lesions (ulcers and papules), diarrhea, splenomegaly, and pericarditis have been reported to be less frequent *(12,21)*. Fungemia is present in the majority of cases *(53)*.

From: Opportunistic Infections: Treatment and Prophylaxis
By: Vassil St. Georgiev © Humana Press Inc., Totowa, NJ

The fungus has been isolated from numerous organs including lung, liver *(54)*, intestine, lymph nodes *(55)*, tonsil, skin *(56)*, bone marrow *(56)*, kidney *(53)*, bone and joints *(36,57)*, and the pericardium *(58)*. Contrary to histoplasmosis, adrenal involvement has been rare in penicilliosis *(59)*.

Hepatosplenomegaly, which is caused by diffuse micro-abscesses not visible on computerized tomography (CT), has been often observed in children *(12,37)*. Mucocutaneous involvement is also a common feature *(12,21,60)*. Usually cutaneous manifestations are presented as generalized small papules, crusted or necrotic papules, chronic ulcers, molluscum contagiosum-like umbillicated papules *(16,18,27)*, abscesses, and cutaneous nodules *(61)*.

Three forms of invasive pulmonary penicilliosis have been described: a subacute to chronic form *(62,63)*, a more acute and rapidly progressive form *(62,64)*, and an invasive pulmonary form caused by *P. marneffei* *(65)*.

Histologic examination of immunocompromised patients have demonstrated the presence of an anergic and necrotizing reaction characterized by a diffuse infiltration of histiocytes saturated with proliferating yeast-like cells *(13)*. Granulomatous and suppurative reaction patterns may also be observed *(13,15,32)*.

Because some clinical and histologic appearances of penicilliosis marneffei may strongly resemble several invasive infectious diseases, it has often been misdiagnosed in the past as tuberculosis *(24,66)* (e.g., suppurative lymphadenopathy *[24]*), histoplasmosis or cryptococcosis *(12,15,21–24,67,68)*, and visceral leishmaniasis *(69)*. To this end, *Histoplasma capsulatum* and *P. marneffei*, by being thermally dimorphic fungi that proliferate within histiocytes, have shown morphologic resemblance during their intrahistiocytic proliferation *(15)*.

Cases of *P. marneffei* osteomyelitis are often misdiagnosed as tuberculosis *(22,58)* and have high mortality rates even with antifungal treatment *(22,24,58)*. Chan and Woo *(70)* described an unusual case in which the patient was afebrile and had no lymphadenopathy but presented with multiple and well-delineated lytic bone lesions. Penicilliosis manifesting as multiple soft-tissue abscesses and infection of the axial skeleton has been reported *(57)*. Early diagnosis and treatment of the infection is essential to prevent bone destruction as well as damage to the spinal cord.

For definitive diagnosis, the pathogen must be isolated on standard mycologic culture media and histologic examination of tissue specimens should be carried out *(12,21)*.

2. TREATMENT OF *PENICILLIUM MARNEFFEI* INFECTION

When diagnosis is made promptly and therapy is instituted immediately, penicilliosis marneffei can be cured *(12)*. Duration of illness may vary between 2 mo and 3 yr, with an average of 10–11 mo, but if left untreated it may become fatal *(15)*.

Nystatin was the first therapeutic agent tried successfully in bamboo rats *(52)*. Owing to its poor systemic absorption *(71)*, however, it is doubtful that oral nystatin would be effective in humans.

Currently, as first choice, mild to moderate cases of penicilliosis marneffei are treated with oral itraconazole at 400 mg daily *(72)*. Amphotericin B parenteral therapy may be required for seriously ill patients. Relapses within 6 mo after the end of amphotericin B therapy have been reported *(18,56)*. Azole antifungals (ketoconazole, fluconazole, and particularly itraconazole) because of lesser toxicities may be considered as first-line maintenance therapy *(16,18,21,34,43,56, 73)*. In a prospective study of HIV-infected children with disseminated penicilliosis marneffei, early diagnosis and appropriate antifungal therapy (amphotericin B, fluconazole, or ketoconazole) reduced the mortality rate to 18% *(37)*.

A combined regimen consisting of intravenous amphotericin B (0.6 mg/kg daily for 2 wk) followed by oral itraconazole (400 mg daily for 10 wk) is recommended for treating disseminated penicilliosis in HIV-infected patients *(74)* (Table 1).

In spite of its relatively moderate in vitro activity *(80)*, intravenous amphotericin B alone (50 mg for 10 d to 8 wk) *(11,21,22,41,49,56,59,75,76)* or in combination with oral 5-fluorocytosine (5-FC),

Table 1
Therapeutic Regimens for treating *Penicillium marneffeii* Infections

Drug	Doses/route of administration	Duration	Refs.
Itraconazole	400 mg daily (oral)	Until resolution	(39,72,74)
Amphotericin B	25–50 mg daily or every other day (i.v.)	10 d–8 wk	(11,21,22,49,56) (59,65,75–77)
Ketoconazole	200–400 mg daily (oral)	Until resolution	(16,78)
Fluconazole	400 mg daily (oral)	2 wk	(61,79)
Flucytosine	150 mg/kg daily (oral)	2–4 wk	(34,51)

fluconazole, and/or ketoconazole *(16,17,22,27,58,77)* has been most beneficial in the treatment of penicilliosis marneffei *(18,21,34)*.

Gelfand et al. *(65)* treated successfully a case of invasive pulmonary penicilliosis marneffei with intravenous amphothericin B at 50 mg given every other day, for a total dose of 1.3 g over a period of 8 wk. Heath et al. *(59)* also treated a case of disseminated penicilliosis marneffei with amphotericin B (only 25 mg daily because of deteriorating renal functions; total dose, 500 mg) for 3 wk, and maintenance therapy with oral itraconazole (200 mg, b.i.d.) for 3 mo.

Swan et al. *(51)* reported a rare case of *Penicillium* species causing endophthalmitis after parenteral drug abuse. The patient was treated with intravenous amphotericin B (total of 510 mg over a 24-d period) and oral flucytosine (150 mg/kg daily, but discontinued after 12 d because of worsening renal function). A similar dose regimen of amphotericin B (total dose 1.4 g, i.v.) and flucytosine (150 mg/kg daily) given over a 20-d period led to a complete resolution of symptoms in a HIV-positive patient with penicilliosis marneffei *(34)*. Afterwards, a maintenance therapy with itraconazole was instituted at daily doses of 400 mg during the first month, followed by 200 mg thereafter *(34)*. Disseminated penicilliosis marneffei infection in a HIV-positive patient who deleloped endophthalmitis responded to a combined treatment with intravenous and intravitreal amphotericin B *(41)*.

A *P. marneffei*-induced retropharyngeal abscess, an unusual case of upper airway obstruction, was treated with amphotericin B (0.35 mg/kg daily, i.v.) and oral fluconazole (400 mg daily). After 6 wk of treatment, the fever subsided, the cervical lymph nodes receded, and the osteolytic lesions responded with gradual radiographic resolution *(79)*.

Peto et al. *(16)* treated successfully an HIV-positive patient with intravenous amphotericin B (1.56 g total dose given over a 22-d period) and oral ketoconazole (200 mg, b.i.d.); the patient continued to receive ketoconazole (200 mg daily) as maintenance therapy. In another report, Sekhon et al. *(78)* described a patient with pulmonary penicilliosis marneffei who responded well to a regimen of amphotericin B (total dose, 1.5 g over a 5-mo period) and ketoconazole (200 mg daily for 5 mo; total dose, approx 30 g). Anti-pencilliosis treatment consisting of intravenous amphotericin B (0.6 mg/kg daily for 2 wk) and oral itraconazole (400 mg daily for 10 wk, and 200 mg daily as maintenance therapy) has also been instituted *(39)*.

Therapy with oral fluconazole alone (100 mg, b.i.d.) for 2 wk was successful in resolving a case of dissiminated penicilliosis marneffei with cutaneous lesions in an HIV-infected patient *(61)*.

The successful use of ketoconazole (200 mg, b.i.d. for 2 mo) *(81)* and itraconazole (200 mg, b.i.d. for 7 mo) *(18)* has also been reported.

3. PROPHYLAXIS AND MAINTENANCE THERAPY AGAINST *PENICILLIUM MARNEFFEI*

Maintenance therapy with 200-mg daily of oral itraconazole is recommended to prevent relapses of penicilliosis *(34,65,72)*. Supparatpinyo et al. *(47)* conducted a double-blind trial in Thailand to evaluate itraconazole as secondary prophylaxis against *P. marneffei* infection in 71 AIDS patients randomly assigned to receive either oral itraconazole (200 mg daily) or placebo. The patients were in complete remission after treatment for culture-proven penicilliosis marneffei infection. None of the 36 patients receiving itraconazole had a relapse within 1 yr, as compared to 20 (out of 35; 57%) patients assigned to placebo that had relapsed.

Ketoconazole (200 mg daily) has also been recommended as maintenance therapy *(16)*.

REFERENCES

1. Raper, K. B. and Thom, C. *A Manual of the Penicillia*. Williams & Wilkins, Baltimore, 1949.
2. Ramirez, C. *Manual and Atlas of the Penicillia*. Elsevier Biomedical Press, New York, 1982.
3. Rippon, J. W. *Medical Mycology: the Pathogenic Fungi and the Pathogenic Actinomycetes*, 2nd ed. W. B. Saunders, Philadelphia, 1982.
4. Gillium, J. S. Jr. and Vest, S. A. *Penicillium* infection of the urinary tract. *J. Urol.*, 65, 484, 1951.
5. Huang, S. N. and Harris, L. S. Acute disseminated penicilliosis: report of a case and review of pertinent literature. *Am. J. Clin. Pathol.*, 39, 167, 1963.
6. Smyth, G. D. L. Fungal infection in otology. *Br. J. Dermatol.*, 76, 425, 1964.
7. Eschete, M. L., King, J. W., West, B. C., and Oberle, A. *Penicillium chrysogenum* endophthalmitis: first reported case. *Mycopathologia*, 74, 125, 1981.
8. Hall III, W. J. *Penicillium* endocarditis following open heart surgery and prosthetic valve insertion. *Am. Heart J.*, 87, 501, 1974.
9. Upshaw, C. B. Jr. *Penicillium* endocarditis of aortic valve prosthesis. *J. Thorac. Cardiovasc. Surg.*, 68, 428, 1974.
10. Del Rossi, A. J., Morse, D., Spagna, P. M., and Lemole, G. M. Successful management of *Penicillium* endocarditis. *J. Thorac. Cardiovasc. Surg.*, 80, 945, 1980.
11. Nouri, M. E. Penicillinose der nasennebenhöhlen. *Laryng. Rhinol. Otol. (Stuttgart)*, 65, 420, 1986.
12. Deng, Z., Ribas, J. L., Gibson, D. W., and Connor, D. H. Infections caused by *Penicillium marneffei* in China and Southeast Asia: review of eighteen published cases and report of four more Chinese cases. *Rev. Infect. Dis.*, 10, 640, 1988.
13. Borradori, L., Schmit, J.-C., Stetzkowski, M., Dussoix, P., Saurat, J.-H., and Filthuth, I. *Penicilliosis marneffei* infection in AIDS. *J. Am. Acad. Dermatol.*, 31, 843, 1994.
14. Di Salvo, A. F., Fickling, A. M., and Ajello, L. Infection caused by *Penicillium marneffei*: description of first natural infection in man. *Am. J. Clin. Pathol.*, 60, 259, 1973.
15. Deng, Z. and Connor, D. H. Progressive disseminated penicilliosis caused by *Penicillium marneffei*: report of eight cases and differentiation of the causative organism from *Histoplasma capsulatum*. *Am. J. Clin. Pathol.*, 84, 323, 1985.
16. Peto, T. E. A., Bull, R., Millard, P. R., et al. Systemic mycosis due to *Penicillium marneffei* in a patient with antibody to human immunodeficiency virus. *J. Infect.*, 16, 285, 1988.
17. Hulshof, C. M. J., van Zanten, R. A. A., Sluiters, J. F., et al. *Penicillium marneffei* infection in an AIDS patient. *Eur. J. Clin. Microbiol. Infect. Dis.*, 9, 370, 1990.
18. Supparatpinyo, K., Chiewchanvit, S., Hirunsri, P., Uthammachai, C., Nelson, K. E., and Sirisanthana, T. *Penicillium marneffei* infection in patients infected with the human immunodeficiency virus. *Clin. Infect. Dis.*, 14, 871, 1992.
19. Tsang, D. N. C., Li, P. C. K., Tsui, M. S., Lau, Y. T., Ma, K. F., and Yeoh, E. K. *Penicillium marneffei*: another pathogen to consider in patients infected with human immunodeficiency virus. *Rev. Infect. Dis.*, 13, 766, 1991.
20. Li, P. C. K., Tsui, M. S., and Ma, K. F. *Penicillium marneffei*: indicator disease for AIDS in East Asia. *AIDS*, 6, 240, 1992.
21. Hilmarsdottir, I., Meynard, J. L., Rogeaux, O., et al. Disseminated *Penicillium marneffei* infection associated with human immunodeficiency virus and a review of 35 published cases. *J. Acquir. Immune Defic. Syndr.*, 6, 466, 1993.
22. Jayanetra, P., Nitiyanant, P., Ajello, L., et al. Penicilliosis marneffei in Thailand: report of five human cases. *Am. J. Trop. Med. Hyg.*, 33, 637, 1984.
23. Pautler, K. B., Padhye, A. A., and Ajello, L. Imported penicilliosis marneffei in the United States: report of a second human infection. *J. Med. Vet. Mycol.*, 22, 433, 1984.
24. Yuen, W. C., Chan, Y. F., Loke, S. L., Seto, W. H., Poon, G. P., and Wong, K. K. Chronic lymphadenopathy caused by *Penicillium marneffei*: a condition mimicking tuberculosis lymphodenopathy. *Br. J. Surg.*, 73, 1007, 1986.
25. Chan, Y. and Chow, T. C. Ultrastructural observations on *Penicillium marneffei* in natural human infection. *Ultrastruct. Pathol.*, 14, 439, 1990.
26. Saadiah, S., Jeffrei, A. H., and Mohamed, A. L. *Penicillium marneffei* infection in a non-AIDS patient: first case report from Malaysia. *Med. J. Malaysia*, 54, 264–266, 1999.
27. Kok, I., Veenstra, J., Rietra, P. J. G. M., Dirks-Go, S., Blaauwgeers, J. L. G., and Weigel, H. M. Disseminated *Penicillium marneffei* infection as an imported disease in HIV-1 infected patients: description of two new cases and a review of the literature. *Neth. J. Med.*, 44, 18, 1994.
28. Rogers, A. L. and Kennedy, M. J. Opportunistic hyaline hyphomycetes, in *Manual of Clinical Microbiology*, 5th ed., Balows, A., Hausler, W. J. Jr., Herrmann, K. L., Isenberg, H. D., and Shadomy, H. J., Eds. American Society for Microbiology, Washington, DC, 659, 1991.
29. Hsueh, P. R., Teng, L. J., Hung, C. C., et al. Molecular evidence for strein dissemination of *Penicillium marneffei*: an emerging pathogen in Taiwan. *J. Infect. Dis.*, 181, 1706–1712, 2000.

30. Dupont, B., Denning, D. W., Marriott, D., Sugar, A., Viviani, M. A., and Sirisanthana, T. Mycoses in AIDS patients. *J. Med. Vet. Mycol.*, 32, 65, 1994.
31. Lo, Y., Tintelnot, K., Lippert, U., and Hoppe, T. Disseminated *Penicillium marneffei* infection in an African AIDS patient. *Trans. R. Soc. Trop. Med. Hyg.*, 94, 187, 2000.
32. Tsui, W. M. S., Ma, K. F., and Tsang, D. N. C. Disseminated *Penicillium marneffei* infection in HIV-infected subject. *Histopathology*, 20, 287, 1992.
33. Jones, P. D. and See, J. *Penicillium marneffei* infection in patients infected with human immunodeficiency virus: late presentation in an area of nonendemicity. *Clin. Infect. Dis.*, 15, 744, 1992.
34. Viviani, M. A., Tortorano, A. M., Rizzardini, G., et al. Treatment and serological studies of an Italian case of penicilliosis marneffei contracted in Thailand by a drug addict infected with the human immunodeficiency virus. *Eur. J. Epidemiol.*, 9, 79, 1993.
35. Supparatpinyo, K., Khamwan, C., Baosoung, V., Nelson, K. E., and Sirisanthana, T. Disseminated *Penicillium marneffei* infection in Southeast Asia. *Lancet*, 344, 110, 1994.
36. Sirisanthana, V. and Sirisanthana, T. *Penicillium marneffei* infection in children infected with human immunodeficiency virus. *Pediatr. Infect. Dis. J.*, 12, 1021, 1993.
37. Sirisanthana, V. and Sirisanthana, T. Disseminated *Penicillium marneffei* infection in human immunodeficiency virus-infected children. *Pediatr. Infect. Dis. J.*, 14, 935, 1995.
38. Viviani, M. A. and Tortorano, A. M. Unusual mycoses in AIDS patients, in *Mycoses in AIDS Patients*, vanden Bossche, H. et al., Eds. Plenum Press, New York, 147, 1990.
39. Rimek, D., Zimmermann, T., Hartmann, M., Prariyachatigul, C., and Kappe, R. Disseminated *Penicillium marneffei* infection in an HIV-positive female from Thailand in Germany. *Mycoses*, 42(Suppl. 2), 25–28, 1999.
40. Fang, C. T., Hung, C. C., Chang, S. C., et al. Pulmonary infection in human immunodeficiency virus-infected patients in Taiwan. *J. Formos. Med. Assoc.*, 99, 123–127, 2000.
41. Vilar, F. J., Hunt, R., Wilkins, E. G., Wilson, G., and Jones, N. P. Disseminated *Penicillium marneffei* in a patient infected with human immunodeficiency virus. *Int. J. STD AIDS*, 11, 126–128, 2000.
42. Mohri, S., Yoshikawa, K., Sagara, H., and Nakajima, H. A case of *Penicillium marneffei* infection in an AIDS patient: the first case in Japan. *Nippon Ishinkin Gakkai Zasshi*, 41, 23–26, 2000.
43. Kurup, A., Leo, Y. S., Tan, A. L., and Wong, S. Y. Disseminated *Penicillium marneffei* infection: a report of five cases in Singapore. *Ann. Acad. Med. Singapore*, 28, 605–609, 2000.
44. Sirisanthana, T. and Supparatpinyo, K. Epidemiology and management of penicilliosis in human immunodeficiency virus-infected patients. *Int. J. Infect. Dis.*, 3, 48–53, 1998.
45. Cooper, C. R., Jr. and Haycocks, N. G. *Penicillium marneffei*: an insurgent species among penicillia. *J. Eukaryot. Microbiol.*, 47, 24–28, 2000.
46. Nittayananta, W. Penicilliosis marneffei: another AIDS defining illness in Southeast Asia *Oral Dis.*, 5, 286–293, 1999 [see also comments in *Oral Dis.*, 5, 269, 1999].
47. Supparatpinyo, K., Perriens, J., Nelson, K. E., and Sirisanthana, T. A controlled trial of itraconazole to prevent relapse of *Penicillium marneffei* infection in patients infected with the human immunodeficiency virus. *N. Engl. J. Med.*, 339, 1739–1743, 1998.
48. Pearson, J. G., McKinney, T. D., and Stone, W. J. *Penicillium* peritonitis in a CAPD patient. *Perit. Dial. Bull.*, 3, 20, 1983.
49. Fahhoum, J. and Gelfand, M. S. Peritonitis due to *Penicillium* sp. in a patient receiving continuous ambulatory peritoneal dialysis. *South. Med. J.*, 89, 87, 1996.
50. Hirst, L. W., Thomas, J. V., and Green, W. R. Endophthalmitis, in *Principles and Practice of Infectious Diseases*, 2nd ed., Mandell, R. L., Douglas, R. G. Jr., and Bennett, J. E., Eds. John Wiley & Sons, New York, 760, 1985.
51. Swan, S. K., Wagner, R. A., Myers, J. P., and Cinelli, A. B. Mycotic endophthalmitis caused by *Penicillium* sp. after parenteral drug abuse. *Am. J. Ophthalmol.*, 100, 408, 1985.
52. Segretain, G. *Penicillium marneffei* n. sp., agent d'une mycose du système réticulo-endothélial. *Mycopathol. Mycol. Appl.*, 11, 327, 1959.
53. Deng, Z., Ribas, J., Gibson, D. W., and Connor, D. H. Infections caused by *Penicillium marneffei* in China and south east Asia: review of eighteen published cases and report of four more Chinese cases. *Rev. Infect. Dis.*, 10, 640, 1988.
54. Kantipong, P., Panich, V., Pongsurachet, V., and Watt, G. Hepatic penicilliosis in patients without skin lesions. *Clin. Infect. Dis.*, 26, 1215–1217, 1998.
55. Ukarapol, N., Sirisanthana, V., and Wongsawasdi, L. *Penicillium marneffei* mesenteric lymphadenitis in human immunodeficiency virus-infected children. *J. Med. Assoc. Thai.*, 81, 637–640, 1998.
56. Piehl, M. R., Kaplan, R. L., and Haber, M. H. Disseminated penicilliosis in a patient with acquired immunodeficiency syndrome. *Arch. Pathol. Lab. Med.*, 112, 1262, 1988.
57. Pun, T. S. and Fang, D. A case of *Penicillium marneffei* osteomyelitis involving the axial skeleton. *Hong Kong Med. J.*, 6, 231–233, 2000.
58. So, S. Y., Chau, P. Y., Jones, B. M., Wu, P. C., Pun, K. K., Lam, W. K., and Lawton, J. W. M. A case of invasive penicilliosis in Hong Kong with immunologic evaluation. *Am. Rev. Respir. Dis.*, 131, 662, 1985.
59. Heath, T. C. B., Patel, A., Fisher, D., Bowden, F. J., and Currie, B. Disseminated *Penicillium marneffei*: presenting illness of advanced HIV infection; a clinicopathological review, illustrated by a case report. *Pathology*, 27, 101, 1995.
60. Chiewchanvit, S., Mahanupab, P., Hirunsri, P., and Vanittanakom, N. Cutaneous manifestations of disseminated *Penicillium marneffei* mycosis in five HIV-infected patients. *Mycoses*, 34, 245, 1991.
61. Liu, M.-T., Wong, C.-K., and Fung, C.-P. Disseminated *Penicillium marneffei* infection with cutaneous lesions in an HIV-positive patient. *Br. J. Dermatol.*, 131, 280, 1994.

62. Huang, S. N. and Harris, L. S. Acute disseminated penicilliosis. *Am. J. Clin. Pathol.*, 39, 167, 1963.
63. Maddoux, G. L., Mohr, J. A., and Muchmore, H. G. Pulmonary penicilliosis. *J. Okla. State Med. Assoc.*, 65, 418, 1972.
64. Shamberger, R. C., Weinstein, H. J., Grier, H. E., and Levey, R. H. The surgical management of fungal pulmonary infections in children with acute myelogenous leukemia. *J. Pediatr. Surg.*, 6, 840, 1985.
65. Gelfand, M. S., Cole, F. H., and Baskin, R. C. Invasive pulmonary penicilliosis successful therapy with amphotericin B. *South. Med. J.*, 83, 701, 1990.
66. Cheng, N. C., Wong, W. W., Fung, C. P., and Liu, C. Y. Unusual pulmonary manifestations of disseminated *Penicillium marneffei* in infections in three AIDS patients. *Med. Mycol.*, 36, 429–432, 1998.
67. Deng, Z. L. Four cases of histoplasmosis in Guangxi. *Guangxi Yi Xue*, 5, 20, 1980.
68. Li, Z. S., Deng, Z. L., Li, E. J., Wei, Z. G., Yue, C. Y., and Wei, X. G. Histoplasmosis in South Guangxi (clinicopathological aspects of five cases). *Chung Hua I Hsueh Tsa Chih*, 62, 267, 1982.
69. Rosenthal, E., Marty, P., Ferrero, C., Le Fichoux, Y., and Cassuto, J. P. Infection a *Penicillium marneffei* evoquant une leishmaniose viscerale chez un patient infecte par le VIH. *Presse Med.*, 29, 363–364, 2000.
70. Chan, Y.-F. and Woo, K. C. *Penicillium marneffei* osteomyelitis. *J. Bone Joint Surg.*, 72-B, 500, 1990.
71. Bennett, J. E. Antifungal agents, in *Principles and Practice of Infectious Diseases*, 2nd ed., Mandell, G. L., Douglas, R. G., and Bennett, J. E., Eds. John Wiley, New York, 263, 1985.
72. Depraetere, K., Colebunders, R., Ieven, M., et al. Two imported cases of *Penicillium marneffei* infection in Belgium. *Acta Clin. Belg.*, 53, 255–258, 1998.
73. Sekhon, A. S., Padhye, A. A., and Garg, A. K. In vitro sensitivity of *Penicillium marneffei* and *Pythium insidiosum* to various antifungal agents. *Eur. J. Epidemiol.*, 8, 427, 1992.
74. Sirisanthana, T., Suppatapinyo, K., Perriens, J., and Nelson, K. E. Amphotericin B and itraconazole for treatment of disseminated *Penicillium marneffei* infection in human immunodeficiency virus-infected patients. *Clin. Infect. Dis.*, 26, 1107–1110, 1998.
75. Kronauer, Ch. M., Schär, G., Barben, M., and Bühler, H. Die HIV-assoziierte *penicillium-marneffei*-infektion. *Schweiz. Med. Wochenschr.*, 123, 385, 1993.
76. Kang, X. M. Penicilliosis marneffei: report of a case and review of literatures. *Chung Hua Chieh Ho Ho Hu Hsi Tsa Chih*, 15, 336, 1992.
77. Ancelle, T., Dupouy-Camet, J., Pujol, F., et al. Un cas de péniciliose disséminée a *Penicillium marneffei* chez un malade atteint d'un syndrome immunodéficitaire acquis. *Presse Med.*, 17, 1095, 1988.
78. Sekhon, A. S., Stein, L., Garg, A. K., Black, W. A., Glezos, J. D., and Wong, C. Pulmonary penicilliosis marneffei: report of the first imported case in Canada. *Mycopathologia*, 128, 3, 1994.
79. Ko, K. F. Retropharyngeal abscess caused by *Penicillium marneffei*: an unusual cause of upper airway obstruction. *Otolaryngol. Head Neck Surg.*, 110, 445, 1994.
80. Supparatpinyo, K., Nelson, K. E., Merz, W. G., et al. Response to antifungal therapy by human immunodeficiency virus-infected patients with disseminated *Penicillium marneffei* infections and in vitro susceptibilities of isolates from clinical specimens. *Antimicrob. Agents Chemother.*, 37, 2407, 1993.
81. Romana, C. A., Stern, M., Chovin, S., Drouhet, E., and Pays, J. F. Peniciliose pulmonaire a *Penicillium marneffei* chez un patient atteint d'un syndrome immunodeficitaire acquis: deuxième cas francais. *Bull. Soc. Fr. Mycol. Med.*, 18, 311, 1989.

34
Zygomycosis (Mucormycosis, Phycomycosis)

1. INTRODUCTION

Zygomycosis is an umbrella term describing acute (rarely chronic) and often fatal opportunistic infections occuring mainly in patients with specific predisposing conditions such as chronic debilitating disease (diabetes, hematologic malignancies, lymphoma), malnutrition, and immunosuppression (organ-transplant recipients, burns) *(1–10)*, as well as in HIV-positive patients *(11–13)*. Mucor infections have also been described in healthy individuals *(14–17)*.

The etiologic agents of zygomycosis are fungi belonging to the class Zygomycetes, which is further subdivided into two orders: Entomophthorales and Mucorales. The latter includes such genera as *Absidia*, *Mucor*, and especially *Rhizopus* (*R. rhizopodiformis*, *R. arrhizus*, and *R. oryzae*) *(18–20)*, which are ubiquitous saprophytic molds residing in decaying matter and soil *(21)*. These infections most often originate in the upper respiratory tract or lungs, in which spores germinate and from which mycelial growths metastasize to other organs.

Cunninghamella spp. (*C. bertholletiae*) in the class Zygomycete and order Mucorales, are unusual opportunistic pathogens that have been identified with increased frequency in immunocompromised patients, especially those with hematologic malignancies *(8,22,23)*.

Apophysomyces elegans, a new genus of the family Mucoraceae (first isolated in 1979) was implicated as the causative agent of rhino-orbital-cerebral mucormycosis in an immunocompetent patient *(14)*. *A. elegans* contrasts with the three genera most commonly responsible for mucomycosis (*Rhizopus*, *Mucor*, and *Absidia*) in that infections with this fungus tend to occur in warm climates, by means of traumatic inoculation, and in immunocompetent patients *(24–28)*.

Saksenaea vasiformis, which was first isolated in 1959, is a zygomycete fungus belonging to the order Mucorales, and found in soils worldwide *(27,29)*. It is the rare but steadily increasing cause of zygomycosis mainly in immunocompromised patients, but immunocompetent individuals as well.

Zygomycosis (the terms phycomycosis and mucormycosis have also been in use) is one of the most acute and fulminant fungal infection known *(30)*. Zygomycosis covers a spectrum of diseases defined by the portal of entry of the pathogen and the kind of predisposing debility of the patient. Two distinct features characterize these infections: (1) an explicit predilection of the fungi to invade major blood vessels resulting in ischemia and necrosis of adjacent tissue (infarction), and (2) the production of "black pus" *(30)*. The zygomycotic infections are usually divided into six major categories: rhinocerebral, pulmonary, gastrointestinal, primary cutaneous, disseminated, and miscellaneous *(2,4,5,31,32)*.

Rhinocerebral mucormycosis is initiated in the paranasal sinuses and frequently progresses to orbital and brain involvement. When diagnosed early, the involvement is usually limited to the nasal cavity and paranasal sinuses. Cases of chronic nasal zygomycosis in otherwise healthy patients are rare *(30)*. A unusual case of craniofacial mucormycosis has also been described *(33)*.

From: Opportunistic Infections: Treatment and Prophylaxis
By: Vassil St. Georgiev © Humana Press Inc., Totowa, NJ

Cardiac mucormycosis has been revealed on X-ray computed tomography *(34)*.

Gupta et al. *(35)* described renal mucormycosis as an underdiagnosed cause of acute renal failure. Cases of mucormycosis occurring in dialysis patients receiving deferoxamine therapy have recently been reported. In addition, deferoxamine has been used in the treatment of iron overload patients with aplastic anemia; a number of cases describing development of mucormycosis in such patients led to the notion that deferoxamine may be a risk factor *(36)*.

2. TREATMENT OF ZYGOMYCOSIS

Before the introduction of amphotericin B therapy, zygomycosis had been almost always fatal *(19,37)*. Also, in the absence of immediate and specific therapy, invasive zygomycosis involving craniofacial structures, lungs, or internal organs is usually fatal *(30)*. Because of its morbidity, the need for early diagnosis (especially in diabetic and other immunosuppressed patients) of zygomycosis as a prerequisite for effective treatment is extremely important.

In the pre-amphotericin B era, treatment of zygomycosis consisted of a combination of surgery and chemotherapy with iodides, nystatin, or cycloheximide *(38)*. Because the chemotherapy has been largely ineffective (based on poorly standardized in vitro susceptibility assays), the accompanying surgery was undoubtedly the major reason for any beneficial response *(30)*.

The azole antimycotics (both imidazoles and triazoles) and 5-fluorocytozine (5-FC) have shown inconsistent in vitro and in vivo activities and have little clinical value as monotherapy for zygomycosis *(39–41)*. Oral nystatin therapy has also been unsuccessful *(42,43)*.

2.1. Amphotericin B Therapy

Intravenous amphotericin B is currently the only recognized single antifungal agent for treatment of zygomycoses. Along with more efficient premortem diagnosis, in recent years, the aggressive therapy with amphotericin B has been credited for the dramatically improved prognosis of zygomycosis *(44–47)*. Since the optimal duration of treatment and total amount of the antibiotic are still not well-determined, the therapeutic regimens should be individualized according to the patient's clinical response and the rate of clearing the infection *(30)*. Favorable outcome in patients with zygomycosis seems to correlate with lack of pulmonary involvement, surgical debridement, neutrophil recovery, and a cumulative total amphotericin B dose of 2.0 g *(7)*.

In most studies, a cumulative dose of 2.0–2.5 g amphotericin B has been recommended, although in some patients as much as 4.0 of the antibiotic was needed to complete the therapy *(38,48–50)*. The rate of administration of amphotericin B is determined by the clinical severity of the disease and the patient's overall conditions *(30)*. It has been recommended that an initial subtherapeutic 1.0-mg dose in 5% glucose solution is administered during the first day of therapy, followed by incremental daily dose increases of 5.0 mg until a daily dose of 1.0 mg/kg is reached *(50,51)*. However, in seriously ill patients with fulminant zygomycosis, such gradual progression in dose schedule may cost valuable time. Instead, the 1.0-mg dose may be followed by larger increments of 10–12 mg every 12 h until a daily dose of 0.7–1.0 mg/kg is achieved *(51)*. Following clinical stabilization, doses of 0.7–1.0 mg/kg may be applied every other day *(49)*.

In another therapeutic approach, the 1.0-mg subtherapeutic dose is avoided altogether; treatment is initiated at 0.25 mg/kg amphotericin B on d 1, followed by a 0.5-mg/kg dose on the 2nd day, and 0.75 mg/kg on the 3rd d of treatment, with a shift to alternate-day administration of 1.0 mg/kg thereafter *(51)*. Each dose, which is injected over a period of 60 min, is adjusted to produce a peak concentration of 2.0–3.0 µg/mL at 5 min after termination of the 60-min injection period of administration *(30)*. Abramson et al. *(48)* used a dose schedule in which the initial dose of 5.0 mg of amphotericin B was increased by 10 mg daily until the patient was receiving 100 mg daily (approx 1.25 mg/kg); the antibiotic was administered intravenously over a 6-h period. Premedication with 600 mg chlorpromazine and 50 mg of diphenylhydramine helped eliminate side effects (chills and fever) *(48)*. Battock et al. *(49)* supported alternate-day amphotericin B therapy at 1.2 mg/kg, which produced at 48 h post-administration adequate serum levels of the antibiotic (0.16–0.69 µg/mL) while reducing its adverse renal side effects as compared to daily treatment.

The therapy of rhinocerebral zygomycosis involved treatment to correct metabolic acidosis, discontinuation of immunosuppressive therapy if possible, adequate dose regimens of amphotericin B, and careful monitoring by CAT scanning of brain involvement combined with successive biopsies to determine the adequacy of treatment *(30,52,53)*. In addition to systemic treatment with amphothericin B, drainage of the sinuses and thorough debridement of infarcted tissue are usually necessary for successful treatment *(26,31,49,54–57)*. Two reports *(31,58)*, have described successful outcomes in patients with intracranial zygomycosis.

Amphotericin B therapy of pulmonary zygomycosis in immunosuppressed patients may be initiated on an empirical basis before diagnosis has been established *(30)*. Alongside amphotericin B therapy, surgical removal of extensive infected tissue has been recommended *(31,59,60)*. Indolent cutaneous mucormycosis with pulmonary dissemination in an asthmatic patient was successfully treated by local surgical debridement of the wound and intravenous amphotericin B. High-dose steroid therapy may have been the major contributing factor *(61)*. Zander et al. *(6)* described a case of mucormycosis involving both the allograft and native lungs in a single lung-transplant recipient with steroid-induced diabetes. Extended intravenous amphotericin B and oral fluconazole therapy, reduction of immunosuppression, and blood glucose control achieved a durable cure without the need for surgical intervention.

Treatment of cutaneous zygomycosis include therapy with amphotericin B *(62,63)*, surgical debridement, and control of the underlying risk factors or disease *(1,2,64)*, especially in diabetic patients *(30,52,65)*. Hall et al. *(66)* presented a rare case of cutaneous mucormycosis in a heart-transplant recipient; successful treatment with amphotericin B was started with 50 mg daily, then gradually increased to reach a total dose of 2.4 g.

Woods and Elewsky *(1)* treated a patient with cutaneous zygomycosis resembling herpes zoster infection (zosteriform zygomycosis) with a combination of amphotericin B and fluconazole. The patient was started with intravenous amphotericin B (60 mg daily) and topical amphotericin B lotion (three times daily) for 3 mo. Only moderate improvement led to the addition of fluconazole (200 mg daily) to the treatment regimen. After 6 mo of combined therapy (100 g total amphotericin B, and 360 g total of fluconazole), there was significant resolution of lesions; areas of persistent fungal granulomas were excised with no recurrence of lesions at 1-yr follow-up examination. It is postulated that by binding to the fungal membrane and compromising its integrity, amphotericin B allows for a better uptake of fluconazole. When internalized, fluconazole inhibits the cytochrome P-450 system and prevents ergosterol biosynthesis and cytochrome respiration necessary for repair of the fungal cell wall *(1)*. In addition to antifungal chemotherapy, surgical excision alone was reported efficient to cure cutaneous zygomycosis *(52,62)*. However, in cases of more widespread infection, surgery should be combined with amphotericin B therapy *(1,18)*.

A case of liver and brain mucormycosis in a diabetic type II patient was successfully resolved by treatment with intravenous liposomal amphotericin B for 40 d followed by itraconazole for 3 mo *(67)*. Hunstad et al. *(35)* used a lipid-complex formulation of amphotericin B to prolong the course of therapy, which was likely critical to the successful eradication of mucormycosis in a pulmonary graft recipient.

The treatment of HIV patients with mucormycosis and renal failure should include hemodialysis, nephrectomy, and intravenous amphotericin B in addition to antiretroviral therapy *(11)*.

In cases of rhinocerebral mucormycosis in immunocompromised patients (diabetics in poor control are at greatest risk), the major therapy consists of reversal of immunosuppression, systemic amphotericin B, and surgical debridement. If not recognized early and/or treated early in its course or if the source of immunosuppression is not reversible, this infection could become potentially fatal *(68)*. Seiff et al. *(69)* recommended conservative orbital debridement with local amphotericin B irrigations as an effective therapy for sino-orbital mucormycosis, especially in patients with reversible immunosuppression and good preoperative visual acuities.

Because rhinocerebral mucormycosis progresses rapidly and is difficult to treat, it necessitates, in addition to surgical excision, large doses of amphotericin B, which in itself can cause significant renal toxicity. To address amphotericin B nephrotoxicity, Moses et al. *(70)* recommended the use of colloidal dispersions of the antibiotic - 1:1 complex of cholesteryl sulfate and amphotericin B. Alternatively, Raj et al. *(71)* described a case of successful treatment of sino-nasal mucormycosis by a combination of aggressive surgical debridement and the use of systemic liposomal amphotericin B and local therapy with nebulized amphotericin B. To this end, Adler et al. *(72)* treated rhinocerebral mucormycosis with intravenous, intracavitary/interstitial, and cerebrospinal fluid (CSF) perfusion delivery of amphotericin B to infected cerebral parenchyma.

The possible role of anticoagulation in the treatment of rhinocerebral mucormycosis was discissed by Hong and Koch *(73)*.

REFERENCES

1. Woods, S. G. and Elewski, B. E. Zosteriform zygomycosis. *J. Am. Acad. Dermatol.*, 32, 357, 1995.
2. Lehrer, R. I. Mucormycosis. *Ann. Intern. Med.*, 93, 93, 1980.
3. Chandler, F. W., Watts, J. C., Kaplan, W., Hendry, A. T., McGinnis, M. R., and Ajello, L. Zygomycosis: report of four cases with formation of chlamydoconidia in tissue. *Am. J. Clin. Pathol.*, 84, 99, 1985.
4. Adrianssens, K., Jorens, P. G., Meuleman, L., Jeuris, W., and Lambert, J. A black skin lesion in an immunocompromised patient. Diagnosis: cutaneous mucormycosis. *Arch. Dermatol.*, 136, 1165–1170, 2000.
5. Zarei, M., Morris, J. Aachi, V, Gregory, R., Meanock, C., and Brito-Babapulle, F. Acute isolated cerebral mucormycosis in a patient with high-grade non-Hodgikin's lymphoma. *Eur. J. Neurol.*, 7, 443–447, 2000.
6. Zander, D. S., Cicale, M. J., and Mergo, P. Durable cure of mucormycosis involving allograft and native lungs. *J. Hearth Lung Transpant.*, 19, 615–618, 2000.
7. Kontoyiannis, D. P., Wessel, V. C., Bodey, G. P., and Rolston, K. V. Zygomycosis in the 1990s in a tertiary-care cancer center. *Clin. Infect. Dis.*, 30, 851–856, 2000.
8. Darrisaw, L., Hanson, G., Vesole, D. H., Kehl, S. C. *Cunninghamella* infection post bone marrow transplant: case report and review of the literature. *Bone Marrow Transplant.*, 25, 1213–1216, 2000.
9. Demirag, A., Elkhammas, E. A., Henry, M. L., Davies, E. A., and Pelletier, R. P. Pulmonary *Rhizopus* infection in a diabetic renal transplant recipient. *Clin. Transplant.*, 14, 8–10, 2000.
10. Joshi, N., Caputo, G. M., Weitekamp, M. R., and Karchmer, A. W. Infections in patients with diabetes mellitus. *N. Engl. J. Med.*, 341, 1906–1912 [see also: *N. Engl. J. Med.*, 342, 895–896, 2000, and *N. Engl. J. Med.*, 342, 896, 2000].
11. Guardia, J. A., Bourgoignie, J., and Diego, J. Renal mucormycosis in the HIV patient. *Am. J. Kidney Dis.*, 35, E24, 2000.
12. Gonzalez Nunez, I., Dosal Caruso, L., Diaz Jidy, M. Torres Gomez De Cadiz Silva, A., and Martinez Machin, G., Pulmonary mucormycosis infection in a boy with AIDS. *Rev. Cubana Med. Trop.*, 49, 218-221, 1997.
13. Scully, C., de Almeida, O. P., and Sposto, M. R. The deep mycoses in HIV infection. *Oral Dis.*, 3(Suppl. 1), S200–S207, 1997.
14. Fairley, C., Sullivan, T. J., Bartley, P., Allworth, T., and Lewandowski, R. Survival after rhino-orbital-cerebral mucormycosis in an immunocompetent patient. *Ophthalmology*, 107, 555–558, 2000.
15. Verma, G. R., Lobo, D. R., Walker, R., Bose, S. M., and Gupta, K. L. Disseminated mucormycosis in healthy adults. *J. Postgrad. Med.*, 41, 40–42, 1995.
16. Sanchez-Recalde, A., Merino, J. L., Dominguez, F., Mate, I., Larrea, J. L., and Sobrino, J. A. Successful treatment of prosthetic aortic valve mucormycosis. *Chest*, 116, 1818–1820, 1999.
17. Carr, E. J., Scott, P., and Gradon, J. D. Fatal gastrointestinal mucormycosis that invaded the postoperative abdominal wall wound in an immunocompetent host. *Clin. Infect. Dis.*, 29, 956–957, 1999.
18. Rippon, J. W. Jr. *Medical Mycology. The Pathogenic Fungi and the Pathogenic Actinomycetes*, 2nd ed. W. B. Saunders, Philadelphia, 615, 1982.
19. Baker, R. D. Mycormycosis (opportunistic phycomycosis), in *Human Infection With Fungi, Actinomycetes and Algae*, Baker, R. D., Ed. Springer-Verlag, 832, 1971.
20. Lehrer, R. I., Howard, D. H., Sypherd, P. S., Edwards, J. E., Segal, G. P., and Winston, D. J. Mucormycosis. *Ann. Intern. Med.*, 93, 93, 1980.
21. Prevoo, P. L. M. A., Starink, T. M., and de Haan, P. Primary cutaneous mucormycosis in a healthy young girl. *J. Am. Acad. Dermatol.*, 24, 882, 1991.
22. Naumann, R., Kerkmann, M. L., Schuler, U., Daniel, W. G., and Ehninger, G. *Cunninghamella bertholletiae* infection mimicking myocardial infarction. *Clin. Infect. Dis.*, 29, 1580–1581, 1999.
23. Mazade, M. A., Margolin, J. F., Rossmann, S. N., Edwards, M. S. Survival from pulmonary infection with *Cunninghamella bertholletiae*: case report and review of the literature. *Pediatr. Infect. Dis.*, 17, 835–839, 1998.

24. Kimura, M., Smith, M. B., and McGinnis, M. R. Zygomycosis due to *Apophysomyces elegans*: report of 2 cases and review of the literature. *Arch. Pathol. Lab. Med.*, 123, 386–390, 1999.
25. Brown, S. R., Shah, I. A., and Grinstead, M. Rhinocerebral mucormycosis caused by *Apophysomyces elegans*. *Am. J. Rhinol.*, 12, 289–292, 1998.
26. Burrell, S. R., Ostlie, D. J., Saubolle, M., Dimler, M., Barbour, S. D. *Apophysomyces elegans* infection associated with cactus spine injury in an immunocompetent pediatric patient. *Pediatr. Infect. Dis.*, 17, 663–664, 1998.
27. Holland, J. Emerging zygomycoses of humans: *Saksenaea vasiformis* and *Apophysomyces elegans*. *Curr. Top. Med. Mycol.*, 8, 27–34, 1997.
28. Chakrabarti, A., Panda, N., Varma, S. C., et al. Craniofacial zygomycosis caused by *Apophysomyces elegans*. *Mycoses*, 40, 419–421, 1997.
29. Solano, T., Atkins, B., Tambosis, E., Mann, S., and Gottlieb, T. Disseminated mucormycosis due to *Saksenaea vasiformis* in an immunocompetent child. *Clin. Infect. Dis.*, 30, 942–943, 2000.
30. Rinaldi, M. G. Zygomycosis. *Infect. Dis. Clin. North Am.*, 3, 19, 1989.
31. Mayer, R. D. and Armstrong, D. Mucormycosis - changing status. *CRC Crit. Rev. Clin. Lab. Sci.*, 4, 412, 1973.
32. Mir, N., Edmonson, R., Yeghen, T., and Rashid, H. Gastrointestinal mucormycosis complicated by arterio-enteric fistula in a patient with non-Hodgkin's lymphoma. *Clin. Lab. Haematol.*, 22, 41–44, 2000.
33. Melsom, S. M. and Khangure, M. S. Craniofacial mucormycosis following assault: an unusual presentation of an unusual disease. *Australas. Radiol.*, 44, 104–106, 2000.
34. Ridley, L., Karunaratne, N., Mann, S., and Solano, T. Cardiac mucormycosis revealed on imaging. *AJR Am. J. Roentgenol.*, 174, 1469, 2000.
35. Hunstad, D. A., Cohen, A. H. and St. Geme, J. W., 3rd. Successful eradication of mucormycosis in a pulmonary allograft. *J. Heart Lung Transplant.*, 18, 801-804, 1999.
36. Miyata, Y., Kajiguchi, T., Saito, M., and Takeyama, H. Development of arterial thrombus of Mucorales hyphae during deferoxamine therapy in a patient with aplastic anemia in transformation to myelodysplastic syndrome. *Rinsho Ketsueki*, 41, 129–134, 2000.
37. Straatsma, B. R., Zimmerman, L. E., and Gass, J. D. M. Phycomycosis: a clinical pathologic study of fifty-one cases. *Lab. Invest.*, 11, 963, 1962.
38. Landau, J. W. and Newcomer, V. D., Acute cerebral phycomycosis (mucormycosis). *J. Pediatr.*, 61, 363, 1962.
39. Hammer, G. S., Bottone, E. J., and Hirschmann, S. Z. Mucormycosis in a transplant recipient. *Am. J. Clin. Pathol.*, 64, 389, 1975.
40. Bennett, J. E. Chemotherapy of systemic mycosis. *N. Engl. J. Med.*, 290, 30, 1974.
41. Stevens, D. A. Miconazole in the treatment of systemic fungal infections. *Am. Rev. Respir. Dis.*, 116, 801, 1977.
42. Neame, P. and Raynor, D. Mucormycosis: a report of twenty-two cases. *Arch. Pathol.*, 70, 261, 1960.
43. Hutter, R. V. P. Phycomycetous infection (mucormycosis) in cancer patients: a complication of therapy. *Cancer*, 12, 330, 1959.
44. Meyers, B. R., Wormser, G., Hirschman, S. Z., and Blitzer, A. Rhinocerebral mucormycosis: premortem diagnosis and therapy. *Arch. Intern. Med.*, 139, 557, 1979.
45. Pastore, P. N. Mucormycosis of the maxillary sinus and diabetes mellitus: report of case with recovery. *South. Med. J.*, 60, 1164, 1967.
46. Pollock, R. A., Pratt, R. C., Shulman, J. A., and Turner, J. S. Nasal mucormycosis: early detection and treatment without radical surgery, or amphotericin B. *South. Med. J.*, 68, 1279, 1979.
47. Sandler, R., Tallman, C. B., Keamy, D. G., and Irving, W. R. Successfully treated rhinocerebral phycomycosis in well controlled diabetes. *N. Engl. J. Med.*, 285, 1180, 1971.
48. Abramson, E., Wilson, D., and Arky, R. A. Rhinocerebral phycomycosis in association with diabetic ketoacidosis: report of two cases and a review of clinical and experimental experience with amphotericin B therapy. *Ann. Intern. Med.*, 66, 735, 1967.
49. Battock, D. J., Grausz, H., Bobrowsky, M., and Littman, M. L. Alternate-day amphotericin B therapy in the treatment of rhinocerebral phycomycosis (mucormycosis). *Ann. Intern. Med.*, 68, 122, 1968.
50. Pillsbury, H. C. and Fischer, N. D. Rhinocerebral mucormycosis. *Arch. Otolaryngol.*, 103, 600, 1977.
51. Hoeprich, P. D. *Infectious Diseases. A Treatise of Infectious Processes*, 3rd ed. Harper and Row, 436, 1983.
52. Tomford, J. W., Whittlesey, D., Ellner, J. J., and Tomaschefski, J. F. Invasive primary cutaneous phycomycosis in diabetic leg ulcers. *Arch. Surg.*, 115, 770, 1980.
53. Hamill, R., Oney, L. A., and Crane, L. R. Successful therapy for rhinocerebral mucormycosis with associated bilateral brain abscesses. *Arch. Intern. Med.*, 143, 581, 1983.
54. Brown, J. F. Jr., Gottlieb, L. S., and McCormick, R. A. Pulmonary and rhinocerebral mucormycosis. Successful outcome with amphotericin B and griseofulvin therapy. *Arch. Intern. Med.*, 137, 936–938, 1977.
55. Berger, C. S., Disque, F. C., and Tapazian, R. G. Rhinocerebral zygomycosis: diagnosis and treatment. *Oral Surg.*, 40, 27, 1975.
56. Ferstenfeld, J. E., Cohen, S. H., and Rytel, M. W. Chronic rhinocerebral phycomycosis in association with diabetes. *Postgrad. Med. J.*, 53, 337, 1977.
57. Halderman, J. H., Cooper, H. S., and Mann, L. Chronic phycomycosis in a controlled diabetic. *Ann. Intern. Med.*, 80, 419, 1974.
58. Lowe, J. T. Jr. and Hudson, W. R. Rhinocerebral phycomycosis and internal carotid artery thrombosis. *Arch. Otolaryngol.*, 101, 100, 1975.

59. DeSouza, R., MacKinnon, S., Spagnola, S. V., and Fossieck, B. E. Jr. Treatment of localized pulmonary phycomycosis. *South. Med. J.*, 72, 609, 1979.
60. Record, N. B. Jr. and Grinder, G. B. Pulmonary phycomycosis without obvious predisposing factors. *J. Am. Med. Assoc.*, 235, 1256, 1976.
61. Wu, C. L., Hsu, W. H., Huang, C. M., and Chiang, C. D. Indolent cutaneous mucormycosis with pulmonary dissemination in an asthmatic patient: survival after local debridement and amphotericin B therapy. *J. Formos. Med. Assos.*, 99, 354–357, 2000.
62. Bruck, H. M., Nash, G., Foley, F. D., and Pruitt, B. A. J. Opportunistic fungal infection of the burn wound with Phycomycetes and *Aspergillus*: a clinical-pathogenic review. *Arch. Surg.*, 102, 476, 1971.
63. Bateman, C. P., Umland, E. T., and Backer, L. E. Cutaneous zygomycosis in a patient with lymphoma. *J. Am. Acad. Dermatol.*, 8, 890, 1983.
64. Ryan, M. E. and Ochs, J. Primary cutaneous mucormycosis: superficial and gangrenous infections. *Pediat. Infect. Dis. J.*, 1, 110, 1982.
65. Baker, R. D. Mucormycosis - a new disease. *J. Am. Med. Assoc.*, 163, 805, 1957.
66. Hall, J. C., Brewer, J. H., Reed, W. A., Steinhaus, D. M., and Watson, K. R. Cutaneous mucormycosis in a heart transplant patient. *Cutis*, 42, 183, 1988.
67. Tsaousis, G., Koutsouri, A., Gatsiou, C., Paniara, O., Peppas, C., and Chalevelakis, G. Liver and brain mucormycosis in a diabetic patient type II successfully trated with amphotericin B. *Scand. J. Infect. Dis.*, 32, 335–337, 2000.
68. Ferguson, B. J. Mucormycosis of the nose and paranasal sinuses. *Otolaryngol. Clin. North Am.*, 33, 349–365, 2000.
69. Seiff, S. R., Choo, P. H., and Carter, S. R. Role of local amphotericin B therapy for sino-orbital fungal infections. *Ophthal. Plast. Reconstr. Surg.*, 15, 28–31, 1999.
70. Moses, A. E., Rahav, G., Barenholz, Y., et al. Rhinocerebral mucormycosis treated with amphotericin B colloidal dispersion in three patients. *Clin. Infect. Dis.*, 26, 1430–1433, 1998.
71. Raj, P., Vella, E. J., and Bickerton, R. C. Successful treatment of rhinocerebral mucormycosis by a combination of aggressive surgical debridement and the use of systemic liposomal amphotericin B and local therapy with nebulized amphotericin: a case report. *J. Laryngol. Otol.*, 112, 367–370, 1998.
72. Adler, D. E., Milhorat, T. H., and Miller, J. I. Treatment of rhinocerebral mucormycosis with intravenous interstitial, and cerebrospinal fluid administration of amphotericin B: case report. *Neurosurgery*, 42, 664–668, 1998 [discussion: pages 648–649].
73. Hong, R. H. and Koch, R. J. Possible role of anticoagulation in the treatment of rhinocerebral mucormycosis. *Otolaryngol. Head Neck Surg.*, 122, 577–578, 2000.

35
Pneumocystis carinii

1. INTRODUCTION

With the advent of the AIDS pandemic in the last 15 years or so, the number of *P. carinii* pneumonia (PCP) cases has risen dramatically *(1–6)*, establishing *P. carinii* pneumonia as the first life-threatening opportunistic infection recognized in AIDS *(3–5,7)*, occuring as the initial manifestation in 50–60% of cases *(8–10)*. It has been estimated that as many as 80% of AIDS patients may develop PCP at least once *(11,12)*.

In addition, the incidence of PCP in patients with malignancies and other immunosuppressive disorders has also been on the rise *(13–19)*. Thus, PCP is one of the most common opportunistic infections in children and adolescents with cancer, leading to considerable mortality in patients with hematologic malignancies and following allogeneic hematopoietic stem-cell transplantations *(20)*.

Other underlying diseases predisposing to *P. carinii* pneumonia include organ *(16,19,21)* and peripheral blood stem *(22)* transplantations, immunodeficiency disorders (affecting either cell-mediated or humoral immunity, or both) *(23–27)*, malnutrition *(28,29)*, lupus erythematosus *(30,31)*, corticosteroid therapy *(32)*, cystic fibrosis (CF) *(33)*, and collagen-vascular diseases *(34)*.

The predominant and most important clinical manifestation of *P. carinii* infection is pneumonia *(35)*. Epidemic pneumocystic pneumonia in infants is generally insidious in onset *(8)*. Among the characteristic symptoms of the disease, restlessness and poor feeding have been observed at the earliest stage of the illness, followed by cyanosis and tachypnea *(36–38)*. Usually, the infection is presented with the same symptoms, whether complicating cancer *(39–41)* or immunodeficiency states *(42–48)*. However, Kingsmore and Schwab *(49)* presented a case of subacute PCP in a transplant recipient with normal arterial oxygen tension and alveolar-arterial oxygen gradient, and normal findings on serial radiographs.

Studies in AIDS *(50)* and heart-transplant *(16)* patients have suggested that recurrences of PCP were more likely the result of new infection than to a relapse of prior disease. The level of immunosuppression has played a critical role in increasing the incidence, especially for long-term (over 2 mo) recipients of corticosteroid therapy.

There has been also a notable increase in the incidence of pneumocystic pneumonia in cancer patients with potential for transmissibility of the infection *(39,40,51)*. Recent data suggested that health-care workers in close occupational contact with patients who had PCP may have become colonized with *P. carinii* *(52)*.

In AIDS patients with pneumocystic pneumonia *(2,53,54)*, the clinical syndrome has an insidious onset with nonspecific symptoms (low-grade fever, chills, shortness of breath, mild, nonproductive cough, and dyspnea on exertion) *(8)*. Additional symptoms may also include weight loss, malaise, and lymphadenopathy *(55)*. Compared to non-AIDS patients, the duration of symptoms in AIDS patients was on average longer (median: 28 d vs 5 d) *(53,56)*. There have been high mortality rates (as high as 50% to no survivors) among HIV-infected patients requiring mechanical ventilation for acute respiratory failure secondary to PCP *(57)*.

PCP has also shown a more aggressive course during pregnancy, with increased morbidity and mortality *(58)*.

It has been shown *(59,60)* that patients with Wagener's granulomatosis undergoing immunosuppressive therapy have an increased risk of developing PCP. In one of the studies *(59)*, the patients, who were all HIV-seronegative, were on a daily medication consisting of glucocorticosteroids and a second immunosuppressive therapy; consequently, lymphocytopenia has appeared in all patients. Lymphocytopenia, coupled with lymphocyte and monocyte functional abnormalities caused by the glucocorticoids *(61)* may have been the most likely factor predisposing to PCP. This observation, which highlights the risk of opportunistic infections secondary to corticosteroid treatment, would make chemoprophylaxis against *P. carinii* exceedingly important.

2. GENETIC DIVERSITY OF *P. CARINII* AND CLINICAL OUTCOME

Molecular techniques have demonstrated extensive heterogeneity among *Pneumocystis carinii* organisms isolated from different host species *(63,63)* Extensive research led to the characterization of various genes and genomes of the *P. carinii* family, which supported the notion that it is comprised of different species rather than strains within the genus. Studying the distribution of *P. carinii* family sp. *hominis* types in the lung of a pediatric patient who died of pneumocystic pneumonia, Ambrose et al. *(64)* identified two different genotypes of *P. carinii* with uneven distribution in the lung, demonstrating that infection of the human lung is not necessarily clonal, and that different *P. carinii* genotypes may predominate in different areas of the lung. The interpretation of genotype data (and in particular the genetic diversity in the internal transcribed spacer region of the nuclear rRNA operon) should be made with caution, because genotyping done on respiratory samples cannot a priori be assumed to represent all genotypes present within the lung *(65)*.

Furthermore, patients infected with *P. carinii* containing mutations in the dihydropteroate synthase (DHPS) gene have a worse outcome than those infected with *P. carinii* containing wild-type DHPS *(66)*.

3. SUBCLINICAL *P. CARINII* INFECTION

Over the years, subclinical infections, although rare, have been well-documented *(67–69)*. As demonstrated by several studies *(70–72)*, most adults and children have shown serologic evidence of occult infections with *P. carinii*.

4. ATYPICAL *P. CARINII* PULMONARY DISEASE

Atypical pneumocystic pneumonia *(53,73,74)* may also present without chest X-ray abnormalities, dyspnea or hypoxia, and with cough being the only symptom *(53)* or with subtle respiratory symptoms and resting or exercise-induced hypoxia but a normal chest X-ray *(8,73,74)*. Some of the more unusual radiologic findings *(75)* associated with atypical PCP include pleural effusion *(76)*, cavitating and noncavitating pulmonary nodules *(77–80)*, lobar pneumonia *(81)*, unilateral hyperlucent lung *(82)*, and bilateral upper lobe infiltrates *(83)*.

PCP with an atypical granulomatous response has been reported in a patient with chronic lymphocytic leukemia *(84)*.

Atypical pulmonary manifestations of *P. carinii* infections in HIV-positive patients have also been associated with long-term prophylactic treatment with aerosolized pentamidine *(85,86)*.

5. EXTRAPULMONARY *P. CARINII* INFECTION

Extrapulmonary disease, usually as a complication of PCP *(23,87–110)*, has been well-documented *(8,51,111)*. In non-AIDS patients, disseminated pneumocystic infections have been reported to involve lymph nodes, blood vessels, liver, spleen, heart, pericardium, thyroid, thymus, colon, small intestine, stomach, pancreas, kidney, adrenals, hard plate, and the retroperitoneum *(23,53,69,73,74, 87–91,94–96)*. Occasionally, dissemination may afflict the bone marrow *(88,99)* and peripheral blood *(92)*, or present as disseminated granulomatous infection *(93)*. Eye involvement due to *P. carinii* has been rarely observed *(103,112–117)*.

In AIDS patients, *P. carinii* pneumonia may very often disseminate to affect virtually all major organs *(8,101)*. Thus, pneumocystic infections complicating AIDS have been associated with otic polyps, otitis media and mastoiditis *(100,102,108,118–120)*, retina *(97)* and choroiditis *(121,122)*, duodenum, esophagus, stomach, heart, pancreas, kidney, apendix renal gland and bone marrow *(123)*, temporal bone osteomyelitis *(109)*, thyroiditis *(107,124)*, and lesions involving the spleen *(104)*, liver, lymph nodes *(103)*, and the skin *(100)*. However, pleural effusions in PCP have been extremely rare *(125)*. There has been one report *(126)* of pleural pneumocystosis in an AIDS patient with PCP and bilateral pneumothorax, and another report *(127)* of an AIDS patient presenting with bilateral pleural effusions and no pneumothorax.

As reported on several occasions *(128–131)*, extrapulmonary *P. carinii* infection may often occur in those AIDS patients who receive aerosolized pentamidine prophylaxis because of its lack of systemic effect. As expected, dissemination has been strongly associated with severe immunosuppression *(132,133)*. Still unexplained low serum albumin levels have been observed in cases of hepatic *C. carinii* involvement *(134,136)*.

Agarwal et al. *(137)* reported an isolated *P. carinii* infection of bilateral adrenal glands in a non-immunocompromised adult patient leading to fatal Addison's disease.

6. *P. CARINII* PNEUMONIA SECONDARY TO METHOTREXATE-TREATED RHEUMATOID ARTHRITIS

Low-dose methotrexate has become an important treatment for rheumatoid and psoriatic arthritis *(138)*. In 1983, Perruquet et al. *(139)* described the first case of *P. carinii* pneumonia in the setting of a low-dose weekly methotrexate therapy of rheumatoid arthritis. Although other corroborating reports followed *(138,140–145)*, the exact pathophysiologic mechanism of this complication is still not known. Subsequently, Wallis et al. *(146)* diagnosed *P. carinii* pneumonia complicating low-dose methotrexate treatment of psoriatic arthropathy.

Kane et al. *(142)* reported a case of pneumocystic pneumonia associated with weekly parenteral methotrexate therapy (20 mg for 20 wk for a total of 500 mg). The patient, who was HIV-negative, had a very low $CD4^+$ count due to stage III squamous cell carcinoma of the larynx. Based on these and other studies *(139,143,144,146,147)*, it has been suggested that in patients with rheumatoid and psoriatic arthritis who receive low-dose (7.5–22.5 mg) weekly methotrexate medication, the possibility of developing PCP exists only when the total dose exceeds 400 mg *(142)*.

The first report of pneumocystic pneumonia secondary to cyclosporin A and methotrexate treatment of rheumatoid arthritis appeared in 1992 *(148)*. Earlier *(149)*, it was suggested that in patients with chronic plaque psoriasis, some cyclosporin A metabolites may be synergistic to the side effects of the parent drug, and in patients with methotrexate-associated impairment of liver functions *(150,151)*, treatment with cyclosporin A would likely increase the likelihood of toxicity. However, the latter, although important in some patients, had not been necessarily the case in patients with no prior methotrexate-induced liver abnormalities *(148)*.

Apparently, methotrexate has the potential to parley more immunosuppressive activity than currently assumed, including effects on certain T lymphocyte subsets, which may result in alterations of immune responses and increased susceptibility to opportunistic pathogens. Thus, Calabrese et al. *(152)* examined peripheral lymphocyte subsets in 15 patients with active rheumatoid arthritis who were not receiving remittive therapy, as well as in 33 controls. The results demonstrated that patients with rheumatoid arthritis not only had a reduced percentage and number of $CD4^+/CD45RA$ naive T lymphocytes, but also a reduced percentage and number of $CD8^+$ cells coexpressing the CD1 1b

Table 1
Drug Therapies for *P. carinii* Infections

Drug	Dose (daily)	Route of administration
Trimethoprim-Sulfamethoxazole	TMP: 15–20 mg/kg SMX: 100 mg/kg	Intravenous or oral (divided into 3-4 doses)
Pentamidine isethionate	3.0–4.0 mg/kg 600 mg	Intravenously[a] or aerosol
Atovaquone	750 mg, t.i.d.	Oral
Dapsone-Trimethoprim[b]	Dapsone: 100 mg TMP: 15–20 mg/kg	Oral (TMP divided into 3–4 doses)
Clindamycin-Primaquine[b]	Clindamycin: 600 mg, t.i.d. Primaquine: 30 mg (as base)	Oral
Trimetrexate-Leucovorin	Trimetrexate: 45 mg/m² Leucovorin: 80 mg/m²	Intravenous

[a]Intramuscular administration may be painful and associated with sterile abscess formation. Higher total doses of parenteral pentamidine may lead to hypoglycemia *(178)*.
[b]Recommended for patients intolerant to TMP-SMX.

marker (suppressor/effector cells). Remarkably, the total number of $CD8^+$ T lymphocytes was significantly lower in patients with rheumatoid arthritis treated for 8 wk with methotrexate than in untreated patients ($p < 0.05$). In another study, Houtman et al. *(153)* determined the T-lymphocyte subsets in a patient with rheumatoid arthritis who developed *P. carinii* pneumonia while receiving treatment with low-dose methotrexate (7.5–15 mg weekly) in addition to D-penicillamine (750 mg daily for persistent high disease activity) and indomethacin (150 mg daily). While the percentage of total T cells ($CD3^+$) and T helper/inducer cells ($CD4^+$) did not differ from those of healthy controls, the number and percentage of naive T lymphocytes ($CD4^+$ cells coexpressing CD45RA) and suppressor/effector T cells ($CD8^+$ coexpressing CD1 1b), were clearly decreased as compared to controls (45 and 17/mm³, respectively, compared to 483 and 214/mm³, respectively, in normal controls). In addition, a significant decrease of the $CD8^+$ subset titer was also observed (95 cells/mm³ vs 524 cells/mm³ in normal controls) *(153)*.

Sohen et al. *(154)* also noted a decreased percentage of $CD8^+/CD45RA$ cells in the peripheral blood of patients with rheumatoid arthritis, even more pronounced in the synovial fluid.

The aforementioned findings have been corroborated in a mouse model where low-dose methotrexate treatment selectively inhibited $Lyt-2^+$ cells in graft-vs-host reactions *(155)*.

7. EVOLUTION OF THERAPIES AND TREATMENT OF *P. CARINII* PNEUMONIA

In spite of the wide use of various antiretroviral agents *(156)* and PCP prophylaxis *(157–159)*, *P. carinii* pneumonia still remains an important opportunistic infection in HIV-positive patients *(160)* as well as in other immunocompromised populations *(16)*. It is often characterized with high morbidity and mortality rates, especially in patients with rapidly progressive respiratory failure *(161–163)*. *P. carinii* organisms have been shown to persist throughout therapy for pneumocystic pneumonia.

Trimethoprim-sulfamethoxazole (TMP-SMX) and parenteral pentamidine isethionate have been the two drugs considered to be most important for the therapy and prophylaxis of *P. carinii* infections in both AIDS and non-AIDS patients (Table 1) *(53,54,164–166)*. Even though TMP-SMX is associated with side effects in a remarkably high number of AIDS patients (60–100%), the observed toxicity is often not severe, allowing for the drug therapy to be continued *(53,165,167–171)*. Hughes et al. *(172,173)* and others *(174–177)* have found that TMP-SMX was also effective against pneumocystic pneumonia in immunocompromised children.

Trimethoprim (TMP), an inhibitor of dihydrofolate reductase, and sulfamethoxazole (SMX), an inhibitor of dihydropteroate synthetase, are administered concurrently either intravenously or orally at daily total doses of 20 mg/kg of TMP and 100 mg/kg of SMX divided in three or four doses. Intravenous administration is preferable as initial treatment of more severe cases of pneumonitis, but oral therapy is feasible after several days as well as in mild cases where there is no gastrointestinal dysfunction to interfere with drug absorption *(169,170,179)*. The adverse effect may be less severe or less frequent when dosage is decreased to 15 mg/kg of TMP and 75 mg/kg of SMX without reducing efficacy *(169)*.

Based on the initial classification of *P. carinii* as a protozoan, pentamidine, an established antitrypanosomal and antileishmanial agent, was the first successful drug used to treat pneumocystic pneumonia *(180)*. It can be safely administered by slow intravenous infusion over 60 min *(181,182)*. Aerosolized pentamidine has been another route of administration that is better tolerated than TMP-SMX but may not be as effective as parenteral treatment in cases of extensive airspace consolidation *(183,184)*. Intramuscular injection, which is painful and may cause sterile abscess formation, is not usually necessary and should be avoided *(8,185)*. The recommended total daily dose of pentamidine is 4.0 mg/kg, given once daily. However, in patients with mild pneumocystic pneumonia, doses of 3.0 mg/kg could be equally effective and less toxic *(182)*.

Aerosolized pentamidine seems to be effective in cases of mild cases of pneumocystic pneumonia because of reduced toxicity compared to parenteral administration *(8)*. However, there has been considerable difference in the recommended total daily dose regimens: 4.0 mg/kg in one report *(182)*, and 600 mg daily in another *(186)*. The response rates to these two regimens were also different: 70% (9 of 13 patients) and 87% (13 of 15 patients) for the 4.0-mg/kg and 600-mg daily regimens, respectively. Furthermore, there were three relapses for the 4.0-mg/kg dose, and none for the 600-mg daily dose. In terms of toxicity, with the exception of bronchospasm (especially in smokers), the aerosolized pentamidine seemed to be devoid of adverse side effects usually associated with parenteral pentamidine therapy *(8)*.

The mode of pentamidine delivery appears to be critically important for therapeutic efficacy because nebulizers that did not produce droplet particles of 2–3 µm in size were unable to deliver adequate drug concentrations to the pulmonary parenchyma *(187)*. Furthermore, the optimal pentamidine dose may also vary with the nebulizer *(136)*. Finally, there have been concerns that aerosolization may increase the incidence of atypical pulmonary disease *(83)* due to *P. carinii* or extrapulmonary pneumocytosis *(169,188)*. Yamamoto et al. *(189)* evaluated in vivo the elimination of aerosolized pentamidine from the bronchial airways following inhalation of 300 mg of the drug. After reaching maximal level on the first day (12 h after inhalation), the pentamidine levels decreased rapidly from the bronchial wall within the first week.

With the exception of one report *(103)*, all other cases of *P. carinii*-induced choroiditis *(112–117)* have developed in the setting of aerosolized pentamidine prophylaxis following PCP. The recommended treatment of pneumocystic choroiditis consisted of intravenous administration of trimethoprim (20 mg/kg daily) together with either SMX (100 mg/kg daily) or pentamidine (4.0 mg/kg daily) *(114,115)*. In most cases, the choroidal lesions gradually decreased in size.

The clinical efficacies and safety of TMP-SMX and pentamidine have been compared in a large prospective, randomized trial in AIDS patients *(190)*. Daily doses of TMP-SMX (20 mg/kg of TMP and 100 mg/kg of SMX) and pentamidine (4.0 mg/kg) were administered intravenously for 3 wk. Failure to complete therapy was common, and survival rates were similar in both groups.

Lentino and Brooks *(191)* described a rare case of HIV-seronegative patient with tuberculosis who developed pneumocystic pneumonia but with no evidence of idiopathic $CD4^+$ T lymphopenia syndrome. The latter immune disorder has been identified in several other patients, which in the absence of HIV infection had developed PCP as a consequence of their lymphopenia *(192–195)*. The patient was successfully treated with TMP-SMX (320 mg and 1,600 mg, respectively, intravenously every 6 h) concurrently with antituberculosis therapy, and remained well 10 yr after the initial presentation with pneumocystic pneumonia *(191)*.

Although extrapulmonary pneumocystosis has been reported in a number of tissues (most often in patients receiving aerosolized pentamidine prophylaxis), Jayes et al. *(196)* reported a unique case of disseminated pneumocystosis presenting as a pleural effusion without apparent lung involvement. The patient was successfully treated with a combination therapy consisting of chest tube drainage, intravenous (4.0 mg/kg daily) and inhaled (600 mg daily) pentamidine, dapsone (100 mg daily, orally), and trimethoprim. The addition of inhaled pentamidine to intravenously administered pentamidine may have increased the pleural fluid levels substantially by transfer across the inflamed pleural membrane, or through air leak of the hydropneumothorax, thus coinciding with the patient's improvement *(196)*.

Price et al. *(197)* observed a dramatic response within 48 h (resolution of X-ray changes and improvement in gas exchange) in an AIDS patient given combined therapy of clarithromycin (500 mg, b.i.d.) and high-dose co-trimoxazole; initial treatment for 2 wk with oxygen, intravenous cotrimoxazole, and steroids provided little objective clinical improvement.

Atovaquone has been approved by the U.S. Food and Drug Administration (FDS) as a second-line therapeutic for use in the treatment of mild to moderate pneumocystic pneumonia in patients intolerant to TMP-SMX *(198)*. An open-label dose-escalation Phase I/II study has confirmed that atovaquone is effective in treating mild to moderate PCP in AIDS patients *(199)*. After a 2-wk therapy, improvement was observed in 85% of patients, and in 79% of them the treatment was considered a success, as defined by successful completion of therapy, improvements in all abnormal signs and symptoms, and no requirement for anti-PCP agent other than atovaquone.

In a multicenter, randomized, double-blind study of 408 AIDS patients lasting for 3 wk, the activity of atovaquone was compared with that of TMP-SMX *(200)*. The patients received either 750 mg of oral atovaquone or oral TMP-SMX (320 mg and 1600 mg, respectively; two double-strength tablets, t.i.d.) The rates of therapeutic success did not differ substantially between the two drug regimens (62 and 64% for atovaquone and TMP-SMX, respectively); the corresponding failure rates were 20 and 7%, respectively ($p = 0.002$). It is important to note that the therapeutic efficacy of atovaquone was closely related to its steady-state concentrations: 97% success rate in patients with plasma concentrations of over 15 μg/mL, and 88% in those with drug levels exceeding 10 μg/mL, as compared with only 65% success rate in patients with drug plasma concentrations of less than 15 μg/mL, and 50% in those with less than 10 μg/mL. It should be emphasized that the best way to achieve maximum bioavailability of atovaquone is to administer the drug with food and in the absence of underlying conditions (diarrhea) that may undermine its absorption. The most common side effects seen with atovaquone include rash, nausea, and diarrhea. Although atovaquone was less effective than TMP-SMX, it has been associated with fewer treatment-limiting adverse effects *(200)*.

The therapeutic efficacies of oral atovaquone (750 mg, t.i.d.) and intravenous pentamidine (3.0–4.0 mg/kg, once daily) were compared in a 3-wk multicenter, randomized, open-label trial involving a small number of AIDS patients with mild to moderate pneumocystic pneumonia *(201)*. The results have shown that the therapeutic efficacies of the two drugs were similar, but atovaquone elicited significantly fewer treatment-limiting adverse side effects. Nevertheless, some investigators *(202)* strongly disagreed with the conclusion that both drugs are comparable, because of the relatively small number of patients involved and because of perceived flaws in determining the failure rate of atovaquone treatment.

In addition to atovaquone and pentamidine, other alternative therapies to treat pneumocystic pneumonia in patients with history of intolerance to TMP-SMX, included trimethoprim-dapsone, clindamycin-primaquine, and rechallenge or disensitization (or both) with TMP-SMX *(203,204)*.

Trimethoprim combined with dapsone (an inhibitor of dihydropteroate synthetase) was also found to be effective as conventional therapy of AIDS patients with mild to moderate *P. carinii* pneumonia *(166,205)*. The enzyme dihydropteroate synthetase has been specifically associated with the *Pneumocystis* organism by blocking the incorporation of *p*-aminobenzoic acid during the first step of the folate biosynthesis *(206,207)*. Although at doses of 25 and 125 mg/kg dapsone showed total efficacy in eradicating extensive pneumonitis in a rat model of pneumocystosis *(208)*, it was ineffective in treating pneumocystic pneumonia in AIDS patients when administered alone *(209)*. However, there has been an excellent clinical response rate of 100% when it was combined with trimethoprim *(166)*.

In a more recent double-blind, randomized study *(210)*, a combination of dapsone (100 mg daily) and trimethoprim (20 mg/kg daily), although as effective as daily administration of TMP(20 mg/kg)-SMX(100 mg/kg) in treating mild to moderate first episodes of PCP, was much better tolerated. Nonetheless, dapsone-associated methemoglobulinemia has been observed in most patients *(210)*.

The anti-pneumocystic clinical efficacy and the response rate of clindamycin in combination with primaquine in both initial and salvage therapy of PCP have been excellent (78–93%) *(211–214)*. Adverse side effects associated with clindamycin-primaquine therapy included bone-marrow depression, maculopapular rashes, increased liver-enzyme levels (serum aspartate transaminase, alanine transaminase, alkaline phosphatase, bilirubin), gastrointestinal disorders, and methemoglobulinemia (usually at daily doses of 30 mg) *(215–217)*. The most serious toxicity of primaquine has been associated with intravascular hemolytic anemia in patients with glucose-6-phosphate dehydrogenase deficiency; it was observed at daily doses of ≥15 mg (primaquine base) *(216)* The side effects of clindamycin were usually associated with diarrhea *(218)*.

In a randomized, double-blind, pilot trial, Toma et al. *(219)* evaluated the toxicity and tolerability of clindamycin-primaquine combination vs TMP-SMX as primary therapy for pneumocystic pneumonia in AIDS patients. Because of the small number of patients (65) studied, the clinical efficacy was not the primary focus of the trial. No significant diferrences were documented in the outcome, duration of survival, length of the PCP-free interval, and the relapse rate. The overall toxicity of the clindamycin-primaquine combination was less than that of TMP-SMX *(219)*.

Noskin et al. *(220)* did a retrospective review of 26 patients who received clindamycin-primaquine therapy for PCP after a conventional treatment had failed or was not tolerated; clindamycin (800 mg every 8 h) was administered intravenously after which oral primaquine (30 mg) was instituted on alternate days. The success rate was 86%, with erythematous rash being the most common adverse effect.

The combination of pyrimethamine and sulfadiazine has also been used in the therapy of PCP based on previously observed activity in a rat model *(221)*. The response was, however, not encouraging with only 31% of treated patients surviving *(222–227)*.

Trimetrexate, one of several inhibitors of *P. carinii* dihydrofolate reductase *(206,228,229)*, elicited a 63–71% response with or without sulfadiazine as initial or salvage therapy in AIDS patients with pneumocystic pneumonia *(230)*. Because of its ability to enter and harm host cells, trimetrexate needs to be administered with calcium leucovorin. The latter, being a reduced folate, is taken preferentially by the host cells, thereby countering the effect of trimetrexate *(8)*. The preferred therapeutic daily regimen of trimetrexate currently under investigation is 30–45 mg/m^3 administered intravenously as a single dose for up to 21 d *(231)*. There has been no specific direction for the dosing of leucovorin, but current protocols recommend 30 mg/m^3 i.v. or orally for 24 d when patients are receiving trimetrexate for 21 d. According to Sattler et al. *(232)* a 45-mg/m^2 daily dose of trimetrexate with 80 mg/m^2 daily of leucovorin resulted in the least dosage-modifying toxicity and excellent efficacy.

Among the side effects of trimetrexate, transient neutropenia or thrombocytopenia, and mild elevation of serum aminotransferase levels have been observed in approx 25% of patients. When used alone as initial therapy for PCP, trimetrexate was associated with high relapse rate (60%) *(8)*. During Phase II trials in cancer patients, Grem et al. *(233)* observed hypersensitivity reactions to trimetrexate. Immediate hypotension with loss of consciousness had occurred in only one patient, whereas immediate systemic effects (facial flushing, fever, shaking, pruritis, bronchospasm, periorbital edema, and difficulty in swallowing) were more common.

α-Difluoromethylornithine (DFMO, eflornithine), a specific inhibitor of ornithine decarboxylase, was found to be moderately effective as salvage therapy against pneumocystic pneumonia in several studies of AIDS patients *(234–237)*. In a compassionate treatment of AIDS patients who were intolerant to and/or unresponsive to conventional TMP-SMX or pentamidine therapy *(238)*, a full course of treatment consisted of daily intravenous administration of 400 mg/kg of eflornithine (but no more than 30 g daily) in four divided doses for 10 d, followed by 4 d of oral administration at 300 mg/kg daily (in four divided doses), and then up to 6 wk at 300 mg/kg daily in four divided oral doses where tolerated. Of the 33 patient-episodes, 15 patients were discharged without need of supplemental oxygen after receiving 10 or more d of parenteral therapy. The most serious side effects of eflornithine were leukopenia, thrombocytopenia (in 12 of 19 patients), as well as anorexia, nausea, and diarrhea *(166,238)*.

In a prospective, open-label trial, co-trimoxazole (3.84 g intravenously, b.i.d.) and eflornithine (400 mg/kg daily as a continuous intravenous infusion) were compared as primary treatment for first-episode PCP in AIDS patients *(239)*. Only 39% of patients treated with eflornithine and 40% of those receiving co-trimoxazole successfully completed therapy; overall, eflornithine was the less effective of the two drugs.

7.1. Adjunctive Corticosteroid Therapy for P. carinii Pneumonia

Even though the exact mechanism of the potential therapeutic effect of corticosteroids has not been elucidated *(240)*, data from various case reports, small series, and several randomized trials *(241–257)* have indicated beneficial effects (lower number of respiratory failures and mortality rates *[242,251–253]*) after using corticosteroids as adjunctive therapy for pneumocystic pneumonia in AIDS patients with moderate to severe pulmonary dysfunctions (initial arterial oxygen partial pressure of less than 70 mm Hg, or an alveolar-arterial gradient greater than 35 mm Hg on room air). Thus, in a prospective, double-blind, placebo-controlled trial in AIDS patients with first episode of mild PCP, Montaner et al. *(258)* assessed the effect of oral prednisone given at 60 mg/kg daily dose for 1 wk, followed by a progressive tapering over 14 d. The oral corticosteroid therapy prevented early deterioration and increased the exercise tolerance of the patients as defined by pulse oximetry.

Studies on the pathogenesis of PCP have suggested the presence of an intense inflammatory component in the disease *(259)*, which may be reduced by the modulatory effects of corticosteroids. The mechanism by which corticosteroids improve the outcome of AIDS patients with severe PCP is still not elucidated. To this end, Huang and Eden *(260)* found that lipopolysaccharide-stimulated alveolar macrophages from patients receiving corticosteroids released significantly less interleukin-1β (IL-1β) and tumor-necrosis factor-α (TNF-α) than alveolar macrophages from nontreated AIDS patients.

A consensus report *(261)* has been isssued backing the use of corticosteroids as adjunctive therapy to pneumocystic pneumonia. However, this recommendation has not been universally accepted and doubts still persist whether adjunctive corticosteroid therapy should be applied to all patients *(262–264)*. The expressed reluctance to use adjunctive corticosteroid therapy has arisen from findings indicating that the known immunosuppressive properties of corticosteroids (reducing the T lymphocyte population by cytokine suppression) have the potential to cause more harm than benefit in already immunocompromised patients, thereby becoming risk factors for pneumocystis pneumonia *(265–267)*, other opportunistic pathogens *(262–264)*, and infections *(242)*. Theoretically, steroids could exacerbate non-PCP pulmonary infections, so it is important to confirm the diagnosis if they are to be used *(268)*. For example, with the increased incidence of multidrug-resistant tuberculosis in HIV-infected patients *(269)*, the empiric use of corticosteroids for undifferentiated pulmonary disease may eventually mask and delay treatment of pulmonary disorders caused by other pathogens, thereby increasing the risk to patients. In addition, corticosteroids have been known to cause malignancies *(270,271)*, as well as to precipitate PCP in animal models *(272–274)*. Additional side effects of corticosteroids include gastrointestinal hemorrhages, hyperglycemia, and neuropsychiatric abnormalities *(268)*.

Walmsley et al. *(268)* presented results from a multicenter, randomized, double-blind, and placebo-controlled trial of AIDS patients with pneumocystic pneumonia that contradicted the aforementioned consensus report *(261)*. The results of this study indicated that corticosteroids (40 mg of parenteral methylprednisolone, b.i.d.) when used as an adjunctive therapy, did not significantly affect the outcome of pneumocystic pneumonia in HIV-positive patients, although they might have lowered the incidence of hypersensitivity reactions (fever and rash) that eventually would require discontinuation of TMP-SMX therapy.

In the majority of studies in which beneficial effects (prevention of death and respiratory failure) have been demonstrated, adjunctive corticosteroid therapy was evaluated in the early treatment of moderate to severe cases of pneumocystic pneumonia *(242,275,276)*. The one study that evaluated the late application of corticosteroids failed to demonstrate meaningful benefit *(277)*. After re-examination of the data obtained in the study by Welmsley et al. *(268)*, Bozzette and Morton *(278)* concluded that although the suggested therapy may have narrowed the scope of potential benefits from early adjunctive corticosteroid treatment in acute pneumocystic pneumonia, it did not provide convincing new evidence suggesting harm from corticosteroids.

In addition to different dose regimens, duration, and timing of corticosteroid therapy, other factors, such as the differences in study populations, entry criteria applied, protocol procedures (blinded vs unblinded *[242,276]*), and the medical care of patients at different hospitals and at different times *(279,280)*, may have influenced the effectiveness of the corticosteroids, thereby explaining the differences in clinical outcome. Furthermore, as demonstrated by univariate and multivariate analyses, specific characteristics of patients may be important in determining the response of PCP to antimicrobial therapy *(268)*.

Infants with congenitally acquired HIV infection who presented with acute respiratory failure (ARF) secondary to pneumocystic pneumonia were reported to have high morbidity and mortality rates (50–90%) *(281–284)*. At present, there is no consensus regarding the use of corticosteroids in infants with pneumocystic pneumonia *(261)*. In two studies by Sleasman et al. *(285)* and Barone et al. *(286)*, the use of early adjunctive corticosteroid therapy did reduce the morbidity and mortality in HIV-infected infants with PCP and ARF. In the study by Barone et al. *(286)*, the four infants (CD4$^+$ counts ranging from 148 cells/mm^3 to 918 cells/mm^3) started to receive adjunctive methylprednisolone therapy (2 mg/kg daily, divided into four doses) immediately after the diagnosis of PCP was confirmed *(286)*. Three of the infants who completed a 21-d course of TMP-SMX, received high-dose corticosteroid for 5 d; the dosage was then tapered over the next 3 wk. The fourth child's treatment was switched to pentamidine (4.0 mg/kg daily) after 9 d because of the clinical failure of treatment with TMP-SMX; the severely ill infant received high-dose corticosteroid for 10 d, followed by a tapered dose over the next 3 wk. No apparent side effects of corticosteroid therapy (gastrointestinal hemorrhage, hyperglycemia) was observed in any of these patients, and all infants from both studies *(285,286)* survived.

7.2. Toxicity of Sulfonamides

It is thought that approx 3% of the general population and 60% of HIV-infected patients will have adverse reactions when treated with sulfonamide antimicrobials such as sulfamethoxazole *(287)*. The most common clinical manifestations of sulfonamide hypersensitivity are fever and a maculopapular rash 7–14 d after intiation of therapy, although various more severe manifestations may also occur. If sulfonamide hypersensitivity is suspected, desensitization protocols are available for use in HIV-infected patients when PCP treatment and prophylaxis is indicated *(287)*.

with acquired immunodeficiency syndrome and acquired immunodeficiency syndrome-related complex. *Pediatrics*, 82, 223, 1988.
285. Sleasman, J. W., Hemenway, C., Klein, A. S., and Barrett, D. J. Corticosteroids improve survival of children with AIDS and *Pneumocystis carinii* pneumonia. *Am. J. Dis. Child.*, 147, 30, 1993.
286. Barone, S. R., Aiuto, L. T., and Krilov, L. R. Increased survival of young infants with *Pneumocystis carinii* pneumonia and acute respiratory failure with early steroid administration. *Clin. Infect. Dis.*, 19, 212, 1994.
287. Tilles, S. A. Practical issues in the management of hypersensitivity reactions: sulfonamides. *South. Med. J.*, 94, 817–824, 2001.
288. Waskin, H., Stehr-Green, J. K., Helmick, C. G., and Sattler, F. R. Risk factors for hypoglycemia associated with pentamidine therapy for *Pneumocystis* pneumonia. *J. Am. Med. Assoc.*, 260, 345, 1988.
289. McSharry, R. J., Kirsch, C. M., Jensen, W. A., and Kagawa, F. T. Prophylaxis of aerosolized pentamidine-induced bronchospasm: a symptom-based approach. *Am. J. Med. Sci.*, 306, 20, 1993.
290. Renzi, P. M., Corbeil, C., Chasse, M., Braidy, J., and Matar, N. Bilateral pneumothoraces hasten mortality in AIDS patients receiving secondary prophylaxis with aerosolized pentamidine: association with a lower Dco prior to receiving aerosolized pentamidine. *Chest*, 102, 491, 1992.
291. Comtois, R., Pouliot, J., Gervais, A., Vinet, B., and Lemieux, C. High pentamidine levels associated with hypoglycemia and azotemia in a patient with *Pneumocystis carinii* pneumonia. *Diagn. Microbiol. Infect. Dis.*, 15, 523, 1992.
292. Comtois, R., Pouliot, J., Vinet, B., Gervais, A., and Lemieux, C. Higher pentamidine levels in AIDS patients with hypoglycemia and azotemia during treatment of *Pneumocystis carinii* pneumonia. *Am. Rev. Respir. Dis.*, 146, 740, 1992.
293. Jones, R. S. Jr., Collier-Brown, C., and Suh, B. Localized cutaneous reaction to intravenous pentamidine. *Clin. Infect. Dis.*, 15, 561, 1992.
294. Klatt, E. C. Pathology of pentamidine-induced pancreatitis. *Arch. Pathol. Lab. Med.*, 116, 162, 1992.
295. Pouwels, A., Eliaszewicz, M., Larrey, D., et al. Pentamidine-induced acute pancreatitis in a patient with AIDS. *J. Clin. Gastroenterol.*, 12, 457, 1990.
296. Murphy, R. L., Noskin, G. A., and Ehrenpreis, E. D. Acute pancreatitis associated with aerosolized pentamidine. *Am. J. Med.*, 88(5N), 53N, 1990.
297. Balslev, U., Berild, D., and Nielsen, T. L., Cardiac arrest during treatment of *Pneumocystis carinii* pneumonia with intravenous pentamidine isethionate. *Scand. J. Infect. Dis.*, 24, 111, 1992.
298. Quadrel, M. A., Atkin, S. H., and Jaker, M. A. Delayed cardiotoxicity during treatment with intravenous pentamidine: two case reports and a review of the literature. *Am. Heart J.*, 123, 1377, 1992.
299. Balslev, U. and Nielsen, T. L. Adverse effects associated with intravenous pentamidine isethionate as treatment of *Pneumocystis carinii* pneumonia. *Dan. Med. Bull.*, 39, 366, 1992.
300. Mani, S., Kocheril, A. G., and Andriole, V. T. Case report: pentamidine and polymorphic ventricular tachycardia revisited. *Am. J. Med. Sci.*, 305, 236, 1993.
301. Cortese, L. M., Gasser, R. A. Jr., Bjornson, D. C., Dacey, M. J., and Oster, C. N. Prolonged recurrence of pentamidine-induced torsades de pointes. *Ann. Pharmacother.*, 26, 1365, 1992.
302. Warton, J. M., Demopulos, P. A., and Goldshlager, N. Torsades de pointes during administration of pentamidine isethionate. *Am. J. Med.*, 83, 571, 1987
303. Harel, Y., Scott, W. A., Szeinberg, A., and Barzilay, Z. Pentamidine-induced torsades de pointes. *Pediatr. Infect. Dis. J.*, 12, 692, 1993.
304. Green, P. T., Reents, S., Harman, F., and Curtis, A. B. Pentamidine-induced torsades de pointes in a renal transplant recipient with *Pneumocystis carinii* pneumonia. *South. Med. J.*, 83, 481, 1990.
305. Mitchell, P., Dodek, P., Lawson, L., Kiess, M., and Russell, J. Torsades de pointes during intravenous pentamidine isethionate therapy. *Can. Med. Assoc. J.*, 140, 173, 1989.
306. Hancock, E. W. Possible torsade in a patient with AIDS. *Hosp. Pract.*, 25, 132, 1990.
307. Engrav, M. B., Coodley, G., and Magnusson, A. R. Torsades de pointes after inhaled pentamidine. *Ann. Emerg. Med.*, 21, 1404, 1992.
308. Vukmir, R. B. Torsades de pointes: a review. *Am. J. Emerg. Med.*, 9, 250, 1991.
309. Stein, K. M., Haronian, H., Mensah, G. A., Acosta, A., Jacobs, J., and Kligfield, P. Ventricular tachycardia and torsades de pointes complicating pentamidine therapy of *Pneumocystis carinii* pneumonia in the acquired immunodeficiency syndrome. *Am. J. Cardiol.*, 66, 888, 1990.
310. Miller, H. C. Cardiac arrest after intravenous pentamidine in an infant. *Pediatr. Infect. Dis. J.*, 12, 694, 1993.
311. Tzivoni, D., Keren, A., Cohen, A. M., et al. Magnesium therapy for torsades de pointes. *Am. J. Cardiol.*, 53, 528, 1984.
312. Sasyniuk, B. I., Valois, M., and Toy, W. Recent advances in understanding the mechanisms of drug-induced torsades de pointes arrhythmias. *Am. J. Cardiol.*, 64, 29J, 1989.
313. Pais, J. R., Cazorla, C., Novo, E., and Viana, A. Massive haemorrhage from rupture of a pancreatic pseudocyst after pentamidine-associated pancreatitis. *Eur. J. Med.*, 1, 251, 1992.
314. Mandrell, B. N. and McCormick, J. N. Dapsone-induced methemoglobinemia in pediatric oncology patients: case examples. *J. Pediatr. Oncol. Nurs.*, 18, 224–228, 2001.
315. DeGowin, R. L., Eppes, B., Powell, R. D., and Carson, P. E. The haemolytic effects of diphenylsulfone (DDS) in normal subjects and in those with glucose-6-phosphate- dehydrogenase deficiency. *Bull. WHO*, 35, 165, 1966.
316. Metroka, C. E., Lewis, N. J., and Jacobus, D. P. Desensitization to dapsone in HIV-positive patients. *J. Am. Med. Assoc.*, 267, 512, 1992.
317. Freund, Y. R., Dousman, L., Riccio, E. S., Sato, B., MacGregor, J. T., and Mohagheghpour, N. Immunohematotoxicity studies with combinations of dapsone. *Int. Immunopharmacol.*, 1, 2131–2141, 2001.

318. Kluge, R. M., Spaulding, D. M., and Spain, A. J. Combination of pentamidine and trimethoprim-sulfamethoxazole in the therapy of *Pneumocystis carinii* pneumonia in rats. *Antimicrob. Agents Chemother.*, 13, 975, 1978.
319. Hughes, W. T., McNabb, P. C., Makres, T. D., and Feldman, S. Efficacy of trimethoprim and sulfamethoxazole in the prevention and treatment of *Pneumocystis carinii* pneumonitis. *Antimicrob. Agents Chemother.*, 5, 289, 1974.
320. Hughes, W. T. and Smith, B. L. Efficacy of diaminodiphenylsulfone and other drugs in murine *Pneumocystis carinii* pneumonitis. *Antimicrob. Agents Chemother.*, 26, 436, 1984.
321. Frenkel, J. K., Good, J. T., and Shultz, J. A. Latent *Pneumocystis* infection of rats, relapse and chemotherapy. *Lab. Invest.*, 15, 1559, 1966.
322. Queener, S. F., Bartlett, M. S., Durkin, M. M., Jay, M. A., and Smith, J. W. Activity of clindamycin with primaquine toward *Pneumocystis carinii* in vitro and in vivo. *Proc. 27th Intersci. Conf. Antimicrob. Agents Chemother.*, American Society for Microbiology, Washington, DC, abstract 574, 1987.
323. Hughes, W. T. and Killmar, J. T. Synergistic anti-*Pneumocystis carinii* effects of erythromycin and sulfisoxazole. *J. Acquir. Immune Defic. Syndr.*, 4, 523, 1991.
324. Walzer, P. D., Foy, J., Steele, P., and White, M. Synergistic combinations of Ro 11-8958 and other dihydrofolate reductase inhibitors with sulfamethoxazole and dapsone for therapy of experimental pneumocystosis. *Antimicrob. Agents Chemother.*, 37, 1436, 1993.
325. U.S. Public Health Service Task Force on anti-pneumocystis prophylaxis in patients with human immunodeficiency virus infection: recommendation for prophylaxis against *Pneumocystis carinii* pneumonia for persons infected with human immunodeficiency virus. *J. Acquir. Immune Defic. Syndr.*, 6, 46, 1993.
326. Hardy, W. D., Feinberg, J., Finkelstein, D. M., et al. A controlled trial of trimethoprim-sulfamethoxazole or aerosolized pentamidine for secondary prophylaxis of *Pneumocystis carinii* pneumonia in patients with acquired immunodeficiency syndrome (AIDS clinical trial group protocol 021). *N. Engl. J. Med.*, 327, 1842, 1992.
327. Arico, M., Molinari, E., Bacchella, L., DeAmici, M., Raiteri, E., and Burgio, G. R. Prospective randomized comparison of toxicity of two prophylactic regimens of cotrimoxazole in leukemic children. *Pediatr. Hematol. Oncol.*, 9, 35, 1992.
328. Badri, M., Ehrlich, R., Wood, R., and Maartens, G. Initiating co-trimoxazole prophylaxis in HIV-infected patients in Africa: an evaluation of the provisional WHO/UNAIDS recommendation. *AIDS*, 15, 1143–1148, 2001.
329. Stearn, B. F. and Polis, M. A. Prophylaxis of opportunistic infections in persons with HIV infection. *Cleve. Clin. J. Med.*, 61, 187, 1994.
330. Nielsen, T. L., Jensen, B. N., Nelsing, S., et al. Prevention of *Pneumocystis carinii* pneumonia relapse in AIDS patients: the efficacy and tolerability of low-dose sulfamethoxazole-trimethoprim. *Dan. Med. Bull.*, 40, 503, 1993.
331. Smulders, Y. M., Spoelstra-de Man, A. M., Slaats, E. H., Weigel, H. M., Stehouwer, C. D., and Jos Frissen P. H. Trimethoprim-sulphamethoxazole as primary *Pneumocystis carinii* prophylaxis does not increase serum homocysteine levels in HIV-positive subjects. *Eur. J. Intern. Med.*, 12, 363–365, 2001.
332. Gifford, A. L., McPhee, S. J., and Fordham, D. Preventive care among HIV-positive patients in a general medicine practice. *Am. J. Prev. Med.*, 10, 5, 1994.
333. Longini, I. M. Jr., Clark, W. S., and Karon, J. M. Effect of routine use of therapy in slowing the clinical course of human immunodeficiency virus (HIV) infection in a population-based cohort. *Am. J. Epidemiol.*, 137, 1229, 1993.
334. Chaisson, R. E., Keruly, J., Richman, D. D., and Moore, R. D. *Pneumocystis* prophylaxis and survival in patients with advanced human immunodeficiency virus infection treated with zidovudine. *Arch. Intern. Med.*, 152, 2009, 1992.
335. Graham, N. M., Zeger, S. L., Park, L. P., et al. The effects on survival of early treatment of human immunodeficiency virus infection. *N. Engl. J. Med.*, 326, 1037, 1992.
336. Mazur, H. Prophylaxis and therapy for *Pneumocystis* pneumonia: where are we? *Infect. Agents Dis.*, 1, 270, 1992.
337. Dworkin, M. S., Williamson, J., Jones, J. L., Kaplan, J. E. Adult and Adolescent Spectrum of HIV Disease Project. *Clin. Infect. Dis.*, 33, 393–398, 2001.
338. Kovacs, J. A., Gill, V. J., Meshnick, S., and Masur, H. New insights into transmission, diagnosis, and drug treatment of *Pneumocystis carinii* pneumonia. *J. Am. Med. Assoc.*, 286, 2450–2460, 2001.
339. Trikalinos, T. A. and Ioannidis, J. P. Discontinuation of *Pneumocystis carinii* prophylaxis in patients infected with human immunodeficiency virus: a meta-analysis and decision analysis. *Clin. Infect. Dis.*, 33, 1901–1909, 2001.
340. Ivez, N. J., Gazzard, B. G., and Esterbrook, P. J. The changing pattern of AIDS-defining illnesses with the introduction of highly active antiretroviral therapy (HAART) in a London clinic. *J. Infect.*, 42, 134–139, 2001.
341. Urschel, S., Schuster, T., Dunsch, D., Wintergerst, U., Hofstetter, R., and Belohradsky, B. H. Discontinuation of primary *Pneumocystis carinii* prophylaxis after reconstitution of CD4 cell counts in HIV-infected children. *AIDS*, 15, 1589–1591, 2001.
342. Koletar, S. L., Heald, A. E., Finkelstein, D., et al. The ACTG 888 Study Team, A prospective study of discontinuing primary and secondary *Pneumocystis carinii* pneumonia prophylaxis after CD4 cell count increase to >200 × 106 /l. *AIDS*, 15, 1509–1515, 2001.
343. Le Moal, G., Breux, J. P., and Roblot, F. Discontinuing prophylaxis against *Pneumocystis carinii* pneumonia. *N. Engl. J. Med.*, 344, 1639–1641, 2001.
344. U.S. Public Health Service (USPHS) and Infectious Diseases Society of America (IDSA). 1999 USPHS/IDSA guidelines for the prevention of opportunistic infections in persons infected with human immunodeficiency virus. *Infect Dis. Obstet. Gynecol.*, 8, 5–74, 2000.
345. Furrer, H., Egger, M., Opravil, M., et al. Discontinuation of primary prophylaxis against *Pneumocystis carinii* pneumonia in HIV-1-infected adults treated with combination antiretroviral therapy. *N. Engl. J. Med.*, 340, 1301–1306, 1999.
346. Weverling, G. J., Mocroft, A., Lederberger, B., et al. Discontinuation of *Pneumocystis carinii* pneumonia prophylaxis after start of highly active antiretroviral therapy in HIV-1 infection. *Lancet*, 353, 1293–1298, 1999.

moniliforme, 349
napiforme, 352–354
nivale, 349
nygamai, 352
oxysporum, 349
poae, 349
proliferatum, 351
solani, 351
sporotrichoides, 349
treatment, 350–353

G

G-CSF. *See* Granulocyte colony-stimulating factor
GM-CSF. *See* Granulocyte-macrophage colony-stimulating factor
Ganciclovir, 5, 6, 13
  toxicity, 5
Geniculosporium spp., 323
Giardia, 143
  lamblia, 184
Globuline, cow's milk, 148
1,3-β-*D*-Glucan synthase, 444
Gordona rubropertincta, 79
  terrae, 79
Graft-vs-host disease, 362
Granulocyte colony-stimulating factor, 247, 361
Granulocyte-macrophage colony-stimulating factor, 245, 250, 351, 352
Graphium, 348

H

HAART. *See* Highly active antiretroviral therapy
Hansenula spp., 281, 303–305
  anomala, 303
  polymorpha, 303
  treatment, 303, 304
    amphotericin B, 303, 304
Hapsidospora, 354
HBC. *See* Colostrums
HCE. *See* Candidiasis, treatment
HCMV, 8–13. *See* Cytomegalovirus
  HAART effects on, 13
  immunotherapy, 13
  in AIDS patients, 8–10
  in bone marrow transplantation, 10, 11
  in solid organ transplantation, 10, 11
  prophylaxis, 11–13
  treatment, 8–11, 13

Helminthosporium, 311
Herpes simplex virus, 33–51
  drug-resistant, 40
    therapy of, 40
  treatment, 34–42
  prophylaxis, 42, 43
Herpes zoster. *See* Varicella-zoster
Herpes zoster ophthalmicus, 27
Herpesviridae, 3
Herpetic geometric glossitis, 34
Highly active antiretroviral therapy (HAART), 13, 84, 107, 150, 175, 256
Histoplasma spp., 383–408
  capsulatum, 383–396, 496
    var. *capsulatum,* 383
    var. *duboisii,* 409–412
  falciminosum, 383
Histoplasmosis, 383–396
  African. *See* African histoplasmosis
  adrenal, 394
  carpal tunnel syndrome, 392
  CNS involvement, 393, 394
  endocarditis, 392
  gastrointestinal, 390
  genitourinary, 394, 395
    prostatic, 395
  host immune defense in, 396
    macrophage blockade, 396
  hypercalcemia in, 384
  in AIDS patients, 386–389
  in childhood, 395, 396
  in transplant patients, 389
  mediastinal, 392, 393
  methotrexate effect on, 384, 385
  musculoskeletal, 394
  ocular manifestations, 391
  orofacial manifestations, 390, 391
  prophylaxis, 386
  pulmonary, 393
    pleural effusions in, 393
  rheumatic manifestations, 391, 392
  skin manifestations, 389, 390
  thyroid involvement, 394
  treatment, 383–396
    amphotericin B, 387, 389, 393–395
    fluconazole, 388, 389
    itraconazole, 387
    ketoconazole, 388
Hormonema dermatioides, 320
HPMPC. *See* Cidofovir
HSV. *See* Herpes simplex virus

HTLV-1. *See* Human T-lymphotropic virus type 1
HuGM-CSF. *See* Human granulocyte-macrophage colony-stimulating factor
Human granulocyte-macrophage colony-stimulating factor, 149
Human histocompatibility complexes (HLA antigens), 485
Human T-lymphotropic virus type 1, 196
Hyalohyphomycosis, 343–382
2-Hydroxystilbamidine, 415

I
IL-2. *See* Interleukin-2
Immune DLE, 149
Immunotherapy
   cryptosporidiosis, 148, 149
   HIV infections, 92
   MAC infections, 103
   toxoplasmosis, 175
IFN-γ. *See* Interferon-γ
Infections
   Acremonium spp., 354, 355
   Acrophialophora fusispora, 361
   bacterial, 55–139
   coccidioidal, 461–473
   cyclosporiasis
     treatment, 206, 207
   dematiaceous fungal, 307–342
   Engyodontium album, 361
   Gore-Tex mesh, 280
   emerging *Candida* spp., 269–290
   enteric, 136, 137
     therapy, 136, 137
     prevention, 137
   Fusarium spp., 349–354
   gastrointestinal, 135–139
     ethiologic pathogens, 136
   HCMV, 8–13
     HAART effects on, 13
     immunotherapy, 13
     in AIDS patients, 8–10
     in bone marrow transplantation, 10, 11
     in solid organ transplantation, 10, 11
     prophylaxis, 11–13
     treatment, 8–11, 13
   herpes simplex virus, 34–44
   fungal, 211–532
   Microascus spp., 357
   nontuberculous mycobacterial, 95–128
     in AIDS, 96

Paecilomyces spp., 358–360
parasitic, 141–208
peritonitis, fungal, 325, 326
   treatment, 325, 326
Phialemonium spp., 354, 355
Pneumocystis carinii, 508–510
   atypical, 508
   extrapulmonary, 508, 509
   secondary to methotrexate, 509, 510
   subclinical, 508
Pseudallescheria boidii, 343–347
Scedosporium spp., 347–349
Scopulariopsis spp., 355–357
varicella-zoster, 23–32
   drug-resistant, management, 27
   pneumonitis, management, 27, 28
   treatment, 25–27
     organ-transplant recipients, 26
     HIV-infected patients, 27
viral, 3–51
Interferon-γ, 213, 344, 443, 484
Interleukin-2, 149
Invasive pulmonary aspergillosis, 429, 436
IPA. *See* Invasive pulmonary aspergillosis
ISIS 2922. *See* Fomivirsen
Isoniazid, 99, 100
   toxicity, 104
Isospora spp., 159
   belli, 159
   hominis, 159
Isosporiasis, 159–162
   treatment, 160, 161
   TMP-SMX, 162
Itraconazole, 187, 215, 225, 226, 250, 312, 315, 387, 410, 419, 420, 441–443, 496
   drug interactions, 226
Ivermectin, 198

K
Ketoconazole, 222, 250, 251, 275, 314, 388, 418, 419, 441

L
LAS. *See* Lymphadenopathy syndrome
Lecythophora, 354
Leprieuria, 322
Listeria monocytogenes, 129–134
Listeriosis, 129–134
   in AIDS patients, 130, 131
   treatment, 131, 132
Lomenospora prolificans, 348

Lymphodenopathy syndrome, persistent, 149
Lymphopenia syndrome, idiopathic CD⁺ T cell, 511, 512

M
MAC, 96–107
  treatment, 97–103
    HAART effects on, 107
    immunotherapy, 103
    prophylaxis, 103–107
Mebendazole, 198
Meningitis
  candidal, 249, 254
  cryptococcal, 214–217
Metronidazole, 250
Miconazole, 221, 222, 252, 420, 439
Microascus spp., 357
  cinereus, 357
  cirrosis, 357
Microsporidia, 183–193
Microsporidiosis, 186–188
  treatment, 186–188
Microsporidium spp., 183
  africanum, 183
  ceylonensis, 183
Monosporium apiospermum, 347
Mucor, 501
Mucorales, 501
Mucormycosis. *See* Zygomycosis
Mycobacterium africanum, 91
Mycobacterium avium-intracellulare scrofulaceum complex. *See* MAC
Mycobacterium bovis, 91–94
  treatment, 92, 93
Mycobacterium celatum, 111
Mycobacterium chelone, 95
Mycobacterium fortuitum, 95, 308
Mycobacterium genavense, 114
Mycobacterium gordonae, 95
Mycobacterium haemophilium, 95, 112, 113
  treatment, 112, 113
Mycobacterium kansasii, 95, 107–110
  treatment, 108–110
Mycobacterium malmoense, 95
Mycobacterium neoaurum, 95
Mycobacterium scrofulaceum, 95
Mycobacterium szulgai, 110
Mycobacterium terrae-triviale, 95
Mycobacterium tuberculosis, 57, 81–89, 433
  in AIDS patients, 81
  drug interactions, 83
  HAART effect on, 84
  drug-resistance, 83, 84
  prophylaxis, 85
  treatment, 82, 83
    adjunctive immunotherapy, 85
    vaccine development, 85, 86
Mycobacterium xenopi, 110–112
  treatment, 111–112
Mycoderma rugosa, 277
Mycoleptodiscus indicus, 321
Muromegalovirus, 3

N
Natamycin, 353
Nippostrongylus brasiliensis, 197
Nitazoxanide, 146, 147
Necator americana, 198
Nectria, 354
Nectriella, 354
Neo-penotran, 250
Nocardia spp., 55–69
  asteroids, 55
  brasiliensis, 55
  co-infections with, 57
    Aspergillus fumigatus, 57
    Exophiala jeanselmei, 57
    Mycobacterium tuberculosis, 57
    Mycobacterium kansasii, 57
    MAC, 57
    Pneumocystis carinii, 57
    Rhodococcus equi, 57
  drug-resistance, 60
  farcinica, 56
  nova, 56
  otitidiscaviarum, 55
  transvalensis, 55
  turbata, 55
Nocardiosis. *See Nocardia* spp.
  in HIV-positive patients, 56, 57
  treatment, 57–60
    antibiotics, 59, 60
    sulfonamides, 58
    sulfonamide-trimethoprim, 58, 59
Nodulisporium spp., 323
Non-*Candida* mycoses
  after transplantation, 362–364
Nontuberculous mycobacteria, 95–128
  in AIDS patients, 96
Nosema spp., 183, 185, 187
  algerae, 185

connori, 183, 185
corneum, 183, 185
oculatum, 183
NTM. *See* Nontuberculous mycobacteria
NTZ. *See* Nitazoxanide
Nyotran. *See* Nystatin
Nystatin, 272, 310
   liposomal (nyotran), 248

O

Ochroconis gallopava, 318, 319, 323
Octeotride, 147
Oerskovia spp., 71, 72
   treatment, 71
   turbata, 71
   xanthineolytica, 71
Onychomycosis, 446
Ornidazole, 160
Orungal, 251
Otomycosis, 446, 447

P

Paecilomyces spp., 358–360
   lilacinus, 359, 360
      treatment, 359
         amphotericin B, 359
         post-transplantation therapy, 360
   javanicus, 358
   marquandii, 358
   variotii, 358
   treatment, 359
      amphotericin B, 359, 360
      post-transplantation therapy, 360
Paracoccidioides brasiliensis, 483–493
Paracoccidioidomycosis, 483–489
   host immune response, 484, 485
   in immunocompromised hosts, 485
   treatment, 486–489
      amphotericin B, 486, 487
      azole derivatives, 487, 488
         in adrenocortical dysfunction, 488
      immunostimulants, 489
Paromomycin, 145, 146
Penciclovir, 35, 38, 39
Penicillium spp., 358
   citrinum, 495
   commune, 495
   crustaceum, 495
   expansum, 495
   glaucum, 495
   spinulosum, 495

Penicillium marneffei, 495–501
   treatment, 496, 497
      amphotericin B, 496, 497
      itraconazole, 496
      prophylaxis, 497, 498
Penicillosis marneffei. *See Penicillium marneffei*
Pentamidine, 511, 512
   toxicity, 516
Petrillidium boydii, 347
Phaeoacremonium spp., 320
   inflatipes, 320
   parasiticum, 320
   rubrigenum, 320
Phaeohyphomycosis, 308–327
   cerebral, 322–325
Phialemonium spp., 354
   curvatum, 354
   dimorphosporum, 354
   obovatum, 354
Phialophora spp., 319, 320, 354
   gougerotii, 312
   parasitica, 319
   pedrosoi, 308
   repens, 319
   richardsiae, 319, 320
   verrucosa, 319
Phoma spp., 321, 322
   cava, 321, 322
   cruris-hominis, 321, 322
   eupyrena, 321
   herbarum, 321
   hibernica, 321
   minutella, 321
   minutispora, 321
   oculo-hominis, 321
   sorghina, 321
Phycomycosis. *See* Zygomycosis
Phylacia, 322
Pichia spp., 303
   anomala, 303
Pichia jadini, 281
Pimaricin, 353
Plasmodium spp., 143
Pleistophora spp., 183, 185, 186
Pleurophomopsis spp., 322
   lignicoca, 322
Pott's disease, 112
Pneumocystis carinii, 507–533
   dihydropteroate synthetase effect on, 513
   genetic diversity, 508